Oncology of CNS Tumors

Jörg-Christian Tonn • David A. Reardon
James T. Rutka • Manfred Westphal
Editors

Oncology of CNS Tumors

Third edition 2019

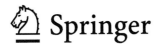 Springer

Editors
Jörg-Christian Tonn
Department of Neurosurgery
University of Munich Department
of Neurosurgery
Munich
Germany

James T. Rutka
SickKids Hospital
University of Toronto
Toronto, ON
Canada

David A. Reardon
Dana-Farber Cancer Institute Center
Harvard University
Boston
USA

Manfred Westphal
Department of Neurosurgery
University of Hamburg
Hamburg
Germany

ISBN 978-3-030-04151-9   ISBN 978-3-030-04152-6   (eBook)
https://doi.org/10.1007/978-3-030-04152-6

Library of Congress Control Number: 2019935556

This Springer imprint is published by the registered company Springer Nature Switzerland AG
The registered company address is: Gewerbestrasse 11, 6330 Cham, Switzerland

Preface

Neurooncology has definitively evolved into a molecular-based medicine as many entities are now being diagnosed and classified using molecular signatures. Their clinical relevance has been validated by numerous large cohort studies. This led to a revision of the WHO Classification with major changes including the incorporation of new entities that are defined by histology and molecular features. Therefore, treatment concepts had to be revised and refined accordingly, reflecting the respective roles of microsurgery, chemo- and immunotherapies, and radiation oncology. Likewise, the progress of imaging techniques within the last years needed to be considered.

Thus, the third edition of this textbook had to be reorganized within the framework of the revised WHO Classification System and most chapters had to be thoroughly revised. We also added new chapters with focus on principal concepts of neurooncology and practical issues of patient care.

We gratefully acknowledge the contribution of all authors who are highly renowned international experts in their field as well as Meike Stoeck and Sushil Kumar Sharma with their team from Springer-Verlag for their excellent support and assistance.

Munich, Germany
Boston, MA, USA
Toronto, ON, Canada
Hamburg, Germany

Jörg-Christian Tonn
David A. Reardon
James T. Rutka
Manfred Westphal

Contents

Part I

General Aspects in Neurooncology

David A. Reardon, Manfred Westphal,
Jörg-Christian Tonn

Pathology and Classification of Tumors of the Central Nervous System

Guido Reifenberger, Ingmar Blümcke, Pieter Wesseling, Torsten Pietsch, and Werner Paulus

1.1 Introduction

1.1.1 Histologic Classification of Central Nervous System Tumors

Rudolf Virchow (1821–1902), the founder of cellular pathology, already separated the gliomas from the "psammomas," the "melanomas," and other "sarcomas" of the nervous system in 1864/1865 [160]. However, it was not before 1926 that Bailey and Cushing developed the first systematic classification scheme for gliomas and introduced the concept of brain tumor grading [5]. The first edition of the World Health Organization (WHO) classification of tumors of the nervous system was published in 1979 [171], followed by consecutive editions in 1993, 2000, and 2007. All these WHO classifications primarily relied on histologic criteria and basically followed the histogenetic principle proposed by Bailey and Cushing [5]. Based on morphologic and immunohistochemical features, each tumor entity was classified according to its presumed cell of origin. In addition to the histologic tumor typing, the WHO classification traditionally comprises a histologic grading according to a four-tiered scheme ranging from WHO grade I (benign) to WHO grade IV (malignant). The WHO grading is not equivalent to the histologic tumor grading commonly used in other fields of surgical pathology, but rather reflects an estimate of the presumed natural course of disease and the prognosis of the patient. In general, WHO grade I lesions include tumors with a minimal proliferative potential and the possibility of cure following surgical resection. Typical examples are pilocytic astrocytomas, subependymomas, myxopapillary

G. Reifenberger (✉)
Institute of Neuropathology, Heinrich Heine University, Düsseldorf, Germany
e-mail: reifenberger@med.uni-duesseldorf.de

I. Blümcke
Department of Neuropathology, University Hospital Erlangen, Erlangen, Germany
e-mail: Ingmar.Bluemcke@uk-erlangen.de

P. Wesseling
Department of Pathology, VU University Medical Center, Amsterdam, The Netherlands

Department of Pathology, Princess Máxima Center for Pediatric Oncology, Utrecht, The Netherlands

University Medical Center, Utrecht, The Netherlands
e-mail: p.wesseling@vumc.nl

T. Pietsch
Department of Neuropathology, University of Bonn Medical Center, Bonn, Germany
e-mail: t.pietsch@uni-bonn.de

W. Paulus
Institute of Neuropathology, University Hospital Münster, Münster, Germany
e-mail: paulusw@uni-muenster.de

© Springer Nature Switzerland AG 2019
J.-C. Tonn et al. (eds.), *Oncology of CNS Tumors*, https://doi.org/10.1007/978-3-030-04152-6_1

ependymomas of the cauda equina, a variety of neuronal and mixed neuronal-glial tumors, schwannomas, and most meningiomas. Tumors of WHO grade II are those with low mitotic activity but a tendency for recurrence. Diffuse astrocytomas, isocitrate dehydrogenase (IDH)-mutant, and oligodendrogliomas, IDH-mutant and 1p/19q-codeleted, are classic examples of WHO grade II tumors. WHO grade III is reserved for neoplasms with histologic evidence of anaplasia, generally in the form of increased mitotic activity, increased cellularity, nuclear pleomorphism, and cellular anaplasia. WHO grade IV is assigned to mitotically active and necrosis-prone highly malignant neoplasms that are typically associated with a rapid pre- and postoperative evolution of the disease. These include the glioblastomas and the various forms of embryonal tumors [88].

1.1.2 The WHO Classification 2016: Integrated Histologic and Molecular Classification

Histology-based classification allowed for meaningful separation of biologically and clinically distinct brain tumor entities and thus represented the diagnostic "gold standard" for many decades. However, the histogenetic concept of central nervous system (CNS) tumor classification has been challenged as for most tumors the actual cell of origin is still unknown. Experimental evidence from mouse models suggests that gliomas, for example, are more likely to arise from neural stem or progenitor cells rather than from terminally differentiated astrocytes or oligodendrocytes [141]. More importantly, it became evident that the rapidly growing knowledge on the diagnostic and/or prognostic value of particular genetic and epigenetic alterations in different tumor types needed to be included in an integrated morphologic and molecular approach for tumor classification [90]. Several studies reported that molecular classification of, e.g., adult gliomas correlates better with clinical outcome than histologic classification. In

addition, it has become clear that certain tumor entities, including glioblastoma, correspond to a spectrum of genetically and biologically distinct tumor groups, whereas oligoastrocytomas lack distinctive genetic alterations but molecularly correspond to either astrocytic or oligodendroglial tumors.

The revised fourth edition of the WHO classification of CNS tumors of 2016 [89, 91] has considered these advances and employs a combination of histologic and molecular characteristics for the definition of several tumor entities, in particular among the gliomas and embryonal tumors (Table 1.1). This integrated "histomolecular" approach represents a paradigm shift and allows for a more reproducible diagnosis but also may cause new challenges, e.g., in terms of the required implementation of molecular diagnostic methods [97]. Moreover, it is important to be aware of the shortcomings of molecular tests. For example, for the diagnosis of "canonical" oligodendroglioma according to the WHO classification 2016, the tumor should have complete loss of both the short arm of chromosome 1 and of the long arm of chromosome 19 (whole arm 1p/19q codeletion), but, e.g., fluorescent *in situ* hybridization (FISH) analysis using one probe on 1p and one on 19q does not allow to discriminate partial from complete losses [164]. In certain situations, the molecular characteristics may actually override the histologic diagnosis in the integrated diagnostic approach. For instance, in a diffuse glioma with the histologic appearance of an astrocytoma, detection of the presence of *IDH1* or *IDH2* hotspot mutation combined with 1p/19q codeletion leads to the diagnosis of oligodendroglioma, IDH-mutant and 1p/19q-codeleted [91].

While tumor typing has been improved by diagnostic molecular markers in the WHO classification 2016, assessment of malignancy grades is still based on traditional morphologic criteria. Table 1.2 shows an overview of WHO grades assigned to major CNS tumor entities [91]. In most instances, WHO grading continues to provide important information on a tumor's malignancy

Table 1.1 WHO classification of tumors of the central nervous system 2016 (adapted from [91])

Diffuse astrocytic and oligodendroglial tumors	**Tumors of the cranial and paraspinal nerves**
Diffuse astrocytoma, IDH-mutant	Schwannoma
Gemistocytic astrocytoma, IDH-mutant	Cellular schwannoma
Diffuse astrocytoma, IDH-wild-type	Plexiform schwannoma
Diffuse astrocytoma, NOS	Melanotic schwannoma
Anaplastic astrocytoma, IDH-mutant	Neurofibroma
Anaplastic astrocytoma, IDH-wild-type	Atypical neurofibroma
Anaplastic astrocytoma, NOS	Plexiform neurofibroma
Glioblastoma, IDH-wild-type	Perineurioma
Giant cell glioblastoma	Hybrid nerve sheath tumors
Gliosarcoma	Malignant peripheral nerve sheath tumor (MPNST)
Epithelioid glioblastoma	Epithelioid MPNST
Glioblastoma, IDH-mutant	MPNST with perineurial differentiation
Glioblastoma, NOS	**Meningiomas**
Diffuse midline glioma, H3-K27M-mutant	Meningioma
Oligodendroglioma, IDH-mutant and 1p/19q-codeleted	Meningothelial meningioma
Oligodendroglioma, NOS	Fibrous meningioma
Anaplastic oligodendroglioma, IDH-mutant and 1p/19q-codeleted	Transitional meningioma
Anaplastic oligodendroglioma, NOS	Psammomatous meningioma
Oligoastrocytoma, NOS	Angiomatous meningioma
Anaplastic oligoastrocytoma, NOS	Microcystic meningioma
Other astrocytic tumors	Secretory meningioma
Pilocytic astrocytoma	Lymphoplasmacyte-rich meningioma
Pilomyxoid astrocytoma	Metaplastic meningioma
Subependymal giant cell astrocytoma	Chordoid meningioma
Pleomorphic xanthoastrocytoma	Clear cell meningioma
Anaplastic pleomorphic xanthoastrocytoma	Atypical meningioma
Ependymal tumors	Papillary meningioma
Subependymoma	Rhabdoid meningioma
Myxopapillary ependymoma	Anaplastic (malignant) meningioma
Ependymoma	**Mesenchymal, non-meningothelial tumors**
Papillary ependymoma	Solitary fibrous tumor/hemangiopericytoma
Clear cell ependymoma	Hemangioblastoma
Tanycytic ependymoma	Hemangioma
Ependymoma, *RELA* fusion-positive	Epithelioid hemangioendothelioma
Anaplastic ependymoma	Angiosarcoma
Other gliomas	Kaposi sarcoma
Chordoid glioma of third ventricle	Ewing sarcoma/peripheral primitive neuroectodermal tumor
Angiocentric glioma	Lipoma
Astroblastoma	Angiolipoma
Choroid plexus tumors	Liposarcoma
Choroid plexus papilloma	Desmoid-type fibromatosis
Atypical choroid plexus papilloma	Myofibroblastoma
Choroid plexus carcinoma	Inflammatory myofibroblastic tumor
Neuronal and mixed neuronal-glial tumors	Benign fibrous histiocytoma
Dysembryoplastic neuroepithelial tumor	Fibrosarcoma
Gangliocytoma	Undifferentiated pleomorphic sarcoma (UPS)/ malignant fibrous histiocytoma (MFH)
Ganglioglioma	Leiomyoma
Anaplastic ganglioglioma	Leiomyosarcoma

(continued)

Table 1.1 (continued)

Dysplastic gangliocytoma of cerebellum (Lhermitte-Duclos)	Rhabdomyoma
Desmoplastic infantile astrocytoma and ganglioglioma	Rhabdomyosarcoma
Papillary glioneuronal tumor	Chondroma
Rosette-forming glioneuronal tumor	Chondrosarcoma
Diffuse leptomeningeal glioneuronal tumor	Osteoma
Central neurocytoma	Osteochondroma
Extraventricular neurocytoma	Osteosarcoma
Cerebellar liponeurocytoma	**Melanocytic lesions**
Paraganglioma	Meningeal melanocytosis
Tumors of the pineal region	Meningeal melanocytoma
Pineocytoma	Meningeal melanoma
Pineal parenchymal tumor of intermediate differentiation	Meningeal melanomatosis
Pineoblastoma	*Lymphomas*
Papillary tumor of the pineal region	Diffuse large B-cell lymphoma (DLBCL) of the CNS
Embryonal tumors	Immunodeficiency-associated lymphoproliferative disorders of the CNS
Medulloblastoma, genetically defined	AIDS-related diffuse large B-cell lymphoma
Medulloblastoma, WNT-activated	EBV-positive diffuse large B-cell lymphoma, NOS
Medulloblastoma, SHH-activated and *TP53*-mutant	Lymphomatoid granulomatosis
Medulloblastoma, SHH-activated and *TP53*-wild-type	Intravascular large B-cell lymphoma
Medulloblastoma, non-WNT/non-SHH	
Medulloblastoma, group 3	Low-grade B-cell lymphomas of the CNS
Medulloblastoma, group 4	T-cell and NK/T-cell lymphomas of the CNS
Medulloblastoma, histologically defined	Anaplastic large cell lymphoma, *ALK*-positive
Medulloblastoma, classic	Anaplastic large cell lymphoma, *ALK*-negative
Medulloblastoma, desmoplastic/nodular	MALT lymphoma of the dura
Medulloblastoma with extensive nodularity	*Histiocytic tumors*
Medulloblastoma, large cell/anaplastic	Langerhans cell histiocytosis
Medulloblastoma, NOS	Erdheim-Chester disease
Embryonal tumor with multilayered rosettes, C19MC-altered	Rosai-Dorfman disease
Embryonal tumor with multilayered rosettes, NOS	Juvenile xanthogranuloma
Medulloepithelioma	Histiocytic sarcoma
CNS neuroblastoma	*Germ cell tumors*
CNS ganglioneuroblastoma	Germinoma
CNS embryonal tumor, NOS	Embryonal carcinoma
Atypical teratoid/rhabdoid tumor	Yolk sac tumor
CNS embryonal tumor with rhabdoid features	Choriocarcinoma
	Teratoma
	Mature teratoma
	Immature teratoma
	Teratoma with malignant transformation
	Mixed germ cell tumor
	Tumors of the sellar region
	Craniopharyngioma
	Adamantinomatous craniopharyngioma
	Papillary craniopharyngioma
	Granular cell tumor
	Pituicytoma
	Spindle cell oncocytoma
	Metastatic tumors

Provisional entities are printed in italics

Table 1.2 WHO grading of tumors of the CNS (adapted from [91])

Tumor group	Tumor entity	WHO grade I	WHO grade II	WHO grade III	WHO grade IV
Diffuse astrocytic and oligodendroglial tumors	Diffuse astrocytoma, IDH-mutant		o		
	Anaplastic astrocytoma, IDH-mutant			o	
	Glioblastoma, IDH-wild-type				o
	Glioblastoma, IDH-mutant				o
	Diffuse astrocytic glioma, IDH-wild-type, with molecular features of glioblastoma				o
	Diffuse midline glioma, H3-K27M-mutant				o
	Oligodendroglioma, IDH-mutant and 1p/19-codeleted		o		
	Anaplastic oligodendroglioma, IDH-mutant and 1p/19q-codeleted			o	
Other astrocytic gliomas	Pilocytic astrocytoma	o			
	Subependymal giant cell astrocytoma	o			
	Pleomorphic xanthoastrocytoma		o		
	Anaplastic pleomorphic xanthoastrocytoma			o	
Ependymal tumors	Myxopapillary ependymoma	o			
	Subependymoma	o			
	Ependymoma		o		
	Ependymoma, *RELA* fusion-positive		o	o	
	Anaplastic ependymoma			o	
Other gliomas	Angiocentric glioma	o			
	Chordoid glioma of the third ventricle		o		
Choroid plexus tumors	Choroid plexus papilloma	o			
	Atypical choroid plexus papilloma		o		
	Choroid plexus carcinoma			o	
Neuronal and mixed neuronal-glial tumors	Gangliocytoma	o			
	Ganglioglioma	o			
	Anaplastic ganglioglioma			o	
	Dysembryoplastic neuroepithelial tumor	o			
	Dysplastic gangliocytoma of the cerebellum	o			
	Desmoplastic infantile ganglioglioma	o			
	Central/extraventricular neurocytoma		o		
	Cerebellar liponeurocytoma		o		
	Papillary glioneuronal tumor	o			
	Rosette-forming glioneuronal tumor	o			
	Paraganglioma of the filum terminale	o			
Pineal parenchymal tumors	Pineocytoma	o			
	Pineal parenchymal tumor of intermediate differentiation		o	o	
	Pineoblastoma				o
	Papillary tumor of the pineal region		o	o	
Embryonal tumors	Medulloblastoma (all subtypes)				o
	ETMR, C19MC-altered				o
	Medulloepithelioma				o
	CNS neuroblastoma/ganglioneuroblastoma				o
	Atypical teratoid/rhabdoid tumor				o
Tumors of the cranial and peripheral nerves	Schwannoma	o			
	Neurofibroma	o			
	Perineurioma	o			
	MPNST		o	o	o

(continued)

Table 1.2 (continued)

Tumor group	Tumor entity	WHO grade I	WHO grade II	WHO grade III	WHO grade IV
Meningiomas	Meningioma	o			
	Atypical meningioma		o		
	Clear cell meningioma		o		
	Chordoid meningioma		o		
	Anaplastic meningioma			o	
	Papillary meningioma			o	
	Rhabdoid meningioma			o	
Mesenchymal, non-meningo-thelial tumors	Capillary hemangioblastoma	o			
	Solitary fibrous tumor/hemangiopericytoma	o[a]	o[a]	o[a]	
Tumors of the sellar region	Craniopharyngioma	o			
	Granular cell tumor	o			
	Pituicytoma	o			
	Spindle cell oncocytoma	o			

[a]Grading according to soft tissue tumor grade 1, 2, or 3

and the patient's prognosis. However, the relevance of histologic grading has been challenged in certain entities, including IDH-mutant diffuse astrocytomas and ependymal tumors [107, 161]. Thus, WHO grading likely needs to be refined by assessment of molecular markers in the future. For example, diffuse astrocytomas, IDH-wild-type, WHO grade II, that carry genetic alterations typical of glioblastoma, such as gain of chromosome 7 and loss of chromosome 10, *TERT* promoter mutation, or *EGFR* amplification, clinically behave like glioblastomas, IDH-wild-type, WHO grade IV [120, 163]. The term "diffuse astrocytic glioma, IDH-wild-type, with molecular features of glioblastoma, WHO grade IV" has been suggested for such cases, indicating that certain molecular markers may override histologic grading.

1.1.3 Immunohistochemistry in the Classification of Central Nervous System Tumors

Immunohistochemical staining for the expression of specific differentiation markers, mutant oncoproteins, as well as proliferation-associated antigens greatly facilitates CNS tumor classification. Table 1.3 provides a list of diagnostically helpful antigens that are commonly used for the differential diagnosis of different tumor entities

or the assessment of proliferative activity. In the routine setting, immunohistochemistry is usually performed on formalin-fixed paraffin-embedded sections. Thereby, important differential diagnostic problems that are impossible to solve by conventional histology alone can be clarified. For example, the challenging differential diagnosis of malignant small, round, and blue cell tumors can often be solved by immunohistochemistry. In case of a metastasis of unknown primary, several markers are available that identify the organ site and type of the primary tumor. However, there are still a number of issues that cannot be solved by immunohistochemistry, such as the classification of oligoastrocytomas, which traditionally suffered from interobserver variability because specific immunohistochemical markers for neoplastic astrocytes or oligodendrocytes are missing [80, 156]. In addition, most markers (including GFAP) are expressed in both neoplastic and non-neoplastic cells, i.e., may not allow for the distinction between neoplastic and nonneoplastic/reactive cells.

To facilitate the histologic assessment of a tumor's malignancy grade, immunohistochemistry for the proliferation-associated antigen Ki-67 using the MIB1 antibody has become common practice. Although the MIB1 index does provide useful information in several circumstances, the fact that staining results and evaluation methods are variable in different laboratories, together with the considerable overlap of MIB1 positivity in tumors of different WHO grades, has so far precluded the definition of defined cutoff values. Therefore, MIB1 staining isn't a criterion for grading in most tumor entities, except for meningioma, where a high MIB1 index is considered as evidence of atypia.

Importantly, immunohistochemistry using antibodies that detect tumor-specific aberrations, such as point mutations, loss of nuclear expression, or nuclear translocation of mutant proteins, may greatly facilitate diagnostics. Mutation-specific antibodies readily allow for the demonstration of relevant mutations like IDH1-R132H, H3-K27M, and BRAF-V600E. Other diagnostically relevant markers include loss of nuclear expression of ATRX, H3-K27me3, SMARCB1/INI1, or

SMARCA4/BRG1, as well as aberrant nuclear staining for p53, STAT6, RELA, β-catenin, and others (Table 1.3). Thus, in many instances immunohistochemical markers allow for an integrated WHO diagnosis without the need of (cyto)genetic analyses [87, 111, 121, 149].

1.1.4 Molecular Markers for Central Nervous System Tumors

Diagnostic markers. WHO classification of CNS tumors requires immunohistochemical and/or molecular assessment of diagnostic markers, including IDH mutation, 1p/19q codeletion and H3-K27M mutation in diffuse gliomas, *C11orf95/RELA* fusion in supratentorial ependymomas, *C19MC* alteration in embryonal tumors

Table 1.3 Selected immunohistochemical markers used in CNS tumor classification

Markers for molecular characteristics of gliomas
Loss of nuclear ATRX staining, BRAF-V600E, H3-K27M nuclear staining, loss of nuclear H3-K27me3 staining, IDH1-R132H, L1CAM, p53 nuclear staining, RELA nuclear staining

Markers for molecular characteristics of embryonal tumors
β-Catenin nuclear staining, YAP1, GAB1, OTX2, p75^{NGFR}, LIN28A, BCOR, loss of nuclear SMARCB1/INI1 or SMARCA4/BRG1 staining

Glial and/or neuronal/neuroendocrine markers
GFAP, MAP2, OLIG2, S-100, synaptophysin, neurofilament proteins, NeuN, chromogranin A

Epithelial markers
Cytokeratins (pan-cytokeratins, various subtypes), desmoplakin, epithelial membrane antigen (EMA), TTF1 (carcinomas of the lung or thyroid, tumors of the neurohypophysis), napsin (bronchial adenocarcinoma), CDX2 (carcinomas of the (lower) gastrointestinal tract), prostate-specific antigen (PSA), thyreoglobulin, GATA3 (carcinomas breast or urothelial tract), estrogen and progesterone receptors, HER2/Neu (receptor status of breast cancer), CD10, PAX8 (renal cell carcinoma)

Melanocytic markers
Melan A, HMB-45

Mesenchymal markers
Vimentin, smooth muscle actin (SMA), desmin, myoglobin, myoD1, myogenin (skeletal muscle), STAT6 nuclear staining (solitary fibrous tumor/hemangiopericytoma), CD31, CD34 (endothelial)

Lymphocytic markers
CD45 (pan-leukocytes), CD19, CD20, CD79, PAX5 (B cells), CD3 (T cells), CD68, CD163, IBA-1, HLA-DR (monocytes, macrophages, microglia), CD138 (plasma cells), kappa/lambda light chains

Germ cell markers
β-HCG, alpha-fetoprotein (AFP), placental alkaline phosphatase (PLAP), human placental lactogen (HPL), OCT4, c-Kit, CD30

Pituitary hormones
Prolactin, ACTH, TSH, FSH, LH, GH

Proliferation marker
Ki-67 (MIB1)

Other useful markers
PD-L1 (predictive for immune checkpoint inhibition, e.g., in non-small cell lung cancer metastases)

Table 1.4 Selected molecular diagnostic tests used in CNS tumor classification

Genetic variables	Tumor type(s)
ATRX mutation*	IDH-mutant diffuse astrocytic gliomas (WHO grades II, III, and IV)
	H3-G34-mutant glioblastoma, IDH-wild-type anaplastic astrocytoma with piloid features
BRAF-V600E mutation*	PXA, ganglioglioma, DNT, pilocytic astrocytoma, glioblastoma, epithelioid, papillary craniopharyngioma
KIAA1549-BRAF fusion	Pilocytic astrocytoma, diffuse leptomeningeal glioneuronal tumor
C11orf95-RELA fusion*	**Ependymoma, RELA fusion-positive**
C19MC alteration*	**ETMR, C19MC-altered**
Chromosome 6 monosomy	Medulloblastoma, WNT-activated
Chromosome 7 gain & 10 loss	Glioblastoma, IDH-wild-type, *diffuse astrocytic glioma, IDH-wild-type, with molecular features of glioblastoma*
1p/19q codeletion	**Oligodendroglial tumors, IDH-mutant and 1p/19q-codeleted**
CTNNB1 mutation*	Medulloblastoma, WNT-activated, adamantinomatous craniopharyngioma
EGFR amplification	Glioblastoma, IDH-wild-type, *diffuse astrocytic glioma, IDH-wild-type, with molecular features of glioblastoma*
GNAQ or *GNA11* mutation	Meningeal (and uveal) melanocytic tumors
H3-K27M mutation*	**Diffuse midline glioma, H3-K27M-mutant**
H3-G34 mutation	*Glioblastoma, IDH-wild-type, H3-G34-mutant*
IDH mutation*	**Diffuse gliomas, IDH-mutant**
MGMT promoter methylation	Predictive marker for better response of glioblastoma, IDH-wild-type to DNA-alkylating chemotherapy
MYC/MYCN amplification	Poor prognosis in (subgroups of) medulloblastoma
NAB2-STAT6 fusion*	Solitary fibrous tumor/hemangiopericytoma
SMARCB1 or SMARCA4 alteration*	**Atypical teratoid/rhabdoid tumors**, peripheral nerve tumors associated with NF2 or schwannomatosis, epithelioid MPNST, poorly differentiated chordoma, CRINET
TERT promoter mutation	Oligodendroglial tumors, IDH-mutant and 1p/19-codeleted, glioblastoma, IDH-wild-type, clinically aggressive meningiomas
TP53 mutation*	**Medulloblastoma, SHH-activated and *TP53*-mutant**, astrocytic gliomas, IDH-mutant or IDH-wild-type

List of genetic variables (left column) and associated tumor type(s). In some situations the genetic variables are part of the WHO 2016 definition of the tumor; these variables and tumors are listed in bold. Asterisks indicate markers that can (to some extent) be assessed by immunohistochemistry (see Table 1.3). Of note, the implications of finding a genetic variable in a CNS tumor should always be carefully interpreted in the clinical, radiological, and histopathological context. For instance, a tumor should only be called a diffuse midline glioma, H3-K27M-mutant when the tumor is a (1) diffusely infiltrative glioma, (2) located in the midline, and (3) carries the H3-K27M mutation. *ETMR* embryonal tumor with multilayered rosettes, *PXA* pleomorphic xanthoastrocytoma, *DNT* dysembryoplastic neuroepithelial tumor. Provisional or novel tumor types are printed in italics

with multilayered rosettes, and *SMARCB1/INI1* or *SMARCA4/BRG1* mutation and/or loss of nuclear expression in atypical teratoid/rhabdoid tumors (Table 1.4). The number of molecular markers providing diagnostic information is steadily increasing, e.g., mutation or loss of nuclear ATRX expression, *TERT* promoter mutation, *EGFR* amplification, gain of chromosome 7 and loss of chromosome 10, BRAF-V600E mutation, *KIAA1549-BRAF* fusions, and H3-G34 mutations (Table 1.4). In case that molecular

analysis for required biomarkers is impossible or remains inconclusive, the term "NOS" (*not otherwise specified*) has been introduced in the WHO classification 2016 (Table 1.1). This term indicates that the diagnosis is based on histology only, i.e., that information on the relevant biomarker(s) is not available for an integrated diagnosis, e.g., due to limited availability of tissue [91]. NOS diagnoses should remain exceptional as they suffer from diagnostic uncertainty and individual treatment decisions may be more difficult [97]. The term "not elsewhere classified (NEC)" has been proposed for tumors that cannot be assigned to any of the accepted WHO entities despite comprehensive molecular analyses were successfully performed [92]. Most commonly, NEC diagnosis is used in case of a mismatch between morphologic and molecular features or when new entities have been identified that are not yet included in the WHO classification 2016. In addition, NEC may be used when genetic findings not yet required for a specific WHO diagnosis are nonetheless considered important for classification [92].

Prognostic and predictive biomarkers. The *MGMT* promoter methylation status has gained clinical significance in neurooncology as a predictive marker for response to chemotherapy with DNA-alkylating drugs, in particular temozolomide, and longer survival of glioblastoma patients [165]. Hegi et al. [52] reported that patients with *MGMT* promoter-methylated glioblastoma responded significantly better to temozolomide treatment and survived longer than patients with *MGMT* promoter-unmethylated glioblastoma. *MGMT* testing is thus used to guide postoperative therapy, in particular in elderly glioblastoma patients, and to stratify patients into clinical trials evaluating novel therapies specifically for either *MGMT* promoter-methylated or promoter-unmethylated gliomas.

In addition to its role as diagnostic marker for oligodendroglioma, 1p/19q codeletion has been linked to benefit from the addition of procarbazine, lomustine, and vincristine (PCV) chemotherapy to upfront radiochemotherapy in anaplastic glioma patients and thus may guide treatment decisions in this patient population [162]. Similarly, detection of an IDH mutation is not only relevant for diagnostic purposes but identifies patients suitable for clinical trials evaluating treatments with mutant IDH inhibitors or peptide-based vaccination strategies [115, 136]. Molecular analyses may also be important to identify various other aberrant genes or signaling pathways that can be therapeutically targeted by small-molecule inhibitors or monoclonal antibodies, e.g., BRAF, MEK, NTRK1, ALK, or FGFR inhibitors, as well as antibodies targeting overexpressed EGFR or the EGFRvIII mutant protein [118].

High-throughput approaches. Due to the increasing demands for diagnostic assessment of more than single molecular markers, high-throughput techniques such as array-based comparative genomic hybridization, next-generation sequencing, as well as DNA methylation profiling have been implemented for parallel detection of multiple diagnostic, prognostic, or predictive markers, and such methods have been successfully evaluated for routine use in neurooncology. These methods allow for rapid, cost-effective, and comprehensive molecular analyses that provide valuable information beyond histology and represent an indispensable tool for individualized patient stratification in ongoing trials on novel molecularly targeted therapies [118]. A particularly powerful approach based on microarray-based DNA methylation profiling coupled with machine learning approaches has been recently reported that refines brain tumor classification to an unprecedented level of accuracy and reproducibility [24].

1.2 Diffuse Astrocytic and Oligodendroglial Tumors

The WHO classification 2016 groups together different entities under this header, including IDH-mutant astrocytic gliomas of WHO grades II, III, or IV, IDH-mutant and 1p/19q-codeleted oligodendroglial tumors of WHO grades II and III, IDH-wild-type glioblastomas, and H3-K27M-mutant diffuse midline gliomas (both WHO grade IV) (Table 1.1). In addition, IDH-wild-type diffuse and anaplastic astrocytomas are listed as provisional categories. Distinction of these different categories involves diagnostic assessments of defined molecular markers, in particular IDH mutation, 1p/19q codeletion, and H3-K27M mutation (Table 1.4). Testing for the most common IDH1-R132H mutation and the H3-K27M mutation can be accomplished by immunohistochemistry with mutation-specific antibodies. In addition, immunohistochemical demonstration of loss of nuclear ATRX expression facilitates the distinction between IDH-mutant astrocytic and oligodendroglial tumors, while loss of nuclear positivity for trimethylated histone 3 lysin 27 (H3-K27me3) is typical for diffuse midline glioma, H3-K27M-mutant [87]. Detection of less common *IDH1* or *IDH2* mutations requires molecular genetic analyses, e.g., by DNA sequencing. Similarly, the 1p/19q codeletion status can only be determined by molecular (cyto)genetic analyses, such as fluorescent *in situ* hybridization (FISH), microsatellite analyses for loss of heterozygosity, multiplex ligation-dependent probe amplification (MLPA), or microarray-based techniques [98]. IDH-wild-type diffuse and anaplastic astrocytomas should be additionally tested for combined gain of chromosome 7 and loss of chromosome 10, *EGFR* amplification, and/or *TERT* promoter mutation to characterize tumors with molecular features of glioblastoma, IDH-wild-type [120]. Figure 1.1 shows an overview of the molecular diagnostic approach used for diffuse astrocytic and oligodendroglial tumors.

1.2.1 Diffuse Astrocytoma, IDH-Mutant

Definition. A slowly growing, diffusely infiltrating astrocytic glioma with a mutation affecting either IDH1 codon 132 or IDH2 codon 172 ("IDH mutation"). These tumors preferentially develop supratentorially in young adults and carry an intrinsic tendency for malignant progression to IDH-mutant anaplastic astrocytoma or IDH-mutant glioblastoma.

Incidence and age distribution. Diffuse astrocytomas, IDH-mutant, account for approximately 5% of CNS tumors and 10–15% of the astrocytic gliomas. They preferentially develop in young adults (age peak, 30–40 years).

Macroscopy and localization. Diffuse astrocytomas, IDH-mutant, predominantly grow in the cerebral hemispheres, in particular the frontal lobes. Macroscopically, they are ill-defined, gray to yellow, usually soft lesions in the white and/or gray matter. They enlarge preexisting struc-

tures and blur anatomical boundaries (Fig. 1.2a). Cystic changes are common.

Histopathology. Microscopy shows a well-differentiated astrocytic tumor of low to moderate cellularity and infiltrative growth. Mitotic activity is low. Necrosis and microvascular proliferation are absent. Most tumors are composed of multipolar neoplastic astrocytes with scant cytoplasm and fine cell processes that build a fibrillar glial matrix, often showing microcystic degeneration (Fig. 1.3a). *Gemistocytic astrocytoma, IDH-mutant*, is a variant characterized by tumor cells with enlarged eosinophilic cytoplasm, eccentric nuclei, and stout processes (Fig. 1.3b). To make the diagnosis, at least 20% of the tumor cells should demonstrate the gemistocytic phenotype. Diffuse astrocytomas (including gemistocytic astrocytoma), IDH-mutant, correspond to WHO grade II. As histologic signs of anaplasia may develop focally, selection of biopsy site and tissue sampling are important issues.

Immunohistochemistry. The tumors stain positive for glial fibrillary acidic protein (GFAP) and protein S-100. More than 90% carry the IDH1-R132H mutation [48] and express this mutant protein (Fig. 1.3d). Most tumors demonstrate widespread nuclear positivity for p53 (Fig. 1.3e) and loss of nuclear ATRX expression (Fig. 1.3f). The MIB1 index is low (<5%).

Differential diagnosis. Diffuse astrocytoma, IDH-mutant, is readily distinguished from reactive astrogliosis as well as IDH-wild-type astrocytic gliomas by the demonstration of an IDH mutation. Immunohistochemistry for ATRX and p53 can be helpful for distinction from oligodendroglial tumors. The differential diagnosis toward anaplastic astrocytoma, IDH-mutant, relies on histologic features of anaplasia, in particular elevated mitotic activity.

Molecular pathology. Missense mutations affecting codon 132 of IDH1 or, less commonly, codon 172 of IDH2 constitute the earliest aberration in these gliomas [23, 25, 147]. Any IDH mutation results in elevated levels of 2-hydroxyglutarate, which in turn leads to aberrant DNA and histone methylation, eventually causing a glioma CpG island methylator pheno-

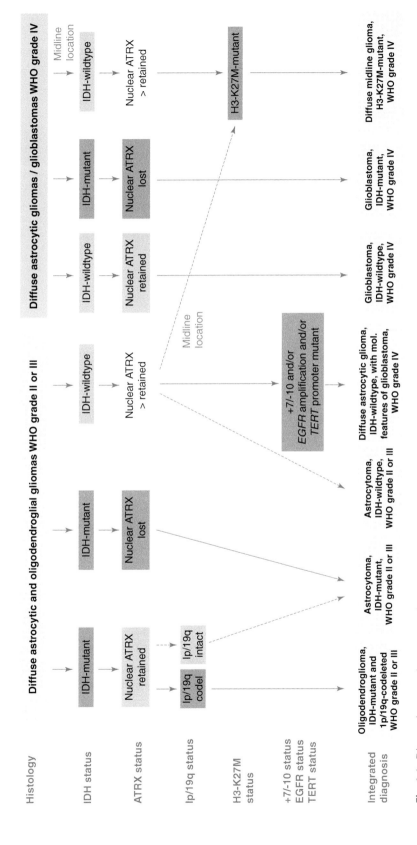

Fig. 1.1 Diagnostic approach commonly followed for WHO classification of diffuse astrocytic and oligodendroglial tumors (modified from [118])

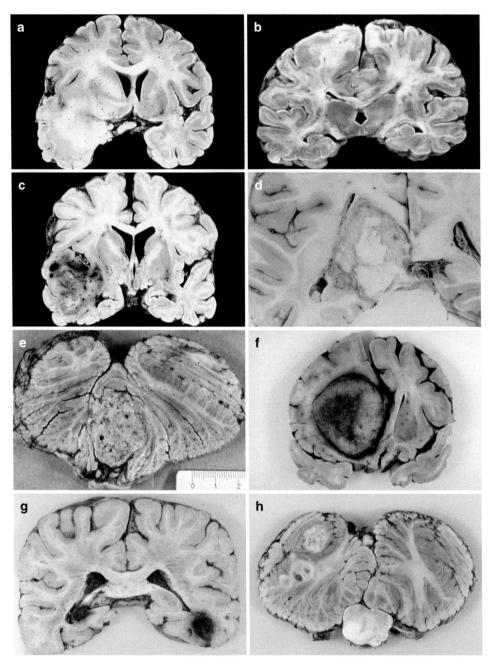

Fig. 1.2 Macroscopic appearance of selected types of primary and metastatic brain tumors. (**a**) Diffuse astrocytoma in the left temporal lobe. Note a diffuse mass lesion in the white matter without any distinct borders and blurring of the border between gray and white matter. (**b**) Oligodendroglioma involving the corpus callosum and cingulated gyrus on the right side. The tumor lacks any clear-cut borders and grows into the cortical gray matter. (**c**) Glioblastoma, IDH-wild-type, in the left temporal lobe with a heterogeneous cut surface demonstrating areas of necrosis and intratumoral hemorrhages. (**d**) Larger magni-fication of a glioblastoma showing large necroses in the tumor center. (**e**) Ependymoma in the fourth ventricle with complete obstruction of the ventricular lumen. Note that the tumor appears well demarcated from the surrounding cerebellar tissue. (**f**) Intraventricular meningioma in the left lateral ventricle. (**g**) Two distinct melanoma metastases in the brain. (**h**) Multiple metastases of a bronchial adeno-carcinoma in the cerebellum and brain stem. (**i**) Dysplastic gangliocytoma of the cerebellum (Lhermitte-Duclos disease). Note enlargement of the cerebellar folia in the right hemisphere. (**j**) Diffuse leptomeningeal melanocytosis

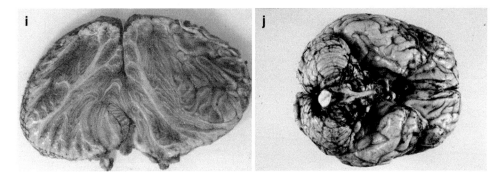

Fig. 1.2 (continued)

type (G-CIMP) [154]. IDH-mutant astrocytomas commonly carry *TP53* mutations associated with loss of heterozygosity on chromosome arm 17p, as well as *ATRX* mutations associated with loss of nuclear ATRX expression (Fig. 1.4a). *TERT* promoter mutations are restricted to a subset of tumors, while 1p/19q codeletion is absent by definition. Copy number gains of chromosome 7 or 7q are a common chromosomal imbalance in diffuse astrocytic gliomas, IDH-mutant, but gains and losses may also affect other chromosomes [163].

1.2.2 Anaplastic Astrocytoma, IDH-Mutant

Definition. An IDH-mutant astrocytic glioma with histologic features of anaplasia, in particular elevated mitotic activity. The tumors may arise from preexisting diffuse astrocytoma, IDH-mutant, but more commonly develop de novo, in the absence of a less malignant precursor lesion. They have an intrinsic tendency for progression to IDH-mutant glioblastoma.

Incidence and age distribution. Anaplastic astrocytomas, IDH-mutant, are similarly frequent as diffuse astrocytoma, IDH-mutant. The age distribution also overlaps, with a slightly later age peak between 35 and 45 years.

Macroscopy and localization. Anaplastic astrocytomas, IDH-mutant, are preferentially located in the cerebral hemispheres. Macroscopically, they are expanding lesions with perifocal edema. The distinction from normal brain tissue may be easier than in diffuse astrocytomas, but the borders are similarly ill-defined.

Histopathology. IDH-mutant anaplastic astrocytomas are characterized by signs of focal or diffuse anaplasia, such as increased cellularity, nuclear atypia, and in particular elevated mitotic activity (Fig. 1.3c). The histologic hallmarks of glioblastoma (microvascular proliferation and necrosis) are absent. Anaplastic astrocytomas, IDH-mutant, correspond to WHO grade III. However, the histologic distinction from diffuse astrocytoma, IDH-mutant, may be difficult in some cases, and grading criteria may need to be refined [161].

Immunohistochemistry. Anaplastic astrocytomas, IDH-mutant, share the immunohistochemical profile of diffuse astrocytoma, IDH-mutant. The MIB1 labeling index is increased (generally >5% positive tumor cells).

Molecular pathology. The mutational and copy number profile is similar to diffuse astrocytoma, IDH-mutant [23, 147, 163] (Fig. 1.4a). Genetic alterations associated with progression from diffuse (WHO grade II) to anaplastic (WHO grade III) astrocytoma are as yet poorly defined. A recent study indicated that *CDK4* amplification, *CDKN2A* deletion, and chromosome 14 loss are linked to less favorable outcome among patients with IDH-mutant astrocytic gliomas [27]. Other authors also reported on mutations, altered DNA methylation, and aberrant expression of cell-cycle regulatory genes as drivers of progression [25].

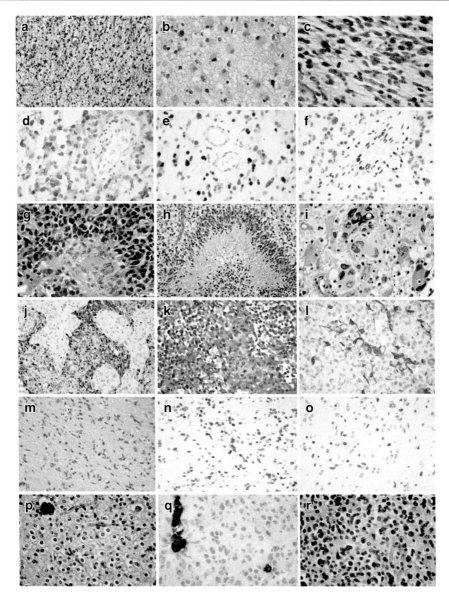

Fig. 1.3 Selected histologic and immunohistochemical findings in diffusely infiltrating astrocytic and oligodendroglial tumors. (**a**) Diffuse astrocytoma, IDH-mutant, WHO grade II (H&E). (**b**) Gemistocytic astrocytoma, IDH-mutant, WHO grade II (H&E). (**c**) Anaplastic astrocytoma, IDH-mutant, WHO grade III (H&E). Note increased cellularity, nuclear pleomorphisms, and mitotic activity. (**d–f**) Expression of IDH1-R132H (**d**) and nuclear p53 (**e**) as well as loss of nuclear ATRX immunopositivity in a diffuse astrocytoma, IDH-mutant. (**g**) Glioblastoma, IDH-wild-type, WHO grade IV. Highly cellular, pleomorphic glioma with mitotic activity and a pathological tumor vessel (H&E). (**h**) Typical necrosis with perinecrotic pseudopalisading in a glioblastoma, IDH-wild-type (H&E). (**i**) Giant cell glioblastoma, IDH-wild-type, WHO grade IV, with numerous multinucleated giant cells (H&E). (**j**) Gliosarcoma, IDH-wild-type, WHO grade IV. Note the biphasic pattern caused by GFAP-positive glial tumor areas and GFAP-negative sarcomatous tissue (GFAP). (**k, l**) Epithelioid glioblastoma, IDH-wild-type, WHO grade IV, composed of epithelioid tumor cells with eccentric nuclei (**k**, H&E) showing variable GFAP positivity (**l**). (**m–o**) Diffuse midline glioma, H3-k27M-mutant, WHO grade IV. Note a diffusely infiltrating astrocytic glioma (**m**, H&E) with nuclear staining for H3-K27M (**n**) and loss of nuclear H3-K27me3 positivity (**o**). (**p, q**) Oligodendroglioma, IDH-mutant and 1p/19q-codeleted, WHO grade II. (**p**) Oligodendroglioma-typical honeycomb appearance of tumor cells in formalin-fixed paraffin-embedded sections (H&E). (**q**) This artifact is not seen on frozen sections (H&E). (**r**) Anaplastic oligodendroglioma, IDH-mutant, WHO grade III. A cellular oligodendroglial tumor with anaplastic features including nuclear pleomorphism and mitotic activity

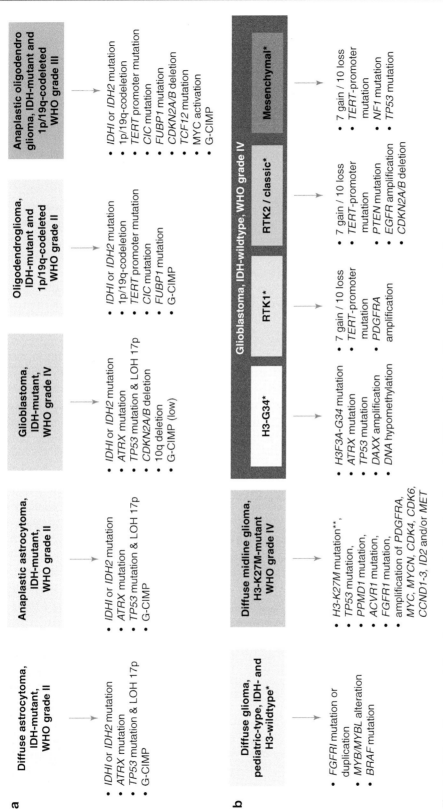

Fig. 1.4 Schematic representation of common genetic alterations detected in IDH-mutant (**a**) and IDH-wild-type (**b**) diffuse astrocytic and oligodendroglial tumors. *G-CIMP* glioma CpG island methylator phenotype, *LOH* loss of heterozygosity.

Asterisk—Glioma entities and variants not yet recognized in the WHO classification 2016. Double asterisk—H3-K27M mutations most commonly affect the *H3F3A* gene but may less commonly alternatively affect the *HIST1H3B* or *HIST1H3C* genes

1.2.3 Glioblastoma, IDH-Mutant

Definition. An IDH-mutant astrocytic glioma with marked histologic features of anaplasia including elevated mitotic activity, microvascular proliferation, and/or spontaneous necrosis. Glioblastoma, IDH-mutant, may arise from a preexisting diffuse or anaplastic astrocytoma, IDH-mutant, but also presents *de novo*, i.e., without a history of a lower-grade precursor tumor.

Incidence and age distribution. Glioblastomas, IDH-mutant, account for less than 10% of all glioblastomas. With a mean age of 45 years at diagnosis, patients are typically younger compared to patients with IDH-wild-type glioblastoma.

Macroscopy and localization. Glioblastoma IDH-mutant preferentially develops in the cerebral hemispheres, most commonly in the frontal lobe. Macroscopically, the tumors are ill-defined lesions that diffusely infiltrate the surrounding brain tissue. Areas of necrosis may be visible but often are less pronounced as in IDH-wild-type glioblastomas.

Histopathology. IDH-mutant glioblastomas are diffusely infiltrating astrocytic gliomas with marked features of anaplasia, including high cellularity, increased nuclear atypia and cellular pleomorphism, mitotic activity, pathologic microvascular proliferation, and/or areas of necrosis, including palisading necroses. Thus, the histologic appearance corresponds to glioblastoma, IDH-wild-type. In cases that have relapsed from pretreated diffuse or anaplastic astrocytomas, distinction between treatment-induced necrosis (radiation necrosis) and spontaneous tumor necrosis may be difficult, and grading may need to rely on the presence of microvascular proliferation. Glioblastoma, IDH-mutant, corresponds to WHO grade IV, although patient survival is longer compared to glioblastoma, IDH-wild-type, and anaplastic astrocytoma, IDH-wild-type [47].

Immunohistochemistry. The immunohistochemical profile corresponds to that of diffuse and anaplastic astrocytomas, IDH-mutant. The MIB1 index is usually high.

Differential diagnosis. Distinction from IDH-wild-type glioblastoma is based on the demonstration of IDH mutation. Anaplastic oligodendroglioma differs by a 1p/19q codeletion in addition to IDH mutation. H3-K27M-mutant diffuse midline gliomas are IDH-wild-type but carry the H3-K27M mutation.

Molecular pathology. Molecular alterations are similar to IDH-mutant diffuse and anaplastic astrocytomas, including IDH mutation as well as frequent *TP53* and *ATRX* mutation (Fig. 1.4a). Alteration of cell-cycle regulatory genes, including *CDKN2A* deletion and *CDK4* amplification, has been associated with poor outcome [27]. Lower DNA methylation levels compared to IDH-mutant lower-grade gliomas have also been associated with more aggressive behavior [25].

1.2.4 Glioblastoma, IDH-Wild-Type

Definition. An IDH-wild-type diffusely infiltrating glioma with predominantly astrocytic differentiation, usually high cellularity, marked cellular pleomorphism, nuclear atypia, brisk mitotic activity, as well as microvascular proliferation and/or necrosis. Glioblastoma, IDH-wild-type, typically presents with a short clinical history and preferentially develops in the cerebral hemispheres.

Incidence and age distribution. Glioblastomas, IDH-wild-type, are the most common gliomas. They account for 10–15% of all intracranial tumors and 50–60% of the astrocytic gliomas. The annual incidence is approximately 3–4 new cases per 100,000 population. Glioblastomas, IDH-wild-type, may develop at any age, but adult patients are most commonly affected (peak incidence, 50–70 years).

Macroscopy and localization. These tumors typically develop in the cerebral hemispheres. Tumor spread into the basal ganglia or to the contralateral hemisphere is not uncommon. Glioblastomas, IDH-wild-type, located in the cerebellum or spinal cord are rare. Macroscopically, IDH-wild-type glioblastomas are largely necrotic masses with a peripheral zone of fleshy gray tumor tissue (Fig. 1.2c, d). Intratumoral hemorrhages are frequent. The surrounding brain tissue usually shows a marked edema.

Histopathology. Microscopy shows a cellular, highly anaplastic glioma that may be composed of cells with various morphologies, including fibrillar and gemistocytic cells, fusiform cells, epithelioid cells, small anaplastic cells, and multinuclear giant cells. Nuclear atypia is usually marked, and mitotic activity, including atypical forms, is prominent (Fig. 1.3g). The presence of microvascular proliferation and/or necrosis is essential for the diagnosis (Fig. 1.3g, h). Microvascular proliferation often results in glomerulum- or garland-like capillary structures. Vascular thrombosis is common. In addition to large ischemic necroses, which are macroscopically visible and appear as the non-enhancing central part of the tumor on neuroimaging, glioblastomas typically demonstrate smaller, often multiple, irregularly shaped band-like or serpiginous foci of palisading necrosis (Fig. 1.3h).

Variants of glioblastoma, IDH-wild-type. The WHO classification distinguishes two variants, namely, *giant cell glioblastoma* and *gliosarcoma*. In addition, *epithelioid glioblastoma* is considered as a provisional variant.

Giant cell glioblastoma is characterized by numerous pleomorphic, multinucleated giant cells that may be extremely bizarre and reach sizes up to 500 μm (Fig. 1.3i). Some giant cell glioblastomas demonstrate a collagen- and reticulin fiber-rich matrix. Lymphocytic infiltration is often prominent. Giant cell glioblastomas may show a more circumscribed growth compared to classic glioblastoma, IDH-wild-type.

Gliosarcomas are characterized by histologically distinct gliomatous and sarcomatous areas (Fig. 1.3j). The glial component corresponds to glioblastoma and is immunohistochemically positive for GFAP. The sarcomatous tumor parts are rich in reticulin fibers and composed of GFAP-negative spindle cells, often resembling fibrosarcoma. Occasional cases may show evidence of chondroid, osseous, or myogenic differentiation. Epithelial metaplasia has also been reported.

Epithelioid glioblastomas are composed of epithelioid and sometimes rhabdoid tumor cells that are variably GFAP-positive (Fig. 1.3k, l). Their histologic features overlap with those of anaplastic pleomorphic xanthoastrocytoma.

Recent data questioned that these tumors are a biologically distinct group but show that they molecularly stratify into three established entities [77].

Grading. Glioblastoma, IDH-wild-type, and its variants correspond to WHO grade IV.

Immunohistochemistry. Glioblastomas are usually positive for GFAP and protein S-100. Nuclear p53 immunoreactivity can be detected in 30–40% of the cases, with giant cell glioblastomas being more commonly p53-positive. Strong expression of the epidermal growth factor receptor (EGFR) is found in about 60% of the tumors. Immunostaining for IDH1-R132H is negative, and nuclear ATRX expression is typically retained; however, it may be lost in rare instances, e.g., the H3-G34-mutant glioblastomas. In patients older than 55 years, absence of IDH1-R132H staining is sufficient for the diagnosis of an IDH-wild-type glioblastoma [91]. In younger patients and patients with a lower-grade precursor tumor, sequencing of *IDH1* and *IDH2* is required to exclude other, less common IDH mutations. The MIB1 index is usually high but may show marked regional heterogeneity.

Differential diagnosis. The presence of microvascular proliferation and/or necrosis distinguishes glioblastoma, IDH-wild-type, from anaplastic astrocytoma, IDH-wild-type, although molecular alterations in the latter commonly correspond to those in glioblastomas (see below). The differential diagnosis toward IDH-mutant astrocytic tumors depends on the IDH status. Giant cell glioblastoma and epithelioid glioblastoma needs to be distinguished from anaplastic pleomorphic xanthoastrocytoma.

Molecular pathology. IDH-wild-type glioblastomas in adults are characterized by frequent gain of chromosome 7, loss of chromosome 10, *TERT* promoter mutations, mutation of the phosphatase and tensin homolog on chromosome 10 (*PTEN*) gene, homozygous deletion of the *CDKN2A/p14^{ARF}* and *CDKN2B* genes, and many other, less common alterations such as mutations in the *TP53*, *PIK3CA*, PI3K regulatory subunit 1 (*PIK3R1*), and neurofibromatosis type 1 (*NF1*) genes [118]. Amplification of *EGFR* is detectable in 40–50% of the tumors, while amplification of *PDGFRA*, *MET*, *CDK4*, *CDK6*, *MDM2*, and *MDM4* is seen in smaller subsets of tumors. About 50% of the *EGFR*-amplified glioblastomas carry on oncogenic deletion rearrangement (EGFRvIII) that encodes a constitutively active receptor lacking the external domain parts encoded by exons 2–7. BRAF-V600E mutation is overall rare in glioblastoma, IDH-wild-type, but found in about 50% of epithelioid glioblastomas [71].

Studies based on large-scale molecular profiling have indicated that glioblastoma, IDH-wild-type, comprises biologically distinct subgroups that can be separated by specific DNA methylation profiles associated with defined signature mutations and gene expression profiles [18, 24, 145]. Figure 1.4b shows a schematic representation of major molecular subgroups of glioblastoma and the most commonly associated genetic alterations.

1.2.5 Diffuse and Anaplastic Astrocytoma, IDH-Wild-Type

IDH-wild-type diffuse astrocytoma, WHO grade II, and anaplastic astrocytoma, WHO grade III, are considered as provisional entities in the WHO classification 2016 [89, 91]. In adults, most of these tumors carry genetic alterations typical for IDH-wild-type glioblastoma, such as gain of chromosome 7 and loss of chromosome 10, *TERT* promoter mutation, *EGFR* amplification, and others [23, 120, 148, 163]. Clinical behavior of these tumors closely corresponds to glioblastoma, IDH-wild-type, indicating that they represent histologically underdiagnosed glioblastomas, and thus may be better classified as *diffuse astrocytic glioma, IDH-wild-type, with molecular features of glioblastoma*. Alternatively, DNA methylation and copy number profiling can readily identify such tumors as distinct types of IDH-wild-type glioblastoma [24]. A smaller subset of IDH-wild-type diffuse astrocytomas, in particular those arising in children, correspond genetically to other entities, including *diffuse gliomas with BRAF, FGFR1, or MYB/MYBL alterations* that usually show an indolent clinical behavior following resection (Fig. 1.4b). In addition, rare tumors may correspond to newly delineated entities like *anaplastic astrocytoma with piloid features* [119].

1.2.6 Diffuse Midline Glioma, H3-K27M-Mutant

Definition. A diffusely infiltrating glioma with predominantly astrocytic differentiation located in CNS midline structures, in particular the thalamus, pons, brain stem and spinal cord, and carrying a K27M missense mutation in a histone 3 protein encoded either by *H3F3A*, *HIST1H3B*, or *HIST1H3C*.

Incidence and age distribution. Data on incidence of this newly defined entity are not available. Most tumors present in children and adolescents. However, adults may also be affected, in particular by thalamic and spinal tumors.

Macroscopy and localization. By definition, these tumors are located in CNS midline structures including the thalamus, pons, brain stem, and spinal cord. Occasional tumors may involve the cerebellum. The tumors are macroscopically ill-defined and cause enlargement of the involved anatomical structures. Areas of necrosis may be present.

Histopathology. The tumors present as diffusely infiltrative gliomas of predominantly astrocytic differentiation (Fig. 1.3m). Some tumors present histologically as low-grade lesions with monomorphic tumor cells, moderate cellularity, and low mitotic activity, while others show features of frank malignancy, including high cellularity and pleomorphism, mitotic activity, microvascular proliferation, and necrosis. Independent of histologic differentiation, diffuse midline glioma, H3-K27M-mutant, corresponds to WHO grade IV.

Immunohistochemistry. The tumor cells demonstrate nuclear immunoreactivity with antibodies against H3-K27M and loss of nuclear immunoreactivity for the trimethylated lysine at codon 27 of histone 3 (H3-K27me3) (Fig. 1.3n, o). Immunoreactivity for OLIG2, S-100, and MAP2 is common, while GFAP positivity may be variable. Loss of nuclear ATRX expression is restricted to a minor subset, while nuclear p53 staining is common. MIB1 labeling is variable depending on cellularity and degree of differentiation.

Differential diagnosis. Other types of diffuse gliomas are distinguished by the absence of the disease-defining H3-K27M mutation. Rare instances of H3-K27M mutations in other types of gliomas, e.g., ependymomas or gliomas located outside of midline structures, do not suffice for the diagnosis of diffuse midline glioma, H3-K27M-mutant [87].

Molecular pathology. The diagnostic hallmark is a K27M mutation in *H3F3A*, *HIST1H3B*, or *HIST1H3C*, with mutations in the latter two genes being mostly restricted to pontine tumors. The H3-K27M mutation leads to aberrant recruitment of the polycomb repressive complex 2 and inhibition of the histone methyltransferase EZH2, which in turn causes loss of H3K27 trimethylation [7, 85]. In addition, mutations in *TP53* or *PPMD1* are frequently present as are amplifications of *PDGFRA*, *MYC*, *MYCN*, *CDK4*, *CDK6*, or cyclin D (*CCND1-3*) genes, *ID2*, or *MET* (Fig. 1.4b). Activin receptor 1 gene (*ACVR1*) mutations are seen in a subset of pontine tumors, while *FGFR1* alterations are found mostly in thalamic tumors [118].

1.2.7 Oligodendroglioma, IDH-Mutant and 1p/19q-Codeleted

Definition. A diffusely infiltrating, slowly growing glioma with IDH mutation and 1p/19q codeletion.

Incidence and age distribution. The annual incidence of oligodendroglial tumors, IDH-mutant and 1p/19q-codeleted (including anaplastic forms), is approximately 0.3 per 100,000 individuals. About 5–10% of all gliomas are oligodendroglial tumors. The incidence peaks between 35 and 45 years of age. These tumors are rare in children.

Macroscopy and localization. Most tumors arise in the cerebral hemispheres, most commonly the frontal lobe. The tumor mass is typically located in the white matter, but extension into the cerebral cortex is common. Rarely, oligodendrogliomas develop in the cerebellum, brain stem, or spinal cord. Macroscopically, the tumors appear as soft masses of grayish-pink color (Fig. 1.2b). Calcifications are frequently found. Areas of mucoid degeneration, cystic changes, and intratumoral hemorrhages are not unusual.

Histopathology. IDH-mutant and 1p/19q-codeleted oligodendrogliomas are moderately cellular, diffusely infiltrating gliomas of WHO grade II that are composed of isomorphic cells with round, hyperchromatic nuclei. After formalin fixation and embedding in paraffin, oligodendroglial tumor cells suffer from artifactual swelling that results in clear cells with central spherical nuclei and well-defined cell borders, the so-called honeycomb appearance (Fig. 1.3p). This diagnostically useful artifact is absent in smear preparations and frozen sections (Fig. 1.3q), thus making a definite intraoperative diagnosis difficult. Oligodendrogliomas may contain small gemistocytic cells that are GFAP-positive. A bona fide astrocytic tumor component may be present and is compatible with the diagnosis when molecular analysis shows IDH mutation and whole arm 1p/19q codeletion. Microcalcifications in the tumor tissue and/or the surrounding brain are common. Other degenerative features include extracellular mucin deposition and microcyst formation. Oligodendroglioma, IDH-mutant and 1p/19q-codeleted, shows a typical vascularization pattern that consists of a dense network of branching capillaries resembling the pattern of chicken wire. Infiltration of the cortex is frequent, with tumor cells forming secondary structures, such as perineuronal satellitosis, perivascular aggregations, and subpial accumulations.

Immunohistochemistry. Oligodendrogliomas are positive for S-100, MAP2, and Olig2. GFAP-positive small gemistocytes and gliofibrillary oligodendrocytes may be present. IDH1-R132H positivity is seen in the majority of tumors, and nuclear ATRX expression is generally retained, while nuclear p53 staining is absent or sparse. The MIB1 index is low (<5%).

Differential diagnosis. Differential diagnosis against macrophage-rich reactive lesions (demyelinating diseases or cerebral infarcts) as well as other tumor types that may present with clear cells, such as clear cell ependymoma, neurocytoma, dysembryoplastic neuroepithelial tumor (DNT), clear cell meningioma, and metastatic clear cell carcinoma, is accomplished by demonstration of IDH mutation and 1p/19q codeletion.

Molecular pathology. The combination of IDH mutation and 1p/19q codeletion defines these tumors. The characteristic whole arm 1p and 19q codeletion is due to an unbalanced t(1;19)(q10;p10) translocation [46, 61]. Losses of chromosome 4 are the second most common chromosomal aberration [27]. Most tumors additionally carry *TERT* promoter mutations (Fig. 1.4a), while *ATRX* and *TP53* mutations are typically absent [23, 25, 147]. Mutations in the *Drosophila homolog of capicua* (*CIC*) gene on 19q are also common, while mutations in the far upstream element-binding protein 1 gene (*FUBP1*) on 1p are restricted to about one third of tumors. IDH-mutant and 1p/19q-codeleted oligodendrogliomas demonstrate G-CIMP and *MGMT* promoter methylation [118].

1.2.8 Anaplastic Oligodendroglioma, IDH-Mutant and 1p/19q-Codeleted

Definition. An oligodendroglioma, IDH-mutant and 1p/19q-codeleted, with focal or diffuse histologic features of anaplasia.

Incidence and age distribution. Anaplastic oligodendrogliomas account for about half of the IDH-mutant and 1p/19q-codeleted oligodendroglial tumors. The age distribution overlaps with oligodendroglioma, IDH-mutant and 1p/19q-codeleted, and peaks in the fifth decade.

Macroscopy and localization. Tumors are usually located in the cerebral hemispheres with a preference for the frontal lobe, followed by the temporal lobe. Macroscopic appearance is similar to WHO grade II oligodendrogliomas. In some cases, areas of necrosis may be seen.

Histopathology. Anaplastic oligodendrogliomas are diffusely infiltrating cellular gliomas with histologic signs of anaplasia, including obvious mitotic activity (Fig. 1.3r), microvascular proliferation, and necrosis with or without pseudopalisading. The typical honeycomb cells and the vascular pattern of oligodendrogliomas are still recognizable. Microcalcifications may be seen. Gliofibrillary oligodendrocytes and minigemistocytes are common. Some cases may show marked cellular pleomorphism. An astrocytic component in an IDH-mutant and 1p/19q-codeleted tumor does not argue against the diagnosis of an oligodendroglial tumor. Anaplastic oligodendroglioma, IDH-mutant and 1p/19q-codeleted, corresponds to WHO grade III and is associated with shorter survival as compared to oligodendroglioma, IDH-mutant and 1p/19q-codeleted [27]. It has been suggested that presence of microvascular proliferation and necrosis is associated with shorter survival within the group of anaplastic oligodendroglioma, IDH-mutant and 1p/19q-codeleted [33].

Immunohistochemistry. The immunohistochemical profile is similar to WHO grade II oligodendrogliomas. GFAP-positive cells are more common and proliferative activity is increased.

Differential diagnosis. The differential diagnosis versus other types of high-grade gliomas, including malignant small cell astrocytic neoplasms, is readily solved by the demonstration of IDH mutation and 1p/19q codeletion.

Molecular pathology. The molecular profile is similar to oligodendroglioma, IDH-mutant and 1p/19q-codeleted (Fig. 1.4a). Alterations that have been linked to aggressive clinical behavior are 9p21 (*CDKN2A/B*) deletion, *TCF12* mutation, and activation of MYC signaling [3, 69, 83].

1.2.9 Oligoastrocytoma and Anaplastic Oligoastrocytoma, NOS

The WHO classification 2016 no longer considers oligoastrocytic gliomas as distinct entities as they lack specific genetic profiles but either carry genotypes of diffuse astrocytic or oligodendroglial gliomas [131]. Only when molecular testing remains inconclusive or not possible and histology shows both astrocytic and oligodendroglial phenotypes, tumors may be classified as oligoastrocytoma, NOS, or anaplastic oligoastrocytoma, NOS. Individual tumors with histologic features of an oligoastrocytoma and genetically distinct cell populations showing molecular features of diffuse astrocytoma, IDH-mutant, or oligodendroglioma, IDH-mutant and 1p/19q-codeleted, have been reported, but these *oligoastrocytomas with dual genotype* are not recognized as distinct WHO entity [89, 91].

1.3 Other Astrocytic Tumors

1.3.1 Pilocytic Astrocytoma

Definition. A slowly growing, well-circumscribed, and frequently cystic astrocytoma of children and young adults. Histologic characteristics include a biphasic growth pattern of loose and compact tissue, Rosenthal fibers, and eosinophilic granular bodies. Biologically, pilocytic astrocytoma constitutes a single pathway disease characterized by genetic alterations in MAPK pathway genes.

Incidence and age distribution. Pilocytic astrocytomas account for 5–6% of all gliomas. Children and young adults are preferentially affected. Pilocytic astrocytomas are the most common primary brain tumors in pediatric patients. Patients with neurofibromatosis type 1 have an increased risk for pilocytic astrocytomas, in particular optic nerve gliomas. However, most pilocytic astrocytomas are sporadic tumors.

Macroscopy and localization. More than 80% are cerebellar tumors. Other typical sites include the optic nerve and optic chiasm, hypothalamus, thalamus, basal ganglia, brain stem, and spinal cord. Rare cases originate in the cerebral hemispheres. Macroscopically, pilocytic astrocytomas are soft, gray, frequently cystic lesions that are well-circumscribed. Local involvement of the leptomeninges may be seen.

Histopathology. Pilocytic astrocytomas are characterized by low to moderate cellularity and a biphasic architecture, consisting of compact areas

with bipolar (piloid) tumor cells and microcystic areas with multipolar tumor cells (Fig. 1.5a). Rosenthal fibers and eosinophilic granular bodies are common (Fig. 1.5b). Capillary proliferation, degenerative cellular pleomorphism, foci of non-palisading necrosis, and occasional mitoses are still consistent with this diagnosis. However, high mitotic activity and palisading necrosis indicate that the tumor behaves more aggressively. Such rare cases may correspond to *anaplastic astrocytoma with piloid features* [119].

Pilomyxoid astrocytoma is a variant characterized by a monomorphic population of bipolar neoplastic astrocytes in a myxoid matrix. The tumor cells form pseudorosette-like angiocentric architectures (Fig. 1.5c). Rosenthal fibers are often missing. Pilomyxoid astrocytomas are predominantly found in the optic chiasms/hypothalamus region of children and associated with a higher risk of local recurrence and CSF seeding [152]. Intermediate forms between pilocytic and pilomyxoid astrocytoma have been reported [66].

Immunohistochemistry. Pilocytic astrocytomas are positive for GFAP, OLIG2, MAP2, and protein S-100. Immunostaining for p53 remains negative or restricted to individual cells. MIB1 labeling is usually low (<5%).

Differential diagnosis. The most important differential diagnosis is piloid gliosis, which may be found as a reaction to slowly growing tumors, such as craniopharyngioma or capillary hemangioblastoma, vascular malformations, as well as other chronic CNS lesions. In the spinal cord, tanycytic ependymoma is a rare differential diagnosis. Gangliogliomas are a common clinical differential diagnosis in long-standing, well-circumscribed lesions of the temporal lobe. However, the histologic demonstration of neoplastic ganglion cells clearly separates ganglioglioma from pilocytic astrocytomas.

Molecular pathology. Pilocytic astrocytomas are characterized by genetic alterations leading to aberrant activation of the MAPK pathway (Fig. 1.6a). Most common are in-frame fusions of the *KIAA1549* gene with the *BRAF* gene that activate BRAF signaling [28]. Less frequent are fusion genes involving other MAPK pathway genes like *RAF1*, *PTPN11*, or *NTRK2* and mutations in

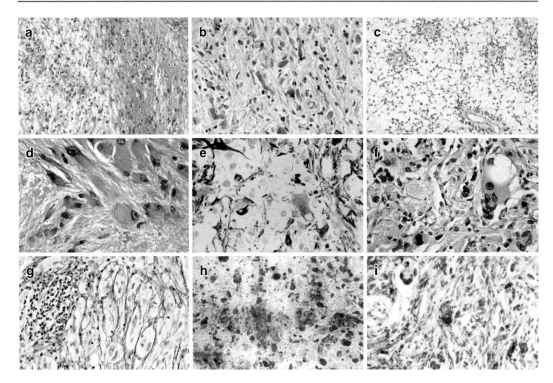

Fig. 1.5 Selected histologic and immunohistochemical features of other astrocytic gliomas. (**a**) Pilocytic astrocytoma, WHO grade I, showing a typical biphasic architecture with compact areas of bipolar (piloid) tumor cells and microcystic areas of multipolar tumor cells (H&E). (**b**) Numerous Rosenthal fibers in a pilocytic astrocytoma (H&E). (**c**) Pilomyxoid astrocytoma with perivascular tumor cell arrangements and myxoid degeneration of the tumor matrix (H&E). (**d**) Subependymal giant cell astrocytoma, WHO grade I. Histology shows a moderately cellular tumor composed of astrocytic cells with abundant eosinophilic cytoplasm and enlarged ganglion cell-like nuclei (H&E). (**e**) Variable expression of GFAP in a subependymal giant cell astrocytoma. (**f–i**) Pleomorphic xanthoastrocytoma, WHO grade II. (**f**) Histology shows pleomorphic tumor cells with cytoplasmic vacuolization (H&E). (**g**) Pericellular reticulin network and lymphocytic infiltrates (Gomori stain). (**h**) Lipidization of tumor cells (oil red stain). (**i**) Strong expression of CD34

BRAF, KRAS, FGFR1, or *NF1* [65]. The combination of MAPK gene alterations with *CDKN2A* deletion and *ATRX* mutation is typical for *anaplastic astrocytoma with piloid features* [119].

1.3.2 Subependymal Giant Cell Astrocytoma

Definition. A slowly growing tumor composed of large ganglionic astrocytes, typically arising in the wall of the lateral ventricles. Subependymal giant cell astrocytoma (SEGA) is closely associated with the tuberous sclerosis complex.

Incidence and age distribution. SEGAs typically manifest in the first two decades of life. Approximately 5–15% of patients with tuberous sclerosis develop SEGAs.

Macroscopy and localization. SEGAs are located in the wall of the lateral ventricles, often adjacent to the foramen of Monro. Hydrocephalus caused by blockade of this foramen is a common feature. Macroscopically, SEGAs are discrete intraventricular masses that frequently contain calcifications. The tumors are well vascularized and may show spontaneous intratumoral hemorrhage.

Histopathology. SEGAs are circumscribed, moderately cellular tumors composed of pleomorphic large astrocytic or ganglioid cells with abundant glassy eosinophilic cytoplasm and round, vesicular nuclei with distinct nucleoli

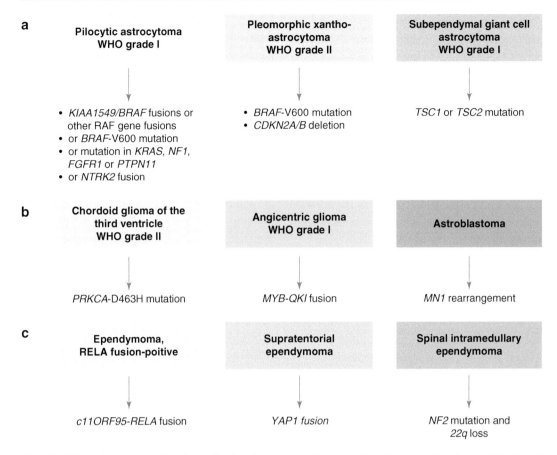

Fig. 1.6 Schematic representation of genetic alterations commonly detected in other astrocytic gliomas (**a**), selected ependymal tumors (**b**), and other gliomas (**c**)

(Fig. 1.5d). In addition, somewhat smaller spindle cells arranged in streams are commonly encountered. Multinucleated cells may be present but true giant cells are rare. Formation of perivascular pseudorosettes mimicking ependymal pseudorosettes is sometimes seen. Calcification is common. Mitotic activity is low. The presence of necrotic areas does not imply malignant behavior. SEGAs correspond to WHO grade I.

Immunohistochemistry. The tumor cells show variable expression of glial (GFAP, S-100) and/or neuronal markers (synaptophysin) (Fig. 1.5e). The MIB1 index is low.

Differential diagnosis. SEGAs primarily need to be distinguished from diffuse astrocytic gliomas, in particular gemistocytic astrocytomas and giant cell glioblastomas. Patients diagnosed with SEGA that are not already known with

tuberous sclerosis should be checked for the presence of other manifestations of this syndrome.

Molecular pathology. SEGAs are characterized by biallelic inactivation of either the *TSC1* or the *TSC2* tumor suppressor gene (Fig. 1.6a). This leads to aberrant activation of mTOR signaling, which represents a target for pharmacologic inhibition [49].

1.3.3 Pleomorphic Xanthoastrocytoma

Definition. A well-circumscribed, slowly growing astrocytic glioma with a superficial (meningocerebral) location, histologically characterized by pronounced cellular pleomorphism, xanthomatous tumor cells, perivascular lymphocytes, a reticulin network around single or grouped cells, and eosinophilic granular bodies. Activating *BRAF* mutation combined with *CDKN2A* deletion is present in most cases.

Incidence and age distribution. Pleomorphic xanthoastrocytomas are rare tumors. Children and young adults are primarily affected. A longstanding history of seizures is common.

Macroscopy and localization. Pleomorphic xanthoastrocytomas are well-circumscribed, often cystic tumors that grow superficially in the cerebral cortex and extend into the adjacent leptomeninges. The temporal lobe is most commonly affected.

Histopathology. Pleomorphic xanthoastrocytomas are relatively compact and well-circumscribed tumors growing in the cerebral cortex and invading the meninges. A fascicular growth pattern is commonly seen. Histologic hallmarks include the presence of pleomorphic, sometimes bizarre, and multinucleated giant cells, lipidized astrocytic tumor cells, eosinophilic protein droplets, often prominent perivascular lymphocytic infiltrates, and a variably dense pericellular/perilobular network of reticulin fibers (Fig. 1.5f–h). The adjacent cortex frequently shows dysplastic features. Rare variants include tumors with angiomatous, epithelioid or gangliocytic/gangliogliomatous components.

Pleomorphic xanthoastrocytoma is a WHO grade II glioma and associated with a relatively favorable prognosis, as indicated by a 10-year survival rate of >70% [158]. However, tumors with five or more mitoses per ten microscopic high-power fields are classified as *anaplastic pleomorphic xanthoastrocytoma WHO grade III* and associate with more aggressive clinical behavior [158].

Immunohistochemistry. GFAP immunoreactivity is generally present but may be variable. S-100 staining is usually strong. Nuclear p53 staining is usually absent or restricted to few cells. A subset of tumors, including rare instances with ganglion cell component, additionally stains for neuronal markers, such as neurofilaments and synaptophysin. Pleomorphic xanthoastrocytomas show frequent expression of CD34 (Fig. 1.5i). Immunoreactivity for BRAF-V600E and loss of

nuclear p16^{INK4a} expression are common [74]. MIB1 labeling is low (<5%) in pleomorphic xanthoastrocytomas but increased in anaplastic tumors.

Differential diagnosis. Their superficial location, preferential occurrence in young patients, and typical histologic features distinguish pleomorphic xanthoastrocytomas from high-grade diffuse astrocytic gliomas. The differential diagnosis between anaplastic pleomorphic xanthoastrocytoma and IDH-wild-type glioblastoma, in particular the epithelioid variant, may be difficult, as both share common BRAF-V600E mutations [77]. On the other end of the spectrum, pleomorphic xanthoastrocytoma needs to be distinguished from pilocytic astrocytoma and ganglioglioma, with occasional cases of combined pleomorphic xanthoastrocytoma/ganglioglioma being reported.

Molecular pathology. The characteristic genetic profile consists in BRAF-V600E mutation combined with homozygous *CDKN2A* deletion and loss of p16^{INK4a} expression [74, 134, 158] (Fig. 1.6a). Losses on chromosomes 14 and 22 are more common in anaplastic tumors [158].

1.4   Ependymal Tumors

Definition. Glial tumors with histologic features of ependymal differentiation, including perivascular pseudorosettes and true ependymal rosettes.

Incidence and age distribution. Ependymal tumors account for 1.8% of all primary CNS tumors and for 6.8% of all gliomas [129]. In children, about 5% of primary CNS tumors are ependymal tumors. They may occur at any age but are proportionally more common in children and adolescents.

Macroscopy and localization. Ependymal tumors typically arise along the ventricular system (Fig. 1.2e), including the central canal of the spinal cord. In adults, the frequency of infratentorial versus supratentorial ependymomas is approximately equal, while in children posterior fossa ependymomas are more common. Subependymomas are usually attached to the wall of the fourth or the lateral ventricles.

Myxopapillary ependymomas are located in the conus/cauda region. Ependymal tumors may occasionally grow without relation to the ventricles or even outside of the brain or spinal cord.

Molecular pathology. Recent studies have revealed nine distinct biological subgroups of ependymal tumors, with three subgroups in each anatomical location, i.e., the spinal cord, posterior fossa, and supratentorial compartment [107]. In each location, one prognostically favorable subgroup was designated as molecular subependymoma group that is composed of subependymomas and a subset of classic ependymomas. Among the supratentorial tumors, two subgroups are characterized by fusion genes involving either the NF-κB downstream intermediate transcription factor p65 (*RELA*) or the YES-associated protein 1 (*YAP1*) gene (Fig. 1.6b) [107, 108]. The *RELA* fusion-positive tumors are associated with less favorable prognosis and constitute a separate entity. Among posterior fossa (PF) tumors, the prognostically unfavorable subgroup A (PF-A ependymoma) mainly occurs in children and is characterized by a stable genome. Immunohistochemically, PF-A ependymomas show loss of nuclear H3-K27me3 expression [106]. The second subgroup (PF-B ependymoma) is characterized by chromosomal instability but more favorable clinical behavior [107]. Spinal intramedullary ependymomas carry chromosome 22 deletions associated with *NF2* gene mutations (Fig. 1.6b), while myxopapillary ependymomas often show multiple numerical chromosome aberrations [107]. *RELA* fusion-positive ependymomas and PF-A ependymomas are associated with the worst outcome among all ependymoma subgroups [107].

1.4.1 Ependymoma

Histopathology. Diagnostic hallmarks are pseudorosettes, i.e., perivascular tumor cells extending radial, fibrillary processes toward the vessel wall, and true ependymal rosettes, i.e., canals and tubuli composed of a single layer of cuboidal tumor cells (Fig. 1.7c). Cellular density is moderate and mitoses are rare, while necroses may occur. Ependymomas are usually well delineated from the brain. The *papillary ependymoma* variant shows marked disintegration of areas remote to vessels, leading to a pseudopapillary pattern (Fig. 1.7d). *Clear cell ependymoma* is largely composed of oligodendroglia-like tumor cells with clear, PAS-positive cytoplasm. *Tanycytic ependymoma* features fascicles of spindle cells with elongated processes (Fig. 1.7e). Ependymomas correspond to WHO grade II.

Immunohistochemistry. Tumor cells are positive for GFAP, preferentially around blood vessels. A dot-like perinuclear EMA positivity is typical, while ring-like staining pattern and linear labeling of luminal surfaces are less common. OLIG2 staining is typically negative or sparse in ependymomas. Loss of nuclear immunoreactivity for H3-K27me3 is typical for posterior fossa type A tumors (Fig. 1.7g).

Differential diagnosis. Papillary ependymoma has to be differentiated from other types of papillary tumors, including choroid plexus papilloma, astroblastoma, papillary meningioma, papillary tumor of the pineal region, and metastatic papillary carcinoma. Clear cell ependymoma closely resembles neurocytoma and oligodendroglioma, and diagnosis may require application of immunohistochemistry to exclude neurocytic differentiation and molecular testing for IDH mutation and 1p/19q codeletion to exclude an oligodendroglial tumor. Tanycytic ependymoma may be difficult to distinguish from pilocytic astrocytoma but in contrast to pilocytic astrocytoma lacks OLIG2 expression.

1.4.2 Anaplastic Ependymoma

Histopathology. The most important criterion for anaplasia in ependymal tumors is high mitotic activity, while high cellular density, microvascular proliferation, and pseudopalisading necrosis being also typically encountered. Pseudorosettes are less prominent, and ependymal rosettes are commonly missing in anaplastic ependymomas.

Immunohistochemistry. The immunohistochemical expression pattern corresponds to that of WHO grade II ependymoma.

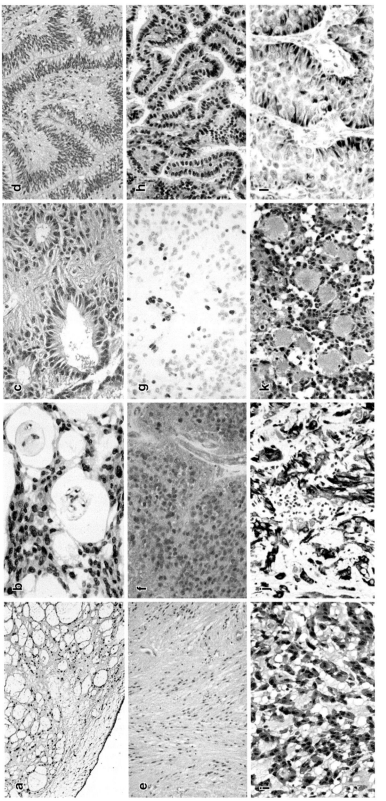

Fig. 1.7 Histology of ependymal tumors, choroid plexus tumors, and other glial tumors. (**a**) Subependymoma, WHO grade I. Note low cellularity with numerous microcysts (H&E). (**b**) Myxopapillary ependymoma, WHO grade I. Ependymal tumor cells are arranged around hyalinized vessels with perivascular mucin deposition (H&E). (**c**) Ependymoma, WHO grade II. Formation of typical ependymal canals (H&E). (**d**) Papillary ependymoma, WHO grade II (H&E). (**e**) Tanycytic ependymoma, WHO grade II, composed of elongated tumor cells (H&E). (**f**) Nuclear RELA positivity in a supratentorial ependymoma, RELA fusion-positive. (**g**) Loss of nuclear H3-K27me3 expression in a posterior fossa group A ependymoma. (**h**) Choroid plexus papilloma, WHO grade I (H&E). (**i**) Chordoid glioma of the third ventricle, WHO grade II with eosinophilic cells forming chordoma-like cords in a strongly mucinous matrix (H&E). (**j**) The same tumor shows strong immunoreactivity for GFAP. (**k**) Astroblastoma with glial tumor cells forming astroblastic pseudorosettes around hyalinized blood vessels (H&E). (**l**) GFAP staining of this tumor highlights perivascular astroblastic cells

Differential diagnosis. Occasionally, distinction from a malignant astrocytic glioma may be difficult. Immunohistochemical detection of EMA dots is more frequent in ependymal tumors, while strong nuclear staining for OLIG2 and p53 as well as a diffusely infiltrative growth pattern would argue for an astrocytic glioma.

1.4.3 Ependymoma, *RELA* Fusion-Positive

Definition. A supratentorial ependymoma characterized by a *C11orf95-RELA* fusion gene.

Histopathology. Ependymoma, *RELA* fusion-positive, most commonly shows histologic features of anaplastic ependymoma, but some tumors may also correspond to ependymoma WHO grade II. A clear cell component is not infrequent, and tumors often have a distinctive vascular pattern of branching capillaries.

Immunohistochemistry. The immunohistochemical profile corresponds to those of other ependymomas. Positivity for L1CAM and nuclear RELA expression is common (Fig. 1.7f).

Molecular pathology. Classification of these tumors requires the demonstration of a *C11orf95-RELA* fusion gene, e.g. by FISH or by RT-PCR analysis.

1.4.4 Myxopapillary Ependymoma

Histopathology. Myxopapillary ependymoma is characterized by cuboidal to elongated ependymal tumor cells arranged in a radial manner around frequently hyalinized blood vessels with perivascular mucoid degeneration (Fig. 1.7b). Mitotic activity is usually low or absent, corresponding to a tumor of WHO grade I.

Immunohistochemistry. Tumor cells are GFAP-positive, while dot-like EMA staining may be sparse. MIB1 index is usually low, although higher values may occur without being related to recurrence or the very rare extraspinal metastases.

Differential diagnosis. Differential diagnostic considerations may include paraganglioma, chordoma, chondroid tumors, adenoid cystic carcinoma, and mucinous adenocarcinoma, but in those less unequivocal cases, immunostaining for GFAP is helpful. More commonly the question arises whether the myxoid and pseudopapillary features of an ependymal tumor are pronounced enough as to justify the diagnosis of myxopapillary ependymoma, although there are no known prognostic or other clinical differences between myxopapillary and WHO grade II lumbosacral ependymomas.

1.4.5 Subependymoma

Histopathology. Histology shows an ependymal tumor of low cellularity characterized by clustering of tumor cell nuclei against a microcystic, fibrillary background (Fig. 1.7a). Perivascular pseudorosettes are indistinct. Mitoses and necrosis are absent. Nuclear pleomorphism, calcification, and hemorrhage are degenerative features. Vessels may undergo hyalinosis.

Immunohistochemistry. Tumor cells express GFAP. Dot-like EMA positivity is less pronounced as in classic ependymomas. The MIB1 index is low.

Differential diagnosis. Some tumors focally comprise areas corresponding to ependymoma, but this is without clinical implication.

1.5 Other Gliomas

1.5.1 Chordoid Glioma of the Third Ventricle

Definition. A well-circumscribed, slowly growing, GFAP-positive glioma in the third ventricle characterized by chordoma-like histologic features.

Incidence and age distribution. Chordoid gliomas are rare tumors that manifest in adults. Females are more commonly affected than males.

Macroscopy and localization. The tumors are located in the anterior part of the third ventricle and may extend to the suprasellar region. Macroscopically, chordoid gliomas are well-circumscribed solid tumors that adhere to the ventricular wall and may cause obstructive hydrocephalus.

Histopathology. Chordoid gliomas are moderately cellular and characterized by clusters and cords of epithelioid tumor cells with prominent eosinophilic cytoplasm, relatively uniform nuclei and inconspicuous nucleoli. The tumor cells are embedded in an alcianophilic, mucinous, and sometimes vacuolated matrix (Fig. 1.7i). Lympho-plasmacellular infiltrates are a regular feature. Mitotic activity is low and signs of anaplasia are absent. The tumors are well demarcated from the surrounding brain tissue, which shows reactive astrogliosis, often with Rosenthal fibers. Chordoid glioma corresponds to WHO grade II.

Immunohistochemistry. The immunohistochemical profile consists in strong positivity for GFAP (Fig. 1.7j), vimentin, CD34, and TTF1, as well as variable expression of S-100, EMA, and cytokeratins. Synaptophysin is negative and nuclear accumulation of p53 is absent. The MIB1 index is low (<5%).

Differential diagnosis. Important differential diagnoses are chordoid meningioma and chordoma. Chordoid meningiomas are positive for EMA but negative for GFAP and CD34. Chordomas stain strongly for cytokeratins and lack immunoreactivity for GFAP and CD34. In addition, chordomas contain physaliphorous cells, which are not seen in chordoid gliomas.

Molecular pathology. Chordoid gliomas are characterized by a recurrent D463H missense mutation in the *PRKCA* gene [42] (Fig. 1.6c).

1.5.2 Angiocentric Glioma

Definition. A slowly growing or stable, chronic epilepsy-associated, cortico-subcortical glioma characterized by monomorphous bipolar cells, angiocentric growth pattern, and features of both astrocytic and ependymal differentiation.

Incidence and age distribution. Angiocentric gliomas are rare tumors that may manifest at any age but are most common in children and young adults. Both sexes are equally affected. Most patients present with a history of long-standing

drug-resistant epilepsy. The prognosis is usually favorable.

Macroscopy and localization. The tumors are typically located superficially in the cerebral cortex with extension into the subcortical white matter. The frontoparietal and temporal lobes are most commonly affected. A stalk-like extension to an adjacent ventricle is often seen on MRI.

Histopathology. Microscopically, angiocentric glioma consists of monomorphous bipolar, spindle-shaped cells with oval or elongated nuclei. The tumor cells grow diffusely in the cortex and subcortical white matter, typically along intracortical vessels. Formation of perivascular pseudorosette-like structures, subpial tumor cell accumulations, and areas with palisading of tumor cells are additional common features. Nonneoplastic, residual neurons are often entrapped in the tumor tissue. Mitoses are rare and signs of anaplasia are absent. Angiocentric glioma corresponds to a WHO grade I lesion.

Immunohistochemistry. The tumor cells stain positively for glial fibrillary acidic protein, vimentin, and protein S-100. Similar to ependymal tumors, EMA-positive microlumen-like cytoplasmic dots are typically seen.

Molecular pathology. Angiocentric gliomas are characterized by rearrangements involving the *MYB* gene, in particular *MYB-QKI* fusions [6] (Fig. 1.6c).

1.5.3 Astroblastoma

Definition. A well-circumscribed glioma with prominent formation of distinctive perivascular pseudorosettes ("astroblastic pseudorosettes"), which are characterized by a single layer of GFAP-positive epithelioid tumor cells sending broad, non-tapering processes toward a central blood vessel. Vascular thickening and hyalinization is another characteristic feature.

Incidence and age distribution. Astroblastomas are extremely rare tumors. Precise data on their incidence are not available. Young adults and children are preferentially affected.

Macroscopy and localization. Astroblastomas may be found throughout the CNS, with the cerebral hemispheres being the most common site. The tumors are often superficially located and macroscopically appear as well-circumscribed, solid, or cystic mass lesions. Areas of necrosis may be discernable.

Histopathology. The histologic hallmark consists in the formation of a distinctive type of perivascular pseudorosette, the astroblastic pseudorosette, which is formed by a single layer of tumor cells with epithelioid cytoplasm and broad, non-tapering processes radiating toward a central vessel (Fig. 1.6k). Artificial tissue shrinkage may give rise to the appearance of pseudopapillae. A second characteristic histologic feature of astroblastomas is the presence of prominent vascular hyalinization and tissue fibrosis. Dystrophic calcifications also may be found. The histogenesis of astroblastoma is unclear, with certain ultrastructural features suggesting a possible origin from tanycytes, i.e., specialized ependymal cells.

Grading. Astroblastomas are not assigned to a definite WHO grade. However, histologic subdivision into low-grade (well-differentiated) and high-grade (malignant) lesions has been suggested [16]. High-grade lesions show increased cellularity and cellular atypia, high mitotic activity, microvascular proliferation, as well as necrosis with ps [16]. The prognosis appears to be favorable for patients with completely resected well-differentiated astroblastomas. In contrast, high-grade lesions frequently recur after resection, thus arguing in favor of adjuvant therapy.

Immunohistochemistry. Astroblastomas are immunoreactive for GFAP (Fig. 1.6l), S-100 protein, and vimentin. Focal staining for EMA is also common.

Differential diagnosis. Astroblastomas need to be distinguished from diffuse astrocytic gliomas, ependymomas, and papillary meningiomas. Astroblastic differentiation with pseudorosette formation occasionally may be seen in diffuse astrocytic gliomas, including some glioblastomas, but is generally restricted to focal areas. The differential diagnosis toward ependymoma relies on the presence of ependymal pseudorosettes as well as true ependymal rosettes in ependymomas. Papillary meningioma usually contains areas of conventional meningioma and is negative for GFAP.

Molecular pathology. A CGH study revealed gains of chromosome arm 20q and chromosome 19 as the most frequent chromosomal alterations [16]. Recurrent losses were found on 9q, 10, and the X chromosome. Recent data implicated *MN1* gene rearrangements in pediatric high-grade neuroepithelial tumors with histologic features of astroblastoma [146].

1.6 Choroid Plexus Tumors

Definition. Intraventricular neuroectodermal tumors with a papillary pattern resembling nonneoplastic choroid plexus.

Incidence and age distribution. Choroid plexus tumors account for 0.5% of all CNS tumors, 2.5% of CNS tumors in children under 15 years of age, and 13% in children under 1 year of age. More than 85% of choroid plexus tumors are papillomas (WHO grade I), while atypical tumors (WHO grade II) and choroid plexus carcinomas (WHO grade III) are less common. Choroid plexus papillomas may occur in all age groups, while the vast majority of choroid plexus carcinomas arise in young children.

Macroscopy and localization. Tumors arise from the choroid plexus of the lateral ventricles (50%), the third ventricle (5%), the fourth ventricle (40%), or from more than one ventricle (5%). Primary manifestation in the cerebellopontine angle is rare. Tumors of the lateral ventricles occur predominantly in children, and 60% manifest in the first decade of life. Age distribution is relatively even in tumors of the fourth ventricle. Macroscopically, the floating cauliflower-like appearance imposed by the papillary structure is characteristic.

1.6.1 Choroid Plexus Papilloma

Histopathology. The histologic appearance closely resembles nonneoplastic choroid plexus. Fibrovascular cores are lined by a single layer of columnar, cuboidal, or flattened epithelial cells (Fig. 1.6h). Nuclei are usually monomorphic and mitoses are rare (<1 mitosis per 20 high-power fields). A variety of degenerative features are common and include nuclear polymorphism, calcification, stromal edema, and accumulation of macrophages. Choroid plexus papillomas correspond to WHO grade I.

Immunohistochemistry. Normal and neoplastic choroid plexus epithelial cells express potassium channel Kir7.1 and stanniocalcin-1, which serve as sensitive and specific diagnostic markers [50]. Immunostaining for NHERF1 and NF2 has also been described as useful diagnostic markers [38]. Most tumors express cytokeratins, vimentin, S-100 protein, and transthyretin. GFAP may be focally positive. The MIB1 index is low (mean, 2%).

Differential diagnosis. In contrast to normal choroid plexus, choroid plexus papilloma usually shows higher cellular density, more frequently flattened epithelial cells, and more irregularities with respect to lining and nuclear morphology. In contrast to choroid plexus tumors, papillary ependymoma exhibits perivascular pseudorosettes, widespread positivity for GFAP, and a dot-like staining pattern for epithelial membrane antigen. For exclusion of highly differentiated papillary carcinoma metastases, immunohistochemistry for antigens expressed by lung, thyroid, colon, and other carcinomas (thyreoglobulin, thyroid transcription factor-1, napsin A, CEA) as well as for choroid plexus antigens, including Kir7.1 and the excitatory amino acid transporter-1 (EAAT-1), is useful.

Molecular pathology. More than 90% of choroid plexus papillomas show numerical chromosomal aberrations [123]. Next-generation sequencing studies have not been performed, but driver mutations are unknown so far. *TP53* mutations are very rare and *hSNF5/INI1* mutations are absent. DNA methylome analysis revealed three subgroups, including methylation low-risk cluster 1 (pediatric papilloma and atypical papilloma of mainly supratentorial location), low-risk cluster 2 (adult papilloma and atypical papilloma of mainly infratentorial location), and high-risk cluster 3 (pediatric papilloma, atypical papilloma, and carcinoma of supratentorial location), providing prognostic information in addition to histopathology [151].

1.6.2 Atypical Choroid Plexus Papilloma

These are tumors with histologic and prognostic features intermediate between WHO grade I and grade III choroid plexus tumors, representing about 10% of choroid plexus tumors. WHO grade II (atypical) choroid plexus papilloma has been defined by increased mitotic index of two or more mitoses per ten high-power fields [60]. Atypical choroid plexus papilloma has a higher likelihood of recurrence, and close follow-up of patients is warranted.

1.6.3 Choroid Plexus Carcinoma

Histopathology. Choroid plexus carcinomas show frank signs of malignancy. At least four of the following five features are present: frequent mitoses, increased cellular density, nuclear pleomorphism, blurring of the papillary pattern, and necrotic areas. Choroid plexus carcinoma corresponds to WHO grade III.

Immunohistochemistry. Most choroid plexus carcinomas express Kir7.1 and are typically positive for cytokeratins, vimentin, and S-100 protein, as well as occasionally for GFAP. They are negative for lung and thyroid carcinoma markers and most tumors stain with the anti-epithelial antibodies HEA125 and BerEP4, which do not stain most metastases. MIB1 index is higher than 5% (mean: 15%).

Differential diagnosis. In children, choroid plexus carcinoma is one of the most difficult diagnoses, in particular in dedifferentiated cases where the papillary pattern has been lost. Atypical teratoid/rhabdoid tumor can be excluded on the basis of immunohistochemical loss of SMARCB1/INI1 or SMARCA4/BRG1. However, there may be genetic, morphologic, and possibly nosologic relationship between the two tumor entities [39], and rare tumors with features of both choroid plexus carcinoma and AT/RT with loss of SMARCB1/INI1 or SMARCA4/BRG1 pose challenges. Immunohistochemistry for germ cell antigens (PLAP, alpha-fetoprotein, β-HCG) is useful for excluding papillary germ cell tumors. Metastatic carcinoma can closely mimic choroid plexus carcinoma but hardly ever occurs in infancy. In contrast, malignant papillary tumors in old patients virtually never are choroid plexus carcinomas, even if located around the ventricles, but usually represent metastatic carcinoma.

Molecular pathology. Almost all choroid plexus carcinomas carry numerical chromosomal changes [123]. No driver mutations have been identified. Choroid plexus carcinoma may occur in the setting of Li-Fraumeni syndrome or rhabdoid predisposition syndrome.

1.7 Neuronal and Mixed Neuronal-Glial Tumors

This group comprises a heterogeneous family of tumors showing neuronal or biphasic neuronal-glial differentiation. Except for anaplastic ganglioglioma (WHO grade III), most tumors are slowly growing and correspond to WHO grade I or II. Clinically, intractable focal seizures are a frequent symptom of supratentorial tumors, with ganglioglioma being the most common tumor found in patients operated on for chronic epilepsy [10].

Incidence and age distribution. Neuronal and mixed neuronal-glial tumors represent less than 2% of all CNS neoplasms [56]. Children and young adults are most frequently affected, except for central and extraventricular neurocytoma, cerebellar liponeurocytoma, dysplastic gangliocytoma of the cerebellum, and paraganglioma, which predominately manifest in adults.

Macroscopy and localization. Neuronal or mixed neuronal-glial tumors may originate at any sites of the CNS. The preferred location of gangliogliomas and DNTs is the temporal lobe [10]. Central neurocytomas are typically located within the supratentorial ventricles, often close to the foramen of Monro. Dysplastic gangliocytoma of the cerebellum and cerebellar liponeurocytomas are infratentorial lesions. Desmoplastic infantile astrocytomas/gangliogliomas are often large lesions involving the cerebral cortex, ventricles, and meninges. Diffuse leptomeningeal

glioneuronal tumors show widespread meningeal growth. Paragangliomas are typically located in the cauda equina region. Rare examples of intracranial paraganglioma are usually extensions from jugulotympanic tumors.

1.7.1 Gangliocytoma and Ganglioglioma

Definition. Slowly growing, benign neuroepithelial tumors either consisting entirely of neuronal cells (gangliocytoma) or, more commonly, of neuronal and glial cells (ganglioglioma).

Histopathology. Gangliocytomas are homogeneously composed of neuronal cells with ganglion cell differentiation (Fig. 1.8a, b). Gangliogliomas are biphasic tumors consisting of dysplastic, sometimes binucleated neurons in irregular anatomical orientations, as well as neoplastic glial cells (Fig. 1.8c, d). The glial component most commonly shows astrocytic differentiation. The fraction of neuronal and glial cells varies from tumor to tumor. Additional histopathological features are calcification, lymphocytic infiltrates, eosinophilic granular or hyaline bodies, areas with stromal reticulin network, as well as microcysts. Some tumors are densely vascularized. Subarachnoid tumor spread is common in superficial lesions.

Immunohistochemistry. Almost 80% of the gangliogliomas are CD34 positive [11]. Immunoreactivity may be found along the cell membrane of glial and neuronal cells, either within the bulk tumor mass or in small clusters in adjacent cortical regions. Dysplastic neurons accumulate neurofilament proteins and/or demonstrate a perisomatic rim of enhanced synaptophysin staining ("corona") (Fig. 1.8b). The glial tumor cells express S-100 protein and often GFAP (Fig. 1.8d), whereas glial MAP2 staining and strong nuclear p53 accumulation are usually absent. The MIB1 index is typically less than 1%. If the glial cell component demonstrates increased MIB1 labeling, atypical or anaplastic variants of gangliogliomas should be considered (see below).

Grading. Among 184 patients with supratentorial gangliogliomas and a median follow-up of

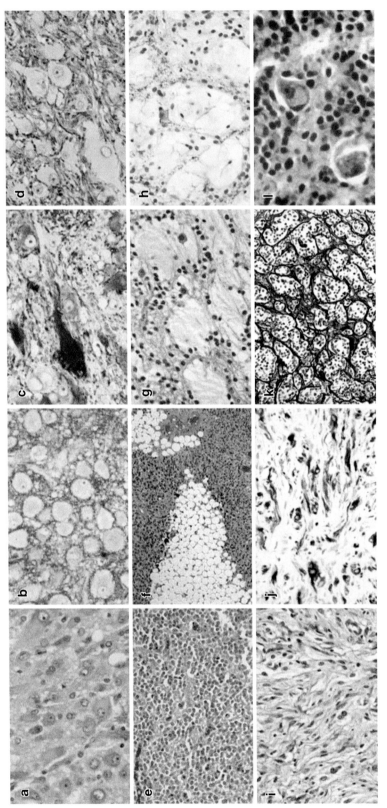

Fig. 1.8 Histologic features of selected neuronal and glioneuronal neoplasms. (**a**, **b**) Gangliocytoma, WHO grade I. The H&E stain (**a**) shows a tumor composed of ganglion cells that are strongly positive for synaptophysin (**b**). (**c**, **d**) Ganglioglioma, WHO grade I is a mixed tumor composed of dysplastic ganglion cells expressing synaptophysin (**c**) and a neoplastic glial component that stains for GFAP (**d**). (**e**) Central neurocytoma, WHO grade II. Note an isomorphic tumor composed of oligodendroglia-like neurocytic cells and neuropil islands (H&E). (**f**) Cerebellar liponeurocytoma, WHO grade II. These rare neoplasms are characterized by neurocytic tumor cells and areas of lipomatous differentiation (H&E). (**g**, **h**) Dysembryoplastic neuroepithelial tumor, WHO grade I. The H&E stain (**g**) shows an area composed of small, oligodendroglia-like cells and individual neurons floating in a myxoid matrix. Staining for synaptophysin shows positivity of a floating neuron (**h**). (**i**, **j**) Desmoplastic infantile astrocytoma, WHO grade I. On H&E, the tumors are characterized by spindle-shaped astrocytic cells in a desmoplastic matrix (**i**). Immunostaining for GFAP highlights the astrocytic tumor cells in a desmoplastic matrix (**j**). (**k**) Paraganglioma of the cauda equina with characteristic "Zellballen" architecture (reticulin stain). (**l**) Gangliocytic differentiation in a paraganglioma (H&E)

8 years, tumor recurrence occurred in only 3% of the patients [95]. However, malignant progression (2%) and death (1%) were occasionally encountered. Tumor location within the temporal lobe, complete surgical resection, history of long-standing epilepsy, and WHO grade I are associated with favorable prognosis. Increased cellularity, nuclear pleomorphism, and proliferative activity (MIB1 > 5%) of the glial component are associated with a higher risk for tumor recurrence [96] corresponding to WHO grade II tumor. A markedly increased proliferation index of more than 10% and the presence of necrosis were regarded as signs of progression to anaplastic ganglioglioma (WHO grade III) [95]. However, secondary glioblastomas were diagnosed in 5 of 11 patients (45%) who underwent surgery for tumor recurrence [96]. Predictors for an adverse clinical course are a gemistocytic cell component, as well as lack of protein droplets and CD34 immunolabeling.

Differential diagnosis. Gangliogliomas need to be distinguished from diffuse astrocytomas and oligodendrogliomas with entrapped residual neurons. Immunohistochemical staining for CD34 and IDH-R132H may help in this respect. Another differential diagnosis is pilocytic astrocytoma, which differs by the absence of a dysplastic neuronal component. The lack of specific glioneuronal elements and the characteristic immunohistochemical profile help to separate ganglioglioma from dysembryoplastic neuroepithelial tumor. The desmoplastic infantile ganglioglioma differs from ordinary ganglioglioma by its age restriction, massive growth, dural attachment, and marked desmoplasia. Extraventricular neurocytic neoplasms with ganglion cell differentiation, i.e., ganglioneurocytomas, are extremely rare. In gangliogliomas with markedly pleomorphic glial component, the differential diagnosis of pleomorphic xanthoastrocytoma may arise, in particular since several cases of pleomorphic xanthoastrocytoma with ganglion cell component and CD34 immunoreactivity have been reported. Gangliocytomas primarily need to be distinguished from cortical dysplasias, which may be difficult in small specimens.

Molecular pathology. An integrated histomorphologic classification is not yet established for ganglioglioma. Gene alterations typically found in diffuse gliomas, e.g., *IDH1* or *IDH2* mutation, 1p/19q codeletion, and *ATRX* and *TP53* mutation, are absent in gangliogliomas. Instead, molecular alterations in the MAPK signaling pathway prevail. BRAF-V600E mutations are found in between 30 and 60% of the cases [19, 134]. Mutant BRAF protein is predominantly expressed in neuronal but also in glial cells [75]. DNA methylation-based classification represents a promising new option [24], in particular when only small or histologically nonrepresentative samples are available.

Multinodular and vacuolating neuronal tumor of the cerebrum (MVNT). This tumor was newly introduced into the WHO classification 2016 as a rare gangliocytoma variant corresponding to WHO grade I. The tumor is characterized by nodular arrangement of neuronal cell clusters showing prominent vacuolation. Patients typically present focal epilepsy [58, 150]. MVNT most commonly occurs in the temporal lobe involving the cortex and/or subcortical white matter. It is composed of small- to medium-sized neuroepithelial cells with large nuclei with vesicular chromatin and distinctive nucleoli resembling small neurons. The cells are arranged in nodules showing prominent intracellular or stromal vacuolation. They express synaptophysin, MAP2, and neurofilaments but usually not NeuN. Prominent labeling of the lesional cells for developmentally regulated proteins (OTX1, TBR1, SOX2, MAP1b, CD34, GFAPδ) and oligodendroglial lineage markers (OLIG2, SMI94) has also been also observed [150]. CD34-positive neural cell elements may be observed in the adjacent cortex. MVNT are molecularly characterized by genetic alterations activating the MAPK pathway [109].

1.7.2 Desmoplastic Infantile Astrocytoma and Desmoplastic Infantile Ganglioglioma

Definition. A benign neuroepithelial tumor that develops in the first 2 years of life and is composed of astrocytes (desmoplastic infantile astrocytoma) or astrocytes and neurons (desmoplastic infantile ganglioglioma) embedded in a markedly desmoplastic stroma. Both entities correspond to WHO grade I.

Macroscopy and localization. Desmoplastic infantile astrocytomas/gangliogliomas are usually large, superficially located, supratentorial lesions with dural attachment. Cyst formation is common. The tumors may occupy large parts of a cerebral hemisphere and cause macrocephaly and increased intracranial pressure.

Histopathology. The histologic picture is characterized by small astrocytes with elongated nuclei in a reticulin and collagen fiber-rich desmoplastic stroma (Fig. 1.8i). In the ganglioglioma variant, intermingled ganglion cells are additionally present. Some tumors contain mitotically active cellular areas resembling a primitive neuroectodermal tumor or a high-grade glioma. Microvascular proliferation and necrosis may occur but do not appear to be invariably associated with malignant behavior.

Immunohistochemistry. The neoplastic astrocytes are positive for GFAP (Fig. 1.8j) and S-100, while neuronal cells, when present, express synaptophysin and neurofilaments.

Differential diagnosis. The young patient age, the superficial tumor localization with dural attachment, as well as the markedly desmoplastic stroma are diagnostic features that allow the distinction from ordinary ganglioglioma and malignant gliomas, such as glioblastoma or gliosarcoma, IDH-wild-type. The demonstration of immunohistochemical positivity for GFAP excludes fibrous lesions like meningeal fibromatosis, solitary fibrous tumor/hemangiopericytoma, and fibrous histiocytoma.

Molecular pathology. Desmoplastic infantile astrocytoma and desmoplastic infantile ganglioglioma show rather stable genotypes and lack distinctive molecular aberrations, suggesting they represent a single entity [41]. BRAF-V600 mutations are rare [45].

1.7.3 Dysembryoplastic Neuroepithelial Tumor (DNT)

Definition. A benign, usually supratentorial, multinodular, predominantly intracortical neuronal-glial tumor composed of monomorphic oligodendrocyte-like cells in a mucinous matrix. Characteristic histologic features are the formation of neuronal-glial elements and the presence of floating neurons. DNT corresponds to WHO grade I.

Macroscopy and localization. The vast majority of DNT are supratentorial lesions, with the temporal cortex being most commonly involved [10]. Patients typically present with a long-standing history of epilepsy. The macroscopic picture may vary but commonly shows a multinodular, intracortical lesion of soft gelatinous consistency that expands the cortex. Extension of tumor tissue into the subcortical white matter may occur. Erosion of the inner table of the overlying skull is not infrequent. DNT-like tumors have also been described in the septum pellucidum and caudate nucleus areas.

Histopathology. Microscopy shows a moderately cellular, multinodular lesion within the cortex that consists of oligodendroglia-like cells within a mucinous matrix (Fig. 1.8g). Mitotic activity is generally low. Microvascular proliferation may be present but is not indicative of anaplasia. Formation of *specific glioneuronal elements*, which consist of vertical columns of neurites sheathed by oligodendroglia-like cells, and the presence of cortical ganglion cells floating in mucin, the *floating neurons* (Fig. 1.8g, h), are characteristic diagnostic features. Dysplastic neurons in the vicinity of the tumor are regarded as a component of its dysontogenetic origin (and not as double pathology). The "complex form" of DNT is characterized by additional histologic features resembling pilocytic astrocytoma, diffuse astrocytoma, oligodendroglioma, or ganglioglioma. The histology of DNTs of the septum pellucidum and caudate nucleus resembles that of cortical DNT, and the biological behavior is similarly indolent.

Immunohistochemistry. The small oligodendroglia-like cells are strongly positive for S-100 but negative for GFAP. Nuclear OLIG2 positivity is common. The lack of CD34 immunoreactivity is a useful marker to differentiate DNT from ganglioglioma. Floating neurons are positive for neurofilament protein and synaptophysin (Fig. 1.8h). The MIB1 index is generally low.

Differential diagnosis. DNT differs from oligodendroglioma by the lack of IDH mutation and 1p/19q codeletion. Distinction from ganglioglioma may sometimes be difficult. The lack of a specific glioneuronal element and positivity for CD34 argue in favor of ganglioglioma; however, mixed DNT and ganglioglioma have also been reported.

Molecular pathology. Somatic alterations of the *FGFR1* gene are detectable in the majority of DNT [125, 144]. Aberrant FGFR1 signaling thus represents the molecular driver in most DNT. BRAF-V600E mutations have also been reported in DNT but appear to be less common than *FGFR1* alterations [125, 144]. Most DNTs are sporadic lesions, but rare instances of familial occurrence [51] or constitutional *FGFR1* mutation have been reported [125].

1.7.4 Central Neurocytoma and Extraventricular Neurocytoma

Definition. A tumor composed of isomorphic round cells with neuronal differentiation, either located in the lateral ventricles, often close to the foramen of Monro (*central neurocytoma*), or in the brain parenchyma (*extraventricular neurocytoma*). The WHO classification considers both as WHO grade II tumors.

Macroscopy and localization. *Central neurocytoma* is located in the ventricles close to the foramen of Monro. The tumors are commonly attached to the septum pellucidum and extend into the lateral and/or third ventricles. Tumors occurring within cerebral hemispheres or spinal cord are classified as *extraventricular neurocytomas*. Macroscopically, neurocytomas are solid or partly cystic lesions that are well demarcated. Calcifications may be seen.

Histopathology. The tumor is composed of small, uniformly shaped oligodendroglia-like cells embedded in a fibrillar matrix (Fig. 1.8e). A honeycomb architecture may present. Nuclei-free neuropil islands and microcalcifications are common features. Rare tumors demonstrate ganglion cell differentiation ("ganglioneurocyto-

mas"). Mitotic activity is usually low. However, a small fraction of central neurocytomas may show obvious mitotic activity and a correspondingly elevated MIB1 index. Such tumors have been designated as "atypical neurocytomas" and carry a higher risk of local recurrence [143]. The histology of extraventricular neurocytomas is closely related to that of central neurocytoma, although astrocytic and/or ganglionic differentiation is more common. Most extraventricular tumors show a good prognosis after complete resection; however, about one third recurs, with "atypical" histologic features (high proliferative activity, vascular proliferation, necrosis), subtotal resection, and older age being associated with a higher likelihood of recurrence [17].

Immunohistochemistry. The tumor cells are positive for synaptophysin, NeuN, and MAP2. Focal expression of GFAP may be detectable in rare cases. The MIB1 index is usually low (<5%), except for the rare "atypical" variants.

Differential diagnosis. Neurocytoma may histologically mimic oligodendroglioma, clear cell ependymoma, or DNT. The lack of IDH mutation and 1p/19q codeletion excludes an oligodendroglioma. The lack of neuronal markers but dot-like EMA positive argues for clear cell ependymoma. Tumor cells in DNT are usually negative for NeuN but positive for OLIG2 and S-100. Pineocytoma is distinguished by its location and the characteristic rosettes.

Molecular pathology. Central neurocytomas carry numerous chromosomal imbalances including gains of the *MYCN* locus [79]. They lack IDH mutation and 1p/19q codeletion.

1.7.5 Cerebellar Liponeurocytoma

Definition. A very rare cerebellar tumor of adults, histologically characterized by isomorphic neurocytic cells, variable astrocytic and focal lipomatous differentiation, as well as low proliferative activity. Cerebellar liponeurocytoma is considered as a WHO grade II lesion.

Histopathology. Cerebellar liponeurocytomas are cellular tumors composed of uniform neurocytic cells with round isomorphic nuclei as well as local accumulations of lipidized tumor cells resembling adipocytes (Fig. 1.8f). Mitotic activity is usually low.

Immunohistochemistry. The neurocytic tumor cells are positive for synaptophysin, NeuN, and MAP2. Focal expression of GFAP and S-100 may be observed.

Differential diagnosis and prognosis. Manifestation in adults, lack of anaplastic features, and the presence of focal lipomatous differentiation separate cerebellar liponeurocytoma from medulloblastomas. Immunohistochemical staining for synaptophysin helps to distinguish oligodendroglial and ependymal tumors. Cerebellar liponeurocytoma usually shows a favorable clinical outcome, but occasional cases may take an aggressive course [62].

Molecular pathology. Molecular investigation of 20 cerebellar liponeurocytomas revealed *TP53* mutation in 20% of the cases [57]. Medulloblastoma-associated alterations, such as isochromosome 17q or mutations in *PTCH*, *APC*, or *CNNTB1*, as well as BRAF-V600E and IDH1-R132H mutations, are absent [116]. Cluster analysis of mRNA expression profiles grouped cerebellar liponeurocytomas close to central neurocytomas but apart from medulloblastomas [57].

1.7.6 Dysplastic Cerebellar Gangliocytoma (Lhermitte-Duclos Disease)

Definition. A rare, benign cerebellar mass composed of dysplastic ganglion cells that conform to the existing cortical architecture. Histologically, the enlarged ganglion cells predominantly replace and expand the internal granular layer of the cerebellar cortex, leading to enlargement of the affected cerebellar folia. Of note, it is still not clear if dysplastic cerebellar gangliocytoma is neoplastic or hamartomatous in nature, but if neoplastic, it corresponds to WHO grade I.

Incidence and age distribution. Dysplastic cerebellar gangliocytoma is a very rare lesion, occurring in about one third of patients with Cowden syndrome (with a prevalence of about 1 in 250,000 in the Dutch population) and very rarely in patients in which Cowden syndrome was or could not be demonstrated [122]. Most patients with dysplastic gangliocytoma present in the second or third decade of life with cerebellar symptoms and/or signs of increased intracranial pressure due to obstructive hydrocephalus.

Macroscopy and localization. The lesion is usually confined to one cerebellar hemisphere, the affected area showing diffuse hypertrophy with thickened cerebellar folia (Fig. 1.2i).

Histopathology. Histology reveals diffuse replacement of especially the internal granule cells by enlarged, dysplastic neurons resembling small ganglion cells. Thereby, the layer's thickness increases up to severalfold. The Purkinje cell layer may also be affected and replaced by the dysplastic neurons. In addition, abnormal bundles of myelinated fibers extend from the internal granule cell layer to the molecular layer. Thus, the affected folia show a distinctive morphology referred to as "inverted cerebellar cortex." Calcifications may be present within the lesion.

Immunohistochemistry. The dysplastic neurons are positive for neuronal markers (synaptophysin, neurofilaments) and show high levels of phospho-AKT, indicating activation of the PTEN/AKT/mTOR pathway [2].

Differential diagnosis. Dysplastic cerebellar gangliocytoma differs from conventional ganglion cell tumors because it predominantly affects and expands the internal granule cell layer of the cerebellar cortex.

Molecular pathology. Patients with dysplastic cerebellar gangliocytoma often show additional features of Cowden syndrome, which is caused by germline mutations in the *PTEN* gene. Accordingly, the vast majority of these patients carry *PTEN* germline mutations [169] and should be counseled similarly to patients with this syndrome.

1.7.7 Papillary Glioneuronal Tumor

Definition. A rare, biphasic cerebral tumor composed of GFAP-positive astrocytic cells lining hyalinized vascular pseudopapillae and synaptophysin-immunoreactive interpapillary clusters of neuronal cells. This tumor corresponds to WHO grade I.

Macroscopy and localization. Macroscopically, these tumors often present as cystic, hemispheric lesion but without considerable mass effects in young adults without sex preference. The temporal lobe is most commonly affected.

Histopathology. Papillary glioneuronal tumors are histologically characterized by a single or pseudostratified layer of flat to cuboidal, GFAP-positive astrocytic tumor cells that cover hyalinized vascular pseudopapillae and by interpapillary sheets of synaptophysin-positive neuronal cells, including neurocytes, large neurons, or intermediate-size ganglion cells. Calcifications may be present.

Immunohistochemistry. The astrocytic cell lining along pseudopapillae is GFAP-positive. Neuronal cell components are always embedded into a synaptophysin-immunoreactive matrix. The MIB1 index is low.

Molecular pathology. These tumors are characterized by a t(9;17)(q31;q24) translocation that results in a *SLC44A1-PRKCA* fusion gene [20].

1.7.8 Rosette-Forming Glioneuronal Tumor

Definition. A rare, slowly growing tumor, predominantly occurring in the fourth ventricular region and in young adults, histologically characterized by neurocytes forming rosettes and/or perivascular pseudorosettes and astrocytes, typically showing pilocytic features. This tumor corresponds to WHO grade I.

Macroscopy. Rosette-forming glioneuronal tumor typically arises in the midline involving the cerebellum and wall or floor of the fourth ventricle. The tumor usually extends into the ventricle and may cause obstructive hydrocephalus. Localization outside the fourth ventricle has been described.

Histopathology. The tumors grow relatively well demarcated, while limited invasion into the adjacent parenchyma of the brain stem or cerebellum is possible. Microscopically, a bipha-

sic architecture comprising a neurocytic and an astrocytic component is seen [76, 113]. The neurocytic cells typically form neurocytic rosettes and/or perivascular pseudorosettes. These structures may lie in a partly microcystic or mucinous matrix. The glial components usually resemble pilocytic astrocytoma, including the presence of Rosenthal fibers and eosinophilic granular bodies. Mitotic activity is low and other features of anaplasia are absent.

Immunohistochemistry. Immunoreactivity for synaptophysin is seen within the center of neurocytic rosettes and the neuropil of perivascular pseudorosettes. The glial component stains positive for GFAP and S-100. The Ki-67 proliferation index is below 3%.

Differential diagnosis. Pilocytic astrocytoma and dysembryoplastic neuroepithelial tumors are challenging differential diagnosis, especially in small biopsy specimens with insufficient sampling of the neurocytic component.

Molecular pathology. Mutations in the *FGFR1* gene have been described [40], challenging its separation as true entity from DNT. *KIAA1549-BRAF* fusions and BRAF-V600E mutations were not detected, helping to differentiate these tumors from pilocytic astrocytomas.

1.7.9 Paraganglioma

Definition. A well-demarcated, usually encapsulated and slowly growing tumor composed of uniform neuroendocrine cells (chief cells) forming nests or lobules ("Zellballen") that are surrounded by sustentacular cells.

Macroscopy and localization. Paragangliomas are thought to originate from specialized neural crest cells in autonomic ganglia. In the CNS, the vast majority of paragangliomas are located in the filum terminale/cauda equina region, where they grow as intradural tumors attached to the filum terminale and/or caudal nerve roots. Paragangliomas of the head and neck typically originate from the glomus jugulare (jugulotympanic paragangliomas) or the glomus caroticum. Intracranial paragangliomas are rare and usually extend from jugulotympanic lesions.

Macroscopically, paragangliomas are encapsulated, soft, and vessel-rich tumors. Cystic areas may be present.

Histopathology. Microscopy shows a cellular neuroendocrine tumor composed of uniform, chief cells growing in a characteristic *Zellballen* architecture (Fig. 1.8k). Sustentacular cells are spindle cells located at the margins of the *Zellballen*. Focal ganglion cell differentiation is detectable in up to 50% of the cauda equina tumors ("gangliocytic variant") (Fig. 1.8l). Paragangliomas are densely vascularized and often contain microcystic areas. Formation of perivascular pseudorosette-like structure mimicking ependymal pseudorosettes can occur. Scattered mitotic figures and foci of hemorrhagic necrosis may be present but are not indicative of malignancy. Paragangliomas of the filum terminale correspond to WHO grade I.

Immunohistochemistry. Immunohistochemical stainings confirm the neuroendocrine nature of this tumor by demonstrating strong expression of chromogranin A and synaptophysin in the chief cells. Most paragangliomas of the cauda equina are additionally positive for vimentin and cytokeratins. The sustentacular cells react with antibodies against S-100 protein and partially GFAP. In addition, S-100 may be variably expressed by chief cells. Ki-67 immunoreactivity should be reported, but its predicting value needs further clarification.

Differential diagnosis. The major clinical differential diagnoses in spinal cases are ependymoma, schwannoma, and meningioma. These entities can be distinguished by histology and immunohistochemistry. Occasionally, a metastasis from an extra-axial neuroendocrine tumor needs to be excluded.

Molecular pathology. It is estimated that half of all tumors in adults and more than 80% of these tumors in children are inherited with autosomal dominant germline mutations described in several genes [34]. Familial paragangliomas of the head and neck are frequently caused by germline mutations in the mitochondrial complex II genes *SDHB*, *SDHC*, or *SDHD* [73]. *VHL* (associated with von Hippel-Lindau disease), *RET* (associated with multiple endocrine neoplasia type 2),

and *NF1* (associated with neurofibromatosis type 1) are other frequently encountered genes. A subset of patients with apparently sporadic paragangliomas, including rare instances of spinal paragangliomas, also carry germline mutations in these genes [99]. Comprehensive mutational profiling identified driver mutations in *CSDE1*, *HRAS*, *RET*, *EPAS1*, and *NF1*, as well as several fusion genes involving *MAML3*, *BRAF*, *NGFR*, and *NF1* in chromaffin tumors including paragangliomas and pheochromocytomas [34].

1.7.10 Diffuse Leptomeningeal Glioneuronal Tumor

Definition. A glioneuronal tumor with predominant and widespread leptomeningeal growth, mostly composed of oligodendroglial-like tumor cells (OLC) and evidence for neuronal differentiation in some cases. Due to limited patient numbers (approximately 60 patients published to date) and inadequate clinical follow-up, the WHO classification has not yet assigned a distinct grade. Patients with this tumor entity were reported, however, with considerable morbidity and decreased survival.

Macroscopy and localization. Postmortem investigations confirmed widespread diffuse leptomeningeal tumor growth in spinal and intracranial compartments [126]. Multifocal extension of tumor tissue along Virchow-Robin spaces and limited brain invasion are common. In the intracranial compartment, leptomeningeal growth is most commonly seen in the posterior fossa, around the brain stem and along the skull base.

Histopathology. Tumors are of low to medium cellularity and composed of OLC with uniform round nuclei. Tumor cells grow diffusely or in small nests in the leptomeninges, with desmoplastic and myxoid changes commonly present. Mitotic activity is low, with only rare examples of progression or primary anaplasia [126].

Immunohistochemistry. OLC typically express OLIG1, MAP2, and S-100 protein [126]. Synaptophysin immunoreactivity may indicate a neuronal component in up to 30%, whereas NeuN and neurofilaments are negative. Immunoreactivity for IDH1-R132H is also negative. Ki-67 proliferation index is in the range of 1–2%.

Differential diagnosis. The differential diagnosis includes mostly oligodendrogliomas and pilocytic astrocytomas with leptomeningeal spread. The characteristic molecular profile with *KIAA1549-BRAF* fusion and 1p deletion suggested that it is a distinct entity [127]. Pleomorphic xanthoastrocytomas and other glioneuronal tumors with leptomeningeal spread may also be taken into consideration.

Molecular pathology. The most frequent genetic alteration observed in 75% of 16 cases studied is a *KIAA1549-BRAF* fusion [127]. No BRAF-V600E or IDH1-R132H mutations were detected. Deletions of 1p were seen in 59% of 17 tumor cases [127], whereas codeletions of 1p and 19q are rare.

1.8   Tumors of the Pineal Region

1.8.1   Pineocytoma

Definition. A well-differentiated pineal parenchymal neoplasm composed of uniform cells forming large pineocytomatous rosettes and/or of pleomorphic cells showing gangliocytic differentiation.

Incidence and age distribution. Pineocytomas are rare intracranial neoplasms representing approximately 0.1% of all intracranial tumors. They do not show a specific predilection for any age group or gender; the mean age at diagnosis is 43 years.

Macroscopy. Pineocytomas are well-circumscribed, homogeneous tumors of the pineal region with gray-brown color. They may contain degenerative changes such as cystic alterations or hemorrhages.

Histopathology. Pineocytomas show moderate cellularity and are composed of isomorphic cells with round nuclei characterized by a granular chromatin and low mitotic activity. The cells form larger, solid nodules. A characteristic feature is the formation of relatively large, sometimes confluent "pineocytomatous" rosettes (Fig. 1.9a). Occasional cases contain large gan-

glionic cells and/or pleomorphic multinucleated giant cells. Pineocytomas correspond to WHO grade I.

Immunohistochemistry. Pineocytomas are strongly positive for synaptophysin. Neurofilament proteins and other neuronal markers may also be expressed. Some tumors show photoreceptor-like differentiation with expression of retinal S-antigen and/or rhodopsin. The MIB1-index is generally low (Fig. 1.9b).

Differential diagnosis. The differential diagnosis includes other pineal parenchymal tumors (pineoblastomas, pineal parenchymal tumors of intermediate differentiation), but these can be separated by their higher proliferative activity and the lack of large pineocytomatous rosettes. If the biopsy material is limited, the distinction between pineocytoma and normal pineal tissue may be difficult although the lobulation pattern is different and proliferative activity is absent in normal pineal tissue. Pineal cyst needs to be distinguished from a cystic pineocytoma.

Molecular pathology. Only few cases have been studied by cytogenetics or molecular genetics. CGH analysis of three cases of pineocytomas did not show any gains or losses of chromosomal material [124].

1.8.2   Pineal Parenchymal Tumor of Intermediate Differentiation

Definition. A pineal parenchymal tumor that is intermediate in malignancy between pineocytoma and pineoblastoma and is composed of diffuse sheets or large lobules of monomorphic round cells that appear more differentiated than those observed in pineoblastoma.

Incidence and age distribution. The WHO classification estimates that pineal parenchymal tumors of intermediate differentiation (PPTID) account for approximately 45% of all pineal parenchymal tumors. The neoplasms may develop at any age, with a peak incidence in adults between 35 and 45 years of age.

Macroscopy. Similar to pineocytoma, most tumors present as localized lesion. CSF

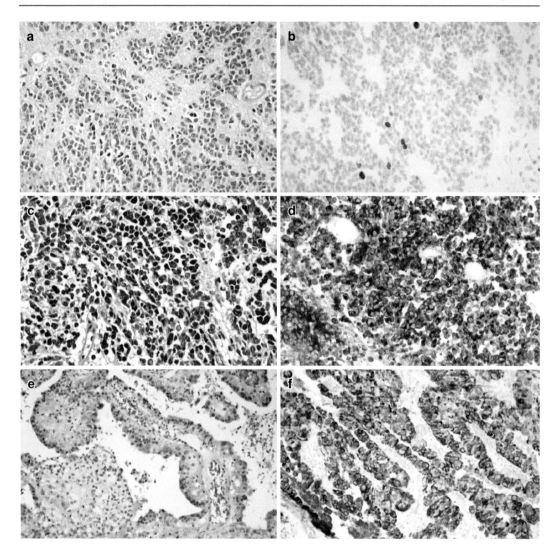

Fig. 1.9 Histologic features of pineal gland tumors. (**a,** **b**) Pineocytoma, WHO grade I. Note large pineocytomatous rosettes (**a,** H&E) and a low MIB1 index (**b**). (**c, d**) Pineoblastoma, WHO grade IV. The H&E picture (**c**) shows a cellular tumor composed of poorly differentiated neuroepithelial cells. The tumor cells are strongly positive for synaptophysin (**d**). (**e, f**) Papillary tumor of the pineal region with papillary growth pattern (**e,** H&E) and positivity for cytokeratins (**f**)

dissemination is less common as compared to pineoblastoma. It can be observed in 10% of cases at the time of diagnosis and in 15% of cases during the course of the disease [32].

Histopathology. Pineal parenchymal tumors of intermediate differentiation are cellular neoplasms that may show a diffuse, neurocytoma-like growth or an endocrine tumor-like lobular arrangement of tumor cells. Some tumors contain both lobular and diffuse areas. Neuroblastic (Homer-Wright) rosettes are sometimes seen,

while large pineocytomatous rosettes are rare or absent. Mitotic activity is usually present but may vary considerably. Areas of necrosis and/or vascular proliferation are detectable in a fraction of tumors. The WHO classification states that these tumors may correspond to WHO grade II or III but grading criteria remain to be defined. Jouvet et al. suggested to use grade II for tumors with strong expression of neurofilament proteins and less than six mitoses per ten high-power fields (HPF), while grade III should be assigned to cases with either six or more mitoses per ten HPF or cases with less than six mitoses per ten HPF that lack neurofilament staining [68]. More recently, the distinction of small cell versus large cell morphological subtypes has been reported to distinguish prognostically different patient subgroups [117].

Immunohistochemistry. The tumor cells are positive for synaptophysin, while expression of neurofilament proteins is variable. Retinal S-antigen and/or the interphotoreceptor retinoid-binding protein may be expressed in some cases.

Molecular pathology. CGH analysis of three cases revealed gains on 4q and 12q as well as losses on 22 in 2 tumors each [124].

1.8.3 Pineoblastoma

Definition. A poorly differentiated, highly cellular, malignant embryonal neoplasm arising in the pineal gland.

Incidence and age distribution. These tumors can arise at any age but most frequently occur in the first two decades of life. They represent approximately 35% of all pineal parenchymal tumors.

Macroscopy. Pineoblastomas are usually soft and poorly demarcated tumors of the pineal region. Hemorrhagic and necrotic areas may be present. They destroy the pineal gland, bulge into the posterior third ventricle, and may compress the aqueduct, resulting in obstructive hydrocephalus. Craniospinal dissemination via the CSF is frequent; approximately 30% of patients present with CFF dissemination at diagnosis.

Histopathology. Pineoblastomas are composed of densely packed small undifferentiated cells with scant cytoplasms and round or irregularly shaped nuclei (Fig. 1.9c). The cells resemble those in other CNS embryonal tumors. The chromatin is usually dense; mitotic figures are frequent. Homer-Wright (neuroblastic) rosettes can be seen, but "pineocytomatous" larger rosettes are usually absent. Pineoblastoma corresponds to WHO grade IV.

Immunohistochemistry. Similar to pineocytomas, pineoblastomas frequently express synaptophysin (Fig. 1.9d). Immunoreactivity for neurofilament proteins and/or chromogranin A is inconsistent and usually restricted to individual tumor cells. Some tumors show expression of retinal S-antigen. Consistent with their potential derivation from undifferentiated progenitor cells of the pineal gland and retina, pineoblastomas express Otx2 and Otx3 (CRX). The Ki-67 proliferation index is high.

Differential diagnosis. The differential diagnosis includes other small round blue cell tumors metastatic to the pineal region as well as embryonal tumors of other regions that can seed to or infiltrate into the pineal region.

Molecular pathology. So far, no consistent molecular alterations have been described for pineoblastomas. Cytogenetic studies showed structural and numerical alterations of chromosomes 1, 9, 13, and 16 [101, 124]. Although most pineoblastomas occur sporadically, the incidence is higher in patients carrying an *RB1* germline mutation. Occasional patients with familial retinoblastoma may develop a pineoblastoma ("trilateral retinoblastoma"). Somatic or germline *DICER1* mutations also have been reported [29].

1.8.4 Papillary Tumor of the Pineal Region

Definition. A neuroepithelial tumor localized in the pineal region and characterized by a combination of papillary and solid areas, with epithelial-like cells and immunoreactivity for cytokeratins (especially cytokeratin 18).

Incidence and age distribution. Papillary tumor of the pineal region (PTPR) is a rare tumor that was first reported in 2003 [67]. Most tumors develop in adults; however, pediatric cases have also been reported. There is no obvious gender preference.

Macroscopy. The tumors appear as large, well-circumscribed masses in the pineal region that macroscopically resemble pineocytomas.

Histopathology. Histology shows a cellular tumor with an epithelial-like growth pattern and prominent formation of papillary features (Fig. 1.9e). Ependymal-like differentiation, including formation of true rosettes or tubes as well as occasional perivascular pseudorosettes may be present. The tumor cells usually show a columnar to cuboidal cytoplasm with a well-defined cytoplasmic membrane. Vacuolated or clear cells, partially positive for PAS, are common. Moderate mitotic activity is usually detectable and necrotic foci are common. The tumors usually lack microvascular proliferation, but vascular hyalinization is frequent. According to the WHO classification, PTPR may correspond to WHO grade II or III. However, definite criteria for grading are not yet established. High mitotic activity ($\geq$5 mitoses per ten high-power fields) has been associated with less favorable outcome.

Immunohistochemistry. PTPR are positive for cytokeratins (Fig. 1.9f), which separates them from pineal parenchymal tumors. Immunoreactivity for protein S-100, vimentin, MAP2, and transthyretin is also common. Expression of chromogranin A and synaptophysin may be focally present. In addition, rare cases feature dot- or ring-like EMA staining. Immunoreactivity for GFAP, neurofilament proteins, retinal S-antigen, and the choroid plexus markers Kir7.1 and stanniocalcin-1 is absent.

Differential diagnosis. PTPR need to be distinguished from several other papillary tumors, including papillary ependymoma, choroid plexus papilloma, papillary meningioma, astroblastoma, and metastatic papillary carcinoma. However, histology and immunohistochemical profiles can usually solve these differential diagnoses. In contrast to pineal parenchymal tumors, PTPR usually do not show strong expression of synaptophysin but demonstrate cytokeratin positivity.

Histogenesis. Electron microscopy revealed ultrastructural features indicative of ependymal differentiation. Therefore, it was suggested that PTPR arise from specialized cytokeratin-positive ependymal cells that are derived from the subcommissural organ [67].

Molecular pathology. Genetic analysis of PTPR showed loss of chromosome 10 in the majority of cases [53]. *PTEN* mutations could be identified in some cases, and the PI3K/AKT/mTOR pathway was found to be activated [43].

1.9   Embryonal Tumors

Embryonal tumors represent a heterogeneous group of highly malignant tumors composed of immature cells resembling neural progenitor cells during embryonal development of the nervous system. These tumors most frequently occur in the pediatric age group. Despite rapid proliferation some tumor cells may differentiate along various neuroectodermal or other lineages. The embryonal tumors include different entities of medulloblastomas, embryonal tumors with multilayered rosettes (ETMR), the group of other embryonal tumors of the central nervous system (CNS-ET), and atypical teratoid/rhabdoid tumors (AT/RT), all histologically corresponding to WHO grade IV.

1.9.1   Medulloblastoma: Genetically and Histologically Defined

General definition. An embryonal neuroepithelial tumor arising in the cerebellum or dorsal brain stem, presenting mainly in childhood and consisting of densely packed small round undifferentiated cells with mild to moderate nuclear pleomorphism and a high mitotic activity.

Incidence and age distribution. Medulloblastomas represent the most frequent malignant brain tumors in childhood. The incidence is approximately six cases/one million children. The incidence peaks at the age of 7 years. However, infants and young adults may also be affected. Approximately 65% of the patients are male.

Macroscopy and localization. The macroscopic findings vary considerably. Many tumors are soft. Others, in particular desmoplastic medulloblastomas, often present as firm tumors. Some medulloblastomas show calcification. The extent of infiltration into adjacent brain structures as well as the tendency to seed along the cerebrospinal fluid pathways is also highly variable. At the time of diagnosis, metastatic disease is seen in approximately 30% of the patients. Most medulloblastomas are located in the midline/cerebellar vermis. Desmoplastic medulloblastomas are more commonly located in the cerebellar hemispheres.

WHO classification of medulloblastoma 2016. It has been recognized that medulloblastomas comprise several distinct tumor entities with different cells of origin, histology, genetic features, pathway activation, and clinical behavior. According to the WHO classification 2016, the definition of medulloblastoma disease entities requires an integration of histologic features and additional molecular information. By this approach, the traditional histologic diagnosis (e.g., "classic medulloblastoma") and the histologic grade ("WHO grade IV") are combined with defined molecular features (e.g., "WNT activation").

Histopathology. Four *histologically defined medulloblastoma entities* are distinguished that correspond to *classic medulloblastoma, desmoplastic/nodular medulloblastoma* (DNMB), *medulloblastoma with extensive nodularity* (MBEN), and *large cell/anaplastic medulloblastoma* (LCA) (Table 1.1). In general, medulloblastomas are composed of densely packed, small round tumor cells with scant cytoplasm, round or carrot-shaped nucleus, and condensed chromatin. The most frequent *classic medulloblastoma* shows a solid growth pattern with or without formation of Homer-Wright (neuroblastic) rosettes (Fig. 1.11a). The mitotic activity is elevated. Nuclear and cellular anaplasia shows a continuum from low nuclear variance to focal anaplastic phenotype with large bizarre nuclei and nuclear molding. Cases showing severe and diffuse anaplasia or a predominant component of large cells with single prominent nucleoli qualify for the diagnosis of *large cell/anaplastic medulloblastoma*. Mitoses and apoptotic figures are abundant, and large areas of necrosis are commonly present. Clinically, this variant is associated with a very aggressive behavior and poor outcome. Approximately 25% of medulloblastomas correspond to the *desmoplastic/nodular medulloblastoma*. These tumors are characterized by a nodular architecture consisting of densely cellular, reticulin-rich (desmoplastic) areas and less cellular, reticulin-free islands (so-called pale islands) (Fig. 1.11c, d). Mitotic activity is highest in the desmoplastic areas. A rare entity occurring in young children during the first years of life is the *medulloblastoma with extensive nodularity*. These tumors show large nodules with advanced neurocytic differentiation and smaller areas resembling desmoplastic medulloblastomas. The prognosis after surgery and chemotherapy appears to be favorable.

Medulloblastoma, genetically defined. Regarding the genetically defined component of the diagnosis, *four genetic medulloblastoma entities* have been defined in the WHO classification 2016 (Table 1.1).

- *Medulloblastomas, WNT-activated,* have mostly classic morphology and show nuclear accumulation of β-catenin protein as surrogate biomarker for WNT activation caused by *CTNNB1*-activating mutations or, less common, mutations in *APC* or other genes encoding components of the WNT signaling pathway [72]. The precise identification of these tumors is important because of their favorable prognosis in the pediatric age (<16 years) [31].
- *Medulloblastoma, SHH-activated and TP53-wild-type.* These tumors occur mostly in adolescents/adults and young children who have a good prognosis if adequately treated. Histology most frequently corresponds to DNMB or MBEN. SHH activation is caused by mutations in *PTCH1, SUFUH, SMOH,* or other components of the SHH signaling pathway. SHH activation can be reliably assessed by different methods including a panel of antibodies against SHH target proteins [112]. A significant fraction of young children with SHH-activated medulloblastomas have underlying germline mutations of *PTCH1* or *SUFUH* which correspond to Gorlin syndrome. These patients and their families should be offered genetic counseling.
- *Medulloblastoma, SHH-activated and TP53-mutant.* These tumors preferentially present in older children and have a poor prognosis [170]. In case that SHH activation is identified in a medulloblastoma, the *TP53* mutation

status has to be determined by sequencing for a precise classification. *TP53*-mutant SHH medulloblastomas can indicate *TP53* germline mutations corresponding to the Li-Fraumeni syndrome.

- *Medulloblastoma, non-WNT/non-SHH.* The fourth genetically defined entity represents the majority of medulloblastomas lacking either WNT or SHH pathway activation (non-WNT/non-SHH medulloblastomas). These tumors seem to lack recurrent mutations but show frequent chromosomal copy number alterations such as isochromosome 17q. They can be further subdivided with DNA methylation profiling or mRNA expression studies in "group 3" and "group 4" medulloblastomas. *MYC* amplification is frequently found in young children with group 3 tumors and is associated with poor outcome. Group 3 and 4 medulloblastomas have so far only been considered as provisional subentities because it is not clear if they represent distinct diseases or variants of a single entity.

All combinations between histologic and genetic parts of the medulloblastoma classification scheme are theoretically possible, but there are frequent associations (Figure 1.10). For example, most WNT-activated medulloblastomas are of classic histology (as are most non-WNT/non-SHH medulloblastomas), most SHH-activated medulloblastomas with *TP53* mutation show an anaplastic phenotype, while desmoplastic/nodular medulloblastomas and medulloblastomas with extensive nodularity are SHH-activated.

Immunohistochemistry. Medulloblastomas consistently express neural markers such as MAP2 and NCAM. The Ki-67/MIB1 index is usually high (Fig. 1.11b). Synaptophysin immunoreactivity is detected in many medulloblastomas. Tumor cells in large cell/anaplastic medulloblastomas often demonstrate a dot-like synaptophysin staining pattern. WNT-activated tumors show nuclear accumulation of β-catenin as well as Yap1 positivity in tumor cells, while SHH-activated tumors express Gab1, p75-NGFR, and Yap1 (Fig. 1.11e, f) but are negative for Otx2. In contrast, non-Wnt/non-SHH tumors are negative for Gab1, p75-NGFR, and Yap1 but express Otx2 [112]. The large islands of medulloblastomas with extensive nodularity are strongly stained for synaptophysin and the neuronal marker NeuN, reflecting an advanced neurocytic or granule cell differentiation.

Differential diagnosis. The differential diagnosis includes various other malignant CNS

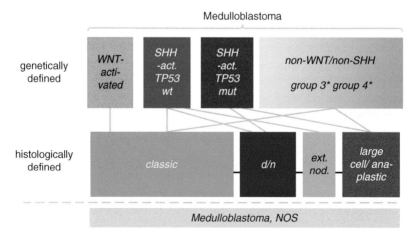

Fig. 1.10 Schematic representation of genetically and histologically defined medulloblastoma variants. Gray lines indicate the most prominent associations between the histologically and genetically defined entities. *d/n* desmoplastic/nodular medulloblastoma, *ext.nod.* medulloblastoma with extensive nodularity, *non-WNT/non-SHH* medulloblastoma, non-WNT/non-SHH, *NOS* not otherwise specified, *SHH-act. TP53wt medulloblastoma*, SHH-activated and *TP53* wild-type, *SHH-act. TP53mut medulloblastoma* SHH-activated and *TP53*-mutant. Asterisk—Provisional subentities

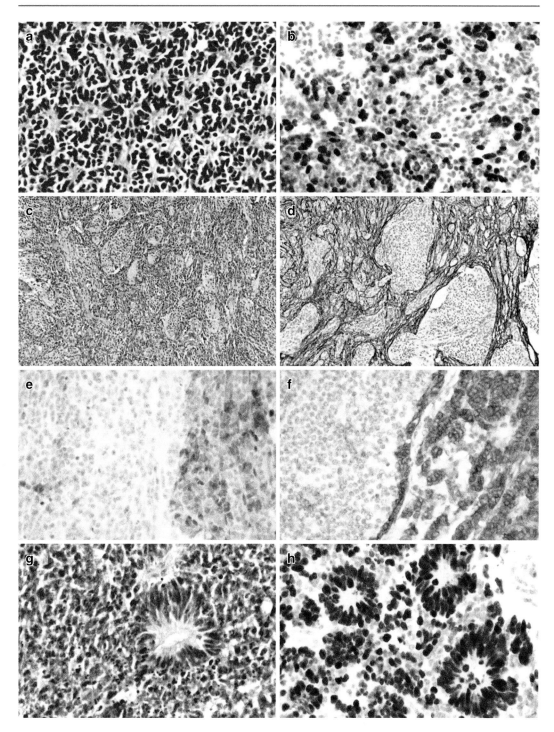

Fig. 1.11 Histologic features of selected embryonal tumors of the central nervous system. (**a**, **b**) Classic medulloblastoma. H&E stain showing a cellular tumor with formation of multiple neuroblastic (Homer-Wright) rosettes (**a**). High proliferative activity determined by MIB1 expression (**b**). (**c–f**) Desmoplastic medulloblastoma. Note a nodular pattern consisting of reticulin-rich, highly proliferative desmoplastic areas and reticulin-free pale island showing neuronal differentiation (**e**, H&E; **f**, reticulin stain). Tumor cells in desmoplastic areas stain positive for YAP1 (**e**) and p75NGFR (**f**), consistent with SHH pathway activation. (**g**, **h**) ETMR, c19MC-altered. The characteristic histologic feature of this rare embryonal tumor is the formation of multilayered, highly proliferative (ependymoblastic) rosettes (**g**, H&E; **h**, MIB1). (**i**, **j**) Atypical teratoid/rhabdoid tumor with expression of vimentin (**i**) and loss of nuclear INI1 immunoreactivity in the tumor cells (**j**)

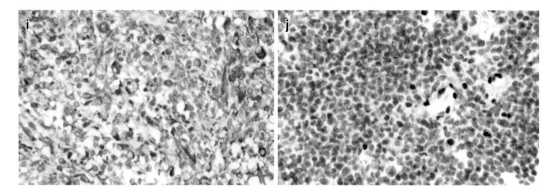

Fig. 1.11 (continued)

tumors, including anaplastic ependymoma, ETMR, atypical teratoid/rhabdoid tumor, as well as malignant gliomas composed of small anaplastic cells. On the other end of the spectrum, medulloblastoma needs to be distinguished from cerebellar neurocytoma/liponeurocytoma. In adult patients, cerebellar metastases from other small, round, and blue cell tumors, e.g., small cell carcinoma, need to be considered in the differential diagnosis.

Molecular pathology. Genetic findings as well as epigenetic and mRNA expression studies indicate that medulloblastoma represents a basket term for distinct disease entities with different histogenesis, genetic events involved in transformation, expression patterns, and different clinical behavior. From a cytogenetic point of view, the MB variants show specific recurrent alterations; WNT-activated medulloblastomas frequently have monosomy of chromosome 6, while SHH-activated tumors carry losses or allelic imbalances of chromosome arm 9q (containing *PTCH1*), associated with 17p deletions in SHH-activated and *TP53*-mutant tumors. The latter are characterized by chromosomal instability and may carry amplifications of *MYCN* and/or *GLI2* or show chromothripsis of individual chromosomes. The most frequent genetic alteration in non-WNT/non-SHH medulloblastomas is the formation of isochromosome 17q. Many of these tumors show an aneuploid karyotype with whole chromosomal gains and losses. In particular the group 3 tumors frequently show *MYCC* amplification related to adverse outcome. *MYCC* amplification is associated with large cell/anaplastic histologic phenotypes that have been associated with poor outcome. The mutational landscape at the genetic level has been extensively studied in large cohorts. Besides driver mutations defining the WNT- and SHH-activated entities, a multitude of mutant genes have been identified in medulloblastoma entities including, e.g., different chromatin modifier genes [103].

1.9.2 Embryonal Tumors with Multilayered Rosettes, C19MC-Altered

Definition. An aggressive CNS embryonal tumor with multilayered rosettes and alterations of the *C19MC* locus at 19q13.42. Most of these tumors have previously been diagnosed as *ependymoblastoma* (highly cellular variants) or *embryonal tumors with abundant neuropil and true rosettes* (variants with a dominant neuropil component).

Incidence and age distribution. The tumor is very rare and occurs in neonates and young children, mostly during the first 2 years of life.

Macroscopy and localization. Embryonal tumors with multilayered rosettes (ETMR) show relatively distinct tumor margins. The tumors are frequently inhomogeneous with formation of intratumoral cysts. Most tumors are located supratentorially and are usually related to the ventricles. However, other locations have been described. Leptomeningeal seeding is common.

Histopathology. ETMR display features of other primitive neuroepithelial tumors. They are composed of densely packed small round blue cells with high mitotic activity. Some cases show a dominant neuropil component. The distinctive histologic feature is the presence of multilayered rosettes with highly proliferating cells arranged around a lumen, so-called "ependymoblastic" rosettes (Fig. 1.11g, h). Some ETMR show tubular and trabecular structures consistent with the histology of medulloepithelioma.

Immunohistochemistry. ETMR is characterized by expression of LIN28A and vimentin. Neuropil islands are positive for synaptophysin, and glial differentiation may occur that can be visualized by immunostaining with antibodies against S-100 protein and GFAP.

Differential diagnosis. The major differential diagnoses are medulloblastoma, other embryonal tumors of the CNS, and anaplastic ependymoma. In contrast to ETMR, these tumors do not contain the multilayered ependymoblastic rosettes. Ependymomas display perivascular pseudorosettes and true ependymal rosettes, but no ependymoblastic rosettes.

Molecular pathology. ETMR are characterized by alterations (amplifications or fusions) of the oncogenic *C19MC* micro-RNA cluster on chromosome 19 [78]. Other chromosomal changes occur, such as frequent chromosome 2 gains.

Other CNS embryonal tumors. In the WHO classification 2016, the term "CNS-PNET" was replaced by the term "other CNS embryonal tumors" to avoid confusion caused by different meanings of primitive neuroectodermal tumor (PNET) in the last decades and also to discriminate these tumors from peripheral tumors belonging to the Ewing tumor family. Other CNS embryonal tumors represent a basket term for a heterogeneous group of tumors composed of poorly differentiated neuroepithelial cells. These tumors can arise in different regions of the CNS including the spinal cord. Tumors with predominant neuroblastic/neuronal differentiation are termed *CNS neuroblastomas* or, if ganglion cells are present, *CNS ganglioneuroblastomas*. Tumors displaying predominant features of neu-

ral tube differentiation are called *medulloepitheliomas* (*if they lack C19MC alteration*). These tumors most frequently occur in early childhood.

1.9.3 Medulloepithelioma

Definition. A CNS embryonal tumor with a prominent pseudostratified neuroepithelium that resembles the embryonic neural tube in addition to poorly differentiated neuroepithelial cells.

Incidence and age distribution. Medulloepithelioma is an extremely rare CNS tumor that either manifests as a congenital neoplasm or develops during the first 5 years of live.

Macroscopy and localization. The tumor most frequently arises in the cerebral hemispheres but can affect almost all CNS structures, including the eye. Medulloepitheliomas are usually bulky tumors that are well demarcated from the adjacent brain. Cysts, hemorrhages, and necrotic areas may be macroscopically visible. Some tumors disseminate in the subarachnoid space.

Histopathology. Medulloepitheliomas are characterized by the formation of pseudostratified neuroepitheliomatous structures resembling the primitive neural tube. The neoplastic neuroepithelium is arranged in tubular, papillary, or trabecular formations with an external limiting basal membrane. The rapidly dividing cells are of cuboid, sometimes elongated shape. The nuclei are oval and have a course chromatin structure. Mitotic figures tend to be located near the luminal surface. In other areas, the tumor cells are often densely packed. These areas may show evidence of divergent lines of differentiation, including an advanced neuronal differentiation. Ependymoblastomatous rosettes can also occur.

Immunohistochemistry. The medulloepithelioma component is positive for LIN28A, nestin and vimentin. Focal expression of cytokeratin or EMA has been described. Various differentiation lineages may be detected by immunohistochemistry, including tumor cells with neuronal (synaptophysin and neurofilament positivity) and glial (GFAP positivity) differentiation.

Differential diagnosis. The differential diagnoses include choroid plexus carcinoma, atypical teratoid/rhabdoid tumor, medulloblastoma, other CNS embryonal tumors, anaplastic ependymoma, and ETMR. Another differential diagnosis is immature teratoma, which additionally contains tissues from non-neuroectodermal germ layers.

Molecular pathology. The molecular genetic alterations in medulloepithelioma are poorly investigated. By definition, medulloepitheliomas should not carry *C19MC* alterations. If these are detected, tumors should be diagnosed as ETMR, *C19MC*-altered.

1.9.4   CNS Neuroblastoma/ Ganglioneuroblastoma

Definition. A CNS embryonal tumor characterized by poorly differentiated neuroepithelial cells, groups of neurocytic cells, and a variable neuropil-rich stroma. CNS ganglioneuroblastomas additionally contain ganglion cells.

Incidence and age distribution. CNS neuroblastomas are very rare tumors of childhood, mostly located in the cerebral hemispheres.

Macroscopy and localization. Most CNS neuroblastomas are of soft consistency. The tumors may contain areas of hemorrhage and/or necrosis. Most commonly these tumors occur in the cerebral hemispheres.

Histopathology. The histology of CNS neuroblastoma resembles that of peripheral neuroblastomas, i.e., the tumor is mainly composed of poorly differentiated or neuroblastic neuroepithelial cells embedded in a neuropil-like matrix. Some CNS neuroblastomas show nodular architectures. Formation of Homer-Wright rosettes may be seen. Cell density and mitotic activity vary. Ganglioneuroblastomas additionally contain variable fractions of ganglion cells.

Immunohistochemistry. These tumors express synaptophysin in varying intensity and Olig2 in fractions of tumors cells. Subpopulations of tumor cells may express NeuN and GFAP. The majority of tumor cells are negative for vimentin. Lin28A is absent.

Differential diagnosis. The differential diagnosis includes glioblastoma, oligodendroglioma, ETMR, and other highly proliferative small cell neoplasms. The differential diagnosis between glioblastoma and CNS neuroblastoma may be particularly difficult. Immunohistochemical evidence for neuronal differentiation and absence of vimentin argues in favor of a CNS neuroblastoma.

Molecular pathology. DNA methylation studies and sequencing showed that a fraction of CNS neuroblastomas show *FOXR2* rearrangements [146]. In addition, single cases with *MYCN* amplification have been identified.

CNS embryonal tumors, NOS. These tumors lack the specific features that define any of the other embryonal tumor entities. It is not clear if these tumors represent an undifferentiated variant of CNS neuroblastoma or an own entity. The differential diagnosis is broad; immunohistologic and molecular analysis are necessary for the exclusion of other entities.

1.9.5   Atypical Teratoid/Rhabdoid Tumor

Definition. A malignant CNS embryonal tumor composed predominantly of poorly differentiated cells, frequently including rhabdoid cells, with inactivation of *SMARCB1/INI1* or (extremely rare) *SMARCA4/BRG1*.

Incidence and age distribution. Atypical teratoid/rhabdoid tumor (AT/RT) accounts for approximately 2% of brain tumors in patients less than 18 years. Most tumors occur in the first 3 years of life or are already present at birth. Adults are only exceptionally affected. AT/RTs can occur sporadically or as part of the "rhabdoid tumor predisposition syndrome."

Macroscopy and localization. The often bulky tumors are soft and of pink or white color. The degree of demarcation from the surrounding brain tissue varies. The tumors may contain hemorrhagic or necrotic areas. Growth and seeding in the leptomeninx are frequently seen already at the time of diagnosis. AT/RTs can arise in any CNS area, but are most common in the posterior fossa, especially the cerebellopontine angle, followed by supratentorial locations.

Histopathology. AT/RTs are characterized by rhabdoid cells with eosinophilic, frequently homogenously stained cytoplasm and an eccentric nucleus with vesicular chromatin structure and prominent nucleolus. Mitotic figures are abundant. In addition to these characteristic rhabdoid cells, AT/RTs often contain areas showing differentiation along glial, epithelial, mesenchymal, and other lineages, i.e., may mimic the appearance of a malignant glioma, carcinoma, or sarcoma, respectively. Furthermore, areas composed of small undifferentiated cells are not infrequent.

Immunohistochemistry. Immunohistochemical studies are very helpful to establish the diagnosis, especially in cases with only rare rhabdoid cells and/or undifferentiated areas. Rhabdoid cells strongly express vimentin (Fig. 1.11i). EMA reactivity is also found in most tumors. Reflecting their variable differentiation potential, neoplastic cells with immunoreactivity for cytokeratins, smooth muscle actin, desmin, GFAP, and/or synaptophysin may be detected in variable amounts. AT/RTs lack nuclear expression of SMARCB1/INI1 (Fig. 1.11j) or in rare cases of SMARCA4/BRG1, which both are ubiquitously expressed in normal tissues. Demonstration of either protein loss is necessary to diagnose an AT/RT but not sufficient. Several other tumor entities may also show loss of nuclear SMARCB1/INI1.

Differential diagnosis. AT/RT needs to be distinguished from medulloblastoma, other CNS embryonal tumors, glioblastoma, and choroid plexus carcinoma. Application of a panel of antibodies, in particular against SMARCB1/INI1 and SMARCA4/BRG1, and molecular studies help to circumvent diagnostic difficulties caused by the lack of a significant rhabdoid cell component and potentially misleading differentiation.

Molecular pathology. The majority of AT/RT show *SMARCB1* gene mutations or deletions of the *SMARCB1* locus at 22q11.2. In rare cases, the *SMARCA4* gene is mutated. The respective proteins INI1 and BRG1 are components of the SWI/SNF chromatin remodelling complex regulating transcription. Some patients carry

de novo germline mutations in *SMARCB1*. It is estimated that germline mutations occur in up to one third of the patients. These patients typically develop tumors early in their life (rhabdoid tumor syndrome). In addition, few familial cases have been described. Three distinct DNA methylation subgroups of AT/RT have been identified [64].

1.10 Tumors of the Cranial and Paraspinal Nerves

This chapter focuses on the most common cranial and paraspinal nerve tumors, namely, *schwannoma, neurofibroma, perineurioma*, and *malignant peripheral nerve sheath tumor (MPNST)*. An important clinical issue of cranial and paraspinal nerve tumors is their potential association with the following familial tumor syndromes (Table 1.6):

- *Neurofibromatosis type 1* (NF1): an autosomal dominant disorder caused by mutations of the *NF1* gene at 17q11.2 and characterized by multiple neurofibromas (with the plexiform variant being almost pathognomonic for NF1), optic glioma, and an increased risk for malignant peripheral nerve sheath tumor (MPNST) and other (nonneural) neoplasms.
- *Neurofibromatosis type 2* (NF2): an autosomal dominant disorder caused by mutations of the *NF2* gene on chromosome 22q12 and characterized by schwannomas in the cerebellopontine angle ("vestibular schwannomas," often bilateral), and schwannomas of other cranial, spinal, and peripheral nerves and the skin, by gliomas (in particular ependymomas in the spinal cord), and by a variety of non-tumoral/dysplastic lesions.
- *Schwannomatosis*: a usually sporadic, sometimes autosomal dominant disorder caused by mutations in *SMARCB1* or *LZTR1*, both on chromosome 22q, and characterized by multiple schwannomas (spinal, cutaneous, cranial, but typically not in the cerebellopontine angle) and multiple cranial and/or spinal meningiomas.

Patients diagnosed with multiple nerve sheath tumors, including particular forms or distribution of these tumors (esp. plexiform neurofibroma, bilateral vestibular schwannoma), or combination with particular other tumor entities should be checked for further clinical features of these familial tumor syndromes (Table 1.6). Of note, in the WHO 2016 classification of CNS tumors, a *hybrid nerve sheath tumor* was introduced for a group of benign, peripheral nerve sheath tumors with combined features of more than one conventional type, such as schwannoma/perineurioma (often occurring sporadically) and schwannoma/neurofibroma (typically associated with NF1, NF2, or schwannomatosis).

1.10.1 Schwannoma

Definition. A benign, usually encapsulated nerve sheath tumor entirely composed of neoplastic Schwann cells. Schwannomas carry *NF2* gene mutations typically causing loss of expression of merlin, the *NF2* gene product.

Incidence and age distribution. Schwannomas (synonyms: neurinoma, neurilemoma) account for about 8% of intracranial 30% of spinal nerve root tumors. They may develop at any age, with a peak of incidence between the fourth and sixth decade. Most studies show no clear sex predilection, although intracranial schwannomas may occur more often in females.

Macroscopy and localization. Schwannomas are usually encapsulated, globular to multinodular masses associated with a nerve or nerve root. Schwannomas located within the brain or spinal cord parenchyma lack encapsulation and obvious association with a parent nerve. On cut surface, schwannomas are light tan to yellow, frequently cystic, and partially hemorrhagic. The vast majority of intracranial schwannomas develop from the vestibular nerve (Fig. 1.12a). Tumors of the trigeminal or facial nerve are far less common. Primary intracerebral, intraventricular, or intramedullary schwannomas are very rare. Spinal schwannomas can originate from any nerve root, with the dorsal (sensory) roots being more commonly affected than the ventral roots. The majority of spinal schwannomas are intradural lesions. However, some tumors extend through the intervertebral foramen and form so-called *dumbbell* or *hourglass schwannomas*.

Histopathology. Schwannomas typically show two distinct histologic patterns designated as *Antoni A* and *B*, respectively. Antoni A areas are relatively compact with closely apposed, spindle-shaped Schwann cells and elongated nuclei arranged in streams and with often dispersed nuclear palisades (*Verocay bodies*) (Fig. 1.12b). Verocay bodies are more common in peripheral and spinal tumors as compared to vestibular tumors. The Antoni B pattern refers to loosely textured, less cellular, and often lipidized tumor areas that are thought to result from a degenerative process. In Antoni B areas, the neoplastic Schwann cells commonly demonstrate more rounded nuclei and stellate processes. Foamy histiocytes may be prominent. Vascular hyalinization is another characteristic feature of schwannomas. In addition, areas with cystic degeneration and intratumoral hemorrhages are frequent. Marked nuclear pleomorphism, including the presence of bizarre nuclei, is a prominent degenerative feature in the so-called ancient schwannomas. Occasional mitotic figures may be present in schwannomas but are not indicative of malignancy. The Gomori stain reveals a dense network of curly reticulin fibers in the tumor tissue, in particular in the Antoni A areas.

Histologic variants listed in the WHO classification are *cellular schwannoma, plexiform schwannoma*, and *melanotic schwannoma*. *Cellular schwannoma* refers to hypercellular tumors with low to moderate mitotic activity, an exclusive or predominant Antoni A growth pattern, and absence of Verocay bodies. Cellular schwannomas are benign tumors that need to be distinguished from MPNST. The risk of recurrence after incomplete resection is higher as compared to conventional schwannoma. *Plexiform schwannomas* are characterized by a multinodular or plexiform growth pattern and most commonly involve dermal or subcutaneous nerves. Most cases are sporadic and solitary. Plexiform schwannomas are (in contrast to plexiform neurofibromas) not associated with NF1 but may be more common in NF2 and schwannomatosis. *Melanotic schwannomas* are characterized by tumor cells containing melanosomes. Two forms can be distinguished, melanotic schwannoma with and without psammoma bodies. Most non-psammomatous tumors affect spinal nerves, whereas psammomatous variants are also found in visceral organs. About half of the psammomatous melanotic schwannomas occur in patients with *Carney complex*, a rare, autosomal dominantly inherited disorder with facial lentigines, cardiac myxoma, endocrine hyperfunction (Cushing syndrome), and Sertoli cell tumors as other characteristics. About 10% of melanotic schwannomas show histologic signs of anaplasia and behave clinically malignant.

Immunohistochemistry. Schwannomas are strongly positive for S-100 and SOX10. Antibodies against collagen IV or laminin stain the pericellular basal lamina. Focal GFAP immunoreactivity may be observed. Melanotic schwannomas may react with antibodies against melan A or HMB-45.

Molecular pathology. The majority of sporadic schwannomas carry somatic mutations in the *NF2* tumor suppressor gene at 22q12, frequently combined with loss of heterozygosity on chromosome 22. Germline *NF2* mutations are underlying the development of often multiple schwannomas in NF2 patients.

Differential diagnosis. Hybrid tumors showing a combination of schwannoma and perineurioma or of schwannoma and neurofibroma features may occur. In particular in patients with NF1, neurofibromas containing schwannoma-like nodules are sometimes encountered. Plexiform schwannomas must not be confused with plexiform neurofibromas; the latter are usually larger and deeper situated lesions. The absence of marked anaplasia and uniform S-100 expression helps to distinguish cellular schwannomas from MPNSTs. The presence of areas with typical schwannoma features and a dense pericellular reticulin network supports the diagnosis melanotic schwannoma over (primary) melanocytic CNS tumor, and testing for *GNAQ* and *GNA11* mutations may distinguish these entities [81].

1.10.2 Neurofibroma

Definition. A benign, well-demarcated intraneural, or diffusely infiltrative extraneural peripheral nerve sheath tumor composed of neoplastic, well-differentiated Schwann cells, intermixed with perineurial-like cells, fibroblasts, mast cells, a variably myxoid to collagenous matrix, and residual axons or ganglion cells.

Incidence and age distribution. Neurofibromas are common tumors that are found at all ages without any gender preference.

Macroscopy and localization. Most neurofibromas present as solitary, slowly growing, circumscribed but not encapsulated cutaneous nodules. These *localized cutaneous neurofibromas* are distinguished from several other variants. *Diffuse cutaneous neurofibromas* are large, ill-defined, plaque-like lesions in the dermis and subcutis. *Localized intraneural neurofibroma* typically presents as fusiform swelling of a spinal or peripheral nerve. *Plexiform neurofibromas* are elongated, multinodular lesions involving multiple fascicles of a large nerve or multiple trunks of a nerve plexus. Their macroscopic appearance often is referred to as corresponding to a "bag of worms." With very rare exceptions, plexiform neurofibromas are pathognomonic of NF1. *Massive soft tissue neurofibromas* ("elephantiasis neuromatosa") are huge lesions closely associated with NF1, leading to localized gigantism of certain regions of the body, such as the shoulder, the pelvic girdle, or a limb. *Visceral neurofibromas* affect inner organs, most commonly the gastrointestinal tract. Neurofibromas of the cranial nerves are rare. Solitary neurofibromas are mostly sporadic tumors, whereas multiple neurofibromas, e.g., multiple diffuse or localized cutaneous tumors or multiple localized intraneural tumors of the spinal roots, are frequently associated with NF1. Plexiform neurofibromas and intraneural neurofibromas of major nerves are associated with an increased risk of progression toward MPNST.

Histopathology. Neurofibromas consist of a mixture of different cell types including neoplastic Schwann cells, perineurial-like cells, and fibroblasts. Mast cells are also commonly seen. The different cells are typically embedded in an alcianophilic myxoid matrix containing thick collagen fibers (Fig. 1.12c). The latter often resemble the picture of "shredded carrots." Mitotic figures are rare. Extraneural tumors lack encapsulation and may diffusely infiltrate into the surrounding soft tissue. Intraneural lesions are generally more or less demarcated and infiltrate along existing axons, which often remain visible within the tumor tissue. Tumors originating from spinal roots frequently infiltrate into the adjacent ganglia. Formation of tactile structures is occasionally seen. Tumors with degenerative nuclear atypia may be referred to as "atypical neurofibroma," while "cellular neurofibromas" show increased cellularity but no definite features of malignancy. All types of neurofibromas correspond to WHO grade I.

Immunohistochemistry. The neoplastic Schwann cells in neurofibromas are positive for S-100 and SOX10.

Differential diagnosis. Schwannoma is the principal differential diagnosis of localized intraneural neurofibroma. Large neurofibromas of major nerves as well as plexiform variants should be carefully screened for the presence of anaplastic features. Perineurioma differs from neurofibroma by the lack of S-100 expression and positivity for EMA.

Molecular pathology. Neurofibromas are caused either by somatic (sporadic tumors) or by germline (NF1-associated tumors) mutations in the *NF1* tumor suppressor gene. Among the different cell types in neurofibromas, the Schwann cells are the neoplastic cells that show biallelic *NF1* inactivation [138].

1.10.3 Perineurioma

Definition. A peripheral nerve sheath tumor composed of neoplastic perineurial cells. Two principal types are distinguished: *intraneural perineurioma* and *soft tissue perineurioma*.

Incidence and age distribution. Perineuriomas account for <1% of all peripheral nerve neoplasms. Intraneural perineuriomas (long mistakenly considered as hypertrophic neuropathy)

predominantly affect adolescents and young adults without a gender preference. Soft tissue perineuriomas are more common in females and preferentially occur in adults.

Macroscopy and localization. Intraneural perineuriomas present as cylindric nerve enlargement, typically affecting peripheral nerves of an extremity. In contrast, soft tissue perineuriomas are not clearly associated with a nerve but present as small, solitary, unencapsulated, subcutaneous nodular lesions of the leg or hand or in deep soft tissues.

Histopathology. Intraneural perineurioma is characterized by perineurial cells that form concentric, multilayered whorls around nerve fibers ("pseudo-onion bulbs"). Mitoses are absent or rare. Intraneural perineuriomas correspond to WHO grade I. Soft tissue perineuriomas consist of spindle-shaped perineurial cells forming fascicles, storiform patterns, and/or loose whorls in a collagen-rich matrix. Markedly sclerotic areas may be seen. Mitotic activity is low in most cases but may be elevated in a fraction of cases. Benign soft tissue perineurioma corresponds to WHO grade I. Soft tissue perineuriomas with hypercellularity, hyperchromasia, and increased, sometimes brisk, mitotic activity correspond to WHO grade II. Additional presence of necrosis is indicative of anaplasia corresponding to WHO grade III.

Immunohistochemistry. Perineuriomas are positive for EMA but negative for S-100, SOX10, and CD34.

Molecular pathology. Intraneural perineuriomas frequently carry *TRAF7* mutations [70].

1.10.4 Hybrid Nerve Sheath Tumors

These benign tumors of WHO grade I are defined by combined features of two distinct peripheral nerve sheath tumor types, most commonly schwannoma/neurofibroma (Fig. 1.12d), which are seen in more than 70% of patients with schwannomatosis and less commonly in NF2 or NF1 patients, and schwannoma/perineurioma. Neurofibroma/perineurioma is rare and often associated with NF1. Multiple peripheral nerve

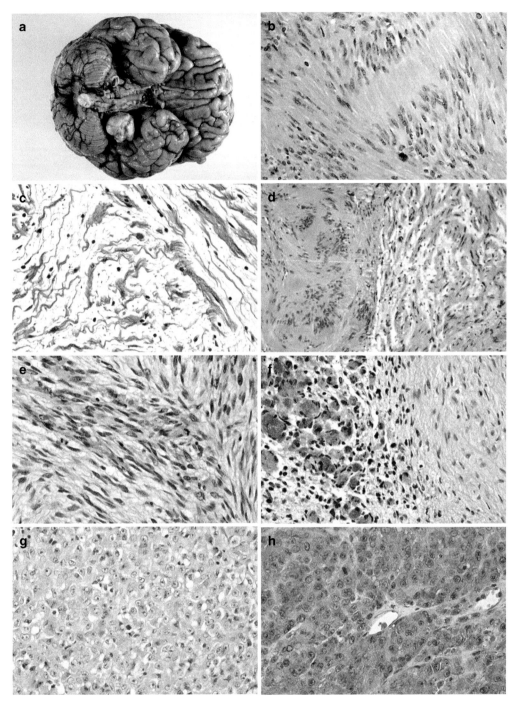

Fig. 1.12 Macroscopic and histologic features of selected tumors of the peripheral nervous system. (**a**) Autopsy finding of a vestibular schwannoma in the right cerebellopontine angle. (**b**) Schwannoma, WHO grade I with typical formation of palisades (*Verocay bodies*) (H&E). (**c**) Neurofibroma, WHO grade I. Note spindle cells and collagen bundles in a myxoid matrix (H&E). (**d**) Hybrid nerve sheath tumor with areas of schwannoma and neurofibroma (H&E). (**e**) Malignant peripheral nerve sheath tumor (MPNST) with fascicular growth and high mitotic activity (H&E). (**f**) MPNST with rhabdomyoblastic differentiation (malignant triton tumor) (H&E). (**g, h**) Epithelioid MPNST composed of epithelioid tumor cells with prominent nucleoli (**g**, H&E) and strong expression of S-100 (**h**). (**i, j**) MPNST with increased expression of EGFR (**i**) and loss of nuclear H3-K27me3 expression (**j**)

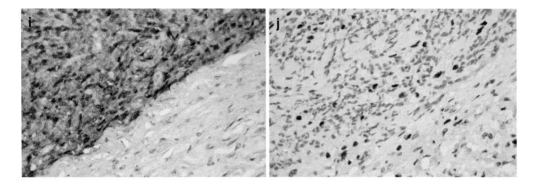

Fig.1. 12 (continued)

sheath tumors are present in more than 50% of patients with a hybrid nerve sheath tumors, indicating frequent hereditary predisposition.

1.10.5 Malignant Peripheral Nerve Sheath Tumor

Definition. A malignant tumor with evidence of Schwann cell or perineurial cell differentiation, commonly arising in a peripheral nerve or in extraneural soft tissue.

Incidence and age distribution. Malignant peripheral nerve sheath tumors (MPNSTs) are estimated to account for less than 5% of all malignant soft tissue tumors. Young and middle-aged adults are primarily affected. More than half of MPNST develop in NF1 patients, often from preexisting neurofibromas of major nerves or plexiform neurofibromas.

Macroscopy and localization. Most MPNSTs arise from medium or large nerves, with the sciatic nerve being most often affected. Development from a precursor lesion, such as a plexiform neurofibroma, is also frequent, in particular in NF1. Less commonly, MPNST presents as a soft tissue mass not associated with a recognizable nerve. Macroscopically, MPNST appears as usually large, fusiform or globoid, pseudoencapsulated tumors with a firm, gray or tan cut surface. Hemorrhagic and necrotic areas are often present.

Histopathology. The classic microscopic picture is a highly cellular spindle cell tumor

with a fibrosarcoma-like fascicular growth pattern (Fig. 1.12e). Most tumor cells have elongated, hyperchromatic nuclei with tapered ends and a bipolar, faintly eosinophilic cytoplasm. Mitotic activity is usually brisk, and necroses with or without pseudopalisading are commonly seen. MPNSTs invade not only the parent nerve but also grow invasively into the surrounding soft tissue. The following histologic variants are distinguished: *MPNST with divergent differentiation* (e.g., glandular MPNST or MPNST with rhabdomyosarcomatous or other mesenchymal differentiation), *epithelioid MPNST*, and *MPNST with perineurial differentiation/ malignant perineurioma*. Epithelioid MPNST (Fig. 1.12g, h) is composed of malignant epithelioid cells, accounts for approximately 5% of all MPNSTs, and is not associated with NF1. The glandular variant is characterized by the presence of epithelial glands, often with mucin production. MPNST with areas of rhabdomyosarcomatous differentiation is also called malignant triton tumor (Fig. 1.12f). Both glandular MPNST and malignant triton tumor are frequently associated with NF1. Occasional MPNSTs may show formation of bone or cartilage or demonstrate areas of both mesenchymal and epithelial differentiation. Robust and validated criteria for grading of MPNSTs are lacking, and (consequently) no firm association between histologic grade and survival has been established. One approach is to divide MPNSTs in low grade (about 15% of cases, showing a well-differentiated phenotype, most often arising in transition from neurofibroma and without marked mitotic activity) and high grade.

Immunohistochemistry. Vimentin is strongly expressed in MPNSTs but of limited diagnostic help. Expression of protein S-100 is found in half of the tumors and, when present, often restricted to only a fraction of tumor cells. In contrast to benign Schwann cell tumors, nuclear accumulation of p53 and increased expression of EGFR (Fig. 1.12i) may be seen in MPNST. In addition, loss of nuclear expression of H3-K27me3 (Fig. 1.12j), p16^{INK4A}, SOX10, and/or SUZ12 has been linked to MPNST [130]. Loss of nuclear SMARCB1/INI1 expression is seen in about half of all epithelioid MPNST [63]. Occasional tumors may show EMA immunoreactivity indicating cells with perineurial differentiation. Epithelial elements in glandular MPNST are positive for cytokeratins and EMA. Rhabdomyoblastic cells in malignant triton tumors react with antibodies against muscle antigens, while melanotic MPNSTs may show expression of melanocytic antigens (HMB-45, melan A). The MIB1 index is generally high.

Molecular pathology. Aberrations of *NF1*, *CDKN2A*, *SUZ12*, and *TP53*, as well as Ras pathway gene mutations, are frequent [21]. DNA methylation profiling distinguished two groups of high-grade MPNST characterized by loss or retention of H3-K27 trimethylation [128].

Differential diagnosis. MPNST needs to be distinguished from the cellular variants of schwannoma and neurofibroma. To identify focal progression toward MPNST in predisposing lesions such as plexiform neurofibroma, careful sampling is important. Several sarcomas, such as fibrosarcoma, leiomyosarcoma, rhabdomyosarcoma, synovial sarcoma, and epithelioid sarcoma, and melanoma have to be considered in the differential diagnosis.

1.11   Meningiomas

Definition. Meningiomas are tumors composed of neoplastic meningothelial (arachnoid) cells. Most meningiomas are slowly growing benign tumors that are attached to the dura mater. Less commonly, meningiomas show atypical or anaplastic histologic features that are associated with an increased likelihood for recurrence and/or aggressive behavior.

Incidence and age distribution. Meningiomas are the most common group of primary CNS tumors. The annual incidence is estimated at approximately 6 per 100,000 population. The tumors preferentially develop in elderly patients (age peak, 50–70 years). Females are more commonly affected than males. Most meningiomas are sporadic tumors. Patients with NF2 have a significantly increased risk, often resulting in multiple meningiomas. Familial meningioma in the absence of NF2 is rare.

Macroscopy and localization. Most meningiomas arise in the intracranial cavity, followed by spinal and intraorbital locations. Typical sites of intracranial meningiomas are the cerebral convexity and falx cerebri, olfactory groove, sphenoid or petrous ridges, parasellar region, optic nerve sheath, tentorium cerebelli, and posterior fossa. Intraventricular meningiomas are rare tumors thought to arise from meningothelial cells located in the choroid plexus or tela choroidea (Fig. 1.2f). Macroscopically, most meningiomas are solid, well-demarcated, often firm tumors that are broadly attached to the dura. The cut surface frequently appears lobulated. Benign meningiomas compress and displace but do not usually invade the adjacent brain tissue. In contrast, even benign meningiomas commonly invade into the dura including dural sinuses. Tumor growth into the skull is not infrequent, with some tumors invading through the skull into the adjacent extracranial soft tissues. Reactive hyperostosis of the skull involved by a meningioma is a typical finding. *Meningioma en plaque* describes a carpet-like flat meningioma, most often found over the sphenoid wing.

Histopathology. The histologic appearance of meningiomas is highly variable. The WHO classification includes nine different histologic variants associated with benign clinical behavior (meningiomas of WHO grade I) and six histologic variants associated with a greater risk for recurrence and/or aggressive clinical behavior (meningiomas of WHO grade II or III) (Table 1.5).

Table 1.5 Meningiomas: clinical behavior, WHO classification, and aberrant genes (modified from 114)

Tumor type and WHO grade	Aberrant genes
Meningiomas with low risk of recurrence and/or aggressive behavior	
Meningothelial meningioma (WHO grade I)	TRAF7, AKT1, PIK3CA, POLR2A, SMOH
Fibrous/fibroblastic meningioma (WHO grade I)	NF2
Transitional (mixed) meningioma (WHO grade I)	NF2, AKT1, PIK3CA
Psammomatous meningioma (WHO grade I)	NF2
Angiomatous meningioma (WHO grade I)	n.d. (polysomy chromosome 5)
Microcystic meningioma (WHO grade I)	n.d.
Secretory meningioma (WHO grade I)	KLF4, TRAF7
Lymphoplasmacyte-rich meningioma (WHO grade I)	n.d.
Metaplastic meningioma (WHO grade I)	n.d.
Meningiomas with greater risk of recurrence and/or aggressive behavior[a]	
Atypical meningioma (WHO grade II)	NF2, TRAF7, AKT1
Clear cell meningioma (WHO grade II)	SMARCE1
Chordoid meningioma (WHO grade II)	n.d.
Rhabdoid meningioma (WHO grade III)	BAP1
Papillary meningioma (WHO grade III)	n.d.
Anaplastic meningioma (WHO grade III)	NF2, CDKN2A, TERT

[a]Also includes meningiomas of any subtype with high proliferation index

In between 85 and 90% of all meningiomas belong to the first group of WHO grade I tumors, with meningothelial, fibrous/fibroblastic, and transitional variants being most common. Atypical meningiomas are the most frequent WHO grade II tumors, which account for approximately 10% of all meningiomas. Malignant meningiomas of WHO grade III are rare tumors (2–3% of all meningiomas).

Meningiomas of WHO grade I. This group of tumors consists of nine different histologic variants. In general, benign meningiomas show low mitotic activity (<4 mitoses per ten high-power fields) and do not fulfill the other histologic criteria indicative of atypical or anaplastic meningiomas (see below). *Meningothelial meningioma* is composed of uniform tumor cells closely resembling normal arachnoid cap cells (Fig. 1.13a). The tumor cells show a syncytially appearing growth in sheets and lobules surrounded by thin stromal septae. Nuclei are rounded to oval and may contain eosinophilic cytoplasmic invagination (pseudoinclusions). Nuclei with central clearing (hole nuclei) are also common. Whorl formations and occasional psammoma bodies may be seen but are less common as compared to transitional and psammomatous variants, respectively. The *fibrous (fibroblastic) meningioma* is characterized by fibroblast-like spindle

cells growing in a collagen- and reticulin fiber-rich matrix (Fig. 1.13b). A vaguely fascicular growth pattern is frequently seen, while whorls and psammoma bodies are rare. The *transitional (mixed) meningioma* shows both meningothelial and fibroblastic features. Whorl formation is often very prominent in this variant (Fig. 1.13c). *Psammomatous meningiomas* are characterized by the presence of abundant psammoma bodies. In some tumors, the psammoma bodies become confluent and form areas of calcification, occasionally leading to rock-hard lesions. The psammomatous variant is particularly common among meningiomas arising in the thoracic spinal region of women. *Angiomatous meningioma* refers to meningiomas showing excessive vascularization by small- to medium-sized, often hyalinized blood vessels with only interspersed meningothelial tumor cells (Fig. 1.13f). *Microcystic meningioma* is composed of bi- and multipolar cells lying in a mucinous matrix characterized by prominent microcystic degeneration (Fig. 1.13d). Occasionally, the tumor cells may be quite pleomorphic. Cytoplasmic vacuolation may also be seen. The *secretory meningioma* shows focal epithelial differentiation with deposition of glycogen-rich, strongly PAS-positive droplets (Fig. 1.13e). These so-called pseudo-psammoma bodies are surrounded by tumor cells expressing epithelial

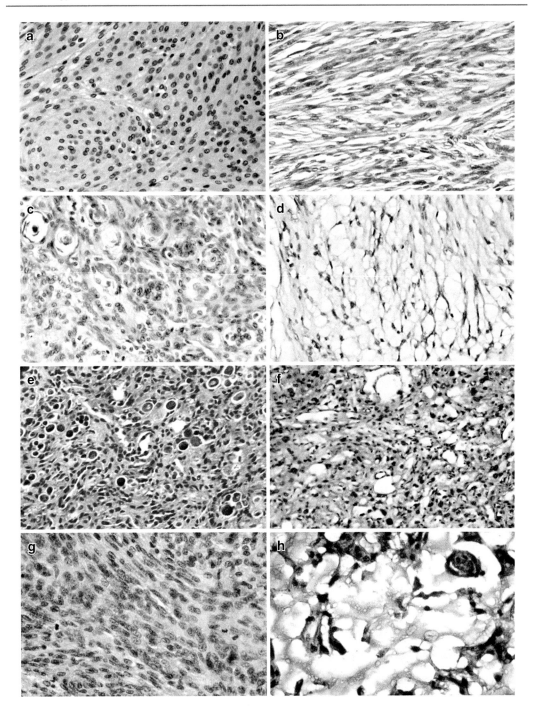

Fig. 1.13 Histologic features of selected meningioma variants (**a–f**). Meningiomas of WHO grade I corresponding to meningothelial (**a**), fibrous (**b**), transitional (**c**), microcystic (**d**), secretory (**e**), and angiomatous (**f**) variants (**a–d**, **f**: H&E; **e**, PAS). Note syncytial growth of meningothelial cells (**a**), fascicular growth of fibroblast-like spindle cells (**b**), formation of multiple meningeal whorls (**c**), prominent microcystic degeneration (**d**), production of PAS-positive pseudo-psammoma bodies (**e**), and numerous densely packed blood vessels (**e**). (**g**) Atypical meningioma, WHO grade II, with increased mitotic activity (H&E). (**h**) Chordoid meningioma showing chordoma-like growth of tumor cells in a myxoid matrix (H&E). (**i**) Anaplastic meningioma, WHO grade III with cellular anaplasia and numerous mitotic figures (H&E). (**j**) Papillary meningioma, WHO grade III demonstrating a pseudopapillary growth pattern (H&E)

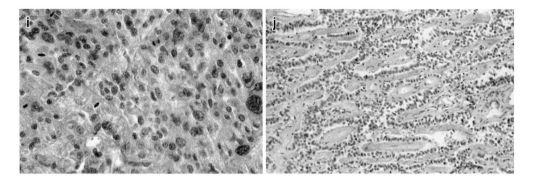

Fig. 1.13 (continued)

antigens, such as cytokeratins and carcinoem-bryonic antigen (CEA). A clinically important feature associated with secretory meningiomas is the induction of a marked peritumoral edema in the adjacent brain tissue. *Lymphoplasmacyte-rich meningioma* is a rare variant showing extensive inflammatory infiltrates and formation of Russell bodies. Recognition of the actual meningioma tissue may be difficult in some of these lesions. *Metaplastic meningioma* refers to tumors show-ing areas of differentiation toward adipose tissue, cartilage, or bone. The WHO classification also lists meningiomas with prominent xanthomatous or myxoid change under this subtype.

Meningiomas of WHO grade II. Three his-tologic meningioma variants are known to be associated with an increased likelihood for local recurrence after operative resection. *Atypical meningioma* (Fig. 1.13g) is the most common representative of WHO grade II meningioma and defined by (1) an increased mitotic count (four or more mitoses per ten high-power fields), (2) brain invasion, or (3) three or more of the follow-ing five histologic criteria: (a) increased cellular-ity, (b) presence of small cells with high nuclear/cytoplasmic ratios, (c) prominent nucleoli, (d) uninterrupted patternless or sheet-like growth, and (e) foci of spontaneous necrosis. *Chordoid meningioma* is a rare meningioma subtype char-acterized by areas histologically resembling chordoma, i.e., consisting of cords and clusters of eosinophilic, sometimes vacuolated cells in a basophilic mucoid matrix (Fig. 1.13h). In con-trast to chordoma, chordoid meningioma lacks

typical physaliphorous cells and usually contains areas showing meningothelial features, such as whorl formation or psammoma bodies. *Clear cell meningioma* is another rare variant composed of glycogen-rich, PAS-positive cells showing a clear cytoplasm on hematoxylin-eosin-stained paraffin sections. The tumors typically lack clas-sic features of meningioma and are preferentially found in the cauda equina region and the cerebel-lopontine angle.

Meningiomas of WHO grade III. This group of tumors includes three histologic vari-ants that show aggressive clinical behavior with locally invasive and destructive growth and the potential of metastasis formation. The prognosis is usually unfavorable as indicated by a mean overall survival of less than 2 years for patients with anaplastic meningiomas. *Anaplastic menin-gioma* (Fig. 1.13i) is histologically defined by a high mitotic count (20 or more mitoses per ten high-power fields) and/or an obviously malig-nant morphology resembling sarcoma, carci-noma, or malignant melanoma. Brain invasion is frequently present. However, brain invasion alone is not sufficient for the diagnosis of ana-plastic meningioma. *Rhabdoid meningioma* is an uncommon variant that is predominantly com-posed of so-called rhabdoid cells, i.e., tumor cells with rounded, eosinophilic cytoplasm and an eccentric nucleus. Mitotic activity is usu-ally high in these tumors, and other histologic features of malignancy, such as necroses, are present. The prognostic significance of focal rhabdoid differentiation in an otherwise ordinary meningioma without other signs of malignancy is questionable. A third variant of WHO grade III meningioma, the *papillary meningioma*, is also very rare and seems to occur more commonly in children. Histology shows a cellular meningeal tumor with prominent formation of perivascular pseudorosette-like structures and pseudopapillae (Fig. 1.13j).

Immunohistochemistry. Meningiomas are generally positive for vimentin and EMA, although membranous EMA expression may sometimes be focal or patchy. Other markers of potential diagnostic value are claudin-1, somatostatin receptor 2A, and desmoplakins. Secretory meningiomas show additional expression of cytokeratins and CEA, typically restricted to cells adjacent to pseudo-psammoma bodies. Immunoreactivity for S-100 or CD34 is seen in some cases. More than half of the benign meningiomas express progesterone receptors, while estrogen receptors are very rarely detectable. The MIB1 index is generally low (<5%) in benign meningiomas. In contrast, atypical meningiomas usually show increased MIB1 labeling of more than 5%, while anaplastic meningiomas are generally characterized by a very high MIB1 index. However, whether or not elevated MIB1 indices represent an independent prognostic variable in meningiomas that should be used for tumor grading is debated. Therefore, the MIB1 index has not been accepted as a grading criterion in the WHO classification. However, it is recognized that a high proliferation index should be considered as an indicator of a greater likelihood of recurrence and/or aggressive behavior (Table 1.5).

Differential diagnosis. The differential diagnosis of meningiomas is complex and, depending on the histologic subtype of meningioma, includes a spectrum of different types of benign and malignant neoplasms. For example, fibrous meningiomas need to be distinguished from other spindle cell tumors, such as schwannoma, solitary fibrous tumor/hemangiopericytoma, or smooth muscle tumors. Immunohistochemistry for EMA, S-100, CD34, and smooth muscle actin (SMA) helps to separate these entities. Immunohistochemistry for EMA and STAT6

also allows to distinguish meningioma from solitary fibrous tumor/hemangiopericytoma. The differential diagnosis of chordoid meningioma primarily includes chordoma and chordoid glioma of the third ventricle. Chordomas strongly stain for cytokeratins and brachyury, while chordoid gliomas are positive for GFAP and CD34. Microcystic meningiomas may be confused with astrocytic gliomas, in particular on frozen section, but are GFAP-negative. Clear cell meningioma lacks immunoreactivity for cytokeratins and thereby differs from metastatic clear cell carcinoma. Papillary meningiomas usually lack GFAP expression. In contrast, papillary ependymoma and astroblastoma, two important differential diagnoses, are GFAP-positive. In occasional cases of lymphoplasmacyte-rich meningioma, the meningeal tumor cells may be difficult to find; hence the differential diagnosis of inflammatory pseudotumor, IgG4-related or unrelated pachymeningitis, MALT-type dural-based lymphoma, or plasmacytoma may arise. Demonstration of monoclonality of kappa and lamba light chains by immunohistochemistry or by in situ hybridization or genetic demonstration of monoclonal immunoglobulin gene rearrangement may be required to confirm the diagnosis of lymphatic tumors. Anaplastic meningioma may mimic metastatic carcinoma, sarcoma, or melanoma. Again, thorough immunohistochemical analysis may be necessary to separate these entities, although problems may arise due to common aberrant expression of antigens in anaplastic meningioma, such as cytokeratins.

Molecular pathology. Meningioma was the first solid neoplasm shown to carry a characteristic cytogenetic alteration, namely, monosomy 22. Subsequent studies revealed the *NF2* gene as the primary target on 22q, whose mutation and/or deletion constitutes the most common early event in meningiomas [114]. *NF2* alterations are particularly common in fibroblastic, transitional, psammomatous, atypical, and anaplastic meningiomas but less common in meningothelial meningiomas. Several meningioma-associated mutant genes have been identified, and these are related to tumor location and histologic subtype (Table 1.5). About 13% of *NF2*-wild-

type meningiomas show *AKT1* hotspot mutations (E17K). Secretory meningiomas carry
combined *KLF4* and *TRAF7* mutations; clear
cell meningiomas show *SMARCE1* mutations,
while *BAP1* mutations are seen in rhabdoid
meningioma [139]. Angiomatous meningiomas
typically demonstrate polysomy of multiple
chromosomes including chromosome 5 [1].
Genes mutated in minor subsets of meningioma include *SMOH*, *SMARCB1*, *PIK3CA*, and
POLR2A [114]. Interestingly, convexity meningiomas frequently carry *NF2* mutations, with
a minor subset showing *SMARCB1* alterations.
Skull-base meningiomas more commonly carry
AKT1, *SMOH*, *KLF4*, *TRAF7*, and *POLR2A*
mutations, while *SMARCE1* mutations prefer
spinal (clear cell) meningiomas [114]. *TERT*
promoter mutations occur in about 6% of meningiomas, predominantly anaplastic variants,
and are associated with poor prognosis [132].
About two thirds of anaplastic meningiomas
demonstrate homozygous deletion, mutation,
or promoter hypermethylation of the *CDKN2A*,
p14^{ARF}, and *CDKN2B* genes on 9p21 [12], and
CDKN2A deletion has been associated with
poor survival [110]. DNA methylation profiling
revealed six DNA methylation classes, providing clinically relevant information beyond histologic grades [133].

1.12   Mesenchymal, Non-meningothelial Tumors

The group of mesenchymal, non-meningothelial
tumors consists of a heterogeneous mixture of
benign and malignant mesenchymal neoplasms
that arise in the meninges or, less commonly,
in the CNS parenchyma or choroid plexus. The
WHO classification lists different types of lipomatous, fibrous, myogenic, osteocartilaginous,
and vascular neoplasms under this category
(Table 1.1). The histologic features of the individual mesenchymal tumor entities correspond
to their respective counterparts arising in soft
tissues or bone, respectively. Here, we will only
address *solitary fibrous tumor/hemangiopericy-
toma* and *hemangioblastoma*.

1.12.1   Solitary Fibrous Tumor/Hemangiopericytoma

Definition. A mesenchymal, densely vascularized, and collagen-rich tumor, usually with
immunoreactivity for CD34 and fusion of the
NAB2 and *STAT6* genes.

Incidence and age distribution. Solitary
fibrous tumors/hemangiopericytomas are about
50 times less common than meningiomas. The
patient age at diagnosis is lower as compared to
meningiomas, with a peak incidence in the fourth
to sixth decades. Males are more commonly
affected than females.

Macroscopy and localization. Most tumors
are solitary and are attached to the intracranial
or spinal dura. They are well-demarcated, solid,
and firm lesions that macroscopically cannot
be distinguished from a meningioma. The cut
surface may appear somewhat lobulated, and
numerous vessels as well as intratumoral hemorrhage may be visible. Some tumors may invade
into the adjacent CNS tissue or nerve roots.
High-grade solitary fibrous tumors/hemangio-
pericytomas represent the most common intracranial tumors with systemic metastases (up to
20% of patients).

Histopathology. Grade I tumors correspond
to the solitary fibrous tumor phenotype in other
locations outside the CNS. The paucicellular
tumors are composed of elongated to spindle-
shaped cells growing in fascicles in a collagen
fiber-rich matrix. Mitotic activity is virtually
absent or low (less than five mitoses per ten
high-power fields). In contrast to meningiomas,
whorls and psammoma bodies are absent. Grade
II and III tumors exhibit the hemangiopericytoma histologic phenotype (Fig. 1.14a). These
moderately to highly cellular tumors are composed of relatively uniform, small cells with oval
nuclei and inconspicuous nucleoli. Mitotic activity is usually present. The tumor tissue is richly
vascularized and contains characteristic slit-like
or staghorn-like sinusoidal vessels. The reticulin stain reveals a dense pericellular network of
reticulin fibers. Less cellular areas of fibrosis are
often present and reflect transitions to the solitary fibrous tumor phenotype. Grade III (ana-

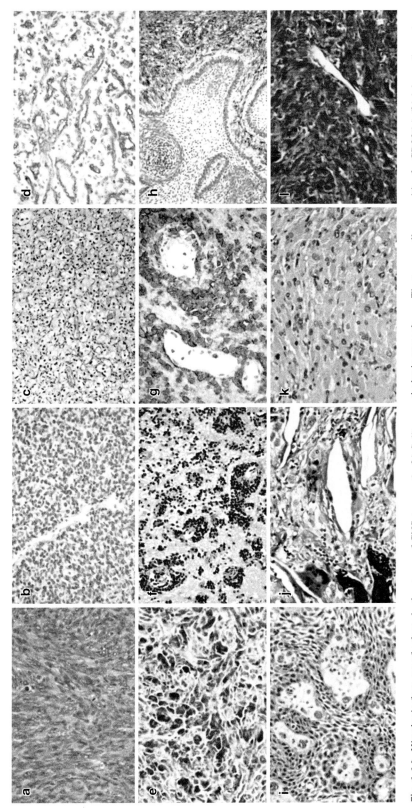

Fig. 1.14 Histologic features of selected other types of CNS tumors. (**a, b**) Solitary fibrous tumor/hemangiopericytoma of the meninges. Note a cellular tumor (**a**, H&E) with nuclear positivity for STAT6 (**b**). (**c, d**) Hemangioblastoma, WHO grade I. On H&E, these tumors are characterized by vacuolated stromal cells located in a dense network of capillary vessels (**c**). Immunostaining for CD34 highlights the dense vascularization (**d**). (**e**) Meningeal melanocytoma composed of isomorphic melanocytic cells with abundant melanin pigmentation (H&E). (**f, g**) Primary intracerebral diffuse large B-cell lymphoma. On H&E (**f**), the tumor shows an angiocentric growth within

the brain parenchyma. The tumor cells are positive for CD20 (**g**). (**h**) Adamantinomatous craniopharyngioma, WHO grade I pushing toward the adjacent brain tissue, which shows a strongly GFAP-positive reactive gliosis (right side). The actual craniopharyngioma tissue (left side) is GFAP-negative. (**i**) Papillary craniopharyngioma with tumor cells forming pseudopapillary structures around hyalinized vessels (H&E). (**j**) Xanthogranuloma of the sellar region (Masson trichrome stain). (**k, l**) Granular cell tumor of the neurohypophysis, WHO grade I. Shown is a moderately cellular tumor composed of granular cells (**k**, H&E) that are strongly PAS positive (**l**)

plastic) tumors are characterized by increased mitotic activity (five or more mitoses per ten high-power fields).

Immunohistochemistry. Most helpful is staining for STAT6 which shows positivity of tumor cell nuclei, because the tumor-specific *NAB2-STAT6* fusion leads to nuclear translocation of STAT6 (Fig. 1.14b). In contrast, virtually all other tumors including meningiomas show cytoplasmic immunoreactivity for STAT6, making nuclear STAT6 a reliable marker for solitary fibrous tumors/hemangiopericytomas. Tumor cells are usually positive for vimentin, CD34, CD99, and bcl2 but lack expression of desmoplakin, progesterone receptor, cytokeratins, desmin, muscle actin, and S-100. EMA is negative or only focally positive. Endothelial antigens such as CD31 are restricted to vessels.

Differential diagnosis. The most common differential diagnosis includes meningiomas which can usually be differentiated by their positivity for EMA and desmoplakin, negativity for CD34, and cytoplasmic (rather than nuclear) positivity for STAT6. Rare (malignant) cases need to be differentiated from other mesenchymal tumors, such as mesenchymal chondrosarcoma and malignant peripheral nerve sheath tumor.

Molecular pathology. Fusion of the *NAB2* and *STAT6* genes represent the diagnostic molecular hallmark, which is invariably present in solitary fibrous tumors/hemangiopericytomas [137]. Homozygous *CDKN2A* deletion has been reported in a subset of tumors [105].

1.12.2 Hemangioblastoma

Definition. A benign, slowly growing tumor of uncertain histogenesis histologically composed of neoplastic stromal cells and abundant small vessels.

Incidence and age distribution. Hemangioblastomas account for less than 2% of all intracranial neoplasms. The tumors usually become manifest in adults, with a peak incidence between the third to fifth decade. Approximately 25–30% of hemangioblastoma patients have von Hippel-Lindau (VHL) disease, with tumors in VHL patients more commonly arising before the age of 30 years. Because of the association with VHL disease, it is recommended that all hemangioblastoma patients should be screened for clinical and radiological features of this disease and that genetic testing for *VHL* gene mutation be offered to hemangioblastoma patients who are younger than 50 years [54].

Macroscopy and localization. Over 80% of the CNS hemangioblastomas are located in the cerebellum. Less common sites include the brain stem and spinal cord, while supratentorial hemangioblastomas are very rare. The combination of retinal and cerebellar hemangioblastoma and of multiple CNS hemangioblastomas is characteristic for VHL disease. Macroscopically, hemangioblastomas are typically presenting as a well-demarcated large cyst with a densely vascularized, red or yellow tumor nodule attached to the cyst wall.

Histopathology. Microscopically, hemangioblastomas are composed of two principal components: a dense network of vascular channels, mostly capillaries, and so-called stromal or interstitial cells, which represent the actual tumor cells (Fig. 1.14c). These latter cells are characterized by a relatively large, often clear and lipidized (vacuolated) cytoplasm. Nuclear pleomorphism may be prominent but mitoses are rare or absent. Mast cells are commonly observed and some tumors may demonstrate foci of intratumoral erythropoiesis. Cystic degeneration is commonly seen, as are areas of fibrosis. The brain parenchyma adjacent to the tumor often shows marked reactive gliosis. Depending on the abundance of stromal cells, cellular and reticular histologic variants may be distinguished.

Immunohistochemistry. The stromal cell is positive for S-100, neuron-specific enolase, and vimentin but negative for cytokeratins and EMA. In addition, EGFR and its ligand TGF-α are strongly coexpressed by the stromal cells. Focal staining for erythropoietin may be observed in some case. The dense vasculature is highlighted by staining for endothelial markers such as CD31 or CD34 (Fig. 1.14d). The MIB1 index is generally low.

Differential diagnosis. On frozen sections, hemangioblastoma may sometimes be difficult to distinguish from a glioma. In addition, the cerebellar tissue adjacent to a hemangioblastoma may demonstrate marked "piloid" gliosis, which should not be mistaken for a pilocytic astrocytoma. The cellular variant of hemangioblastoma needs to be distinguished from a metastatic renal clear cell carcinoma by lack of immunoreactivity for cytokeratins, EMA, inhibin A, and CD10.

Molecular pathology. Familial cases of hemangioblastoma uniformly result from mutations in the VHL gene. In the vast majority of sporadic cases, inactivation of the VHL gene can be demonstrated as well [140]. VHL gene alterations are restricted to the stromal cells, supporting the hypothesis that these cells are the neoplastic elements in hemangioblastomas [84]. Loss of VHL protein function in the stromal cells leads to stabilization of hypoxia-inducible factors (HIFs) and constitutive upregulation of HIF-regulated genes, including the genes for vascular endothelial growth factor (VEGF) and erythropoietin. The receptors for VEGF, i.e., VEGFR-1 and VEGFR-2, are expressed on the capillary endothelial cells, suggesting that angiogenesis and cyst formation in hemangioblastomas is stimulated via a paracrine mechanism [166].

1.13 Melanocytic Tumors

Definition. A spectrum of benign to malignant, primary melanocytic tumors presumably arising from leptomeningeal melanocytes. Diffuse benign lesions without forming macroscopic masses are termed *meningeal melanocytosis*, diffuse malignant lesions *meningeal melanomatosis*, benign or intermediate-grade tumoral lesions *meningeal melanocytoma*, and malignant tumors *meningeal melanoma*.

Incidence and age distribution. Primary melanocytic tumors of the meninges are rare neoplasms. *Meningeal melanocytosis* is most common in pediatric patients and may be combined with giant and/or numerous congenital cutaneous nevi (*neurocutaneous melanosis*). Congenital nevus of Ota may also be associated.

Meningeal melanocytoma and *melanoma* may manifest at any age but are preferentially found in adults [81].

Macroscopy and localization. *Meningeal melanocytosis* and *melanomatosis* typically cause black discoloration and variable thickening of large parts of the intracranial and spinal leptomeninges (Fig. 1.2j). *Melanocytomas* are usually solitary, circumscribed tumors attached to the dura mater. Preferential locations of *meningeal melanocytoma and melanoma* include regions where leptomeningeal melanocytes are physiologically present at highest density, such as the base of the brain and posterior fossa, as well as the upper cervical cord [81].

Histopathology. *Meningeal melanocytosis* is histologically characterized by a diffuse proliferation of uniform melanocytic cells in the leptomeninges. Tumor cells often spread along vessels in the Virchow-Robin spaces but do not infiltrate into the brain parenchyma. However, progression to melanoma and/or melanomatosis may occur, and the prognosis is often poor, even in the absence of histologic malignancy. The morphology of tumor cells in *meningeal melanocytoma* is quite variable, ranging from epithelioid cells growing in a nested pattern to spindle cells forming fascicular architectures. Melanin pigmentation is also variable, with some tumors being heavily melanotic (Fig. 1.14e) and others containing large amelanotic areas. Nucleoli may be prominent but mitotic activity is low. Histologic features of anaplasia are absent. It has been suggested that cases with bland cytologic features but with increased mitotic activity or ingrowth in CNS parenchyma should be designated as intermediate-grade melanocytoma. *Meningeal melanomas* histologically resemble melanomas in other locations. In contrast to melanocytomas, the tumors cytologically show features of malignancy, such as marked cellular and nuclear pleomorphism, high mitotic activity, areas of necrosis, and intratumoral hemorrhage, often combined with invasion into CNS tissue. Occasionally, melanocytoma may show progression to meningeal melanoma on recurrence. Secondary diffuse subarachnoid tumor spread of a malignant melanoma may cause *meningeal melanomatosis* [81].

Immunohistochemistry. Like other melanocytic tumors, primary meningeal melanocytic lesions generally stain strongly for S-100. In addition, immunoreactivity for melanocytic markers, such as melan A and HMB-45, is usually present. The MIB1 index is low in meningeal melanocytoma and melanocytosis, but high in meningeal melanoma and melanomatosis.

Molecular characteristics. Similar to uveal melanomas but unlike those of the skin, both benign and malignant primary melanocytic CNS tumors in adult patients frequently carry activating *GNAQ* or *GNA11* hotspot mutations, while *BRAF* mutations are exceedingly rare. More recently, mutations in *SF3B1*, *EIF1AX*, *CYSLTR2*, and *PLCB4* were reported to occur especially in (uveal and) CNS melanocytic tumors [81, 82, 155]. In children, primary melanocytic CNS tumors more frequently harbor *NRAS* mutations, especially in the context of neurocutaneous melanosis [81].

Differential diagnosis. Meningeal melanocytoma can generally be distinguished from primary meningeal or metastatic melanoma by its low mitotic activity and the absence of other histologic signs of high-grade malignancy. Histology and immunohistochemistry cannot reliably distinguish between melanoma metastasis and primary meningeal melanoma. However, demonstration of mutation of, e.g., *GNAQ* or *GNA11* argues for the latter diagnosis. Similarly, in the differential diagnosis of melanotic schwannoma versus melanocytoma, such mutations argue for the latter, while the presence of areas with typical schwannoma features and a dense pericellular reticulin network favor the diagnosis of melanotic schwannoma [81].

1.14 Lymphomas

The nervous system may be affected by a variety of lymphoid tumors. In addition to primary CNS lymphomas (PCNSLs), systemic lymphomas and leukemias may secondarily involve the nervous system by metastatic spread or continuous growth from adjacent structures. These secondary tumor manifestations prefer the dura and leptomeninges, while intraparenchymal CNS seeding from systemic lymphomas or leukemias is rare.

1.14.1 Diffuse Large B-Cell Lymphoma of the Central Nervous System

Definition. A diffuse large B-cell lymphoma (DLBCL) primarily manifesting in the CNS. These tumors account for the vast majority of primary central nervous system lymphomas (PCNSLs).

Incidence and age distribution. CNS-DLBCL account for about 3% of all brain tumors. Their incidence increased over the past decades. Sporadic CNS-DLBCL preferentially affect elderly with an age peak in the sixth and seventh decade. Tumors arising in immunodeficient patients more commonly affect younger individuals.

Macroscopy and localization. The majority of CNS-DLBCL present as supratentorial, homogenously contrast-enhancing lesions located in the deep white matter that often abut the ventricular walls. Multiple intracerebral lesions are commonly seen. The macroscopic appearance of CNS-DLBCL is highly variable, ranging from rather well-circumscribed masses to diffusely growing lesions with indistinct borders. Areas of necrosis are more common in Epstein-Barr virus (EBV)-associated CNS-DLBCL of immunodeficient patients.

Histopathology. Histology shows a highly malignant non-Hodgkin lymphoma of B-cell type morphologically corresponding to a diffuse large B-cell lymphoma. Tumors are highly cellular and composed of lymphoid blasts with enlarged nuclei and often prominent nucleoli. The tumor cells grow in perivascular cuffs (Fig. 1.14f) and solid sheets blending into a diffuse infiltration of the adjacent brain parenchyma. Mitotic activity is high. Reactive changes are common, including marked reactive astrogliosis and sometimes prominent infiltrates of T cells.

CNS-DLBCL is usually diagnosed by means of stereotactic biopsy. Preoperative corticosteroid treatment should be avoided because the tumor cells rapidly undergo apoptosis. Thus, biopsies taken after corticosteroid treatment may remain diagnostically inconclusive because the tumor cells have disappeared, while only reactive infiltrates consisting of macrophages and small T cells are remaining.

About one third of PCNSLs show tumor cell dissemination into the cerebrospinal fluid (CSF). Thus, cytologic and immunocytochemical investigation of CSF may help to establish the diagnosis.

Immunohistochemistry. CNS-DLBCL are positive for B-cell markers, including CD19, CD20 (Fig. 1.14g), and PAX5, while expression of CD3 is restricted to small reactive T cells. Most tumors stain positive for MUM1, BCL2, and BCL6. Proliferative activity is high, with MIB1 indices often exceeding 70%. PD1 and PD-L1 expression is frequent in CNS-DLBCL [8]. Tumors arising in immunodeficient patients including AIDS patients are frequently positive for EBV antigens. In contrast, sporadic tumors usually do not stain for EBV antigens.

Differential diagnosis. Immunohistochemical analysis allows for the distinction of CNS-DLBCL from malignant gliomas and other tumors, such as small cell carcinomas and malignant melanomas. In cases treated with corticosteroids, the differential diagnosis of infarction or demyelinating disease often arises. Lymphomas in immunosuppressed patients need to be distinguished from opportunistic infections, such as toxoplasmosis or progressive multifocal leukoencephalopathy.

Molecular pathology. Molecular analyses have revealed that CNS-DLBCL are derived from highly mutated, late germinal center B cells homing to the CNS [102]. The tumor cells show a preferential usage of the immunoglobulin V4-34 gene segment and are targeted by aberrant somatic hypermutation. Frequently mutated genes include *BCL6*, *PIM1*, *BTG2*, *MYD88*, *CD79B*, *CARD11*, *PRDM1*, and others [13, 35, 157]. Translocations involving immunoglobulin genes or *BCL6* are present in subsets of tumors, while *MYC* and *BCL2* translocations are rare. Homozygous deletion or promoter methylation of *CDKN2A* is frequent [13]. *MGMT* promoter methylation has been detected in about half of the cases [26].

1.14.2 Less Common Lymphomas of the Central Nervous System

Besides the common CNS-DLBCL, miscellaneous types of lymphomas may occur in the CNS but are overall rare. These include cases of *intravascular large B-cell lymphoma, low-grade B-cell lymphomas, T-cell and NK/T-cell lymphomas*, and *anaplastic large cell lymphoma*. Primary intracerebral *Hodgkin lymphoma* is a rarity. *Extranodal marginal zone lymphoma of mucosa-associated lymphoid tissue (MALT lymphoma) of the dura* is a rare meningeal tumor that needs to be distinguished from lymphoplasmacyte-rich meningioma and inflammatory lesions of the meninges. *Lymphomatoid granulomatosis* is an EBV-associated lesion that may affect the brain of immunodeficient patients including AIDS patients.

1.15 Histiocytic Lesions Affecting the Central Nervous System and Its Coverings

Definition. A heterogeneous group of tumors and tumor-like lesions composed of histiocytic cells, including Langerhans cell histiocytosis and various forms of non-Langerhans cell histiocytoses.

Incidence and age distribution. The majority of histiocytic lesions involving the CNS and its coverings are rare and preferentially occur in children and young adults. An exception is the so-called xanthogranuloma of the choroid plexus, which is a common incidental finding at autopsy but usually remains asymptomatic during lifetime. Erdheim-Chester disease and Rosai-Dorfman disease are rare non-Langerhans cell histiocytoses that preferentially manifest in adults.

1.15.1 Langerhans Cell Histiocytosis

Macroscopy and localization. Langerhans cell histiocytosis (LCH) comprises a spectrum of diseases ranging from solitary benign lesions to a disseminated disease with visceral involvement and poor outcome. Most commonly, LCH presents in the form of solitary or multifocal osteolytic lesions of the skull (*eosinophilic granuloma*). *Hand-Schüller-Christian disease* refers to multifocal LCH involving bones and the hypothalamus. *Abt-Letterer-Siwe disease* is a multifocal LCH involving the lymph nodes, skin, and viscera. The most common intracranial location of LCH is the hypothalamus and infundibulum, often resulting in the development of diabetes insipidus. Rarely, LCH presents with lesions in the cerebral hemispheres, choroid plexus, or brain stem. Macroscopically, eosinophilic granuloma appears as on osteolytic, soft, gray-tan to yellow lesion that extends through the skull bone.

Histopathology. LCH lesions are composed of a mixture of different cell types, including large, pleomorphic histiocytes (Langerhans cells) with folded and indented nuclei. These are accompanied by a reactive inflammatory infiltrate consisting of eosinophils, lymphocytes, and plasma cells. Foamy macrophages are also commonly present. Occasional multinucleated giant cells may also be observed. Long-standing and regressing eosinophilic granulomas may be largely fibrotic.

Immunohistochemistry. Langerhans cells are positive for CD1a, CD207 (langerin), CD68, and S-100 protein.

Molecular pathology. Most LCH lesions carry mutations in MAPK pathway genes, most commonly affecting *BRAF* (V600) or *MAP2K1* [4]. *CDKN2A/B* deletion and double-hit MAPK pathway gene mutations have been associated with more aggressive behavior [167].

Differential diagnosis. The differential diagnosis includes the various forms of non-Langerhans cell histiocytoses (see below) as well as other xanthomatous or xanthogranulomatous lesions. Occasional cases of eosinophilic granuloma may be heavily infiltrated by polymorphonuclear leukocytes, thereby raising the differential diagnosis of acute osteomyelitis.

1.15.2 Non-Langerhans Cell Histiocytoses

The non-LCH comprise a heterogeneous group of lesions showing macrophage but no Langerhans

cell differentiation. The WHO classification lists the following entities under this category that may present with CNS involvement: *Rosai-Dorfman disease*, *Erdheim-Chester disease*, *familial hemophagocytic lymphohistiocytosis*, *juvenile xanthogranuloma*, *xanthoma disseminatum*, and *malignant histiocytic disorders*. *Rosai-Dorfman disease* typically presents as an intracranial, dural-based mass mimicking a meningioma. The prognosis is good after resection. The classic clinical features of the disease, i.e., cervical lymphadenopathy, fever, and weight loss, are present in only a subset of the patients with intracranial lesions. *Erdheim-Chester disease* develops preferentially in adults and can involve multiple organs. Intracranial lesions are most commonly located in the cerebellum, the pituitary region, and the meninges. Spinal and orbital manifestations are also known. Bone lesions are usually present. *Familial hemophagocytic lymphohistiocytosis* is a rare autosomal recessive disorder characterized by defective immune response. Aberrantly activated T-lymphocytes and macrophages infiltrate multiple organs including the CNS, resulting in a rapidly progressive multisystem disorder of early infancy. Without treatment (bone marrow transplantation), median survival is in the range of only 2 months. The disease is caused by germline mutations in different genes, including *UNC13D*, *PRF1*, and *STX11*. *Juvenile xanthogranuloma* usually presents as a solitary skin nodule in children, but visceral involvement, including the brain and meninges, may occur, even in the absence of any cutaneous manifestation. *Xanthoma disseminatum* refers to lesions composed of lipidized (xanthomatous) histiocytes and is believed to represent a disseminated form of juvenile xanthogranuloma. Intracranial lesions are preferentially located in the pituitary/hypothalamic region or associated with the dura mater. A potential differential diagnosis is *choroid plexus xanthogranuloma*, which is a benign intraventricular lesion, most commonly located in the lateral ventricles, that occasionally may become symptomatic by obstructing CSF flow. Microscopy shows a granulomatous lesion composed of foamy macrophages, chronic inflammatory infiltrates, cholesterol clefts, and foreign body giant cells. In contrast, *choroid plexus xanthoma* consists only of foamy macrophages. *Malignant histiocytic tumors* of the nervous system are exceptionally rare high-grade neoplasms that include *histiocytic sarcoma* and *follicular dendritic cell sarcoma*. Except for classical cases of LCH, neuropathological work-up of histiocytic lesions tends to be difficult and elaborate, because histology may differ from systemic histiocytic lesions and because a wide variety of immunohistochemical and molecular markers needs to be applied in order to prove histiocytic differentiation and to exclude many other lineages that may mimic histiocytic lesions.

1.16 Germ Cell Tumors of the Central Nervous System

Definition. Germ cell tumors arising in the CNS that are homologous to germ cell tumors in the gonads or in extragonadal sites outside the CNS. The histologic classification of CNS germ cell tumors follows the classification of gonadal germ cell neoplasms, with the following entities being distinguished: *germinoma, embryonal carcinoma, endodermal sinus tumor (yolk sac tumor), choriocarcinoma, mature teratoma, immature teratoma, teratoma with malignant transformation*, and *mixed germ cell tumor*.

Incidence and age distribution. In western countries, CNS germ cell tumors account for approximately 0.5% of all primary brain tumors. In Asia, their incidence is markedly higher. For example, germ cell tumors account for up to 3% of all primary intracranial tumors in Japan. CNS germ cell tumors most frequently develop in children and young adults, with an incidence peak between 10 and 12 years of age. Overall, males are approximately twice as often affected as females. Germinoma accounts for up to 50% of all germ cell tumors in the pineal region and thus is the most common type of intracranial germ cell tumor, followed by mixed germ cell tumors and teratomas.

Macroscopy and localization. Germ cell tumors preferentially develop in midline structures of the CNS, with more than 80% of the cases arising in the pineal and third ventricular region. Other sites include the suprasellar region, basal ganglia, thalamus, cerebral hemispheres, and spinal cord. Bifocal tumors often involve both the pineal and suprasellar regions. The macroscopic appearance depends on the type of germ cell tumor.

Histopathology. The typical histologic features of the various germ cell tumor types can be described as follows:

Germinomas are the CNS homologs to testicular seminomas and ovarian dysgerminomas, respectively. They are typically composed of two cell populations, large neoplastic cells and small reactive lymphocytes. The large tumor cells are relatively uniform, round cells with large vesicular nuclei, prominent nucleoli, and pale, often vacuolated, glycogen-rich (PAS-positive) cytoplasm. Mitoses are frequent, while necrosis is uncommon. The tumor tissue is densely infiltrated by reactive lymphocytes, mostly T cells and cells of the macrophage lineages suggesting inflammatory as well as immunosuppressive mechanisms in germinomas [168]. Some germinomas demonstrate such a prominent inflammation, that the actual germinoma cells may be difficult to identify. Occasionally, syncytiotrophoblastic giant cells are present in otherwise typical germinomas.

Yolk sac tumors (synonym: *endodermal sinus tumors*) are highly malignant germ cell tumors composed of primitive epithelial cells in a myxoid matrix. Formation of so-called *Schiller-Duval bodies* is a characteristic finding. These are small glomeruloid or papilla-like structures formed by small vessels covered with epithelium and projecting into epithelium-lined channels resembling endodermal sinuses. The presence of eosinophilic hyaline bodies that are PAS positive and strongly react with antibodies against alpha-fetoprotein is another diagnostically important feature.

Embryonal carcinomas consist of large, cuboidal to columnar epithelial cells that grow in sheets or cords and may form abortive papillae or gland-like structures. The tumor cell nuclei are enlarged and contain prominent nucleoli. Mitotic activity is high and areas of coagulation necrosis are common. Formation of so-called embryoid bodies showing early embryonic or extraembryonic differentiation is occasionally seen.

Choriocarcinomas are highly malignant tumors that demonstrate extraembryonic differentiation as evidenced by the presence of malignant cytotrophoblastic cells and syncytiotrophoblastic giant cells. Choriocarcinomas often show large areas of hemorrhagic necrosis and are prone to intratumoral bleedings.

Teratomas are germ cell tumors that contain areas corresponding to endodermal, mesodermal, and ectodermal differentiation. *Mature teratomas* are benign tumors with low or absent mitotic activity that are composed of fully differentiated tissues derived from all three germ layers, including most commonly skin and brain tissue (ectodermal derivatives), cartilage, bone, fat and muscle (mesodermal derivatives), and cystic structures lined by enteric or respiratory epithelia (endodermal derivatives). More frequent among the CNS germ cell tumors are *immature teratomas*, which are characterized by the presence of incompletely differentiated, embryonic or fetal tissues. Most commonly observed are hypercellular stromal areas resembling immature mesenchyme as well as highly cellular primitive neuroectodermal tissue, often with formation of neuroepithelial rosettes or canals. *Teratoma with malignant transformation* refers to a teratoma that gives rise to the development of a malignant cancer of somatic type, most commonly a sarcoma, such as rhabdomyosarcoma or not otherwise specified sarcoma, and less commonly a squamous cell carcinoma or an adenocarcinoma.

Mixed germ cell tumors are composed of more than one of the different entities listed above. Mixed tumors composed of a teratoma component and one or several malignant GCT components are common among the CNS germ cell neoplasms. Since both sensitivity to therapy and prognosis differ markedly between the different germ cell tumor entities, it is important to identify the components of mixed lesions. In particular, teratomas show a markedly better outcome as compared to mixed germ cell tumors composed of teratoma and a malignant non-germinomatous

tumor component. When intracranial germ cell tumors are diagnosed by means of stereotactic biopsy, one has to be aware of the risk of missing small malignant areas in an otherwise well-differentiated teratoma.

Immunohistochemistry. Teratoma components can be differentiated with antibodies against epithelial, mesenchymal, and neural antigens. Germinomas are positive for placental alkaline phosphatase (PLAP), KIT, podoplanin (D2-40), and OCT4 [86]. PLAP positivity may also be seen in embryonal carcinoma and, less consistently, yolk sac tumor and choriocarcinoma. Yolk sac tumors are positive for alpha-fetoprotein and cytokeratins and frequently express glypican-3. Embryonal carcinomas express OCT4, CD30, cytokeratins, and often PLAP. Choriocarcinomas are positive for cytokeratins, beta-HCG, and human placental lactogen.

Differential diagnosis. Germ cell tumors of the pineal region need to be distinguished from pineal parenchymal neoplasms. Histologically, this distinction is usually no problem. The distinction of malignant germ cell tumors as well as the identification of mixed variants requires immunohistochemical analyses as detailed above. Similarly, immunohistochemistry allows for the distinction of embryonal carcinomas and choriocarcinomas from metastases of somatic type carcinomas. The immature neural component in immature teratomas shows tube formation resembling ependymoblastic rosettes in ETMR. However the prototypic alteration of the *C19MC* micro-RNA cluster of ETMR is absent in teratomas.

Molecular pathology. Teratomas are diploid and characterized by general chromosomal integrity. Gains of hypomethylated, active X chromosomes have been detected in the vast majority of malignant intracranial germ cell tumors, regardless of histologic subtype, while gains of 12p, including formation of isochromosome 12p, and losses on 13q were found to be restricted to subsets of the cases [104]. Mutations in the *c-KIT* gene or *RAS* genes are common in germinomas [36]. Recent comprehensive genetic studies in germinomas identified marked genetic instability and frequent mutational events both in the KIT/

RAS and the AKT/mTOR pathways [59, 135]. DNA methylation profiles indicate a primordial germ cell origin for germinomas [37, 135].

1.17 Familial Tumor Syndromes

The majority of tumors of the nervous system are sporadic lesions that arise in patients without a hereditary cancer predisposition syndrome. However, there are a number of familial tumor syndromes that are associated with a markedly increased risk of nervous system tumors, especially *neurofibromatosis type 1* (NF1) and *neurofibromatosis type 2* (NF2), *schwannomatosis*, *von Hippel-Lindau disease*, *tuberous sclerosis*, *Li-Fraumeni syndrome*, *Cowden syndrome*, *Turcot syndrome*, *nevoid basal cell carcinoma syndrome* (*Gorlin syndrome*), and *rhabdoid tumor*

predisposition syndrome. Nowadays, Turcot syndrome (the association of brain tumors with gastrointestinal polyps and cancers) is considered to constitute two different syndromes with distinct inheritance and cancer spectrums: mismatch repair cancer syndrome (brain tumor-polyposis syndrome 1, BTP1) and familial adenomatous polyposis (brain tumor-polyposis syndrome 2, BTP2). Table 1.6 provides an overview of the responsible genes, the associated nervous system lesions, as well as other clinical features of the major familial tumor syndromes involving the nervous system. For a more detailed account of the pathogenetic and clinicopathologic characteristics of each syndrome, the reader is referred to the "WHO 2016 classification 'blue book'" [91]. Characteristic manifestations outside the nervous system such as skin abnormalities facilitate identification of patients with some of these familial

Table 1.6 Familial tumor syndromes of the nervous system

Syndrome	Gene(s)	Chr.	Nervous system tumors	Other CNS manifestations	Skin lesions	Lesions in other organs
Neurofibromatosis type 1 (NF1)	*NF1*	17q11	Neurofibromas, plexiform neurofibroma, MPNST, optic glioma/pilocytic astrocytoma, diffuse glioma (less common)	Aqueductal stenosis, epilepsy, learning deficits, macrocephaly	Neurofibromas, café au lait spots, axillar/inguinal freckling	Osseous malformation, Lisch nodules, pheochromocytoma, duodenal/thyroid endocrine neoplasm, GIST, juvenile CML, rhabdomyosarcoma
Neurofibromatosis type 2 (NF2)	*NF2*	22q12	Bilateral vestibular schwannoma, spinal root schwannoma, meningioma, spinal ependymoma, astrocytoma	Glial hamartomas, cerebral calcifications, meningioangiomatosis, spinal schwannosis	–	Posterior lens opacities, retinal hamartomas
Schwannomatosis	*SMARCB1* *LZTR1*	22q11 22q11	Schwannomas (typically not vestibular)	–	–	–
von Hippel-Lindau disease	*VHL*	3p25	Hemangioblastoma (cerebellar, brain stem, spinal, often multiple)	–	–	Retinal hemangioblastoma, renal cell carcinoma, pheochromocytoma, endolymphatic sac tumor, kidney cyst, pancreas cyst, cystadenoma epididymis/broad ligament

(continued)

Table 1.6 (continued)

Syndrome	Gene(s)	Chr.	Nervous system tumors	Other CNS manifestations	Skin lesions	Lesions in other organs
Tuberous sclerosis complex	TSC1 TSC2	9q34 16p13	Subependymal giant cell astrocytoma (SEGA)	Cortical tubers, subependymal nodules, white matter hamartoma/heterotopia, epilepsy, mental retardation	Facial angiofibroma (adenoma sebaceum), shagreen patch, forehead plaque, peri- and subungual fibroma	Cardiac rhabdomyoma, renal angiomyolipoma, hamartoma of the liver/retina, hamartomatous rectal polyp, hypopigmented iris spot, cyst of the kidney/liver/lung/bone, gingival fibroma, pitting of dental enamel, retinal giant cell astrocytoma
Li-Fraumeni syndrome	TP53	17p13	Astrocytoma, embryonal tumor/medulloblastoma, choroid plexus carcinoma	–	–	Breast carcinoma, sarcomas, adrenal cortical carcinoma, osteosarcoma
Cowden syndrome	PTEN	10q23	Dysplastic cerebellar gangliocytoma (Lhermitte-Duclos)	Megalencephaly, gray matter heterotopias	Multiple facial trichilemmomas, fibromas	Breast carcinoma, thyroid cancer (esp. follicular), sarcomas, leukemias, other cancers, hamartomatous intestinal polyps
"Turcot 1" Mismatch repair cancer syndrome	MLH1 PSM2 MSH2 MSH6	3p22 7p22 2p47 2p16	Malignant glioma/(giant cell) glioblastoma, low(er)-grade glioma, embryonal tumor/medulloblastoma	–	Café au lait spots	Gastrointestinal polyposis and cancer, T-cell lymphoma, other cancers (urinary tract, sarcomas)
"Turcot 2" Familial adenomatous polyposis syndrome	APC	5q21	Medulloblastoma, WNT-activated	–	–	Multiple colon polyps, colon carcinoma, osteoma, aggressive fibromatosis, thyroid cancer, hepatoblastoma
Gorlin syndrome (nevoid basal cell carcinoma syndrome)	PTCH1 PTCH2	9q22 1p34	Medulloblastoma, SHH-activated (desmoplastic/nodular or extensive nodularity variant)	Intracranial (dural) calcifications, corpus callosum dysgenesis	Basal cell carcinomas, palmar and plantar pits, epidermal cysts	Odontogenic keratocysts, skeletal malformations, ovarian fibroma
Rhabdoid tumor predisposition syndrome (RTPS)	SMARCB1 SMARCA4	22q11 19p13	Atypical teratoid/rhabdoid tumor	–	–	Malignant rhabdoid tumor (mostly in the kidney); in SMARCA4 RTPS: small cell carcinoma of the ovary of hypercalcemic type

tumor syndromes, which is of paramount importance for prevention and genetic counseling.

1.18 Tumors of the Sellar Region

1.18.1 Craniopharyngioma

Definition. Craniopharyngiomas are benign epithelial tumor of the sellar region related to Rathke's pouch, occurring in two histologically and biologically distinct types, namely, adamantinomatous and papillary craniopharyngiomas. Adamantinomatous craniopharyngiomas carry CTNNB1 mutations leading to aberrant WNT pathway activation and nuclear localization of β-catenin. In contrast, papillary craniopharyngiomas are characterized by BRAF-V600E mutation.

Incidence and age distribution. Craniopharyngioma represents approximately 3% of all intracranial tumors and 5–10% of pediatric intracranial tumors. Adamantinomatous craniopharyngioma occurs in all age groups, with age peaks in children and adults between 45 and 60 years, while the papillary form is virtually restricted to adults (mean age 40–55 years).

Macroscopy and localization. Adamantinomatous craniopharyngioma is most commonly localized in the suprasellar region (95%), with most tumors comprising an additional intrasellar component. Purely intrasellar location is found in only 5% of cases. Papillary craniopharyngioma typically involves the third ventricle. Only the adamantinomatous form is frequently cystic and calcified.

Histopathology. *Adamantinomatous craniopharyngioma* (Fig. 1.14h) resembles odontogenic tumors, particularly calcifying odontogenic cyst and ameloblastoma. A basal layer of palisading cuboidal tumor cells merges with stratified epithelial cells arranged in a reticular pattern. Cuboidal cells form tubuli and larger cysts. The upper layers of the epithelium undergo keratinization, typically with recognizable cell borders, and calcification. Cholesterol clefts may occur, but they are more typical of xanthogranuloma of the sellar region. *Papillary craniopharyn-*

gioma shows multilayered squamous epithelial cells covering fibrovascular cores (Fig. 1.14i). Infiltration of neutrophilic granulocytes among epithelial cells is common, whereas keratinization and calcification are absent.

Immunohistochemistry. Given the distinct histologic appearance, immunostaining is not required for making the diagnosis of craniopharyngioma. Like all epithelial tumors, they are positive for cytokeratins, in particular the squamous epithelial cytokeratin 5/6. In line with their odontogenic appearance, adamantinomatous but not papillary tumors express enamel proteins (amelogenin, enamelin, enamelysin). Nuclear immunoreactivity for β-catenin is typical for adamantinomatous craniopharyngiomas, while immunostaining for mutant BRAF is seen in papillary craniopharyngiomas. MIB1 proliferation indices are relatively high for a benign tumor with a mean of 9%, but they are not strictly related to recurrence.

Differential diagnosis. *Xanthogranuloma of the sellar region* (Fig. 1.14j) is a benign, typically intrasellar lesion of young adults that is histologically composed of cholesterol clefts, xanthoma cells, chronic inflammatory cells, necroses, hemosiderin deposits, and occasionally a few epithelial cells. Rathke's cleft cyst may be distinguished from cystic craniopharyngioma by lack of immunostaining for β-catenin and BRAF-V600E.

Molecular pathology. Numerical chromosomal changes have been found in a minority of adamantinomatous craniopharyngiomas, while the papillary tumors studied so far showed a normal karyotype. *CNNTB1* exon 3 mutations are detectable in most adamantinomatous craniopharyngiomas, while papillary craniopharyngiomas carry BRAF-V600E mutations [15, 44, 55]. DNA methylation profiles are also distinct between the two variants [55].

1.18.2 Pituitary Adenoma

Definition. A neuroendocrine tumor of the sellar region originating from a neoplastic proliferation of hormone-producing adenohypophysial cells.

Most pituitary adenomas are benign, but invasive adenomas may grow locally aggressive.

General comment. Pituitary adenomas are included in the WHO classification of tumors of endocrine organs [93]. However, since pituitary adenomas are tumors commonly encountered by neuropathologists, their most important features are briefly summarized here.

Incidence and age distribution. In autopsy and MRI series, pituitary adenomas occur in up to 25% of the general population, the vast majority being asymptomatic. Symptomatic tumors are far less common and account for approximately 15% of intracranial tumors. They usually occur in adults, with only 5% being diagnosed before the age of 20 years.

Macroscopy. Based on the largest tumor diameter, pituitary adenomas may be radiologically classified into microadenomas (<10 mm diameter), macroadenomas with a diameter of 10–40 mm, and *giant adenomas* with a diameter of more than 40 mm.

Histopathology. Tumor cells usually show monomorphic, round or oval nuclei and well-delineated cytoplasm. The tinctorial properties of the cytoplasm no longer represent the basis for histologic classification, but typically they are to some degree correlated with immunohistochemistry in that eosinophilic cells often express HGH, basophilic cells often express ACTH, and chromophobic cells may express prolactin, gonadotrophins, or no routinely detectable hormone. Mitotic figures are rare. Common histologic patterns include small cell nests surrounded by capillaries, trabecules, pseudopapillae, or perivascular pseudorosettes. Some adenomas present with radiologic, histologic, and immunohistochemical features suggestive of more aggressive behavior, such as locally invasive growth, elevated mitotic activity, and a high MIB1 index. While the term *atypical pituitary adenoma* is no longer recommended for such tumors, these cases have a higher risk for clinically more aggressive behavior and thus should be followed up more closely [94].

Immunohistochemistry. Tumor cells express neuronal and neuroendocrine antigens such as chromogranin and synaptophysin. The expression of pituitary hormones and certain transcription factors forms the basis of adenoma subtyping. *Gonadotroph adenomas* are positive for FSH and/or LH as well as the transcription factors SF1 and GATA2, *corticotroph adenomas* express ACTH and TPIT, *thyrotroph adenomas* stain for TSH and PIT1, *lactotroph adenomas* react for prolactin and PIT1, and *somatotroph adenomas* are positive for hGH and PIT1. Somatotroph adenomas are subdivided into sparsely or densely granulated variants, with low molecular weight cytokeratins showing a typical dot-like staining pattern corresponding to fibrous bodies in sparsely granulated tumors. Coexpression of prolactin and hGH, together with PIT1, may be seen in subsets of somatotroph adenomas, corresponding to *mammosomatotroph adenomas* when both hormones are expressed in the same cells or *mixed somatotroph and lactotroph adenoma* when the hormones are expressed in distinct cell populations. *Acidophil stem cell adenoma* is a variant of lactotroph adenoma with focal positivity for hGH. *Plurihormonal PIT1-positive adenomas* express various combinations of hormones, typically hGH, prolactin, and TSH. Tumors with coexpression of prolactin and ACTH may also be seen. All of these adenoma types may be associated with endocrine manifestations (clinically functioning), or they may be nonfunctioning. *Null cell adenomas* are clinically nonfunctioning tumors that are immunohistochemically negative for pituitary hormones and lineage-specific transcription factors PIT1, TPIT, SF1, and GATA2. A subtype of null cell adenoma is oncocytoma, being composed of cells with an abundance of mitochondria which can be immunohistochemically verified by using anti-mitochondrial antibodies.

Differential diagnosis. *Pituitary carcinoma* is exceedingly rare and defined as adenoma undergoing metastasis, implying that the diagnosis cannot be made on the basis of a surgical specimen derived from the sellar region. It often but not necessarily exhibits anaplastic histologic features, such as numerous mitoses, high cellular density, cellular pleomorphism, necrosis, and diffuse brain invasion. *Pituitary hyperplasia* represents an increased number of secretory cells in response to a physiological or pathological stimulus; it is histologically characterized by the lack of the typical lobulation of the normal adenohypophysis. Various *cysts*, most commonly Rathke's cleft cyst and colloid cyst of the intermediate lobe, and *inflammatory lesions*, most commonly lymphocytic hypophysitis and granulomatous hypophysitis, may present as mass lesions. Finally, a wide variety of tumors that are histogenetically unrelated to the pituitary gland may occasionally grow in the sellar region.

Molecular pathology. The molecular pathogenesis of pituitary adenomas is complex and involves alterations in hormone regulation, growth factor stimulation, cell-cycle control, and cell-stromal interactions that result from genetic mutations, genomic copy number changes, or epigenetic inactivation of various genes [9, 22]. Mutations in *GNAS1* have been identified in about 40% of somatotroph adenomas, while *USP8* are seen in more than half of the corticotroph adenomas. Several tumor suppressor genes such as *CDKN2A* and *RB1* may be downregulated due to promoter hypermethylation. Two distinct groups of pituitary adenomas could be stratified based on genomic copy number aberrations: one group of genomically instable tumors with frequent losses of chromosome arm 1p or chromosome 11 and a second group of genomically quiet tumors with only rare copy number imbalances [9]. Large-scale sequencing revealed relatively low overall mutation rates, with rare mutations affecting several genes in addition to those mentioned above [9, 22].

Germline mutations of the *MEN1* tumor suppressor gene are responsible for multiple endocrine neoplasia type 1, which in 10–50% comprises pituitary adenoma, whereas sporadic pituitary adenomas rarely show *MEN1* mutations. Several other hereditary cancer predisposition syndromes are associated with increased risk for pituitary adenomas, including SDH mutation-related familial pheochromocytoma and paraganglioma, MEN type 4 due to *CDKN1B* mutation, Carney complex, McCune-Albright syndrome, DICER 1 syndrome, and neurofibromatosis type 1 [22]. Mutations in the aryl hydrocarbon receptor-interacting protein-coding gene AIP are the most common germline mutations in familial pituitary adenoma and particularly seen in younger patients with somatotroph adenoma [159]. In addition, microduplication or mutation of the *GPR101* or *GNAS* on chromosome X has been identified as a cause of familial somatotroph adenoma causing acromegaly [22, 153].

1.18.3 Granular Cell Tumor of the Sellar Region

Definition. A tumor of the sellar region composed of epithelioid to spindle-shaped eosinophilic granular cells that are strongly PAS positive due to abundant intracytoplasmic lysosomes.

Incidence and age distribution. Granular tumors are rare lesions that manifest in adults.

Macroscopy and localization. The tumor presents as an intrasellar and/or infundibular/suprasellar, well-circumscribed mass lesion with a granular, gray to yellow cut surface.

Histopathology. Granular cell tumors are composed of polygonal or elongated cells with small nuclei and abundant, granular, strongly PAS-positive cytoplasm (Fig. 1.14k, l). Ultrastructural studies showed that the cytoplasmic granularity and PAS positivity are due to dense accumulation of lysosomes. Mitotic activity is low or absent. Perivascular lymphocytic cuffs are often seen. The tumors correspond to WHO grade I. Occasional tumors showing nuclear pleomorphism and increased mitotic and proliferative activity have been reported and referred to as atypical granular cell tumors. However, the clinical significance of these atypical histologic features is still unknown. The histogenesis of granular cell tumors of the sellar region is unclear. They are supposed to arise from the neurohypophysis or infundibulum, with pituicytes being considered as a possible cellular origin shared with other TTF1-positive sellar region tumors like pituicytoma and spindle cell oncocytoma [30, 94].

Immunohistochemistry. Granular cell tumors are positive for TTF1, vimentin, and S-100. Immunoreactivity for CD68 may be present, while expression of GFAP is variable.

Neuronal and epithelial markers, as well as pituitary hormones, are not expressed. The MIB1 index is low (<5%).

Differential diagnosis. Granular tumors of sellar region need to be differentiated from pituitary adenomas, pituicytomas, and spindle cell oncocytoma of the adenohypophysis, with the latter three possibly representing a continuous histologic spectrum of a single nosologic entity.

1.18.4 Pituicytoma

Pituicytoma (*WHO grade I*) is a low-grade neuroepithelial tumor that is supposed to arise from pituicytes, i.e., specialized glial cells of the posterior lobe and the stalk of the pituitary gland [30]. A possible origin from specialized stromal folliculo-stellate cells of the adenohypophysis has also been suggested. Pituicytomas are slowly growing tumors of the sellar and suprasellar regions that occur in adult patients and are associated with a favorable prognosis following total resection. Malignant progression or metastasis has not been reported to date. Histologically, pituicytomas consist of sheets and fascicles of spindle cells with oval-to-elongated nuclei and pinpoint nucleoli. Mitotic activity is low. In contrast to pilocytic astrocytomas, Rosenthal fibers and eosinophilic granular bodies are absent. Immunohistochemistry shows nuclear TTF1 positivity as well as strong staining for vimentin and S-100. GFAP expression is variable and may be negative. Neuronal markers are negative, while patchy staining for EMA may be observed. The MIB1 index is low (<2%).

1.18.5 Spindle Cell Oncocytoma

Spindle cell oncocytoma (SCO) is a rare, slowly growing, benign tumor of the pituitary gland that predominantly affects adults and macroscopically cannot be distinguished from pituitary adenoma. Histologically, SCO is characterized by interlacing fascicles of spindled to epithelioid cells with eosinophilic, variably oncocytic cytoplasm. Focal areas of increased cellular pleomor-

phism may be present; however, mitotic activity is generally low, and features of anaplasia are absent. Immunohistochemistry shows nuclear expression of TTF1 as well as cytoplasmic positivity with antibodies against vimentin, S-100 protein, EMA, and galectin-3, as well as with the anti-mitochondrial antibody 113-1. Neuronal markers, pituitary hormones, and GFAP are negative. The MIB1 index is low. Exome sequencing revealed an overall low mutation rate with evidence for a role of mutational activation of MAPK pathway genes [100]. The histogenesis of SCO is unclear. Nuclear TTF1 positivity may indicate a shared origin from pituicytes with sellar granular cell tumor and pituicytoma [30, 94]. The prognosis after resection is favorable, corresponding to a WHO grade I lesion.

1.19 Metastatic Tumors of the Central Nervous System

Definition. Malignant tumors involving the CNS and/or its coverings that originate from primary cancers in other organs. Most CNS metastases originate from hematogenous spread, while direct invasion from neighboring anatomical sites is far less common.

Incidence and age distribution. Altogether, metastatic tumors are the most common tumors of the CNS (approximately 3–10 times more common than primary brain tumors). Autopsy series reported on intracranial metastases in approximately 25% and spinal metastases in 5–10% of all cancer patients. The incidence markedly increases with age, i.e., metastatic lesions are rare in children and young adults but common in elderly patients.

Origin. Metastatic tumors reach the CNS and/or its coverings by hematogenous spread of tumor cells from primary tumors in other organs. Tumors that most commonly metastasize into the brain are carcinomas of the lung (in particular bronchial adenocarcinomas and small cell neuroendocrine lung carcinomas), which account for approximately 50% of all CNS metastases, followed by carcinomas of the breast, malignant melanomas, and renal carcinomas. In at least 10% of the patients operated on metastatic brain tumors, the corresponding primary tumors are unknown at the time of brain surgery. Diffuse infiltration of the leptomeninges (*leptomeningeal carcinomatosis/leptomeningeal blastomatosis*) is most commonly seen in patients suffering from leukemia or lymphoma, melanoma, and carcinomas of the breast, lung, or gastrointestinal tract.

Macroscopy and localization. Most CNS metastases are located in the brain parenchyma itself, most commonly at the cortical/subcortical border in the cerebral hemispheres and in the cerebellum (Fig. 1.2g, h). Dural metastases often compress rather than infiltrate the adjacent brain and may be macroscopically mistaken for meningiomas. Spinal metastases are most commonly located in the epidural space and frequently extend from metastatic lesions in the vertebral bodies. Spinal intramedullary metastases are rare. Leptomeningeal tumor spread may be found in patients with and without intraparenchymal metastases. Macroscopically, intracerebral metastases are either solitary or multiple, usually well-demarcated lesions surrounded by edematous brain tissue. The tumor's cut surface is inhomogeneous, with gray, white, or tan areas of vital tumor tissue, hemorrhagic zones, as well as frequently large areas of necrosis. Intratumoral bleeding is particularly common in metastases from renal cell carcinoma, choriocarcinoma, and malignant melanoma. Dural metastases may present as nodular or plaque-like lesions. Leptomeningeal carcinomatosis may lead to circumscribed or diffuse thickening of the meninges.

Histopathology. The histologic appearance and immunohistochemical profile of metastatic lesions in the CNS usually correspond to those of the respective primary tumor. However, many metastases of carcinomas are histologically poorly differentiated. In contrast to malignant gliomas and primary CNS lymphomas, carcinoma metastases typically show histologically well-defined borders toward the adjacent brain tissue. However, metastases of small cell carcinomas and malignant melanomas may also demonstrate a locally infiltrative growth. Areas of necrosis are usually present and may be quite large, with vital tumor tissue often restricted to perivascular tumor cuffs within the necrotic zones.

Immunohistochemistry. Carcinoma metastases are generally positive for epithelial antigens such as cytokeratins and EMA. A specific expression pattern of cytokeratin subtypes may help to distinguish carcinomas of different types, e.g., adenocarcinoma and squamous cell carcinoma, and origin. Neuroendocrine carcinomas are revealed by their positivity for synaptophysin and chromogranin A. When positive, specific markers such as TTF1 (thyroid and bronchial carcinomas), prostate-specific antigen (PSA, prostate carcinoma), HepPar (hepatocellular carcinoma), thyreoglobulin (thyroid carcinoma), Cdx2 (gastrointestinal carcinomas), and PAX8 (renal cell carcinoma) may help to clarify tumor origin. Expression of GATA3, as well as estrogen and progesterone receptors, may help to identify metastatic breast carcinoma. Melanoma metastases show positivity for melanocytic markers (HMB-45, melan A). Immunohistochemical staining for PD-L1 expression is frequently performed to identify patients potentially eligible for treatment with immune checkpoint inhibitors, in particular among patients with non-small cell lung cancer and melanoma metastases.

Differential diagnosis. The differential diagnosis of metastases in the cerebral hemispheres primarily includes malignant glioma and primary CNS lymphoma. Dural metastases need to be distinguished from anaplastic meningiomas. Among cerebellar metastases, small cell carcinomas must be separated from medulloblastomas, while clear cell carcinoma metastases may mimic capillary hemangioblastoma. Because metastatic papillary adenocarcinomas are primarily tumors of adults, the differential diagnosis of choroid plexus carcinoma, which mostly present in young children, rarely arises. In case of a pineal tumor, the papillary tumor of the pineal region needs to be distinguished from a metastatic adenocarcinoma.

Molecular pathology. Molecular analysis for potentially druggable mutations has become of major clinical relevance, in particular in patients with brain metastases from non-small cell lung carcinoma (e.g., *EGFR* mutations, rearrangements of *ALK*, *ROS*, *RET*, or *NTRK1*), breast carcinoma (e.g., *HER2* amplification/overexpression), and melanoma (e.g., BRAF-V600E mutation) [142]. Large-scale DNA sequencing revealed evidence for branched evolution of brain metastases, i.e., shared origin of primary tumor and brain metastases from a common ancestor but independent further progression [14]. Thus, brain metastases may frequently carry clinically informative alterations not detectable in the matched primary tumors [14].

References

1. Abedalthagafi MS, Merrill PH, Bi WL, Jones RT, Listewnik ML, Ramkissoon SH, Thorner AR, Dunn IF, Beroukhim R, Alexander BM, Brastianos PK, Francis JM, Folkerth RD, Ligon KL, Van Hummelen P, Ligon AH, Santagata S (2014) Angiomatous meningiomas have a distinct genetic profile with multiple chromosomal polysomies including polysomy of chromosome 5. Oncotarget 5(21):10596–10606

2. Abel TW, Baker SJ, Fraser MM, Tihan T, Nelson JS, Yachnis AT, Bouffard JP, Mena H, Burger PC, Eberhart CG (2005) Lhermitte-Duclos disease: a report of 31 cases with immunohistochemical analysis of the PTEN/AKT/mTOR pathway. J Neuropathol Exp Neurol 64(4):341–349

3. Alentorn A, Dehais C, Ducray F, Carpentier C, Mokhtari K, Figarella-Branger D, Chinot O, Cohen-Moyal E, Ramirez C, Loiseau H, Elouahdani-Hamdi S, Beauchesne P, Langlois O, Desenclos C, Guillamo JS, Dam-Hieu P, Ghiringhelli F, Colin P, Godard J, Parker F, Dhermain F, Carpentier AF, Frenel JS, Menei P, Bauchet L, Faillot T, Fesneau M, Fontaine D, Motuo-Fotso MJ, Vauleon E, Gaultier C, Le Guerinel C, Gueye EM, Noel G, Desse N, Durando X, Barrascout E, Wager M, Ricard D, Carpiuc I, Delattre JY, Idbaih A, POLA Network (2015) Allelic loss of 9p21.3 is a prognostic factor in 1p/19q codeleted anaplastic gliomas. Neurology 85(15):1325–1331

4. Badalian-Very G, Vergilio JA, Fleming M, Rollins BJ (2013) Pathogenesis of Langerhans cell histiocytosis. Annu Rev Pathol 8:1–20

5. Bailey P, Cushing H (1926) A classification of the tumors of the glioma group on a histogenetic basis with a correlated study of prognosis. J.B. Lippincott, Philadelphia

6. Bandopadhayay P, Ramkissoon LA, Jain P, Bergthold G, Wala J, Zeid R, Schumacher SE, Urbanski L, O'Rourke R, Gibson WJ, Pelton K, Ramkissoon SH, Han HJ, Zhu Y, Choudhari N, Silva A, Boucher K, Henn RE, Kang YJ, Knoff D, Paolella BR, Gladden-Young A, Varlet P, Pages M, Horowitz PM, Federation A, Malkin H, Tracy AA, Seepo S, Ducar M, Van

Hummelen P, Santi M, Buccoliero AM, Scagnet M, Bowers DC, Giannini C, Puget S, Hawkins C, Tabori U, Klekner A, Bognar L, Burger PC, Eberhart C, Rodriguez FJ, Hill DA, Mueller S, Haas-Kogan DA, Phillips JJ, Santagata S, Stiles CD, Bradner JE, Jabado N, Goren A, Grill J, Ligon AH, Goumnerova L, Waanders AJ, Storm PB, Kieran MW, Ligon KL, Beroukhim R, Resnick AC (2016) MYB-QKI rearrangements in angiocentric glioma drive tumorigenicity through a tripartite mechanism. Nat Genet 48(3):273–282

7. Bender S, Tang Y, Lindroth AM, Hovestadt V, Jones DT, Kool M, Zapatka M, Northcott PA, Sturm D, Wang W, Radlwimmer B, Højfeldt JW, Truffaux N, Castel D, Schubert S, Ryzhova M, Seker-Cin H, Gronych J, Johann PD, Stark S, Meyer J, Milde T, Schuhmann M, Ebinger M, Monoranu CM, Ponnuswami A, Chen S, Jones C, Witt O, Collins VP, von Deimling A, Jabado N, Puget S, Grill J, Helin K, Korshunov A, Lichter P, Monje M, Plass C, Cho YJ, Pfister SM (2013) Reduced H3K27me3 and DNA hypomethylation are major drivers of gene expression in K27M mutant pediatric high-grade gliomas. Cancer Cell 24(5):660–672

8. Berghoff AS, Ricken G, Widhalm G, Rajky O, Hainfellner JA, Birner P, Raderer M, Preusser M (2014) PD1 (CD279) and PD-L1 (CD274, B7H1) expression in primary central nervous system lymphomas (PCNSL). Clin Neuropathol 33(1):42–49

9. Bi WL, Horowitz P, Greenwald NF, Abedalthagafi M, Agarwalla PK, Gibson WJ, Mei Y, Schumacher SE, Ben-David U, Chevalier A, Carter S, Tiao G, Brastianos PK, Ligon AH, Ducar M, MacConaill L, Laws ER Jr, Santagata S, Beroukhim R, Dunn IF (2017) Landscape of genomic alterations in pituitary adenomas. Clin Cancer Res 23(7):1841–1851

10. Blümcke I, Spreafico R, Haaker G, Coras R, Kobow K, Bien CG, Pfäfflin M, Elger C, Widman G, Schramm J, Becker A, Braun KP, Leijten F, Baayen JC, Aronica E, Chassoux F, Hamer H, Stefan H, Rössler K, Thom M, Walker MC, Sisodiya SM, Duncan JS, AW ME, Pieper T, Holthausen H, Kudernatsch M, Meencke HJ, Kahane P, Schulze-Bonhage A, Zentner J, Heiland DH, Urbach H, Steinhoff BJ, Bast T, Tassi L, Lo Russo G, Özkara C, Oz B, Krsek P, Vogelgesang S, Runge U, Lerche H, Weber Y, Honavar M, Pimentel J, Arzimanoglou A, Ulate-Campos A, Noachtar S, Hartl E, Schijns O, Guerrini R, Barba C, Jacques TS, Cross JH, Feucht M, Mühlebner A, Grunwald T, Trinka E, Winkler PA, Gil-Nagel A, Toledano Delgado R, Mayer T, Lutz M, Zountsas B, Garganis K, Rosenow F, Hermsen A, von Oertzen TJ, Diepgen TL, Avanzini G, EEBB Consortium (2017) Histopathological findings in brain tissue obtained during epilepsy surgery. N Engl J Med 377(17):1648–1656

11. Blümcke I, Wiestler OD (2002) Gangliogliomas: an intriguing tumor entity associated with focal epilepsies. J Neuropathol Exp Neurol 61(7):575–584

12. Boström J, Meyer-Puttlitz B, Wolter M, Blaschke B, Weber RG, Lichter P, Ichimura K, Collins VP,

Reifenberger G (2001) Alterations of the tumor suppressor genes CDKN2A (p16(INK4a)), p14(ARF), CDKN2B (p15(INK4b)), and CDKN2C (p18(INK4c)) in atypical and anaplastic meningiomas. Am J Pathol 159(2):661–669

13. Braggio E, Van Wier S, Ojha J, McPhail E, Asmann YW, Egan J, da Silva JA, Schiff D, Lopes MB, Decker PA, Valdez R, Tibes R, Eckloff B, Witzig TE, Stewart AK, Fonseca R, O'Neill BP (2015) Genome-wide analysis uncovers novel recurrent alterations in primary central nervous system lymphomas. Clin Cancer Res 21(17):3986–3994

14. Brastianos PK, Carter SL, Santagata S, Cahill DP, Taylor-Weiner A, Jones RT, Van Allen EM, Lawrence MS, Horowitz PM, Cibulskis K, Ligon KL, Tabernero J, Seoane J, Martinez-Saez E, Curry WT, Dunn IF, Paek SH, Park SH, McKenna A, Chevalier A, Rosenberg M, Barker FG II, Gill CM, Van Hummelen P, Thorner AR, Johnson BE, Hoang MP, Choueiri TK, Signoretti S, Sougnez C, Rabin MS, Lin NU, Winer EP, Stemmer-Rachamimov A, Meyerson M, Garraway L, Gabriel S, Lander ES, Beroukhim R, Batchelor TT, Baselga J, Louis DN, Getz G, Hahn WC (2015) Genomic characterization of brain metastases reveals branched evolution and potential therapeutic targets. Cancer Discov 5(11):1164–1177

15. Brastianos PK, Taylor-Weiner A, Manley PE, Jones RT, Dias-Santagata D, Thorner AR, Lawrence MS, Rodriguez FJ, Bernardo LA, Schubert L, Sunkavalli A, Shillingford N, Calicchio ML, Lidov HG, Taha H, Martinez-Lage M, Santi M, Storm PB, Lee JY, Palmer JN, Adappa ND, Scott RM, Dunn IF, Laws ER Jr, Stewart C, Ligon KL, Hoang MP, Van Hummelen P, Hahn WC, Louis DN, Resnick AC, Kieran MW, Getz G, Santagata S (2014) Exome sequencing identifies BRAF mutations in papillary craniopharyngiomas. Nat Genet 46(2):161–165

16. Brat DJ, Hirose Y, Cohen KJ, Feuerstein BG, Burger PC (2000) Astroblastoma: clinicopathologic features and chromosomal abnormalities defined by comparative genomic hybridization. Brain Pathol 10(3):342–352

17. Brat DJ, Scheithauer BW, Eberhart CG, Burger PC (2001) Extraventricular neurocytomas: pathologic features and clinical outcome. Am J Surg Pathol 25(10):1252–1260

18. Brennan CW, Verhaak RG, McKenna A, Campos B, Noushmehr H, Salama SR, Zheng S, Chakravarty D, Sanborn JZ, Berman SH, Beroukhim R, Bernard B, Wu CJ, Genovese G, Shmulevich I, Barnholtz-Sloan J, Zou L, Vegesna R, Shukla SA, Ciriello G, Yung WK, Zhang W, Sougnez C, Mikkelsen T, Aldape K, Bigner DD, Van Meir EG, Prados M, Sloan A, Black KL, Eschbacher J, Finocchiaro G, Friedman W, Andrews DW, Guha A, Iacocca M, O'Neill BP, Foltz G, Myers J, Weisenberger DJ, Penny R, Kucherlapati R, Perou CM, Hayes DN, Gibbs R, Marra M, Mills GB, Lander E, Spellman P, Wilson R, Sander C, Weinstein J, Meyerson M, Gabriel S, Laird PW, Haussler D, Getz G, Chin L, TCGA Research Network (2013) The somatic genomic landscape of glioblastoma. Cell 155(2):462–477

19. Breton Q, Plouhinec H, Prunier-Mirebeau D, Boisselier B, Michalak S, Menei P, Rousseau A (2017) BRAF-V600E immunohistochemistry in a large series of glial and glial-neuronal tumors. Brain Behav 7(3):e00641

20. Bridge JA, Liu XQ, Sumegi J, Nelson M, Reyes C, Bruch LA, Rosenblum M, Puccioni MJ, Bowdino BS, McComb RD (2013) Identification of a novel, recurrent SLC44A1-PRKCA fusion in papillary glioneuronal tumor. Brain Pathol 23(2):121–128

21. Brohl AS, Kahen E, Yoder SJ, Teer JK, Reed DR (2017) The genomic landscape of malignant peripheral nerve sheath tumors: diverse drivers of Ras pathway activation. Sci Rep 7(1):14992

22. Caimari F, Korbonits M (2016) Novel genetic causes of pituitary adenomas. Clin Cancer Res 22(20):5030–5042

23. Cancer Genome Atlas Research Network, Brat DJ, Verhaak RG, Aldape KD, Yung WK, Salama SR, Cooper LA, Rheinbay E, Miller CR, Vitucci M, Morozova O, Robertson AG, Noushmehr H, Laird PW, Cherniack AD, Akbani R, Huse JT, Ciriello G, Poisson LM, Barnholtz-Sloan JS, Berger MS, Brennan C, Colen RR, Colman H, Flanders AE, Giannini C, Grifford M, Iavarone A, Jain R, Joseph I, Kim J, Kasaian K, Mikkelsen T, Murray BA, O'Neill BP, Pachter L, Parsons DW, Sougnez C, Sulman EP, Vandenberg SR, Van Meir EG, von Deimling A, Zhang H, Crain D, Lau K, Mallery D, Morris S, Paulauskis J, Penny R, Shelton T, Sherman M, Yena P, Black A, Bowen J, Dicostanzo K, Gastier-Foster J, Leraas KM, Lichtenberg TM, Pierson CR, Ramirez NC, Taylor C, Weaver S, Wise L, Zmuda E, Davidsen T, Demchok JA, Eley G, Ferguson ML, Hutter CM, Mills Shaw KR, Ozenberger BA, Sheth M, Sofia HJ, Tarnuzzer R, Wang Z, Yang L, Zenklusen JC, Ayala B, Baboud J, Chudamani S, Jensen MA, Liu J, Pihl T, Raman R, Wan Y, Wu Y, Ally A, Auman JT, Balasundaram M, Balu S, Baylin SB, Beroukhim R, Bootwalla MS, Bowlby R, Bristow CA, Brooks D, Butterfield Y, Carlsen R, Carter S, Chin L, Chu A, Chuah E, Cibulskis K, Clarke A, Coetzee SG, Dhalla N, Fennell T, Fisher S, Gabriel S, Getz G, Gibbs R, Guin R, Hadjipanayis A, Hayes DN, Hinoue T, Hoadley K, Holt RA, Hoyle AP, Jefferys SR, Jones S, Jones CD, Kucherlapati R, Lai PH, Lander E, Lee S, Lichtenstein L, Ma Y, Maglinte DT, Mahadeshwar HS, Marra MA, Mayo M, Meng S, Meyerson ML, Mieczkowski PA, Moore RA, Mose LE, Mungall AJ, Pantazi A, Parfenov M, Park PJ, Parker JS, Perou CM, Protopopov A, Ren X, Roach J, Sabedot TS, Schein J, Schumacher SE, Seidman JG, Seth S, Shen H, Simons JV, Sipahimalani P, Soloway MG, Song X, Sun H, Tabak B, Tam A, Tan D, Tang J, Thiessen N, Triche T Jr, Van Den Berg DJ, Veluvolu U, Waring S, Weisenberger DJ, Wilkerson MD, Wong T, Wu J, Xi L, Xu AW, Yang L, Zack TI, Zhang J, Aksoy BA, Arachchi H, Benz C, Bernard B, Carlin D, Cho J, DiCara D, Frazer S, Fuller GN,

Gao J, Gehlenborg N, Haussler D, Heiman DI, Iype L, Jacobsen A, Ju Z, Katzman S, Kim H, Knijnenburg T, Kreisberg RB, Lawrence MS, Lee W, Leinonen K, Lin P, Ling S, Liu W, Liu Y, Liu Y, Lu Y, Mills G, Ng S, Noble MS, Paull E, Rao A, Reynolds S, Saksena G, Sanborn Z, Sander C, Schultz N, Senbabaoglu Y, Shen R, Shmulevich I, Sinha R, Stuart J, Sumer SO, Sun Y, Tasman N, Taylor BS, Voet D, Weinhold N, Weinstein JN, Yang D, Yoshihara K, Zheng S, Zhang W, Zou L, Abel T, Sadeghi S, Cohen ML, Eschbacher J, Hattab EM, Raghunathan A, Schniederjan MJ, Aziz D, Barnett G, Barrett W, Bigner DD, Boice L, Brewer C, Calatozzolo C, Campos B, Carlotti CG Jr, Chan TA, Cuppini L, Curley E, Cuzzubbo S, Devine K, DiMeco F, Duell R, Elder JB, Fehrenbach A, Finocchiaro G, Friedman W, Fulop J, Gardner J, Hermes B, Herold-Mende C, Jungk C, Kendler A, Lehman NL, Lipp E, Liu O, Mandt R, McGraw M, Mclendon R, McPherson C, Neder L, Nguyen P, Noss A, Nunziata R, Ostrom QT, Palmer C, Perin A, Pollo B, Potapov A, Potapova O, Rathmell WK, Rotin D, Scarpace L, Schilero C, Senecal K, Shimmel K, Shurkhay V, Sifri S, Singh R, Sloan AE, Smolenski K, Staugaitis SM, Steele R, Thorne L, Tirapelli DP, Unterberg A, Vallurupalli M, Wang Y, Warnick R, Williams F, Wolinsky Y, Bell S, Rosenberg M, Stewart C, Huang F, Grimsby JL, Radenbaugh AJ, Zhang J (2015) Comprehensive, integrative genomic analysis of diffuse lower-grade gliomas. N Engl J Med 372(26):2481–2498

24. Capper D, Jones DTW, Sill M, Hovestadt V, Schrimpf D, Sturm D, Koelsche C, Sahm F, Chavez L, Reuss DE, Kratz A, Wefers AK, Huang K, Pajtler KW, Schweizer L, Stichel D, Olar A, Engel NW, Lindenberg K, Harter PN, Braczynski AK, Plate KH, Dohmen H, Garvalov BK, Coras R, Hölsken A, Hewer E, Bewerunge-Hudler M, Schick M, Fischer R, Beschorner R, Schittenhelm J, Staszewski O, Wani K, Varlet P, Pages M, Temming P, Lohmann D, Selt F, Witt H, Milde T, Witt O, Aronica E, Giangaspero F, Rushing E, Scheurlen W, Geisenberger C, Rodriguez FJ, Becker A, Preusser M, Haberler C, Bjerkvig R, Cryan J, Farrell M, Deckert M, Hench J, Frank S, Serrano J, Kannan K, Tsirigos A, Brück W, Hofer S, Brehmer S, Seiz-Rosenhagen M, Hänggi D, Hans V, Rozsnoki S, Hansford JR, Kohlhof P, Kristensen BW, Lechner M, Lopes B, Mawrin C, Ketter R, Kulozik A, Khatib Z, Heppner F, Koch A, Jouvet A, Keohane C, Mühleisen H, Mueller W, Pohl U, Prinz M, Benner A, Zapatka M, Gottardo NG, Driever PH, Kramm CM, Müller HL, Rutkowski S, von Hoff K, Frühwald MC, Gnekow A, Fleischhack G, Tippelt S, Calaminus G, Monoranu CM, Perry A, Jones C, Jacques TS, Radlwimmer B, Gessi M, Pietsch T, Schramm J, Schackert G, Westphal M, Reifenberger G, Wesseling P, Weller M, Collins VP, Blümcke I, Bendszus M, Debus J, Huang A, Jabado N, Northcott PA, Paulus W, Gajjar A, Robinson GW, Taylor MD, Jaunmuktane Z, Ryzhova M, Platten M, Unterberg A, Wick W, Karajannis MA, Mittelbronn M, Acker T, Hartmann C, Aldape K, Schüller U, Buslei R, Lichter P, Kool M, Herold-Mende C, Ellison DW, Hasselblatt M, Snuderl M, Brandner S, Korshunov A, von Deimling A, Pfister SM (2018) DNA methylation-based classification of central nervous system tumours. Nature 555(7697):469–474

25. Ceccarelli M, Barthel FP, Malta TM, Sabedot TS, Salama SR, Murray BA, Morozova O, Newton Y, Radenbaugh A, Pagnotta SM, Anjum S, Wang J, Manyam G, Zoppoli P, Ling S, Rao AA, Grifford M, Cherniack AD, Zhang H, Poisson L, Carlotti CG Jr, Tirapelli DP, Rao A, Mikkelsen T, Lau CC, Yung WK, Rabadan R, Huse J, Brat DJ, Lehman NL, Barnholtz-Sloan JS, Zheng S, Hess K, Rao G, Meyerson M, Beroukhim R, Cooper L, Akbani R, Wrensch M, Haussler D, Aldape KD, Laird PW, Gutmann DH, Research Network TCGA, Noushmehr H, Iavarone A, Verhaak RG (2016) Molecular profiling reveals biologically discrete subsets and pathways of progression in diffuse glioma. Cell 164(3):550–563

26. Chu LC, Eberhart CG, Grossman SA, Herman JG (2006) Epigenetic silencing of multiple genes in primary CNS lymphoma. Int J Cancer 119(10):2487–2491

27. Cimino PJ, Zager M, McFerrin L, Wirsching HG, Bolouri H, Hentschel B, von Deimling A, Jones D, Reifenberger G, Weller M, Holland EC (2017) Multidimensional scaling of diffuse gliomas: application to the 2016 World Health Organization classification system with prognostically relevant molecular subtype discovery. Acta Neuropathol Commun 5(1):39

28. Collins VP, Jones DT, Giannini C (2015) Pilocytic astrocytoma: pathology, molecular mechanisms and markers. Acta Neuropathol 129(6):775–788

29. de Kock L, Sabbaghian N, Druker H, Weber E, Hamel N, Miller S, Choong CS, Gottardo NG, Kees UR, Rednam SP, van Hest LP, Jongmans MC, Jhangiani S, Lupski JR, Zacharin M, Bouron-Dal Soglio D, Huang A, Priest JR, Perry A, Mueller S, Albrecht S, Malkin D, Grundy RG, Foulkes WD (2014) Germ-line and somatic DICER1 mutations in pineoblastoma. Acta Neuropathol 128(4):583–595

30. El Hussein S, Vincentelli C (2017) Pituicytoma: review of commonalities and distinguishing features among TTF-1 positive tumors of the central nervous system. Ann Diagn Pathol 29:57–61

31. Ellison DW, Onilude OE, Lindsey JC, Lusher ME, Weston CL, Taylor RE, Pearson AD, Clifford SC, United Kingdom Children's Cancer Study Group Brain Tumour Committee (2005) beta-Catenin status predicts a favorable outcome in childhood medulloblastoma: the United Kingdom Children's Cancer Study Group Brain Tumour Committee. J Clin Oncol 23(31):7951–7957

32. Fauchon F, Jouvet A, Paquis P, Saint-Pierre G, Mottolese C, Ben Hassel M, Chauveinc L, Sichez JP, Philippon J, Schlienger M, Bouffet E (2000) Parenchymal pineal tumors: a clinicopathological study of 76 cases. Int J Radiat Oncol Biol Phys 46(4):959–968

33. Figarella-Branger D, Mokhtari K, Dehais C, Carpentier C, Colin C, Jouvet A, Uro-Coste E, Forest F, Maurage CA, Vignaud JM, Polivka M, Lechapt-Zalcman E, Eimer S, Viennet G, Quintin-Roué I, Aubriot-Lorton MH, Diebold MD, Loussouarn D, Lacroix C, Rigau V, Laquerrière A, Vandenbos F, Michalak S, Sevestre H, Peoch M, Labrousse F, Christov C, Kemeny JL, Chenard MP, Chiforeanu D, Ducray F, Idbaih A, Delattre JY, Network POLA (2016) Mitotic index, microvascular proliferation, and necrosis define 3 pathological subgroups of prognostic relevance among 1p/19q co-deleted anaplastic oligodendrogliomas. Neuro Oncol 18(6):888–890

34. Fishbein L, Leshchiner I, Walter V, Danilova L, Robertson AG, Johnson AR, Lichtenberg TM, Murray BA, Ghayee HK, Else T, Ling S, Jefferys SR, de Cubas AA, Wenz B, Korpershoek E, Amelio AL, Makowski L, Rathmell WK, Gimenez-Roqueplo AP, Giordano TJ, Asa SL, Tischler AS; Cancer Genome Atlas Research Network, Pacak K, Nathanson KL, Wilkerson MD (2017) Comprehensive molecular characterization of pheochromocytoma and paraganglioma. Cancer Cell 31(2):181–193

35. Fukumura K, Kawazu M, Kojima S, Ueno T, Sai E, Soda M, Ueda H, Yasuda T, Yamaguchi H, Lee J, Shishido-Hara Y, Sasaki A, Shirahata M, Mishima K, Ichimura K, Mukasa A, Narita Y, Saito N, Aburatani H, Nishikawa R, Nagane M, Mano H (2016) Genomic characterization of primary central nervous system lymphoma. Acta Neuropathol 131(6):865–875

36. Fukushima S, Otsuka A, Suzuki T, Yanagisawa T, Mishima K, Mukasa A, Saito N, Kumabe T, Kanamori M, Tominaga T, Narita Y, Shibui S, Kato M, Shibata T, Matsutani M, Nishikawa R, Ichimura K, Intracranial Germ Cell Tumor Genome Analysis Consortium (iGCT Consortium) (2014) Mutually exclusive mutations of KIT and RAS are associated with KIT mRNA expression and chromosomal instability in primary intracranial pure germinomas. Acta Neuropathol 127(6):911–925

37. Fukushima S, Yamashita S, Kobayashi H, Takami H, Fukuoka K, Nakamura T, Yamasaki K, Matsushita Y, Nakamura H, Totoki Y, Kato M, Suzuki T, Mishima K, Yanagisawa T, Mukasa A, Saito N, Kanamori M, Kumabe T, Tominaga T, Nagane M, Iuchi T, Yoshimoto K, Mizoguchi M, Tamura K, Sakai K, Sugiyama K, Nakada M, Yokogami K, Takeshima H, Kanemura Y, Matsuda M, Matsumura A, Kurozumi K, Ueki K, Nonaka M, Asai A, Kawahara N, Hirose Y, Takayama T, Nakazato Y, Narita Y, Shibata T, Matsutani M, Ushijima T, Nishikawa R, Ichimura K, Intracranial Germ Cell Tumor Genome Analysis Consortium (The iGCTConsortium) (2017) Genome-wide methylation profiles in primary intracranial germ cell tumors indicate a primordial germ cell origin for germinomas. Acta Neuropathol 133(3):445–462

38. Georgescu MM, Mobley BC, Orr BA, Shang P, Lehman NL, Zhu X, O'Neill TJ, Rajaram V, Hatanpaa KJ, Timmons CF, Raisanen JM (2016) NHERF1/ EBP50 and NF2 as diagnostic markers for choroid plexus tumors. Acta Neuropathol Commun 4(1):55

39. Gessi M, Giangaspero F, Pietsch T (2003) Atypical teratoid/rhabdoid tumors and choroid plexus tumors: when genetics "surprise" pathology. Brain Pathol 13(3):409–414

40. Gessi M, Moneim YA, Hammes J, Goschzik T, Scholz M, Denkhaus D, Waha A, Pietsch T (2014) FGFR1 mutations in Rosette-forming glioneuronal tumors of the fourth ventricle. J Neuropathol Exp Neurol 73(6):580–584

41. Gessi M, Zur Mühlen A, Hammes J, Waha A, Denkhaus D, Pietsch T (2013) Genome-wide DNA copy number analysis of desmoplastic infantile astrocytomas and desmoplastic infantile gangliogliomas. J Neuropathol Exp Neurol 72(9):807–815

42. Goode B, Mondal G, Hyun M, Ruiz DG, Lin YH, Van Ziffle J, Joseph NM, Onodera C, Talevich E, Grenert JP, Hewedi IH, Snuderl M, Brat DJ, Kleinschmidt-DeMasters BK, Rodriguez FJ, Louis DN, Yong WH, Lopes MB, Rosenblum MK, Butowski N, Tihan T, Bollen AW, Phillips JJ, Wiita AP, Yeh I, Jacobson MP, Bastian BC, Perry A, Solomon DA (2018) A recurrent kinase domain mutation in PRKCA defines chordoid glioma of the third ventricle. Nat Commun 9(1):810

43. Goschzik T, Gessi M, Denkhaus D, Pietsch T (2014) PTEN mutations and activation of the PI3K/Akt/mTOR signaling pathway in papillary tumors of the pineal region. J Neuropathol Exp Neurol 73(8):747–751

44. Goschzik T, Gessi M, Dreschmann V, Gebhardt U, Wang L, Yamaguchi S, Wheeler DA, Lauriola L, Lau CC, Müller HL, Pietsch T (2017) Genomic alterations of adamantinomatous and papillary craniopharyngioma. J Neuropathol Exp Neurol 76(2):126–134

45. Greer A, Foreman NK, Donson A, Davies KD, Kleinschmidt-DeMasters BK (2017) Desmoplastic infantile astrocytoma/ganglioglioma with rare BRAF V600D mutation. Pediatr Blood Cancer 64(6). https://doi.org/10.1002/pbc.26350

46. Griffin CA, Burger P, Morsberger L, Yonescu R, Swierczynski S, Weingart JD, Murphy KM (2006) Identification of der(1;19)(q10;p10) in five oligodendrogliomas suggests mechanism of concurrent 1p and 19q loss. J Neuropathol Exp Neurol 65(10):988–994

47. Hartmann C, Hentschel B, Wick W, Capper D, Felsberg J, Simon M, Westphal M, Schackert G, Meyermann R, Pietsch T, Reifenberger G, Weller M, Loeffler M, von Deimling A (2010) Patients with IDH1 wild type anaplastic astrocytomas exhibit worse prognosis than IDH1-mutated glioblastomas, and IDH1 mutation status accounts for the unfavorable prognostic effect of higher age: implications for classification of gliomas. Acta Neuropathol 120(6):707–718

48. Hartmann C, Meyer J, Balss J, Capper D, Mueller W, Christians A, Felsberg J, Wolter M, Mawrin C, Wick W, Weller M, Herold-Mende C, Unterberg A, Jeuken JW, Wesseling P, Reifenberger G, von Deimling A (2009) Type and frequency of IDH1 and IDH2 mutations are related to astrocytic and oligodendroglial

differentiation and age: a study of 1,010 diffuse gliomas. Acta Neuropathol 118(4):469–474

49. Hasbani DM, Crino PB (2018) Tuberous sclerosis complex. Handb Clin Neurol 148:813–822

50. Hasselblatt M, Böhm C, Tatenhorst L, Dinh V, Newrzella D, Keyvani K, Jeibmann A, Buerger H, Rickert CH, Paulus W (2006) Identification of novel diagnostic markers for choroid plexus tumors: a microarray-based approach. Am J Surg Pathol 30(1):66–74

51. Hasselblatt M, Kurlemann G, Rickert CH, Debus OM, Brentrup A, Schachenmayr W, Paulus W (2004 23) Familial occurrence of dysembryoplastic neuroepithelial tumor. Neurology 62(6):1020–1021

52. Hegi ME, Diserens AC, Gorlia T, Hamou MF, de Tribolet N, Weller M, Kros JM, Hainfellner JA, Mason W, Mariani L, Bromberg JE, Hau P, Mirimanoff RO, Cairncross JG, Janzer RC, Stupp R (2005) MGMT gene silencing and benefit from temozolomide in glioblastoma. N Engl J Med 352(10):997–1003

53. Heim S, Sill M, Jones DT, Vasiljevic A, Jouvet A, Fèvre-Montange M, Wesseling P, Beschorner R, Mittelbronn M, Kohlhof P, Hovestadt V, Johann P, Kool M, Pajtler KW, Korshunov A, Ruland V, Sperveslage J, Thomas C, Witt H, von Deimling A, Paulus W, Pfister SM, Capper D, Hasselblatt M (2016) Papillary tumor of the pineal region: a distinct molecular entity. Brain Pathol 26(2):199–205

54. Hes FJ, McKee S, Taphoorn MJ, Rehal P, van Der Luijt RB, McMahon R, van Der Smagt JJ, Dow D, Zewald RA, Whittaker J, Lips CJ, MacDonald F, Pearson PL, Maher ER (2000) Cryptic von Hippel-Lindau disease: germline mutations in patients with haemangioblastoma only. J Med Genet 37(12):939–943

55. Hölsken A, Sill M, Merkle J, Schweizer L, Buchfelder M, Flitsch J, Fahlbusch R, Metzler M, Kool M, Pfister SM, von Deimling A, Capper D, Jones DT, Buslei R (2016) Adamantinomatous and papillary craniopharyngiomas are characterized by distinct epigenomic as well as mutational and transcriptomic profiles. Acta Neuropathol Commun 4:20

56. Holthausen H, Blümcke I (2016) Epilepsy-associated tumours: what epileptologists should know about neuropathology, terminology, and classification systems. Epileptic Disord 18(3):240–251

57. Horstmann S, Perry A, Reifenberger G, Giangaspero F, Huang H, Hara A, Masuoka J, Rainov NG, Bergmann M, Heppner FL, Brandner S, Chimelli L, Montagna N, Jackson T, Davis DG, Markesbery WR, Ellison DW, Weller RO, Taddei GL, Conti R, Del Bigio MR, Gonzalez-Campora R, Radhakrishnan VV, Soylemezoglu F, Uro-Coste E, Qian J, Kleihues P, Ohgaki H (2004) Genetic and expression profiles of cerebellar liponeurocytomas. Brain Pathol 14(3):281–289

58. Huse JT, Edgar M, Halliday J, Mikolaenko I, Lavi E, Rosenblum MK (2013) Multinodular and vacuolating neuronal tumors of the cerebrum: 10 cases of a distinctive seizure-associated lesion. Brain Pathol 23(5):515–524

59. Ichimura K, Fukushima S, Totoki Y, Matsushita Y, Otsuka A, Tomiyama A, Niwa T, Takami H, Nakamura T, Suzuki T, Fukuoka K, Yanagisawa T, Mishima K, Nakazato Y, Hosoda F, Narita Y, Shibui S, Yoshida A, Mukasa A, Saito N, Kumabe T, Kanamori M, Tominaga T, Kobayashi K, Shimizu S, Nagane M, Iuchi T, Mizoguchi M, Yoshimoto K, Tamura K, Maehara T, Sugiyama K, Nakada M, Sakai K, Kanemura Y, Nonaka M, Asai A, Yokogami K, Takeshima H, Kawahara N, Takayama T, Yao M, Kato M, Nakamura H, Hama N, Sakai R, Ushijima T, Matsutani M, Shibata T, Nishikawa R, Intracranial Germ Cell Tumor Genome Analysis Consortium (2016) Recurrent neomorphic mutations of MTOR in central nervous system and testicular germ cell tumors may be targeted for therapy. Acta Neuropathol 131(6):889–901

60. Jeibmann A, Hasselblatt M, Gerss J, Wrede B, Egensperger R, Beschorner R, Hans VH, Rickert CH, Wolff JE, Paulus W (2006) Prognostic implications of atypical histologic features in choroid plexus papilloma. J Neuropathol Exp Neurol 65(11):1069–1073

61. Jenkins RB, Blair H, Ballman KV, Giannini C, Arusell RM, Law M, Flynn H, Passe S, Felten S, Brown PD, Shaw EG, Buckner JC (2006 15) A t(1;19)(q10;p10) mediates the combined deletions of 1p and 19q and predicts a better prognosis of patients with oligodendroglioma. Cancer Res 66(20):9852–9861

62. Jenkinson MD, Bosma JJ, Du Plessis D, Ohgaki H, Kleihues P, Warnke P, Rainov NG (2003) Cerebellar liponeurocytoma with an unusually aggressive clinical course: case report. Neurosurgery 53(6):1425–1427

63. Jo VY, Fletcher CDM (2017) SMARCB1/INI1 loss in epithelioid schwannoma: a clinicopathologic and immunohistochemical study of 65 cases. Am J Surg Pathol 41(8):1013–1022

64. Johann PD, Erkek S, Zapatka M, Kerl K, Buchhalter I, Hovestadt V, Jones DT, Sturm D, Hermann C, Segura Wang M, Korshunov A, Rhyzova M, Gröbner S, Brabetz S, Chavez L, Bens S, Gröschel S, Kratochwil F, Wittmann A, Sieber L, Geörg C, Wolf S, Beck K, Oyen F, Capper D, van Sluis P, Volckmann R, Koster J, Versteeg R, von Deimling A, Milde T, Witt O, Kulozik AE, Ebinger M, Shalaby T, Grotzer M, Sumerauer D, Zamecnik J, Mora J, Jabado N, Taylor MD, Huang A, Aronica E, Bertoni A, Radlwimmer B, Pietsch T, Schüller U, Schneppenheim R, Northcott PA, Korbel JO, Siebert R, Frühwald MC, Lichter P, Eils R, Gajjar A, Hasselblatt M, Pfister SM, Kool M (2016) Atypical teratoid/rhabdoid tumors are comprised of three epigenetic subgroups with distinct enhancer landscapes. Cancer Cell 29(3):379–393

65. Jones DT, Hutter B, Jäger N, Korshunov A, Kool M, Warnatz HJ, Zichner T, Lambert SR, Ryzhova M, Quang DA, Fontebasso AM, Stütz AM, Hutter S, Zuckermann M, Sturm D, Gronych J, Lasitschka B, Schmidt S, Seker-Cin H, Witt H, Sultan M, Ralser M, Northcott PA, Hovestadt V, Bender S, Pfaff E, Stark S, Faury D, Schwartzentruber J, Majewski J, Weber UD, Zapatka M, Raeder B, Schlesner M,

Worth CL, Bartholomae CC, von Kalle C, Imbusch CD, Radomski S, Lawerenz C, van Sluis P, Koster J, Volckmann R, Versteeg R, Lehrach H, Monoranu C, Winkler B, Unterberg A, Herold-Mende C, Milde T, Kulozik AE, Ebinger M, Schuhmann MU, Cho YJ, Pomeroy SL, von Deimling A, Witt O, Taylor MD, Wolf S, Karajannis MA, Eberhart CG, Scheurlen W, Hasselblatt M, Ligon KL, Kieran MW, Korbel JO, Yaspo ML, Brors B, Felsberg J, Reifenberger G, Collins VP, Jabado N, Eils R, Lichter P, Pfister SM, International Cancer Genome Consortium PedBrain Tumor Project (2013) Recurrent somatic alterations of FGFR1 and NTRK2 in pilocytic astrocytoma. Nat Genet 45(8):927–932

66. Johnson MW, Eberhart CG, Perry A, Tihan T, Cohen KJ, Rosenblum MK, Rais-Bahrami S, Goldthwaite P, Burger PC (2010) Spectrum of pilomyxoid astrocytomas: intermediate pilomyxoid tumors. Am J Surg Pathol 34(12):1783–1791

67. Jouvet A, Fauchon F, Liberski P, Saint-Pierre G, Didier-Bazes M, Heitzmann A, Delisle MB, Biassette HA, Vincent S, Mikol J, Streichenberger N, Ahboucha S, Brisson C, Belin MF, Fèvre-Montange M (2003) Papillary tumor of the pineal region. Am J Surg Pathol 27(4):505–512

68. Jouvet A, Saint-Pierre G, Fauchon F, Privat K, Bouffet E, Ruchoux MM, Chauveinc L, Fèvre-Montange M (2000) Pineal parenchymal tumors: a correlation of histological features with prognosis in 66 cases. Brain Pathol 10(1):49–60

69. Kamoun A, Idbaih A, Dehais C, Elarouci N, Carpentier C, Letouzé E, Colin C, Mokhtari K, Jouvet A, Uro-Coste E, Martin-Duverneuil N, Sanson M, Delattre JY, Figarella-Branger D, de Reyniès A, Ducray F, POLA Network (2016) Integrated multiomics analysis of oligodendroglial tumours identifies three subgroups of 1p/19q co-deleted gliomas. Nat Commun 7:11263

70. Klein CJ, Wu Y, Jentoft ME, Mer G, Spinner RJ, Dyck PJ, Dyck PJ, Mauermann ML (2017) Genomic analysis reveals frequent TRAF7 mutations in intraneural perineuriomas. Ann Neurol 81(2):316–321

71. Kleinschmidt-DeMasters BK, Aisner DL, Birks DK, Foreman NK (2013) Epithelioid GBMs show a high percentage of BRAF V600E mutation. Am J Surg Pathol 37(5):685–698

72. Koch A, Waha A, Tonn JC, Sörensen N, Berthold F, Wolter M, Reifenberger J, Hartmann W, Friedl W, Reifenberger G, Wiestler OD, Pietsch T (2001) Somatic mutations of WNT/wingless signaling pathway components in primitive neuroectodermal tumors. Int J Cancer 93(3):445–449

73. Koch CA, Vortmeyer AO, Zhuang Z, Brouwers FM, Pacak K (2002) New insights into the genetics of familial chromaffin cell tumors. Ann N Y Acad Sci 970:11–28

74. Koelsche C, Sahm F, Wöhrer A, Jeibmann A, Schittenhelm J, Kohlhof P, Preusser M, Romeike B, Dohmen-Scheufler H, Hartmann C, Mittelbronn M, Becker A, von Deimling A, Capper D (2014) BRAF-mutated pleomorphic xanthoastrocytoma is associated with temporal location, reticulin fiber deposition and CD34 expression. Brain Pathol 24(3):221–229

75. Koelsche C, Wöhrer A, Jeibmann A, Schittenhelm J, Schindler G, Preusser M, Lasitschka F, von Deimling A, Capper D (2013) Mutant BRAF V600E protein in ganglioglioma is predominantly expressed by neuronal tumor cells. Acta Neuropathol 125(6):891–900

76. Komori T, Scheithauer BW, Hirose T (2002) A rosette-forming glioneuronal tumor of the fourth ventricle: infratentorial form of dysembryoplastic neuroepithelial tumor? Am J Surg Pathol 26(5):582–591

77. Korshunov A, Chavez L, Sharma T, Ryzhova M, Schrimpf D, Stichel D, Capper D, Sturm D, Kool M, Habel A, Kleinschmidt-DeMasters BK, Rosenblum M, Absalyamova O, Golanov A, Lichter P, Pfister SM, Jones DTW, Perry A, von Deimling A (2017) Epithelioid glioblastomas stratify into established diagnostic subsets upon integrated molecular analysis. Brain Pathol. https://doi.org/10.1111/bpa.12566. [Epub ahead of print]

78. Korshunov A, Sturm D, Ryzhova M, Hovestadt V, Gessi M, Jones DT, Remke M, Northcott P, Perry A, Picard D, Rosenblum M, Antonelli M, Aronica E, Schüller U, Hasselblatt M, Woehrer A, Zheludkova O, Kumirova E, Puget S, Taylor MD, Giangaspero F, Peter Collins V, von Deimling A, Lichter P, Huang A, Pietsch T, Pfister SM, Kool M (2014) Embryonal tumor with abundant neuropil and true rosettes (ETANTR), ependymoblastoma, and medulloepithelioma share molecular similarity and comprise a single clinicopathological entity. Acta Neuropathol 128(2):279–289

79. Korshunov A, Sycheva R, Golanov A (2007) Recurrent cytogenetic aberrations in central neurocytomas and their biological relevance. Acta Neuropathol 113(3):303–312

80. Kros JM, Gorlia T, Kouwenhoven MC, Zheng PP, Collins VP, Figarella-Branger D, Giangaspero F, Giannini C, Mokhtari K, Mørk SJ, Paetau A, Reifenberger G, van den Bent MJ (2007) Panel review of anaplastic oligodendroglioma from European Organization For Research and Treatment of Cancer Trial 26951: assessment of consensus in diagnosis, influence of 1p/19q loss, and correlations with outcome. J Neuropathol Exp Neurol 66(6):545–551

81. Küsters-Vandevelde HV, Küsters B, van Engen-van Grunsven AC, Groenen PJ, Wesseling P, Blokx WA (2015) Primary melanocytic tumors of the central nervous system: a review with focus on molecular aspects. Brain Pathol 25(2):209–226

82. Küsters-Vandevelde HV, Creytens D, van Engen-van Grunsven AC, Jeunink M, Winnepenninckx V, Groenen PJ, Küsters B, Wesseling P, Blokx WA, Prinsen CF (2016) SF3B1 and EIF1AX mutations occur in primary leptomeningeal melanocytic neoplasms; yet another similarity to uveal melanomas. Acta Neuropathol Commun 4:5

83. Labreche K, Simeonova I, Kamoun A, Gleize V, Chubb D, Letouzé E, Riazalhosseini Y, Dobbins SE,

Elarouci N, Ducray F, de Reyniès A, Zelenika D, Wardell CP, Frampton M, Saulnier O, Pastinen T, Hallout S, Figarella-Branger D, Dehais C, Idbaih A, Mokhtari K, Delattre JY, Huillard E, Mark Lathrop G, Sanson M, Houlston RS, POLA Network (2015) TCF12 is mutated in anaplastic oligodendroglioma. Nat Commun 6:7207

84. Lee JY, Dong SM, Park WS, Yoo NJ, Kim CS, Jang JJ, Chi JG, Zbar B, Lubensky IA, Linehan WM, Vortmeyer AO, Zhuang Z (1998) Loss of heterozygosity and somatic mutations of the VHL tumor suppressor gene in sporadic cerebellar hemangioblastomas. Cancer Res 58(3):504–508

85. Lewis PW, Müller MM, Koletsky MS, Cordero F, Lin S, Banaszynski LA, Garcia BA, Muir TW, Becher OJ, Allis CD (2013) Inhibition of PRC2 activity by a gain-of-function H3 mutation found in pediatric glioblastoma. Science 340(6134): 857–861

86. Looijenga LH, Stoop H, de Leeuw HP, de Gouveia Brazao CA, Gillis AJ, van Roozendaal KE, van Zoelen EJ, Weber RF, Wolffenbuttel KP, van Dekken H, Honecker F, Bokemeyer C, Perlman EJ, Schneider DT, Kononen J, Sauter G, Oosterhuis JW (2003) POU5F1 (OCT3/4) identifies cells with pluripotent potential in human germ cell tumors. Cancer Res 63(9):2244–2250

87. Louis DN, Giannini C, Capper D, Paulus W, Figarella-Branger D, Lopes MB, Batchelor TT, Cairncross JG, van den Bent M, Wick W, Wesseling P (2018) cIMPACT-NOW update 2: diagnostic clarifications for diffuse midline glioma, H3 K27M-mutant and diffuse astrocytoma/anaplastic astrocytoma, IDH-mutant. Acta Neuropathol. https://doi.org/10.1007/s00401-018-1826-y. [Epub ahead of print]

88. Louis DN, Ohgaki H, Wiestler OD, Cavenee WK (eds) (2007) WHO classification of tumours of the central nervous system, 4th edn. IARC, Lyon

89. Louis DN, Ohgaki H, Wiestler OD, Cavenee WK (eds) (2016) WHO classification of tumours of the central nervous system (Revised 4th ed). IARC, Lyon

90. Louis DN, Perry A, Burger P, Ellison DW, Reifenberger G, von Deimling A, Aldape K, Brat D, Collins VP, Eberhart C, Figarella-Branger D, Fuller GN, Giangaspero F, Giannini C, Hawkins C, Kleihues P, Korshunov A, Kros JM, Beatriz Lopes M, Ng HK, Ohgaki H, Paulus W, Pietsch T, Rosenblum M, Rushing E, Soylemezoglu F, Wiestler O, Wesseling P, International Society of Neuropathology, Haarlem. International Society of Neuropathology (2014) Haarlem consensus guidelines for nervous system tumor classification and grading. Brain Pathol 24(5):429–435

91. Louis DN, Perry A, Reifenberger G, von Deimling A, Figarella-Branger D, Cavenee WK, Ohgaki H, Wiestler OD, Kleihues P, Ellison DW (2016) The 2016 World Health Organization classification of tumors of the central nervous system: a summary. Acta Neuropathol 131(6):803–820

92. Louis DN, Wesseling P, Paulus W, Giannini C, Batchelor TT, Cairncross JG, Capper D, Figarella-Branger D, Lopes MB, Wick W, van den Bent M (2018) cIMPACT-NOW update 1: not otherwise specified (NOS) and not elsewhere classified (NEC). Acta Neuropathol 135(3):481–484

93. Lloyd RV, Osamura RY, Klöppel G, Rosai J (2017) WHO classification of tumours of endocrine organs. In: World Health Organization classification of tumours, vol 10, 4th edn. IARC, Lyon

94. Lopes MBS (2017) The 2017 World Health Organization classification of tumors of the pituitary gland: a summary. Acta Neuropathol 134(4):521–535

95. Luyken C, Blümcke I, Fimmers R, Urbach H, Wiestler OD, Schramm J (2004) Supratentorial gangliogliomas: histopathologic grading and tumor recurrence in 184 patients with a median follow-up of 8 years. Cancer 101(1):146–155

96. Majores M, von Lehe M, Fassunke J, Schramm J, Becker AJ, Simon M (2008) Tumor recurrence and malignant progression of gangliogliomas. Cancer 113(12):3355–3363

97. Malzkorn B, Reifenberger G (2016) Practical implications of integrated glioma classification according to the World Health Organization classification of tumors of the central nervous system 2016. Curr Opin Oncol 28(6):494–501

98. Masui K, Mischel PS, Reifenberger G (2016) Molecular classification of gliomas. Handb Clin Neurol 134:97–120

99. Masuoka J, Brandner S, Paulus W, Soffer D, Vital A, Chimelli L, Jouvet A, Yonekawa Y, Kleihues P, Ohgaki H (2001) Germline SDHD mutation in paraganglioma of the spinal cord. Oncogene 20(36):5084–5086

100. Miller MB, Bi WL, Ramkissoon LA, Kang YJ, Abedalthagafi M, Knoff DS, Agarwalla PK, Wen PY, Reardon DA, Alexander BM, Laws ER, Dunn IF, Beroukhim R, Ligon KL, Ramkissoon SH (2016) MAPK activation and HRAS mutation identified in pituitary spindle cell oncocytoma. Oncotarget 7(24):37054–37063

101. Miller S, Rogers HA, Lyon P, Rand V, Adamowicz-Brice M, Clifford SC, Hayden JT, Dyer S, Pfister S, Korshunov A, Brundler MA, Lowe J, Coyle B, Grundy RG (2011) Genome-wide molecular characterization of central nervous system primitive neuroectodermal tumor and pineoblastoma. Neuro Oncol 13(8):866–879

102. Montesinos-Rongen M, Brunn A, Bentink S, Basso K, Lim WK, Klapper W, Schaller C, Reifenberger G, Rubenstein J, Wiestler OD, Spang R, Dalla-Favera R, Siebert R, Deckert M (2008) Gene expression profiling suggests primary central nervous system lymphomas to be derived from a late germinal center B cell. Leukemia 22(2):400–405

103. Northcott PA, Buchhalter I, Morrissy AS, Hovestadt V, Weischenfeldt J, Ehrenberger T, Gröbner S, Segura-Wang M, Zichner T, Rudneva VA, Warnatz HJ, Sidiropoulos N, Phillips AH, Schumacher S, Kleinheinz

K, Waszak SM, Erkek S, Jones DTW, Worst BC, Kool M, Zapatka M, Jäger N, Chavez L, Hutter B, Bieg M, Paramasivam N, Heinold M, Gu Z, Ishaque N, Jäger-Schmidt C, Imbusch CD, Jugold A, Hübschmann D, Risch T, Amstislavskiy V, Gonzalez FGR, Weber UD, Wolf S, Robinson GW, Zhou X, Wu G, Finkelstein D, Liu Y, Cavalli FMG, Luu B, Ramaswamy V, Wu X, Koster J, Ryzhova M, Cho YJ, Pomeroy SL, Herold-Mende C, Schuhmann M, Ebinger M, Liau LM, Mora J, McLendon RE, Jabado N, Kumabe T, Chuah E, Ma Y, Moore RA, Mungall AJ, Mungall KL, Thiessen N, Tse K, Wong T, Jones SJM, Witt O, Milde T, Von Deimling A, Capper D, Korshunov A, Yaspo ML, Kriwacki R, Gajjar A, Zhang J, Beroukhim R, Fraenkel E, Korbel JO, Brors B, Schlesner M, Eils R, Marra MA, Pfister SM, Taylor MD, Lichter P (2017) The whole-genome landscape of medulloblastoma subtypes. Nature 547(7663):311–317

104. Okada Y, Nishikawa R, Matsutani M, Louis DN (2002) Hypomethylated X chromosome gain and rare isochromosome 12p in diverse intracranial germ cell tumors. J Neuropathol Exp Neurol 61(6):531–538

105. Ono Y, Ueki K, Joseph JT, Louis DN (1996) Homozygous deletions of the *CDKN2/p16* gene in dural hemangiopericytomas. Acta Neuropathol (Berl) 91(3):221–225

106. Panwalkar P, Clark J, Ramaswamy V, Hawes D, Yang F, Dunham C, Yip S, Hukin J, Sun Y, Schipper MJ, Chavez L, Margol A, Pekmezci M, Chung C, Banda A, Bayliss JM, Curry SJ, Santi M, Rodriguez FJ, Snuderl M, Karajannis MA, Saratsis AM, Horbinski CM, Carret AS, Wilson B, Johnston D, Lafay-Cousin L, Zelcer S, Eisenstat D, Silva M, Scheinemann K, Jabado N, McNeely PD, Kool M, Pfister SM, Taylor MD, Hawkins C, Korshunov A, Judkins AR, Venneti S (2017) Immunohistochemical analysis of H3K27me3 demonstrates global reduction in group-A childhood posterior fossa ependymoma and is a powerful predictor of outcome. Acta Neuropathol 134(5):705–714

107. Pajtler KW, Witt H, Sill M, Jones DT, Hovestadt V, Kratochwil F, Wani K, Tatevossian R, Punchihewa C, Johann P, Reimand J, Warnatz HJ, Ryzhova M, Mack S, Ramaswamy V, Capper D, Schweizer L, Sieber L, Wittmann A, Huang Z, van Sluis P, Volckmann R, Koster J, Versteeg R, Fults D, Toledano H, Avigad S, Hoffman LM, Donson AM, Foreman N, Hewer E, Zitterbart K, Gilbert M, Armstrong TS, Gupta N, Allen JC, Karajannis MA, Zagzag D, Hasselblatt M, Kulozik AE, Witt O, Collins VP, von Hoff K, Rutkowski S, Pietsch T, Bader G, Yaspo ML, von Deimling A, Lichter P, Taylor MD, Gilbertson R, Ellison DW, Aldape K, Korshunov A, Kool M, Pfister SM (2015) Molecular classification of ependymal tumors across all CNS compartments, histopathological grades, and age groups. Cancer Cell 27(5):728–743

108. Parker M, Mohankumar KM, Punchihewa C, Weinlich R, Dalton JD, Li Y, Lee R, Tatevossian RG, Phoenix TN, Thiruvenkatam R, White E, Tang B, Orisme W, Gupta K, Rusch M, Chen X, Li Y, Nagahawhatte P, Hedlund E, Finkelstein D, Wu G, Shurtleff S, Easton J, Boggs K, Yergeau D, Vadodaria B, Mulder HL, Becksfort J, Gupta P, Huether R, Ma J, Song G, Gajjar A, Merchant T, Boop F, Smith AA, Ding L, Lu C, Ochoa K, Zhao D, Fulton RS, Fulton LL, Mardis ER, Wilson RK, Downing JR, Green DR, Zhang J, Ellison DW, Gilbertson RJ (2014) C11orf95-RELA fusions drive oncogenic NF-κB signalling in ependymoma. Nature 506(7489):451–455

109. Pekmezci M, Stevers M, Phillips JJ, Van Ziffle J, Bastian BC, Tsankova NM, Kleinschmidt-DeMasters BK, Rosenblum MK, Tihan T, Perry A, Solomon DA (2018) Multinodular and vacuolating neuronal tumor of the cerebrum is a clonal neoplasm defined by genetic alterations that activate the MAP kinase signaling pathway. Acta Neuropathol 135(3):485–488

110. Perry A, Banerjee R, Lohse CM, Kleinschmidt-DeMasters BK, Scheithauer BW (2002) A role for chromosome 9p21 deletions in the malignant progression of meningiomas and the prognosis of anaplastic meningiomas. Brain Pathol 12(2):183–190

111. Pickles JC, Hawkins C, Pietsch T, Jacques TS (2018) CNS embryonal tumours: WHO 2016 and beyond. Neuropathol Appl Neurobiol 44(2):151–162

112. Pietsch T, Haberler C (2016) Update on the integrated histopathological and genetic classification of medulloblastoma - a practical diagnostic guideline. Clin Neuropathol 35(6):344–352

113. Preusser M, Dietrich W, Czech T, Prayer D, Budka H, Hainfellner JA (2003) Rosette-forming glioneuronal tumor of the fourth ventricle. Acta Neuropathol 106(5):506–508

114. Preusser M, Brastianos PK, Mawrin C (2018) Advances in meningioma genetics: novel therapeutic opportunities. Nat Rev Neurol 14(2):106–115

115. Pusch S, Krausert S, Fischer V, Balss J, Ott M, Schrimpf D, Capper D, Sahm F, Eisel J, Beck AC, Jugold M, Eichwald V, Kaulfuss S, Panknin O, Rehwinkel H, Zimmermann K, Hillig RC, Guenther J, Toschi L, Neuhaus R, Haegebart A, Hess-Stumpp H, Bauser M, Wick W, Unterberg A, Herold-Mende C, Platten M, von Deimling A (2017) Pan-mutant IDH1 inhibitor BAY 1436032 for effective treatment of IDH1 mutant astrocytoma in vivo. Acta Neuropathol 133(4):629–644

116. Radke J, Gehlhaar C, Lenze D, Capper D, Bock A, Heppner FL, Jödicke A, Koch A (2015) The evolution of the anaplastic cerebellar liponeurocytoma: case report and review of the literature. Clin Neuropathol 34(1):19–25

117. Raleigh DR, Solomon DA, Lloyd SA, Lazar A, Garcia MA, Sneed PK, Clarke JL, McDermott MW, Berger MS, Tihan T, Haas-Kogan DA (2017) Histopathologic review of pineal parenchymal tumors identifies novel morphologic subtypes

and prognostic factors for outcome. Neuro Oncol 19(1):78–88

118. Reifenberger G, Wirsching HG, Knobbe-Thomsen CB, Weller M (2017) Advances in the molecular genetics of gliomas - implications for classification and therapy. Nat Rev Clin Oncol 14(7):434–452

119. Reinhardt A, Stichel D, Schrimpf D, Sahm F, Korshunov A, Reuss DE, Koelsche C, Huang K, Wefers AK, Hovestadt V, Sill M, Gramatzki D, Felsberg J, Reifenberger G, Koch A, Thomale UW, Becker A, Hans VH, Prinz M, Staszewski O, Acker T, Dohmen H, Hartmann C, Mueller W, Tuffaha MSA, Paulus W, Heß K, Brokinkel B, Schittenhelm J, Monoranu CM, Kessler AF, Loehr M, Buslei R, Deckert M, Mawrin C, Kohlhof P, Hewer E, Olar A, Rodriguez FJ, Giannini C, NageswaraRao AA, Tabori U, Nunes NM, Weller M, Pohl U, Jaunmuktane Z, Brandner S, Unterberg A, Hänggi D, Platten M, Pfister SM, Wick W, Herold-Mende C, Jones DTW, von Deimling A, Capper D (2018) Anaplastic astrocytoma with piloid features, a novel molecular class of IDH wildtype glioma with recurrent MAPK pathway, CDKN2A/B and ATRX alterations. Acta Neuropathol. Acta Neuropathol. 136(2): 273–291

120. Reuss DE, Kratz A, Sahm F, Capper D, Schrimpf D, Koelsche C, Hovestadt V, Bewerunge-Hudler M, Jones DT, Schittenhelm J, Mittelbronn M, Rushing E, Simon M, Westphal M, Unterberg A, Platten M, Paulus W, Reifenberger G, Tonn JC, Aldape K, Pfister SM, Korshunov A, Weller M, Herold-Mende C, Wick W, Brandner S, von Deimling A (2015) Adult IDH wild type astrocytomas biologically and clinically resolve into other tumor entities. Acta Neuropathol 130(3):407–417

121. Reuss DE, Sahm F, Schrimpf D, Wiestler B, Capper D, Koelsche C, Schweizer L, Korshunov A, Jones DT, Hovestadt V, Mittelbronn M, Schittenhelm J, Herold-Mende C, Unterberg A, Platten M, Weller M, Wick W, Pfister SM, von Deimling A (2015) ATRX and IDH1-R132H immunohistochemistry with subsequent copy number analysis and IDH sequencing as a basis for an "integrated" diagnostic approach for adult astrocytoma, oligodendroglioma and glioblastoma. Acta Neuropathol 129(1):133–146

122. Riegert-Johnson DL, Gleeson FC, Roberts M, Tholen K, Youngborg L, Bullock M, Boardman LA (2010) Cancer and Lhermitte-Duclos disease are common in Cowden syndrome patients. Hered Cancer Clin Pract 8(1):6

123. Rickert CH, Paulus W (2004) Comparative genomic hybridization in central and peripheral nervous system tumors of childhood and adolescence. J Neuropathol Exp Neurol 63(5):399–417

124. Rickert CH, Simon R, Bergmann M, Dockhorn-Dworniczak B, Paulus W (2001) Comparative genomic hybridization in pineal parenchymal tumors. Genes Chromosomes Cancer 30(1):99–104

125. Rivera B, Gayden T, Carrot-Zhang J, Nadaf J, Boshari T, Faury D, Zeinieh M, Blanc R, Burk DL, Fahiminiya S, Bareke E, Schüller U, Monoranu CM, Sträter R, Kerl K, Niederstadt T, Kurlemann G, Ellezam B, Michalak Z, Thom M, Lockhart PJ, Leventer RJ, Ohm M, MacGregor D, Jones D, Karamchandani J, Greenwood CM, Berghuis AM, Bens S, Siebert R, Zakrzewska M, Liberski PP, Zakrzewski K, Sisodiya SM, Paulus W, Albrecht S, Hasselblatt M, Jabado N, Foulkes WD, Majewski J (2016) Germline and somatic FGFR1 abnormalities in dysembryoplastic neuroepithelial tumors. Acta Neuropathol 131(6):847–863

126. Rodriguez FJ, Perry A, Rosenblum MK, Krawitz S, Cohen KJ, Lin D, Mosier S, Lin MT, Eberhart CG, Burger PC (2012) Disseminated oligodendroglial-like leptomeningeal tumor of childhood: a distinctive clinicopathologic entity. Acta Neuropathol 124(5):627–641

127. Rodriguez FJ, Schniederjan MJ, Nicolaides T, Tihan T, Burger PC, Perry A (2015) High rate of concurrent BRAF-KIAA1549 gene fusion and 1p deletion in disseminated oligodendroglioma-like leptomeningeal neoplasms (DOLN). Acta Neuropathol 129(4):609–610

128. Röhrich M, Koelsche C, Schrimpf D, Capper D, Sahm F, Kratz A, Reuss J, Hovestadt V, Jones DT, Bewerunge-Hudler M, Becker A, Weis J, Mawrin C, Mittelbronn M, Perry A, Mautner VF, Mechtersheimer G, Hartmann C, Okuducu AF, Arp M, Seiz-Rosenhagen M, Hänggi D, Heim S, Paulus W, Schittenhelm J, Ahmadi R, Herold-Mende C, Unterberg A, Pfister SM, von Deimling A, Reuss DE (2016) Methylation-based classification of benign and malignant peripheral nerve sheath tumors. Acta Neuropathol 131(6):877–887

129. Rudà R, Reifenberger G, Frappaz D, Pfister SM, Laprie A, Santarius T, Roth P, Tonn JC, Soffietti R, Weller M, Moyal EC (2017) EANO guidelines for the diagnosis and treatment of ependymal tumors. Neuro Oncol. Neuro Oncol. 20(4):445–456

130. Sahm F, Reuss DE, Giannini C (2018) WHO 2016 classification: changes and advancements in the diagnosis of miscellaneous primary CNS tumours. Neuropathol Appl Neurobiol 44(2):163–171

131. Sahm F, Reuss D, Koelsche C, Capper D, Schittenhelm J, Heim S, Jones DT, Pfister SM, Herold-Mende C, Wick W, Mueller W, Hartmann C, Paulus W, von Deimling A (2014) Farewell to oligoastrocytoma: in situ molecular genetics favor classification as either oligodendroglioma or astrocytoma. Acta Neuropathol 128(4):551–559

132. Sahm F, Schrimpf D, Olar A, Koelsche C, Reuss D, Bissel J, Kratz A, Capper D, Schefzyk S, Hielscher T, Wang Q, Sulman EP, Adeberg S, Koch A, Okuducu AF, Brehmer S, Schittenhelm J, Becker A, Brokinkel B, Schmidt M, Ull T, Gousias K, Kessler AF, Lamszus K, Debus J, Mawrin C, Kim YJ, Simon M, Ketter R, Paulus W, Aldape KD, Herold-Mende C, von Deimling A (2015) TERT promoter mutations and risk of recurrence in meningioma. J Natl Cancer Inst 108(5). https://doi.org/10.1093/jnci/djv377

133. Sahm F, Schrimpf D, Stichel D, Jones DTW, Hielscher T, Schefzyk S, Okonechnikov K, Koelsche C, Reuss DE, Capper D, Sturm D, Wirsching HG, Berghoff AS, Baumgarten P, Kratz A, Huang K, Wefers AK, Hovestadt V, Sill M, Ellis HP, Kurian KM, Okuducu AF, Jungk C, Drueschler K, Schick M, Bewerunge-Hudler M, Mawrin C, Seiz-Rosenhagen M, Ketter R, Simon M, Westphal M, Lamszus K, Becker A, Koch A, Schittenhelm J, Rushing EJ, Collins VP, Brehmer S, Chavez L, Platten M, Hänggi D, Unterberg A, Paulus W, Wick W, Pfister SM, Mittelbronn M, Preusser M, Herold-Mende C, Weller M, von Deimling A (2017) DNA methylation-based classification and grading system for meningioma: a multicentre, retrospective analysis. Lancet Oncol 18(5):682–694

134. Schindler G, Capper D, Meyer J, Janzarik W, Omran H, Herold-Mende C, Schmieder K, Wesseling P, Mawrin C, Hasselblatt M, Louis DN, Korshunov A, Pfister S, Hartmann C, Paulus W, Reifenberger G, von Deimling A (2011) Analysis of BRAF V600E mutation in 1,320 nervous system tumors reveals high mutation frequencies in pleomorphic xanthoastrocytoma, ganglioglioma and extracerebellar pilocytic astrocytoma. Acta Neuropathol 121(3):397–405

135. Schulte SL, Waha A, Steiger B, Denkhaus D, Dörner E, Calaminus G, Leuschner I, Pietsch T (2016) CNS germinomas are characterized by global demethylation, chromosomal instability and mutational activation of the Kit-, Ras/Raf/Erk- and Akt-pathways. Oncotarget 7(34):55026–55042

136. Schumacher T, Bunse L, Pusch S, Sahm F, Wiestler B, Quandt J, Menn O, Osswald M, Oezen I, Ott M, Keil M, Balß J, Rauschenbach K, Grabowska AK, Vogler I, Diekmann J, Trautwein N, Eichmüller SB, Okun J, Stevanović S, Riemer AB, Sahin U, Friese MA, Beckhove P, von Deimling A, Wick W, Platten M (2014) A vaccine targeting mutant IDH1 induces antitumour immunity. Nature 512(7514):324–327

137. Schweizer L, Koelsche C, Sahm F, Piro RM, Capper D, Reuss DE, Pusch S, Habel A, Meyer J, Göck T, Jones DT, Mawrin C, Schittenhelm J, Becker A, Heim S, Simon M, Herold-Mende C, Mechtersheimer G, Paulus W, König R, Wiestler OD, Pfister SM, von Deimling A (2013) Meningeal hemangiopericytoma and solitary fibrous tumors carry the NAB2-STAT6 fusion and can be diagnosed by nuclear expression of STAT6 protein. Acta Neuropathol 125(5):651–658

138. Serra E, Rosenbaum T, Winner U, Aledo R, Ars E, Estivill X, Lenard HG, Lazaro C (2000) Schwann cells harbor the somatic NF1 mutation in neurofibromas: evidence of two different Schwann cell subpopulations. Hum Mol Genet 9(20):3055–3064

139. Shankar GM, Abedalthagafi M, Vaubel RA, Merrill PH, Nayyar N, Gill CM, Brewster R, Bi WL, Agarwalla PK, Thorner AR, Reardon DA, Al-Mefty O, Wen PY, Alexander BM, van Hummelen P, Batchelor TT, Ligon KL, Ligon AH, Meyerson M, Dunn IF, Beroukhim R, Louis DN, Perry A, Carter SL, Giannini C, Curry WT Jr, Cahill DP, Barker FG 2nd, Brastianos PK, Santagata S (2017) Germline and somatic BAP1 mutations in high-grade rhabdoid meningiomas. Neuro Oncol 19(4):535–545

140. Shankar GM, Taylor-Weiner A, Lelic N, Jones RT, Kim JC, Francis JM, Abedalthagafi M, Borges LF, Coumans JV, Curry WT, Nahed BV, Shin JH, Paek SH, Park SH, Stewart C, Lawrence MS, Cibulskis K, Thorner AR, Van Hummelen P, Stemmer-Rachamimov AO, Batchelor TT, Carter SL, Hoang MP, Santagata S, Louis DN, Barker FG, Meyerson M, Getz G, Brastianos PK, Cahill DP (2014) Sporadic hemangioblastomas are characterized by cryptic VHL inactivation. Acta Neuropathol Commun 2:167

141. Shih AH, Holland EC (2004) Developmental neurobiology and the origin of brain tumors. J Neurooncol 70(2):125–135

142. Soffietti R, Abacioglu U, Baumert B, Combs SE, Kinhult S, Kros JM, Marosi C, Metellus P, Radbruch A, Villa Freixa SS, Brada M, Carapella CM, Preusser M, Le Rhun E, Rudà R, Tonn JC, Weber DC, Weller M (2017) Diagnosis and treatment of brain metastases from solid tumors: guidelines from the European Association of Neuro-Oncology (EANO). Neuro Oncol 19(2):162–174

143. Soylemezoglu F, Scheithauer BW, Esteve J, Kleihues P (1997) Atypical central neurocytoma. J Neuropathol Exp Neurol 56(5):551–556

144. Stone TJ, Keeley A, Virasami A, Harkness W, Tisdall M, Izquierdo Delgado E, Gutteridge A, Brooks T, Kristiansen M, Chalker J, Wilkhu L, Mifsud W, Apps J, Thom M, Hubank M, Forshew T, Cross JH, Hargrave D, Ham J, Jacques TS (2018) Comprehensive molecular characterisation of epilepsy-associated glioneuronal tumours. Acta Neuropathol 135(1):115–129

145. Sturm D, Witt H, Hovestadt V, Khuong-Quang DA, Jones DT, Konermann C, Pfaff E, Tönjes M, Sill M, Bender S, Kool M, Zapatka M, Becker N, Zucknick M, Hielscher T, Liu XY, Fontebasso AM, Ryzhova M, Albrecht S, Jacob K, Wolter M, Ebinger M, Schuhmann MU, van Meter T, Frühwald MC, Hauch H, Pekrun A, Radlwimmer B, Niehues T, von Komorowski G, Dürken M, Kulozik AE, Madden J, Donson A, Foreman NK, Drissi R, Fouladi M, Scheurlen W, von Deimling A, Monoranu C, Roggendorf W, Herold-Mende C, Unterberg A, Kramm CM, Felsberg J, Hartmann C, Wiestler B, Wick W, Milde T, Witt O, Lindroth AM, Schwartzentruber J, Faury D, Fleming A, Zakrzewska M, Liberski PP, Zakrzewski K, Hauser P, Garami M, Klekner A, Bognar L, Morrissy S, Cavalli F, Taylor MD, van Sluis P, Koster J, Versteeg R, Volckmann R, Mikkelsen T, Aldape K, Reifenberger G, Collins VP, Majewski J, Korshunov A, Lichter P, Plass C, Jabado N, Pfister SM (2012) Hotspot mutations in H3F3A and IDH1 define distinct epigenetic and biological subgroups of glioblastoma. Cancer Cell 22(4):425–437

146. Sturm D, Orr BA, Toprak UH, Hovestadt V, Jones DTW, Capper D, Sill M, Buchhalter I, Northcott PA, Leis I, Ryzhova M, Koelsche C, Pfaff E, Allen SJ, Balasubramanian G, Worst BC, Pajtler KW, Brabetz S, Johann PD, Sahm F, Reimand J, Mackay A, Carvalho DM, Remke M, Phillips JJ, Perry A, Cowdrey C, Drissi R, Fouladi M, Giangaspero F, Łastowska M, Grajkowska W, Scheurlen W, Pietsch T, Hagel C, Gojo J, Lötsch D, Berger W, Slavc I, Haberler C, Jouvet A, Holm S, Hofer S, Prinz M, Keohane C, Fried I, Mawrin C, Scheie D, Mobley BC, Schniederjan MJ, Santi M, Buccoliero AM, Dahiya S, Kramm CM, von Bueren AO, von Hoff K, Rutkowski S, Herold-Mende C, Frühwald MC, Milde T, Hasselblatt M, Wesseling P, Rößler J, Schüller U, Ebinger M, Schittenhelm J, Frank S, Grobholz R, Vajtai I, Hans V, Schneppenheim R, Zitterbart K, Collins VP, Aronica E, Varlet P, Puget S, Dufour C, Grill J, Figarella-Branger D, Wolter M, Schuhmann MU, Shalaby T, Grotzer M, van Meter T, Monoranu CM, Felsberg J, Reifenberger G, Snuderl M, Forrester LA, Koster J, Versteeg R, Volckmann R, van Sluis P, Wolf S, Mikkelsen T, Gajjar A, Aldape K, Moore AS, Taylor MD, Jones C, Jabado N, Karajannis MA, Eils R, Schlesner M, Lichter P, von Deimling A, Pfister SM, Ellison DW, Korshunov A, Kool M (2016) New brain tumor entities emerge from molecular classification of CNS-PNETs. Cell 164(5):1060–1072

147. Suzuki H, Aoki K, Chiba K, Sato Y, Shiozawa Y, Shiraishi Y, Shimamura T, Niida A, Motomura K, Ohka F, Yamamoto T, Tanahashi K, Ranjit M, Wakabayashi T, Yoshizato T, Kataoka K, Yoshida K, Nagata Y, Sato-Otsubo A, Tanaka H, Sanada M, Kondo Y, Nakamura H, Mizoguchi M, Abe T, Muragaki Y, Watanabe R, Ito I, Miyano S, Natsume A, Ogawa S (2015) Mutational landscape and clonal architecture in grade II and III gliomas. Nat Genet 47(5):458–468

148. Tabouret E, Nguyen AT, Dehais C, Carpentier C, Ducray F, Idbaih A, Mokhtari K, Jouvet A, Uro-Coste E, Colin C, Chinot O, Loiseau H, Moyal E, Maurage CA, Polivka M, Lechapt-Zalcman E, Desenclos C, Meyronet D, Delattre JY, Figarella-Branger D, Network FPOLA (2016) Prognostic impact of the 2016 WHO classification of diffuse gliomas in the French POLA cohort. Acta Neuropathol 132(4):625–634

149. Tanboon J, Williams EA, Louis DN (2016) The diagnostic use of immunohistochemical surrogates for signature molecular genetic alterations in gliomas. J Neuropathol Exp Neurol 75(1):4–18

150. Thom M, Liu J, Bongaarts A, Reinten RJ, Paradiso B, Jäger HR, Reeves C, Somani A, An S, Marsdon D, McEvoy A, Miserocchi A, Thorne L, Newman F, Bucur S, Honavar M, Jacques T, Aronica E (2018) Multinodular and vacuolating neuronal tumors in epilepsy: dysplasia or neoplasia? Brain Pathol 28(2):155–171

151. Thomas C, Sill M, Ruland V, Witten A, Hartung S, Kordes U, Jeibmann A, Beschorner R, Keyvani K, Bergmann M, Mittelbronn M, Pietsch T, Felsberg J, Monoranu CM, Varlet P, Hauser P, Olar A, Grundy RG, Wolff JE, Korshunov A, Jones DT, Bewerunge-Hudler M, Hovestadt V, von Deimling A, Pfister SM, Paulus W, Capper D, Hasselblatt M (2016) Methylation profiling of choroid plexus tumors reveals 3 clinically distinct subgroups. Neuro Oncol 18(6):790–796

152. Tihan T, Fisher PG, Kepner JL, Godfraind C, McComb RD, Goldthwaite PT, Burger PC (1999) Pediatric astrocytomas with monomorphous pilomyxoid features and a less favorable outcome. J Neuropathol Exp Neurol 58(10):1061–1068

153. Trivellin G, Daly AF, Faucz FR, Yuan B, Rostomyan L, Larco DO et al (2014) Gigantism and acromegaly due to Xq26 microduplications and GPR101 mutation. N Engl J Med 371:2363–2374

154. Turcan S, Rohle D, Goenka A, Walsh LA, Fang F, Yilmaz E, Campos C, Fabius AW, Lu C, Ward PS, Thompson CB, Kaufman A, Guryanova O, Levine R, Heguy A, Viale A, Morris LG, Huse JT, Mellinghoff IK, Chan TA (2012) IDH1 mutation is sufficient to establish the glioma hypermethylator phenotype. Nature 483(7390):479–483

155. van de Nes JAP, Koelsche C, Gessi M, Möller I, Sucker A, Scolyer RA, Buckland ME, Pietsch T, Murali R, Schadendorf D, Griewank KG (2017) Activating CYSLTR2 and PLCB4 mutations in primary leptomeningeal melanocytic tumors. J Invest Dermatol 137(9):2033–2035

156. van den Bent MJ (2010) Interobserver variation of the histopathological diagnosis in clinical trials on glioma: a clinician's perspective. Acta Neuropathol 120(3):297–304

157. Vater I, Montesinos-Rongen M, Schlesner M, Haake A, Purschke F, Sprute R, Mettenmeyer N, Nazzal I, Nagel I, Gutwein J, Richter J, Buchhalter I, Russell RB, Wiestler OD, Eils R, Deckert M, Siebert R (2015) The mutational pattern of primary lymphoma of the central nervous system determined by whole-exome sequencing. Leukemia 29(3): 677–685

158. Vaubel RA, Caron AA, Yamada S, Decker PA, Eckel Passow JE, Rodriguez FJ, Nageswara Rao AA, Lachance D, Parney I, Jenkins R, Giannini C (2018) Recurrent copy number alterations in low-grade and anaplastic pleomorphic xanthoastrocytoma with and without BRAF V600E mutation. Brain Pathol 28(2):172–182

159. Vierimaa O, Georgitsi M, Lehtonen R, Vahteristo P, Kokko A, Raitila A, Tuppurainen K, Ebeling TM, Salmela PI, Paschke R, Gündogdu S, De Menis E, Mäkinen MJ, Launonen V, Karhu A, Aaltonen LA (2006) Pituitary adenoma predisposition caused by germline mutations in the AIP gene. Science 312(5777):1228–1230

160. Virchow R (1864) Die krankhaften Geschwülste. Achtzehnte Vorlesung: Psammome, Melanome, Gliome, vol 65. Verlag von August Hirschwald, Berlin, pp 106–169

161. von Deimling A, Ono T, Shirahata M, Louis DN (2018) Grading of diffuse astrocytic gliomas: a review of studies before and after the advent of IDH testing. Semin Neurol 38(1):19–23

162. Weller M, van den Bent M, Tonn JC, Stupp R, Preusser M, Cohen-Jonathan-Moyal E, Henriksson R, Le Rhun E, Balana C, Chinot O, Bendszus M, Reijneveld JC, Dhermain F, French P, Marosi C, Watts C, Oberg I, Pilkington G, Baumert BG, Taphoorn MJB, Hegi M, Westphal M, Reifenberger G, Soffietti R, Wick W, European Association for Neuro-Oncology (EANO) Task Force on Gliomas (2017) European Association for Neuro-Oncology (EANO) guideline on the diagnosis and treatment of adult astrocytic and oligodendroglial gliomas. Lancet Oncol 18(6):e315–e329

163. Weller M, Weber RG, Willscher E, Riehmer V, Hentschel B, Kreuz M, Felsberg J, Beyer U, Löffler-Wirth H, Kaulich K, Steinbach JP, Hartmann C, Gramatzki D, Schramm J, Westphal M, Schackert G, Simon M, Martens T, Boström J, Hagel C, Sabel M, Krex D, Tonn JC, Wick W, Noell S, Schlegel U, Radlwimmer B, Pietsch T, Loeffler M, von Deimling A, Binder H, Reifenberger G (2015) Molecular classification of diffuse cerebral WHO grade II/III gliomas using genome- and transcriptome-wide profiling improves stratification of prognostically distinct patient groups. Acta Neuropathol 129(5):679–693

164. Wesseling P, van den Bent M, Perry A (2015) Oligodendroglioma: pathology, molecular mechanisms and markers. Acta Neuropathol 129(6):809–827

165. Wick W, Weller M, van den Bent M, Sanson M, Weiler M, von Deimling A, Plass C, Hegi M, Platten M, Reifenberger G (2014) MGMT testing--the challenges for biomarker-based glioma treatment. Nat Rev Neurol 10(7):372–385

166. Wizigmann-Voos S, Breier G, Risau W, Plate KH (1995) Up-regulation of vascular endothelial growth factor and its receptors in von Hippel-Lindau disease-associated and sporadic hemangioblastomas. Cancer Res 55(6):1358–1364

167. Xerri L, Adélaïde J, Popovici C, Garnier S, Guille A, Mescam-Mancini L, Laurent C, Brousset P, Coze C, Michel G, Chaffanet M, Bouabdallah R, Coso D, Bertucci F, Birnbaum D (2018) CDKN2A/B deletion and double-hit mutations of the MAPK pathway underlie the aggressive behavior of Langerhans cell tumors. Am J Surg Pathol 42(2):150–159

168. Zapka P, Dörner E, Dreschmann V, Sakamato N, Kristiansen G, Calaminus G, Vokuhl C, Leuschner I, Pietsch T (2018) Type, frequency, and spatial distribution of immune cell infiltrates in CNS germinomas: evidence for inflammatory and immunosuppressive mechanisms. J Neuropathol Exp Neurol 77(2):119–127

169. Zhou XP, Marsh DJ, Morrison CD, Chaudhury AR, Maxwell M, Reifenberger G, Eng C (2003) Germline inactivation of PTEN and dysregulation of the phosphoinositol-3-kinase/Akt pathway cause human Lhermitte-Duclos disease in adults. Am J Hum Genet 73(5):1191–1198

170. Zhukova N, Ramaswamy V, Remke M, Pfaff E, Shih DJ, Martin DC, Castelo-Branco P, Baskin B, Ray PN, Bouffet E, von Bueren AO, Jones DT, Northcott PA, Kool M, Sturm D, Pugh TJ, Pomeroy SL, Cho YJ, Pietsch T, Gessi M, Rutkowski S, Bognar L, Klekner A, Cho BK, Kim SK, Wang KC, Eberhart CG, Fevre-Montange M, Fouladi M, French PJ, Kros M, Grajkowska WA, Gupta N, Weiss WA, Hauser P, Jabado N, Jouvet A, Jung S, Kumabe T, Lach B, Leonard JR, Rubin JB, Liau LM, Massimi L, Pollack IF, Shin Ra Y, Van Meir EG, Zitterbart K, Schüller U, Hill RM, Lindsey JC, Schwalbe EC, Bailey S, Ellison DW, Hawkins C, Malkin D, Clifford SC, Korshunov A, Pfister S, Taylor MD, Tabori U (2013) Subgroup-specific prognostic implications of TP53 mutation in medulloblastoma. J Clin Oncol 31(23):2927–2935

171. Zülch KJ (1979) Histological typing of tumors of the central nervous system. In: International histological classification of tumors, vol 21. World Health Organization, Geneva

Etiological and Epidemiological Aspects

2

Daniel I. Jacobs, E. Susan Amirian,
Elizabeth B. Claus, Robert B. Jenkins,
Melissa L. Bondy, and Margaret R. Wrensch

2.1 Introduction

Globally, brain and other central nervous system tumors account for approximately 1.8% of incident cancer cases and 2.3% of cancer deaths [1]. Nearly 80,000 new cases of brain and other central nervous system tumors are estimated to be newly diagnosed in the United States in 2017 [2]. Meningiomas are the most common primary brain tumor, while gliomas are the most common primary malignant brain tumor. Incidence and survival patterns of these tumors vary characteristically by demographic factors and tumor subtype. Gliomas cause significant morbidity and mortality due to their aggressive behavior and limited treatment options. While much remains to be discovered, major advances in molecular classification for gliomas and in discovering risk factors for brain tumors have been made in recent years through large-scale epidemiology, genetics, and neuropathology collaborations. This chapter provides an overview of the epidemiology and current understanding of the genetic and environmental risk factors for primary brain tumors, with a focus on glioma and meningioma in adults. We also highlight important unresolved questions in this field.

2.2 Molecular Classification and Integrated Subtypes of Diffuse Glioma

Traditional classification of diffuse glioma relied primarily on histopathological assessment, entailing evaluation of tumor cells for their resemblance to supposed cells-of-origin (i.e., astrocytes and/or oligodendrocytes) and designation of grade according to criteria including tumor infiltration, nuclear atypia, mitotic activity, necrosis, and vascularity [3]. Such criteria led to regional differences in classifications of glioma entities, especially for lower-grade and the so-called mixed tumors [4], and often unaccounted for variability in survival within certain categories. In an effort to address these deficiencies, the WHO updated the criteria for diffuse glioma classification in 2016 that integrated histopathological review with important tumor molecular alterations [5].

D. I. Jacobs · E. S. Amirian · M. L. Bondy
Department of Medicine, Dan L. Duncan
Comprehensive Cancer Center, Baylor College of
Medicine, Houston, TX, USA

E. B. Claus
Department of Biostatistics, Yale School of Public
Health, New Haven, CT, USA

Department of Neurosurgery, Brigham and Women's
Hospital, Boston, MA, USA

R. B. Jenkins
Department of Laboratory Medicine and Pathology,
Mayo Clinic Comprehensive Cancer Center, Mayo
Clinic, Rochester, MN, USA

M. R. Wrensch (✉)
Department of Neurological Surgery, University of
California, San Francisco, San Francisco, CA, USA
e-mail: Margaret.Wrensch@ucsf.edu

© Springer Nature Switzerland AG 2019
J.-C. Tonn et al. (eds.), *Oncology of CNS Tumors*, https://doi.org/10.1007/978-3-030-04152-6_2

Several recent studies provided the evidence and impetus for this new classification. These landmark studies have proposed glioma classification schemes in an effort to define more molecularly and clinically homogenous subgroups of glioma, as summarized in Fig. 2.1. An analysis from the TCGA network used unsupervised clustering of genomic, transcriptomic, epigenomic, and proteomic data from 293 lower-grade gliomas to define three disease subgroups according to *IDH* mutation and 1p/19q status [6]: (1) patients with *IDH* mutation and 1p/19q codeletion, (2) patients with *IDH* mutation and no 1p/19q codeletion, and (3) patients without *IDH* mutation. Group 1 was also characterized by *TERT* promoter mutation and oligodendroglial histology, *ATRX* and *TP53* mutations were commonly seen in Group 2, and Group 3 tumors were molecularly and clinically comparable

to primary glioblastoma. In a separate report, Eckel-Passow et al. classified 1087 gliomas into 5 subgroups according to *IDH* mutation, 1p/19q codeletion, and *TERT* promoter mutation status [7]. The scheme is similar to that proposed by the TCGA study but refines TCGA Groups 2 and 3 as described above by incorporating *TERT* promoter mutation status. This comprehensive classification also incorporates high-grade glioma and generates subgroups with characteristic somatic mutations and copy number changes, TCGA expression subtypes [8], and germline risk alleles.

Most recently, through multi-platform profiling of 1122 diffuse gliomas (grades II–IV), Ceccarelli et al. described seven glioma subtypes that were predominantly defined by their methylation and gene expression signatures [9]. Cases fell into seven groups including:

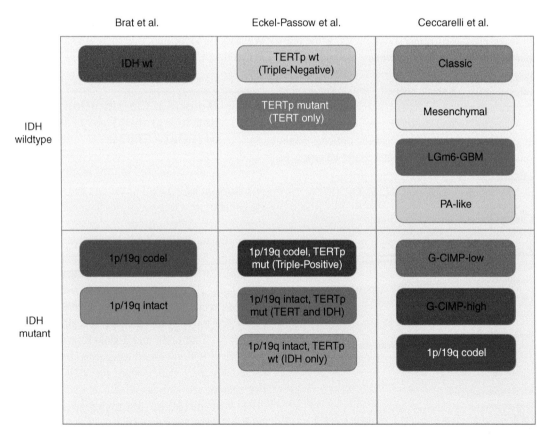

Fig. 2.1 Comparison of integrated molecular subtypes of glioma from recent publications by Brat et al. [6], Eckel-Passow et al. [7], and Ceccarelli et al. [9]

1. IDH-mutant gliomas with 1p/19q codeletion (18% of population)
2. IDH-mutant gliomas without 1p/19q codeletion and a hypermethylator phenotype (G-CIMP) [10] (25%)
3. IDH-mutant non-codeleted gliomas with low methylation levels and poor survival relative to the hypermethylated group (3% of total population)
4. IDH-wild-type glioblastomas with a classical gene expression profile (18%)
5. IDH-wild-type glioblastomas with a mesenchymal gene expression profile (27%)
6. IDH-wild-type glioblastomas characterized by a distinct methylation pattern and stable telomeres (5% of population)
7. Tumors resembling pilocytic astrocytoma with young age-at-onset and favorable survival (3% of population)

In the updated WHO model (as illustrated in Fig. 2.2), all tumors are evaluated for IDH mutations (typically in *IDH1*), which occur in more than 80% of low-grade gliomas [11, 12]. IDH-mutant tumors are further tested for codeletion of chromosome arms 1p and 19q, a feature that is diagnostic for oligodendroglioma [13]. Tumor grade is judged according to histopathological criteria, and while tumors are still evaluated for their histologic appearance (i.e., astrocytic and/or oligodendroglial cell populations), in the event of a discrepancy between histology and molecular features, genotype supersedes phenotype in the diagnostic schema. For example, a tumor that is astrocytic in appearance with IDH mutation and 1p/19q codeletion would nonetheless be classified as *oligodendroglioma, IDH-mutant*, and *1p/19q-codeleted*. The designation "not otherwise specified" (NOS) is used in conjunction with histologic appearance in the absence of definitive molecular profiling. The resulting WHO classification categories are presented in Table 2.1.

2.3 Descriptive Epidemiology

2.3.1 Glioma

2.3.1.1 Incidence
The incidence of glioma varies considerably by tumor histology, age, and sex. In the United States, the average annual age-adjusted incidence

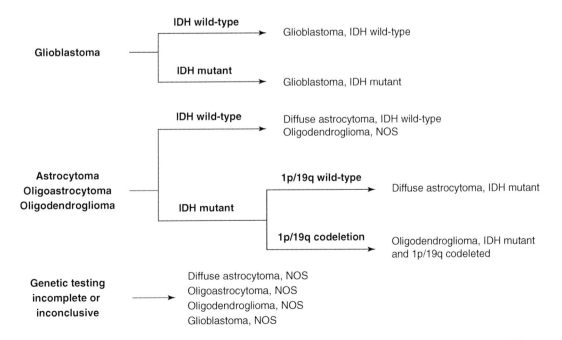

Fig. 2.2 Diffuse glioma classification algorithm according to new WHO guidelines (adapted from Louis et al. [5])

Table 2.1 Updated classification and grading of diffuse gliomas (from Louis et al. [5])

Glioma classification	ICD-O morphology code	WHO grade
Diffuse astrocytoma, IDH-mutant	9400/3	II
Diffuse astrocytoma, IDH-wild-type		
Diffuse astrocytoma, NOS		
Anaplastic astrocytoma, IDH-mutant	9401/3	III
Anaplastic astrocytoma, IDH-wild-type		
Anaplastic astrocytoma, NOS		
Oligodendroglioma, IDH-mutant and 1p/19q-codeleted	9450/3	II
Oligodendroglioma, NOS		
Anaplastic oligodendroglioma, IDH-mutant and 1p/19q-codeleted	9451/3	III
Anaplastic oligodendroglioma, NOS		
Glioblastoma, IDH-mutant	9445/3	IV
Glioblastoma, IDH-wild-type	9440/3	
Glioblastoma, NOS		

Fig. 2.3 Distribution of gliomas by histology in the United States. Data are from Ostrom et al. [2]

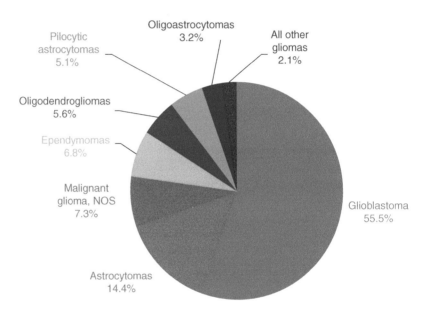

rate of glioma is 6.26 cases per 100,000 population [2]. The most common glioma histology is glioblastoma, accounting for 55.5% of gliomas and occurring at an average annual age-adjusted incidence rate of 3.20 cases per 100,000 population, followed by lower-grade astrocytomas (as defined by traditional histological classification), accounting for 14.4% of gliomas (Fig. 2.3). While the overall incidence of glioma in adults increases sharply with age (from ~2.8 cases among those aged 20–34 years to a peak of ~19.3 cases per 100,000 population among those aged 75–84 years), this is driven primarily by increasing incidence of glioblastoma with age (Fig. 2.4).

Gliomas occur approximately 1.4 times as frequently in males as compared to females (7.37 vs. 5.30 cases per 100,000 population annually), and glioblastoma specifically occurs approximately 1.6 times as frequently [2].

Differences in glioma incidence are also observed across ethnic groups and around the globe. Higher incidence rates of all glioma histologies (traditional classifications) are observed in White populations as compared to other racial/ethnic groups in the United States; glioblastoma occurs approximately 1.9 times and 2.1 times as frequently in White as compared to Black and Asian populations, respectively (Fig. 2.5).

Fig. 2.4 Average annual incidence rate of (**a**) all glioma and (**b**) non-glioblastoma glioma in the United States by tumor histology and age group. Data are from Ostrom et al. [2]

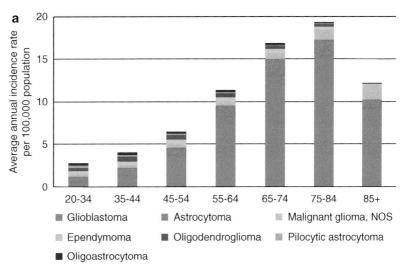

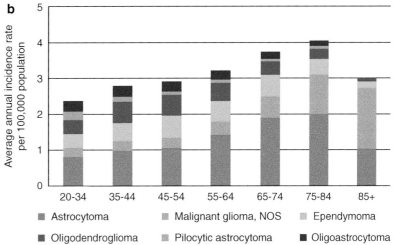

Fig. 2.5 Average annual incidence rate of gliomas in the United States by tumor histology. Data are from Ostrom et al. [2]

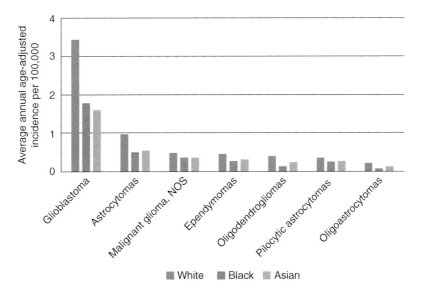

Table 2.2 Average age-adjusted annual incidence of glioma per 100,000 population in select countries by sex

Country	Average age-adjusted rate	
	Male	Female
Israel	5.5	3.7
France	5.5	3.2
Sweden	5.3	4.0
Denmark	5.1	3.4
Australia	5.1	3.4
United States	5.0	3.5
Italy	5.0	3.3
Spain	5.0	3.3
Germany	4.9	3.8
Canada	4.8	3.3
England	4.3	2.7
Czech Republic	4.2	3.2
India	2.9	1.9
Brazil	2.8	1.8
Argentina	2.8	2.1
Egypt	2.3	1.7
Tunisia	2.1	1.3
Costa Rica	2.1	1.5
China	2.0	1.5
South Korea	1.6	1.3
Japan	1.2	1.0

Data are from the Cancer Incidence in Five Continents, Volume X [1]

Patterns of glioma incidence around the world follow a similar pattern as seen in the United States. Although differences in case ascertainment and reporting limit the comparability of worldwide incidence data, rates tend to be highest in the United States, Israel, and European countries and the lowest in Asian countries (Table 2.2).

Due to the recent update of WHO classification guidelines, population-based incidence data are not yet available according to molecularly defined subtypes of glioma. However, an estimate of the annual distribution of gliomas in the United States according to histology and molecular subtype, as defined by Eckel-Passow et al. [14], has been reported and is illustrated in Fig. 2.6. According to these estimates, approximately 55% of gliomas are expected to be molecularly classified in the TERT-only subgroup (comprised predominantly of glioblastoma histology), 20% as IDH-only (predominantly astrocytoma grade II/III), 14% as triple-negative (predominantly glioblastoma), 6% as triple-positive (predominantly oligodendroglioma), and 4% as TERT and

IDH-mutated (roughly equal distribution of glioblastoma and astrocytoma grade II/III).

2.3.1.2 Survival

While all diffuse gliomas are incurable in current practice, survival following glioma diagnosis varies distinctly by tumor grade, histology, sex, and ethnicity. Ten-year relative survival for glioblastoma in the United States is estimated at 2.9%, while 10-year survival for lower-grade diffuse gliomas ranges from 20.9% for grade III astrocytomas up to 65.0% for grade II oligodendrogliomas (Fig. 2.7) [2]. For all glioma subtypes combined, females have improved survival as compared to males (28.2% vs. 24.4% 10-year relative survival, respectively); this discrepancy is greater among glioblastoma patients specifically (Table 2.3) [15]. With respect to race/ethnicity, relative survival is lowest among non-Hispanic White patients with glioma and/or glioblastoma.

Furthermore, glioma prognosis is closely linked with the molecular nature of the tumor. Key prognostic features include *IDH1* and *IDH2* mutations, which are associated with improved overall survival, and may also predict improved response to treatment with temozolomide [16, 17] and codeletion of chromosomes 1p and 19q, which is also predictive of significantly improved survival [18, 19]. Recently defined glioma subgroupings reflect the association of these molecular features with survival: in the three-group classification scheme described above, the co-occurrence of IDH mutation and 1p/19q codeletion portends the best survival, tumors without an IDH mutation confer the worst survival, and those with an IDH mutation but not codeletion confer intermediate survival [6]. Other classification schemes offer finer stratification of molecular markers and clinical course, such as that described by Eckel-Passow et al. In this scheme, the presence or absence of TERT promoter mutation further refines the IDH-wildtype and IDH-mutant/1p/19q-intact groups [7]. Additional work from this group has demonstrated the prognostic value of alterations in *ATRX* specifically among IDH-wildtype glioblastomas, where such alterations were

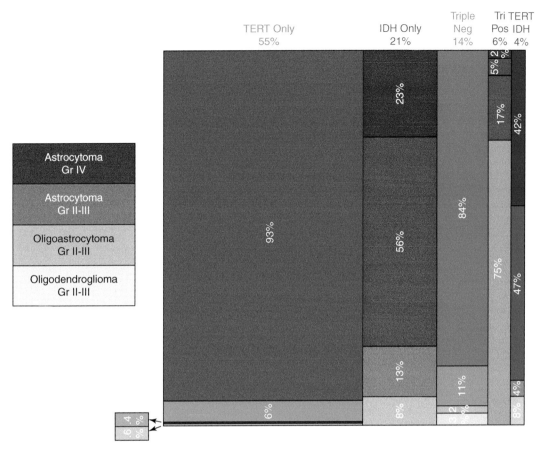

Fig. 2.6 Estimated population proportions of glioma by histology and molecular subtype. Percentages on top denote the estimated proportions of each molecular subtype, and percentages within boxes denote estimated proportions of each histological subtype within a given molecular subtype. Shading corresponds to glioma histology as illustrated in the legend. Proportions were estimated utilizing data from Eckel-Passow et al. [7] and CBTRUS [119] and calculated according to the method described by Rice et al. [14]

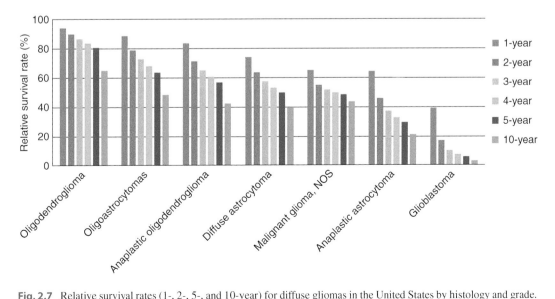

Fig. 2.7 Relative survival rates (1-, 2-, 5-, and 10-year) for diffuse gliomas in the United States by histology and grade. Data are from Ostrom et al. [2]

Table 2.3 Relative survival after diagnosis with a malignant brain tumor in the United States by ethnicity, sex, and histological type

	Glioma relative survival (95% CI)			Glioblastoma relative survival (95% CI)		
	1-Year	5-Year	10-Year	1-Year	5-Year	10-Year
Male	57.0 (56.5–57.5)	29.9 (29.4–30.5)	24.4 (23.9–25.0)	37.9 (37.2–38.6)	4.8 (4.5–5.2)	2.2 (1.9–2.6)
White, non-Hispanic	55.1 (54.5–55.8)	27.7 (27.1–28.3)	22.5 (21.8–23.1)	37.4 (36.6–38.2)	4.4 (4.0–4.8)	1.9 (1.6–2.3)
White, Hispanic	63.5 (61.9–65.0)	39.7 (38.0–41.4)	33.3 (31.4–35.3)	39.2 (36.8–41.6)	7.5 (6.0–9.1)	4.4 (2.9–6.3)
Black	61.3 (59.2–63.4)	33.1 (30.9–35.3)	28.2 (25.8–30.6)	40.1 (37.0–43.2)	5.3 (3.7–7.2)	3.8 (2.4–5.7)
Asian Pacific Islander	62.3 (59.9–64.7)	34.3 (31.8–36.8)	27.1 (24.5–29.9)	42.0 (38.5–45.5)	6.5 (4.6–8.9)	1.7 (0.5–4.2)
Female	56.2 (55.6–56.8)	33.3 (32.6–33.8)	28.2 (27.6–28.9)	34.3 (33.4–35.1)	4.8 (4.4–5.3)	2.9 (2.5–3.3)
White, non-Hispanic	53.4 (52.7–54.1)	30.3 (29.6–31.0)	25.7 (25.0–26.5)	33.0 (32.1–33.9)	4.1 (3.7–4.6)	2.5 (2.1–3)
White, Hispanic	64.8 (63.1–66.5)	43.1 (41.2–45.0)	36.6 (34.6–38.7)	39.1 (36.3–41.9)	7.3 (5.7–9.1)	4.2 (2.8–6.2)
Black	60.0 (57.7–62.2)	37.8 (35.4–40.2)	32.4 (29.8–35.0)	35.0 (31.6–38.3)	6.4 (4.6–8.6)	3.5 (2.0–5.7)
Asian Pacific Islander	67.0 (64.4–69.4)	41.2 (38.3–44.0)	35.3 (32.3–38.4)	44.5 (40.3–48.6)	10.1 (7.4–13.4)	6.5 (4.0–10.0)

Data are from the Surveillance, Epidemiology, and End Results Program, 1995–2012 [15]

associated with more favorable outcomes [20]. Pekmezci et al. [21] applied the new WHO 2016 criteria to a large number of historical glioma cases. Although the cases were not population-based, this study provided a good indication of the survival differences among the five major groups of glioma using the WHO 2016 criteria for the first time. The seven-group scheme proposed by Ceccarelli et al. is largely consistent with other reports but adds additional resolution to the survival differences by molecular profile, such as noting the uncharacteristically poor survival of patients with IDH-mutant, noncodeleted tumors without a hypermethylator phenotype [9].

Additional characteristics related to glioma survival include promoter methylation of DNA repair gene *MGMT*, which is an important marker of temozolomide response and overall survival in glioblastoma [21], and presence of the glioma risk allele at rs55705857 on chromosome 8q24.21, which has been associated with improved progression-free survival for patients treated with procarbazine, lomustine, and vincristine [22]. Finally, other well-established

prognostic factors for glioblastoma include extent of resection, age at diagnosis, and performance status [2, 23, 24].

2.3.2 Meningioma

2.3.2.1 Incidence

Meningioma is the most common primary brain tumor, occurring in the United States at a rate of 8.03 cases per 100,000 and accounting for 37% of brain and central nervous system (CNS) tumors overall [2]. Meningioma incidence increases sharply with age (Fig. 2.8); the median age at diagnosis is 66 years, and the incidence rate is doubled among adults 40 years or older relative to the overall population (16.3 cases per 100,000 population). These tumors occur more than twice as often in females as in males, and in contrast to the incidence patterns by ethnicity observed for glioma, meningioma occurs more frequently among Black than White individuals. While there have been some data suggesting that the incidence of nonmalignant and malignant

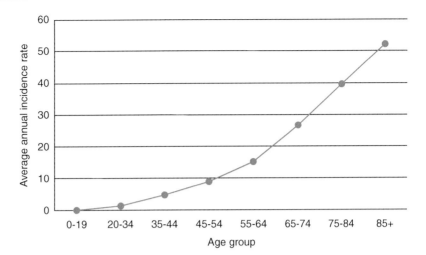

Fig. 2.8 Average annual meningioma incidence rate in the United States by age group per 100,000. Data are from Ostrom et al. [2]

meningioma has increased and decreased, respectively, in the past decade, these fluctuations are likely attributable to changes in reporting and tumor definitions [2, 25].

2.3.2.2 Survival

Nearly 99% of meningiomas are benign; however, they are nonetheless a cause of significant morbidity and mortality. Five-year relative survival after nonmalignant meningioma diagnosis is 86.4%, as compared to 5-year survival of 64.9% for malignant meningioma [2]. Survival has been shown to be higher for younger patients, female patients, those with unilateral tumors, and those treated with resection [26]. Recurrence occurs in 18% and 26% of patients at 5 and 10 years after initial treatment, respectively, and long-term neurological deficits are common [27].

2.4 Genetic Risk Factors

2.4.1 Familial Predisposition Syndromes and High-Risk Mutations

It is estimated that 5–10% of gliomas occur in families with two or more affected relatives, and studies have indicated that individuals with a family history of the disease carry approximately twice the risk of glioma development as compared to the general population [28–32]. As few exposures are known that may contribute to increased risk of tumor development due to shared environmental factors, inherited genetic risk factors are likely to be the primary basis for familial aggregation of tumors.

A small fraction of gliomas are caused by single-gene hereditary cancer syndromes including Li-Fraumeni syndrome, neurofibromatosis type I/II, Lynch syndrome, melanoma-neural system tumor syndrome, and Ollier disease [33–35] (Table 2.4). Several syndromes also increase risk of meningioma development, most notably neurofibromatosis type 2 as mutations in the *NF2* tumor suppressor are the most frequent genetic alteration in meningiomas. Meningiomas have also been reported in families with germline defects in *NF1*, *VHL*, *PTEN*, *PTCH*, and *CREBBP* [36, 37].

Linkage analyses have been conducted in order to identify putative glioma risk loci in non-syndromic families, with an early study detecting a potential familial glioma locus at 15q23-q26 [38]. A larger linkage analysis conducted by the Gliogene Consortium found a significant linkage peak for gliomas of all grades on chromosome 17q [39, 40], and subsequent sequencing of the 17q region identified candidate variants implicating four genes (*MYO19*, *KIF18B*, *SPAG9*, and *RUNDC1*) of potential importance to gliomagenesis [41]; however, the basis for this signal is not fully understood.

Table 2.4 Familial syndromes associated with increased risk of glioma

Syndrome	Gene(s)	Mode of inheritance	Other features/ predispositions	Associated glioma subtypes
Li-Fraumeni syndrome	*TP53*	Dominant	Breast, brain cancer, soft-tissue sarcoma, other cancers	All glioma
Lynch syndrome	*MSH2, MLH1, MSH6, PMS2*	Dominant	Gastrointestinal, endometrial, other cancers	All glioma
Melanoma-neural system tumor syndrome	*CDKN2A*	Dominant	Malignant melanoma	All glioma
Melanoma-oligodendroglioma susceptibility syndrome	*POT1*	Dominant with reduced penetrance	Malignant melanoma	Oligodendroglioma and oligoastrocytoma
Neurofibromatosis 1	*NF1*	Dominant	Neurofibromas, schwannomas, café-au-lait macules	Astrocytoma
Ollier disease/Maffucci syndrome	*IDH1/IDH2*	Dominant with reduced penetrance	Intraosseous benign cartilaginous tumors, other cancers	All glioma

Table adapted from [34, 118]

More recently, whole exome sequencing of germline DNA was performed in 90 members of 55 families with glioma aggregation in an effort to detect germline mutations associated with glioma risk. Three families were identified to harbor three different mutations in *protection of telomeres protein 1 (POT1)* [42], which is a telomere shelterin complex member involved in telomere maintenance and DNA damage response [43–45]. While this study was the first to specifically identify mutations in *POT1* as being related to glioma predisposition, it added to a growing literature indicating that disruption of normal telomere maintenance is a hallmark of gliomagenesis [9, 46].

2.4.2 Common Inherited Susceptibility Variants

Genome-wide association studies (GWAS) since 2009 have detected 27 single-nucleotide polymorphisms (SNPs) that were significantly associated with glioma risk [47–51]. The largest and most recent study reported associations with 25 of these SNPs [52] (Fig. 2.9). In this study, 6 loci were associated with GBM only and 14 with non-GBM only (grade II/III glioma), 5 loci were significant for both GBM and non-GBM, and 2

previously identified loci were not statistically significant. Of the loci associated with risk of GBM, the strongest effects have been observed in regions encoding *TERT, EGFR*, and *TP53* genes that are each also frequently somatically altered in glioma. The strongest association for risk of non-GBM tumors is observed in the 8q24.21 region, which maps to long-intergenic noncoding RNA *CCDC26* [48, 53–55]. Fine-mapping of the region has pinpointed rs55705857 as the strongest risk allele, yielding strikingly large odds ratios (>3-fold increased risk) for risk of IDH-mutant tumor development [7, 56, 57]. Variants in five regions have been associated with the development of all glioma grades and have been among the strongest and most consistent findings in glioma GWAS. These sites include chromosome 5p15.33 near *TERT*, 7p11.2 near *EGFR*, 9p21.3 near *CDKN2A/B*, 17p13.1 near *TP53*, and 20q13.33 near *RTEL1* [7, 34, 47, 48, 58–60].

With respect to GWAS of meningioma development, a 2011 study by Dobbins et al. reported that rs11012732 on chromosome 10p12.31 was associated with a 46% increased risk [61]. This SNP is located in the third intron of *MLLT10*, which is a component in several gene fusions resulting in forms of leukemia [62]. Efforts to identify additional meningioma-predisposing polymorphisms are underway.

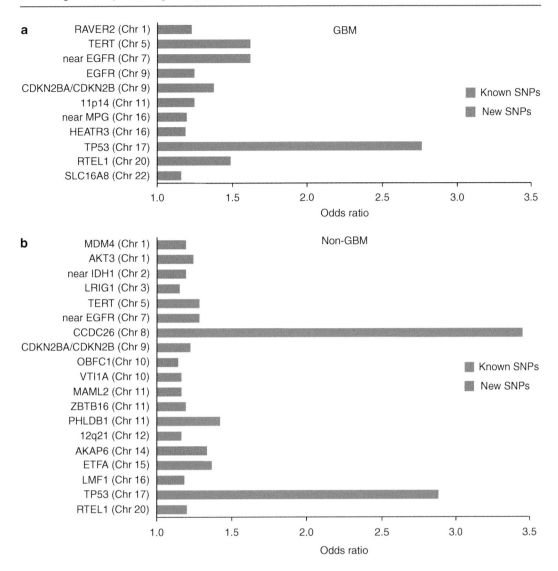

Fig. 2.9 Gene regions and effect sizes of (**a**) GBM- and (**b**) non-GBM-associated single-nucleotide polymorphisms (SNPs). Known and new SNPs refer to those identified prior to or from the most recent GWAS by Melin et al. [52]

2.5   Nongenetic Risk Factors

Many different types of exposures have been explored in epidemiological studies of brain tumor risk; however, results have been inconsistent for most factors studied [34, 63]. This may be attributable to the rare and often rapidly fatal nature of these tumors, as well as the frequent pooling of molecularly heterogeneous tumors, particularly in the study of malig-

nant glioma. Thus, large studies with detailed exposure histories and molecularly annotated biospecimens will be required to more conclusively study risk factors for which evidence has been limited. Currently established and potential risk factors for glioma and meningioma development are summarized in Table 2.5, and well-studied exposures are discussed below with respect to their association with brain tumor development.

Table 2.5 Nongenetic risk factors for glioma and meningioma

Established risk factors
  High-dose ionizing radiation (increased glioma and meningioma risk)
  Male vs. female gender (increased glioma risk, decreased meningioma risk)
  White vs. African American ethnicity (increased glioma risk, decreased meningioma risk)
Probable risk factors
  History of allergies/asthma (decreased glioma risk)
Probably not risk factors
  Alcohol and tobacco use
  Antihistamine use
  Cellular phone use
  Head injury
  Low-frequency magnetic fields
More research required
  NSAID use
  Diagnostic radiation
  Varicella zoster virus
  BMI, height

2.5.1 Radiation

The most established nongenetic cause of brain tumors is therapeutic or high-dose ionizing radiation to the CNS [64]. Studies of second primary cancers in the Childhood Cancer Survivor Study have demonstrated clear dose-response relationships between the dose of therapeutic radiation received and the subsequent development of CNS tumors [65, 66]. Further, any radiation exposure to the CNS was linked with a nearly seven- and tenfold increased risk of glioma and meningioma development, respectively. Similar patterns have been reported among children who had received radiotherapy for treatment of tinea capitis, a fungal infection of the scalp. In a study of over 10,000 tinea capitis patients with 30 years of follow-up, relative risks of 1.98 and 4.63 per Gy of radiation exposure were observed for development of malignant CNS tumors and nonmalignant meningioma, respectively [67].

With regard to medical diagnostic radiation exposure, small increases in brain tumor risks have been reported, but results have been largely inconclusive. In a large cohort of children and young adults who were examined with CT scans, one additional brain tumor case was expected to occur in a 10-year period per 10,000 CT scans of the head [68]. A separate study that evaluated the relationship between self-reported history of CT scans (three or more scans as compared to no scans) and glioma diagnosis did not identify a significant association, though there was a suggestive association among cases with a family history of cancer [69]. Occupational exposures among medical radiation workers have been associated with approximately twice the risk of brain cancer mortality, though individual-level radiation exposure data were not available [70]. While early studies were somewhat inconsistent regarding a link between dental X-rays and meningioma [71, 72], larger and more recent studies suggest that individuals who have received full-mouth dental X-rays have approximately twice the risk of meningioma development [73, 74].

With respect to the impact of nonionizing radiation from cell phones, the association between this widespread exposure and brain cancer has been the subject of much research and speculation. Radiofrequency fields were classified by the International Agency for Research on Cancer in 2007 as a possible carcinogen following the observation of increased glioma risk among heavy cell phone users [75]. This conclusion was driven primarily by results of the INTERPHONE study, which reported a 40% increase in glioma risk for the highest decile of mobile phone use as well as increased risk of tumor development on the side of the head to which the phone is typically held; significantly increased risk was also reported for heavy mobile phone users in a separate study by Hardell et al. [76, 77]. However, considerable concerns exist regarding the validity of these studies owing to potential reporting and selection biases and other methodological issues; in fact, subsequent studies have largely not supported an association between cell phone use and glioma development [34]. In particular, two large studies with long follow-up and use of cell phone subscription records for exposure assessment reported no increase in glioma risk [78, 79]. Given the ubiquitous nature of this exposure, it would be expected that overall brain tumor incidence would increase following a sufficiently long latency period if use of mobile phones in general, or of a specific class of mobile phone, was related to brain tumor development. While such increases in incidence have not yet been observed [2, 80, 81], continued surveillance of incidence patterns is necessary.

2.5.2   Allergies and Viruses

Epidemiologic studies have indicated that allergic conditions are inversely associated with glioma risk with remarkable consistency across study designs (single-site, multisite, and nested case control; prospective cohort; meta-analysis) and exposure definitions [82–85]. However, there has been some inconsistency in the effect of allergy history by glioma grade; some studies have reported comparable associations between allergy or asthma history and both low-grade glioma and higher-grade glioma development [86, 87], while others have reported weaker protective effects of allergy history against low-grade glioma than for high-grade glioma [88, 89]. In the largest and most recent study on this subject, an analysis in the Glioma International Case-Control Study (GICC) demonstrated a borderline significant reduction in glioma risk associated with a history of having any allergy (OR = 0.79, 95% CI 0.61–1.02), and this association was significant for high-grade (OR = 0.75, 95% CI 0.58–0.98) but not low-grade (OR = 0.84, 95% CI 0.63–1.11) glioma [85]. When restricting to respiratory allergies specifically, the study reported a significant ~30% reduction in risk (OR = 0.72, 95% CI 0.58–0.90) overall; the association was comparable for high-grade glioma (OR = 0.70, 95% CI 0.57–0.85) but attenuated for low-grade glioma (OR = 0.80, 95% CI 0.62–1.03) when stratifying by grade. Asthma and eczema history were also associated with decreased glioma risk in this study. Inverse associations with allergy history have also been observed for other CNS tumors, including meningiomas [89].

Varicella zoster virus (VZV) infection has also been inversely linked with glioma susceptibility using an array of exposure metrics including self-reported history of chicken pox [90, 91], anti-VZV immunoglobulin G levels [91, 92], and

antibodies against specific VZV proteins [93]. In the GICC, self-reported history of chickenpox was associated with a ~20% reduced glioma risk (OR = 0.79, 95% CI 0.65–0.96), supporting previous findings in the largest study to date to address this association [94]. The biological mechanisms by which allergies and VZV exposure confer protection against glioma are not yet known, though it has been suggested that both may augment antitumor immune surveillance.

2.5.3   Diet, Alcohol, and Tobacco Use

Dietary factors that promote or inhibit oxidative damage have been examined in a series of studies as potential modulators of brain tumor risk and progression. This hypothesis has been bolstered by studies such as those demonstrating that N-nitroso compounds, which are found in processed meat, have neurocarcinogenic properties in vivo and cause DNA damage in vitro [95, 96]. A case-control study from 1997 reported that glioma cases reported higher consumption of cured meats and lower consumption of vitamin-rich fruits and vegetables relative to controls [97]. However, no association was found in two large subsequent prospective studies between processed meat or N-nitroso compound consumption and glioma risk [98, 99]. Thus, studies have not generated compelling evidence of associations between dietary factors and glioma risk, though it must be kept in mind that accurate measurements of dietary exposures are difficult to ascertain, particularly retrospectively.

Similarly, the relationships between alcohol or tobacco use and glioma risk have been examined in numerous studies but have not been demonstrated to be risk factors for gliomagenesis. The association between alcohol consumption and glioma risk has been quite inconsistent across studies, with some studies suggesting increased risk and others suggesting decreased risk associated with alcohol consumption. A meta-analysis of 19 studies on the subject reported no association between alcohol consumption and glioma risk among moderate drinkers, heavy drinkers, or for specific alcohol classes [100]. Alcohol consumption also appears to be unrelated to meningioma risk [101]. In a recent meta-analysis including 24 studies of smoking and adult glioma risk, no associations were found between any smoking history and glioma risk [102]; the same conclusion was drawn following a meta-analysis of 9 studies investigating smoking and meningioma risk [103].

2.5.4 Anthropometric/Reproductive Factors and Medication Use

Anthropometric factors, including obesity and height, have been examined for association with brain tumor risk in multiple studies. In a meta-analysis of 22 studies, including over ten million subjects, obesity was associated with glioma among females and meningiomas overall [104]. However, in a large Norwegian cohort in which a greater number of incident glioma cases were observed than included in the meta-analysis, no association between overweight or obesity and glioma risk was found [105]. Epidemiologic studies have been more consistent in suggesting that taller height is a risk factor for glioma, particularly among males [105–107]. Taller height has also been associated with significantly increased risk of meningioma [101]. However, additional research is needed to draw definitive conclusions on the relationship between these anthropometric factors and brain tumor risk.

Owing to the observed differences in glioma and meningioma incidence by gender (higher glioma incidence among males; higher meningioma incidence among females), the role of hormonal and reproductive factors in risk of these tumors has been considered. Older age at menarche and older age at first pregnancy have both been associated with increased glioma risk, and exogenous hormone use has been shown to reduce glioma risk [108, 109]. In contrast, the number of pregnancies and age at first pregnancy appear to have protective effects against meningioma, and hormone replacement therapy may increase meningioma risk [110, 111]. While there has been a suggestion from this literature

that female sex hormones may protect against glioma while increasing risk of meningioma, further study is needed as results have not been entirely consistent.

With regard to the impact of the use of specific medications and supplements on the risk of CNS tumors, some studies have suggested that certain vitamin supplements, specifically those containing vitamin C and E, are protective against glioma [112, 113]. Some studies have also found that antihistamine use is associated with increased risk of glioma [114, 115]; another analysis detected protective effects of antihistamine use on glioma risk [86], yet the largest study to date to address this question found no association [85]. Studies have also investigated the role of nonsteroidal anti-inflammatory drugs (NSAIDs) on glioma risk, indicating that long-term use may be protective against glioma development [115, 116]. However, a recent meta-analysis did not support an association between NSAID use and glioma risk, a result that was driven primarily by several prospective studies in which a protective effect of NSAID use was not observed [117]. An analysis of aspirin and non-aspirin NSAID use with respect to glioma risk in the GICC is ongoing and will provide additional information on this association in a large international population.

2.6 Conclusion and Future Directions

Brain tumor epidemiology has greatly informed our understanding of the patterns of disease and potential risk factors for glioma and meningioma, the two most common types of primary brain tumors. Analyses of the variation in disease incidence by gender, ethnicity, and geographic location have offered interesting clues as to the factors involved in brain tumor etiology and require further investigation. Additionally, careful surveillance of brain tumor incidence rates in the United States and other countries continues on an annual basis, which will yield information on trends in disease occurrence that may be attributable to emerging risk factors. The application of high-throughput genomic technology in increasingly large population-based studies has also yielded enormous gains for our understanding of glioma etiology, from the identification of new genetic variants that predispose to familial glioma to the characterization of clinically meaningful molecular subclasses of tumors. Genome-wide association studies have pinpointed genetic loci that are associated with the development of glioma and meningioma; however, the specific functional variants and mechanisms through which tumorigenesis is modulated are not yet understood and will be the subject of the next wave of molecular epidemiologic research. Additionally, other risk variants will likely emerge as tumor subgroups are analyzed in more molecularly homogenous sets.

Epidemiologic studies have also identified nongenetic factors that affect risk of brain tumor development, including ionizing radiation exposure and allergy history. However, many exposures have not been adequately studied or have yielded conflicting results; large populations with well-annotated biospecimens and detailed exposure histories will be required to rigorously investigate potential risk factors. Furthermore, understanding of the interactions of genetic and nongenetic risk factors will offer additional insight into tumorigenic processes but will require large sample sizes to be adequately studied. Although much has been learned through epidemiologic investigations of brain tumors, additional research in this field is required to further understand mechanisms of tumor etiology that may ultimately offer new paths to targeted screening, prevention, and therapy.

Funding The work by DIJ was supported by the CPRIT Post-Graduate Training Program in Integrative Cancer Epidemiology (Award ID RP160097). The work was also supported by grants from the US National Institutes of Health R01CA119215 (MLB), R01CA070917 (MLB), R01CA139020 (MLB), P50CA097257 (MRW), P50CA108961 (RBJ), and RC1NS068222Z (RBJ), as well as the Loglio Collective and the Stanley D. Lewis and Virginia S. Lewis Endowed Chair in Brain Tumor Research (MRW) and the Bernie and Edith Waterman Foundation and the Ting Tsung and Wei Fong Chao Family Foundation (RBJ).

References

1. Ferlay J, Soerjomataram I, Ervik M, Dikshit R, Eser S, Mathers C et al (2013) GLOBOCAN 2012 v1. 0, cancer incidence and mortality worldwide: IARC cancer base no. 11 [Internet]. Lyon, International Agency for Research on Cancer. globocaniarcfr 2014

2. Ostrom QT, Gittleman H, Xu J, Kromer C, Wolinsky Y, Kruchko C et al (2016) CBTRUS statistical report: primary brain and other central nervous system tumors diagnosed in the United States in 2009–2013. Neurooncol 18(suppl 5):v1–v75

3. Louis DN, Ohgaki H, Wiestler OD, Cavenee WK, Burger PC, Jouvet A et al (2007) The 2007 WHO classification of tumours of the central nervous system. Acta Neuropathol (Berl) 114(2):97–109

4. van den Bent MJ (2010) Interobserver variation of the histopathological diagnosis in clinical trials on glioma: a clinician's perspective. Acta Neuropathol (Berl) 120(3):297–304

5. Louis DN, Perry A, Reifenberger G, von Deimling A, Figarella-Branger D, Cavenee WK et al (2016) The 2016 World Health Organization classification of tumors of the central nervous system: a summary. Acta Neuropathol (Berl) 131(6):803–820

6. Cancer Genome Atlas Research Network et al (2015) Comprehensive, integrative genomic analysis of diffuse lower-grade gliomas. N Engl J Med 372(26):2481–2498

7. Eckel-Passow JE, Lachance DH, Molinaro AM, Walsh KM, Decker PA, Sicotte H et al (2015) Glioma groups based on 1p/19q, IDH, and TERT promoter mutations in tumors. N Engl J Med 372(26):2499–2508

8. Verhaak RG, Hoadley KA, Purdom E, Wang V, Qi Y, Wilkerson MD et al (2010) Integrated genomic analysis identifies clinically relevant subtypes of glioblastoma characterized by abnormalities in *PDGFRA*, *IDH1*, *EGFR*, and *NF1*. Cancer Cell 17(1):98–110

9. Ceccarelli M, Barthel FP, Malta TM, Sabedot TS, Salama SR, Murray BA et al (2016) Molecular profiling reveals biologically discrete subsets and pathways of progression in diffuse glioma. Cell 164(3):550–563

10. Noushmehr H, Weisenberger DJ, Diefes K, Phillips HS, Pujara K, Berman BP et al (2010) Identification of a CpG island methylator phenotype that defines a distinct subgroup of glioma. Cancer Cell 17(5):510–522

11. Watanabe T, Nobusawa S, Kleihues P, Ohgaki H (2009) IDH1 mutations are early events in the development of astrocytomas and oligodendrogliomas. Am J Pathol 174(4):1149–1153

12. Yan H, Parsons DW, Jin G, McLendon R, Rasheed BA, Yuan W et al (2009) IDH1 and IDH2 mutations in gliomas. N Engl J Med 360(8):765–773

13. Kim Y-H, Nobusawa S, Mittelbronn M, Paulus W, Brokinkel B, Keyvani K et al (2010) Molecular classification of low-grade diffuse gliomas. Am J Pathol 177(6):2708–2714

14. Rice T, Lachance DH, Molinaro AM, Eckel-Passow JE, Walsh KM, Barnholtz-Sloan J et al (2016)

Understanding inherited genetic risk of adult glioma–a review. Neurooncol Pract 3(1):10–16

15. Howlader N, Noone A, Krapcho M, Neyman N, Aminou R, Altekruse S, et al (2012) SEER cancer statistics review, 1975–2009. National Cancer Institute, Bethesda. http://seer.cancer.gov/csr/1975_2009_pops09/

16. Hartmann C, Hentschel B, Tatagiba M, Schramm J, Schnell O, Seidel C et al (2011) Molecular markers in low-grade gliomas: predictive or prognostic? Clin Cancer Res 17(13):4588–4599

17. Houillier C, Wang X, Kaloshi G, Mokhtari K, Guillevin R, Laffaire J et al (2010) IDH1 or IDH2 mutations predict longer survival and response to temozolomide in low-grade gliomas. Neurology 75(17):1560–1566

18. Jenkins RB, Blair H, Ballman KV, Giannini C, Arusell RM, Law M et al (2006) A t (1; 19)(q10; p10) mediates the combined deletions of 1p and 19q and predicts a better prognosis of patients with oligodendroglioma. Cancer Res 66(20):9852–9861

19. Sabha N, Knobbe CB, Maganti M, Al Omar S, Bernstein M, Cairns R et al (2014) Analysis of IDH mutation, 1p/19q deletion, and PTEN loss delineates prognosis in clinical low-grade diffuse gliomas. Neuro Oncol 16(7):914–923

20. Pekmezci M, Rice T, Molinaro AM, Walsh KM, Decker PA, Hansen H et al (2017) Adult infiltrating gliomas with WHO 2016 integrated diagnosis: additional prognostic roles of ATRX and TERT. Acta Neuropathol (Berl) 133(6):1001–1016

21. Hegi ME, Diserens A-C, Gorlia T, Hamou M-F, de Tribolet N, Weller M et al (2005) MGMT gene silencing and benefit from temozolomide in glioblastoma. N Engl J Med 352(10):997–1003

22. Cairncross JG, Wang M, Jenkins RB, Shaw EG, Giannini C, Brachman DG et al (2014) Benefit from procarbazine, lomustine, and vincristine in oligodendroglial tumors is associated with mutation of IDH. J Clin Oncol 32(8):783–790

23. Bauchet L, Mathieu-Daudé H, Fabbro-Peray P, Rigau V, Fabbro M, Chinot O et al (2010) Oncological patterns of care and outcome for 952 patients with newly diagnosed glioblastoma in 2004. Neuro Oncol 12(7):725–735

24. Lacroix M, Abi-Said D, Fourney DR, Gokaslan ZL, Shi W, DeMonte F et al (2001) A multivariate analysis of 416 patients with glioblastoma multiforme: prognosis, extent of resection, and survival. J Neurosurg 95(2):190–198

25. Kshettry VR, Ostrom QT, Kruchko C, Al-Mefty O, Barnett GH, Barnholtz-Sloan JS (2015) Descriptive epidemiology of World Health Organization grades II and III intracranial meningiomas in the United States. Neuro Oncol 17(8):1166–1173

26. Cahill KS, Claus EB (2011) Treatment and survival of patients with nonmalignant intracranial meningioma: results from the Surveillance, Epidemiology, and End Results Program of the National Cancer Institute. J Neurosurg 115(2):259–267

27. van Alkemade H, de Leau M, Dieleman EM, Kardaun JW, van Os R, Vandertop WP et al (2012) Impaired survival and long-term neurological problems in benign meningioma. Neuro Oncol 14(5):658–666

28. Wrensch M, Lee M, Miike R, Newman B, Bargar G, Davis R et al (1997) Familial and personal medical history of cancer and nervous system conditions among adults with glioma and controls. Am J Epidemiol 145(7):581–593

29. Scheurer ME, Etzel CJ, Liu M, El-Zein R, Airewele GE, Malmer B et al (2007) Aggregation of cancer in first-degree relatives of patients with glioma. Cancer Epidemiol Biomarkers Prev 16(11):2491–2495

30. Malmer B, Grönberg H, Bergenheim AT, Lenner P, Henriksson R (1999) Familial aggregation of astrocytoma in northern Sweden: an epidemiological cohort study. Int J Cancer 81(3):366–370

31. Blumenthal DT, Cannon-Albright LA (2008) Familiality in brain tumors. Neurology 71(13): 1015–1020

32. Robertson LB, Armstrong GN, Olver BD, Lloyd AL, Shete S, Lau C et al (2010) Survey of familial glioma and role of germline p16 INK4A/p14 ARF and p53 mutation. Familial Cancer 9(3):413–421

33. Louis DN, Deimling A (1995) Hereditary tumor syndromes of the nervous system: overview and rare syndromes. Brain Pathol 5(2):145–151

34. Ostrom QT, Bauchet L, Davis FG, Deltour I, Fisher JL, Langer CE et al (2014) The epidemiology of glioma in adults: a "state of the science" review. Neuro Oncol 16(7):896–913

35. Ceccarelli M, Barthel Floris P, Malta Tathiane M, Sabedot Thais S, Salama Sofie R, Murray Bradley A et al (2016) Molecular profiling reveals biologically discrete subsets and pathways of progression in diffuse glioma. Cell 164(3):550–563

36. Simon M, Boström JP, Hartmann C (2007) Molecular genetics of meningiomas: from basic research to potential clinical applications. Neurosurgery 60(5):787–798

37. Wiemels J, Wrensch M, Claus EB (2010) Epidemiology and etiology of meningioma. J Neurooncol 99(3): 307–314

38. Paunu N, Lahermo P, Onkamo P, Ollikainen V, Rantala I, Helén P et al (2002) A novel low-penetrance locus for familial glioma at 15q23-q26.3. Cancer Res 62(13):3798–3802

39. Shete S, Lau CC, Houlston RS, Claus EB, Barnholtz-Sloan J, Lai R et al (2011) Genome-wide high-density SNP linkage search for glioma susceptibility loci: results from the Gliogene Consortium. Cancer Res 71(24):7568–7575

40. Sun X, Vengoechea J, Elston R, Chen Y, Amos CI, Armstrong G et al (2012) A variable age of onset segregation model for linkage analysis, with correction for ascertainment, applied to glioma. Cancer Epidemiol Biomarkers Prev 21(12):2242–2251

41. Jalali A, Amirian ES, Bainbridge MN, Armstrong GN, Liu Y, Tsavachidis S et al (2015) Targeted sequencing in chromosome 17q linkage region identifies familial

glioma candidates in the Gliogene Consortium. Sci Rep 5:8278

42. Bainbridge MN, Armstrong GN, Gramatges MM, Bertuch AA, Jhangiani SN, Doddapaneni H et al (2015) Germline mutations in shelterin complex genes are associated with familial glioma. J Natl Cancer Inst 107(1):dju384

43. Baumann P, Cech TR (2001) Pot1, the putative telomere end-binding protein in fission yeast and humans. Science 292(5519):1171–1175

44. Hockemeyer D, Sfeir AJ, Shay JW, Wright WE, de Lange T (2005) POT1 protects telomeres from a transient DNA damage response and determines how human chromosomes end. EMBO J 24(14):2667–2678

45. Ramsay AJ, Quesada V, Foronda M, Conde L, Martínez-Trillos A, Villamor N et al (2013) POT1 mutations cause telomere dysfunction in chronic lymphocytic leukemia. Nat Genet 45(5):526–530

46. Walsh KM, Wiencke JK, Lachance DH, Wiemels JL, Molinaro AM, Eckel-Passow JE et al (2015) Telomere maintenance and the etiology of adult glioma. Neuro Oncol 17(11):1445–1452

47. Wrensch M, Jenkins RB, Chang JS, Yeh R-F, Xiao Y, Decker PA et al (2009) Variants in the CDKN2B and RTEL1 regions are associated with high-grade glioma susceptibility. Nat Genet 41(8):905–908

48. Shete S, Hosking FJ, Robertson LB, Dobbins SE, Sanson M, Malmer B et al (2009) Genome-wide association study identifies five susceptibility loci for glioma. Nat Genet 41(8):899–904

49. Walsh KM, Codd V, Smirnov IV, Rice T, Decker PA, Hansen HM et al (2014) Variants near TERT and TERC influencing telomere length are associated with high-grade glioma risk. Nat Genet 46(7):731–735

50. Kinnersley B, Labussière M, Holroyd A, Di Stefano A-L, Broderick P, Vijayakrishnan J et al (2015) Genome-wide association study identifies multiple susceptibility loci for glioma. Nat Commun 6:8559

51. Sanson M, Hosking FJ, Shete S, Zelenika D, Dobbins SE, Ma Y et al (2011) Chromosome 7p11.2 (EGFR) variation influences glioma risk. Hum Mol Genet 20(14):2897–2904

52. Melin BS, Barnholtz-Sloan JS, Wrensch MR, Johansen C, Il'yasova D, Kinnersley B et al (2017) Genome-wide association study of glioma subtypes identifies specific differences in genetic susceptibility to glioblastoma and non-glioblastoma tumors. Nat Genet 49(5):789–794

53. Jenkins RB, Wrensch MR, Johnson D, Fridley BL, Decker PA, Xiao Y et al (2011) Distinct germ line polymorphisms underlie glioma morphologic heterogeneity. Cancer Genet 204(1):13–18

54. Egan KM, Thompson RC, Nabors L, Olson JJ, Brat DJ, LaRocca RV et al (2011) Cancer susceptibility variants and the risk of adult glioma in a US case–control study. J Neurooncol 104(2):535–542

55. Simon M, Hosking FJ, Marie Y, Gousias K, Boisselier B, Carpentier C et al (2010) Genetic risk profiles identify different molecular etiologies for glioma. Clin Cancer Res 16(21):5252–5259

56. Jenkins RB, Xiao Y, Sicotte H, Decker PA, Kollmeyer TM, Hansen HM et al (2012) A low-frequency variant at 8q24. 21 is strongly associated with risk of oligodendroglial tumors and astrocytomas with IDH1 or IDH2 mutation. Nat Genet 44(10): 1122–1125

57. Enciso-Mora V, Hosking FJ, Kinnersley B, Wang Y, Shete S, Zelenika D et al (2013) Deciphering the 8q24. 21 association for glioma. Hum Mol Genet 22(11):2293–2302

58. Stacey SN, Sulem P, Jonasdottir A, Masson G, Gudmundsson J, Gudbjartsson DF et al (2011) A germline variant in the TP53 polyadenylation signal confers cancer susceptibility. Nat Genet 43(11):1098–1103

59. Enciso-Mora V, Hosking F, Di Stefano A, Zelenika D, Shete S, Broderick P et al (2013) Low penetrance susceptibility to glioma is caused by the TP53 variant rs78378222. Br J Cancer 108(10):2178–2185

60. Egan KM, Nabors LB, Olson JJ, Monteiro AN, Browning JE, Madden MH et al (2012) Rare TP53 genetic variant associated with glioma risk and outcome. J Med Genet 49(7):420–421

61. Dobbins SE, Broderick P, Melin B, Feychting M, Johansen C, Andersson U et al (2011) Common variation at 10p12. 31 near MLLT10 influences meningioma risk. Nat Genet 43(9):825–827

62. Brandimarte L, Pierini V, Di Giacomo D, Borga C, Nozza F, Gorello P et al (2013) New MLLT10 gene recombinations in pediatric T-acute lymphoblastic leukemia. Blood 121(25):5064–5067

63. Bauchet L (2013) Epidemiology of diffuse low-grade gliomas. In: Duffau H (ed) Diffuse low-grade gliomas in adults. Springer, London, pp 9–30

64. Bondy ML, Scheurer ME, Malmer B, Barnholtz-Sloan JS, Davis FG, Il'yasova D et al (2008) Brain tumor epidemiology: consensus from the Brain Tumor Epidemiology Consortium. Cancer 113(S7):1953–1968

65. Neglia JP, Robison LL, Stovall M, Liu Y, Packer RJ, Hammond S et al (2006) New primary neoplasms of the central nervous system in survivors of childhood cancer: a report from the Childhood Cancer Survivor Study. J Natl Cancer Inst 98(21):1528–1537

66. Inskip PD, Sigurdson AJ, Veiga L, Bhatti P, Ronckers C, Rajaraman P et al (2016) Radiation-related new primary solid cancers in the Childhood Cancer Survivor Study: comparative radiation dose response and modification of treatment effects. Int J Radiat Oncol Biol Phys 94(4):800–807

67. Sadetzki S, Chetrit A, Freedman L, Stovall M, Modan B, Novikov I (2005) Long-term follow-up for brain tumor development after childhood exposure to ionizing radiation for tinea capitis. Radiat Res 163(4):424–432

68. Pearce MS, Salotti JA, Little MP, McHugh K, Lee C, Kim KP et al (2012) Radiation exposure from CT scans in childhood and subsequent risk of leukaemia and brain tumours: a retrospective cohort study. Lancet 380(9840):499–505

69. Davis F, Il'yasova D, Rankin K, McCarthy B, Bigner DD (2011) Medical diagnostic radiation exposures and risk of gliomas. Radiat Res 175(6): 790–796

70. Rajaraman P, Doody MM, Yu CL, Preston DL, Miller JS, Sigurdson AJ et al (2016) Cancer risks in US radiologic technologists working with fluoroscopically guided interventional procedures, 1994–2008. Am J Roentgenol 206(5):1101–1109

71. Ryan P, Lee MW, North B, McMichael AJ (1992) Amalgam fillings, diagnostic dental x-rays and tumours of the brain and meninges. Eur J Cancer B Oral Oncol 28(2):91–95

72. Schlehofer B, Blettner M, Becker N, Martinsohn C, Wahrendorf J (1992) Medical risk factors and the development of brain tumors. Cancer 69(10):2541–2547

73. Longstreth W, Phillips LE, Drangsholt M, Koepsell TD, Custer BS, Gehrels JA et al (2004) Dental X-rays and the risk of intracranial meningioma. Cancer 100(5):1026–1034

74. Claus EB, Calvocoressi L, Bondy ML, Schildkraut JM, Wiemels JL, Wrensch M (2012) Dental x-rays and risk of meningioma. Cancer 118(18): 4530–4537

75. Baan R, Grosse Y, Lauby-Secretan B, El Ghissassi F, Bouvard V, Benbrahim-Tallaa L et al (2011) Carcinogenicity of radiofrequency electromagnetic fields. Lancet Oncol 12(7):624–626

76. Cardis E, Deltour I, Vrijheid M, Combalot E, Moissonnier M, Tardy H et al (2010) Brain tumour risk in relation to mobile telephone use: results of the INTERPHONE international case–control study. Int J Epidemiol 39(3):675–694

77. Hardell L, Carlberg M, Hansson Mild K (2011) Pooled analysis of case-control studies on malignant brain tumours and the use of mobile and cordless phones including living and deceased subjects. Int J Oncol 38(5):1465–1474

78. Frei P, Poulsen AH, Johansen C, Olsen JH, Steding-Jessen M, Schüz J (2011) Use of mobile phones and risk of brain tumours: update of Danish cohort study. BMJ 343:d6387

79. Benson VS, Pirie K, Schüz J, Reeves GK, Beral V, Green J et al (2013) Mobile phone use and risk of brain neoplasms and other cancers: prospective study. Int J Epidemiol 42(3):792–802

80. Barchana M, Margaliot M, Liphshitz I (2012) Changes in brain glioma incidence and laterality correlates with use of mobile phones-a nationwide population based study in Israel. Asian Pac J Cancer Prev 13(11):5857–5863

81. Deltour I, Auvinen A, Feychting M, Johansen C, Klaeboe L, Sankila R et al (2012) Mobile phone use and incidence of glioma in the Nordic countries 1979–2008: consistency check. Epidemiology 23(2):301–307

82. Chen C, Xu T, Chen J, Zhou J, Yan Y, Lu Y et al (2011) Allergy and risk of glioma: a meta-analysis. Eur J Neurol 18(3):387–395

83. Linos E, Raine T, Alonso A, Michaud D (2007) Atopy and risk of brain tumors: a meta-analysis. J Natl Cancer Inst 99(20):1544–1550

84. Zhao H, Cai W, Su S, Zhi D, Lu J, Liu S (2014) Allergic conditions reduce the risk of glioma: a meta-analysis based on 128,936 subjects. Tumor Biol 35(4):3875–3880

85. Amirian ES, Zhou R, Wrensch MR, Olson SH, Scheurer ME, Il'Yasova D et al (2016) Approaching a scientific consensus on the association between allergies and glioma risk: a report from the Glioma International Case-Control Study. Cancer Epidemiol Biomarkers Prev 25(2):282–290

86. McCarthy BJ, Rankin K, Il'yasova D, Erdal S, Vick N, Ali-Osman F et al (2011) Assessment of type of allergy and antihistamine use in the development of glioma. Cancer Epidemiol Biomarkers Prev 20(2):370–378

87. Scheurer ME, Amirian ES, Davlin SL, Rice T, Wrensch M, Bondy ML (2011) Effects of antihistamine and anti-inflammatory medication use on risk of specific glioma histologies. Int J Cancer 129(9):2290–2296

88. Schlehofer B, Siegmund B, Linseisen J, Schüz J, Rohrmann S, Becker S et al (2011) Primary brain tumours and specific serum immunoglobulin E: a case–control study nested in the European Prospective Investigation into Cancer and Nutrition cohort. Allergy 66(11):1434–1441

89. Turner MC, Krewski D, Armstrong BK, Chetrit A, Giles GG, Hours M et al (2013) Allergy and brain tumors in the INTERPHONE study: pooled results from Australia, Canada, France, Israel, and New Zealand. Cancer Causes Control 24(5):949–960

90. Wrensch M, Weinberg A, Wiencke J, Masters H, Miike R, Barger G et al (1997) Does prior infection with varicella-zoster virus influence risk of adult glioma? Am J Epidemiol 145(7):594–597

91. Wrensch M, Weinberg A, Wiencke J, Miike R, Sison J, Wiemels J et al (2005) History of chickenpox and shingles and prevalence of antibodies to varicella-zoster virus and three other herpesviruses among adults with glioma and controls. Am J Epidemiol 161(10):929–938

92. Wrensch M, Weinberg A, Wiencke J, Miike R, Barger G, Kelsey K (2001) Prevalence of antibodies to four herpesviruses among adults with glioma and controls. Am J Epidemiol 154(2):161–165

93. Lee ST, Bracci P, Zhou M, Rice T, Wiencke J, Wrensch M et al (2014) Interaction of allergy history and antibodies to specific varicella-zoster virus proteins on glioma risk. Int J Cancer 134(9):2199–2210

94. Amirian ES, Scheurer ME, Zhou R, Wrensch MR, Armstrong GN, Lachance D et al (2016) History of chickenpox in glioma risk: a report from the glioma international case–control study (GICC). Cancer Med 5(6):1352–1358

95. Berleur M-P, Cordier S (1995) The role of chemical, physical, or viral exposures and health factors in neurocarcinogenesis: implications for epidemio-

logic studies of brain tumors. Cancer Causes Control 6(3):240–256

96. Dietrich M, Block G, Pogoda JM, Buffler P, Hecht S, Preston-Martin S (2005) A review: dietary and endogenously formed N-nitroso compounds and risk of childhood brain tumors. Cancer Causes Control 16(6):619–635

97. Lee M, Wrensch M, Miike R (1997) Dietary and tobacco risk factors for adult onset glioma in the San Francisco Bay Area (California, USA). Cancer Causes Control 8(1):13–24

98. Michaud DS, Holick CN, Batchelor TT, Giovannucci E, Hunter DJ (2009) Prospective study of meat intake and dietary nitrates, nitrites, and nitrosamines and risk of adult glioma. Am J Clin Nutr 90(3):570–577

99. Dubrow R, Darefsky AS, Park Y, Mayne ST, Moore SC, Kilfoy B et al (2010) Dietary components related to N-nitroso compound formation: a prospective study of adult glioma. Cancer Epidemiol Biomarkers Prev 19(7):1709–1722

100. Galeone C, Malerba S, Rota M, Bagnardi V, Negri E, Scotti L et al (2012) A meta-analysis of alcohol consumption and the risk of brain tumours. Ann Oncol 24(2):514–523

101. Benson VS, Pirie K, Green J, Casabonne D, Beral V (2008) Lifestyle factors and primary glioma and meningioma tumours in the Million Women Study cohort. Br J Cancer 99(1):185

102. Li HX, Peng XX, Zong Q, Zhang K, Wang MX, Liu YZ et al (2016) Cigarette smoking and risk of adult glioma: a meta-analysis of 24 observational studies involving more than 2.3 million individuals. Onco Targets Ther 9:3511–3523

103. Fan Z, Ji T, Wan S, Wu Y, Zhu Y, Xiao F et al (2013) Smoking and risk of meningioma: a meta-analysis. Cancer Epidemiol 37(1):39–45

104. Sergentanis TN, Tsivgoulis G, Perlepe C, Ntanasis-Stathopoulos I, Tzanninis I-G, Sergentanis IN et al (2015) Obesity and risk for brain/CNS tumors, gliomas and meningiomas: a meta-analysis. PLoS One 10(9):e0136974

105. Wiedmann MK, Brunborg C, Di Ieva A, Lindemann K, Johannesen TB, Vatten L et al (2016) The impact of body mass index and height on the risk for glioblastoma and other glioma subgroups: a large prospective cohort study. Neuro Oncol 19(7):976–985

106. Moore SC, Rajaraman P, Dubrow R, Darefsky AS, Koebnick C, Hollenbeck A et al (2009) Height, body mass index, and physical activity in relation to glioma risk. Cancer Res 69(21):8349–8355

107. Kitahara CM, Gamborg M, Rajaraman P, Sørensen TI, Baker JL (2014) A prospective study of height and body mass index in childhood, birth weight, and risk of adult glioma over 40 years of follow-up. Am J Epidemiol 180(8):821–829

108. Hatch EE, Linet MS, Zhang J, Fine HA, Shapiro WR, Selker RG et al (2005) Reproductive and hormonal factors and risk of brain tumors in adult females. Int J Cancer 114(5):797–805

109. Qi Z-Y, Shao C, Zhang X, Hui G-Z, Wang Z (2013) Exogenous and endogenous hormones in relation to glioma in women: a meta-analysis of 11 case-control studies. PLoS One 8(7):e68695

110. Lee E, Grutsch J, Persky V, Glick R, Mendes J, Davis F (2006) Association of meningioma with reproductive factors. Int J Cancer 119(5): 1152–1157

111. Qi Z-Y, Shao C, Huang Y-L, Hui G-Z, Zhou Y-X, Wang Z (2013) Reproductive and exogenous hormone factors in relation to risk of meningioma in women: a meta-analysis. PLoS One 8(12): e83261

112. Kyritsis AP, Bondy ML, Levin VA (2011) Modulation of glioma risk and progression by dietary nutrients and antiinflammatory agents. Nutr Cancer 63(2):174–184

113. Sheweita SA, Sheikh BY (2011) Can dietary antioxidants reduce the incidence of brain tumors? Curr Drug Metab 12(6):587–593

114. Amirian ES, Marquez-Do D, Bondy ML, Scheurer ME (2013) Antihistamine use and immunoglobulin E levels in glioma risk and prognosis. Cancer Epidemiol 37(6):908–912

115. Scheurer ME, El-Zein R, Thompson PA, Aldape KD, Levin VA, Gilbert MR et al (2008) Long-term anti-inflammatory and antihistamine medication use and adult glioma risk. Cancer Epidemiol Biomarkers Prev 17(5):1277–1281

116. Gaist D, Garcia-Rodriguez L, Sørensen H, Hallas J, Friis S (2013) Use of low-dose aspirin and non-aspirin nonsteroidal anti-inflammatory drugs and risk of glioma: a case–control study. Br J Cancer 108(5):1189

117. Liu Y, Lu Y, Wang J, Xie L, Li T, He Y et al (2014) Association between nonsteroidal anti-inflammatory drug use and brain tumour risk: a meta-analysis. Br J Clin Pharmacol 78(1):58–68

118. Goodenberger ML, Jenkins RB (2012) Genetics of adult glioma. Cancer Genet 205(12):613–621

119. Ostrom QT, Gittleman H, Fulop J, Liu M, Blanda R, Kromer C et al (2015) CBTRUS statistical report: primary brain and central nervous system tumors diagnosed in the United States in 2008–2012. Neuro Oncol 17(suppl 4):iv1–iv62

Imaging of Central Nervous System Tumors

3

K. Ina Ly, Nathalie L. Albert,
and Elizabeth R. Gerstner

3.1 Introduction

Imaging has become indispensable to the field of neuro-oncology and has proven to be an invaluable tool to help answer important biologic and clinical questions. While computed tomography (CT) is the imaging modality of choice to evaluate acute conditions such as intracranial hemorrhage, herniation, and hydrocephalus, structural or anatomical magnetic resonance imaging (MRI) constitutes the current gold standard in the initial diagnostic and long-term follow-up management of patients with central nervous system (CNS) tumors. However, while it provides excellent resolution and tissue contrast, anatomical MRI has a number of limitations, including its ability to depict tumor heterogeneity, delineate tumor boundaries of diffuse gliomas, and differentiate between tumor tissue and therapy-related changes. The advances made in

the field of physiologic MR imaging in recent decades have enabled us to study more complex biologic and clinical questions. Functional MRI provides a more accurate way to distinguish neoplastic from inflammatory, demyelinating, and infectious processes; differentiates between different tumor types, their histologic subgroups, and tumor grade; aids in surgical and radiotherapy planning; assesses treatment response; and offers insights into the underlying molecular makeup of the tumor. In addition to functional MRI, positron emission tomography (PET) has assumed increasing importance in the clinical workup of oncologic diseases. The use of radioactively labeled tracer substances can help visualize processes at the molecular level such as glucose consumption or amino acid metabolism, thus providing a useful complementary diagnostic tool [1–5]. Given the higher spatial resolution of PET instrumentation and the availability of relevant radiotracers, PET has prevailed over single-photon emission computed tomography (SPECT).

In this chapter, we provide an overview of the physical principles and clinical applications of structural and functional MR and PET imaging. We also discuss new cutting-edge techniques such as vessel caliber imaging and iron nanoparticle-based perfusion MRI and provide an outlook on the challenges and future directions in the field.

K. Ina Ly · E. R. Gerstner (✉)
Stephen E. and Catherine Pappas Center for
Neuro-Oncology, Massachusetts General Hospital,
Boston, MA, USA
e-mail: ily@partners.org;
egerstner@mgh.harvard.edu

N. L. Albert
Department of Nuclear Medicine,
Ludwig-Maxilimians-University,
Munich, Germany
e-mail: Nathalie.Albert@med.uni-muenchen.de

© Springer Nature Switzerland AG 2019
J.-C. Tonn et al. (eds.), *Oncology of CNS Tumors*, https://doi.org/10.1007/978-3-030-04152-6_3

3.2 Magnetic Resonance Imaging of CNS Tumors

3.2.1 Standard Anatomical MRI

All MRI techniques are based on the fundamental principle that hydrogen nuclei of water molecules become magnetized when exposed to a strong static magnetic field [6]. Using radiofrequency wave pulses at a resonant frequency, this magnetization can be manipulated or "excited," in turn leading the magnetized nuclei to re-emit radiofrequency waves that are received through a coil as a signal [7]. The type of signal depends on the biological, chemical, and physical properties of the nuclei and their environment and is thus unique for different types of tissue.

Standard anatomical MRI sequences in neuro-oncology include pre- and post-contrast T1-weighted (T1W), T2W, and fluid-attenuated inversion recovery (FLAIR) sequences. Most institutions also add diffusion and gradient-echo sequences to standardized brain tumor acquisition protocols. Post-contrast T1W and FLAIR sequences constitute the gold standard for diagnosis and response assessment [8]. In general, contrast-enhancing areas are thought to reflect more aggressive and malignant processes. This is because a growing neoplasm that undergoes malignant transformation typically promotes angiogenesis and disrupts the blood-brain barrier (BBB) [9], thus permitting extravasation of contrast agent into the interstitial space which generates the hyperintense signal on post-contrast T1W images. FLAIR sequences, on the other hand, are a type of T2W pulse sequence that suppresses the signal from cerebrospinal fluid (CSF). FLAIR is most useful in assessing the extent of non-enhancing tumor, vasogenic edema, and gliosis. Figures 3.1, 3.2, 3.3, and 3.4 show representative characteristic MR images of common brain tumors.

Post-contrast T1W and FLAIR sequences form the cornerstone of the Response Assessment in Neuro-Oncology (RANO) criteria, an imaging- and clinically based response assessment in CNS tumor patients. The RANO criteria have largely been adopted as a standardized assessment and monitoring tool, particularly in the setting of clinical trials [8]. Similar to the older Macdonald criteria [10], the RANO criteria use the two-dimensional change in enhancing tumor diameters, stability of corticosteroid dosing, and the patient's clinical status to categorize response. Since enhancing tumor is primarily seen in high-grade but not low-grade tumors, the RANO Working Group has recently added response criteria for low-grade gliomas (LGGs) by including the change in the non-enhancing FLAIR area as an important factor in response assessment [11].

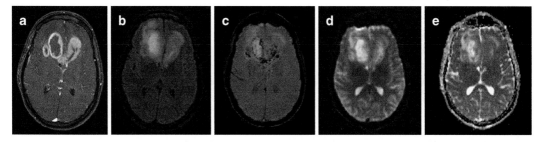

Fig. 3.1 Characteristic axial MR images of a high-grade glioma from a 49-year-old woman who presented with behavioral changes. T1-weighted post-contrast images (**a**) demonstrate an enhancing lesion in the bilateral frontal lobes and involving the genu of the corpus callosum; this "butterfly appearance" is classic for glioblastomas. There is associated T2/FLAIR hyperintensity (**b**), likely representing a mix of non-enhancing infiltrating tumor and vasogenic edema. Associated microhemorrhages are seen on susceptibility-weighted images (**c**). Diffusion-weighted images (**d**) reveal patchy restricted diffusion as evidenced by dark areas at the medial tumor margins on the ADC maps (**e**), indicative of areas of high cellularity. Biopsy revealed an *IDH*-wild-type, *MGMT*-unmethylated glioblastoma

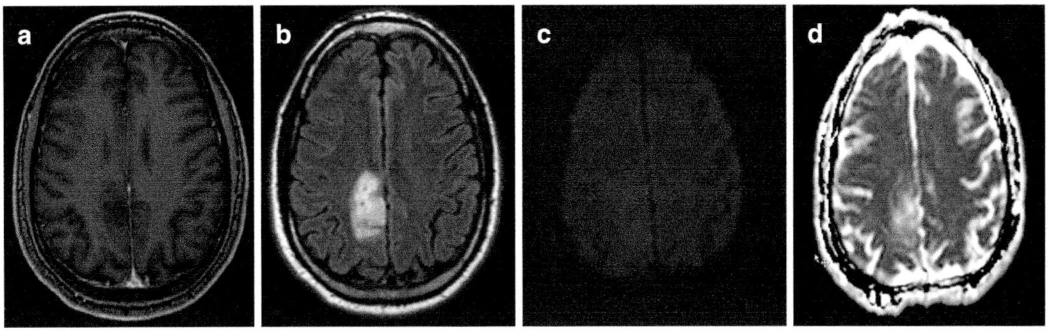

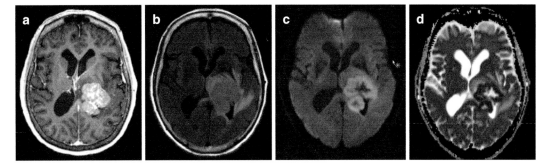

Fig. 3.2 Characteristic axial MR images of a low-grade glioma from a 60-year-old man with incidental finding of a mass lesion. T1-weighted post-contrast (**a**) and T2-weighted FLAIR images (**b**) reveal a non-enhancing T2/FLAIR-hyperintense lesion in the right parieto-occipital lobe, which does not demonstrate restricted diffusion on diffusion-weighted imaging (**c**) and corresponding ADC maps (**d**). Biopsy revealed an *IDH*-mutant grade II oligodendroglioma

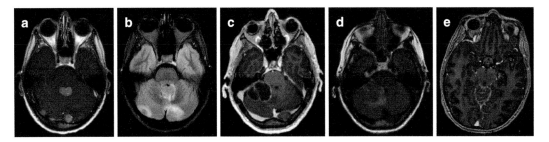

Fig. 3.3 Axial MR images of a 68-year-old woman who was diagnosed with primary CNS lymphoma. T1-weighted post-contrast images (**a**) reveal a heterogeneously enhancing lesion in the left thalamus and atrium of the left lateral ventricle with associated T2/FLAIR hyperintensity (**b**) and obstructive hydrocephalus. There is restricted diffusion on diffusion-weighted imaging (**c**) and corresponding ADC maps (**d**), which is typical of lymphomas

Fig. 3.4 Representative axial MR images of heterogeneous appearance of brain metastases. T1-weighted post-contrast (**a**) and T2-weighted FLAIR images (**b**) in a 46-year-old woman with non-small cell lung cancer (NSCLC) show multiple homogeneously enhancing lesions with associated T2/FLAIR hyperintensity in the posterior fossa, representing solid metastases. Metastases can also be solitary and have a cystic component as seen in a 66-year-old woman with NSCLC (**c** (T1-weighted post-contrast), **d** (T2-weighted FLAIR)). Lastly, metastatic disease can manifest solely in the leptomeninges (**e**); note the leptomeningeal enhancement in the cerebellar folia in this 36-year-old woman with widespread metastatic breast cancer

Furthermore, response criteria have been developed for other tumor entities such as parenchymal and leptomeningeal metastases and meningiomas and recommendations proposed on how to classify response in the setting of immunotherapy (iRANO) [8].

Despite the widespread use of post-contrast T1W and FLAIR sequences, they also have significant shortcomings in certain clinical contexts. For one, contrast enhancement is not specific to malignancy or tumor progression as treatment-induced inflammation can also disrupt the BBB and cause contrast enhancement. These treatment-related MRI changes reflect a spectrum of biologic processes, including pseudoprogression and radiation necrosis. *Pseudoprogression* is a subacute inflammatory process that usually occurs within the first 3 months after completion of chemoradiation and can persist up to 6 months following treatment completion [12]. It is observed in 10–20% of patients with newly diagnosed GBM treated with radiotherapy and temozolomide [13, 14] and more commonly in patients with *MGMT*-methylated gliomas [15] (Fig. 3.5). *Radiation necrosis* typically occurs 3–12 months after completion of radiotherapy but has been observed even years later [16]. It represents a more severe form of treatment-induced inflammation characterized by the presence of necrosis, which is absent in pseudoprogression [17]. Most recently, treatment-related MRI changes have also been increasingly observed after provision of immunotherapy. Immunotherapy stimulates the host's immune system to attack tumor cells and results in a heightened inflammatory response, which is visualized as increased contrast enhancement and FLAIR hyperintensity on MRI [18]. In contrast to pseudoprogression, the opposite MRI effects are seen with anti-angiogenic agents such as bevacizumab, which normalize the tumor vasculature and decrease contrast enhancement, thereby creating the false impression of improved tumor burden [18]. This is referred to as *pseudoresponse* (Fig. 3.6).

FLAIR sequences, while sensitive to most pathologic processes, cannot reliably distinguish between non-enhancing infiltrating tumor, edema, and treatment effect (i.e., gliosis).

Although frequently used to assess the burden of non-enhancing disease in patients on anti-angiogenic therapy, FLAIR does not have prognostic utility [19].

In light of the limitations of T1W post-contrast and FLAIR sequences, a plethora of research has been dedicated to develop more sophisticated MRI techniques that provide a more accurate reflection of the underlying tumor biology. Some of these are becoming more routinely incorporated into clinical practice (e.g., diffusion- and perfusion-weighted MRI and MR spectroscopy), while others are primarily used in the research setting only (e.g., novel perfusion MRI techniques and machine learning).

3.2.2 Diffusion-Weighted and Diffusion Tensor Imaging

3.2.2.1 Diffusion-Weighted Imaging

Principles of Diffusion-Weighted Imaging

Diffusion-weighted imaging (DWI) uses MR sequences sensitized to the intrinsic random (Brownian) motion of water molecules [20, 21]. Using bipolar pulsed gradient methods, this microscopic diffusion is detected by changes in the magnitude of moving spins. The most commonly used method is echo-planar imaging, an ultrafast imaging technique that can acquire images in the range of milliseconds. In biologic tissues, diffusion exists in three modes: free, hindered, and restricted diffusion. Free diffusion, as it occurs in the CSF, refers to the Brownian motion of water molecules due to thermal agitation in the absence of any obstacles [6]. Hindered diffusion describes the delay of passage of water molecules in the extracellular space (e.g. the tumor interstitium) as they navigate around cellular obstacles. This delay is influenced by a variety of factors such as extracellular matrix composition, extracellular volume fraction, and shape of cells [6]. For instance, the extracellular volume fraction tends to be increased in the tumor interstitium due to the presence of vasogenic edema and necrosis, thus giving rise to increased hindered diffusion. Restricted diffusion

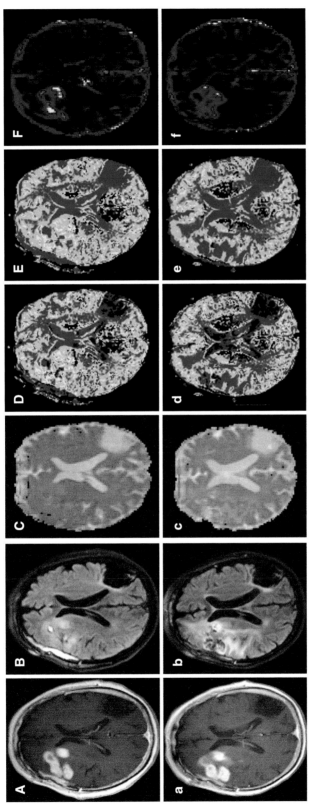

Fig. 3.5 Axial MR images of a patient with a right frontal glioblastoma before (**A–F**) and 4 weeks after treatment with chemoradiation (**a–f**). Pre-treatment T1-weighted post-contrast (**A**) and T2-weighted FLAIR (**B**) images show an enhancing lesion with a mild degree of associated T2/FLAIR hyperintensity in the right frontal lobe. There is little restricted diffusion on the ADC maps (**C**). Perfusion imaging reveals some areas of elevated rCBV (**D**) and rCBF (**E**) on spin-echo sequences as well as increased K^{trans} (**F**). After treatment, there is an increase in the contrast-enhancing (**a**) and FLAIR (**b**) volumes. However, a concomitant increase in ADC values (**c**) and decrease in rCBV (**d**), rCBF (**e**), and K^{trans} (**f**) argue against tumor progression. Overall, these features are suggestive of pseudoprogression

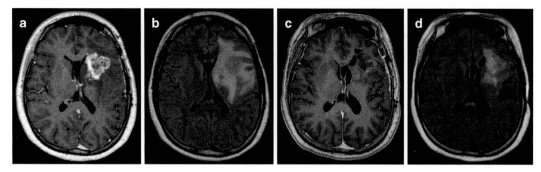

Fig. 3.6 Axial MR images demonstrating pseudo-response in a 30-year-old woman with secondary *IDH*-mutant glioblastoma. T1-weighted post-contrast (**a**) and T2-weighted FLAIR images (**b**) before initiation of bevacizumab reveal avid enhancement (**a**) and extensive T2/FLAIR hyperintensity (**b**) in the left frontotemporal lobe, respectively. Post-contrast (**c**) and FLAIR (**d**) images 4 months after treatment with bevacizumab demonstrate near-complete resolution of enhancement (**c**) and significant reduction in T2/FLAIR hyperintensity (**d**), consistent with pseudoresponse due to bevacizumab-induced normalization of the blood-brain barrier

refers to the trapping of water molecules within a cell bounded by a plasma membrane [6, 22]. Given the increased cellularity in high-grade tumors, restricted diffusion tends to be increased in malignancy.

From a practical standpoint, diffusion is quantitatively expressed by the apparent diffusion coefficient (ADC), which characterizes the rate of diffusional motion (measured in mm^2/s). In tumor imaging, ADC values are typically inversely correlated with cellularity: low ADC values imply increased cellularity and restricted diffusion (as seen in high-grade tumors), while high ADC values are associated with relatively unrestricted diffusion [23]. However, tumor regions tend to contain a mix of tumor cells, edema, and necrosis, therefore making it difficult to interpret ADC values [6, 24, 25]. Thus, although widely used in clinical imaging practice, the ADC lacks specificity for the underlying tumor biology. Much effort is thus being devoted to develop new modeling techniques that more accurately mirror the three-compartment model of diffusion and fit tissue-specific parameters, such as cell size and density, directly to the diffusion signal [26].

Applications of DWI

Despite the abovementioned shortcomings of DWI-derived ADC values, they can still provide important information about tumor biology. For instance, ADC values tend to be decreased in highly cellular tumors such as high-grade gliomas, CNS lymphomas, and medulloblastomas [27–29]. Very low ADC has also been observed in patients with high-grade gliomas [30–33] and metastases treated with bevacizumab [34]. In many patients who underwent additional imaging studies and/or biopsy of the ADC-dark area, hypoperfusion on perfusion MRI, hypometabolism on PET imaging, and areas of necrosis but no viable tumor or radiation effect were seen, suggesting that the low ADC may be a result of bevacizumab-induced chronic hypoxia. ADC values may also be useful in differentiating tumor grades [35, 36]. For example, the mean minimum ADC has been shown to be significantly lower in GBMs than grade III anaplastic astrocytomas [36].

Multiple studies have evaluated the predictive and prognostic utility of DWI. In patients with primary CNS lymphoma, low ADC values in the enhancing region of interest (ROI) correlated with shorter progression-free survival (PFS) and overall survival (OS), whereas the total volume of the enhancing lesion and the number of enhancing lesions did not [27]. Similarly, low pre-treatment tumor ADC in low- and high-grade glioma patients was associated with shorter OS [37, 38], and ADC values were lower in high-grade glioma patients with progressive disease than those with stable disease [36], likely reflecting the more aggressive behavior of tumors with higher cellularity. In addition to absolute ADC values, functional diffusion maps (fDMs) have increasingly been applied to study voxel-wise changes over time. fDMs use co-registered scans from multiple time points and measure ADC changes on a voxel-wise basis, thus enabling quantification of regional tumor changes over time, which is particularly important in heterogeneous tumors like high-grade gliomas [39]. A multitude of studies have shown that increased ADC on fDMs before and after treatment with chemoradiation or adjuvant temozolomide (TMZ) in high-grade glioma patients predicted better PFS and/or OS [40–42].

DWI may also have a role in distinguishing true tumor progression from pseudoprogression: patients with recurrent tumor typically have a lower mean ADC value or ADC ratio (defined as the ratio of the ADC of the enhancing lesion and ADC of the contralateral white matter) than those with pseudoprogression [43–45]. In addition, increasing data suggest that multimodal imaging including DWI can significantly increase the diagnostic accuracy. For example, the addition of perfusion imaging to post-contrast T1W and DW imaging significantly improved the area under the receiver operating characteristic curve from a range of 0.81–0.84 to 0.93–0.96 [46]. Others have reported enhanced discrimination between true progression and pseudoprogression when combining diffusion and perfusion imaging and MR spectroscopy [47, 48]: the diagnostic accuracy was greater than 96% with all three modalities compared to 79–90% with single or dual parameter imaging [47].

3.2.2.2 Diffusion Tensor Imaging (DTI)

Principles of Diffusion Tensor Imaging

The DTI model extends the ADC concept to three-dimensional space and measures ADCs along and perpendicular to the principal axis of diffusion [49], hence interrogating the motion of water with multiple gradient directions [21]. A number of imaging parameters can be calculated from DTI, including fractional anisotropy (FA), mean diffusivity (the average of the three diffusivities in the three orthogonal directions), radial

diffusion (RD; an increase in RD is associated with demyelination), and axial diffusion (AD; a decrease in AD is associated with axonal degeneration and gliosis) [21, 50]. The general concept is that water readily diffuses parallel to the long axis of axons, while diffusion perpendicular to axons is restricted.

Applications of DTI

The most powerful clinical application of DTI lies in the analysis and visualization of neuronal fiber pathways (tractography), which is highly relevant for surgical planning and navigational purposes [21]. In addition, as DTI metrics are generally considered markers of white matter integrity, DTI has the potential to characterize early treatment-induced changes that may not be captured on conventional MRI. For instance, DTI in pediatric medulloblastoma patients treated with combination therapy revealed a reduction in FA by up to 18% in multiple anatomic sites [51]. The magnitude of change in white matter FA was also an independent predictor of IQ scores after adjusting for clinical parameters, suggesting a role for FA as a biomarker to predict treatment-related neurotoxicity in childhood cancer survivors [52]. In adult patients with primary and secondary brain tumors, a transient decrease in FA in normal-appearing white matter (NAWM) was detected as early as 3 months after radiation therapy (RT) [53, 54] with a concomitant reduction in the NAA/Cr ratio on MR spectroscopy [53], possibly reflecting neuronal disruption due to demyelination. More recently, increased radial diffusion in the parahippocampal cingulum at 18 months after completion of RT was identified as an independent predictive marker of cognitive decline in low-grade tumor patients [50].

3.2.3 Perfusion-Weighted Imaging

The utility of perfusion-weighted MR imaging (PWI) in neuro-oncology is based on the notion that tumor vasculature is different from that of normal brain tissue. As tumor cells replicate, they quickly outgrow their existing blood supply and produce pro-angiogenic factors to sustain their growth and metabolic demands. The new tumor vasculature is highly heterogeneous and characterized by dilated, tortuous, and more permeable blood vessels [9, 55].

PWI is most commonly performed in two ways: (1) dynamic imaging of the passage of a contrast agent (accomplished with dynamic susceptibility contrast (DSC) and dynamic contrast enhancement (DCE) techniques) and (2) imaging of magnetically labeled endogenous protons in blood (accomplished with arterial spin labeling (ASL)) [20]. A number of parameters can be quantified with each PWI method, including cerebral blood volume (CBV), cerebral blood flow (CBF), mean transit time, and vessel permeability. Collectively, these parameters provide complementary information about the tumor vasculature and different biologic processes [56].

3.2.3.1 Dynamic Susceptibility Contrast (DSC) MRI

Principles of DSC MRI
DSC MRI is a T2- or T2*-weighted technique based on the acquisition of gradient-echo or spin-echo-planar images during first-pass transit of an exogenous, paramagnetic contrast agent through the brain. This contrast agent produces a decrease in signal intensity. Using signal-time curves and tracer kinetic modeling, voxel-wise changes in contrast agent concentration can be determined and various metrics calculated [57]. The most commonly reported DSC metrics are relative cerebral blood volume (rCBV) and cerebral blood flow (rCBF). CBV reflects the volume of blood in tissue, while CBF measures the speed of blood flow through tissue [56]. CBV is typically elevated in tumors due to an increase in vessel number and size and correlates strongly with tumor grade and response to therapy [56]. Of note, areas of elevated CBV do not necessarily correlate with elevated CBF as blood flow may be slowed in the more tortuous tumor vasculature and as a result of mechanical vessel compression [58, 59].

While DSC MRI may be available in clinical practice and quick to perform, it has a number of shortcomings. DSC MRI is based on the assumption that the contrast agent remains intravascular which is frequently not the case with brain tumors as breakdown of the BBB permits contrast leakage into the extravascular-extracellular space. This contrast extravasation produces a "T1 shine-through effect" and causes underestimation of the CBV [20]. To adjust for T1 shine-through effects, a preload of contrast can be administered before acquiring the dynamic data, followed by model-based post-processing leakage correction [60]. Other methods include the use of low flip angles or longer repetition times and echo times to reduce T1 contamination although this occurs at the expense of a lower signal-to-noise ratio of the CBV maps [20, 57, 61].

Applications of DSC MRI
Tumor rCBV values are typically higher in high-grade than low-grade gliomas [62] although rCBV does not appear to be sufficiently sensitive to reliably distinguish between grade III and IV gliomas [20]. rCBV may help distinguish between low-grade glioma subtypes: grade II oligodendrogliomas have demonstrated higher maximum rCBV values than grade II astrocytoma [63]. Furthermore, peritumoral rCBV has been shown to be higher in gliomas than metastases [62, 64].

rCBV may be superior than standard T1W post-contrast and FLAIR sequences in assessing treatment response. For instance, mean rCBV at 1 month after completion of chemoradiation in GBM patients was a strong predictor of OS, while a change in size of the enhancing tumor was not [65]. Similar to functional diffusion maps in DWI, parametric response maps (PRMs) may represent a more accurate method to assess spatial and temporal voxel-wise changes than whole-tumor mean or median values, given that heterogeneous changes in blood volume and flow are not captured by averaging values on whole-tumor measurements. For instance, the mean change in tumor perfusion did not predict OS, whereas rCBV and rCBF PRMs at 1 and 3 weeks post-chemoradiation did [66].

Given the effects of anti-angiogenic therapy on tumor vasculature, rCBV has been shown to be a more reliable measure of treatment response to these agents compared to anatomical imaging. Using leakage correction and standardized rCBV values (stdRCBV; a method that takes into account variabilities in measurement across MR scanner models and field strength), Schmainda et al. found that increased pre- and post-bevacizumab stdRCBV were predictive of shorter OS in recurrent high-grade glioma patients [67]. Furthermore, in the ACRIN 6677 trial (a collaboration with the RTOG 0625 trial in which recurrent GBM patients received either bevacizumab plus irinotecan or TMZ), a reduction in stdRCBV and normalized rCBV (to normal-appearing white matter) at 2 and 16 weeks after initiating bevacizumab was associated with improved OS [68]. By contrast, rCBV changes at 8 weeks did not correlate with OS [68, 69]. Contrary to the aforementioned data, a study of patients with newly diagnosed GBM treated with cediranib (a pan-VEGF receptor tyrosine kinase inhibitor) revealed that OS was 6 months longer in the group with an early increase in subnormal tumor perfusion than in the group with stable or decreased perfusion [70, 71]. The authors argued that this may be related to improved drug and oxygen delivery early during the critical time period of chemoradiation. Overall, however, these studies support the notion that the interpretation of perfusion MRI strongly depends on the timing of imaging, given that vascular remodeling is a highly dynamic and complex process, as well as on the specific parameter measured.

Lastly, rCBV can help distinguish between tumor progression and pseudoprogression. In one study comparing pre- and posttreatment rCBVs, patients with pseudoprogression had a mean rCBV decrease of 41%, whereas those with progressive disease had a mean rCBV increase of 12% following treatment [65]. In addition, as more immunotherapy agents are being tested in brain tumor patients, DSC MRI may assume an increasingly important role in characterizing immunotherapy-associated imaging changes. An early retrospective report of GBM patients treated with a dendritic cell vaccine, for instance, showed that rCBV ratios were higher in those with progressive disease than pseudoprogression [72].

Despite the numerous strengths of DSC MRI, its practical and universal implementation has been hampered by the uncertainty about the optimal standardization approach, especially pertaining to post-processing methods [56, 73]. The Jump Starting Brain Tumor Coalition and National Institutes of Health-funded Quantitative Imaging Network are collaborative groups that aim to create a standardized start-to-end analysis pipeline to facilitate the translation of perfusion imaging beyond the research setting and optimize imaging protocols for clinical trials [74].

3.2.3.2 Dynamic Contrast-Enhanced (DCE) MRI

Principles of DCE MRI
DCE MRI uses dynamic T1-weighted sequences to measure changes in signal intensity before, during, and after the passage of contrast agent, thus providing a quantitative measure of leakage of contrast agent across the BBB [57]. The most commonly applied pharmacokinetic model is based on the presence of two compartments (plasma and extravascular-extracellular spaces) and the modeling of three main imaging biomarkers: extravascular-extracellular (v_e) and plasma (v_p) space volume fractions and the transfer constant coefficient (K^{trans}). K^{trans} is a composite marker of vascular permeability, vessel surface area, and blood flow. Under conditions of low permeability where there is limited contrast agent leakage, K^{trans} is considered a surrogate marker of microvascular permeability. In the setting of high permeability, however, K^{trans} also reflects blood flow since permeability is limited by the blood flow to a particular area [75]. Theoretically, DCE MRI has numerous advantages over DSC MRI, including higher spatial and temporal resolution, the ability to measure permeability, and less sensitivity to susceptibility artifacts, but the optimal model of the contrast bolus needs to be established [76, 77].

Applications of DCE MRI
K^{trans} can help predict tumor grade, with higher-grade tumors demonstrating higher K^{trans} than lower-grade tumors, presumably due to increased

capillary permeability associated with more malignant lesions [78–80]. In addition, numerous studies in recurrent GBM patients have underpinned the potential of pre-treatment or early decrease in K^{trans} to predict response to anti-angiogenic therapy [71, 81, 82]. For example, a decrease in K^{trans} as early as 24 hours within cediranib administration correlated positively with OS and/or PFS [81].

Given that K^{trans} reflects vascular permeability and thus BBB permeability, it may be the optimal tool to study critical time points when chemotherapy delivery to the tumor is most efficacious. This is particularly relevant when administering cytotoxic chemotherapy with concomitant anti-angiogenic therapy which may normalize the tumor vasculature and improve blood flow to underperfused tumor areas, thus theoretically enhancing drug delivery. Unfortunately, the dose-response relationship appears to differ between different anti-angiogenic agents and complicates the interpretation of the biologic effects of these agents on tumor vasculature. For instance, a reduction in K^{trans} seems to correlate with the administered dose of cediranib, vatalanib, pazopanib, and sorafenib, but this linear relationship does not apply to other agents such as telatinib and motesanib [83]. Further studies will be required to help elucidate critical time windows for enhanced drug delivery.

Recent work has demonstrated potential long-term retention of gadolinium-based contrast agents (GBCA) in various brain regions after repeated GBCA injections for contrast-enhanced MRIs, including the dentate nucleus and globus pallidus [84–88]. This has raised concerns about the safety of multiple GBCA injections as would occur, for instance, in the setting of a DSC MRI study with a pre-dose to aid in leakage correction. The use of multiple spin- and gradient-echo (SAGE) echo-planar imaging (EPI) potentially allows for simultaneous measurement of CBV and CBF as well as DCE MRI-derived parameters such as K^{trans} and v_e [61, 89, 90]. SAGE EPI may thus represent a promising tool to simultaneously compute perfusion and permeability data while limiting GBCA exposure to one contrast bolus. However, the clinical significance of GBCA accumulation is unknown, and data with newer GBCA agents is lacking.

3.2.3.3 Arterial Spin Labeling (ASL)

ASL uses magnetic labeling of endogenous inflowing protons in arterial blood to quantify CBF and thus does not require administration of an exogenous contrast agent. The label is created by applying a radiofrequency pulse that inverts the bulk magnetization of protons in blood [91]. After the labeling and inflow period, images are obtained through rapid acquisition techniques such as echo-planar imaging and gradient- and spin-echo imaging [91]. These images are always acquired as a pair of a labeled image (in which the blood water magnetization is inverted) and a control image (in which the blood water magnetization is not inverted) [91]. Subtraction of these labeled and control images will subsequently generate CBF maps. The potential advantage of ASL over DSC MRI is that it does not depend on accurate estimation of a rapid intravascular bolus of contrast and does not require application of complicated post-processing leakage-correction algorithms [91]. However, while ASL can provide relatively accurate measures of absolute CBF in normal brain tissue, this ability is compromised in tumors due to irregular and nonlinear blood flow patterns [20]. In addition, ASL sequences have a relatively poor signal-to-noise ratio which can lead to inaccuracies in CBF measurements [20]. While some sites routinely incorporate ASL in their clinical imaging protocols, others primarily use it as a research tool.

3.2.3.4 Vessel Caliber MRI

The theoretical basis of vessel caliber MRI dates back to the early 1990s [92, 93], but its implementation beyond the research setting has in part been prevented by its relatively complex acquisition protocol. It requires both gradient (GE) and spin-echo (SE) protocols which combined capture large- and small-caliber vessels. Vessel caliber MRI provides estimates of average vessel diameters and vessel densities of arteries, capillaries, and veins per image voxel, commonly referred to as the vessel size index (VSI) [94]. It can be performed using DSC MRI, super-paramagnetic iron oxide nanoparticles (see below), or blood-oxy-gen-level-dependent (BOLD) MRI [94]. Each of these techniques is based on specific biologic a priori assumptions and has inherent advantages and/or limitations with regard to temporal and spatial resolution and signal-to-noise ratio [94]. Vessel caliber MRI has revealed larger vessel calibers and a wider spectrum of caliber size with increasing tumor grade [94–96], reflecting the highly abnormal vasculature of cancers. A special type of vessel caliber MRI, termed vessel architectural imaging (VAI), measures the relative difference between arteriole and venule oxygen saturation and thus provides an estimate of oxygen consumption. In newly diagnosed and recurrent GBM patients treated with cediranib monotherapy or in combination with chemoradiation, there was a reduction in vessel caliber as early as 1 day after initiation of treatment [70, 97]. In addition, those with a reduction in vessel caliber and improved SO_2 concentrations had improved OS and PFS compared to those who did not manifest these changes [97]. Thus, vessel caliber imaging may serve as a useful imaging biomarker in future clinical trials.

3.2.3.5 Estimation of Capillary Transit Time Heterogeneity

Another novel technique that attempts to quantify the heterogeneity of tumor vasculature and differential distribution of microvascular flow patterns is capillary transit time heterogeneity (CTTH). Unlike in normal tissue, where regional availability of oxygen is a function of cerebral blood flow and arterial oxygen concentration, blood flow and oxygen extraction from tumor capillaries is altered due to due to differences in transit times through these capillaries [98, 99]. CTTH can be estimated using DSC or DCE MRI [100, 101]. Further validation studies could potentially advance our understanding of the complex underlying tumor biology and tumor response to treatment, particularly anti-angiogenic agents.

3.2.3.6 Iron Oxide Nanoparticles

Ferumoxytol is an ultrasmall supermagnetic iron oxide with a large particle size (molecular weight approximately 750 kD, compared to 600 D for gadoteridol [102]) which prevents it from significantly leaking across a damaged BBB [103], thus bypassing the challenges associated with extravascular gadolinium-based contrast agent (GBCA) leakage in conventional DSC MRI. Ferumoxytol enhancement is based on its intracellular uptake by phagocytic white blood cells, reactive astrocytes, microglia, and dendritic cells in pathologic tissue [102]. Compared to GBCA where enhancement is immediate after injection, ferumoxytol enhancement peaks around 24–48 h [103]. It has been used to create steady-state CBV maps, which demonstrated good consistency with conventional DSC MRI-derived CBV maps as well as improved contrast-to-noise ratios and less motion artifact [104]. Preliminary data also suggest a role of ferumoxytol rCBV to help distinguish between true progression and pseudoprogression after chemoradiation [105]. Unlike GBCA, ferumoxytol is not renally cleared and may be a useful MRI contrast agent in patients with renal impairment. However, it currently carries a boxed warning due to potentially fatal allergic reactions, which has limited enthusiasm for its use [106].

3.2.4   Chemical MR Imaging

3.2.4.1 Magnetic Resonance Spectroscopy

Principles of Magnetic Resonance Spectroscopy

While water is the most abundant molecule in brain tissue and generates the strongest signal on MR imaging, other protons bound to macromolecules also produce signals albeit on a much smaller scale, reflecting their low concentration in tissue [20]. These macromolecule-bound protons demonstrate small variations in the Larmor frequency which are expressed in parts per million (ppm) in relation to a known reference frequency [20]. MR spectroscopy (MRS) is a technique that detects these frequency peaks by suppressing the large water peak, thus providing information about the chemical composition of the brain. The most important molecular spectra measured with ^{1}H (proton) MRS are *N*-acetylaspartate (NAA; a measure of neuronal integrity), choline (Cho; a marker of cell membrane turnover), creatinine (Cr; a marker of energy metabolism), lactate (a surrogate for non-oxidative glycolysis, necrosis, and hypoxia), myoinositol (related to astrocytic integrity and regulation of brain osmosis), and lipid (a marker of cellular necrosis) [107–109].

MRS can be performed using a single-voxel technique to an ROI (single-voxel spectroscopy) vs. a 2D or 3D technique that captures a larger target region (chemical shift imaging (CSI)). The latter requires longer acquisition times although recent advances in the field have enabled shortening of scan times [107]. Of note, the presence of bone or air-tissue interfaces can significantly decrease the technical quality of the spectra and should thus be excluded from the ROI during image acquisition [107].

Other MRS techniques include ^{31}P (phosphorus) and ^{13}C (carbon) MRS but are less commonly used than ^{1}H MRS [107]. In addition, with the discovery of the prognostic significance of isocitrate dehydrogenase (*IDH*) mutations in gliomas, much interest in the field has focused on CSI of the oncometabolite of the *IDH* mutation, 2-hydroxyglutarate (2HG).

Applications of MR Spectroscopy

There is ample evidence that MRS can distinguish between low- and high-grade tumors since high-grade lesions are associated with elevated Cho/NAA and Cho/Cr ratios [110–113] and decreased NAA levels [112, 113] and NAA/Cr ratios [110]. MRS has also been studied as a tool to differentiate between intratumoral vs. peritumoral areas. For instance, peritumoral Cho/Cr and Cho/NAA ratios are higher in high-grade gliomas than brain metastases [114], likely reflecting the infiltrating nature of gliomas into the surrounding brain parenchyma and disruption of the normal neuronal architecture. This is biologically distinct from the peritumoral region in metastases which primarily consists of vasogenic edema and few tumor cells.

MRS has demonstrated some utility in distinguishing between tumor progression and radiation-induced changes. Characteristically, progressive tumors exhibit higher Cho/Cr and Cho/NAA ratios and lower Cho/NAA ratios than radiation injury [44, 115, 116]. However, the spectral patterns may be less definitive when the ROI contains a mix of both tumor and necrosis, e.g., after provision of RT. A recent meta-analysis found that the ability of MRS to differentiate tumor recurrence from radiation necrosis was moderate at best and advocated for a combined multimodal imaging approach to improve diagnostic accuracy [117].

2HG MRS is an advanced method to noninvasively probe the presence of 2HG, the oncometabolite of the *IDH* mutation, which accumulates in high concentrations in *IDH*-mutant gliomas [118]. Given that 2HG is only present at trace levels in cells lacking the *IDH* mutation and 99% of *IDH*-mutant tumors express 2HG at significantly higher levels, 2HG appears to be a highly sensitive and specific marker of *IDH*-mutant gliomas [119]. Multiple studies have confirmed the reliable *in vivo* detection of 2HG in *IDH*-mutant-gliomas using CSI [120, 121]. At some institutions, including ours, 2HG MRS has been used as a research tool to guide neurosurgical planning. For example, a gross total resection of an *IDH*-mutant glioma is considered a good prognostic factor in young patients [122], and pre-surgical confirmation of this mutation may help in surgical decision-making. It has also been shown that 2HG levels decrease significantly after treatment with radiation and TMZ, raising the exciting potential of 2HG as a more accurate marker of true tumor burden than contrast enhancement [123]. Furthermore, investigators have begun to routinely incorporate 2HG MRS as an additional response assessment tool in *IDH* inhibitor trials; the final results of these trials have yet to be announced. A few caveats should be highlighted, however. MRS can occasionally fail to detect 2HG if 2HG concentrations are very low as can occur in tumors with low cellularity or following treatment [119]. In addition, accurate localization of the 2HG signal is heavily technique-dependent and requires customized *in vivo* MRS sequences such as localized adiabatic spin-echo refocusing (LASER), J-difference spectroscopy, and 2D correlation spectroscopy [119].

3.2.4.2 pH-Weighted Molecular MRI

Tumor tissue is characterized by a markedly abnormal microenvironment both in the intra- and extracellular space. The extracellular pH value is in the acidic range (6.2–6.9) compared to normal tissue (7.3–7.4) [124], which leads to decreased immune function and promotes tumor invasion, angiogenesis, and resistance to therapy [125, 126]. Chemical exchange-dependent saturation transfer (CEST) MRI is a novel imaging technique sensitive to the chemical exchange between protons on the functional groups of metabolites such as hydroxyls, amides, and amines [127]. The chemical exchange rate varies with alterations in hydrogen ion activity as occurs in the tumor microenvironment and is reflected by changes in the CEST contrast [127]. Amide proton transfer (APT) MRI, a CEST MRI method which detects amide protons of endogenous mobile proteins and peptides in tissue, has been applied successfully to distinguish between glioma grades in humans [128] and between radiation necrosis and viable glioma tissue in rat models [129]. Specifically, APT signal intensity was shown to increase with higher histologic grade [128]. Analogously, radiation necrosis appears APT-hypo- to isointense, while true tumor is APT-hyperintense [129]. A more recently developed CEST MRI technique targets amine protons on glutamine (which is produced at higher concentrations in tumor tissue [130]) and demonstrated that those with stable or growing acidic lesions after surgery recurred more quickly after chemoradiation than those with lower acidity lesions [127]. As with APT MRI, amine CEST MRI demonstrated increasing signal intensity with higher tumor grade [131].

3.2.5 Radiomics and Machine Learning

3.2.5.1 Principles of Radiomics and Machine Learning

One of the main challenges in tumor imaging is to adequately capture and characterize tumor heterogeneity. While standard radiology reports often contain subjective descriptors such as "moderate heterogeneity," "highly spiculated," and "significant enhancement," these do not provide any reliable information about the underlying tumor biology. Radiomics refers to the comprehensive quantification of tumor phenotypes by extracting and mining a large number of quantitative image features from CT, PET, or MR imaging via a high-throughput approach [132]. These data are then used to relate image characteristics to phenotypes or gene-protein signatures and to provide diagnostic, prognostic, and predictive information [132]. The general process of radiomics is reviewed in detail elsewhere but includes (1) image acquisition and reconstruction, (2) image segmentation and rendering, (3) feature extraction and feature qualification, (4) database formation and data sharing, and (5) ad hoc informatics analyses [132]. Common features that are routinely extracted are tumor intensity histograms (e.g., high vs. low contrast), tumor shape (e.g., round vs. spiculated), texture patterns (e.g., homogeneous vs. heterogeneous), and tumor location. Once extracted, the imaging features from the development or discovery cohort are then validated in an independent validation cohort, e.g., data from The Cancer Genome Atlas (TCGA) [132, 133].

Machine learning is a form of artificial intelligence which uses computer algorithms to learn complex relationships or patterns [134]. It can be applied to a number of scenarios such as image segmentation, image registration, and functional image analysis (e.g., using physiologic MR images) to improve diagnostic, predictive, and prognostic accuracy compared to that of an expert radiology reader [134, 135].

3.2.5.2 Applications of Radiomics and Machine Learning

There is emerging evidence that radiomics may provide clinically useful information in GBM patients. Itakura et al. identified three distinct "clusters" in newly diagnosed GBM based on tumor shape, texture, and edge sharpness, named "pre-multifocal," "spherical," and "rim-enhancing" [133]. Importantly, each of these clusters was associated with distinct up- or downregulation of specific molecular pathways and correlated significantly with survival probabilities [133]. The potential to build a risk stratification model based on radiomic signature was further underscored in a later study [136]. Using a similar radiomics approach, a prediction and risk stratification model to predict response to bevacizumab and OS was generated in recurrent GBM patients [137].

Machine learning has also been increasingly explored in the clinical setting. Zacharaki et al. applied multiple machine learning techniques to classify brain tumors by attributes extracted from neoplastic, necrotic, and edematous regions of interest on conventional and perfusion MRI. Using this method, they achieved a 97% and 95% classification accuracy for primary vs. secondary brain tumors and low- vs. high-grade gliomas, respectively [138]. The ability of machine learning to predict molecular glioma subgroups remains to be established. A recent machine learning-based classification study only demonstrated moderate accuracy in predicting *EGFR* amplification status (61%) and *RTK II* subgroups (63%) [139]. Similarly, an algorithm aimed to predict *IDH* status based on MR imaging and clinical features only achieved accuracies of 86% and 89% in the training and validation cohort, respectively [140]. Although this approach may be useful in the pre-surgical setting, it remains inferior to the sensitivity of 94% and specificity of 100% of *IDH1* testing by immunohistochemistry [141]. From a prognostic value standpoint, Emblem et al. demonstrated that the use of presurgical whole-tumor rCBV maps combined with a support vector machine model had higher diagnostic accuracy than expert reader values for 6-month to 3-year survival associations in glioma patients [135]. Similarly, using a prediction model consisting of extent of resection, mass effect, contrast-enhancing volume, maximum B0 intensity, and mean trace intensity in the non-enhancing region, survival could be predicted with 85% accuracy. Importantly, this prediction model appeared to correlate more accurately with survival than histopathology [142].

As with other advanced MRI techniques, radiomics and machine learning are largely research tools, and their utility in clinical practice remains to be validated within larger-scale

multi-institutional studies. In addition, *how* the computer algorithm determines patterns and associations and makes specific decisions is an area of active research. While these techniques will unlikely replace standard histopathology in the initial diagnosis of most brain tumors, they may prove valuable in the diagnosis of surgically inaccessible lesions (e.g., in the brainstem) and monitoring of tumors.

3.3 Positron Emission Tomography (PET) Imaging of CNS Tumors

3.3.1 General Principles of PET

Positron emission tomography (PET) is a functional imaging technique which registers pairs of gamma rays emitted indirectly by a positron-emitting radionuclide. In brief, a radionuclide undergoes positive beta decay by emitting a positron, which travels in tissue for a very short distance until it interacts with an electron. This leads to the annihilation of both positron and electron and the consecutive emission of a pair of gamma photons, which are moving in approximately $180°$ direction and are coincidentally registered by a detector ring. Most modern PET scanners have an integrated CT scanner, which enables simultaneous acquisition of morphological information.

PET uses radioisotopes with relatively short half-lives, in particular ^{18}F (110 min), ^{68}Ga (68 min), or ^{11}C (20 min), which are incorporated into compounds that are either used in metabolic pathways or bind to receptors. Due to the radioactive label, these compounds and their distribution within the body can be traced after intravenous injection, thus explaining the expression "PET tracer."

3.3.2 Commonly Used PET Tracers and Clinical Applications

The choice of the PET tracer for a study depends on the underlying type of neoplasm (Table 3.1). While radioactive-labeled amino acids are

Table 3.1 Overview of main clinical indications of PET imaging for different types of brain tumors, used radiopharmaceuticals, and depicted metabolic function

Brain tumor type	Indication	Radiopharmaceutical	Metabolic function depicted
Glioma	• Differential diagnostics and tumor grading • Biopsy planning, including demarcation of "hot spots" • Delineation of tumor boundaries for treatment planning • Evaluation of therapy response (including detection of pseudoresponse) • Differentiation between post-therapeutic changes and tumor tissue (including detection of pseudo-progression)	• ^{18}F-FET • ^{18}F-FDOPA • ^{11}C-MET	Amino acid transport
Meningioma	• Registering tumor extension (in particular bone infiltration) • Detection of additional meningiomas in multifocal cases • Differentiation between recurrence and post-therapeutic changes/gliosis • Registering the occupancy at receptors for evaluation of possible ^{177}Lu-DOTA-TATE/-TOC therapy	• ^{68}Ga-DOTATATE • ^{68}Ga-DOTATOC	Somatostatin receptor expression
Metastases	• Differentiation between radionecrosis and recurrence	• ^{18}F-FET • ^{18}F-FDOPA • ^{11}C-MET	Amino acid transport
CNS lymphoma	• Differential diagnosis • Evaluation of therapy response	• ^{18}F-FDG • ^{18}F-FET • ^{18}F-FDOPA • ^{11}C-MET	Glucose metabolism Amino acid transport

Adapted with permission from [211]

particularly useful in gliomas as well as brain metastases, labeled somatostatin receptor ligands find use for meningiomas, and labeled glucose is preferred for CNS lymphomas. PET investigations can provide complementary information to MRI about tumor biology, for example, regarding metabolic rate and vitality of tumor cells or the expression of particular receptors.

3.3.2.1 ^{18}F-FDG

Principles of ^{18}F-FDG PET
The most widely available and frequently used PET tracer in general oncology is the radioactively labeled sugar 2-deoxy-2-[^{18}F]fluoro-D-glucose (^{18}F-FDG), which is incorporated into cells by glucose-specific transporters and trapped intracellularly due to phosphorylation processes [143]. As tumor cells characteristically display increased glucose consumption, tumors can be visualized by enhanced ^{18}F-FDG uptake.

Applications of ^{18}F-FDG PET
Although ^{18}F-FDG PET has evolved as a helpful imaging tool for a broad range of oncologic diseases, it is not of great value in neuro-oncologic diagnostics [144]. The reason for this lies in the physiologically high cerebral metabolic rate and consequently high ^{18}F-FDG trapping in healthy brain tissue, which imparts poor visualization of tumor boundaries and a limited sensitivity for tumor detection, particularly for low-grade gliomas (Fig. 3.7). Furthermore, the specificity of ^{18}F-FDG for brain tumor diagnostics is significantly limited, given that inflammatory processes such as abscesses or postradiation changes also show increased glucose consumption and can consequently not be reliably differentiated from tumor tissues [144]. Therefore, the use of ^{18}F-FDG for brain tumor imaging is limited to aggressive CNS lymphomas and rarely GBMs.

Due to their high cell density and their massively increased glucose metabolic rate, CNS

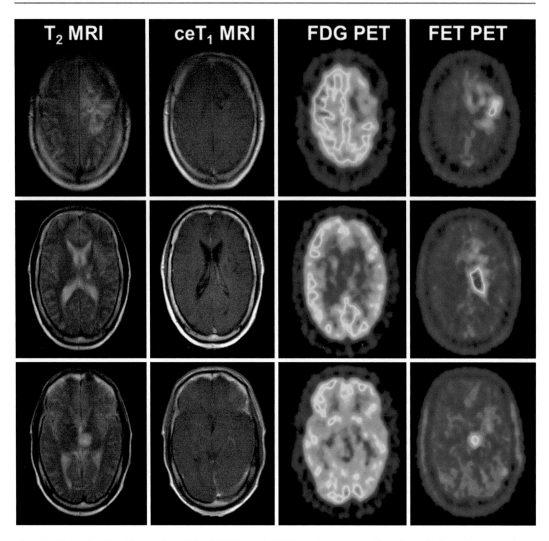

T₂ MRI **ceT₁ MRI** **FDG PET** **FET PET**

Fig. 3.7 Example of a patient with multifocal WHO grade III oligoastrocytoma in the left hemisphere: the tumor shows high amino acid uptake on the FET PET images, while no glucose uptake is found on the FDG PET scan

lymphomas typically show an ^{18}F-FDG uptake that is distinctly higher than the intrinsically high physiological background activity of cerebral cortex. The uptake of ^{18}F-FDG in lymphomas is also significantly higher than in inflammatory lesions and GBMs although this can vary depending on whether or not the patient is receiving steroids [3]. During ongoing steroid therapy, ^{18}F-FDG uptake declines and becomes comparable to that in GBM. The response to therapy can be well ascertained on the basis of ^{18}F-FDG PET, which reveals a therapeutic response by virtue of a normalization of glucose metabolism that precedes changes to exclusively morphologic

imaging techniques [145]. Lymphomas also show an elevated uptake of amino acid tracers albeit to a lesser extent than with ^{18}F-FDG PET. Similar to gliomas, amino acid PET permits better demarcation of healthy brain tissue, likewise showing a similarly high sensitivity for the detection of lymphoma tissue [146].

Due to improvements in oncologic treatments in recent years and the resultant improved life expectancy of cancer patients, the occurrence of cerebral metastases has increased. In the context of routine whole-body staging with ^{18}F-FDG PET/CT diagnostics, for example, in cases with bronchial cancer or malignant melanoma, the brain is often included in the staging examination, although the physiologically high ^{18}F-FDG uptake in healthy brain tissue limits the ability to detect intracerebral metastases [147]. Therefore, the use of amino acid tracers is more useful than ^{18}F-FDG for imaging of brain metastases but, thus far, there have only been few amino acid PET studies evaluating cerebral metastases.

3.3.2.2 Amino Acid Tracers

Principles of Amino Acid PET

Due to the abovementioned limited value of ^{18}F-FDG, amino acid tracers have gained increasing importance for brain tumor PET imaging [148] as they show low physiologic uptake in healthy brain tissue and minor uptake in inflammatory lesions [2, 3, 5]. Of note, amino acid PET has been used more widely in Europe than in the USA, which is partly related to reimbursement issues from insurance companies. The most widely used amino acid PET tracers in the clinic are O-(2-[^{18}F]fluoroethyl)-L-tyrosine (^{18}F-FET), [^{11}C]-methionine (^{11}C-MET), and 3,4-dihydroxy-6-[^{18}F]-fluoro-L-phenylalanine (^{18}F-FDOPA). Because of the short physical half-life of [11]C (20 min), the use of ^{11}C-MET is limited to centers with an on-site cyclotron, while the long-lived ^{18}F-labeled tracers (half-life 110 min) are more widely available and applicable [3].

The uptake of amino acid tracers into the tumor cells is mediated via the L-amino acid transporter system, which is overexpressed in neoplastic cells but not in nonneoplastic cells. In contrast to ^{18}F-FDG, amino acids therefore provide a high contrast between tumor and healthy brain tissue even in low-grade malignancies such as grade II oligodendroglial tumors [149] (Fig. 3.7). Although tumoral uptake in static PET images is reported to be comparable using the different amino acid tracers, ^{18}F-FDOPA is characterized by physiologically increased uptake in the striatum, therefore limiting its use for glioma delineation in patients with tumors in close proximity to the striatum.

Applications of Amino Acid PET in Gliomas

Gliomas are the main brain tumors investigated with amino acid PET in clinical practice, both at the time of diagnosis and during the course of the disease [148]. Amino acid PET can be helpful in a variety of settings, including narrowing down the differential diagnosis, tumor grading, biopsy and therapy planning, assessment of treatment response, and prognostication.

Gliomas usually present with distinctly elevated amino acid tracer uptake, which, in part, correlates with the WHO histologic tumor grade [150–152]. Of note, high-grade tumors display heightened uptake in about 95% of cases, whereas this is the case in only around 70% of low-grade tumors [153, 154]. Thus, an inconspicuous PET finding does not exclude a low-grade tumor, while elevated uptake makes the presence of a glioma very likely. Intense tracer uptake has only rarely been described in nonneoplastic acutely inflamed lesions such as active demyelinated plaque of multiple sclerosis or abscesses [155, 156].

Even though the tracer uptake in high-grade gliomas is significantly elevated compared to low-grade gliomas, there is considerable overlap in the uptake values (measured as tumor-to-background ratio) between groups, which limits the accuracy of tumor grading based on *static* tumor-to-background values [150]. With *dynamic* data acquisition lasting 40–50 min, however, high- and low-grade gliomas can be distinguished by characteristic time courses. This is accomplished by analyzing uptake behavior during the recording period (defined as the "time-activity curve"): low-grade gliomas typically display increasing time-dependent uptake kinetics, whereas high-grade gliomas show declining kinetics [149, 157, 158]. Through this kinetic analysis, high-grade tumors can be detected with a sensitivity of more than 90% [159]. The validity of kinetics in dynamic recordings has only been demonstrated for ^{18}F-FET but not for ^{11}C-MET or ^{18}F-FDOPA [160, 161]. One must note, however, that dynamic ^{18}F-FET recording and evaluation are time-consuming compared to conventional static ^{18}F-FET recordings (approximately 40–50 min vs. 20 min) and have thus far only been employed in a few specialized centers.

PET as an additional imaging procedure to conventional MRI has particular significance for biopsy planning of tumors that do not enhance on MRI and thus may fail to depict the most malignant tumor area. Consequently, a heterogeneous glioma can be "undergraded." Amino acid PET may reliably reveal regions of increased metabolism [157, 162–164]. In particular, additional dynamic ^{18}F-FET PET evaluation was valuable for the identification of most aggressive tumor regions within a heterogeneous glioma, as measured by decreased kinetics, and can thus guide biopsy planning [157].

In addition to biopsy planning, amino acid PET can be useful for therapy planning. Numerous studies have shown that tumor extent on conventional MR imaging does not always correspond to the true histologic tumor extent [165]. In comparative studies of biologic and morphologic tumor volumes of high-grade gliomas, the PET volume frequently extends beyond the territory of pathologic contrast enhancement, with the implication that PET can reliably depict tumor regions lacking a disturbance of the BBB [162, 166]. Also, in gliomas without contrast enhancement, the detection of tumor boundaries with MR presents a challenge, as the separation of tumor tissue and peritumoral edema can be difficult. Moreover, areas with high-grade tumor tissue might not be depicted [167]. In surgical planning, an accurate delineation of tumor boundaries plays a decisive role, especially when eloquent brain areas are involved [168]. The postoperative biologic tumor volume exposed to chemoradiation has prognostic value, and a small residual tumor volume is associated with improved survival. As such, knowledge of the preoperative tumor volume should be incorporated into surgical planning to afford maximal resection [169, 170]. Studies focusing on recurrence after radiation therapy suggest that the inclusion of biologic PET volume is helpful for determining the correct target volume [171, 172]. Whether PET-based radiation therapy is associated with improved survival is a matter of ongoing studies.

As outlined previously in this chapter, multiple factors, including pseudoprogression and pseudoresponse, can make it challenging to accurately guide response assessment with conventional MR

imaging [2, 173]. Unlike gadolinium-based contrast agent, uptake of radiolabeled amino acids is not a function of BBB integrity, and the use of amino acid PET thus represents an efficient complementary imaging modality to assess disease course and treatment response [2]. For instance, by means of ^{18}F-FET PET, malignant progression of low-grade gliomas can be detected independent of any concomitant changes in MR contrast enhancement [174, 175], such that timely application of appropriate therapeutic measures can be undertaken.

Chemotherapy presents an important therapy option for patients with a low-grade glioma, especially when resection or irradiation of the tumor cannot be performed due to its location. The treatment response assessment in gliomas without contrast enhancement is usually based on changes of the tumor size on T2/FLAIR-weighted MR images. Such changes of tumor size can indeed be detected with a remarkable time delay after initiation of therapy, while changes of the metabolically active tumor volume on amino acid PET can be seen earlier, resulting in an earlier assessment of treatment response [176]. Also, in high-grade gliomas, a reduction in the metabolically active tumor volume shortly after (radio-)chemotherapy is associated with therapeutic response and improved patient survival [177].

Amino acid PET is of particular significance in the assessment of treatment response after anti-angiogenic therapy and may help overcome the problem of interpreting pseudoresponse. With PET, the regions containing vital tumor tissue will be reliably revealed by pathologic tracer uptake, notwithstanding any treatment-related effects on BBB integrity [178]. Similarly, amino acid PET can be helpful to differentiate pseudoprogression from true tumor progression. Since regions of reactive changes usually show little or no PET tracer uptake, vital remaining or recurrent tumor tissue can be discriminated with high reliability from reactive, therapy-induced changes [2, 3]. This is important in cases of progression so that a timely intervention can be made as well as to avoid the premature cessation of an effective therapy due to pseudoprogression.

The reported high sensitivity of dynamic ^{18}F-FET PET investigations for tumor grading is accompanied by rather moderate specificity [159]. Thus, some low-grade gliomas show declining kinetics more characteristic of high-grade tumors. Interestingly, this kind of kinetics seems to be diagnostically ominous, in that these types of low-grade gliomas have a distinctly worse clinical course in comparison to those with more typical increasing kinetics and are associated with faster malignant progression to high-grade gliomas and earlier death [154]. There may therefore be an association between the dynamic course of tracer uptake in the tumor and an inherently aggressive tumor biology in molecular terms, which can probably not be detected on the basis of histology alone [154]. In support of this hypothesis is the phenomenon that in the course of the malignant transformation of low-grade gliomas, the time course of the PET time-activity curves changes from ascending to declining kinetics with earlier attainment of the peak uptake [174]. Also, in cases of high-grade gliomas, the shape of the time-activity curve plays a prognostic role, in that increasing aggressiveness of the tumor shows a shift in the time-to-peak uptake to earlier values [153].

In addition to kinetics, the magnitude of the intensity of tracer uptake, expressed as the tumor-to-brain uptake quotient (tumor-to-brain ratio; TBR), and the metabolically active "biologic" tumor volume as depicted by PET are also considered prognostic indicators [179]. For GBMs treated with radiation therapy or chemoradiation, it seems that the pre-therapeutic biologic tumor volume has an especially high prognostic value, such that this index merits special attention in surgical planning [169, 170].

Applications of Amino Acid PET in Brain Metastases

In contrast to infiltrating gliomas, in which the tumor boundaries are often ill-defined on MR imaging, metastases are sharply delineated such that MRI only has a subordinate role in the depiction of metastatic tumor extent. PET has greater significance in brain metastases diagnostics for the differentiation between post-therapeutic changes and vital tumor tissue. In addition to whole-brain irradiation, stereotactic irradiation is an important therapy option that finds frequent clinical use especially when there are fewer than five metastases. The MRI signal changes that frequently occur after therapy, along with the sometimes long-lasting disturbances of the BBB, often impede a reliable delineation of vital residual or recurrent tumor tissue. According to first comprehensive study results, amino acid PET reliably aids in the classification of such lesions not just in cases of gliomas but also in cases of metastases [180, 181].

3.3.2.3 Somatostatin Receptor Ligands

Principles of Somatostatin Receptor PET

Tumors characterized by an overexpression of somatostatin receptors can be visualized with PET using radiolabeled ligands to the somatostatin receptor. The most frequently used radiopharmaceuticals in clinical routine are ^{68}Ga-DOTATOC, ^{68}Ga-DOTATATE, and ^{68}Ga-DOTANOC. Meningiomas typically show high levels of somatostatin receptor expression and are therefore depicted with high sensitivity [182–185]. Due to extremely low uptake in healthy brain tissue and unaffected bone, somatostatin receptor ligands provide an excellent tumor-to-background contrast [186, 187]. While somatostatin receptor ligands are most frequently used to image meningiomas, rare cases of brain metastases with overexpression of somatostatin receptors have also been reported [188]. Comparing the tracers ^{68}Ga-DOTATOC and ^{68}Ga-DOTATATE, the latter seems to have slightly superior sensitivity for the detection of meningiomas, given its higher receptor affinity and binding [189].

Applications of Somatostatin Receptor PET

Somatostatin receptor PET can help narrow down the differential diagnosis and, additionally, discern with high sensitivity small lesions that would otherwise go undetected on conventional imaging [187] (Fig. 3.8). Furthermore, somatostatin PET can detect osseous involvement

[190]. Above and beyond this, PET with ^{68}Ga-DOTATATE/^{68}Ga-DOTA-TOC can differentiate with high diagnostic reliability between vital meningioma tissue and post-therapeutic scar tissue [191], such that this imaging procedure constitutes a sensible tool for monitoring disease course and for early detection of recurrence of meningioma. Only in rare cases, and more as a coincidence, can somatostatin receptor ligands be used to visualize cerebral metastases of neuroendocrine tumors or other tumors with increased somatostatin receptor expression.

A further aspect of somatostatin PET imaging that is assuming an increasing interest in the clinic is expressed in the term "theranostics." This term refers to the dual aspect of radiolabeling, a process by which a somatosta-

tin receptor ligand is labeled with a PET radionuclide. This can then be applied not only for imaging of a meningioma but also for therapeutic irradiation, in the context of peptide radiotherapy using ligands labeled with a (β-) emitting radionuclide such as ^{177}Lu or ^{90}Y. An advantage presented by this approach lies in the pre-therapeutic imaging of the target, which allows furthermore the calculation of the therapeutic target dose to be expected on the basis of the PET result [192]. By the same token, this also allows post-therapeutic monitoring as it reliably shows the actual target in a way that is not affected by non-specific alterations in the BBB arising after the treatment [191]. The most recent study results indicate that pre-therapeutic somatostatin receptor PET investigation has

Fig. 3.8 Example of a patient with multifocal meningioma: even small meningioma lesions that are difficult to detect with CT alone are visualized by high uptake on the DOTA-TATE PET scan

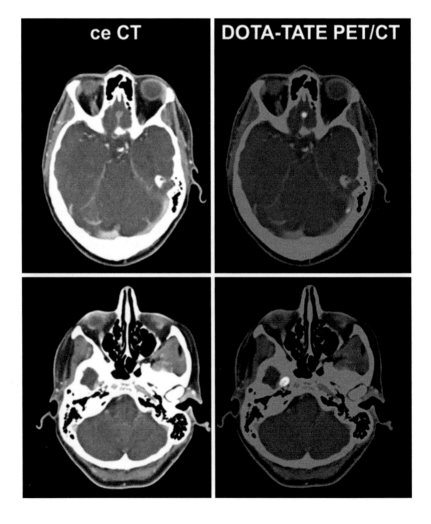

Fig. 38 (continued)

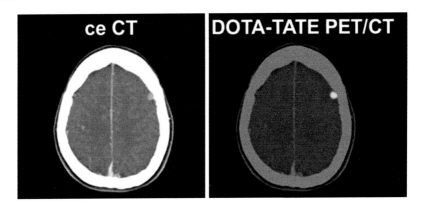

prognostic or predictive value and can most likely identify meningiomas that are not suitable for targeted radiotherapy on the basis of their lower ^{68}Ga-DOTATATE/^{68}Ga-DOTA-TOC uptake [193]. By this means, future patient-specific therapy decisions may be reached based on the biochemical properties of the underlying lesions. Prospective studies of this concept remain to be undertaken.

3.3.3 Other Tracers

3.3.3.1 Principles of Other Tracers and Applications

There are an increasing number of interesting tracers for brain tumor imaging, addressing different metabolic pathways or processes. These tracers, however, are mostly used in experimental settings and not in clinical routine.

Thymidine analogues such as 2-[^{11}C]-thymidine [194] or 3'-deoxy-3'-[^{18}F]-fluorothymidine (^{18}F-FLT) [195] quantify tumoral proliferation rates mediated via the enzyme thymidine kinase-1 in the process of DNA synthesis [196]. ^{18}F-FLT uptake was found to be correlated with glioma cell proliferation rate [196–198], but discrimination of tumoral proliferation from background activity might be difficult because of high variability in ^{18}F-FLT uptake in normal white matter tissue [199]. Furthermore, the tumoral ^{18}F-FLT uptake was reported to depend on the increased permeability, intracellular transport, and influx after the disruption of the BBB [200]. These challenges, along with a relatively difficult synthesis

process, have limited the use of ^{18}F-FLT to certain academic and research institutions. Other tracers address the increased phospholipid synthesis in tumor cells [201], such as ^{11}C-Choline, or tumor hypoxia (e.g., [^{18}F]-fluoromisonidazole; ^{18}F-FMISO [202]).

A highly promising target for PET visualization of glioma cells is the 18 kDa translocator protein (TSPO), which is upregulated in high-grade gliomas and correlates with malignancy [203]. However, most published studies thus far are preclinical studies, and more studies in humans are needed to evaluate whether TSPO-directed radioligands might visualize different tumor areas than amino acid PET, as suggested by preliminary data from a small case series [204].

Another interesting candidate for brain tumor PET is presented by radioligands to the prostate-specific membrane antigen (PSMA), which is not only overexpressed in prostate cancer cells but also in the neovasculature of different malignancies [205, 206]. Preliminary small studies and case reports show an increased tracer binding to high-grade gliomas and lymphomas [207, 208] as well as in brain metastases of primary prostate cancer [209].

3.4 Outlook

Over the last few decades, tumor imaging has evolved from the simple visualization of abnormal brain tissue to our ability to acquire detailed information about structural, biological, and physical processes in real time, thus providing a solid basis for informed decision-making and personalized medicine. The field of MR imaging has seen tremendous progress in the quantity and quality of available imaging modalities. Similarly, nuclear medicine diagnostic PET procedures currently established in clinical practice can be powerful tools for accurate pre- and posttreatment visualization of tumor tissue.

Our biggest challenge will be to establish the true validity and utility of these novel imaging techniques and to extend their application from the research to the clinical setting. Sophisticated combined-modality imaging, such as combined PET and perfusion-weighted MRI to study the direct correlation of regional ^{18}F-FET kinetics with perfusion data [210] or combined DSC and DCE MRI, could provide new insights into underlying tumor biology. In addition, combined-modality imaging and the implementation of standardized acquisition protocols could substantially lower the logistical challenges and the time demand for patients and study staff alike. Lastly, in the current era of molecular target-driven clinical trials, incorporating relevant novel imaging techniques should be considered as has been done for 2HG MRS in the evaluation of *IDH* inhibitor trials.

Acknowledgments Parts of the PET chapter were edited and translated from German by Inglewood Biomedical Editing.

References

1. Dhermain FG, Hau P, Lanfermann H, Jacobs AH, van den Bent MJ (2010) Advanced MRI and PET imaging for assessment of treatment response in patients with gliomas. Lancet Neurol 9(9):906–920. https://doi.org/10.1016/S1474-4422(10)70181-2

2. Galldiks N, Langen KJ, Pope WB (2015) From the clinician's point of view—what is the status quo of positron emission tomography in patients with brain tumors? Neuro Oncol 17(11):1434–1444. https://doi.org/10.1093/neuonc/nov118

3. Suchorska B, Tonn JC, Jansen NL (2014) PET imaging for brain tumor diagnostics. Curr Opin Neurol 27(6):683–688. https://doi.org/10.1097/WCO.0000000000000143

4. Pauleit D, Floeth F, Hamacher K, Riemenschneider MJ, Reifenberger G, Muller HW et al (2005) O-(2-[18F]fluoroethyl)-L-tyrosine PET combined with MRI improves the diagnostic assessment of cerebral gliomas. Brain 128(Pt 3):678–687. https://doi.org/10.1093/brain/awh399. awh399 [pii]

5. la Fougere C, Suchorska B, Bartenstein P, Kreth FW, Tonn JC (2011) Molecular imaging of gliomas with PET: opportunities and limitations. Neuro Oncol 13(8):806–819. https://doi.org/10.1093/neuonc/nor054

6. White NS, McDonald C, Farid N, Kuperman J, Karow D, Schenker-Ahmed NM et al (2014) Diffusion-weighted imaging in cancer: physical foundations and applications of restriction spectrum imaging. Cancer Res 74(17):4638–4652. https://doi.org/10.1158/0008-5472.CAN-13-3534

7. Le Bihan D, Iima M (2015) Diffusion magnetic resonance imaging: what water tells us about biological tissues. PLoS Biol 13(7):e1002203. https://doi.org/10.1371/journal.pbio.1002203

8. Okada H, Weller M, Huang R et al (2015) Immunotherapy response assessment in neuro-oncology: a report of the RANO working group. Lancet Oncol 16(15):e534–e542

9. Carmeliet P, Jain RK (2011) Molecular mechanisms and clinical applications of angiogenesis. Nature 473(7347):298–307. https://doi.org/10.1038/nature10144

10. Macdonald DR, Cascino TL, Schold SC Jr, Cairncross JG (1990) Response criteria for phase II studies of supratentorial malignant glioma. J Clin Oncol 8(7):1277–1280. https://doi.org/10.1200/JCO.1990.8.7.1277

11. van den Bent MJ, Wefel JS, Schiff D, Taphoorn MJ, Jaeckle K, Junck L et al (2011) Response assessment in neuro-oncology (a report of the RANO group): assessment of outcome in trials of diffuse low-grade gliomas. Lancet Oncol 12(6):583–593. https://doi.org/10.1016/S1470-2045(11)70057-2

12. Linhares P, Carvalho B, Figueiredo R, Reis RM, Vaz R (2013) Early pseudoprogression following chemoradiotherapy in glioblastoma patients: the value of RANO evaluation. J Oncol 2013:690585. https://doi.org/10.1155/2013/690585

13. Radbruch A, Fladt J, Kickingereder P, Wiestler B, Nowosielski M, Baumer P et al (2015) Pseudoprogression in patients with glioblastoma: clinical relevance despite low incidence. Neuro Oncol 17(1):151–159. https://doi.org/10.1093/neuonc/nou129

14. Brandsma D, Stalpers L, Taal W, Sminia P, van den Bent MJ (2008) Clinical features, mechanisms, and management of pseudoprogression in malignant gliomas. Lancet Oncol 9(5):453–461. https://doi.org/10.1016/S1470-2045(08)70125-6

15. Brandes AA, Franceschi E, Tosoni A, Blatt V, Pession A, Tallini G et al (2008) MGMT promoter methylation status can predict the incidence and outcome of pseudoprogression after concomitant radiochemotherapy in newly diagnosed glioblastoma patients. J Clin

Oncol 26(13):2192–2197. https://doi.org/10.1200/JCO.2007.14.8163

16. O'Brien BJ, Colen RR (2014) Post-treatment imaging changes in primary brain tumors. Curr Oncol Rep 16(8):397. https://doi.org/10.1007/s11912-014-0397-x

17. Siu A, Wind JJ, Iorgulescu JB, Chan TA, Yamada Y, Sherman JH (2012) Radiation necrosis following treatment of high grade glioma—a review of the literature and current understanding. Acta Neurochir (Wien) 154(2):191–201; discussion 201. https://doi.org/10.1007/s00701-011-1228-6

18. Huang RY, Neagu MR, Reardon DA, Wen PY (2015) Pitfalls in the neuroimaging of glioblastoma in the era of antiangiogenic and immuno/targeted therapy—detecting illusive disease, defining response. Front Neurol 6:33. https://doi.org/10.3389/fneur.2015.00033

19. Boxerman JL, Zhang Z, Safriel Y, Larvie M, Snyder BS, Jain R et al (2013) Early post-bevacizumab progression on contrast-enhanced MRI as a prognostic marker for overall survival in recurrent glioblastoma: results from the ACRIN 6677/RTOG 0625 Central Reader Study. Neuro Oncol 15(7):945–954. https://doi.org/10.1093/neuonc/not049

20. Pope WB, Djoukhadar I, Jackson A (2016) Neuroimaging. Handb Clin Neurol 134:27–50. https://doi.org/10.1016/B978-0-12-802997-8.00003-7

21. Mabray MC, Cha S (2016) Advanced MR imaging techniques in daily practice. Neuroimaging Clin N Am 26(4):647–666. https://doi.org/10.1016/j.nic.2016.06.010

22. Zhang H, Schneider T, Wheeler-Kingshott CA, Alexander DC (2012) NODDI: practical in vivo neurite orientation dispersion and density imaging of the human brain. Neuroimage 61(4):1000–1016. https://doi.org/10.1016/j.neuroimage.2012.03.072

23. Sugahara T, Korogi Y, Kochi M, Ikushima I, Shigematu Y, Hirai T et al (1999) Usefulness of diffusion-weighted MRI with echo-planar technique in the evaluation of cellularity in gliomas. J Magn Reson Imaging 9(1):53–60

24. Chenevert TL, Sundgren PC, Ross BD (2006) Diffusion imaging: insight to cell status and cytoarchitecture. Neuroimaging Clin N Am 16(4):619–632. , viii-ix. https://doi.org/10.1016/j.nic.2006.06.005

25. Nicholson C (2005) Factors governing diffusing molecular signals in brain extracellular space. J Neural Transm (Vienna) 112(1):29–44. https://doi.org/10.1007/s00702-004-0204-1

26. Panagiotaki E, Schneider T, Siow B, Hall MG, Lythgoe MF, Alexander DC (2012) Compartment models of the diffusion MR signal in brain white matter: a taxonomy and comparison. Neuroimage 59(3):2241–2254. https://doi.org/10.1016/j.neuroimage.2011.09.081

27. Barajas RF Jr, Rubenstein JL, Chang JS, Hwang J, Cha S (2010) Diffusion-weighted MR imaging derived apparent diffusion coefficient is predictive of clinical outcome in primary central nervous system lymphoma. AJNR Am J Neuroradiol 31(1):60–66. https://doi.org/10.3174/ajnr.A1750

28. Herneth AM, Guccione S, Bednarski M (2003) Apparent diffusion coefficient: a quantitative parameter for in vivo tumor characterization. Eur J Radiol 45(3):208–213

29. Rumboldt Z, Camacho DL, Lake D, Welsh CT, Castillo M (2006) Apparent diffusion coefficients for differentiation of cerebellar tumors in children. AJNR Am J Neuroradiol 27(6):1362–1369

30. LaViolette PS, Mickevicius NJ, Cochran EJ, Rand SD, Connelly J, Bovi JA et al (2014) Precise ex vivo histological validation of heightened cellularity and diffusion-restricted necrosis in regions of dark apparent diffusion coefficient in 7 cases of high-grade glioma. Neuro Oncol 16(12):1599–1606. https://doi.org/10.1093/neuonc/nou142

31. Farid N, Almeida-Freitas DB, White NS, McDonald CR, Muller KA, Vandenberg SR et al (2013) Restriction-spectrum imaging of bevacizumab-related necrosis in a patient with GBM. Front Oncol 3:258. https://doi.org/10.3389/fonc.2013.00258

32. Rieger J, Bahr O, Muller K, Franz K, Steinbach J, Hattingen E (2010) Bevacizumab-induced diffusion-restricted lesions in malignant glioma patients. J Neurooncol 99(1):49–56. https://doi.org/10.1007/s11060-009-0098-8

33. Futterer SF, Nemeth AJ, Grimm SA, Ragin AB, Chandler JP, Muro K et al (2014) Diffusion abnormalities of the corpus callosum in patients receiving bevacizumab for malignant brain tumors: suspected treatment toxicity. J Neurooncol 118(1):147–153. https://doi.org/10.1007/s11060-014-1409-2

34. Sivasundaram L, Hazany S, Wagle N, Zada G, Chen TC, Lerner A et al (2014) Diffusion restriction in a non-enhancing metastatic brain tumor treated with bevacizumab—recurrent tumor or atypical necrosis? Clin Imaging 38(5):724–726. https://doi.org/10.1016/j.clinimag.2014.04.014

35. Bulakbasi N, Guvenc I, Onguru O, Erdogan E, Tayfun C, Ucoz T (2004) The added value of the apparent diffusion coefficient calculation to magnetic resonance imaging in the differentiation and grading of malignant brain tumors. J Comput Assist Tomogr 28(6):735–746

36. Higano S, Yun X, Kumabe T, Watanabe M, Mugikura S, Umetsu A et al (2006) Malignant astrocytic tumors: clinical importance of apparent diffusion coefficient in prediction of grade and prognosis. Radiology 241(3):839–846. https://doi.org/10.1148/radiol.2413051276

37. Hilario A, Sepulveda JM, Perez-Nunez A, Salvador E, Millan JM, Hernandez-Lain A et al (2014) A prognostic model based on preoperative MRI predicts overall survival in patients with diffuse gliomas. AJNR Am J Neuroradiol 35(6):1096–1102. https://doi.org/10.3174/ajnr.A3837

38. Saraswathy S, Crawford FW, Lamborn KR, Pirzkall A, Chang S, Cha S et al (2009) Evaluation of

MR markers that predict survival in patients with newly diagnosed GBM prior to adjuvant therapy. J Neurooncol 91(1):69–81. https://doi.org/10.1007/s11060-008-9685-3

39. Moffat BA, Chenevert TL, Lawrence TS, Meyer CR, Johnson TD, Dong Q et al (2005) Functional diffusion map: a noninvasive MRI biomarker for early stratification of clinical brain tumor response. Proc Natl Acad Sci U S A 102(15):5524–5529. https://doi.org/10.1073/pnas.0501532102

40. Hamstra DA, Chenevert TL, Moffat BA, Johnson TD, Meyer CR, Mukherji SK et al (2005) Evaluation of the functional diffusion map as an early biomarker of time-to-progression and overall survival in high-grade glioma. Proc Natl Acad Sci U S A 102(46):16759–16764. https://doi.org/10.1073/pnas.0508347102

41. Ellingson BM, Cloughesy TF, Lai A, Nghiemphu PL, Liau LM, Pope WB (2013) Quantitative probabilistic functional diffusion mapping in newly diagnosed glioblastoma treated with radiochemotherapy. Neuro Oncol 15(3):382–390. https://doi.org/10.1093/neuonc/nos314

42. Ellingson BM, Cloughesy TF, Zaw T, Lai A, Nghiemphu PL, Harris R et al (2012) Functional diffusion maps (fDMs) evaluated before and after radiochemotherapy predict progression-free and overall survival in newly diagnosed glioblastoma. Neuro Oncol 14(3):333–343. https://doi.org/10.1093/neuonc/nor220

43. Lee WJ, Choi SH, Park CK, Yi KS, Kim TM, Lee SH et al (2012) Diffusion-weighted MR imaging for the differentiation of true progression from pseudoprogression following concomitant radiotherapy with temozolomide in patients with newly diagnosed high-grade gliomas. Acad Radiol 19(11):1353–1361. https://doi.org/10.1016/j.acra.2012.06.011

44. Zeng QS, Li CF, Liu H, Zhen JH, Feng DC (2007) Distinction between recurrent glioma and radiation injury using magnetic resonance spectroscopy in combination with diffusion-weighted imaging. Int J Radiat Oncol Biol Phys 68(1):151–158. https://doi.org/10.1016/j.ijrobp.2006.12.001

45. Hein PA, Eskey CJ, Dunn JF, Hug EB (2004) Diffusion-weighted imaging in the follow-up of treated high-grade gliomas: tumor recurrence versus radiation injury. AJNR Am J Neuroradiol 25(2):201–209

46. Kim HS, Goh MJ, Kim N, Choi CG, Kim SJ, Kim JH (2014) Which combination of MR imaging modalities is best for predicting recurrent glioblastoma? Study of diagnostic accuracy and reproducibility. Radiology 273(3):831–843. https://doi.org/10.1148/radiol.14132868

47. Di Costanzo A, Scarabino T, Trojsi F, Popolizio T, Bonavita S, de Cristofaro M et al (2014) Recurrent glioblastoma multiforme versus radiation injury: a multiparametric 3-T MR approach. Radiol Med 119(8):616–624. https://doi.org/10.1007/s11547-013-0371-y

48. Matsusue E, Fink JR, Rockhill JK, Ogawa T, Maravilla KR (2010) Distinction between glioma progression and post-radiation change by combined physiologic MR imaging. Neuroradiology 52(4):297–306. https://doi.org/10.1007/s00234-009-0613-9

49. Basser PJ, Mattiello J, LeBihan D (1994) MR diffusion tensor spectroscopy and imaging. Biophys J 66(1):259–267. https://doi.org/10.1016/S0006-3495(94)80775-1

50. Chapman CH, Zhu T, Nazem-Zadeh M, Tao Y, Buchtel HA, Tsien CI et al (2016) Diffusion tensor imaging predicts cognitive function change following partial brain radiotherapy for low-grade and benign tumors. Radiother Oncol 120(2):234–240. https://doi.org/10.1016/j.radonc.2016.06.021

51. Khong PL, Kwong DL, Chan GC, Sham JS, Chan FL, Ooi GC (2003) Diffusion-tensor imaging for the detection and quantification of treatment-induced white matter injury in children with medulloblastoma: a pilot study. AJNR Am J Neuroradiol 24(4):734–740

52. Khong PL, Leung LH, Fung AS, Fong DY, Qiu D, Kwong DL et al (2006) White matter anisotropy in post-treatment childhood cancer survivors: preliminary evidence of association with neurocognitive function. J Clin Oncol 24(6):884–890. https://doi.org/10.1200/JCO.2005.02.4505

53. Kitahara S, Nakasu S, Murata K, Sho K, Ito R (2005) Evaluation of treatment-induced cerebral white matter injury by using diffusion-tensor MR imaging: initial experience. AJNR Am J Neuroradiol 26(9):2200–2206

54. Haris M, Kumar S, Raj MK, Das KJ, Sapru S, Behari S et al (2008) Serial diffusion tensor imaging to characterize radiation-induced changes in normal-appearing white matter following radiotherapy in patients with adult low-grade gliomas. Radiat Med 26(3):140–150

55. Folkman J (1971) Tumor angiogenesis: therapeutic implications. N Engl J Med 285(21):1182–1186. https://doi.org/10.1056/NEJM197111182852108

56. Gerstner ER, Emblem KE, Sorensen GA (2015) Vascular magnetic resonance imaging in brain tumors during antiangiogenic therapy—are we there yet? Cancer J 21(4):337–342. https://doi.org/10.1097/PPO.0000000000000128

57. Shiroishi MS, Boxerman JL, Pope WB (2016) Physiologic MRI for assessment of response to therapy and prognosis in glioblastoma. Neuro Oncol 18(4):467–478. https://doi.org/10.1093/neuonc/nov179

58. Jain RK, Martin JD, Stylianopoulos T (2014) The role of mechanical forces in tumor growth and therapy. Annu Rev Biomed Eng 16:321–346. https://doi.org/10.1146/annurev-bioeng-071813-105259

59. Chauhan VP, Boucher Y, Ferrone CR, Roberge S, Martin JD, Stylianopoulos T et al (2014) Compression of pancreatic tumor blood vessels by hyaluronan is caused by solid stress and not intersti-

tial fluid pressure. Cancer Cell 26(1):14–15. https://doi.org/10.1016/j.ccr.2014.06.003

60. Boxerman JL, Schmainda KM, Weisskoff RM (2006) Relative cerebral blood volume maps corrected for contrast agent extravasation significantly correlate with glioma tumor grade, whereas uncorrected maps do not. AJNR Am J Neuroradiol 27(4):859–867

61. Quarles CC, Gore JC, Xu L, Yankeelov TE (2012) Comparison of dual-echo DSC-MRI- and DCE-MRI-derived contrast agent kinetic parameters. Magn Reson Imaging 30(7):944–953. https://doi.org/10.1016/j.mri.2012.03.008

62. Rollin N, Guyotat J, Streichenberger N, Honnorat J, Tran Minh VA, Cotton F (2006) Clinical relevance of diffusion and perfusion magnetic resonance imaging in assessing intra-axial brain tumors. Neuroradiology 48(3):150–159. https://doi.org/10.1007/s00234-005-0030-7

63. Cha S, Tihan T, Crawford F, Fischbein NJ, Chang S, Bollen A et al (2005) Differentiation of low-grade oligodendrogliomas from low-grade astrocytomas by using quantitative blood-volume measurements derived from dynamic susceptibility contrast-enhanced MR imaging. AJNR Am J Neuroradiol 26(2):266–273

64. Law M, Cha S, Knopp EA, Johnson G, Arnett J, Litt AW (2002) High-grade gliomas and solitary metastases: differentiation by using perfusion and proton spectroscopic MR imaging. Radiology 222(3):715–721. https://doi.org/10.1148/radiol.2223010558

65. Mangla R, Singh G, Ziegelitz D, Milano MT, Korones DN, Zhong J et al (2010) Changes in relative cerebral blood volume 1 month after radiation-temozolomide therapy can help predict overall survival in patients with glioblastoma. Radiology 256(2):575–584. https://doi.org/10.1148/radiol.10091440

66. Galban CJ, Chenevert TL, Meyer CR, Tsien C, Lawrence TS, Hamstra DA et al (2009) The parametric response map is an imaging biomarker for early cancer treatment outcome. Nat Med 15(5):572–576. https://doi.org/10.1038/nm.1919

67. Schmainda KM, Prah M, Connelly J, Rand SD, Hoffman RG, Mueller W et al (2014) Dynamic-susceptibility contrast agent MRI measures of relative cerebral blood volume predict response to bevacizumab in recurrent high-grade glioma. Neuro Oncol 16(6):880–888. https://doi.org/10.1093/neuonc/not216

68. Schmainda KM, Zhang Z, Prah M, Snyder BS, Gilbert MR, Sorensen AG et al (2015) Dynamic susceptibility contrast MRI measures of relative cerebral blood volume as a prognostic marker for overall survival in recurrent glioblastoma: results from the ACRIN 6677/RTOG 0625 multicenter trial. Neuro Oncol 17(8):1148–1156. https://doi.org/10.1093/neuonc/nou364

69. Kickingereder P, Wiestler B, Burth S, Wick A, Nowosielski M, Heiland S et al (2015) Relative cerebral blood volume is a potential predictive imaging biomarker of bevacizumab efficacy in recurrent glioblastoma. Neuro Oncol 17(8):1139–1147. https://doi.org/10.1093/neuonc/nov028

70. Batchelor TT, Gerstner ER, Emblem KE, Duda DG, Kalpathy-Cramer J, Snuderl M et al (2013) Improved tumor oxygenation and survival in glioblastoma patients who show increased blood perfusion after cediranib and chemoradiation. Proc Natl Acad Sci U S A 110(47):19059–19064. https://doi.org/10.1073/pnas.1318022110

71. Batchelor TT, Sorensen AG, di Tomaso E, Zhang WT, Duda DG, Cohen KS et al (2007) AZD2171, a pan-VEGF receptor tyrosine kinase inhibitor, normalizes tumor vasculature and alleviates edema in glioblastoma patients. Cancer Cell 11(1):83–95. https://doi.org/10.1016/j.ccr.2006.11.021

72. Vrabec M, Van Cauter S, Himmelreich U, Van Gool SW, Sunaert S, De Vleeschouwer S et al (2011) MR perfusion and diffusion imaging in the follow-up of recurrent glioblastoma treated with dendritic cell immunotherapy: a pilot study. Neuroradiology 53(10):721–731. https://doi.org/10.1007/s00234-010-0802-6

73. Pope WB (2015) Predictive imaging marker of bevacizumab efficacy: perfusion MRI. Neuro Oncol 17(8):1046–1047. https://doi.org/10.1093/neuonc/nov067

74. Wen PY, Cloughesy TF, Ellingson BM, Reardon DA, Fine HA, Abrey L et al (2014) Report of the Jumpstarting Brain Tumor Drug Development Coalition and FDA clinical trials neuroimaging endpoint workshop (January 30, 2014, Bethesda MD). Neuro Oncol 16(Suppl 7):vii36–vii47. https://doi.org/10.1093/neuonc/nou226

75. Tofts PS, Brix G, Buckley DL, Evelhoch JL, Henderson E, Knopp MV et al (1999) Estimating kinetic parameters from dynamic contrast-enhanced T(1)-weighted MRI of a diffusable tracer: standardized quantities and symbols. J Magn Reson Imaging 10(3):223–232

76. Shin KE, Ahn KJ, Choi HS, Jung SL, Kim BS, Jeon SS et al (2014) DCE and DSC MR perfusion imaging in the differentiation of recurrent tumour from treatment-related changes in patients with glioma. Clin Radiol 69(6):e264–e272. https://doi.org/10.1016/j.crad.2014.01.016

77. Alcaide-Leon P, Pareto D, Martinez-Saez E, Auger C, Bharatha A, Rovira A (2015) Pixel-by-pixel comparison of volume transfer constant and estimates of cerebral blood volume from dynamic contrast-enhanced and dynamic susceptibility contrast-enhanced MR imaging in high-grade gliomas. AJNR Am J Neuroradiol 36(5):871–876. https://doi.org/10.3174/ajnr.A4231

78. Roberts HC, Roberts TP, Bollen AW, Ley S, Brasch RC, Dillon WP (2001) Correlation of microvascular permeability derived from dynamic contrast-enhanced MR imaging with histologic grade and tumor labeling index: a study in human brain tumors. Acad Radiol 8(5):384–391. https://doi.org/10.1016/S1076-6332(03)80545-7

79. Patankar TF, Haroon HA, Mills SJ, Baleriaux D, Buckley DL, Parker GJ et al (2005) Is volume transfer coefficient (K(trans)) related to histologic grade in human gliomas? AJNR Am J Neuroradiol 26(10):2455–2465

80. Roberts HC, Roberts TP, Brasch RC, Dillon WP (2000) Quantitative measurement of microvascular permeability in human brain tumors achieved using dynamic contrast-enhanced MR imaging: correlation with histologic grade. AJNR Am J Neuroradiol 21(5):891–899

81. Sorensen AG, Batchelor TT, Zhang WT, Chen PJ, Yeo P, Wang M et al (2009) A "vascular normalization index" as potential mechanistic biomarker to predict survival after a single dose of cediranib in recurrent glioblastoma patients. Cancer Res 69(13):5296–5300. https://doi.org/10.1158/0008-5472.CAN-09-0814

82. Kickingereder P, Wiestler B, Graf M, Heiland S, Schlemmer HP, Wick W et al (2015) Evaluation of dynamic contrast-enhanced MRI derived microvascular permeability in recurrent glioblastoma treated with bevacizumab. J Neurooncol 121(2):373–380. https://doi.org/10.1007/s11060-014-1644-6

83. O'Connor JP, Jackson A, Parker GJ, Roberts C, Jayson GC (2012) Dynamic contrast-enhanced MRI in clinical trials of antivascular therapies. Nat Rev Clin Oncol 9(3):167–177. https://doi.org/10.1038/nrclinonc.2012.2

84. Radbruch A, Weberling LD, Kieslich PJ, Eidel O, Burth S, Kickingereder P et al (2015) Gadolinium retention in the dentate nucleus and globus pallidus is dependent on the class of contrast agent. Radiology 275(3):783–791. https://doi.org/10.1148/radiol.2015150337

85. Ramalho J, Castillo M, AlObaidy M, Nunes RH, Ramalho M, Dale BM et al (2015) High signal intensity in globus pallidus and dentate nucleus on unenhanced T1-weighted MR images: evaluation of two linear gadolinium-based contrast agents. Radiology 276(3):836–844. https://doi.org/10.1148/radiol.2015150872

86. Kanda T, Ishii K, Kawaguchi H, Kitajima K, Takenaka D (2014) High signal intensity in the dentate nucleus and globus pallidus on unenhanced T1-weighted MR images: relationship with increasing cumulative dose of a gadolinium-based contrast material. Radiology 270(3):834–841. https://doi.org/10.1148/radiol.13131669

87. Kanda T, Osawa M, Oba H, Toyoda K, Kotoku J, Haruyama T et al (2015) High signal intensity in dentate nucleus on unenhanced T1-weighted MR images: association with linear versus macrocyclic gadolinium chelate administration. Radiology 275(3):803–809. https://doi.org/10.1148/radiol.14140364

88. Adin ME, Kleinberg L, Vaidya D, Zan E, Mirbagheri S, Yousem DM (2015) Hyperintense dentate nuclei on T1-weighted MRI: relation to repeat gadolinium administration. AJNR Am J Neuroradiol 36(10):1859–1865. https://doi.org/10.3174/ajnr.A4378

89. Skinner JT, Moots PL, Ayers GD, Quarles CC (2016) On the use of DSC-MRI for measuring vascular permeability. AJNR Am J Neuroradiol 37(1):80–87. https://doi.org/10.3174/ajnr.A4478

90. Skinner JT, Robison RK, Elder CP, Newton AT, Damon BM, Quarles CC (2014) Evaluation of a multiple spin- and gradient-echo (SAGE) EPI acquisition with SENSE acceleration: applications for perfusion imaging in and outside the brain. Magn Reson Imaging 32(10):1171–1180. https://doi.org/10.1016/j.mri.2014.08.032

91. Haller S, Zaharchuk G, Thomas DL, Lovblad KO, Barkhof F, Golay X (2016) Arterial spin labeling perfusion of the brain: emerging clinical applications. Radiology 281(2):337–356. https://doi.org/10.1148/radiol.2016150789

92. Rosen BR, Belliveau JW, Aronen HJ, Kennedy D, Buchbinder BR, Fischman A et al (1991) Susceptibility contrast imaging of cerebral blood volume: human experience. Magn Reson Med 22(2):293–299; discussion 300–3

93. Rosen BR, Belliveau JW, Buchbinder BR, McKinstry RC, Porkka LM, Kennedy DN et al (1991) Contrast agents and cerebral hemodynamics. Magn Reson Med 19(2):285–292

94. Emblem KE, Farrar CT, Gerstner ER, Batchelor TT, Borra RJ, Rosen BR et al (2014) Vessel caliber—a potential MRI biomarker of tumour response in clinical trials. Nat Rev Clin Oncol 11(10):566–584. https://doi.org/10.1038/nrclinonc.2014.126

95. Donahue KM, Krouwer HG, Rand SD, Pathak AP, Marszalkowski CS, Censky SC et al (2000) Utility of simultaneously acquired gradient-echo and spin-echo cerebral blood volume and morphology maps in brain tumor patients. Magn Reson Med 43(6):845–853

96. Schmainda KM, Rand SD, Joseph AM, Lund R, Ward BD, Pathak AP et al (2004) Characterization of a first-pass gradient-echo spin-echo method to predict brain tumor grade and angiogenesis. AJNR Am J Neuroradiol 25(9):1524–1532

97. Emblem KE, Mouridsen K, Bjornerud A, Farrar CT, Jennings D, Borra RJ et al (2013) Vessel architectural imaging identifies cancer patient responders to anti-angiogenic therapy. Nat Med 19(9):1178–1183. https://doi.org/10.1038/nm.3289

98. Ostergaard L, Tietze A, Nielsen T, Drasbek KR, Mouridsen K, Jespersen SN et al (2013) The relationship between tumor blood flow, angiogenesis, tumor hypoxia, and aerobic glycolysis. Cancer Res 73(18):5618–5624. https://doi.org/10.1158/0008-5472.CAN-13-0964

99. Jespersen SN, Ostergaard L (2012) The roles of cerebral blood flow, capillary transit time heterogeneity, and oxygen tension in brain oxygenation and metabolism. J Cereb Blood Flow Metab 32(2):264–277. https://doi.org/10.1038/jcbfm.2011.153

100. Mouridsen K, Hansen MB, Ostergaard L, Jespersen SN (2014) Reliable estimation of capillary transit time distributions using DSC-MRI. J Cereb Blood Flow Metab 34(9):1511–1521. https://doi.org/10.1038/jcbfm.2014.111

101. Larsson HBW, Vestergaard MB, Lindberg U, Iversen HK, Cramer SP (2017) Brain capillary transit time heterogeneity in healthy volunteers measured by dynamic contrast-enhanced T1-weighted perfusion MRI. J Magn Reson Imaging 45(6):1809–1820. https://doi.org/10.1002/jmri.25488

102. Hamilton BE, Nesbit GM, Dosa E, Gahramanov S, Rooney B, Nesbit EG et al (2011) Comparative analysis of ferumoxytol and gadoteridol enhancement using T1- and T2-weighted MRI in neuroimaging. AJR Am J Roentgenol 197(4):981–988. https://doi.org/10.2214/AJR.10.5992

103. Neuwelt EA, Varallyay CG, Manninger S, Solymosi D, Haluska M, Hunt MA et al (2007) The potential of ferumoxytol nanoparticle magnetic resonance imaging, perfusion, and angiography in central nervous system malignancy: a pilot study. Neurosurgery 60(4):601–11; discussion 11–2. https://doi.org/10.1227/01.NEU.0000255350.71700.37

104. Varallyay CG, Nesbit E, Fu R, Gahramanov S, Moloney B, Earl E et al (2013) High-resolution steady-state cerebral blood volume maps in patients with central nervous system neoplasms using ferumoxytol, a superparamagnetic iron oxide nanoparticle. J Cereb Blood Flow Metab 33(5):780–786. https://doi.org/10.1038/jcbfm.2013.36

105. Gahramanov S, Raslan AM, Muldoon LL, Hamilton BE, Rooney WD, Varallyay CG et al (2011) Potential for differentiation of pseudoprogression from true tumor progression with dynamic susceptibility-weighted contrast-enhanced magnetic resonance imaging using ferumoxytol vs. gadoteridol: a pilot study. Int J Radiat Oncol Biol Phys 79(2):514–523. https://doi.org/10.1016/j.ijrobp.2009.10.072

106. FDA (2015) Feraheme (ferumoxytol): drug safety communication—warnings strengthened and prescribing instructions changed. https://www.fda.gov/safety/medwatch/safetyinformation/safetyalertsforhumanmedicalproducts/ucm440479.htm. Accessed 29 Aug 2017

107. Rapalino O, Ratai EM (2016) Multiparametric imaging analysis: magnetic resonance spectroscopy. Magn Reson Imaging Clin N Am 24(4):671–686. https://doi.org/10.1016/j.mric.2016.06.001

108. Howe FA, Barton SJ, Cudlip SA, Stubbs M, Saunders DE, Murphy M et al (2003) Metabolic profiles of human brain tumors using quantitative in vivo 1H magnetic resonance spectroscopy. Magn Reson Med 49(2):223–232. https://doi.org/10.1002/mrm.10367

109. Horska A, Barker PB (2010) Imaging of brain tumors: MR spectroscopy and metabolic imaging. Neuroimaging Clin N Am 20(3):293–310. https://doi.org/10.1016/j.nic.2010.04.003

110. Zeng Q, Liu H, Zhang K, Li C, Zhou G (2011) Noninvasive evaluation of cerebral glioma grade by using multivoxel 3D proton MR spectroscopy. Magn Reson Imaging 29(1):25–31. https://doi.org/10.1016/j.mri.2010.07.017

111. Yang D, Korogi Y, Sugahara T, Kitajima M, Shigematsu Y, Liang L et al (2002) Cerebral gliomas: prospective comparison of multivoxel 2D chemical-shift imaging proton MR spectroscopy, echoplanar perfusion and diffusion-weighted MRI. Neuroradiology 44(8):656–666. https://doi.org/10.1007/s00234-002-0816-9

112. Stadlbauer A, Gruber S, Nimsky C, Fahlbusch R, Hammen T, Buslei R et al (2006) Preoperative grading of gliomas by using metabolite quantification with high-spatial-resolution proton MR spectroscopic imaging. Radiology 238(3):958–969. https://doi.org/10.1148/radiol.2382041896

113. Fountas KN, Kapsalaki EZ, Vogel RL, Fezoulidis I, Robinson JS, Gotsis ED (2004) Noninvasive histologic grading of solid astrocytomas using proton magnetic resonance spectroscopy. Stereotact Funct Neurosurg 82(2-3):90–97. https://doi.org/10.1159/000077458

114. Server A, Josefsen R, Kulle B, Maehlen J, Schellhorn T, Gadmar O et al (2010) Proton magnetic resonance spectroscopy in the distinction of high-grade cerebral gliomas from single metastatic brain tumors. Acta Radiol 51(3):316–325. https://doi.org/10.3109/02841850903482901

115. Weybright P, Sundgren PC, Maly P, Hassan DG, Nan B, Rohrer S et al (2005) Differentiation between brain tumor recurrence and radiation injury using MR spectroscopy. AJR Am J Roentgenol 185(6):1471–1476. https://doi.org/10.2214/AJR.04.0933

116. Smith EA, Carlos RC, Junck LR, Tsien CI, Elias A, Sundgren PC (2009) Developing a clinical decision model: MR spectroscopy to differentiate between recurrent tumor and radiation change in patients with new contrast-enhancing lesions. AJR Am J Roentgenol 192(2):W45–W52. https://doi.org/10.2214/AJR.07.3934

117. Zhang H, Ma L, Wang Q, Zheng X, Wu C, Xu BN (2014) Role of magnetic resonance spectroscopy for the differentiation of recurrent glioma from radiation necrosis: a systematic review and meta-analysis. Eur J Radiol 83(12):2181–2189. https://doi.org/10.1016/j.ejrad.2014.09.018

118. Dang L, White DW, Gross S, Bennett BD, Bittinger MA, Driggers EM et al (2009) Cancer-associated IDH1 mutations produce 2-hydroxyglutarate. Nature 462(7274):739–744. https://doi.org/10.1038/nature08617

119. Andronesi OC, Rapalino O, Gerstner E, Chi A, Batchelor TT, Cahill DP et al (2013) Detection of oncogenic IDH1 mutations using magnetic resonance spectroscopy of 2-hydroxyglutarate. J Clin Invest 123(9):3659–3663. https://doi.org/10.1172/JCI67229

120. Choi C, Ganji SK, DeBerardinis RJ, Hatanpaa KJ, Rakheja D, Kovacs Z et al (2012) 2-hydroxyglutarate detection by magnetic resonance spectroscopy

in IDH-mutated patients with gliomas. Nat Med 18(4):624–629. https://doi.org/10.1038/nm.2682

121. Andronesi OC, Kim GS, Gerstner E, Batchelor T, Tzika AA, Fantin VR et al (2012) Detection of 2-hydroxyglutarate in IDH-mutated glioma patients by in vivo spectral-editing and 2D correlation magnetic resonance spectroscopy. Sci Transl Med 4(116):116ra4. https://doi.org/10.1126/scitranslmed.3002693

122. Buckner J, Giannini C, Eckel-Passow J, Lachance D, Parney I, Laack N et al (2017) Management of diffuse low-grade gliomas in adults—use of molecular diagnostics. Nat Rev Neurol 13(6):340–351. https://doi.org/10.1038/nrneurol.2017.54

123. Andronesi OC, Loebel F, Bogner W, Marjanska M, Vander Heiden MG, Iafrate AJ et al (2016) Treatment response assessment in IDH-mutant glioma patients by noninvasive 3D functional spectroscopic mapping of 2-hydroxyglutarate. Clin Cancer Res 22(7):1632–1641. https://doi.org/10.1158/1078-0432.CCR-15-0656

124. Gillies RJ (2001) Causes and consequences of acidic pH in tumors. John Eiley and Sons, Ltd., West Sussex, UK

125. Martinez-Zaguilan R, Seftor EA, Seftor RE, Chu YW, Gillies RJ, Hendrix MJ (1996) Acidic pH enhances the invasive behavior of human melanoma cells. Clin Exp Metastasis 14(2):176–186

126. Lardner A (2001) The effects of extracellular pH on immune function. J Leukoc Biol 69(4):522–530

127. Harris RJ, Cloughesy TF, Liau LM, Prins RM, Antonios JP, Li D et al (2015) pH-weighted molecular imaging of gliomas using amine chemical exchange saturation transfer MRI. Neuro Oncol 17(11):1514–1524. https://doi.org/10.1093/neuonc/nov106

128. Togao O, Yoshiura T, Keupp J, Hiwatashi A, Yamashita K, Kikuchi K et al (2014) Amide proton transfer imaging of adult diffuse gliomas: correlation with histopathological grades. Neuro Oncol 16(3):441–448. https://doi.org/10.1093/neuonc/not158

129. Zhou J, Tryggestad E, Wen Z, Lal B, Zhou T, Grossman R et al (2011) Differentiation between glioma and radiation necrosis using molecular magnetic resonance imaging of endogenous proteins and peptides. Nat Med 17(1):130–134. https://doi.org/10.1038/nm.2268

130. Souba WW (1993) Glutamine and cancer. Ann Surg 218(6):715–728

131. Harris RJ, Cloughesy TF, Liau LM, Nghiemphu PL, Lai A, Pope WB et al (2016) Simulation, phantom validation, and clinical evaluation of fast pH-weighted molecular imaging using amine chemical exchange saturation transfer echo planar imaging (CEST-EPI) in glioma at 3 T. NMR Biomed 29(11):1563–1576. https://doi.org/10.1002/nbm.3611

132. Kumar V, Gu Y, Basu S, Berglund A, Eschrich SA, Schabath MB et al (2012) Radiomics: the process and the challenges. Magn Reson Imaging 30(9):1234–1248. https://doi.org/10.1016/j.mri.2012.06.010

133. Itakura H, Achrol AS, Mitchell LA, Loya JJ, Liu T, Westbroek EM et al (2015) Magnetic resonance image features identify glioblastoma phenotypic subtypes with distinct molecular pathway activities. Sci Transl Med 7(303):303ra138. https://doi.org/10.1126/scitranslmed.aaa7582

134. Wang S, Summers RM (2012) Machine learning and radiology. Med Image Anal 16(5):933–951. https://doi.org/10.1016/j.media.2012.02.005

135. Emblem KE, Pinho MC, Zollner FG, Due-Tonnessen P, Hald JK, Schad LR et al (2015) A generic support vector machine model for preoperative glioma survival associations. Radiology 275(1):228–234. https://doi.org/10.1148/radiol.14140770

136. Kickingereder P, Burth S, Wick A, Gotz M, Eidel O, Schlemmer HP et al (2016) Radiomic profiling of glioblastoma: identifying an imaging predictor of patient survival with improved performance over established clinical and radiologic risk models. Radiology 280(3):880–889. https://doi.org/10.1148/radiol.2016160845

137. Kickingereder P, Gotz M, Muschelli J, Wick A, Neuberger U, Shinohara RT et al (2016) Large-scale radiomic profiling of recurrent glioblastoma identifies an imaging predictor for stratifying anti-angiogenic treatment response. Clin Cancer Res 22(23):5765–5771. https://doi.org/10.1158/1078-0432.CCR-16-0702

138. Zacharaki EI, Kanas VG, Davatzikos C (2011) Investigating machine learning techniques for MRI-based classification of brain neoplasms. Int J Comput Assist Radiol Surg 6(6):821–828. https://doi.org/10.1007/s11548-011-0559-3

139. Kickingereder P, Bonekamp D, Nowosielski M, Kratz A, Sill M, Burth S et al (2016) Radiogenomics of glioblastoma: machine learning-based classification of molecular characteristics by using multiparametric and multiregional MR imaging features. Radiology 281(3):907–918. https://doi.org/10.1148/radiol.2016161382

140. Zhang B, Chang K, Ramkissoon S, Tanguturi S, Bi WL, Reardon DA et al (2017) Multimodal MRI features predict isocitrate dehydrogenase genotype in high-grade gliomas. Neuro Oncol 19(1):109–117. https://doi.org/10.1093/neuonc/now121

141. Capper D, Weissert S, Balss J, Habel A, Meyer J, Jager D et al (2010) Characterization of R132H mutation-specific IDH1 antibody binding in brain tumors. Brain Pathol 20(1):245–254. https://doi.org/10.1111/j.1750-3639.2009.00352.x

142. Zacharaki EI, Morita N, Bhatt P, O'Rourke DM, Melhem ER, Davatzikos C (2012) Survival analysis of patients with high-grade gliomas based on data mining of imaging variables. AJNR Am J Neuroradiol 33(6):1065–1071. https://doi.org/10.3174/ajnr.A2939

143. Alavi A, Dann R, Chawluk J, Alavi J, Kushner M, Reivich M (1986) Positron emission tomography imaging of regional cerebral glucose metabolism. Semin Nucl Med 16(1):2–34

144. Gulyas B, Halldin C (2012) New PET radiopharmaceuticals beyond FDG for brain tumor imaging. Q J Nucl Med Mol Imaging 56(2):173–190

145. Palmedo H, Urbach H, Bender H, Schlegel U, Schmidt-Wolf IG, Matthies A et al (2006) FDG-PET in immunocompetent patients with primary central nervous system lymphoma: correlation with MRI and clinical follow-up. Eur J Nucl Med Mol Imaging 33(2):164–168. https://doi.org/10.1007/s00259-005-1917-6

146. Kawase Y, Yamamoto Y, Kameyama R, Kawai N, Kudomi N, Nishiyama Y (2011) Comparison of 11C-methionine PET and 18F-FDG PET in patients with primary central nervous system lymphoma. Mol Imaging Biol 13(6):1284–1289. https://doi.org/10.1007/s11307-010-0447-1

147. Manohar K, Bhattacharya A, Mittal BR (2013) Low positive yield from routine inclusion of the brain in whole-body 18F-FDG PET/CT imaging for noncerebral malignancies: results from a large population study. Nucl Med Commun 34(6):540–543. https://doi.org/10.1097/MNM.0b013e32836066c0

148. Albert NL, Weller M, Suchorska B, Galldiks N, Soffietti R, Kim MM et al (2016) Response Assessment in Neuro-Oncology working group and European Association for Neuro-Oncology recommendations for the clinical use of PET imaging in gliomas. Neuro Oncol 18(9):1199–1208. https://doi.org/10.1093/neuonc/now058

149. Jansen NL, Schwartz C, Graute V, Eigenbrod S, Lutz J, Egensperger R et al (2012) Prediction of oligodendroglial histology and LOH 1p/19q using dynamic [(18)F]FET-PET imaging in intracranial WHO grade II and III gliomas. Neuro Oncol 14(12):1473–1480. https://doi.org/10.1093/neuonc/nos259

150. Popperl G, Kreth FW, Mehrkens JH, Herms J, Seelos K, Koch W et al (2007) FET PET for the evaluation of untreated gliomas: correlation of FET uptake and uptake kinetics with tumour grading. Eur J Nucl Med Mol Imaging 34(12):1933–1942. https://doi.org/10.1007/s00259-007-0534-y

151. Singhal T, Narayanan TK, Jacobs MP, Bal C, Mantil JC (2012) 11C-methionine PET for grading and prognostication in gliomas: a comparison study with 18F-FDG PET and contrast enhancement on MRI. J Nucl Med 53(11):1709–1715. https://doi.org/10.2967/jnumed.111.102533

152. Fueger BJ, Czernin J, Cloughesy T, Silverman DH, Geist CL, Walter MA et al (2010) Correlation of 6-18F-fluoro-L-dopa PET uptake with proliferation and tumor grade in newly diagnosed and recurrent gliomas. J Nucl Med 51(10):1532–1538. https://doi.org/10.2967/jnumed.110.078592

153. Jansen NL, Suchorska B, Wenter V, Schmid-Tannwald C, Todica A, Eigenbrod S et al (2015) Prognostic significance of dynamic 18F-FET PET in newly diagnosed astrocytic high-grade glioma. J Nucl Med 56(1):9–15. https://doi.org/10.2967/jnumed.114.144675

154. Jansen NL, Suchorska B, Wenter V, Eigenbrod S, Schmid-Tannwald C, Zwergal A et al (2014) Dynamic 18F-FET PET in newly diagnosed astrocytic low-grade glioma identifies high-risk patients. J Nucl Med 55(2):198–203. https://doi.org/10.2967/jnumed.113.122333

155. Floeth FW, Pauleit D, Sabel M, Reifenberger G, Stoffels G, Stummer W et al (2006) 18F-FET PET differentiation of ring-enhancing brain lesions. J Nucl Med 47(5):776–782. 47/5/776 [pii]

156. Hutterer M, Nowosielski M, Putzer D, Jansen NL, Seiz M, Schocke M et al (2013) [18F]-fluoro-ethyl-L-tyrosine PET: a valuable diagnostic tool in neuro-oncology, but not all that glitters is glioma. Neuro Oncol 15(3):341–351. https://doi.org/10.1093/neuonc/nos300

157. Kunz M, Thon N, Eigenbrod S, Hartmann C, Egensperger R, Herms J et al (2011) Hot spots in dynamic (18)FET-PET delineate malignant tumor parts within suspected WHO grade II gliomas. Neuro Oncol 13(3):307–316. https://doi.org/10.1093/neuonc/noq196. noq196 [pii]

158. Calcagni ML, Galli G, Giordano A, Taralli S, Anile C, Niesen A et al (2011) Dynamic O-(2-[18F]fluoroethyl)-L-tyrosine (F-18 FET) PET for glioma grading: assessment of individual probability of malignancy. Clin Nucl Med 36(10):841–847. https://doi.org/10.1097/RLU.0b013e3182291b40. 00003072-201110000-00001 [pii]

159. Jansen NL, Graute V, Armbruster L, Suchorska B, Lutz J, Eigenbrod S et al (2012) MRI-suspected low-grade glioma: is there a need to perform dynamic FET PET? Eur J Nucl Med Mol Imaging 39(6):1021–1029. https://doi.org/10.1007/s00259-012-2109-9

160. Moulin-Romsee G, D'Hondt E, de Groot T, Goffin J, Sciot R, Mortelmans L et al (2007) Non-invasive grading of brain tumours using dynamic amino acid PET imaging: does it work for 11C-methionine? Eur J Nucl Med Mol Imaging 34(12):2082–2087. https://doi.org/10.1007/s00259-007-0557-4

161. Kratochwil C, Combs SE, Leotta K, Afshar-Oromieh A, Rieken S, Debus J et al (2014) Intra-individual comparison of (1)(8)F-FET and (1)(8)F-DOPA in PET imaging of recurrent brain tumors. Neuro Oncol 16(3):434–440. https://doi.org/10.1093/neuonc/not199

162. Pafundi DH, Laack NN, Youland RS, Parney IF, Lowe VJ, Giannini C et al (2013) Biopsy validation of 18F-DOPA PET and biodistribution in gliomas for neurosurgical planning and radiotherapy target delineation: results of a prospective pilot study. Neuro Oncol 15(8):1058–1067. https://doi.org/10.1093/neuonc/not002

163. Plotkin M, Blechschmidt C, Auf G, Nyuyki F, Geworski L, Denecke T et al (2010) Comparison of F-18 FET-PET with F-18 FDG-PET for biopsy planning of non-contrast-enhancing gliomas. Eur Radiol 20(10):2496–2502. https://doi.org/10.1007/s00330-010-1819-2

164. Ewelt C, Floeth FW, Felsberg J, Steiger HJ, Sabel M, Langen KJ et al (2011) Finding the anaplastic focus in diffuse gliomas: the value of Gd-DTPA enhanced MRI, FET-PET, and intraoperative, ALA-derived tissue fluorescence. Clin Neurol Neurosurg 113(7):541–547. https://doi.org/10.1016/j.clineuro.2011.03.008

165. Watanabe M, Tanaka R, Takeda N (1992) Magnetic resonance imaging and histopathology of cerebral gliomas. Neuroradiology 34(6):463–469

166. Munck Af Rosenschold P, Costa J, Engelholm SA, Lundemann MJ, Law I, Ohlhues L et al (2015) Impact of [18F]-fluoro-ethyl-tyrosine PET imaging on target definition for radiation therapy of high-grade glioma. Neuro Oncol 17(5):757–763. https://doi.org/10.1093/neuonc/nou316

167. Kracht LW, Miletic H, Busch S, Jacobs AH, Voges J, Hoevels M et al (2004) Delineation of brain tumor extent with [11C]L-methionine positron emission tomography: local comparison with stereotactic histopathology. Clin Cancer Res 10(21):7163–7170. https://doi.org/10.1158/1078-0432.CCR-04-0262. 10/21/7163 [pii]

168. Tonn JC, Thon N, Schnell O, Kreth FW (2012) Personalized surgical therapy. Ann Oncol 23(Suppl 10):x28–x32. https://doi.org/10.1093/annonc/mds363. mds363 [pii]

169. Suchorska B, Jansen NL, Linn J, Kretzschmar H, Janssen H, Eigenbrod S et al (2015) Biological tumor volume in 18FET-PET before radiochemotherapy correlates with survival in GBM. Neurology 84(7):710–719. https://doi.org/10.1212/WNL.0000000000001262

170. Piroth MD, Holy R, Pinkawa M, Stoffels G, Kaiser HJ, Galldiks N et al (2011) Prognostic impact of postoperative, pre-irradiation (18)F-fluoroethyl-l-tyrosine uptake in glioblastoma patients treated with radiochemotherapy. Radiother Oncol 99(2):218–224. https://doi.org/10.1016/j.radonc.2011.03.006

171. Lee IH, Piert M, Gomez-Hassan D, Junck L, Rogers L, Hayman J et al (2009) Association of 11C-methionine PET uptake with site of failure after concurrent temozolomide and radiation for primary glioblastoma multiforme. Int J Radiat Oncol Biol Phys 73(2):479–485. https://doi.org/10.1016/j.ijrobp.2008.04.050

172. Niyazi M, Schnell O, Suchorska B, Schwarz SB, Ganswindt U, Geisler J et al (2012) FET-PET assessed recurrence pattern after radio-chemotherapy in newly diagnosed patients with glioblastoma is influenced by MGMT methylation status. Radiother Oncol 104(1):78–82. https://doi.org/10.1016/j.radonc.2012.04.022

173. Brandes AA, Tosoni A, Spagnolli F, Frezza G, Leonardi M, Calbucci F et al (2008) Disease progression or pseudoprogression after concomitant radiochemotherapy treatment: pitfalls in neurooncology. Neuro Oncol 10(3):361–367. https://doi.org/10.1215/15228517-2008-008. 15228517-2008-008 [pii]

174. Galldiks N, Stoffels G, Ruge MI, Rapp M, Sabel M, Reifenberger G et al (2013) Role of O-(2-18F-fluoroethyl)-L-tyrosine PET as a diagnostic tool for detection of malignant progression in patients with low-grade glioma. J Nucl Med 54(12):2046–2054. https://doi.org/10.2967/jnumed.113.123836

175. Unterrainer M, Schweisthal F, Suchorska B, Wenter V, Schmid-Tannwald C, Fendler WP et al (2016) Serial 18F-FET PET imaging of primarily 18F-FET-negative glioma: does it make sense? J Nucl Med 57(8):1177–1182. https://doi.org/10.2967/jnumed.115.171033

176. Wyss M, Hofer S, Bruehlmeier M, Hefti M, Uhlmann C, Bartschi E et al (2009) Early metabolic responses in temozolomide treated low-grade glioma patients. J Neurooncol 95(1):87–93. https://doi.org/10.1007/s11060-009-9896-2

177. Piroth MD, Pinkawa M, Holy R, Klotz J, Nussen S, Stoffels G et al (2011) Prognostic value of early [18F]fluoroethyltyrosine positron emission tomography after radiochemotherapy in glioblastoma multiforme. Int J Radiat Oncol Biol Phys 80(1):176–184. https://doi.org/10.1016/j.ijrobp.2010.01.055. S0360-3016(10)00229-4 [pii]

178. Hutterer M, Hattingen E, Palm C, Proescholdt MA, Hau P (2015) Current standards and new concepts in MRI and PET response assessment of antiangiogenic therapies in high-grade glioma patients. Neuro Oncol 17(6):784–800. https://doi.org/10.1093/neuonc/nou322

179. Smits A, Westerberg E, Ribom D (2008) Adding 11C-methionine PET to the EORTC prognostic factors in grade 2 gliomas. Eur J Nucl Med Mol Imaging 35(1):65–71. https://doi.org/10.1007/s00259-007-0531-1

180. Galldiks N, Stoffels G, Filss CP, Piroth MD, Sabel M, Ruge MI et al (2012) Role of O-(2-(18)F-fluoroethyl)-L-tyrosine PET for differentiation of local recurrent brain metastasis from radiation necrosis. J Nucl Med 53(9):1367–1374. https://doi.org/10.2967/jnumed.112.103325

181. Glaudemans AW, Enting RH, Heesters MA, Dierckx RA, van Rheenen RW, Walenkamp AM et al (2013) Value of 11C-methionine PET in imaging brain tumours and metastases. Eur J Nucl Med Mol Imaging 40(4):615–635. https://doi.org/10.1007/s00259-012-2295-5

182. Dutour A, Kumar U, Panetta R, Ouafik L, Fina F, Sasi R et al (1998) Expression of somatostatin receptor subtypes in human brain tumors. Int J Cancer 76(5):620–627

183. Reubi JC, Maurer R, Klijn JG, Stefanko SZ, Foekens JA, Blaauw G et al (1986) High incidence of somatostatin receptors in human meningiomas: biochemical characterization. J Clin Endocrinol Metab 63(2):433–438. https://doi.org/10.1210/jcem-63-2-433

184. Menke JR, Raleigh DR, Gown AM, Thomas S, Perry A, Tihan T (2015) Somatostatin receptor 2a is a more sensitive diagnostic marker of

meningioma than epithelial membrane antigen. Acta Neuropathol 130(3):441–443. https://doi.org/10.1007/s00401-015-1459-3

185. Galldiks N, Albert NL, Sommerauer M, Grosu AL, Ganswindt U, Law I et al (2017) PET imaging in patients with meningioma—report of the RANO/PET group. Neuro Oncol 19(12):1576–1587. https://doi.org/10.1093/neuonc/nox112

186. Rachinger W, Stoecklein VM, Terpolilli NA, Haug AR, Ertl L, Poeschl J et al (2015) Increased 68Ga-DOTATATE uptake in PET imaging discriminates meningioma and tumor-free tissue. J Nucl Med 56(3):347–353. https://doi.org/10.2967/jnumed.114.149120

187. Afshar-Oromieh A, Giesel FL, Linhart HG, Haberkorn U, Haufe S, Combs SE et al (2012) Detection of cranial meningiomas: comparison of (68)Ga-DOTATOC PET/CT and contrast-enhanced MRI. Eur J Nucl Med Mol Imaging 39(9):1409–1415. https://doi.org/10.1007/s00259-012-2155-3

188. Unterrainer M, Ilhan H, Todica A, Bartenstein P, Albert NL (2017) Epidural metastases from follicular thyroid cancer mimicking meningiomas in 68Ga-DOTATATE PET. Clin Nucl Med 42(10):805–806. https://doi.org/10.1097/RLU.0000000000001793

189. Velikyan I, Sundin A, Sorensen J, Lubberink M, Sandstrom M, Garske-Roman U et al (2014) Quantitative and qualitative intrapatient comparison of 68Ga-DOTATOC and 68Ga-DOTATATE: net uptake rate for accurate quantification. J Nucl Med 55(2):204–210. https://doi.org/10.2967/jnumed.113.126177

190. Kunz WG, Jungblut LM, Kazmierczak PM, Vettermann FJ, Bollenbacher A, Tonn JC et al (2017) Improved detection of transosseous meningiomas using 68Ga-DOTATATE PET-CT compared to contrast-enhanced MRI. J Nucl Med 58(10):1580–1587. https://doi.org/10.2967/jnumed.117.191932

191. Rachinger W, Stoecklein VM, Terpolilli NA, Haug AR, Ertl L, Poschl J et al (2015) Increased 68Ga-DOTATATE uptake in PET imaging discriminates meningioma and tumor-free tissue. J Nucl Med 56(3):347–353. https://doi.org/10.2967/jnumed.114.149120

192. Hanscheid H, Sweeney RA, Flentje M, Buck AK, Lohr M, Samnick S et al (2012) PET SUV correlates with radionuclide uptake in peptide receptor therapy in meningioma. Eur J Nucl Med Mol Imaging 39(8):1284–1288. https://doi.org/10.1007/s00259-012-2124-x

193. Seystahl K, Stoecklein V, Schuller U, Rushing E, Nicolas G, Schafer N et al (2016) Somatostatin receptor-targeted radionuclide therapy for progressive meningioma: benefit linked to 68Ga-DOTATATE/-TOC uptake. Neuro Oncol 18(11):1538–1547. https://doi.org/10.1093/neuonc/now060

194. Eary JF, Mankoff DA, Spence AM, Berger MS, Olshen A, Link JM et al (1999) 2-[C-11]thymidine imaging of malignant brain tumors. Cancer Res 59(3):615–621

195. Chen W, Cloughesy T, Kamdar N, Satyamurthy N, Bergsneider M, Liau L et al (2005) Imaging proliferation in brain tumors with 18F-FLT PET: comparison with 18F-FDG. J Nucl Med 46(6):945–952. 46/6/945 [pii]

196. Rasey JS, Grierson JR, Wiens LW, Kolb PD, Schwartz JL (2002) Validation of FLT uptake as a measure of thymidine kinase-1 activity in A549 carcinoma cells. J Nucl Med 43(9):1210–1217

197. Backes H, Ullrich R, Neumaier B, Kracht L, Wienhard K, Jacobs AH (2009) Noninvasive quantification of 18F-FLT human brain PET for the assessment of tumour proliferation in patients with high-grade glioma. Eur J Nucl Med Mol Imaging 36(12):1960–1967. https://doi.org/10.1007/s00259-009-1244-4

198. Ullrich R, Backes H, Li H, Kracht L, Miletic H, Kesper K et al (2008) Glioma proliferation as assessed by 3′-fluoro-3′-deoxy-L-thymidine positron emission tomography in patients with newly diagnosed high-grade glioma. Clin Cancer Res 14(7):2049–2055. https://doi.org/10.1158/1078-0432.CCR-07-1553. 14/7/2049 [pii]

199. Harris RJ, Cloughesy TF, Pope WB, Nghiemphu PL, Lai A, Zaw T et al (2012) 18F-FDOPA and 18F-FLT positron emission tomography parametric response maps predict response in recurrent malignant gliomas treated with bevacizumab. Neuro-Oncology 14(8):1079–1089. https://doi.org/10.1093/neuonc/nos141. nos141 [pii]

200. Nikaki A, Angelidis G, Efthimiadou R, Tsougos I, Valotassiou V, Fountas K et al (2017) 18F-fluorothymidine PET imaging in gliomas: an update. Ann Nucl Med 31(7):495–505. https://doi.org/10.1007/s12149-017-1183-2

201. Krause BJ, Souvatzoglou M, Treiber U (2013) Imaging of prostate cancer with PET/CT and radioactively labeled choline derivates. Urol Oncol 31(4):427–435. https://doi.org/10.1016/j.urolonc.2010.08.008

202. Bell C, Dowson N, Fay M, Thomas P, Puttick S, Gal Y et al (2015) Hypoxia imaging in gliomas with 18F-fluoromisonidazole PET: toward clinical translation. Semin Nucl Med 45(2):136–150. https://doi.org/10.1053/j.semnuclmed.2014.10.001

203. Su Z, Roncaroli F, Durrenberger PF, Coope DJ, Karabatsou K, Hinz R et al (2015) The 18-kDa mitochondrial translocator protein in human gliomas: an 11C-(R)PK11195 PET imaging and neuropathology study. J Nucl Med 56(4):512–517. https://doi.org/10.2967/jnumed.114.151621

204. Jensen P, Feng L, Law I, Svarer C, Knudsen GM, Mikkelsen JD et al (2015) TSPO imaging in glioblastoma multiforme: a direct comparison between 123I-CLINDE SPECT, 18F-FET PET, and gadolinium-enhanced MR imaging. J Nucl Med 56(9):1386–1390. https://doi.org/10.2967/jnumed.115.158998

205. Nomura N, Pastorino S, Jiang P, Lambert G, Crawford JR, Gymnopoulos M et al (2014) Prostate specific membrane antigen (PSMA) expression in primary gliomas and breast cancer brain metastases. Cancer Cell Int 14(1):26. https://doi.org/10.1186/1475-2867-14-26

206. Haffner MC, Laimer J, Chaux A, Schafer G, Obrist P, Brunner A et al (2012) High expression of prostate-specific membrane antigen in the tumor-associated neo-vasculature is associated with worse prognosis in squamous cell carcinoma of the oral cavity. Mod Pathol 25(8):1079–1085. https://doi.org/10.1038/modpathol.2012.66

207. Sasikumar A, Joy A, Pillai MR, Nanabala R, Anees KM, Jayaprakash PG et al (2017) Diagnostic value of 68Ga PSMA-11 PET/CT imaging of brain tumors-preliminary analysis. Clin Nucl Med 42(1):e41–ee8. https://doi.org/10.1097/RLU.0000000000001451

208. Schwenck J, Tabatabai G, Skardelly M, Reischl G, Beschorner R, Pichler B et al (2015) In vivo visualization of prostate-specific membrane antigen in glioblastoma. Eur J Nucl Med Mol Imaging 42(1):170–171. https://doi.org/10.1007/s00259-014-2921-5

209. Chakraborty PS, Kumar R, Tripathi M, Das CJ, Bal C (2015) Detection of brain metastasis with 68Ga-labeled PSMA ligand PET/CT: a novel radiotracer for imaging of prostate carcinoma. Clin Nucl Med 40(4):328–329. https://doi.org/10.1097/RLU.0000000000000709

210. Pichler BJ, Kolb A, Nagele T, Schlemmer HP (2010) PET/MRI: paving the way for the next generation of clinical multimodality imaging applications. J Nucl Med 51(3):333–336. https://doi.org/10.2967/jnumed.109.061853

211. Tonn JC, Kreth FW, Schnell O, Meyer B, Belka C, Combs SE, Lumenta C (2016) Hirntumoren und spinale Tumoren. 4th edn. Munich, Germany: Zuckschwerdt Verlag

Tumor Biology

4

Farshad Nassiri, Laureen Hachem, and Gelareh Zadeh

4.1 Introduction

The advent of new molecular analyses over the past several decades has greatly enhanced our understanding of central nervous system (CNS) tumor biology. In recent years, the emergence of DNA sequencing and molecular profiling has ushered in an era of molecular-based tumor subtyping that has paved the way for personalized cancer therapies. Research into the cellular composition of CNS tumors and understanding of the heterogeneity of the tumor microenvironment have revealed a range of cell types, including a population of supportive and neoplastic cells with complex cellular hierarchy. Interactions between the various cells (cancer, stromal and local host environment) has been shown to be critical contributors of the tumor microenvironment that in turn promote tumor growth and progression. Moreover, examining these complex interactions has helped elucidate key drivers of treatment resistance and disease recurrence.

In this chapter, we aim to highlight the evolution of CNS tumor biology by providing a broad overview of key cellular and genetic factors that play a role in one of the most lethal and well-studied brain tumor—gliomas. We first discuss the cellular origins of tumorigenesis, specifically highlighting the role of cancer stem cells. Next, we outline the key factors of the tumoral microenvironment which contribute to tumor propagation and growth. We then discuss advances in elucidating the genomic landscape of GBM tumors, highlighting important biomarkers and their implications for guiding prognostication and treatment. As a field we strive to build a comprehensive understanding of tumor biology and the underlying genetic alterations that lead to glioma formation so that we can ultimately find treatments that have increased durability in managing gliomas. Where relevant, lessons learned from other tumor types, for example, medulloblastomas and ependymomas, will be highlighted.

4.2 Tumor Cell Populations

Historically, tumor cells were thought to be derived from a clonal expansion of a mutated cell. However, with increasing analyses highlighting the significant degree of cellular and genetic heterogeneity, it has become evident that the evolution of cancer is more complex than we previously appreciated. The application of stem cell biology and genomic profiling to the field of neuro-oncology has led to the establishment of

F. Nassiri · L. Hachem · G. Zadeh (✉)
Division of Neurosurgery, University Health Network and Princess Margaret Cancer Center,
Toronto, ON, Canada
e-mail: farshad.nassiri@mail.utoronto.ca;
laureen.hachem@mail.utoronto.ca;
Gelareh.zadeh@uhn.ca

© Springer Nature Switzerland AG 2019
J.-C. Tonn et al. (eds.), *Oncology of CNS Tumors*, https://doi.org/10.1007/978-3-030-04152-6_4

the cancer stem cell hypothesis to explain the intratumoral heterogeneity seen in many CNS tumors and particularly glioblastomas.

4.2.1 Cancer Stem Cells

Populations of cells with self-renewing properties have been isolated from a number of CNS tumor types including gliomas, medulloblastomas, and ependymomas [1–4]. These cells, known as cancer stem cells (CSCs), have been shown to induce secondary tumor formation in in vivo orthotopic transplantation models and are thought to be a key determinant in tumor growth and progression [1, 4, 5]. CSCs reside in perivascular and perinecrotic/hypoxic niches that serve to maintain the self-renewal capacity of these cells. Within the perivascular niche (PVN), endothelial cells play a critical role in regulating CSC proliferation through various mechanisms including Notch signaling and secretion of soluble factors such as nitric oxide. CSCs in turn have the capacity to differentiate into endothelial cells resulting in a positive feedback cycle that promotes tumorigenesis. Pericytes and smooth muscle cells are further recruited to the PVN and lead to enhanced angiogenesis [6, 7]. The perinecrotic/hypoxic niche also serves to maintain CSCs as hypoxic conditions lead to the activation of hypoxia-inducible factor (HIF) pathways which regulate the undifferentiated phenotype of CSCs [8].

CSCs may be identified by unique cell surface markers with CD133 being the first marker established in glioma CSCs [1, 9, 10]. This population of CD133+ CSCs is thought to contribute to treatment resistance and tumor recurrence in gliomas [9]. CSCs can evade standard therapies through the activation of DNA repair mechanisms and the expression of anti-apoptotic or drug-resistant genes [9, 11]. As such, these CSCs have the potential to recapitulate the tumor mass with resistant progeny that may display a mutational profile different from the initial tumor cell population [12]. The concept of cellular plasticity has also emerged in recent years to further explain the role of CSCs in disease recurrence. Non-CSCs have demonstrated the capacity to dedifferentiate into cells with CSC-like properties in response to radio- or chemotherapy exposure [13, 14].

The importance of this population of CD133+ CSCs on tumor biology is borne out by findings that the proportion of CD133+ cells in glioma tissue is a poor prognostic factor for progression-free survival and overall survival and a risk factor for time to malignant progression [15]. Despite this, emerging evidence suggests that some CD133-negative cells may also take on a CSC-like phenotype, and therefore further research into the unique profiling of this population of stem cells is necessary before CD133 may be used as a prognostic marker [16, 17].

4.2.2 Intratumoral Cellular Heterogeneity

Cellular and genomic analyses have revealed the significant extent of intratumoral heterogeneity seen in many gliomas [18]. Regional differences in chromosomal mutations and genetic and epigenetic signatures have been shown to occur within a single tumor [18, 19]. Emerging techniques in single-cell genomic sequencing coupled with DNA barcoding have helped improve our understanding of the mechanisms underlying the intratumoral heterogeneity seen in gliomas [20, 21]. Single-cell fate mapping using DNA barcoding of glioblastoma cells has recently revealed a stem cell hierarchy to explain the growth of subclones within a single tumor sample [22]. Moreover, single-cell profiling of oligodendroglioma has suggested a tri-potent stem/progenitor cell origin of tumor growth. Through establishment of a stemness expression profile in individual cells, a developmental hierarchy has now been outlined for oligodendroglioma [21].

This intratumoral heterogeneity has significant diagnostic and therapeutic implications. As mutations may not be uniformly expressed within a single tumor sample, technical cutoff must be established when attempting to stratify tumors by mutational status. Determining a reliable and clinically meaningful cutoff requires validation in large cohort studies. Intratumoral heterogeneity may account for treatment failure or disease recurrence as different subclones of tumor cells may have a differential response to a given therapy [23, 24]. This consequently leads to the selection of populations of tumor cells that are treatment-resistant and display a more aggressive phenotype. As selection pressures from both treatment exposure and the tumor microenvironment change over time, the mutational profile of gliomas does not remain static and can also display significant temporal heterogeneity [12, 24]. Mutational analysis of recurrent glioma samples has revealed that in many cases the majority of mutations at initial diagnosis are not detected on recurrence. Moreover, specific treatments like temozolomide chemotherapy may be associated with a distinct pattern of mutations in recurrent tumors [12]. Genetic differences between therapy-naïve tumors and treated recurrences may underlie the lack of treatment effect observed in many previous clinical trials on recurrent disease. Ultimately, understanding the mechanisms of clonal selection which drives divergence in recurrent tumors will be paramount in establishing effective treatment paradigms for recurrent GBM.

4.3 Tumor Microenvironment

Neoplastic cells do not exist in the environment alone. Rather, they are intimately integrated with a network of supportive cells that make up a large portion of the tumor mass, often referred to as the stromal cell population that combine to form the tumor microenvironment. This microenvironment plays a critical role in glioma progression and response to treatment. Alterations in local immune response and vascular networks have been shown to facilitate tumor growth. An understanding of these processes which promote tumorigenesis has now led to the development of many experimental therapies aimed at targeting the underlying molecular and cellular mediators which drive tumor progression. The role of each of these factors on tumor biology is highlighted in this section.

4.3.1 Immune Cells

Aberrations in the local immune and inflammatory response have been shown to play a key role in gliomagenesis. It is recognized that GBMs signal recruitment of bone marrow derived cells, the majority of which differentiate into immune and inflammatory cell population. In fact, it has been shown that the majority of tumoral inflammatory cell populations are bone marrow-derived rather than brain-resident cells. Approximately 30% of the brain tumor mass is comprised of tumor-associated macrophages (TAMs), derived from the activation of CNS microglia or peripheral monocytes [25, 26]. Macrophages have the potential to differentiate into two distinct phenotypes depending on surrounding environmental cues: M1 macrophages are pro-inflammatory, whereas M2 macrophages are anti-inflammatory and promote tissue repair. Secreted tumor factors from gliomas are thought to drive TAMs to an anti-inflammatory M2 phenotype that promotes tumorigenesis [27]. In fact, the proportion of M2 macrophages has been shown to correlate with tumor proliferation and histological grade in human gliomas [28].

Investigations into the mechanisms by which glioma cells induce microglial and macrophage activation and their downstream effect on tumorigenesis have led to the identification of candidate molecular targets for new therapies. Colony-stimulating factor-1 (CSF-1), released by glioma cells, is an important chemoattractant which promotes microglia polarization to an M2 phenotype. CSF-1 receptor inhibitors have been shown to reduce M2 polarization and improve response to radiotherapy and survival in preclinical models of glioblastoma [29, 30]. Moreover, TAMs have been shown to secrete various pro-oncogenic factors such as TGFβ [31] and matrix metalloproteinases [32] that promote tumor invasion. Moving forward, inhibiting factors that regulate the recruitment and differentiation of TAMs and microglia hold potential as adjunct therapies and will require further investigation. The potential to harness recruited bone marrow-derived cells, specifically TAMs and microglia, for delivery of therapeutics will offer an important strategy as they have the inherent ability to infiltrate and reach the tumor microenvironment more effectively than systemic delivered therapeutics.

4.3.2 Tumor Neovascularization

Most CNS tumors rely on a robust vascular supply and therefore induce angiogenesis by upregulating the expression of pro-angiogenic factors. It has been long recognized that vascular endothelial growth factor (VEGF) is highly expressed in malignant gliomas and is a key regulator of angiogenesis and vascular permeability. A large body of preclinical data that supported the role of VEGF blockade in the treatment of malignant gliomas together with a promise in some early clinical applications led the FDA to approve the use of the anti-VEGF monoclonal antibody, bevacizumab (Avastin), in 2009 as salvage therapy for recurrent glioblastoma [33]. However, as bevacizumab failed to demonstrate an effect in improving overall survival in newly diagnosed glioblastoma [34, 35], a search for other drivers of angiogenesis has ensued. Emerging evidence has suggested an important role of angiopoietin-2 (Ang-2) in tumor angiogenesis that may be implicated in tumor resistance to anti-VEGF therapy, and thus investigations into the role of dual inhibition of VEGF and Ang-2 are underway [36]. The putative mechanisms of anti-angiogenic therapy (AATx) failure are thought to be driven by perivascular cells, some in part derived from recruited bone marrow cells and inflammatory cells and some in part from CSCs. These perivascular cells provide an endothelial protective mechanism and resistance against AATx. Upregulation of a number of other angiogenic factors that are part of the robust cascade that regulate tumor neovascularization is thought to also be key in resistance to the single-factor inhibition approach of AATx. Increase in hypoxia and the clonal evolution of cancer cells that themselves have angiogenic potential are also among some of the key perspectives on resistance to AATx. With disappointing results from RTOG and AVAglio trials on bevacizumab, the enthusiasm to pursue effective anti-angiogenic therapy

(AATx) has dampened to some extent. However, understanding predictors of response to AATx, to be able to identify subpopulation of GBMs that have effective response to treatment is important to keep in sight for ongoing investigation.

4.4 The Genomic Landscape of CNS Tumors

Examining the molecular and genomic landscape of gliomas has greatly informed our understanding of glioma biology and pathogenesis. The introduction of DNA sequencing and epigenetic profiling has enabled the identification of various mutations that may serve as biomarkers to help guide prognostication and treatment of gliomas. Collectively, advances in genomic and molecular technology have transformed the way in which glial tumors are classified, allowing for genetic- and molecular-based subtyping that can inform personalized cancer therapies. This section will outline some of the major biomarkers identified across gliomas and highlight their clinical utility in guiding treatment (Table 4.1).

4.4.1 Aberrations in Cell Signaling Pathways Drive Malignant Transformation

Multiple checkpoints exist in normal cells to maintain cellular homeostasis and prevent dysregulated growth. Genetic mutations in cellular signaling pathways that regulate the cell cycle are key drivers of neoplastic transformation in gliomas. In 2008 The Cancer Genome Atlas published a genomic characterization of glioblastoma identifying driver mutations in three canonical cell signaling pathways: RTK/PI3K, p53, and Rb pathways [37].

4.4.1.1 RTK/PI3K Pathway
The RTK/PI3K pathway transduces extracellular signals via receptor tyrosine kinases to regulate cell growth. Mutations in EGFR, a type of receptor tyrosine kinase within this pathway, are seen in upward of 50% of malignant gliomas [38].

Table 4.1 CNS tumor biomarkers

Biomarker	Tumor type	Clinical significance	Targeted therapies under investigation
IDH-1/IDH-2 mutation	Astrocytoma (WHO II/WHO III) Oligodendroglioma (WHO II/WHO III) Secondary glioblastoma	Diagnostic, positive prognostic marker for survival, positive predictive marker for treatment response	IDH-1/IDH-2 inhibitors
1p/19q co-deletion	Oligodendroglioma	Diagnostic, positive prognostic marker for survival, positive predictive marker for treatment response	–
MGMT promoter methylation	Glioblastoma	Positive prognostic marker for survival, positive predictive marker for response to temozolomide and radiotherapy	–
BRAF fusion	Infratentorial PA	May be positive prognostic factor	RAF/MEK inhibitors
BRAF V600E mutation	PXA (most common) Ganglioglioma Supratentorial PA Papillary craniopharyngioma	May be positive prognostic factor	RAF/MEK inhibitors
H3.K27M mutations	Pediatric HGG	Poor prognostic factor	HDAC inhibitors

Abbreviations: *HDAC* histone deacetylase, *HGG* high-grade glioma, *IDH* isocitrate dehydrogenase, *MGMT* O6-methylguanine-DNA methyltransferase, *PA* pilocytic astrocytoma, *PXA* pleomorphic xanthoastrocytoma, *WHO* World Health Organization

The most common mutant, EGFRvIII, resulting from deletion of exons 2–7 leads to constitutive receptor activation ultimately promoting proliferation and tumor invasion [39, 40]. Moreover, PTEN is a tumor suppressor gene located on chromosome 10q that encodes a protein which negatively regulates PI3K downstream signaling. PTEN mutations are seen in nearly 40% of adult glioblastomas but are rare in low-grade gliomas [41]. It is believed that PTEN mutations are associated with malignant progression and are correlated with poor prognosis in patients with gliomas [42].

4.4.1.2 p53 and Rb Pathways

p53 is a nuclear transcription factor involved in initiating cellular apoptosis and maintaining genomic stability. Mutations that impair the normal apoptotic processes within host cells can further drive tumorigenesis. Loss of function mutations in p53 are seen in 67% of anaplastic astrocytomas and 40–70% of glioblastomas [37, 43]. In addition, Rb is another key tumor suppressor protein that inhibits cell cycle progression by binding and inhibiting the transcription

factor E2F, thereby repressing transcription of genes required for the synthesis phase of the cell cycle [44]. Mutations in Rb have been seen in close to 80% of glioblastomas [37].

4.4.2 IDH-1 and IDH-2 Mutations in Diffuse Gliomas and Secondary Glioblastomas

Over the past decade, our improved understanding of the impact of mutations in the isocitrate dehydrogenase (IDH) gene in gliomas has revolutionized how we categorized these tumors. Mutations in IDH-1 and IDH-2 genes are thought to be critical alterations in gliomagenesis and important events in the development of secondary gliomas. Genomic analyses of patient-derived tumor samples have revealed mutations in the IDH-1 gene in almost 80% of grades II and III oligodendrogliomas and astrocytomas along with secondary glioblastomas [45–47].

IDH proteins catalyze the oxidative decarboxylation of isocitrate to α-KG which in turn reduces NADP+ to NADPH. Most IDH mutations in gliomas are missense mutations occurring at arginine 132 (R132) in IDH-1 and R140 or R172 in IDH-2 [47]. The biological significance of IDH mutations in gliomagenesis is thought to be due to a gain of function in mutant IDH proteins which preferentially converts α-KG to the oncometabolite R-2-hydroxyglutarate (2-HG). 2-HG has been found in high levels in human glioma samples with IDH mutations [48] and is thought to drive tumorigenesis through inhibition of cellular differentiation [49] and activation of the mTOR pathway leading to cell growth [50].

Our understanding of the role of IDH mutations in tumor biology has led to significant advances in the classification and prognostication of gliomas. The 2016 WHO classification of CNS tumors has now incorporated IDH mutation status as one of the main molecular diagnostic criteria for secondary glioblastomas along with diffuse astrocytomas and oligodendrogliomas [51]. IDH mutation status also has clear prognostic implications as multiple studies have found that IDH mutations in gliomas portend improved survival and response to treatment compared to IDH wild-type tumors [52–54].

4.4.3 1p/19q Co-Deletion in Oligodendrogliomas

Early studies into the genetic basis of glial tumors revealed that 1p/19q co-deletion was a hallmark of oligodendrogliomas seen in 60–90% of grade II and III subtypes [55, 56]. 1p/19q co-deletion has also been shown to portend a more favorable clinical course and better response to either chemotherapy or radiotherapy [57]. IDH-1 mutations are nearly ubiquitous in 1p/19q co-deleted oligodendrogliomas [58], and genomic studies have revealed that IDH-1 mutations likely occur prior to the acquisition of 1p/19q co-deletion. This finding has led to the hypothesis that low-grade gliomas may originate from precursor cells harboring an IDH-1 mutation and 1p/19q co-deletion may drive it toward an oligodendroglial phenotype, distinct from astrocytomas which rarely harbor this mutation but

instead often possess mutations in ATRX and p53 [59]. Indeed, 1p/19q mutations have been found to be mutually exclusive with ATRX or p53 mutations; the latter often defining astrocytic tumors [60]. The combination of IDH-1 mutation and 1p/19q co-deletion has therefore now been incorporated into the diagnostic criteria for oligodendrogliomas [51].

4.4.4 MGMT Promotor Methylation in Glioblastomas

MGMT promotor methylation is now considered an important predictor of temozolomide chemotherapy response in glioblastoma [61, 62]. O6-Methylguanine-DNA methyltransferase (MGMT) is a DNA repair protein which reverses O6-alkylguanine lesions induced by alkylating chemotherapeutic agents. Methylation of CpG islands in the MGMT gene promoter leads to silencing of the MGMT expression and in turn enhances sensitivity to temozolomide [63].

Approximately 40% of primary glioblastomas are methylated at the MGMT promotor region [61]. There is strong evidence to support the predictive role of MGMT methylation status and response to temozolomide chemotherapy [61]. It has also been suggested that MGMT promoter methylation may be a predictive biomarker of response to radiotherapy [64]. Therefore, it is possible that MGMT promoter methylation may be a general prognostic indicator in glioblastoma regardless of treatment undertaken. Combining MGMT methylation status with other tumor biomarkers may further enhance its prognostic ability. For example, combined IDH-1 mutation and MGMT methylation were associated with the longest survival in glioblastoma patients compared to patients with either IDH-1 mutation or MGMT methylation alone [65].

4.4.5 BRAF Mutations

The potential role of BRAF mutations in gliomas has been raised through the recent interest in a different subtype of CNS tumors—craniopharyngiomas. Exome sequencing analysis has shown that papillary craniopharyngiomas, but not other subtypes of craniopharyngiomas, may be defined by the BRAF V600E mutation [66]. BRAF is a proto-oncogene in the RAF family of serine/threonine kinases and an important regulator of the MAPK signaling pathway that controls cell growth. It has been shown that mutations in the BRAF gene lead to cell cycle dysregulation and have been implicated in the pathogenesis of pediatric low-grade gliomas, first in 2008 with the discovery of a tandem duplication at 7q34 resulting in a fusion oncogene, BRAF/KIAA1549, found in a subset of pilocytic astrocytomas (PAs) [67]. This fusion resulted in constitutive activation of the MAPK pathway and was thus implicated in tumor growth. BRAF fusions are found in approximately 60% of PAs and appear to define a subset of tumors with a less aggressive clinical course [68]. Fusion-positive PAs are more commonly seen in younger patients and in tumors that arise in the posterior fossa [69]. BRAF fusions have also been found in glioneuronal tumors and pleomorphic xanthoastrocytomas (PXA), albeit at lower rates [70].

Constitutive activation of the BRAF gene also results from the canonical BRAF V600E mutation found in many types of low-grade gliomas, most commonly pleomorphic xanthoastrocytoma, ganglioglioma, and supratentorial pilocytic astrocytomas [71, 72]. BRAF V600E mutation has recently been shown to correlate with poor outcomes after chemotherapy and radiotherapy in pediatric low-grade gliomas [73]. As such, BRAF inhibitors are currently under investigation for the treatment of pediatric gliomas harboring the BRAF V600E mutation (clinicaltrials. gov: NCT01677741).

4.4.6 H3.K27M Mutations in Pediatric High-Grade Gliomas

Continued research into the genetic underpinnings of malignant gliomas has revealed that many of the hallmark mutations frequently seen in adult glioblastoma occur at a much lower rate in pediatric glioblastoma [74]. This has sparked a growing interest in identifying distinct mutations within this group of tumors. Exon sequencing of pediatric glioblastoma samples has identified a K27M mutation in the H3F3A gene in approximately 30% of tumors [75], with a considerably lower rate (3%) in adult glioblastoma. Moreover, close to 80% of pediatric diffuse intrinsic pontine gliomas (DIPG) have been found to harbor this mutation [76]. The 2016 WHO classification has now defined the clinical entity of "diffuse midline glioma, H3 K27M-mutant" characterized by tumors primarily occurring in the pediatric population with H3 K27M mutation, a diffuse growth pattern, and midline location.

H3F3A encodes the H3.3 replication-independent histone protein, which is important for chromatin remodeling and DNA replication [77]. K27 represses chromatin and gene expression, and it is believed that K27M mutation may lead to a gain-of-function event; however, further investigation into the exact molecular effects of this mutation is necessary. Importantly, pediatric gliomas with the H3.K27M mutation were found to have significantly worse overall survival compared to H3.3 wildtypes [78].

4.5 Conclusion

The last decade has witnessed a paradigm shift in our understanding of CNS tumor biology and pathogenesis. Technological and biomedical advancements have led to an unprecedented growth in genomic-based analyses that have helped elucidate the underlying mechanisms of adult and pediatric brain and spine tumor formation and progression. The identification of a number of genomic biomarkers has revolutionized the classification of CNS tumors and offered novel tools to guide prognostication and ultimately better inform clinical treatment paradigms. As the field of neuro-oncology continues to remain at the forefront of the molecular and genomic era, the coming years will likely witness continued advancements in tumor genome sequencing and personalized treatment pathways.

References

1. Singh SK, Clarke ID, Terasaki M, Bonn VE, Hawkins C, Squire J et al (2003) Identification of a cancer stem cell in human brain tumors. Cancer Res 63(18):5821–5828

2. Meco D, Servidei T, Lamorte G, Binda E, Arena V, Riccardi R (2014) Ependymoma stem cells are highly sensitive to temozolomide in vitro and in orthotopic models. Neuro Oncol 16(8):1067–1077

3. Manoranjan B, Venugopal C, McFarlane N, Doble BW, Dunn SE, Scheinemann K et al (2012) Medulloblastoma stem cells: where development and cancer cross pathways. Pediatr Res 71(4 Pt 2):516–522

4. Galli R, Binda E, Orfanelli U, Cipelletti B, Gritti A, De Vitis S et al (2004) Isolation and characterization of tumorigenic, stem-like neural precursors from human glioblastoma. Cancer Res 64(19): 7011–7021

5. Singh SK, Hawkins C, Clarke ID, Squire JA, Bayani J, Hide T et al (2004) Identification of human brain tumour initiating cells. Nature 432(7015):396–401

6. Charles NA, Holland EC, Gilbertson R, Glass R, Kettenmann H (2011) The brain tumor microenvironment. Glia 59(8):1169–1180

7. Calabrese C, Poppleton H, Kocak M, Hogg TL, Fuller C, Hamner B et al (2007) A perivascular niche for brain tumor stem cells. Cancer Cell 11(1):69–82

8. Plaks V, Kong N, Werb Z (2015) The cancer stem cell niche: how essential is the niche in regulating stemness of tumor cells? Cell Stem Cell 16(3):225–238

9. Bao S, Wu Q, McLendon RE, Hao Y, Shi Q, Hjelmeland AB et al (2006) Glioma stem cells promote radioresistance by preferential activation of the DNA damage response. Nature 444(7120):756–760

10. Bao S, Wu Q, Sathornsumetee S, Hao Y, Li Z, Hjelmeland AB et al (2006) Stem cell-like glioma cells promote tumor angiogenesis through vascular endothelial growth factor. Cancer Res 66(16):7843–7848

11. Liu G, Yuan X, Zeng Z, Tunici P, Ng H, Abdulkadir IR et al (2006) Analysis of gene expression and chemoresistance of CD133+ cancer stem cells in glioblastoma. Mol Cancer 5:67

12. Johnson BE, Mazor T, Hong C, Barnes M, Aihara K, McLean CY et al (2014) Mutational analysis reveals the origin and therapy-driven evolution of recurrent glioma. Science (New York, NY) 343(6167):189–193

13. Auffinger B, Tobias AL, Han Y, Lee G, Guo D, Dey M et al (2014) Conversion of differentiated cancer cells into cancer stem-like cells in a glioblastoma model after primary chemotherapy. Cell Death Differ 21(7):1119–1131

14. Dahan P, Martinez Gala J, Delmas C, Monferran S, Malric L, Zentkowski D et al (2014) Ionizing radiations sustain glioblastoma cell dedifferentiation to a stem-like phenotype through survivin: possible involvement in radioresistance. Cell Death Dis 5:e1543

15. Zeppernick F, Ahmadi R, Campos B, Dictus C, Helmke BM, Becker N et al (2008) Stem cell marker CD133 affects clinical outcome in glioma patients. Clin Cancer Res 14(1):123–129

16. Beier D, Hau P, Proescholdt M, Lohmeier A, Wischhusen J, Oefner PJ et al (2007) CD133(+) and CD133(−) glioblastoma-derived cancer stem cells show differential growth characteristics and molecular profiles. Cancer Res 67(9):4010–4015

17. Rich JN, Eyler CE (2008) Cancer stem cells in brain tumor biology. Cold Spring Harb Symp Quant Biol 73:411–420

18. Vartanian A, Singh SK, Agnihotri S, Jalali S, Burrell K, Aldape KD et al (2014) GBM's multifaceted landscape: highlighting regional and microenvironmental heterogeneity. Neuro Oncol 16(9):1167–1175

19. Sottoriva A, Spiteri I, Piccirillo SG, Touloumis A, Collins VP, Marioni JC et al (2013) Intratumor heterogeneity in human glioblastoma reflects cancer evolutionary dynamics. Proc Natl Acad Sci U S A 110(10):4009–4014

20. Patel AP, Tirosh I, Trombetta JJ, Shalek AK, Gillespie SM, Wakimoto H et al (2014) Single-cell RNA-seq highlights intratumoral heterogeneity in primary glioblastoma. Science (New York, NY) 344(6190):1396–1401

21. Tirosh I, Venteicher AS, Hebert C, Escalante LE, Patel AP, Yizhak K et al (2016) Single-cell RNA-seq supports a developmental hierarchy in human oligodendroglioma. Nature 539(7628):309–313

22. Lan X, Jorg DJ, Cavalli FMG, Richards LM, Nguyen LV, Vanner RJ et al (2017) Fate mapping of human glioblastoma reveals an invariant stem cell hierarchy. Nature 549(7671):227–232

23. Szerlip NJ, Pedraza A, Chakravarty D, Azim M, McGuire J, Fang Y et al (2012) Intratumoral heterogeneity of receptor tyrosine kinases EGFR and PDGFRA amplification in glioblastoma defines subpopulations with distinct growth factor response. Proc Natl Acad Sci U S A 109(8):3041–3046

24. Nickel GC, Barnholtz-Sloan J, Gould MP, McMahon S, Cohen A, Adams MD et al (2012) Characterizing mutational heterogeneity in a glioblastoma patient with double recurrence. PLoS One 7(4):e35262

25. Graeber MB, Scheithauer BW, Kreutzberg GW (2002) Microglia in brain tumors. Glia 40(2): 252–259

26. De Palma M (2016) Origins of brain tumor macrophages. Cancer Cell 30(6):832–833

27. Sica A, Schioppa T, Mantovani A, Allavena P (2006) Tumour-associated macrophages are a distinct M2 polarised population promoting tumour progression: potential targets of anti-cancer therapy. Eur J Cancer 42(6):717–727

28. Komohara Y, Ohnishi K, Kuratsu J, Takeya M (2008) Possible involvement of the M2 anti-inflammatory macrophage phenotype in growth of human gliomas. J Pathol 216(1):15–24

29. Pyonteck SM, Akkari L, Schuhmacher AJ, Bowman RL, Sevenich L, Quail DF et al (2013) CSF-1R

inhibition alters macrophage polarization and blocks glioma progression. Nat Med 19(10):1264–1272

30. Stafford JH, Hirai T, Deng L, Chernikova SB, Urata K, West BL et al (2016) Colony stimulating factor 1 receptor inhibition delays recurrence of glioblastoma after radiation by altering myeloid cell recruitment and polarization. Neuro Oncol 18(6):797–806

31. Wesolowska A, Kwiatkowska A, Slomnicki L, Dembinski M, Master A, Sliwa M et al (2008) Microglia-derived TGF-beta as an important regulator of glioblastoma invasion—an inhibition of TGF-beta-dependent effects by shRNA against human TGF-beta type II receptor. Oncogene 27(7):918–930

32. Markovic DS, Vinnakota K, Chirasani S, Synowitz M, Raguet H, Stock K et al (2009) Gliomas induce and exploit microglial MT1-MMP expression for tumor expansion. Proc Natl Acad Sci U S A 106(30):12530–12535

33. Field KM, Jordan JT, Wen PY, Rosenthal MA, Reardon DA (2015) Bevacizumab and glioblastoma: scientific review, newly reported updates, and ongoing controversies. Cancer 121(7):997–1007

34. Gilbert MR, Dignam JJ, Armstrong TS, Wefel JS, Blumenthal DT, Vogelbaum MA et al (2014) A randomized trial of bevacizumab for newly diagnosed glioblastoma. N Engl J Med 370(8):699–708

35. Chinot OL, Wick W, Mason W, Henriksson R, Saran F, Nishikawa R et al (2014) Bevacizumab plus radiotherapy-temozolomide for newly diagnosed glioblastoma. N Engl J Med 370(8):709–722

36. Peterson TE, Kirkpatrick ND, Huang Y, Farrar CT, Marijt KA, Kloepper J et al (2016) Dual inhibition of Ang-2 and VEGF receptors normalizes tumor vasculature and prolongs survival in glioblastoma by altering macrophages. Proc Natl Acad Sci U S A 113(16):4470–4475

37. Cancer Genome Atlas Research Network (2008) Comprehensive genomic characterization defines human glioblastoma genes and core pathways. Nature 455(7216):1061–1068

38. Watanabe K, Tachibana O, Sata K, Yonekawa Y, Kleihues P, Ohgaki H (1996) Overexpression of the EGF receptor and p53 mutations are mutually exclusive in the evolution of primary and secondary glioblastomas. Brain Pathol 6(3):217–223; discussion 23–24

39. Lal A, Glazer CA, Martinson HM, Friedman HS, Archer GE, Sampson JH et al (2002) Mutant epidermal growth factor receptor up-regulates molecular effectors of tumor invasion. Cancer Res 62(12):3335–3339

40. Wong AJ, Bigner SH, Bigner DD, Kinzler KW, Hamilton SR, Vogelstein B (1987) Increased expression of the epidermal growth factor receptor gene in malignant gliomas is invariably associated with gene amplification. Proc Natl Acad Sci U S A 84(19):6899–6903

41. Brennan CW, Verhaak RG, McKenna A, Campos B, Noushmehr H, Salama SR et al (2013) The somatic genomic landscape of glioblastoma. Cell 155(2):462–477

42. Han F, Hu R, Yang H, Liu J, Sui J, Xiang X et al (2016) PTEN gene mutations correlate to poor prognosis in glioma patients: a meta-analysis. Onco Targets Ther 9:3485–3492

43. Tada M, Iggo RD, Waridel F, Nozaki M, Matsumoto R, Sawamura Y et al (1997) Reappraisal of p53 mutations in human malignant astrocytic neoplasms by p53 functional assay: comparison with conventional structural analyses. Mol Carcinog 18(3):171–176

44. Du W, Pogoriler J (2006) Retinoblastoma family genes. Oncogene 25(38):5190–5200

45. Balss J, Meyer J, Mueller W, Korshunov A, Hartmann C, von Deimling A (2008) Analysis of the IDH1 codon 132 mutation in brain tumors. Acta Neuropathol 116(6):597–602

46. Hartmann C, Meyer J, Balss J, Capper D, Mueller W, Christians A et al (2009) Type and frequency of IDH1 and IDH2 mutations are related to astrocytic and oligodendroglial differentiation and age: a study of 1,010 diffuse gliomas. Acta Neuropathol 118(4):469–474

47. Yan H, Parsons DW, Jin G, McLendon R, Rasheed BA, Yuan W et al (2009) IDH1 and IDH2 mutations in gliomas. N Engl J Med 360(8):765–773

48. Dang L, White DW, Gross S, Bennett BD, Bittinger MA, Driggers EM et al (2009) Cancer-associated IDH1 mutations produce 2-hydroxyglutarate. Nature 462(7274):739–744

49. Lu C, Ward PS, Kapoor GS, Rohle D, Turcan S, Abdel-Wahab O et al (2012) IDH mutation impairs histone demethylation and results in a block to cell differentiation. Nature 483(7390):474–478

50. Carbonneau M, M Gagné L, Lalonde ME, Germain MA, Motorina A, Guiot MC et al (2016) The oncometabolite 2-hydroxyglutarate activates the mTOR signalling pathway. Nat Commun 7:12700

51. Louis DN, Perry A, Reifenberger G, von Deimling A, Figarella-Branger D, Cavenee WK et al (2016) The 2016 World Health Organization classification of tumors of the central nervous system: a summary. Acta Neuropathol 131(6):803–820

52. Nobusawa S, Watanabe T, Kleihues P, Ohgaki H (2009) IDH1 mutations as molecular signature and predictive factor of secondary glioblastomas. Clin Cancer Res 15(19):6002–6007

53. Sanson M, Marie Y, Paris S, Idbaih A, Laffaire J, Ducray F et al (2009) Isocitrate dehydrogenase 1 codon 132 mutation is an important prognostic biomarker in gliomas. J Clin Oncol 27(25):4150–4154

54. Houillier C, Wang X, Kaloshi G, Mokhtari K, Guillevin R, Laffaire J et al (2010) IDH1 or IDH2 mutations predict longer survival and response to temozolomide in low-grade gliomas. Neurology 75(17):1560–1566

55. Reifenberger J, Reifenberger G, Liu L, James CD, Wechsler W, Collins VP (1994) Molecular genetic analysis of oligodendroglial tumors shows preferential allelic deletions on 19q and 1p. Am J Pathol 145(5):1175–1190

56. von Deimling A, Louis DN, von Ammon K, Petersen I, Wiestler OD, Seizinger BR (1992) Evidence for a

tumor suppressor gene on chromosome 19q associated with human astrocytomas, oligodendrogliomas, and mixed gliomas. Cancer Res 52(15):4277–4279

57. Cairncross JG, Ueki K, Zlatescu MC, Lisle DK, Finkelstein DM, Hammond RR et al (1998) Specific genetic predictors of chemotherapeutic response and survival in patients with anaplastic oligodendrogliomas. J Natl Cancer Inst 90(19):1473–1479

58. Wang XW, Ciccarino P, Rossetto M, Boisselier B, Marie Y, Desestret V et al (2014) IDH mutations: genotype-phenotype correlation and prognostic impact. Biomed Res Int 2014:540236

59. Watanabe T, Nobusawa S, Kleihues P, Ohgaki H (2009) IDH1 mutations are early events in the development of astrocytomas and oligodendrogliomas. Am J Pathol 174(4):1149–1153

60. Wiestler B, Capper D, Holland-Letz T, Korshunov A, von Deimling A, Pfister SM et al (2013) ATRX loss refines the classification of anaplastic gliomas and identifies a subgroup of IDH mutant astrocytic tumors with better prognosis. Acta Neuropathol 126(3):443–451

61. Hegi ME, Diserens AC, Gorlia T, Hamou MF, de Tribolet N, Weller M et al (2005) MGMT gene silencing and benefit from temozolomide in glioblastoma. N Engl J Med 352(10):997–1003

62. Stupp R, Hegi ME, Mason WP, van den Bent MJ, Taphoorn MJ, Janzer RC et al (2009) Effects of radiotherapy with concomitant and adjuvant temozolomide versus radiotherapy alone on survival in glioblastoma in a randomised phase III study: 5-year analysis of the EORTC-NCIC trial. Lancet Oncol 10(5):459–466

63. Hegi ME, Liu L, Herman JG, Stupp R, Wick W, Weller M et al (2008) Correlation of O6-methylguanine methyltransferase (MGMT) promoter methylation with clinical outcomes in glioblastoma and clinical strategies to modulate MGMT activity. J Clin Oncol 26(25):4189–4199

64. Rivera AL, Pelloski CE, Gilbert MR, Colman H, De La Cruz C, Sulman EP et al (2010) MGMT promoter methylation is predictive of response to radiotherapy and prognostic in the absence of adjuvant alkylating chemotherapy for glioblastoma. Neuro Oncol 12(2):116–121

65. Molenaar RJ, Verbaan D, Lamba S, Zanon C, Jeuken JW, Boots-Sprenger SH et al (2014) The combination of IDH1 mutations and MGMT methylation status predicts survival in glioblastoma better than either IDH1 or MGMT alone. Neuro Oncol 16(9):1263–1273

66. Brastianos PK, Taylor-Weiner A, Manley PE, Jones RT, Dias-Santagata D, Thorner AR et al (2014) Exome sequencing identifies BRAF mutations in papillary craniopharyngiomas. Nat Genet 46(2):161–165

67. Jones DT, Kocialkowski S, Liu L, Pearson DM, Backlund LM, Ichimura K et al (2008) Tandem dupli-

cation producing a novel oncogenic BRAF fusion gene defines the majority of pilocytic astrocytomas. Cancer Res 68(21):8673–8677

68. Hawkins C, Walker E, Mohamed N, Zhang C, Jacob K, Shirinian M et al (2011) BRAF-KIAA1549 fusion predicts better clinical outcome in pediatric low-grade astrocytoma. Clin Cancer Res 17(14):4790–4798

69. Jacob K, Albrecht S, Sollier C, Faury D, Sader E, Montpetit A et al (2009) Duplication of 7q34 is specific to juvenile pilocytic astrocytomas and a hallmark of cerebellar and optic pathway tumours. Br J Cancer 101(4):722–733

70. Lin A, Rodriguez FJ, Karajannis MA, Williams SC, Legault G, Zagzag D et al (2012) BRAF alterations in primary glial and glioneuronal neoplasms of the central nervous system with identification of 2 novel KIAA1549:BRAF fusion variants. J Neuropathol Exp Neurol 71(1):66–72

71. Schindler G, Capper D, Meyer J, Janzarik W, Omran H, Herold-Mende C et al (2011) Analysis of BRAF V600E mutation in 1,320 nervous system tumors reveals high mutation frequencies in pleomorphic xanthoastrocytoma, ganglioglioma and extracerebellar pilocytic astrocytoma. Acta Neuropathol 121(3):397–405

72. Dias-Santagata D, Lam Q, Vernovsky K, Vena N, Lennerz JK, Borger DR et al (2011) BRAF V600E mutations are common in pleomorphic xanthoastrocytoma: diagnostic and therapeutic implications. PLoS One 6(3):e17948

73. Lassaletta A, Zapotocky M, Mistry M, Ramaswamy V, Honnorat M, Krishnatry R et al (2017) Therapeutic and prognostic implications of BRAF V600E in pediatric low-grade gliomas. J Clin Oncol 35(25):2934–2941

74. Sturm D, Bender S, Jones DT, Lichter P, Grill J, Becher O et al (2014) Paediatric and adult glioblastoma: multiform (epi)genomic culprits emerge. Nat Rev Cancer 14(2):92–107

75. Schwartzentruber J, Korshunov A, Liu XY, Jones DT, Pfaff E, Jacob K et al (2012) Driver mutations in histone H3.3 and chromatin remodelling genes in paediatric glioblastoma. Nature 482(7384):226–231

76. Wu G, Broniscer A, McEachron TA, Lu C, Paugh BS, Becksfort J et al (2012) Somatic histone H3 alterations in pediatric diffuse intrinsic pontine gliomas and non-brainstem glioblastomas. Nat Genet 44(3):251–253

77. Talbert PB, Henikoff S (2010) Histone variants—ancient wrap artists of the epigenome. Nat Rev Mol Cell Biol 11(4):264–275

78. Khuong-Quang DA, Buczkowicz P, Rakopoulos P, Liu XY, Fontebasso AM, Bouffet E et al (2012) K27M mutation in histone H3.3 defines clinically and biologically distinct subgroups of pediatric diffuse intrinsic pontine gliomas. Acta Neuropathol 124(3):439–447

Concepts of Personalized Medicine in Neuro-oncology

5

Michael Weller, Manfred Westphal, and David A. Reardon

5.1 Introduction

Personalized medicine has become an overarching concept across medicine that is not always clearly defined. Notably in neuro-oncology, neurosurgeons might rightly claim that every surgical intervention touching the brain is a highly personalized procedure. Furthermore, the concept of personalized medicine is not as new as many supporters claim. In fact, the enthusiasm regarding personalized, that is, also individualized, medicine should not make us forget that neuro-oncology has benefited significantly from standardization rather than individualization of various procedures, including mainly radiotherapy with associated quality assurance procedures, but also standard neurosurgical operating procedures as well as how to handle chemotherapy-associated toxicities, and there are many more such examples. Having these caveats in mind, the overall idea of personalized medicine in neuro-oncology largely focusses around increasingly deeper characterization of the tumor tissue initially mostly at genomic but more recently also at transcriptomic, proteomic, and even metabolomic levels. The overall promise of personalized medicine is that deeper understanding of the molecular genetics and pathology results in more targeted and thus more effective approaches with potentially fewer toxicities. Nonetheless, with few exceptions, personalized medicine and the resulting overarching treatment concept of targeted therapy have not met the great expectations yet that the field has put into these developments. Yet, on a more modest level, we have seen the stepwise integration of genetic information derived from thorough tumor tissue characterization, making its way into the clinic first and more recently also into the new WHO classification [1]. Currently, targeted therapy and immunotherapy are the major domains of pharmacological oncological treatment where personalized medicine may assume a role, and these developments are at different stages of evolution in different disease areas, as outlined below.

M. Weller (✉)
Department of Neurology, University Hospital and University of Zurich, Zurich, Switzerland
e-mail: michael.weller@usz.ch

M. Westphal
Department of Neurosurgery, University of Hamburg, University Hospital Eppendorf, Hamburg, Hamburg, Germany
e-mail: westphal@uke.de

D. A. Reardon
Department of Medical Oncology, Center for Neuro-Oncology, Dana-Farber Cancer Institute, Boston, MA, USA
e-mail: david_reardon@dfci.harvard.edu

5.2 Targeted Therapy

The introduction of imatinib for subsets of leukemias or of BRAF inhibitors for subsets of melanomas has demonstrated that targeted therapy

© Springer Nature Switzerland AG 2019
J.-C. Tonn et al. (eds.), *Oncology of CNS Tumors*, https://doi.org/10.1007/978-3-030-04152-6_5

can work in liquid and solid cancers and has also demonstrated how quickly novel diagnostic tests can be implemented, if the potential clinical benefit is of a certain magnitude. There are only few such success stories in neuro-oncology, but they exist: the introduction and approval of the mTOR inhibitor, everolimus, for the treatment of subependymal giant cell astrocytoma associated with tuberous sclerosis is one such example [2], detection of BRAF mutations in papillary craniopharyngioma is another one [3], and evidence accumulates that the few BRAF-mutant glial tumors may also respond to BRAF inhibitors [4]. Yet, it has also become clear that only a minority of primary brain tumors may essentially depend on an alteration of a single pathway.

5.3 Immunotherapy

Compared with some other solid cancers, the overall results obtained with immunotherapy in primary brain tumors have remained disappointing. As with other failed therapeutic approaches in brain tumors, clinical trials were commonly not enriched for candidate biomarkers predicting benefit from immunotherapy although these have not been fully elucidated. Thus, it remains uncertain today whether, e.g., expression of programmed death ligand 1 in the tumor tissue might be a prerequisite for benefit from immune checkpoint inhibition or whether patients for immunotherapy trials should be selected based on tumor mutational burden. Furthermore, even features of the host, e.g., HLA genotype or prevalence of specific immune cell populations in tumor or peripheral blood, could be explored as potential biomarkers to individualize immunotherapy approaches for brain tumor patients.

Attempts to personalize immunotherapeutic approaches for malignant glioma patients are in early stages of development, but there is significant enthusiasm for their pursuit. Some strategies to sensitize the immune system to tumor-expressed targets have used a whole-tumor lysate approach such as DCVax®-L [5], while other therapies are attempting to sensitize the immune system to defined tumor-expressed anti-

gens. Tumor antigens fall into two major categories. Tumor-associated antigens (TAA), although typically upregulated by tumor cells, are also expressed in some normal tissues and thus are subject to central tolerance which may therefore lead to relatively less robust immune responses. In contrast, tumor-specific antigens (TSA) are uniquely expressed by tumor cells, are not subject to central tolerance, and thus are capable of eliciting robust immune responses. Vaccines targeting either tumor-associated or tumor-specific antigens can be appropriately considered personalized therapy. Examples of vaccines targeting either single tumor-associated antigens or combinations thereof that were or are currently in clinical trials for glioblastoma patients include ICT-107, SL-701, and SurVaxM. Vaccines targeting tumor-specific antigens also include those against a single target such as EGFRvIII or the isocitrate dehydrogenase (IDH) 1-mutant peptide as well as those against a panel of expressed tumor-specific mutations also referred to as neoantigens. Although a randomized phase II trial of rindopepimut, an EGFRvIII peptide vaccination, demonstrated encouraging benefit among recurrent glioblastoma patients [6], this vaccine failed to generate a survival benefit among newly diagnosed glioblastoma patients treated on a placebo-controlled, randomized phase III study [7]. The reason underlying the discordant results observed with rindopepimut among recurrent versus newly diagnosed glioblastoma patients remains unclear, but it is well regarded that tumors can evade immune responses against a single tumor-expressed target by downregulating expression of the target, a phenomenon known as immune escape due to immunoediting [8]. Immunotherapy strategies targeting tumor neoantigens are of growing interest based on encouraging immunogenicity as well as therapeutic benefit reported in early trials [9–11]. Ongoing trials are evaluating neoantigen vaccination for glioblastoma patients (NCT02287428 and NCT03422094).

Another personalized immunotherapy approach that is early in development for glioblastoma patients utilizes adoptive T cell approaches such as chimeric antigen receptor (CAR) T cells. Several trials are ongoing utilizing CARs that are engineered to attack tumor antigens for glioblastoma. Initial results of a systemically administered CAR T cell therapy against EGFRvIII generated encouraging evidence of immune reactivity, but did not demonstrate therapeutic benefit [12], while a CAR T cell therapy targeting IL13Rα2, which utilized intratumoral and intraventricular administration, demonstrated a highly encouraging radiographic response in a heavily pretreated, multifocal glioblastoma patient that persisted for 8 months [13]. Personalized immunotherapeutic strategies for neuro-oncology patients are currently in very early stages, and much work remains to be done in order to determine their therapeutic value.

5.4 Gliomas

The most urgent medical need for more personalized medicine approaches in neuro-oncology is commonly perceived for diffuse gliomas of adulthood. The introduction of IDH mutations and 1p19q codeletion as the overruling molecular parameters guiding diagnostic classification of gliomas has undoubtedly enriched for more homogeneous patient populations for clinical trials and helps to adapt treatment approaches and patient counseling in clinical practice, too. Yet, we have still not been successful in using either IDH as a target or understanding what the 1p19q codeletion means on a biochemical level that would allow to exploit this lesion as a target. One of the more successful small steps toward personalized medicine was the stepwise acceptance that O^6-methylguanine DNA methyltransferase (MGMT) promotor methylation is a major prognostic factor for patients exposed to alkylating agent chemotherapy, resulting in the dichotomy that we consider it now unethical to withhold such treatment from patients with tumors showing these molecular alterations, whereas we are readily prepared to omit such chemotherapy in the context of a clinical trial if promising alternatives are available.

Genetic alterations of the epidermal growth factor receptor (EGFR) gene are one of the most dominant molecular alterations in glioblastoma.

Although very well characterized for decades, multiple efforts at exploiting this molecular lesion to establish a more targeted (personalized) approach for glioblastoma have failed, including various unarmed or armed antibodies, pathway inhibitors, or vaccination, with the potentially notable exception of the antibody drug conjugate, ABT-414, which is undergoing exploration for activity in randomized phase II and III trials in EGFR-amplified glioblastoma (NCT02573324, NCT01800695).

5.5 Meningiomas

Although meningiomas have traditionally been a domain for surgery and radiotherapy, there has been tremendous progress in the last 5 years regarding the delineation of the molecular genetic landscape in meningioma, with the identification of several potential new targets for therapy [14, 15]. The most frequent mutations affecting 50% or more of all meningiomas involve the mutational inactivation of the neurofibromatosis (NF) 2 gene which encodes merlin. Furthermore, mutations in the TRAF7, KLF4, AKT1, and SMO genes can be detected in small subsets mostly of skull base meningiomas. A single case report confirms that AKT1 inhibition may become a therapeutic strategy in AKT1-mutant meningioma [16]. It can be anticipated that the systemic treatment approach to meningioma will experience major advances in the next 5–10 years.

5.6 Medulloblastomas

Medulloblastoma has become a paradigmatic tumor where large-scale efforts have been undertaken successfully to dissect the histologically defined entity of medulloblastoma, with the aims, beyond a better understanding of the underlying molecular pathogenesis, of defining risk groups that may allow for therapy de-escalation in some subgroups, but therapy escalation in others. Currently, there are by consensus at least four subgroups of medulloblastoma designated WNT/β-catenin, sonic hedgehog, group 3, and group 4 tumors [17]. While this has allowed for targeted treatment mainly in the sonic hedgehog group, more advanced molecular genetic profiling has resulted in the identification of less prevalent but also potentially therapeutically relevant subgroups of patients with medulloblastoma [18].

5.7   Biomarkers

As astrocytomas grade 2 and above and oligodendrogliomas invariably recur or progress after gross total or partial resection, the therapeutic target is not only the newly diagnosed but also the recurrent tumor situation.

For newly diagnosed glial tumors, comprehensive information will be obtained from the tissue and elaborate high-resolution molecular analyses. IDH mutation, 1p/19q loss, MGMT promotor methylation, and EGFR amplification may also be called biomarkers in this context. Some of these factors may contribute to treatment considerations for many patients including selection of therapeutic drugs that might individually be "repurposed."

To assess and follow the efficacy of treatment, mostly imaging parameters but also subsequent biopsies are currently used in neuro-oncology, especially when imaging changes accompanying immunological therapies or local oncolytic therapies (see Chap. 6) are difficult to interpret. To monitor therapy noninvasively, medical oncology has established the concept of "liquid biopsies" which allows for therapy adaptation based on the individual treatment response in the sense of personalized medicine. This also finds its way into neuro-oncology [19].

Liquid biopsy comprises the analysis of circulating tumor cells (CTC) and circulating DNA mostly isolated from exosomes or extracellular vesicles [19]. Although circulating tumor cells can be found in glioblastoma patients [20], they are infrequent and in such small numbers that they have not attained the same clinical relevance as in other cancers like breast cancer [21] where, as to be expected for glioblastoma, tumor heterogeneity may limit the concordance of molecular markers obtained from tissue and liquid biopsy [22].

The current potential utilization of liquid biopsy for the glioma field includes individualized assessment of EGFR amplification and mutation status [23] or status of MGMT expression in recurrent/progressive tumors [24, 25] which otherwise would need to be biopsied. In the future, predictive parameters of efficacy for local therapies which need to be known at the time of surgery may become a domain for personalized treatment decisions based on liquid biopsy.

5.8   Outlook

Personalized approaches to brain tumor therapy will undoubtedly assume a broader relevance in the treatment of patients with central nervous system neoplasms. Refined tissue diagnostics and inclusion of the aforementioned biomarkers will increase cost and will widen the gap between regions of the world where patients will not or will have access to personalized treatment approaches based thereon. The recent demonstration of the diagnostic power of DNA methylation profiling in distinguishing brain tumor entities represents a challenge to classical histopathology-based classification of brain tumors developed by the WHO [1], and the outcome of the potential competition in this *man* versus *machine* concept of diagnosing brain tumors remains open at present. Moreover, access to novel agents will remain challenging, notably since brain tumors are primarily not common, and their respective incidence artifactually decreases as we dissect more and more brain tumor entities into smaller, molecularly defined subgroups. Furthermore, while the call for patient enrichment in clinical trials is justified, mainly based on many failed trials where no patient selection was foreseen, the conduct of such studies becomes more challenging because international cooperation is required, tissues need to be shipped, and the diversity of regulatory systems, e.g., between the USA and Europe and within Europe, needs to be faced. There are extensive efforts to adapt the clinical trial landscape to these challenges, e.g., the *Screening Cancer Patients for Efficient Clinical*

Trial Access (SPECTA) program of the European Organisation for Research and Treatment of Cancer [26] or, specifically in the context of glioblastoma, the *Adaptive Global Innovative Learning Environment for Glioblastoma* (AGILE) concept which is supposed to become a dynamic clinical trial platform allowing to close arms and to open new arms for experimental treatments whenever new targets or agents emerge [27]. While academically very appealing, several logistical and regulatory problems need to be resolved, especially if these efforts are set up as international programs, and for many brain tumors, we lack appropriate targets, or we cannot even assume that they are single-pathway diseases amenable to simple targeted therapy.

References

1. Louis DN, Perry A, Reifenberger G et al (2016) The 2016 World Health Organization classification of tumors of the central nervous system: a summary. Acta Neuropathol 131:803–820
2. Franz DN, Belousova E, Sparagana S et al (2013) Efficacy and safety of everolimus for subependymal giant cell astrocytomas associated with tuberous sclerosis complex (EXIST-1): a multicentre, randomised, placebo-controlled phase 3 trial. Lancet 381: 125–132
3. Brastianos PK, Taylor-Weiner A, Manley PE et al (2014) Exome sequencing identifies BRAF mutations in papillary craniopharyngiomas. Nat Genet 46:161–165
4. Lassaletta A, Zapotocky M, Mistry M et al (2017) Therapeutic and prognostic implications of BRAF V600E in pediatric low-grade gliomas. J Clin Oncol 35:2934–2941
5. Liau LM, Ashkan K, Tran DD et al (2018) First results on survival from a large phase 3 clinical trial of an autologous dendritic cell vaccine in newly diagnosed glioblastoma. J Transl Med 16:142
6. Reardon DA, Desjardins A, Schuster J et al (2015) ReACT: long-term survival from a randomized phase II study of rindopepimut (CDX-110) plus bevacizumab in relapsed glioblastoma. In: 20th Annual Scientific Meeting and Education Day of the Society for Neuro-Oncology, Oxford University Press, San Antonio
7. Weller M, Butowski N, Tran DD et al (2017) Rindopepimut with temozolomide for patients with newly diagnosed, EGFRvIII-expressing glioblastoma (ACT IV): a randomised, double-blind, international phase 3 trial. Lancet Oncol 18: 1373–1385
8. Schreiber RD, Old LJ, Smyth MJ (2011) Cancer immunoediting: integrating immunity's roles in cancer suppression and promotion. Science 331: 1565–1570
9. Carreno BM, Magrini V, Becker-Hapak M et al (2015) Cancer immunotherapy. A dendritic cell vaccine increases the breadth and diversity of melanoma neoantigen-specific T cells. Science 348: 803–808
10. Sahin U, Derhovanessian E, Miller M et al (2017) Personalized RNA mutanome vaccines mobilize poly-specific therapeutic immunity against cancer. Nature 547:222–226
11. Ott PA, Hu Z, Keskin DB et al (2017) An immunogenic personal neoantigen vaccine for patients with melanoma. Nature 547:217–221
12. O'Rourke DM, Nasrallah MP, Desai A et al (2017) A single dose of peripherally infused EGFRvIII-directed CAR T cells mediates antigen loss and induces adaptive resistance in patients with recurrent glioblastoma. Sci Transl Med 9
13. Brown CE, Alizadeh D, Starr R et al (2016) Regression of glioblastoma after chimeric antigen receptor T-cell therapy. N Engl J Med 375:2561–2569
14. Sahm F, Schrimpf D, Stichel D et al (2017) DNA methylation-based classification and grading system for meningioma: a multicentre, retrospective analysis. Lancet Oncol 18:682–694
15. Preusser M, Brastianos PK, Mawrin C (2018) Advances in meningioma genetics: novel therapeutic opportunities. Nat Rev Neurol 14:106–115
16. Weller M, Roth P, Sahm F et al (2017) Durable control of metastatic AKT1-mutant WHO grade 1 meningothelial meningioma by the AKT inhibitor, AZD5363. J Natl Cancer Inst 109:1–4
17. Taylor MD, Northcott PA, Korshunov A et al (2012) Molecular subgroups of medulloblastoma: the current consensus. Acta Neuropathol 123:465–472
18. Northcott PA, Buchhalter I, Morrissy AS et al (2017) The whole-genome landscape of medulloblastoma subtypes. Nature 547:311–317
19. Shankar GM, Balaj L, Stott SL, Nahed B, Carter BS (2017) Liquid biopsy for brain tumors. Expert Rev Mol Diagn 17:943–947
20. Muller C, Holtschmidt J, Auer M et al (2014) Hematogenous dissemination of glioblastoma multiforme. Sci Transl Med 6:247ra101
21. Krawczyk N, Fehm T, Banys-Paluchowski M, Janni W, Schramm A (2016) Liquid biopsy in metastasized breast cancer as basis for treatment decisions. Oncol Res Treat 39:112–116
22. Chae YK, Davis AA, Jain S et al (2017) Concordance of genomic alterations by next-generation sequencing in tumor tissue versus circulating tumor DNA in breast cancer. Mol Cancer Ther 16: 1412–1420
23. Figueroa JM, Skog J, Akers J et al (2017) Detection of wild-type EGFR amplification and EGFRvIII mutation in CSF-derived extracellular vesicles of glioblastoma patients. Neuro Oncol 19:1494–1502

24. Garnier D, Meehan B, Kislinger T et al (2018) Divergent evolution of temozolomide resistance in glioblastoma stem cells is reflected in extracellular vesicles and coupled with radiosensitization. Neuro Oncol 20:236–248

25. Shao H, Chung J, Lee K et al (2015) Chip-based analysis of exosomal mRNA mediating drug resistance in glioblastoma. Nat Commun 6:6999

26. Lacombe D, Tejpar S, Salgado R et al (2014) European perspective for effective cancer drug development. Nat Rev Clin Oncol 11: 492–498

27. Alexander BM, Ba S, Berger MS et al (2018) Adaptive global innovative learning environment for glioblastoma: GBM AGILE. Clin Cancer Res 24: 737–743

Local Therapies

6

Rachel Grossmann, Zvi Ram,
Michael A. Vogelbaum, E. Antonio Chiocca,
Manfred Westphal, Jörg-Christian Tonn,
Friedrich Kreth, and Niklas Thon

6.1 Definition

Local therapies in the context of cranial tumor encompass the concept of local application or local delivery, respectively. Apart from surgical resection which is the most obvious form of local therapy, radiation is also targeted to the field of the tumor, the residual tumor, or the resection cavity but is dealt within the respective chapters as is the surgical aspect. Here the focus is on therapies which are applied at the time of surgery either into the resection cavity or into the surrounding tissue or are delivered by surgical means like catheters into tumor tissue without resection.

6.2 Intracavitary Chemotherapy

A prototypic local therapy is the instillation of chemotherapeutic agents into a resection cavity. Using biodegradable polymers as a carrier matrix, many different drugs with many permutations of carries have been tried [7]. These agents are placed into the cavity, preferentially attached to the resection walls, and therefore no extra procedure or burden is added for the patient. A wafer formulation containing carmustine (BCNU) was evaluated in the only placebo-controlled phase III local therapy trials for recurrent [8] and newly diagnosed high-grade glioma [79], and the results of both trials came out positive so that the BCNU wafer (Gliadel) is in clinical routine use since a long time and is part of many guidelines and recommendations in clinical neuro-oncology.

R. Grossmann (✉) · Z. Ram
Department of Neurosurgery, Tel Aviv Sourasky
Medical Center, TASMC, Tel Aviv, Israel
e-mail: zviram@tlvmc.gov.il

M. A. Vogelbaum
Rose Ella Burkhardt Brain Tumor and
NeuroOncology Center, Cleveland Clinic Lerner
College of Medicine of Case Western Reserve
University, Cleveland, OH, USA
e-mail: vogelbm@ccf.org

E. A. Chiocca
Department of Neurosurgery, Brigham and Women's
Hospital, Harvard Medical School,
Boston, MA, USA
e-mail: EAChiocca@BWH.harvard.edu

M. Westphal
Department of Neurosurgery, University of Hamburg,
University Hospital Eppendorf, Hamburg,
Hamburg, Germany
e-mail: westphal@uke.de

J.-C. Tonn
Department of Neurosurgery, University Hospital
Ludwig Maximilian University Munich,
Munich, Germany
e-mail: Joerg.Christian.Tonn@med.uni-muenchen.de

F. Kreth · N. Thon
Department of Neurosurgery, LMU, Campus
Grosshadern, Munich, Germany
e-mail: Friedrich-Wilhelm.Kreth@med.uni-muenchen.de;
Niklas.Thon@med.uni-muenchen.de

© Springer Nature Switzerland AG 2019
J.-C. Tonn et al. (eds.), *Oncology of CNS Tumors*, https://doi.org/10.1007/978-3-030-04152-6_6

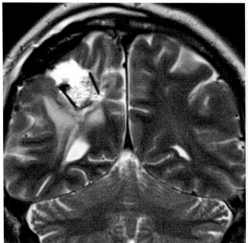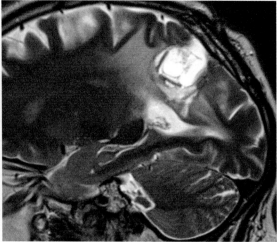

Fig. 6.1 T2-weighted coronal and sagittal postoperative MRI scans after glioblastoma resection and intraoperative insertion of carmustine containing slow-release wafers which impress as thick black linear structures apposed to the wall of the resection cavity

The effectiveness is correlated to the extent of resection, so that the positive result in the trial for newly diagnosed glioblastoma was almost exclusively due to the maximally resected patient group [73]. Most of the BCNU is released within the first 2 weeks, usually for newly diagnosed patients the time which elapses between surgery and radiation and a time period otherwise without treatment, and therefore this is also called a "gap treatment." An inflammatory reaction around the cavity with edema (Fig. 6.1) may need to be countered with steroids [24], and experience and patient selection are important for the clinical benefit [31] but may also contribute to an environment beneficial for immune reaction so that currently the combination of Gliadel wafers and immune checkpoint inhibitors [47] is in early clinical trial testing. The combination with temozolomide seems to be safe [26], and the effects seem to be additive [70].

6.3 Intraparenchymal Drug Delivery: Convection-Enhanced Delivery (CED)

The blood-brain barrier is in the way of delivery for many small molecules with the wrong biophysical properties and for almost all large molecules which need to get into the tumor and not only to the vascular tree. Therefore, a direct intraparenchymal drug delivery modality was developed which uses stereotactically placed catheters and a constant low-pressure infusion [5]. Delivering large molecules reverses the deterring properties of the blood-brain barrier because after delivery beyond the blood-brain barrier, the large molecules cannot escape [17]. Prototypically for the use of that technique in neuro-oncology, targeted toxins were generated which are chimeric molecules binding to a selectively overexpressed cell surface molecule and by virtue of receptor internalization deliver the toxin part into the cell. TGF-alpha binding to the EGF-R, interleukin-4, and interleukin-13 have been linked with the pseudomonas exotoxin (PSET) and been in phase I/II, TGF-alpha-PSET, also known as TP38 [64], and IL-4-PSET [78], or phase III (IL-13-PSET) [38, 52]. While the phase I/II reagents appeared to hold promise, especially with improving convection techniques [18], the IL-13 reagent (cintredekin besudotox) was more formally tested in a randomized trial compared to Gliadel® wafers. This trial involved the use of perilesional multiple site convection in the postresection period for newly diagnosed patients with glioblastoma. In the end, the results failed to show superior survival benefit compared to the control arm (Gliadel® wafers) [37]. Another phase III trial involving the use of intratumoral delivery of transferrin linked to diphtheria-toxin in non-resectable recurrent GBM patients was prematurely closed with only very limited signs of efficacy in this difficult disease stage (Laske et al., unpublished results).

Subsequent retrospective analyses of these trials raised substantial questions as to whether the investigational agents were effectively delivered [50, 65]. Regulatory challenges led the sponsors and investigators to depend upon the reliability as CED delivery devices of already approved catheters ("off-the-shelf" use) that were not specifically designed for delivery of therapeutics into brain tissue. Compounding this problem were both regulator and practical challenges associated with the co-administration of radiographic tracers, and hence there was no ability to perform even indirect "pharmacokinetic" studies. Subsequent, more limited work with a variety of tracers showed that the "off-the-shelf" catheters were not reliable as CED delivery devices.

The challenges associated with the design of reliable CED delivery devices had been identified early in the course of the development of this field. One of the key design features required for avoidance of "backflow" around a CED catheter is that the diameter of the infusion catheter endport be as small as possible, typically smaller than 1 mm [32]. Design of a device that includes a very small diameter infusion tip into a specific location in the brain can be challenging. Nonetheless, there are several devices designed to achieve reliable CED that are now available. Two devices, the MRI Interventions SmartFlow Cannula and the Alcyone MEMS Cannula, are structurally rigid in design and hence for intraoperative use only. They have each been radiographically validated in the clinical setting, via co-infusion of a tracer, to provide reflux-free delivery [6]. However, the intraoperative use restriction coupled with the low infusion rates associated with CED (microliters per minute) combines to limit the total infusion volume to less than about 10 cm³, which may be sufficient for localized delivery to deep nuclei, but less likely to provide complete coverage of enhancing and/or non-enhancing portions of gliomas. Two additional devices, the Brainlab Infusion Cannula and the Infuseon CMC, also feature infusion tips with diameters less than 1 mm, but these devices have flexible shafts and can be left in place for days to allow for more prolonged, higher-volume infusions. Each of these devices also has been clinically validated to provide backflow-resistant delivery [76].

The advent of more reliable delivery devices and more straightforward integration of imaging tracers into clinical trial design has led to a resurgence in interest in the use of CED as a delivery approach. Multiple phase I and II clinical trials are now open, and others planned including oncolytic virus delivery [40].

A pertinent example of the benefits of advanced delivery technology coupled with imaging of delivery comes from an ongoing clinical trial of a radioimmunotherapy agent delivered locally to treat pediatric brain stem glioma. This single-center trial involved the implantation of a single CED optimized cannula followed by infusion of a radiolabelled antibody which was visualized by PET imaging [69]. This phase I study showed that CED in the brain stem was safe and resulted in substantial local delivery of the therapeutic and that there was negligible systemic distribution of the agent. A phase II study is planned.

6.3.1 Viral Therapies: Gene Therapy, Prodrug Conversion, Immunotherapy, and Oncolysis

Over the least two decades, there have been several clinical trials utilizing viral vectors to deliver cytotoxic genes into cancer cells [42]. This process is also thought to generate an active immune response against tumor antigens [10]. Two general types of technologies have been used: (1) replication-defective viral vectors that only deliver a cytotoxic and usually immunostimulatory payload into the cancer cell and (2) replication-competent viruses (tumor-selective, oncolytic, replication-conditional) that can still selectively replicate and generate a productive infection with subsequent waves of viral progeny production. Both of these technologies lead to inflammation and ultimately an adaptive immune response. Selectivity of these virotherapies is provided by molecules expressed specifically on the cell surface (such as integrins) or by aberrant tumor signalling pathways that complement expression of the engineered viruses.

For example, p53 and RB gene mutations have been characterized over almost 20 years [3], and therapeutic intervention has been developed for these pathway aberrancies. Some oncolytic viruses can be targeted to glioma cells because they conditionally replicate in characteristic genetic contexts like the mutation or deletion of p53 [23], a disrupted RB pathway [19], or homozygous deletions of p16. Early clinical trials of these replication-competent adenoviruses have been completed and found safe [9, 75].

Neurosurgically, virotherapies have been administered mostly in recurrent GBM, but some trials have used these as adjuvants in newly diagnosed GBM. Administration has occurred by (a) direct stereotactic inoculation in the GBM [45] or (b) direct injection into the peritumoral area after tumor resection [9] (Chiocca et al., Molecular Therapy, 2004) or (c) direct stereotactic injection followed several days later by resection of the tumor (with the injected virus which can then be studied in the resected tissue) and peritumoral injection of the virotherapy [27, 39, 40].

Over recent years, there have been several clinical trials (phase I and II) published with encouraging results. In fact, one virotherapy is now FDA approved for melanoma, and it has been shown in human melanomas that this is an effective manner to increase cytotoxic T cell infiltrate into tumors [62]. Recent published virotherapies have included (A) replication-defective viruses, such as adenoviral vectors that deliver the herpes simplex thymidine kinase gene which activates drugs such as ganciclovir which was evaluated in a randomized phase III trial [80] or valacyclovir which was evaluated in a phase II clinical trial [81] or adenovirus delivering human interleukin-12 under control of a drug-regulatable promoter (E.A. Chiocca, personal communica-

tion), and (B) oncolytic viruses such as poliovirus [14], adenovirus [40] reovirus [46], herpes simplex virus type 1 (HSV-1), retroviruses [12], parvovirus [22], vaccinia virus, and measles virus. Discussion of all these trials is beyond the scope of this chapter, but several conclusions can be made. In general, patient tolerability has been excellent with little evidence for viral-induced toxicities which cannot be managed. Toxicities are usually related to brain edema or liver function anomalies. Tissues show both evidence of expression of viral gene products and evidence of infiltration by immune cells, including CD8+, CD4+ lymphocytes and plasma cells and transcriptomics consistent with innate and inflammatory gene products [9, 12, 22, 40, 44, 66]. Preliminary evidence of efficacy has also been reported in these trials when compared to historical controls [12, 14, 22, 40] or to concurrent prospective control cohorts accrued during the trial [81]. Several trials are currently open (Table 6.1) for patients, according to clinicaltrials.gov. Yet, only randomized prospective trials with the power to detect efficacy will establish whether any of these virotherapies will become a standard of care.

6.4 Radioimmunotherapy with Specific Ligands for "Oncoproteins"

Part of the glioma cell lineage is a "mesenchymal" phenotype [54] which expresses molecules used for the interaction of the cells with the extracellular matrix of the environment. One of these molecules is tenascin, which has been found overexpressed in many analyses. Antibodies to tenascin have been developed long time ago and have been used for radioimmunotherapy via direct intraparenchymal application with proof of principle and acceptable safety but still outstanding randomized phase III trials as for efficacy [25, 58, 59]. Late results of a study using I-131- or Y-90-labelled anti-tenascin antibody in 15 patients with anaplastic astrocytoma and 40 patients with glioblastoma showed impressively superior results over historical controls [61].

Table 6.1 Currently open clinical trials for gene and viral-therapies (clinicaltrials.gov)

Virus	Name	Major modifications	NCT#
HSV-1	G207	Inactivation of *ICP6* and *γ34.5* genes restricts replication to dividing cells	NCT02457845
	rQNestin34.5v.2	Has *γ34.5* reinserted under nestin promoter control	NCT03152318
	M032	Like HSV-G207 and expresses human IL-12	NCT02062827
Adenovirus	DNX-2401	*E1A* gene deletion restricts replication to Rb/p16 pathway-deficient cells and fiber-modified for infectivity	NCT02798406, NCT03178032
	NSC-CRAd-S-pk7	Neural stem cells loaded with virus where survivin promoter drives *E1A* expression and fiber-modified for infectivity	NCT03072134
	Ad-hCMV-TK Ad-hCMV-Flt3L	*E1A* gene deletion and inserted HSV TK enzyme sensitizes tumor cells to antivirals Combined with Ad-hCMV-TK; expresses *Flt3L* under CMV promoter	NCT01811992
	Ad-RTS-hIL-12	Encodes human IL-12, under inducible RheoSwitch Therapeutic System transcriptional control	NCT02026271
	Ad-TK	Combined with immune checkpoint blockade; inserted HSV TK enzyme sensitizes tumor cells to antivirals	NCT03576612
Retrovirus	Toca511	Replication-competent retrovirus that delivers CD to catalyze prodrug 5-FC into cytotoxic 5-FU	NCT02414165
Vaccinia	TG6002	Inserted CD and UPRT catalyze prodrug 5-FC into cytotoxic 5-FU and 5-FUMP	NCT03294486
Poliovirus	PVSRIPO	PVSRIPO combined with lomustine	NCT02986178, NCT03043391
Reovirus	Pelareorep	Wild-type strain virus	NCT02444546

Basically any molecule which is specifically overexpressed in gliomas lends itself to such radioimmunotherapy, but compared to tenascin, all other developments which also include a broad array of radionuclides (reviewed in [77]) are much delayed, with the development of anti-EGF-R vIII-based therapies being probably the farthest.

6.5 Targeting Through Motile Delivery Systems (Neural Stem Cell Delivery)

As invasiveness of single cells over large distances from the tumors leads inadvertently to treatment failure, thought has been given to the development of disseminated drug delivery or motile therapy targeting this invasive population and that has led to the evaluation of neural stem cells (NSCs) as delivery vehicle [1]. This methodology is very complex as the cells are still artificially immortalized and the reagents delivered will be HSV-Tk or cytosine deaminase as the paradigmatic prodrug-converting enzymes which phosphorylate ganciclovir or convert 5-FC to 5-FU. Especially the production of such cells as a stable and easily handled reagent is very involved, and so many regulatory hurdles need to be resolved [21], but after many years, a first in man study based on neural stem cells transducing cytosine deaminase has been completed showing that the injected cells indeed migrated toward distant tumor [56]. The reagent is rather non-specific, but the targeting of the delivery is highly specific because, theoretically, even single cells can be traced and destroyed. Current developments look at intranasal delivery of such programmed NSCs [60], and phase I trials are being designed.

6.6 Stereotactic Brachytherapy in Low-Grade Gliomas

The aim of highly localized therapies, such as stereotactic brachytherapy (interstitial radiation), is to devitalize a well-defined treatment volume and to avoid damage of the surrounding tissue. Conventional fractionated irradiation is delivered to brain tumors at dose rates in the range of 180–200 cGy/min. In contrast, interstitial irradiation is administered much more slowly. Due to continuous low-dose-rate irradiation, the therapeutic ratio is increased: Ongoing repair of sublethal damage during irradiation has been shown to be more effective in nonneoplastic tissue than in tumor tissue, and neoplastic tumor cells tend to synchronize to the radiosensitive G2 and M phases of the cell cycle at dose-rate levels >60 cGy/h. However, because repopulation and redistribution during the treatment are of minor importance in patients harboring low-grade glioma, a much more protracted course of irradiation with extremely low dose rates (in the range of 10 cGy/h calculated to the boundary of the target volume) appears to be a rational treatment strategy. Thus, on the one hand, stereotactic brachytherapy fulfills one major definition of radiosurgery as given by Larsson [41], i.e., the accurate application of a highly focused necrotizing intratumoral dose with a steep dose decreases from the center to the periphery. A typical (inhomogeneous) dose distribution of iodine-125 brachytherapy is described in Fig. 6.2 (left): 100% of the defined tumor volume received the prescribed treatment dose of 54 Gy, 60% at least 100 Gy, 32% 150 Gy, and 20% at least 200 Gy.

Accurate histological and molecular genetic characterization has to be achieved upfront to enable risk-adapted localized treatment strategies. To obtain representative biopsy trajectories, inclusion of metabolic/molecular imaging data has been shown to be an essential step [16]. Multimodal planning following co-registration of CT (1-mm contrast-enhanced axial images), MRI (2-mm T1-weighted gadolinium-enhanced axial images, 2-mm T2-weighted axial and MR angiography sequences), and metabolic imaging data [e.g., positron emission tomography with amino acid tracers such as methionine or O-(2-[^{18}F] fluoroethyl)-L-tyrosine (FET)] allows the definition of serial tissue samples along representative trajectories which includes the biologically active hot spots if present [16, 55].

Interstitial brachytherapy was initially considered to be indicated for patients with a circumscribed tumor with a maximum diameter of 5 cm, but due to the results of risk analyses, the treatment is now limited to small, circumscribed tumors with a diameter not larger than 3.5 cm.

Iodine-125 seeds are used for preferentially temporary implants, and exclusively low-activity iodine-125 seeds (<20 mCi) should be implanted which deliver a total dose of 50–60 Gy to the tumor margin at a dose rate of approximately 10 cGy/h. Usually, one to four seeds (isocenters) are used to achieve a conformal interstitial irradiation of the tumor volume. One long-term study—conducted within the CT era—concerned stereotactic iodine-125 brachytherapy as the initial treatment concept for 239 patients with eloquently located, circumscribed, supratentorial WHO grade II glioma [33]. Patients had to have either clinical or radiographic progression to be considered candidates for interstitial irradiation. The median follow-up was 10.3 years for the survivors. Five-, 10-, and 15-year progression-free survivals were 45%, 21%, and 14%, respectively. The corresponding survival rates were 51%, 32%, and 22%, respectively. High-performance scores (median Karnofsky score: 80) were generally maintained throughout the follow-up period; tumor progression, however, was associated with a decline on the Karnofsky scale. The results after stereotactic brachytherapy of WHO grade II low-grade gliomas with respect to overall and progression-free survival are comparable to those after microsurgical resection and/or percutaneous radiotherapy: A meta-analysis (own unpublished data) including ten studies from the CT era (of at least 50 patients) with different therapeutic approaches (surgery alone, surgery and radiotherapy, radiotherapy alone, primary stereotactic brachytherapy) showed the 5- and 10-year survival rates to be in the range of 55–70% (61% after stereotactic brachytherapy [36]) and 40–53% (51% after stereotactic brachytherapy [36]), respectively. There was no statistically significant difference between the survival curves of the different therapeutic approaches of primary stereotactic brachytherapy [36] and surgery and radiotherapy [29] as determined in EORTC study

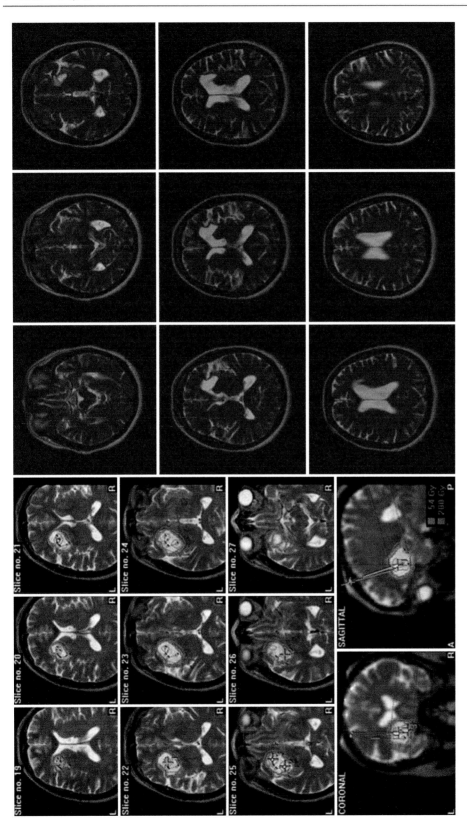

Fig. 6.2 Representative example for treatment planning (*left*, MRI: stereotactic view) and result (*right*, 5-year follow-up, complete response) in a left-sided astrocytoma WHO grade II of the insula of Reil. Tumor volume (as defined by the *pink line*) was 14.5 mL. Three temporary iodine-125 seeds (activity 10.88 mCi) were stereotactically implanted in the rostral and caudal areas of the tumor (seed position indicated by the *green intratumoral crosses*). The *violet line* represents the reference dose of 54 Gy. The dose rate was 12.0 cGy/h

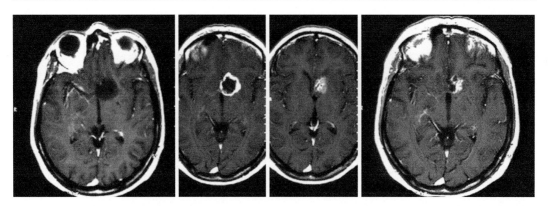

Fig. 6.3 Example documenting the typical imaging changes after stereotactic brachytherapy (left, preoperative; middle two panels, 3 months)

22,844. A representative treatment plan of an insular WHO grade II astrocytoma is given in Fig. 6.2 and a typical follow-up MRI in Fig. 6.3.

Stereotactic brachytherapy is also an effective treatment modality for children with unresectable pilocytic astrocytomas which are frequently seen in highly eloquent areas. It was previously shown in a series of 45 hypothalamic pilocytic astrocytomas (as part of a large series of 97 pilocytic and 358 WHO grade II glioma) [36] that stereotactic brachytherapy is associated with low risk and high efficacy in this tumor entity. The 5- and 10-year survival rates for all 97 patients with pilocytic astrocytomas in that series were 84.9% and 83%, respectively. Unfortunately, detailed functional outcome data were not given, and the median follow-up was only 5 years. Thus, not surprisingly, stereotactic brachytherapy is seldom mentioned or discussed as a valuable treatment option for selected pediatric patients. In a pilot study, Peraud et al. hypothesized the favorable radiobiology of stereotactic brachytherapy with effects of superfractionation at the boundary of the treatment volume and recommend stereotactic brachytherapy for minimally invasive low-risk treatment of complex located glioma (WHO grade I or II) to be either the initial treatment or to be added after previously performed partial tumor resection [53]. Tumor location was lobar (three patients), hypothalamic/suprasellar (four patients), thalamic/pineal (two patients), and mesencephalic/pontine (two patients). None of the patients exhibited tumor progression or tumor recurrence at the time of last follow-up evaluation (median follow-up: 31.5 months), and no radiogenic complications (including cyst formation) occurred. Functional outcome scores were favorable: significant improvement of hemiparesis (three of three patients), improvement of endocrine deficits (one of two patients), and improvement of visual function (one of three patients). Visual and endocrine deficits remained unchanged in two patients and in one patient, respectively, and no child exhibited functional deterioration during the follow-up period. Another study (Ruge et al.) recently reported on their experiences with stereotactic brachytherapy with iodine-125 seeds for the treatment of inoperable low-grade gliomas in children [63]. This long-term outcome analysis included 147 pediatric patients. No procedure-related mortality and a low transient morbidity of 5.4% were reported. Survival rates at 5 and 10 years were 93% and 82%, respectively, with no difference between WHO grade I and II tumors.

Overall, stereotactic brachytherapy has been shown to be a safe method. Those patients with transient symptoms (commonly headache) can usually be rapidly stabilized with steroids (dexamethasone, dose range between 2 and 12 mg/day) within 4 weeks. Very rarely, radiation necrosis that cannot be controlled with steroids might occur, making surgical decompression necessary [33–36, 49]. The estimated rate of radiogenic complications within the first 2 years in a series of 515 patients by Kreth et al. [34] was 7.5%, and no long-term complications were observed beyond this time interval. It was shown that these complications are mostly generated within the treatment volume and are strongly correlated to the tumor volume. Accordingly, the volume has been shown to be the most important risk factor, i.e., beyond a cutoff of 3.5 cm in tumor diameter (tumor volume of 22.4 mL).

An expansion of the concept of stereotactic brachytherapy is a combination with microsurgery where, after primary microsurgical resection of easily accessible parts of the tumor, the residual part is destined for iodine-125 seed implantation. This combined approach might very well spare the patient from the increased risk of suffering a neurological deficit due to attempted radical resection as well as the increased risk for a radiogenic complication linked to interstitial irradiation of tumors with diameters >3.5 cm [49, 53, 67]. Two recently published pilot studies have been performed demonstrating in principle the feasibility and safety of that approach [53, 67].

6.7   Photodynamic Therapy

Oral application of 5-aminolevulinic acid (ALA) leads to a highly specific accumulation of fluorescent protoporphyrin IX (PPIX) in malignant glioma tissue. This is widely used for fluorescence-guided resection within the concept of intraoperative augmentation of tumor identification and visualization. In addition, high intracellular PPIX concentrations in conjunction with white light application lead to apoptosis and subsequent cell death even in cells with stem cell-like properties [20, 28, 71]. As PPIX selectively accumulates in glioma cells in contrast to normal brain, photodynamic therapy (PDT) with ALA seems to be a promising concept. Whereas direct illumination of the resection cavity is less effective due to limited light penetration and reflection phenomena at the surface, interstitial PDT with stereotactically placed light fibers is a more promising concept. Several studies and reports about prolongation of survival exist; however, data from prospective (randomized) trials have to be awaited [2, 4, 72].

6.8   Alternating Electrical Fields (Tumor-Treating Field, TTF)

Tumor-treating fields (TTFields) is a recently approved novel treatment modality that is also referred to as the fourth modality of cancer treatment in addition to surgery, radiation therapy, and chemotherapy [51]. TTFields affect dividing cells by utilizing low-intensity (1–3 V/cm), intermediate-frequency (100–500 kHz) alternating electrical fields that physically interfere with cell division by disrupting cytokinesis in rapidly dividing cells, resulting in apoptosis [30]. TTFields were particularly suited to a trial in patients with glioblastoma since the tumor recurs locally and does not send distant metastases to other organs, thereby enabling full TTFields coverage of the sick organ's volume. Also, the brain has minimal numbers of noncancerous dividing cells, making TTFields potentially safe for use.

A phase III trial in patients with recurrent GBM compared NovoTTF-100A monotherapy to best active chemotherapy according to the physician's best choice (active treatment control group) [74]. Patients treated with TTFields alone had comparable OS to that of patients who received investigator's choice chemotherapy with various agents as monotherapy or in combination, including bevacizumab (31%), irinotecan (31%), nitrosourea (25%), carboplatin (13%), or TMZ (11%), leading to approved TTFields therapy for recurrent glioblastoma in 2011. This was followed by an international, randomized, phase III clinical trial with newly diagnosed glioblastoma into one of two arms: TTFields plus adjuvant TMZ versus adjuvant TMZ alone [9] following standard radiotherapy. Comparison between the results of the TTFields plus TMZ arm with those of TMZ alone showed significantly improved PFS (7.1 vs. 4.0 months, respectively, $P = 0.001$) and OS (20.5 vs. 15.6 months, respectively, $P = 0.004$). Currently, there are several additional ongoing trials of TTFields in patients with glioblastoma, especially when it is administered in combination with radiation therapy and other potential therapeutic agents, such as bevacizumab. TTFields is now being tested for other brain tumor types, such as brain metastases and recurrent atypical and anaplastic meningiomas.

6.9   Focused Ultrasound

Transcranial focused ultrasound (FUS) can non-invasively transmit acoustic energy with a high degree of accuracy and safety to targets and regions within the brain. Using magnetic resonance (MR), MR-guided FUS (MRgFUS) has primarily been investigated for its thermal lesioning capabilities in several fields in the brain, including ablation procedures in functional neurosurgery and neuro-oncology, opening of the blood-brain barrier (BBB) to facilitate delivery of therapeutic agents, neuromodulation, and thrombolysis of blood clots [68]. Here, we review the preclinical and clinical work that has been carried out in the exploration of applying MRgFUS for generating cytotoxicity within tumor tissue, enhancing the delivery or activity of therapeutic agents, and modulating the tumor microenvironment to refine immune recognition and clearance.

Heat deposition resulting in thermal ablation is the most direct mechanism by which FUS can be used to treat brain tumors. Continuous exposures result in high rates of energy deposition, producing progressive elevations in temperature. At temperatures above 55 °C, cellular death occurs as a result of coagulative necrosis, accompanied by protein denaturation and the disruption of cellular membranes [11, 15]. In the field of neuro-oncology, the only clinical experience of FUS is limited to small case series [13, 43, 48]. In an early experience, MRgFUS was used to treat three patients with recurrent glioblastoma through a craniectomy which was required to create an acoustic window [57]. Posttreatment imaging and histopathology revealed evidence of thermocoagulation in two of the three tumors. Most recently, Coluccia et al. [13] reported applying FUS ablation in a patient with thalamic glioblastoma as part of an ongoing clinical phase I study aimed at evaluating the feasibility and safety of transcranial MRgFUS for brain tumor ablation. Applying high-power sonications under MR imaging guidance, partial tumor ablation could be achieved without provoking neurological deficits or other adverse effects in that patient [13]. Three phase I clinical trials (NCT01698437,

NCT00147056, NCT01473485) are currently ongoing to verify the safety of the device and the feasibility of thermal ablation of brain tumors.

6.10   Conclusion

Numerous local therapies exist and are at various stages of clinical development, and validation which either at the time of resection, instead of resection, or in the immediate follow-up can augment the effect of surgical treatment of intrinsic brain tumors and possibly also brain metastases.

References

1. Aboody KS, Najbauer J, Danks MK (2008) Stem and progenitor cell-mediated tumor selective gene therapy. Gene Ther 15:739–752
2. Akimoto J (2016) Photodynamic therapy for malignant brain tumors. Neurol Med Chir 56:151–157
3. Anker L, Ohgaki H, Ludeke BI, Herrmann HD, Kleihues P, Westphal M (1993) p53 protein accumulation and gene mutations in human glioma cell lines. Int J Cancer 55:982–987
4. Beck TJ, Kreth FW, Beyer W, Mehrkens JH, Obermeier A, Stepp H, Stummer W, Baumgartner R (2007) Interstitial photodynamic therapy of nonresectable malignant glioma recurrences using 5-aminolevulinic acid induced protoporphyrin IX. Lasers Surg Med 39:386–393
5. Bobo RH, Laske DW, Akbasak A, Morrison PF, Dedrick RL, Oldfield EH (1994) Convection-enhanced delivery of macromolecules in the brain. Proc Natl Acad Sci U S A 91:2076–2080
6. Brady ML, Raghavan R, Singh D, Anand PJ, Fleisher AS, Mata J, Broaddus WC, Olbricht WL (2014) In vivo performance of a microfabricated catheter for intraparenchymal delivery. J Neurosci Methods 229:76–83
7. Brem H, Gabikian P (2001) Biodegradable polymer implants to treat brain tumors. J Control Release 74:63–67
8. Brem H, Piantadosi S, Burger PC, Walker M, Selker R, Vick NA, Black K, Sisti M, Brem S, Mohr G et al (1995) Placebo-controlled trial of safety and efficacy of intraoperative controlled delivery by biodegradable polymers of chemotherapy for recurrent gliomas. The Polymer-brain Tumor Treatment Group. Lancet 345:1008–1012
9. Chiocca EA, Abbed KM, Tatter S, Louis DN, Hochberg FH, Barker F, Kracher J, Grossman SA, Fisher JD, Carson K, Rosenblum M, Mikkelsen T, Olson J, Markert J, Rosenfeld S, Nabors LB, Brem

S, Phuphanich S, Freeman S, Kaplan R, Zwiebel J (2004) A phase I open-label, dose-escalation, multi-institutional trial of injection with an E1B-Attenuated adenovirus, ONYX-015, into the peritumoral region of recurrent malignant gliomas, in the adjuvant setting. Mol Ther 10:958–966

10. Chiocca EA, Rabkin SD (2014) Oncolytic viruses and their application to cancer immunotherapy. Cancer Immunol Res 2:295–300

11. Cline HE, Hynynen K, Watkins RD, Adams WJ, Schenck JF, Ettinger RH, Freund WR, Vetro JP, Jolesz FA (1995) Focused US system for MR imaging-guided tumor ablation. Radiology 194:731–737

12. Cloughesy TF, Landolfi J, Hogan DJ, Bloomfield S, Carter B, Chen CC, Elder JB, Kalkanis SN, Kesari S, Lai A, Lee IY, Liau LM, Mikkelsen T, Nghiemphu PL, Piccioni D, Walbert T, Chu A, Das A, Diago OR, Gammon D, Gruber HE, Hanna M, Jolly DJ, Kasahara N, McCarthy D, Mitchell L, Ostertag D, Robbins JM, Rodriguez-Aguirre M, Vogelbaum MA (2016) Phase 1 trial of vocimagene amiretrorepvec and 5-fluorocytosine for recurrent high-grade glioma. Sci Transl Med 8:341ra375

13. Coluccia D, Fandino J, Schwyzer L, O'Gorman R, Remonda L, Anon J, Martin E, Werner B (2014) First noninvasive thermal ablation of a brain tumor with MR-guided focused ultrasound. J Ther Ultrasound 2:17

14. Desjardins A, Gromeier M, Herndon JE II, Beaubier N, Bolognesi DP, Friedman AH, Friedman HS, McSherry F, Muscat AM, Nair S, Peters KB, Randazzo D, Sampson JH, Vlahovic G, Harrison WT, McLendon RE, Ashley D, Bigner DD (2018) Recurrent glioblastoma treated with recombinant poliovirus. N Engl J Med 379:150–161

15. Dewhirst MW, Viglianti BL, Lora-Michiels M, Hanson M, Hoopes PJ (2003) Basic principles of thermal dosimetry and thermal thresholds for tissue damage from hyperthermia. Int J Hyperth 19:267–294

16. Eigenbrod S, Trabold R, Brucker D, Eros C, Egensperger R, La Fougere C, Gobel W, Ruhm A, Kretzschmar HA, Tonn JC, Herms J, Giese A, Kreth FW (2014) Molecular stereotactic biopsy technique improves diagnostic accuracy and enables personalized treatment strategies in glioma patients. Acta Neurochir 156:1427–1440

17. Ferguson S, Lesniak MS (2007) Convection enhanced drug delivery of novel therapeutic agents to malignant brain tumors. Curr Drug Deliv 4:169–180

18. Fiandaca MS, Forsayeth JR, Dickinson PJ, Bankiewicz KS (2008) Image-guided convection-enhanced delivery platform in the treatment of neurological diseases. Neurotherapeutics 5:123–127

19. Fueyo J, Alemany R, Gomez-Manzano C, Fuller GN, Khan A, Conrad CA, Liu TJ, Jiang H, Lemoine MG, Suzuki K, Sawaya R, Curiel DT, Yung WK, Lang FF (2003) Preclinical characterization of the antiglioma activity of a tropism-enhanced adenovirus targeted to the retinoblastoma pathway. J Natl Cancer Inst 95:652–660

20. Fujishiro T, Nonoguchi N, Pavliukov M, Ohmura N, Park Y, Kajimoto Y, Ishikawa T, Nakano I, Kuroiwa T (2018) 5-aminolevulinic acid-mediated photodynamic therapy can target human glioma stem-like cells refractory to antineoplastic agents. Photodiagn Photodyn Ther 24:58–68

21. Gad SC (2014) Safety and regulatory requirements and challenge for CNS drug development. Neurobiol Dis 61:39–46

22. Geletneky K, Hajda J, Angelova AL, Leuchs B, Capper D, Bartsch AJ, Neumann JO, Schoning T, Husing J, Beelte B, Kiprianova I, Roscher M, Bhat R, von Deimling A, Bruck W, Just A, Frehtman V, Lobhard S, Terletskaia-Ladwig E, Fry J, Jochims K, Daniel V, Krebs O, Dahm M, Huber B, Unterberg A, Rommelaere J (2017) Oncolytic H-1 parvovirus shows safety and signs of immunogenic activity in a first phase I/IIa glioblastoma trial. Mol Ther 25:2620–2634

23. Geoerger B, Grill J, Opolon P, Morizet J, Aubert G, Lecluse Y, van Beusechem VW, Gerritsen WR, Kirn DH, Vassal G (2003) Potentiation of radiation therapy by the oncolytic adenovirus dl1520 (ONYX-015) in human malignant glioma xenografts. Br J Cancer 89:577–584

24. Giese A, Bock HC, Kantelhardt SR, Rohde V (2010) Risk management in the treatment of malignant gliomas with BCNU wafer implants. Cen Eur Neurosurg 71:199–206

25. Goetz CM, Rachinger W, Decker M, Gildehaus FJ, Stocker S, Jung G, Tatsch K, Tonn JC, Reulen HJ (2005) Distribution of labelled anti-tenascin antibodies and fragments after injection into intact or partly resected C6-gliomas in rats. Cancer Immunol Immunother 54:337–344

26. Gutenberg A, Lumenta CB, Braunsdorf WE, Sabel M, Mehdorn HM, Westphal M, Giese A (2013) The combination of carmustine wafers and temozolomide for the treatment of malignant gliomas. A comprehensive review of the rationale and clinical experience. J Neuro-Oncol 113:163–174

27. Harsh GR, Deisboeck TS, Louis DN, Hilton J, Colvin M, Silver JS, Qureshi NH, Kracher J, Finkelstein D, Chiocca EA, Hochberg FH (2000) Thymidine kinase activation of ganciclovir in recurrent malignant gliomas: a gene-marking and neuropathological study. J Neurosurg 92:804–811

28. Johansson A, Faber F, Kniebuhler G, Stepp H, Sroka R, Egensperger R, Beyer W, Kreth FW (2013) Protoporphyrin IX fluorescence and photobleaching during interstitial photodynamic therapy of malignant gliomas for early treatment prognosis. Lasers Surg Med 45:225–234

29. Karim AB, Maat B, Hatlevoll R, Menten J, Rutten EH, Thomas DG, Mascarenhas F, Horiot JC, Parvinen LM, van Reijn M, Jager JJ, Fabrini MG, van Alphen AM, Hamers HP, Gaspar L, Noordman E, Pierart M, van Glabbeke M (1996) A randomized trial on dose-response in radiation therapy of low-grade cerebral glioma: European Organization for Research and

Treatment of Cancer (EORTC) Study 22844. Int J Radiat Oncol Biol Phys 36:549–556

30. Kirson ED, Dbaly V, Tovarys F, Vymazal J, Soustiel JF, Itzhaki A, Mordechovich D, Steinberg-Shapira S, Gurvich Z, Schneiderman R, Wasserman Y, Salzberg M, Ryffel B, Goldsher D, Dekel E, Palti Y (2007) Alternating electric fields arrest cell proliferation in animal tumor models and human brain tumors. Proc Natl Acad Sci U S A 104:10152–10157

31. Kleinberg L (2016) Polifeprosan 20, 3.85% carmustine slow release wafer in malignant glioma: patient selection and perspectives on a low-burden therapy. Patient Prefer Adherence 10:2397–2406

32. Krauze MT, Saito R, Noble C, Tamas M, Bringas J, Park JW, Berger MS, Bankiewicz K (2005) Reflux-free cannula for convection-enhanced high-speed delivery of therapeutic agents. J Neurosurg 103:923–929

33. Kreth FW, Faist M, Grau S, Ostertag CB (2006) Interstitial 125I radiosurgery of supratentorial de novo WHO Grade 2 astrocytoma and oligoastrocytoma in adults: long-term results and prognostic factors. Cancer 106:1372–1381

34. Kreth FW, Faist M, Rossner R, Birg W, Volk B, Ostertag CB (1997) The risk of interstitial radiotherapy of low-grade gliomas. Radiother Oncol 43:253–260

35. Kreth FW, Faist M, Rossner R, Volk B, Ostertag CB (1997) Supratentorial World Health Organization Grade 2 astrocytomas and oligoastrocytomas. A new pattern of prognostic factors. Cancer 79:370–379

36. Kreth FW, Faist M, Warnke PC, Rossner R, Volk B, Ostertag CB (1995) Interstitial radiosurgery of low-grade gliomas. J Neurosurg 82:418–429

37. Kunwar S, Chang S, Westphal M, Vogelbaum M, Sampson J, Barnett G, Shaffrey M, Ram Z, Piepmeier J, Prados M, Croteau D, Pedain C, Leland P, Husain SR, Joshi BH, Puri RK (2010) Phase III randomized trial of CED of IL13-PE38QQR vs Gliadel for recurrent glioblastoma. Neuro-Oncology 12:871–881

38. Kunwar S, Prados MD, Chang SM, Berger MS, Lang FF, Piepmeier JM, Sampson JH, Ram Z, Gutin PH, Gibbons RD, Aldape KD, Croteau DJ, Sherman JW, Puri RK (2007) Direct intracerebral delivery of cintredekin besudotox (IL13-PE38QQR) in recurrent malignant glioma: a report by the Cintredekin Besudotox Intraparenchymal Study Group. J Clin Oncol 25:837–844

39. Lang FF, Bruner JM, Fuller GN, Aldape K, Prados MD, Chang S, Berger MS, McDermott MW, Kunwar SM, Junck LR, Chandler W, Zwiebel JA, Kaplan RS, Yung WK (2003) Phase I trial of adenovirus-mediated p53 gene therapy for recurrent glioma: biological and clinical results. J Clin Oncol 21:2508–2518

40. Lang FF, Conrad C, Gomez-Manzano C, Yung WKA, Sawaya R, Weinberg JS, Prabhu SS, Rao G, Fuller GN, Aldape KD, Gumin J, Vence LM, Wistuba I, Rodriguez-Canales J, Villalobos PA, Dirven CMF, Tejada S, Valle RD, Alonso MM, Ewald B, Peterkin JJ, Tufaro F, Fueyo J (2018) Phase I study of DNX-2401 (Delta-24-RGD) oncolytic adenovirus: replication and immunotherapeutic effects in recurrent malignant glioma. J Clin Oncol 36:1419–1427

41. Larsson B (1992) Radiological fundamentals in radiosurgery. In: Steiner L (ed) Radiosurgery: baseline and trends. Raven, New York, pp 3–14

42. Lawler SE, Speranza MC, Cho CF, Chiocca EA (2017) Oncolytic viruses in cancer treatment: a review. JAMA Oncol 3:841–849

43. Liberman B, Gianfelice D, Inbar Y, Beck A, Rabin T, Shabshin N, Chander G, Hengst S, Pfeffer R, Chechick A, Hanannel A, Dogadkin O, Catane R (2009) Pain palliation in patients with bone metastases using MR-guided focused ultrasound surgery: a multicenter study. Ann Surg Oncol 16:140–146

44. Markert JM, Liechty PG, Wang W, Gaston S, Braz E, Karrasch M, Nabors LB, Markiewicz M, Lakeman AD, Palmer CA, Parker JN, Whitley RJ, Gillespie GY (2009) Phase Ib trial of mutant herpes simplex virus G207 inoculated pre-and post-tumor resection for recurrent GBM. Mol Ther 17:199–207

45. Markert JM, Medlock MD, Rabkin SD, Gillespie GY, Todo T, Hunter WD, Palmer CA, Feigenbaum F, Tornatore C, Tufaro F, Martuza RL (2000) Conditionally replicating herpes simplex virus mutant, G207 for the treatment of malignant glioma: results of a phase I trial. Gene Ther 7:867–874

46. Markert JM, Razdan SN, Kuo HC, Cantor A, Knoll A, Karrasch M, Nabors LB, Markiewicz M, Agee BS, Coleman JM, Lakeman AD, Palmer CA, Parker JN, Whitley RJ, Weichselbaum RR, Fiveash JB, Gillespie GY (2014) A phase 1 trial of oncolytic HSV-1, G207, given in combination with radiation for recurrent GBM demonstrates safety and radiographic responses. Mol Ther 22:1048–1055

47. Mathios D, Kim JE, Mangraviti A, Phallen J, Park CK, Jackson CM, Garzon-Muvdi T, Kim E, Theodros D, Polanczyk M, Martin AM, Suk I, Ye X, Tyler B, Bettegowda C, Brem H, Pardoll DM, Lim M (2016) Anti-PD-1 antitumor immunity is enhanced by local and abrogated by systemic chemotherapy in GBM. Sci Transl Med 8:370ra180

48. McDannold N, Clement GT, Black P, Jolesz F, Hynynen K (2010) Transcranial magnetic resonance imaging- guided focused ultrasound surgery of brain tumors: initial findings in 3 patients. Neurosurgery 66:323–332; discussion 332

49. Mehrkens JH, Kreth FW, Muacevic A, Ostertag CB (2004) Long term course of WHO grade II astrocytomas of the Insula of Reil after I-125 interstitial irradiation. J Neurol 251:1455–1464

50. Mueller S, Polley MY, Lee B, Kunwar S, Pedain C, Wembacher-Schroder E, Mittermeyer S, Westphal M, Sampson JH, Vogelbaum MA, Croteau D, Chang SM (2011) Effect of imaging and catheter characteristics on clinical outcome for patients in the PRECISE study. J Neuro-Oncol 101:267–277

51. Mun EJ, Babiker HM, Weinberg U, Kirson ED, Von Hoff DD (2018) Tumor-treating fields: a fourth modality in cancer treatment. Clin Cancer Res 24:266–275

52. Mut M, Sherman JH, Shaffrey ME, Schiff D (2008) Cintredekin besudotox in treatment of malignant glioma. Expert Opin Biol Ther 8:805–812

53. Peraud A, Goetz C, Siefert A, Tonn JC, Kreth FW (2007) Interstitial iodine-125 radiosurgery alone or in combination with microsurgery for pediatric patients with eloquently located low-grade glioma: a pilot study. Childs Nerv Syst 23:39–46

54. Phillips HS, Kharbanda S, Chen R, Forrest WF, Soriano RH, Wu TD, Misra A, Nigro JM, Colman H, Soroceanu L, Williams PM, Modrusan Z, Feuerstein BG, Aldape K (2006) Molecular subclasses of high-grade glioma predict prognosis, delineate a pattern of disease progression, and resemble stages in neurogenesis. Cancer Cell 9:157–173

55. Popperl G, Kreth FW, Mehrkens JH, Herms J, Seelos K, Koch W, Gildehaus FJ, Kretzschmar HA, Tonn JC, Tatsch K (2007) FET PET for the evaluation of untreated gliomas: correlation of FET uptake and uptake kinetics with tumour grading. Eur J Nucl Med Mol Imaging 34:1933–1942

56. Portnow J, Synold TW, Badie B, Tirughana R, Lacey SF, D'Apuzzo M, Metz MZ, Najbauer J, Bedell V, Vo T, Gutova M, Frankel P, Chen M, Aboody KS (2017) Neural stem cell-based anticancer gene therapy: a first-in-human study in recurrent high-grade glioma patients. Clin Cancer Res 23: 2951–2960

57. Ram Z, Cohen ZR, Harnof S, Tal S, Faibel M, Nass D, Maier SE, Hadani M, Mardor Y (2006) Magnetic resonance imaging-guided, high-intensity focused ultrasound for brain tumor therapy. Neurosurgery 59:949–955; discussion 955–946

58. Reardon DA, Akabani G, Coleman RE, Friedman AH, Friedman HS, Herndon JE II, Cokgor I, McLendon RE, Pegram CN, Provenzale JM, Quinn JA, Rich JN, Regalado LV, Sampson JH, Shafman TD, Wikstrand CJ, Wong TZ, Zhao XG, Zalutsky MR, Bigner DD (2002) Phase II trial of murine (131)I-labeled antitenascin monoclonal antibody 81C6 administered into surgically created resection cavities of patients with newly diagnosed malignant gliomas. J Clin Oncol 20:1389–1397

59. Reardon DA, Zalutsky MR, Akabani G, Coleman RE, Friedman AH, Herndon JE II, McLendon RE, Pegram CN, Quinn JA, Rich JN, Vredenburgh JJ, Desjardins A, Guruangan S, Boulton S, Raynor RH, Dowell JM, Wong TZ, Zhao XG, Friedman HS, Bigner DD (2008) A pilot study: 131I-antitenascin monoclonal antibody 81c6 to deliver a 44-Gy resection cavity boost. Neuro-Oncology 10:182–189

60. Reitz M, Demestre M, Sedlacik J, Meissner H, Fiehler J, Kim SU, Westphal M, Schmidt NO (2012) Intranasal delivery of neural stem/progenitor cells: a noninvasive passage to target intracerebral glioma. Stem Cells Transl Med 1:866–873

61. Reulen HJ, Poepperl G, Goetz C, Gildehaus FJ, Schmidt M, Tatsch K, Pietsch T, Kraus T, Rachinger W (2015) Long-term outcome of patients with WHO Grade III and IV gliomas treated by fraction-ated intracavitary radioimmunotherapy. J Neurosurg 123:760–770

62. Ribas A, Dummer R, Puzanov I, VanderWalde A, Andtbacka RHI, Michielin O, Olszanski AJ, Malvehy J, Cebon J, Fernandez E, Kirkwood JM, Gajewski TF, Chen L, Gorski KS, Anderson AA, Diede SJ, Lassman ME, Gansert J, Hodi FS, Long GV (2017) Oncolytic virotherapy promotes intratumoral T cell infiltration and improves anti-PD-1 immunotherapy. Cell 170:1109–1119 e1110

63. Ruge MI, Simon T, Suchorska B, Lehrke R, Hamisch C, Koerber F, Maarouf M, Treuer H, Berthold F, Sturm V, Voges J (2011) Stereotactic brachytherapy with iodine-125 seeds for the treatment of inoperable low-grade gliomas in children: long-term outcome. J Clin Oncol 29:4151–4159

64. Sampson JH, Akabani G, Archer GE, Berger MS, Coleman RE, Friedman AH, Friedman HS, Greer K, Herndon JE II, Kunwar S, McLendon RE, Paolino A, Petry NA, Provenzale JM, Reardon DA, Wong TZ, Zalutsky MR, Pastan I, Bigner DD (2008) Intracerebral infusion of an EGFR-targeted toxin in recurrent malignant brain tumors. Neuro-Oncology 10:320–329

65. Sampson JH, Archer G, Pedain C, Wembacher-Schroder E, Westphal M, Kunwar S, Vogelbaum MA, Coan A, Herndon JE, Raghavan R, Brady ML, Reardon DA, Friedman AH, Friedman HS, Rodriguez-Ponce MI, Chang SM, Mittermeyer S, Croteau D, Puri RK (2010) Poor drug distribution as a possible explanation for the results of the PRECISE trial. J Neurosurg 113:301–309

66. Samson A, Scott KJ, Taggart D, West EJ, Wilson E, Nuovo GJ, Thomson S, Corns R, Mathew RK, Fuller MJ, Kottke TJ, Thompson JM, Ilett EJ, Cockle JV, Appleton ES, Migneco G, Rose AS, Coffey MC, Beirne DA, Collinson FJ, Ralph C, Alan Anthoney D, Twelves CJ, Furness AJ, Quezada SA, Wurdak H, Errington-Mais F, Pandha H, Harrington KJ, Selby PJ, Vile RG, Griffin SD, Stead LF, Short SC, Melcher AA (2018) Intravenous delivery of oncolytic reovirus to brain tumor patients immunologically primes for subsequent checkpoint blockade. Sci Transl Med 10:eaam7577

67. Schnell O, Scholler K, Ruge M, Siefert A, Tonn JC, Kreth FW (2008) Surgical resection plus stereotactic 125I brachytherapy in adult patients with eloquently located supratentorial WHO grade II glioma—feasibility and outcome of a combined local treatment concept. J Neurol 255:1495–1502

68. Sloan AE, Ahluwalia MS, Valerio-Pascua J, Manjila S, Torchia MG, Jones SE, Sunshine JL, Phillips M, Griswold MA, Clampitt M, Brewer C, Jochum J, McGraw MV, Diorio D, Ditz G, Barnett GH (2013) Results of the NeuroBlate System first-in-humans Phase I clinical trial for recurrent glioblastoma: clinical article. J Neurosurg 118:1202–1219

69. Souweidane MM, Kramer K, Pandit-Taskar N, Zhou Z, Haque S, Zanzonico P, Carrasquillo JA,

Lyashchenko SK, Thakur SB, Donzelli M, Turner RS, Lewis JS, Cheung NV, Larson SM, Dunkel IJ (2018) Convection-enhanced delivery for diffuse intrinsic pontine glioma: a single-centre, dose-escalation, phase 1 trial. Lancet Oncol 19:1040–1050

70. Spiegel BM, Esrailian E, Laine L, Chamberlain MC (2007) Clinical impact of adjuvant chemotherapy in glioblastoma multiforme: a meta-analysis. CNS Drugs 21:775–787

71. Stepp H, Stummer W (2018) 5-ALA in the management of malignant glioma. Lasers Surg Med 50:399–419

72. Stummer W, Beck T, Beyer W, Mehrkens JH, Obermeier A, Etminan N, Stepp H, Tonn JC, Baumgartner R, Herms J, Kreth FW (2008) Long-sustaining response in a patient with non-resectable, distant recurrence of glioblastoma multiforme treated by interstitial photodynamic therapy using 5-ALA: case report. J Neuro-Oncol 87:103–109

73. Stummer W, van den Bent MJ, Westphal M (2011) Cytoreductive surgery of glioblastoma as the key to successful adjuvant therapies: new arguments in an old discussion. Acta Neurochir 153:1211–1218

74. Stupp R, Wong ET, Kanner AA, Steinberg D, Engelhard H, Heidecke V, Kirson ED, Taillibert S, Liebermann F, Dbaly V, Ram Z, Villano JL, Rainov N, Weinberg U, Schiff D, Kunschner L, Raizer J, Honnorat J, Sloan A, Malkin M, Landolfi JC, Payer F, Mehdorn M, Weil RJ, Pannullo SC, Westphal M, Smrcka M, Chin L, Kostron H, Hofer S, Bruce J, Cosgrove R, Paleologous N, Palti Y, Gutin PH (2012) NovoTTF-100A versus physician's choice chemotherapy in recurrent glioblastoma: a randomised phase III trial of a novel treatment modality. Eur J Cancer 48:2192–2202

75. Vecil GG, Lang FF (2003) Clinical trials of adenoviruses in brain tumors: a review of Ad-p53 and oncolytic adenoviruses. J Neuro-Oncol 65:237–246

76. Vogelbaum MA, Brewer C, Barnett GH, Mohammadi AM, Peereboom DM, Ahluwalia MS, Gao S (2018) First-in-human evaluation of the Cleveland Multiport Catheter for convection-enhanced delivery of topotecan in recurrent high-grade glioma: results of pilot trial 1. J Neurosurg 1–10

77. von Neubeck C, Seidlitz A, Kitzler HH, Beuthien-Baumann B, Krause M (2015) Glioblastoma multiforme: emerging treatments and stratification markers beyond new drugs. Br J Radiol 88:20150354

78. Weber F, Asher A, Bucholz R, Berger M, Prados M, Chang S, Bruce J, Hall W, Rainov NG, Westphal M, Warnick RE, Rand RW, Floeth F, Rommel F, Pan H, Hingorani VN, Puri RK (2003) Safety, tolerability, and tumor response of IL4-Pseudomonas exotoxin (NBI-3001) in patients with recurrent malignant glioma. J Neuro-Oncol 64:125–137

79. Westphal M, Hilt DC, Bortey E, Delavault P, Olivares R, Warnke PC, Whittle IR, Jaaskelainen J, Ram Z (2003) A phase 3 trial of local chemotherapy with biodegradable carmustine (BCNU) wafers (Gliadel wafers) in patients with primary malignant glioma. Neuro-Oncology 5:79–88

80. Westphal M, Yla-Herttuala S, Martin J, Warnke P, Menei P, Eckland D, Kinley J, Kay R, Ram Z (2013) Adenovirus-mediated gene therapy with sitimagene ceradenovec followed by intravenous ganciclovir for patients with operable high-grade glioma (ASPECT): a randomised, open-label, phase 3 trial. Lancet Oncol 14:823–833

81. Wheeler LA, Manzanera AG, Bell SD, Cavaliere R, McGregor JM, Grecula JC, Newton HB, Lo SS, Badie B, Portnow J, Teh BS, Trask TW, Baskin DS, New PZ, Aguilar LK, Aguilar-Cordova E, Chiocca EA (2016) Phase II multicenter study of gene-mediated cytotoxic immunotherapy as adjuvant to surgical resection for newly diagnosed malignant glioma. Neuro-Oncology 18:1137–1145

Part II

Neurooncology of the Cranial Space

David A. Reardon, Manfred Westphal,
Jörg-Christian Tonn

Tumors of the Skull Including Chordoma

7

Roland Goldbrunner, Jörg-Christian Tonn, and Volker Neuschmelting

7.1 Epidemiology

Skull tumors comprise a wide variety of entities, ranging from chronic inflammatory diseases to primary and secondary neoplasms. There are no valid data about the incidence of skull tumors in general, but the epidemiology of single entities has been assessed.

Besides intraosseous meningioma, which is described elsewhere in this textbook, osteoma is the most common diagnosis in benign skull neoplasms [1] and may be accompanied by Gardner's syndrome [2]. In most series, the second most common finding in benign calvarian tumors is hemangioma [3]. Benign osteoblastoma represents about 1% of all bone tumors, and a craniofacial localization is found in 15% of all osteoblastomas [2]. The most common primary malignant skull tumors are osteogenic sarcoma and chondrosarcoma. The former—in general—is the second most common primary malignant bone tumor after plasmocytoma. Osteogenic sar-

coma occurs in all ages with a peak within the first two decades; 85% of osteogenic sarcoma arises before the age of 30 [4]. The main cranial locations are the maxilla and mandible, while manifestation in the calvaria is less common. In contrast, cranial chondrosarcoma arises preferentially at the skull base, accounting for 6% of all skull base tumors [5]. The highest incidence is found in the second decade; however, chondrosarcomas may be found at any age.

The incidence of secondary malignant tumors is on the rise with extended survival of cancer patients so that especially for breast cancer and prostate cancer skull metastases are seen more frequently.

7.2 Symptoms and Clinical Signs

Most entities can be found in any cranial bone; therefore, the clinical presentation varies according to the site of tumor origin. Tumors involving the paranasal sinuses may present with frontal headache and recurrent sinusitis. Intracranial extension of large skull tumors can cause epidural compression and symptoms of elevated intracranial pressure, such as headache and nausea. Tumors of the skull base may present with cranial nerve symptoms, such as diplopia, visual or hearing loss, olfactory sensations, or impaired swallowing function. However, the most common symptom is a painless, slowly growing

R. Goldbrunner (✉) · V. Neuschmelting
Klinik für Allgemeine Neurochirurgie, Zentrum für Neurochirurgie, Uniklinikum Köln, Köln, Germany
e-mail: Roland.Goldbrunner@uk-koeln.de; volker.neuschmelting@uk-koeln.de

J.-C. Tonn
Department of Neurosurgery, University Hospital Ludwig Maximilian University Munich, Munich, Germany
e-mail: joerg.christian.tonn@med.uni-muenchen.de

© Springer Nature Switzerland AG 2019
J.-C. Tonn et al. (eds.), *Oncology of CNS Tumors*, https://doi.org/10.1007/978-3-030-04152-6_7

epicranial mass, which may vary widely in size and velocity of growth. Localized pain is a typical symptom for benign osteoid osteoma, aneurysmal bone cyst, or all types of rapidly growing malignant tumors.

7.3 Diagnostics

7.3.1 Synopsis

Simple calvarian tumors are sufficiently diagnosed by CT. The modern assessment of skull base tumors or complex calvarian tumors is multimodal: MRI is mandatory to evaluate soft-tissue structures and CT for visualizing bone alterations. In some cases, there are indications for angiography or radionuclide scans.

The basic method for diagnostics in skull tumors is still CT. It is superior to MRI in assessing the bony structures and can display bone destruction as well as bone formation or intratumoral calcification in a proper way. Similar information may also be provided by plain skull X-ray films if the tumor is localized at the calvaria. Altogether, CT may be sufficient for the diagnosis of small calvarian tumors without intracranial growth. MRI, including T2-weighted images and contrast-enhanced T1-weighted images, is important for the investigation of tumors at the skull base, where CT diagnosis of soft-tissue structures is impaired by artifacts. Involvement of cranial nerves, which are surrounded by CSF during their intradural extension, is best visualized by constructive interference in steady-state (CISS) sequences. Additionally, in case of intracranial growth of skull tumors, MRI provides more valuable information about the involvement of intracranial structures. MRI angiography may be helpful if the venous sinuses or arterial structures at the skull base are involved. Sometimes an invasive digital subtraction angiography may be indicated, particularly in cases where interventional procedures, such as embolization, are discussed. Radionuclide scans using technetium-99 (99mTc) may provide additional information in diffusely growing lesions, such as fibrous dysplasia [6].

7.4 Staging and Classification

7.4.1 Synopsis

There is a wide variety of histopathological diagnoses in tumors of the skull. These neoplasms comprise tumors of bony, cartilaginous, fibrous, histiocytic, or hematological origin. In several types of skull tumors, the tissue of origin is still a matter of debate among pathologists. This chapter does not intend to provide a complete list of all tumorous disorders of the cranium, but will concentrate on the most common and best characterized entities.

7.5 Tumors of Bony Origin

Osteomas are the most common primary tumors in the craniofacial bones. Skull osteomas are slowly growing, benign entities usually arising from the tabula externa and growing outward. Therefore, intracranial extension is rare. Two distinct subtypes can be differentiated histopathologically: the compact ("ivory") and the spongy osteoma, with the former being the more common variety. Compact osteoma consists of dense lamellar bone, whereas spongy osteoma is characterized by a trabecular architecture with a peripheral bony margin.

Osteoid osteoma is another benign lesion, which is common in the skeleton in general but is found extremely rarely within the skull. It consists of a well-defined osteolytic nidus, comprised of osteoid matrix, bony trabeculae, and vessels. The nidus is surrounded by dense cortical sclerosis [3].

Osteoblastoma is a rare, benign entity with strong histopathological similarities to osteoid osteoma. Therefore, it has also been termed "giant osteoid osteoma." Compared with osteoid osteoma, osteoblastomas are usually larger and possess more fibrous stroma, many multinucleated giant cells, extravasated blood, and less osteoid. Local recurrence after subtotal excision as well as malignant transformation has been reported; therefore, complete excision should be preferred to curettage of the nidus [7].

Osteogenic sarcoma is a highly malignant tumor occurring before the age of 30 in 85% and after the age of 60 in 10% of patients. It is the second most common bone tumor after multiple myeloma. Involvement of craniofacial bones is seen more often in elderly patients, and growth within the skull accounts for less than 1% of all osteogenic sarcomas. These tumors may grow in an osteolytic or osteoblastic pattern. The histological diagnosis is based on the identification of a malignant spindle-cell stroma that produces osteoid or immature bone. Fibroblastic, chondroblastic, and osteoblastic subtypes of osteogenic sarcoma can be distinguished, but these types do not correspond with the prognosis. In elderly patients, more than half of all osteogenic sarcomas arise secondary to fibrous dysplasia or Paget's disease [3]. Previous radiation therapy or occurrence of retinoblastoma is also a known risk factor for secondary osteosarcoma. The 500-fold increased risk of developing an osteogenic sarcoma for retinoblastoma patients might be due to a common mutation of the retinoblastoma tumor suppressor gene, which is observed in a variety of malignancies [8].

7.6 Tumors of Cartilaginous Origin

Benign, well-circumscribed *chondromas* and locally aggressive *chondroblastomas* are very rare tumors of the skull. The latter accounts for only 1% of primary bone tumors and rarely occurs in the craniofacial region. Data are, thus, limited to a few dozen case series reported in the literature. Therein, it predominantly occurs in the temporal bone [9, 10]. Both entities may expand in the cortex of the bone and typically show intralesional calcifications, which may display a pathognomonic "chicken wire" arrangement in chondroblastomas.

Chondrosarcoma is the third most common malignant tumor of the bone, following multiple myeloma and osteogenic sarcoma. Patients with cranial manifestations of chondrosarcoma are usually younger (peak second decade) than patients with extracranial manifestations (peak fourth decade). Some 80% of cranial chondrosarcomas arise in the skull base, representing 6% of all skull base tumors [5]. Three subtypes can be differentiated histologically based upon nuclear size, staining, chromatic pattern, mitotic activity, and cellularity: Grade I chondrosarcoma was reclassified in 2013 in the updated WHO classification for soft and bone tissue tumors as "atypical cartilaginous tumor" and, thus, down classified to an intermediate malignant type of tumor ("locally aggressive") due to the low rate of local recurrences and low risk of metastases observed [11]. Grade 2 chondrosarcoma is more cellular with less chondroid matrix with mitoses present but widely scattered. It is classified as a malignant disease; the metastatic potential is considered to be intermediate (10–15%). The dedifferentiated chondrosarcoma (WHO grade 3) is highly cellular with nuclear pleomorphism and high mitotic index, absence of cartilage lobules, and presence of spindle-cell sarcomatous areas with high metastatic potential and the poorest prognosis of the three subtypes (10-year overall survival rate of 29–55%) [11–13].

7.7 Chordoma

Chordomas arise from remnants of the primitive notochord at the spheno-occipital synchondrosis of the skull base and are rare tumors usually located in the midline. Often, chordomas and chondrosarcomas are considered together despite the fact that they are separate pathological entities with a different clinical course. Both entities can be differentiated by immunohistochemical staining: Chordoma and chondroid chordoma are immunopositive for epithelial markers including cytokeratin and epithelial membrane antigen (EMA), whereas chondrosarcoma is negative for both [14]. The annual incidence of these rare tumors is 0.2–0.5 per 100,000 persons; they account for 0.1–0.7% of intracranial and 6% of skull base tumors [15].

Typical symptoms are lower cranial nerve pareses, diplopia, and headache. Pain which can be provoked by bending/flexing/tilting or rotating the head indicates potential involvement of the condyles with subsequent instability.

Both MRI and CT are necessary for imaging as the latter can visualize bony destruction including the condylar region and hyperostosis whereas MRI depicts the extent of the lesion [15, 16].

Therapy consists of maximal surgical resection albeit with preservation of function. Safe margins, however, are often hard to obtain due to the anatomical sites of origin and the highly infiltrative growth [14, 17]. Adjuvant treatment of residual tumors frequently includes proton beam radiation therapy, fractionated stereotactic radiation therapy, carbon beam radiation therapy, and radiosurgery [15, 18]. The 5-year rates for tumor recurrence and overall survival after initial surgery have been reported to be highly variable ranging from 15 to 80% and 61 to 100% and can be improved by adjuvant radiotherapy [14, 15, 19–24].

7.8 Tumors of Histiocytotic Origin

One of the most common benign lesions found in the calvaria is *eosinophilic granuloma*. It is a proliferative disease of Langerhans-type histiocytes and may be one manifestation of histiocytosis X. Eosinophilic granuloma may present as a single lesion or as part of the Hand-Schüller-Christian syndrome, which is characterized by the triad of diabetes insipidus, exophthalmos, and bony lesions, located in the skull. Eosinophilic granuloma in general may involve any bone, but the skull is the most commonly affected site. Some 34% of patients with eosinophilic granuloma are younger than 4 years of age; 74% are younger than 20 years [3]. The radiological appearance is an osteolytic lesion without peripheral sclerosis (Fig. 7.1). Small eosinophilic granulomas may shrink or even disappear after local injection of corticosteroids, which therefore should be the first choice of therapy. If resection is performed, brownish masses are found, which may contain cysts or hemorrhagic fluid.

Histiocytes are also involved in locally aggressive or malignant tumors, such as *giant-cell tumor* of the bone, *Ewing's sarcoma*, or *malignant fibrous histiocytoma*. However, skull manifestations of these entities are extremely uncommon. Thus, these tumors represent very rare differential diagnoses of skull tumors.

7.9 Fibrous Dysplasia

Fibrous dysplasia is characterized by the excess presence and proliferation of woven bone that has not transformed to lamellar bone during normal evolutionary development. It accounts for approximately 5% of benign bone tumors and occurs sporadically (non-inherited) caused by activating mutations of guanine nucleotide binding protein and alpha stimulating (GNAS) encoding the alpha subunit of G(s) protein [25, 26]. Fibrous dysplasia occurs in the monostotic form or polyostotic form involving multiple bone sites. Of all patients with fibrous dysplasia, 3–12% have McCune-Albright syndrome, which is characterized by precocious puberty, hyperpigmented maculae, and polyostotic fibrous dysplasia. The typical histological appearance of fibrous dysplasia is anvil-shaped trabeculae of woven bone surrounded by swirls of abundant fibrous tissue. The radiological appearance may be cystic, sclerotic, or mixed. The cystic form is usually present in the calvaria with a thinned and bulged outer table and a thickened but preserved inner table. The sclerotic form is typical for fibrous dysplasia of the skull base, mostly present in the anterior and middle fossa, ignoring any suture lines. The mixed form, which is also called "pagetoid" form, is found in patients older than 30 years of age, whereas the other forms are observed in younger individuals. Therefore, the pagetoid form is considered a natural progression of the cystic and sclerotic form. Patients with fibrous dysplasia are considered to have a 400-fold increased risk of developing malignant bone tumors, with osteogenic sarcoma being the most common entity in this patient population [27]. *Paget's disease* is an important differential diag-

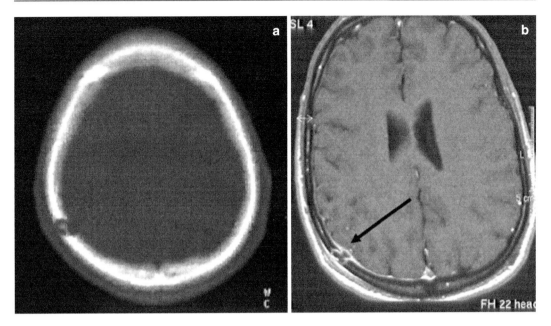

Fig. 7.1 (**a**) CT scan of a parietal eosinophilic granuloma showing a small, osteolytic lesion without any space-occupying effect or any sclerotic reaction. (**b**) T1-weighted MRI of the same patient showing slight contrast enhancement around the lesion (*arrow*)

nosis to fibrous dysplasia. Paget's disease is a premalignant condition with increased bone resorption and bone formation [28]. Woven bone replaces lamellar bone in contrast to fibrous dysplasia where not even lamellar bone develops. Paget's disease occurs in elderly patients, and malignant transformation into osteogenic sarcoma (50%), fibrosarcoma (30%), chondrosarcoma (16%), or other malignancies occurs in about 2% of patients [3].

7.10 Miscellaneous

Besides tumors of well-defined, bony, chondroid, or histiocytic origin, a variety of tumors arise from connective tissue or poorly differentiated mesenchymal structures. Tumors arising from vascular structures are found in the calvaria as well, such as the most common malignant neoplasm of the bone in adults, plasmocytoma.

Multiple myeloma, also formerly known as *plasmocytoma*, may involve any bone, but the vertebral bodies, ribs, pelvic bones, and skull are most frequently involved. Plasmocytoma usually produces multiple osteolytic lesions that may be pathognomonic on skull X-ray. These lesions are highly vascularized, with the blood supply derived from scalp arteries. Solitary plasmocytoma of the skull is an extremely rare lesion representing a single mass of plasma cells without any sign of systemic disease.

Hemangioma is the second most common skull tumor—after osteoma—in several series comprising 10% of benign skull neoplasms [29, 30]. The incidence of calvarian hemangioma increases with age, with a peak between the fourth and sixth decade. Two distinct subtypes are differentiated: the more common sessile hemangioma, which causes an expansion of the diploe and represents a well-demarcated, lytic lesion, and the globular type, which arises from the skull base and acts like a space-occupying lesion. Remnants of the bony trabecular structure are usually seen in hemangioma, but the pathognomonic bony "sunburst" striations occur in only 10–15% of hemangiomas. Hemangiomas are classified according to their vessel size, with cavernous hemangiomas being the most common entity within the skull. Important differential diagnoses for hemangioma are giant-cell tumor and—in particular—*aneurysmal bone cyst*. The latter entity is characterized by a multiloculated, painful swelling and a thin-walled bone cyst filled with unclotted blood.

Dermoid cysts. These are rare congenital lesions resulting from entrapment of the surface ectoderm in the skull bone [31]. They are best removed early. Compression of a sinus can cause pseudotumor cerebri.

One of the most common neoplasms within the skull is *intraosseous meningioma*, which usually grows in an osteoplastic pattern and arises within the anterior fossa. This entity is described in detail elsewhere in this textbook.

An important differential diagnosis to any primary bone tumor is *metastatic carcinoma*. These lesions, derived from breast, prostate, ovarian, or many other types of cancer, may arise in any bone and have to be treated within a comprehensive treatment concept (Fig. 7.2).

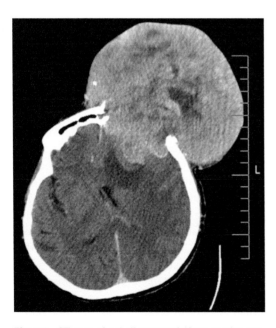

Fig. 7.2 CT scan of a skull metastasis from ovarian cancer. This mass lesion has been growing for more than 6 months in parallel to systemic bone metastases. The tumor displays a sharp demarcation toward the brain, significant perifocal edema, and no evidence of intratumoral sclerosis

7.11 Treatment

7.11.1 Synopsis

Total surgical resection is the standard treatment for benign and most malignant tumors of the skull. Radiation and chemotherapy may be indicated as adjuvant options in case of metastatic or incompletely resected tumors. Local injection of corticosteroids might be considered in the case of small eosinophilic granuloma [32].

7.11.2 Surgery

The standard treatment for benign skull tumors or tumors of unknown etiology is total surgical resection. Most calvarian tumors are palpable, and therefore, a straight skin incision above the tumor can be made depending on the size of the tumor. In small, nonpalpable tumors, neuronavigation or marking of the lesion during CT scanning may be useful to ensure a minimal approach. If a complete resection is accomplished, the bone defect should be covered by cranioplasty, e.g., by artificial polymers. For large lesion with a bone defect which can be pre-defined, a custom-made cranioplasty can be manufactured prior to the planned lesion-bearing craniectomy which is then done exactly in the shape of the implant so that a perfect fit reconstruction can be accomplished. If the craniocervical junction is involved, additional surgical instrumentation needs to be assessed to maintain the craniocervical, axial, and subaxial stability. In those cases the use of modern carbon-derived spondylodesis material needs to to be weighed up the biomechanical durability of standard titanium material to reduce MRI artifacts and enhance readability in necessary follow-up diagnostics. Skull base tumors still represent a major surgical challenge in many cases. Even locally aggressive or malignant tumors like chondrosarcomas may be cured by total excision [13]. Therefore, transfrontal, transsphenoidal, midfacial, pterional, or transzygomatic approaches to the anterior skull base may be used for en bloc resection of these tumors. The risk of cranial nerve impairment or even sacrifice of one carotid artery to enable complete removal has to be discussed with the patient before the procedure (please see Chap. 17). In large skull base neoplasms or bone-forming conditions like fibrous dysplasia, decompression of single cranial nerves may be indicated to improve or prevent nerve dysfunctions, such as visual loss or trigeminal neuralgia [33, 34].

7.11.3 Radiotherapy

The vast majority of skull tumors are cured by surgery alone. However, adjuvant radiotherapy may be indicated in malignant tumors of the skull after incomplete resection or in recurrent disease. In large skull base tumors, commonly chondrosarcomas, which often are nonresectable despite sophisticated skull base approaches, a combined treatment regime consisting of surgery and radiation may be the therapy of choice. Conventional radiotherapy is, however, often dose-limited by adjacent critical structures to preserve (brain stem, optic nerves, spinal cord). Reports suggest local control rates to positively relate to applied radiation dosage [35]. Various centers have, thus, proposed the use of proton beam therapy or carbion ions in raster scan techniques which enable the delivery of higher doses than by conventional radiotherapy. But prospective randomized controlled data are scarce, a phase-2 trial comparing both treatment regimens are currently underway (clinicaltrials.gov identifier: NCT01811394). Another competing treatment option is radiosurgery by Gamma Knife or CyberKnife which enables spatially precise dose delivery and sparing of toxic doses to critical brain and nerve tissue [35, 36]. While protons deliver less dose beyond the target tissue than the latter, there are no randomized data comparing radiosurgery vs. protons or carbon ion boost in those chordoma or chondrosarcoma patients. But both radiosurgery and proton as well as carbon ion beam techniques seem to be a valuable adjunct to surgery for chordomas and chondrosarcomas according to recent retrospective case series reports summarized in [35].

In premalignant bone-forming conditions, such as Paget's disease or fibrous dysplasia, radiation is even contraindicated, since radiation increases the risk of secondary malignancies [37].

7.11.4 Chemotherapy/Medical Therapy

There are only a few indications for chemotherapy in the treatment of skull tumors. High-dose chemo- and immunotherapeutic regimes combined with autologous stem-cell transplantation and currently anti-angiogenic therapy are standard treatment for multiple myeloma. Metastatic malignancies primarily located at the skull, such as osteogenic sarcoma or Ewing's sarcoma, also have to be treated by chemotherapy within a multimodality concept. Medical treatment is required in conditions with increased bone turnover, such as fibrous dysplasia and—even more—Paget's disease. Second- or third-generation bisphosphonates have been shown to inhibit bone turnover in these conditions effectively [28]. However, in general the majority of tumors of the skull are successfully treated by surgical resection and do not need any adjunctive therapy.

7.12 Prognosis/Quality of Life

The prognosis of skull base tumors is defined by the tumor entity. All benign, totally removed tumors have an excellent prognosis. The same is true for locally aggressive or malignant nonmetastatic tumors that have been resected completely. In metastatic tumors and multiple myeloma, the prognosis depends on the systemic control of the disease with increasing overall survival rates due to new developments in the chemo- and immunotherapeutics. Quality of life may be impaired by the degree of resection, particularly in the frontal or skull base area. Cranial nerve dysfunction may lead to a significant worsening in the quality of life. Cosmetic alterations due to large bone defects should be avoided by adequate plastic techniques, e.g., polymer plastic in calvarian defects or autologous bone grafts in skull base surgery.

7.13 Follow-Up/Specific Problems and Measures

If a benign tumor of the skull is excised completely, as documented by postoperative imaging, no further follow-up is mandatory. However, an intense local and systemic follow-up has to be performed in possibly metastatic or incompletely resected malignant skull tumors. In incompletely resected chondrosarcomas, MRI and CT are recommended every 6 months; highly malignant tumors, such as osteogenic sarcoma, need local checks every 3 months for the first 2 years, followed by further checks twice a year.

7.14 Future Perspectives

Modern skull base surgery has already provided the chance to cure even complex processes by total resection or to improve local control of these lesions. Improving imaging modalities based on MRI, CT, or radionuclide scans will allow better demarcation of skull base processes. Implementation of this imaging information in modern neuronavigation systems will provide the basis for more extensive curative surgical approaches. This allows for custom-made implants for cranioplasty to become routine. On the other hand, further developments in radiation protocols based on proton beam or carbon ion techniques may enhance the chance of local control of nonresectable neoplasms [35]. Sparing toxic doses to specific functional structures, such as cranial nerves or brain stem, by the ability to distinctly delineate the radiation target volume is of utmost importance for these patients. Therefore, Gamma Knife- or CyberKnife-based radiosurgery may continue to play an increasing role in the multimodal therapy of skull base tumors [5]. Highly vascularized skull base tumors may be more routinely treated adjunct prior to surgery by the advancing field of different embolization techniques in interventional neuroradiology [38]. Currently, these procedures are performed preoperatively to decrease blood loss during surgery; however, many tumors may be completely controlled by these techniques alone [39].

References

1. Tucker WS, Nasser-Sharif FJ (1997) Benign skull lesions. Can J Surg 40:449–455
2. Bilkay U, Erdem O, Ozek C, Helvaci E, Kilic K, Ertan Y, Gurler T (2004) Benign osteoma with Gardner syndrome: review of the literature and report of a case. J Craniofac Surg 15:506–509
3. Huvos AG (1991) Bone tumors: diagnosis, treatment and prognosis. W.B. Saunders, Philadelphia
4. Vege DS, Borges AM, Aggrawal K, Balasubramaniam G, Parikh DM, Bhaser B (1991) Osteosarcoma of the craniofacial bones. A clinico-pathological study. J Craniomaxillofac Surg 19:90–93
5. Kveton JF, Brackmann DE, Glasscock ME III, House WF, Hitselberger WE (1986) Chondrosarcoma of the skull base. Otolaryngol Head Neck Surg 94:23–32
6. Zhibin Y, Quanyong L, Libo C, Jun Z, Hankui L, Jifang Z, Ruisen Z (2004) The role of radionuclide bone scintigraphy in fibrous dysplasia of bone. Clin Nucl Med 29:177–180
7. Low Y, Foo CL, Seow WT (2000) Childhood temporal bone osteoblastoma: a case report. J Pediatr Surg 35:1127–1129
8. Shen WP, Young RF, Walter BN, Choi BH, Smith M, Katz J (1990) Molecular analysis of a myxoid chondrosarcoma with rearrangements of chromosomes 10 and 22. Cancer Genet Cytogenet 45:207–215
9. Gaudet EL Jr, Nuss DW, Johnson DH Jr, Miranne LS Jr (2004) Chondroblastoma of the temporal bone involving the temporomandibular joint, mandibular condyle, and middle cranial fossa: case report and review of the literature. Cranio 22:160–168
10. Park SW, Kim JH, Park JH, Moon KC, Paeng JC, Choi BS, Lee Y, Kim JH, Yoo RE, Kang KM, Kim SC, Choi SH, Yun TJ, Sohn CH (2017) Temporal bone chondroblastoma: imaging characteristics with pathologic correlation. Head Neck 39:2171–2179
11. Jo VY, Fletcher CD (2014) WHO classification of soft tissue tumours: an update based on the 2013 (4th) edition. Pathology 46:95–104
12. Hassounah M, Al Mefty O, Akhtar M, Jinkins JR, Fox JL (1985) Primary cranial and intracranial chondrosarcoma. A survey. Acta Neurochir 78:123–132
13. Neff B, Sataloff RT, Storey L, Hawkshaw M, Spiegel JR (2002) Chondrosarcoma of the skull base. Laryngoscope 112:134–139
14. Almefty K, Pravdenkova S, Colli BO, Al-Mefty O, Gokden M (2007) Chordoma and chondrosarcoma: similar, but quite different, skull base tumors. Cancer 110:2457–2467
15. Wasserman JK, Gravel D, Purgina B (2018) Chordoma of the head and neck: a review. Head Neck Pathol 12:261–268
16. Santegoeds RGC, Temel Y, Beckervordersandforth JC, Van Overbeeke JJ, Hoeberigs CM (2018) State-of-the-art imaging in human chordoma of the skull base. Curr Radiol Rep 6:16

17. Samii A, Gerganov VM, Herold C, Hayashi N, Naka T, Mirzayan MJ, Ostertag H, Samii M (2007) Chordomas of the skull base: surgical management and outcome. J Neurosurg 107:319–324

18. Leah P, Dower A, Vescovi C, Mulcahy M, Al Khawaja D (2018) Clinical experience of intracranial chordoma—a systematic review and meta-analysis of the literature. J Clin Neurosci 53:6–12

19. Stacchiotti S, Gronchi A, Fossati P, Akiyama T, Alapetite C, Baumann M, Blay JY, Bolle S, Boriani S, Bruzzi P, Capanna R, Caraceni A, Casadei R, Colia V, Debus J, Delaney T, Desai A, Dileo P, Dijkstra S, Doglietto F, Flanagan A, Froelich S, Gardner PA, Gelderblom H, Gokaslan ZL, Haas R, Heery C, Hindi N, Hohenberger P, Hornicek F, Imai R, Jeys L, Jones RL, Kasper B, Kawai A, Krengli M, Leithner A, Logowska I, Martin Broto J, Mazzatenta D, Morosi C, Nicolai P, Norum OJ, Patel S, Penel N, Picci P, Pilotti S, Radaelli S, Ricchini F, Rutkowski P, Scheipl S, Sen C, Tamborini E, Thornton KA, Timmermann B, Torri V, Tunn PU, Uhl M, Yamada Y, Weber DC, Vanel D, Varga PP, Vleggeert-Lankamp CLA, Casali PG, Sommer J (2017) Best practices for the management of local-regional recurrent chordoma: a position paper by the Chordoma Global Consensus Group. Ann Oncol 28:1230–1242

20. Ito E, Saito K, Okada T, Nagatani T, Nagasaka T (2010) Long-term control of clival chordoma with initial aggressive surgical resection and gamma knife radiosurgery for recurrence. Acta Neurochir 152:57–67

21. Colli B, Al-Mefty O (2001) Chordomas of the craniocervical junction: follow-up review and prognostic factors. J Neurosurg 95:933–943

22. Dassoulas K, Schlesinger D, Yen CP, Sheehan J (2009) The role of gamma knife surgery in the treatment of skull base chordomas. J Neurooncol 94:243–248

23. Tzortzidis F, Elahi F, Wright D, Natarajan SK, Sekhar LN (2006) Patient outcome at long-term follow-up after aggressive microsurgical resection of cranial base chordomas. Neurosurgery 59:230–237

24. Takahashi S, Kawase T, Yoshida K, Hasegawa A, Mizoe JE (2009) Skull base chordomas: efficacy of surgery followed by carbon ion radiotherapy. Acta Neurochir 151:759–769

25. Parekh SG, Donthineni-Rao R, Ricchetti E, Lackman RD (2004) Fibrous dysplasia. J Am Acad Orthop Surg 12:305–313

26. Benhamou J, Gensburger D, Messiaen C, Chapurlat R (2016) Prognostic factors from an epidemiologic evaluation of fibrous dysplasia of bone in a modern cohort: the FRANCEDYS study. J Bone Miner Res 31(12):2167–2172

27. Chen YR, Noordhoff MS (1990) Treatment of craniomaxillofacial fibrous dysplasia: how early and how extensive? Plast Reconstr Surg 86:835–842

28. Langston AL, Ralston SH (2004) Management of Paget's disease of bone. Rheumatology (Oxford) 43:955–959

29. Hamilton HB, Voorhies RM (2004) Tumors of the skull. In: Wilkins RH, Rengechary SS (eds) Neurosurgery. McGraw-Hill, New York, pp 1503–1528

30. Thomas JE, Baker HL Jr (1975) Assessment of roentgeno-graphic lucencies of the skull: a systematic approach. Neurology 25:99–106

31. Khalid S, Ruge J (2016) Considerations in the management of congenital cranial dermoid cysts. J Neurosurg Pediatr 20:30–34

32. Angelini A, Mavrogenis AF, Rimondi E, Rossi G, Ruggieri P (2017) Current concepts for the diagnosis and management of eosinophilic granuloma of bone. J Orthop Traumatol 18:83–90

33. Chen YR, Breidahl A, Chang CN (1997) Optic nerve decompression in fibrous dysplasia: indications, efficacy, and safety. Plast Reconstr Surg 99:22–30

34. Ricalde P, Horswell BB (2001) Craniofacial fibrous dysplasia of the fronto-orbital region: a case series and literature review. J Oral Maxillofac Surg 59:157–167

35. De Amorim Bernstein K, DeLaney T (2016) Chordomas and chondrosarcomas—the role of radiation therapy. J Surg Oncol 114:564–569

36. Martin JJ, Niranjan A, Kondziolka D, Flickinger JC, Lozanne KA, Lunsford LD (2007) Radiosurgery for chordomas and chondrosarcomas of the skull base. J Neurosurg 107:758–764

37. Mortensen A, Bojsen-Moller M, Rasmussen P (1989) Fibrous dysplasia of the skull with acromegaly and sarcomatous transformation. Two cases with a review of the literature. J Neurooncol 7:25–29

38. Turowski B, Zanella FE (2003) Interventional neuroradiology of the head and neck. Neuroimaging Clin N Am 13:619–645

39. Bendszus M, Martin-Schrader I, Schlake HP, Solymosi L (2003) Embolisation of intracranial meningiomas without subsequent surgery. Neuroradiology 45:451–455

40. Nguyen QN, Chang EL (2008) Emerging role of proton beam radiation therapy for chordoma and chondrosarcoma of the skull base. Curr Oncol Rep 10:338–343

41. Schulz-Ertner D, Nikoghosyan A, Thilmann C, Haberer T, Jakel O, Karger C, Kraft G, Wannenmacher M, Debus J (2004) Results of carbon ion radiotherapy in 152 patients. Int J Radiat Oncol Biol Phys 58:631–640

Meningiomas and Meningeal Tumors

8

Manfred Westphal, Katrin Lamszus,
and Jörg-Christian Tonn

8.1 Definition

Meningiomas are tumors arising from the arachnoidal coverings of the brain [64]. They are responsible for the vast majority of meningeal tumors and occur anywhere on the brain surface including the skull base and rarely also in the ventricular system.

Other than meningiomas, hemangiopericytomas and meningeal sarcomas belong to the group of mesenchymal, non-meningothelial tumors [4]. As with every other tissue, metastases and lymphoma can also occur in the meninges.

M. Westphal (✉)
Department of Neurosurgery, University of Hamburg,
University Hospital Eppendorf, Hamburg,
Hamburg, Germany
e-mail: westphal@uke.de

K. Lamszus
Department of Neurosurgery, University of Hamburg,
Hamburg, Germany
e-mail: lamszus@uke.de

J.-C. Tonn
Department of Neurosurgery, University Hospital
Ludwig Maximilian University Munich,
Munich, Germany
e-mail: joerg.christian.tonn@med.uni.muenchen.de

8.2 Epidemiology

Epidemiological data for most tumors of the central nervous system are difficult to obtain as cancer registries tend to be regional or at best national as in the Scandinavian countries [16]. A very comprehensive source is the statistical report published by CBTRUS (Central Brain Tumor Registry of the United States) of which the latest 2017 edition covers the data collection time of 2010–2014 [60].

Meningiomas show a rising incidence with age. In unselected autopsy series, 2.7% of the male and 6.2% of the female population over the age of 80 have meningiomas which up to that point were undiscovered. The reported incidence is variable between different investigations but disregarding the changing proportions from the growing incidence of cerebral metastases with better oncological therapies; one can assume that meningiomas are responsible for about 15% of all male intracranial tumors and 30% of the females. Meningiomas make up 36.8% of the gross total of adult tumors of the CNS [60]. Not considering the autoptic cases, the numbers which are reported on a population base vary between 1.6 and 5.5 per 100,000. CBTRUS reports an age-adjusted incidence rate of 8.41 per 100,000 of the US standard population and 0.25 for the age group up to 19 years demonstrating the relation to age [60] . As a rule the tumors are reported to be 1.5–3 times more frequent in

© Springer Nature Switzerland AG 2019
J.-C. Tonn et al. (eds.), *Oncology of CNS Tumors*, https://doi.org/10.1007/978-3-030-04152-6_8

Table 8.1 Meningiomas in an unselected departmental series over 10 years ($N = 679$)[a]

Location	n	Histology[b]	n	Age	n
Convexity	291				
Skull base	153				
Posterior fossa/tentorium	93				
Orbit	28				
Ventricular	5				
		Meningiotheliomatous	250		
		Fibrillary	142		
		Transitional	163		
				0–30 years	35
				31–50 years	190
				51–70 years	361
				71–90 years	93

[a]Courtesy of P. Emami, Dept. of Neurosurgery UKE
[b]The three most frequent histological subtypes

females. In the 2010–2014 period, the rate given by CBTRUS is 4.86 for males and 11.01 for females showing an increase over the years which however may be a reflection of broader availability of and access to diagnostic procedures as well as a reflection of an aging population with growing life expectancy. Peak incidence is the sixth decade in life (median age at diagnosis at CBTRUS is 66 years). Pediatric meningiomas are very rare making up 6.7% in the age group between 0 and 19 years in this report [60] with others putting the number as 2% of all tumors in that population [62].

There does not seem to be any association with race or any geographical preference which cannot be explained with access to medical care or pattern of reporting.

An unselected 10-year series from the university department of neurosurgery in Hamburg reflects these demographics with a female/male ratio of 507:172 (2.9:1) (Table 8.1).

8.3 Molecular Genetics

The majority of patients who suffer from neurofibromatosis type 2 (NF2) develop meningiomas [46, 48, 73]. In sporadic meningiomas *NF2* gene mutations are detectable in up to 60% and thus represent the most frequent gene alteration. The *NF2* tumor suppressor gene is located on chromosome arm 22q, and mutations in one allele are typically associated with either monosomy 22 or large deletions involving the other allele. Absent or strongly reduced immunoreactivity of the NF2 gene product merlin (schwannomin) has also been demonstrated in meningiomas. Merlin belongs to the 4.1 family of structural proteins that link the cytoskeleton to proteins of the cytoplasmic membrane. Recently, another member of this family, the 4.1B/DAL-1 protein, has been implicated in meningioma pathogenesis. 4.1B/DAL-1 expression is lost in 70–80% of meningiomas. No mutations were detected in the *4.1B/DAL-1* gene which is located on chromosome arm 18p. However, loss of heterozygosity (LOH) involving the *4.1B/DAL-1* region on 18p was identified in 70% of meningiomas [45].

Inactivation of the *NF2* and *4.1B/DAL-1* genes occurs with approximately equal frequency in benign (WHO grade I), atypical (WHO grade II), and anaplastic (WHO grade III) meningiomas, suggesting that both represent relatively early events in tumorigenesis. In contrast, several other most likely random genetic alterations have been identified more frequently in the more malignant tumor forms and are therefore believed to be associated with meningioma progression [91]. In the approximate order of their frequency, these alterations are allelic losses on chromosome arms 1p, 14q, 10q, 9p, and 17q. However, with the exception of the *CDKN2A, p14^{ARF}*, and *CDKN2B* genes on 9p which display alterations in the majority of malignant meningiomas and spell for particularly shortened survival ([61], no other tumor suppressor genes could consistently be identified as altered in meningiomas. Recent mutations found in NF2-intact meningiomas affect the AKT1 (involved in PI3K signaling), SMO (Hedgehog activation), KLF4 (transcription factor), and TRAF7 (a ubiquitin ligase) genes [17]. Interestingly these meningiomas were found to be clinically more benign and stable and appeared to have a preference for the medial skull base. Another new mutation affecting the TERT promotor seems to be associated with highly aggressive biological behavior [75].

Gene expression analyses by array-based techniques have been used also in meningioma research and in a series where spinal and cranial meningiomas were compared that way; a distinct set of 35 genes distiguishing between these entities was identified [76], but as such there are no surprising new insights from microarray techniques in the analysis of meningioma.

8.4 Etiology and Prevention

Meningiomas should be considered spontaneous tumors. Very early they have been found to be associated with a complete or partial loss of chromosome 22 [90], but that has so far not provided any clues as for the origin of these tumors. The only established association is with ionizing radiation, and that has been obtained from the large series of immigrants into Palestine in the early 1950s who were regularly irradiated for tinea capitis and then had a much higher than normal incidence of meningiomas with a delay of about 35 years [74]. Likewise has the follow-up from citizens of Hiroshima and Nagasaki who were exposed to the atomic blasts shown that in this population, there was a higher incidence of meningiomas with a very similar delay [65]. The doses producing meningioma with this long delay are to be considered rather low as high doses of therapeutic radiation for neoplasm produces meningiomas with a shorter delay (around 5 years [84]) or rather induces anaplastic gliomas. The indications about the role of diagnostic exposure to radiation are most likely limited to specific dental procedures [49].

As meningiomas occur most frequently in postmenopausal women [85] and meningiomas are known to have high levels of steroid hormone receptors, it has been attempted for a long time to establish a relationship between steroid hormones and the growth of meningiomas [33, 35]. The only vague association comes from the observation that, in some cases, meningiomas which had gone undetected became symptomatic during pregnancy [90] (Fig. 8.1) and even grew so rapidly that they spontaneously hemorrhaged (personal observation). In that context there is a constantly ongoing debate whether women who are known to have a meningioma or have had a meningioma removed should be on hormonal replacement therapy. Currently there does not appear to be a risk in respect to contraceptives, but there is a hint

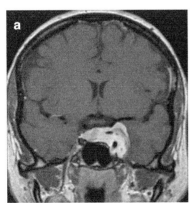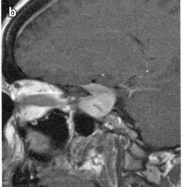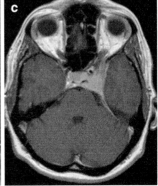

Fig. 8.1 Cavernous sinus meningioma of a 30-year-old woman (**a–c**) which during two pregnancies caused transient visual problems on the left eye. Despite extension into the sellar lumen (**a**), there is no endocrine dysfunction. The tumor has been biopsied and is under observation with the option of radiotherapy in case of progressive symptoms

of an indication that hormonal replacement therapy may increase the risk for meningioma [18]. As, however, no study has been done up to date in which the use of steroid replacement has been evaluated in a randomized controlled prospective fashion in these patients and likely never will be, the management of these patients will remain in the hands of individually deciding physicians who have to closely observe the patient and decide what is best. More recent studies failed to demonstrate any hormonal clues in women [20] and in men found that estrogen-like dietary components of soy and tofu are somewhat reducing the risk, while a high body mass index is associated with a higher incidence of meningioma [78]. A considerable number of meningiomas express progesterone receptors; however proliferating cells shut down the receptor which explains the failure of anti-progesterone therapies in meningiomas [21].

There is a weak indication that there may be an inherited susceptibility as in one epidemiological study, a first degree relative with a meningioma increases the risk 4.4-fold to also develop such lesion [19].

8.5 Signs and Symptoms

There are no typical signs or symptoms which are unequivocally specific for meningiomas. The clinical symptomatology is basically determined by the location of the lesion, the size, and the impact on its immediate surroundings. For clinical purposes, meningiomas are subspecified according to their site of origin, and this classification allows the description of the most frequent signs associated with the typical locations (Table 8.2).

Table 8.2 Symptoms of meningiomas according to location

Location	Typical symptoms
Convexity	
Frontal	Affective disorders
Parietal	Seizures
	Motor or sensory disorder, hemiparesis
Temporal	Speech disorders, memory impairment
Parasagittal	Seizures
	Motor or sensory disturbance
Olfactory meningioma	Loss of olfaction
	Affective disorders
	Loss of activity
Tuberculum sellae meningioma	Visual field or visual acuity loss
Clinoid process meningioma	Visual field or visual acuity loss
Cavernous sinus meningioma	Diplopia
	Facial pain or numbness
	Ocular venous congestion
Optic sheath meningioma	Loss of vision
Orbital meningioma	Exophthalmos
Sphenoid wing meningioma	
Medial	Loss of vision, diplopia
	Psychomotor seizures
	Schizoaffective disorders
Lateral	Seizures
	Speech problems
Tentorial meningioma	Hydrocephalus, seizures, visual field loss
	Ataxia
Cerebellar meningioma	Ataxia, vertigo, hydrocephalus
Foramen magnum meningioma	Hydrocephalus, symptoms of dorsal, lateral or ventral brain stem compression
Cerebellopontine angle meningioma	Unilateral cranial nerve dysfunction
Petroclival or clivus meningioma	Unilateral or bilateral cranial nerve dysfunction and symptoms of ventral brain stem compression
Ventricular meningioma	Partial hydrocephalus

The direct symptoms also depend very much on the size of the tumor and the growth rate. Large tumors which have grown over many years may have produced only very few symptoms because the surrounding brain had a chance to adapt while slowly becoming displaced (Fig. 8.2). In cases of caudal skull base meningiomas, this may lead to extreme brain stem compression without almost any symptoms (Fig. 8.3) or in the case of perisellar meningiomas absence of endocrinopathies. Meningiomas also differ in their respect for the arachnoidal boundary, independent of size. As arachnoid infiltration is related to edematous brain reaction, tumors respecting the arachnoid tend to be larger because of lack of brain reaction.

Seizures may be a presenting sign and were seen in 22.7% of patients preoperatively in one large series [15]. Seizures are more frequent in the typical ictogenic regions, particularly when lesions extend exophytically into the temporomesial region or the perirolandic area.

There are many ways for meningiomas to also indirectly affect the brain and produce symptoms. Meningiomas at the tentorial edge, be they supra- or infratentorial, can lead to compression of the CSF pathways and thus result in occlusive hydrocephalus as do large meningiomas in the posterior fossa (Fig. 8.4). Meningiomas which produce an extraordinary amount of edema (frequently of the secretory type [10, 55]) cause an indirect mass effect exceeding their own mass severalfold and can cause drowsiness and even loss of consciousness up to the extreme of herniation (Fig. 8.5). Meningiomas occluding a major sinus such as the falcine meningiomas or parasagittal meningiomas or those of the torcular or transverse sinus can cause venous congestion and generalized edema to the extreme of chronic intracranial hypertension with papilloedema and impairment of visual acuity and the development of pseudotumor cerebri especially when the occluded sinus is dominant (Fig. 8.6a, b). It is

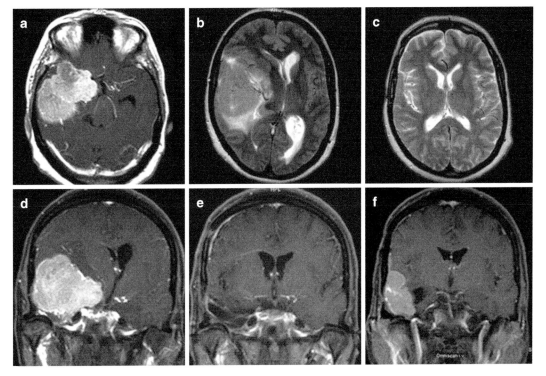

Fig. 8.2 Large temporal meningioma with impressive midline shift but no specific symptoms (**a–c**). The diagnosis was made after lack of concentration and inability to complete simple tasks in daily life lead to cranial imaging. Despite the appearance of encased large vessels, the tumor was completely removed without any deficits (**d, e**). The minimal perilesional edema was reflected by a good dissection plane over most of the tumor surface. The definitive diagnosis being an atypical meningioma, the tumor recurred with more extensive perilesional edema 4 years later (**f**)

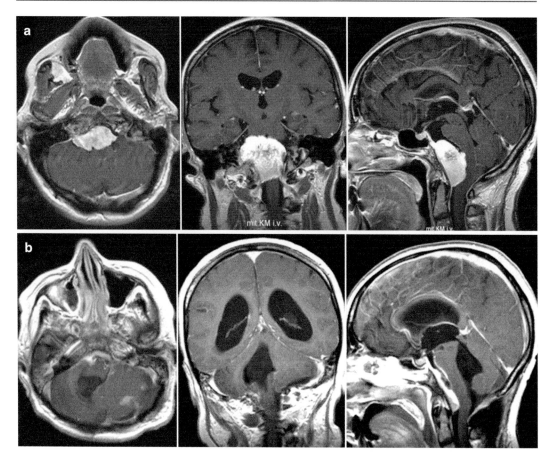

Fig. 8.3 Large meningioma of the clivus extending mostly into the right CP angle (**a**, upper panel). The removal required approaches from both sides because of encasement of the caudal cranial nerves on both sides. The dura of the clivus was completely invaded and was left in place after extensive coagulation (**b**). The course has been stable with no indication of growth of the possible extradural tumor layer seen at the level of the foramen magnum (bottom right). Postoperatively the patient developed a malresorptive hydrocephalus which required shunting

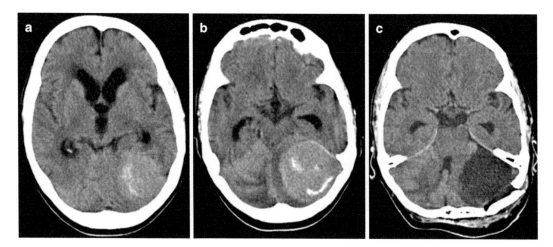

Fig. 8.4 CT of a large meningioma in the posterior fossa which has over months leads to occlusive hydrocephalus which is seen to result in distended temporal horns and peri-ventricular capping over the frontal part of the lateral ventricles (**a**, **b**). A few days after removal, the fourth ventricle is again visible, and the temporal distension is slowly regressing (**c**)

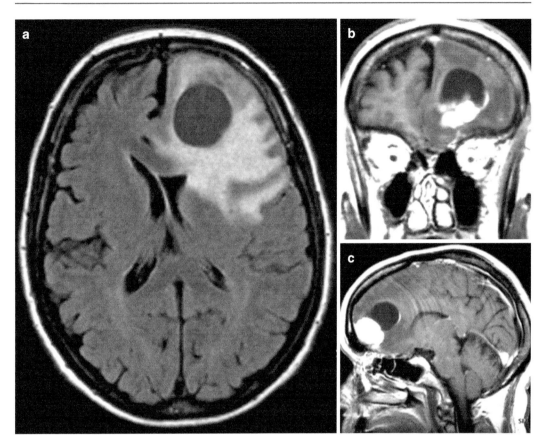

Fig. 8.5 MRI of a patient with a massive edema (**a**) resulting from a cystic meningioma of the secretory type (**b**, **c**). As seen in the T2 images (**a**), the amount of space occupation is mostly due to the edema and not so much due to the mass effect of the tumor

frequently seen that even after complete resection of a meningioma, an edema-like change in signal intensity in the MRI can remain for many years (Fig. 8.6).

It is a general rule that the risk of surgical treatment of a meningioma can be very well assessed when neurological deficits are related to edema. When appropriate treatment with steroids (see below) causes symptoms to dissappear, the surgery will be much less likely to result in additional or increased neurological deficit than when the symptoms persist despite edema resolution.

8.6   Staging and Classification

As described in the chapter on histopathology of CNS tumors, meningiomas are graded according to the WHO grading system into well-differentiated meningiomas of the WHO grade I, atypical meningiomas WHO grade II, and anaplastic meningiomas WHO grade III. According to the most recent revision of the WHO classification system, brain invasion alone qualifies for classification as WHO grade II [62]. In addition there are several subtypes of which two in themselves are equivalent to a higher grade [63]. Due to serially acquired genetic aberrations, progression from a lower grade to the next higher grade is possible [46] (Fig. 8.7a) but rare, and that is also accompanied by increasing production of angiogenic factors [47] and the late incidence of metastasis in the situation of anaplastic meningioma [39]. Meningioma may become a chronic disease in some patients spreading throughout the cranium including the skull bone and spread also to extracranial sites like the spine (Fig. 8.7b).

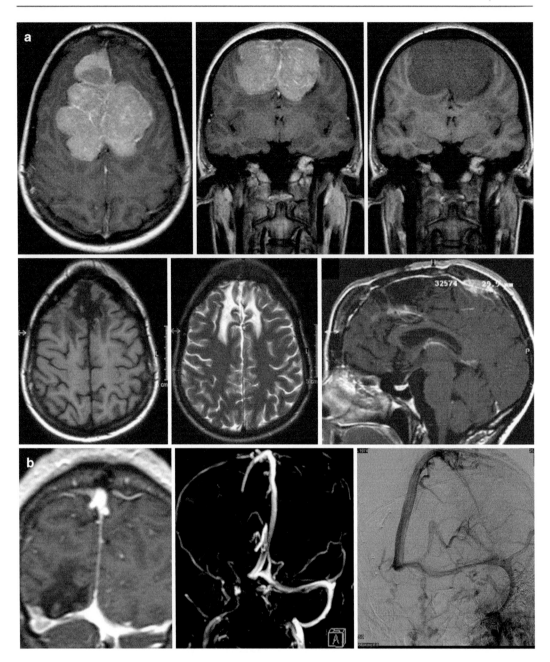

Fig. 8.6 (**a**) Very sharply demarcated bilateral falx meningioma of a 28-year-old woman who had papill-edema and developed optic nerve atrophy from constant pressure. The sinus was removed in its occluded parts. The edema which was present only in the most central aspects around the tumor was still present 5 years after follow-up (top) at which time also a recurrence was seen in the distal part of the sagittal sinus (bottom) which was eventually resected as well as further recurrences toward the frontal as well as the dorsal aspects. (**b**) Progressive meningioma of the wall of the right transverse sinus (left) which despite radiosurgery to that aspect continued to occlude the sinus which could not be removed because of stenosis and partial thrombosis of the contralateral left sinus (MR angiogram middle panel) so that eventually venous congestion as seen by the massive collaterals towards the cerebellar veins and occipital bridging veins seen upon digital subtraction angiography (right panel) became so severe that pseudotumor cerebri required permanent ventriculoperitoneal shunt

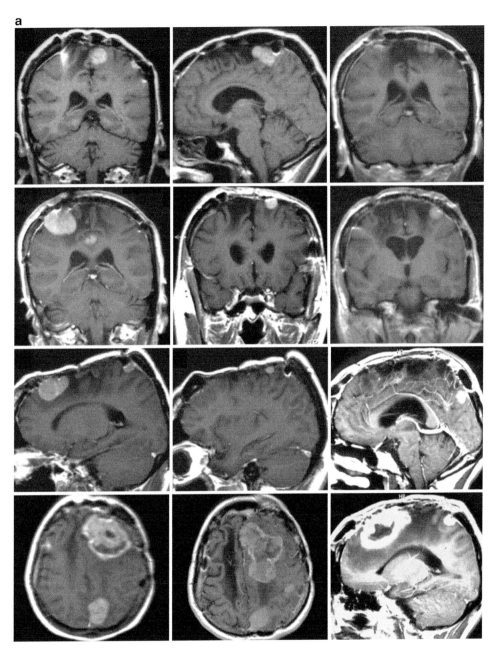

Fig. 8.7 (**a**) Progressive dedifferentiation of a meningioma which was originally operated in 1978. Altogether six operations with increasingly difficult wound conditions followed for recurrences occurring at increasingly short intervals (top two rows). This was correlated to accumulation of additional genetic alterations. After the removal of the bone flap had become necessary and a cranioplasty was placed in the context of further recurrences (third row of panels) the patient received radiosurgical treatment (fourth row) whereupon the lesions rapidly expanded with the development of a steroid dependence and with further progression and severe disability, the patient declined any further treatment in 2003, after 25 years of struggle with a clinically increasingly aggressive meningioma. (**b**) Multiple recurrences of a chronic meningioma disease in a 75-year-old female after 15 years and several resections (left two panels). Sensory and motor radicular symptoms of C7 and C8 beginning on the left side lead to the diagnosis of spinal involvement (middle panel sagittal MRI showing the extensive bone involvement) which was histologically proven to be meningioma with epidural filling of the neuroforamen (right panels) as well as bone infiltration. Due to frail health, the overall situation deteriorated rapidly, and no measures were taken beyond palliation

b

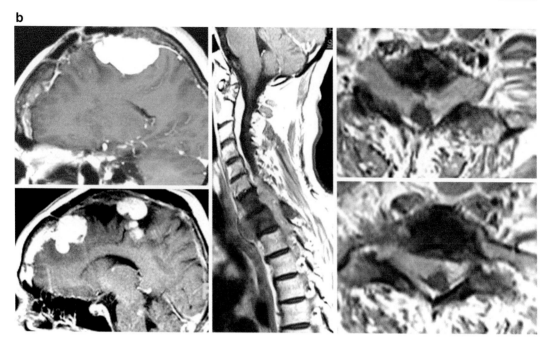

Fig. 8.7 (continued)

Although it would be desirable to clinically stage meningiomas for the extent of the disease, chronicity, or the aggressiveness of the tumor, such distinction is lacking. But there is a classification for the resection (see below). The significance of the histological grading is related to the decision-making for adjuvant therapies (see below) and the follow-up regimen. In general there is a correlation of the grades with survival but only when the tumors are in comparable locations and similar extents of resection can be achieved. On the other hand, there is a much better prognosis for a completely resected atypical meningioma (WHO grade II) of the convexities compared to a non-resectable meningioma grade WHO I of the skull base (Fig. 8.8).

8.7 Diagnostic Procedures

Many meningiomas are found incidentally because of unrelated complaints such as a dizzy spell, a transient ischemic attack, and uncharacteristic headache or because after a minor trauma, an MRI has been performed (Fig. 8.9). Otherwise any of the symptoms summarized in Table 8.2 above may have specifically led to some kind of neuroimaging. Recently, guidelines for diagnosis and therapy of meningiomas have been published [29].

Computed tomography (CT): CT shows meningiomas usually as well as described mass lesions with uniform contrast enhancement located at the surface of the brain, either at the convexity or the base of the skull. A non-enhanced scan must be obtained in the first place because it may show extensive calcification which is mostly associated with very slow growth and thus only relative indications for therapy. Especially in fronto-orbital tumors, it is important to have thin sections and a series of bone windows because that defines the borders of infiltration and resection if not even resectability. CT is the optimal modality to assess intraosseous components of frontobasal skull base meningiomas (Fig. 8.10) or to detect primary intraosseous meningiomas (Fig. 8.11). The extent of edema is shown equally well in CT and MRI.

Magnetic resonance imaging (MRI): MRI is the major modality for the diagnosis of meningiomas, especially as many lesions have some skull

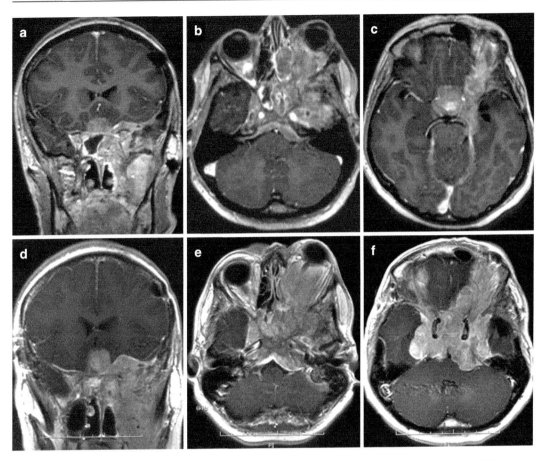

Fig. 8.8 Surgically not manageable, extensive fibrillary meningioma WHO I of the skull base (**a–f**) which was partially decompressed twice to save vision on the right eye. The tumor was rapidly progressive and failed radiosurgery, bromocriptine, anti-progesterone and hydroxyurea tratments

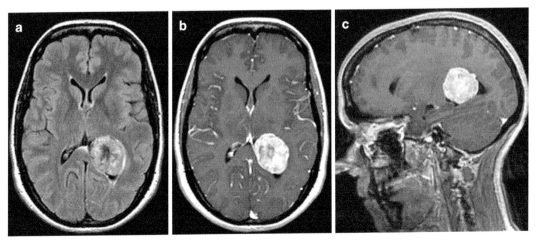

Fig. 8.9 MRI in three planes of a ventricular meningioma which was diagnosed because of intermittent headache which is completely nonreactive in the brain. The intact, non-invaded ependymal surface allowed for unrestricted CSF passage so that not even a partial hydrocephalus had developed

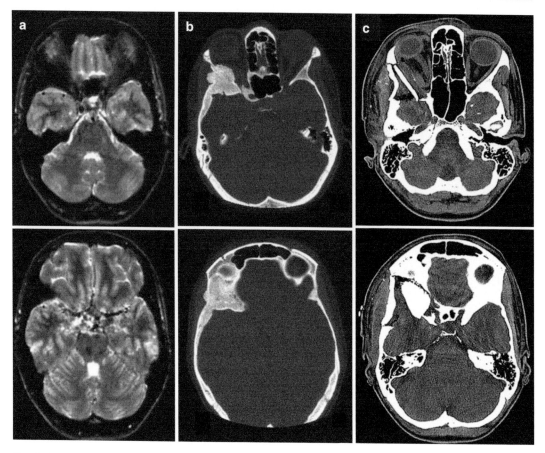

Fig. 8.10 Osseous meningioma of the lateral sphenoid wing, completely taking up the lateral wall of the orbit (**a, b**). No soft tissue components are present. Removal requires extensive drilling of the bone and decompression of the optic canal. The bone is reconstructed with methyl methacrylate providing an orbital roof (**c**) and a lateral wall (right bottom)

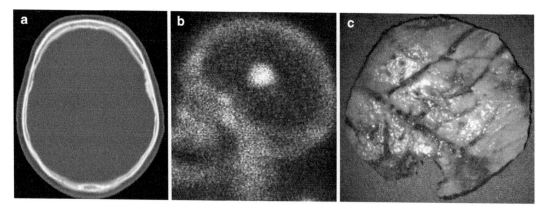

Fig. 8.11 Primary intraosseous meningioma (**a**) which was found because of a staging for prostate carcinoma involving a whole skeletal scintigraphy (**b**). The only sign of the tumor was a slight thickening of the bone and a changed bone structure. The tumor itself could be seen as pale sclerotic bone (**c**). The dura underneath the tumor was completely free of tumor and unreactive. There was no indication for any metastatic involvement

base component or extensions into compartments which are not as well visualized or differentiated in the CT. Again, the mass of the tumor will show homogeneous contrast enhancement, but also tail-like extensions in the meninges will be seen (the so-called "meningeal tail sign" (Fig. 8.12) and infiltration of neighboring structures such as the sinuses). Meningiomas of the medial skull base can be assessed whether they are limited to the cavernous sinus or, for example, can be assessed anatomically for their complex extension towards the optic canal or into the cerebellopontine angle (Figs. 8.13 and 8.14) which leads to various degrees of brain stem compression and is extensive in typical petroclival meningiomas. The carotid artery which is regularly encased by

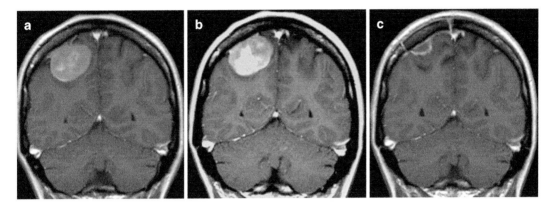

Fig. 8.12 Typical convexity meningioma with the broad dural attachment which extends further than the tumor (meningeal tail sign). Removal of the tumor (right) should include all the infiltrated zone which is to be replaced with periosteum

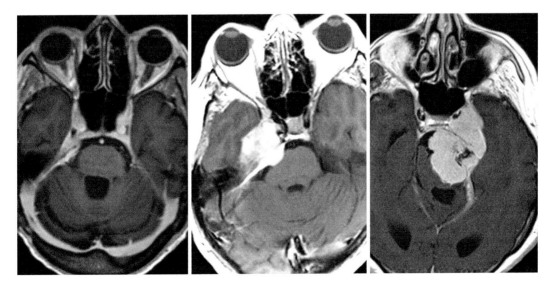

Fig. 8.13 Three examples of meningiomas involving the cavernous sinus. The lesion limited to the cavernous sinus (left) is an a priori nonsurgical lesion and will only be considered for radiation therapy when symptomatic and when discovered incidentally be followed with MRI. A lesion extending into the middle and posterior fossa (mid- dle panel) will require treatment because of cranial nerve symptoms and affection of the brain stem. The strategy can be a combination of reductive surgery and radiation (Fig. 8.14). When expanding for a long time (right panel), the petroclival aspect warrants extensive resection to decompress the brainstem

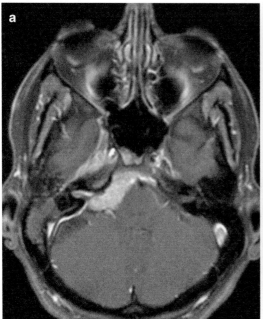
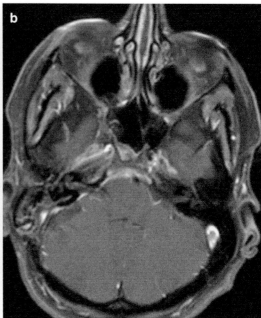

Fig. 8.14 (**a**) Extensive, non-resectable meningioma of the clivus, CP angle, cavernous sinus, sellar lumen, and jugular foramen with extracranial extension (partially not shown). (**b**) Removal of the intracranial parts to decompress the brainstem and free the cranial nerves together with coagulation of the clival and posterior petrosal dura was performed, and the whole residual has been irradiated by fractionated stereotactic radiation

petroclival meningiomas can be judged for its width and shape and patency. When considerable narrowing is present, a "time to peak" analysis after gadolinium application comparing the timing of gadolinium arrival in the two hemispheres already allows to estimate the hemodynamic relevance of the stenosis and indication for bypass surgery (Fig. 8.15). Frontobasal meningiomas are occasionally not much more than a thin layer of contrast enhancement and that is especially true for optic sheath meningiomas which other than on thin-sliced MRI with special attention to all three planes will be missed (Fig. 8.16). When close to a sinus or originating from a sinus wall, extension of the tumor into the sinus or patency of the sinus can be seen on T2-weighted images and MR angiography (Fig. 8.17).

Some differential diagnosis at first imaging is to be considered. In the first place, meningiomas may be taken for a solid metastatic lesion because the age groups with the peak incidence overlap. Clues to decide for meningioma would be the extent of dural involvement and especially a reaction of the bone-like hyperostosis (Fig. 8.18). Meningiomas may also occur in multiple locations in the same patient (Fig. 8.19), but multiplicity is much more common in metastasis, and for three metastatic lesions, it would be very unusual to have all of them on the surface of the brain. Metastases also tend to be cystic from necrosis after a certain size. In patients with a known neoplastic disease, direct metastasis to the meningioma is possible and has to qualify any reservation about surgery in an incidental finding. Most common intrameningiomatous metastases are from mammary carcinoma [77] and second most are from the lung [69].

In tumors over 1 cm^3, MR spectroscopy is an additional tool which shows a characteristic spectrum of metabolites which can provide an increasingly reliable estimate of the nature of the lesion [26]. Diagnostic pitfalls are the rare cystic meningiomas which are from their appearance like a pilocytic astrocytoma or a cystic metastasis (Fig. 8.5).

Angiography: This diagnostic tool is only used to answer specific questions related to the

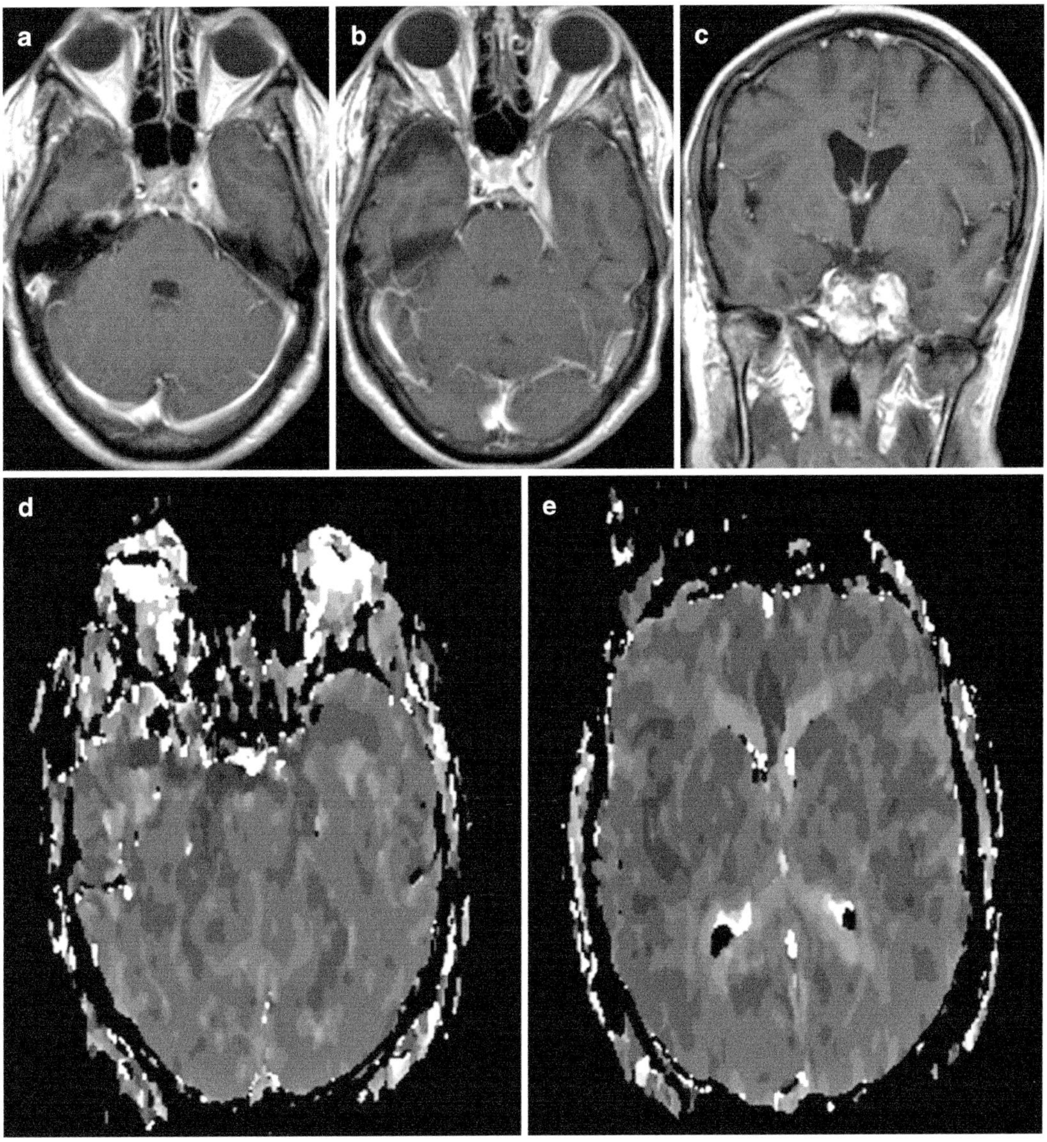

Fig. 8.15 Very compact meningioma of the anterior part of the cavernous sinus with significant narrowing of the left carotid but no symptoms of ischemia (**a–c**). In these situations further progression of the tumor or the sequelae of radiosurgery may lead to "silent" occlusion of the carotid in case of sufficient collateralization. To assess the risk, a very easy screening method is the so-called "time to peak" measurement of the gadolinium distribution in both hemispheres in perfusion-weighted MRI (**d, e**). In case the peaks are reached simultaneously, there is no hemodynamic relevance of the stenosis, and bypass surgery is not indicated

surgical strategy and has no use in the diagnosis itself. It is indicated to answer the question of patency of sinuses, collateralizations, and the hemodynamic relevance of a stenosis within a sinus. It provides a good overview of the vascularization (Fig. 8.20) and in some cases will provide an opportunity for preoperative embolization, especially when there is major blood supply from tentorial or mastoidal meningeal arteries which during surgery will be caught only later during the procedure.

Meningiomas have been found to have several interesting hormone receptors, none of which however have led to targeted therapeutics except

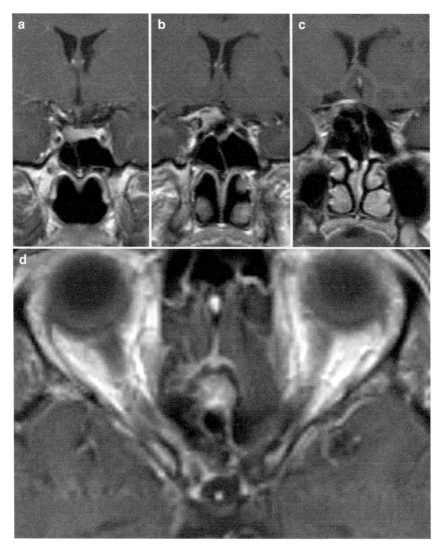

Fig. 8.16 Very small meningioma of the right optic nerve which has led to visual impairment. Only in the coronal view one can see the enhancement which is minimal in the other planes (**d**). The only option is decompression of the optic canal

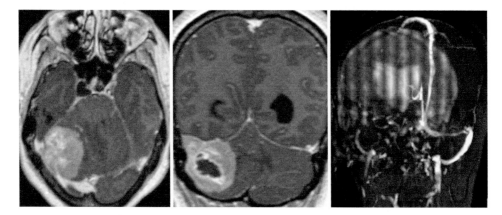

Fig. 8.17 Posterior fossa meningioma which has invaded the sinus and completely fills the niche of the transverse/sigmoid junction, and MR angiography (right panel) confirms the complete obliteration

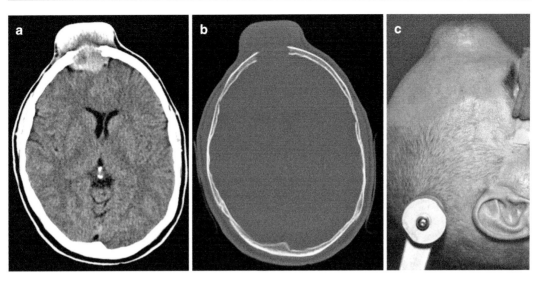

Fig. 8.18 Meningioma which has grown through the bone and can be seen extracranially as a deformity of the skull

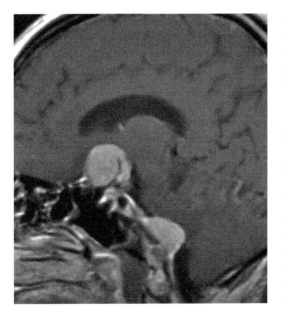

Fig. 8.19 Multiple meningiomas of a patient who was seen because of visual problems on the right eye as a result of a suprasellar meningioma. The MRI revealed a second, non-connected lesion in the right CP angle which was removed in a separate session

for the somatostatin receptor type 2 (SSTR2) [23], which is explored for radiotherapy (see below) or imaging. To determine in cases of inoperable tumors, residuals, or recurrence of the optimal treatment volumes for radiotherapy, a radiolabeled compound, ^{68}Ga-DOTATATE, a positron emitter, is used to delineate active tumor and follow treatment effects (Fig. 8.21) [67]. The place for PET imaging in meningiomas is currently being defined by its increasing use [27].

8.8 Therapy

8.8.1 Surgery

Therapy of meningiomas generally involves surgery [1, 2]. Especially for the skull base locations, over the last decade, it has become more interdisciplinary [32] with additional treatment opportunities also for radiotherapists and neuroradiologists with their improving tools [41]. The refinement of microsurgical approaches offers a resective option, at least partial for almost all locations of meningiomas [1, 2]. Again, as for the symptoms, there are different strategies of surgical management according to location.

The most important question is whether a meningioma needs to be treated at all or can be left to observation, keeping in mind that many lesions are found incidentally. Especially with incidental, calcified meningiomas in the elderly, a repeated imaging within 6 months or even a year is justified, and when no increase in size is

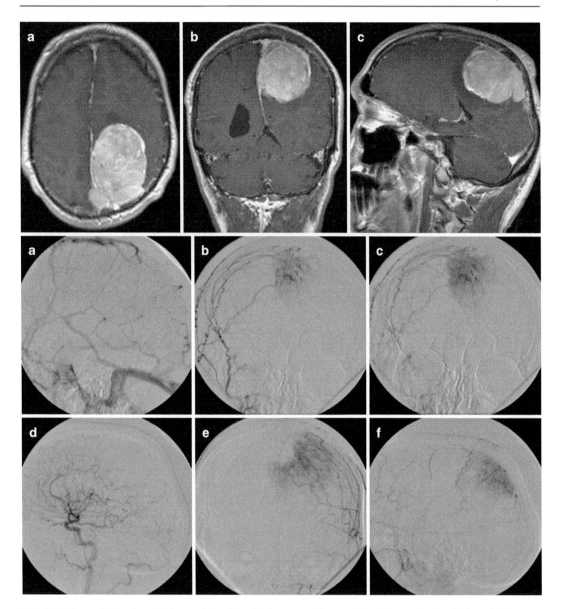

Fig. 8.20 Large bilateral meningioma of the falx which has occluded the sinus and results in pronounced edema (**a–c**) which was the cause of the neurological deficit and which completely resolved within a week of surgery. The vascularization is exclusively via the external carotid artery (**a–c, e, f**) and is completely eliminated when performing the dural circumcision as the first part of the surgery. Consequently, this tumor was an avascular mass during the removal without preoperative embolization. There is no contribution from the internal carotid (**d**)

seen, the lesion is left to observation. In a recent survey, the observation periods to decide for treatment were even 5–10 years [54]. Calcification in CT as such does not indicate a priori slow growth as the tumor upon resection may still be well vascularized and vital and all the hyperdensity due to microcalcification (Fig. 8.22). Tumors may even change their growth characteristics over time. A tumor may recur or a residual may slowly grow in higher age and then slow down and remain constant for many years (Fig. 8.23).

The classical, typical meningioma of the convexity or lateral sphenoid wing will be resected including its origin, likewise meningiomas of the

Fig. 8.21 Recurrent multifocal meningioma in a chronic course where anaplastic transformation took place and a pre-resection DOTATATE-PET was performed to find out whether the tumor cells of all foci actively label with the tracer so that after resection a radioisotope therapy is possible. Two manifestations of the tumor show strong enhancement

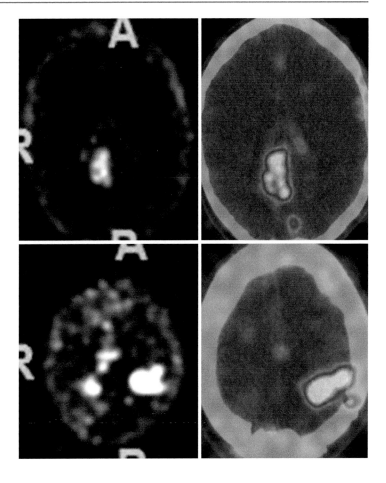

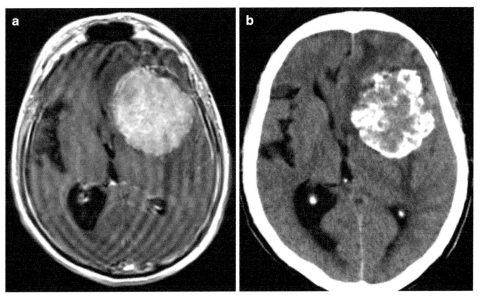

Fig. 8.22 Large sphenoid wing meningioma hyperdense on CT suggesting extensive calcification (**a**). The enhancement on MRI (**b**) already indicates that the tumor may consist mostly of vital tissue, and indeed this was a soft meningioma in which the calcification apparently was microscopic

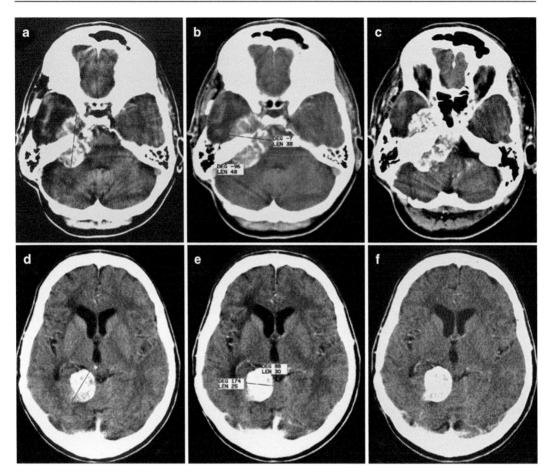

Fig. 8.23 Residuals of a meningioma which was operated 10 years before the first CT scan seen in this follow-up (**a**, **d**). The patient felt no symptoms at the time and had other health problems which resulted in the decision to remain in follow-up without any surgical therapy. Further follow-up at 2 years (**b**, **e**) and after 5 years (**c**, **f**) showed that there was almost no further growth and the patient remained in stable condition without neurological deficits and passed of unrelated cause 5 more years later

falx or the frontal skull base. Excision of the dura should be performed as far as the preoperative imaging showed any enhancement (meningeal tail sign). In most cases there will be sufficient periosteum to substitute the resected dura. If not, artificial materials exist which may be used instead. When the bone appears to be affected, it might be drilled out at the suspicious site, and if it is completely infiltrated, it has to be replaced as well. Thus, in some cases the reconstruction is more laborious than the resection itself, especially in fronto-orbital meningiomas or olfactory grove meningiomas where it may be necessary to close a bony destruction of the frontal skull base with split bone and periosteum [11].

Involvement of sinuses pose a specific problem. When the sagittal sinus in its frontal part is involved or a transverse sinus which has hemodynamically become irrelevant and is compensated by the other side, it can be sacrificed for the sake of a radical resection as there are good collaterals. If the sagittal sinus in its parietal aspect or the confluens or a dominant transverse sinus is involved and still patent and infiltrated to an extent which is beyond what can be easily patched during surgery, the wall and any intra-sinusoidal part should be left. It can be irradiated or left to slowly grow on and slowly occlude the sinus while forming collaterals which usually happens over years and as a rule goes unnoticed.

Then the whole residual can be removed in one block if there are sufficient symptoms or growth over time to justify surgery. There are reports about sinus repair, but the rates of complication exceed that of this "wait and see" and "second look" approach [81] although it is advocated to attempt a venous repair after radical resection if not too risky, which means in selected individual cases [82]. Many reports about focal irradiation have now emerged which state that local control is achieved in a high percentage (see below) either arresting the tumor or leading to a longer delay until the sinus is closed.

The use of preoperative embolization has not become standard [6, 66]. Although many meningiomas would lend themselves to this approach, it is an unnecessary risk for the patient because with most tumors, the surgical approach to the lesion already involves extensive devascularization and achieves the same result as embolization. A large series reports a low complication rate of 3.7% and reduced necessity of blood transfusions, but there is no mention of conversion of an inoperable case to a surgical case [9]. Fibrin glue and particles have been used mostly as embolic materials, and this leads to necrosis in the tumor which can make histopathological classification more difficult. Also there may be swelling with ensuing neurological deficits necessitating more urgent surgical intervention than anticipated. The indication for preoperative embolization should be very strict and limited to cases where there is a clear surgical advantage or a situation in which blood transfusions are anticipated but cannot be done for medical or nonmedical reasons [71]. In one small series, the lesion shrunk considerably so that surgery was delayed for several months or canceled [57].

8.8.2 Radiation

Radiation therapy has a long history as part of meningioma management, either as external beam fractionated radiotherapy (RT) or stereotactic radiation of small volumes with high intensity either as single dose or in very few fractions (stereotactic radiosurgery, SRS). The inclusion of radiosurgery has been the most consequential new therapeutic development over the last decades.

For several tumor locations the treatment paradigms over the last years have shifted and the extensive skull base approaches with bypass surgery and cranial nerve interpositions have been left in favor of a radiosurgical treatment component (Figs. 8.14 and 8.24). It is now common to approach large skull base meningiomas which involve the whole cavernous sinus or parts opportunistically. That applies to petroclival meningiomas and some lesions of the clivus and cerebellopontine angle or fronto-orbital meningiomas where remnants may be left behind deliberately in critical areas to be then treated with preconceived radiotherapy [88]. Any exophytic parts will be aggressively removed and the tumor reduced to the part containing encased cranial nerves and blood vessels which will be left. That part can then be treated with conformal fractionated radiation or radiosurgery with any of the radiosurgical tools [32]. With growing experience the possible risks of radiosurgery become apparent [22, 56] and lead to the conclusion that radical surgery should really be attempted wherever possible so that radiation treatment is only applied when surgical risks are too high. In particular the possibility of an accelerated aggressive growth after radiotherapy is troublesome [22].

Recently, somatostatin receptor-targeted radionuclide therapy has been shown to be quite effective in a multi-institutional series of heavily pretreated progressive meningiomas [79], but further confirmatory studies are pending.

Another specific situation occurs in optic sheath meningiomas (Fig. 8.25a, b) [58]. These meningiomas are usually very difficult to treat and pose a major dilemma. In an attempt to temporarily stabilize the disease, surgery may for some cases be limited to decompression of the optic nerve canal and splitting of the sheath as much as the tumor infiltration allows (Fig. 8.25b). Attempts at resection almost always result in severe immediate deterioration of vision. With decompression only, visual loss will come gradually and may be

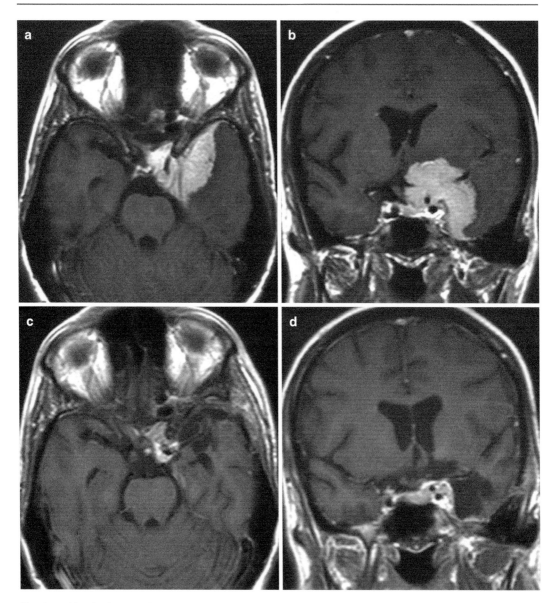

Fig. 8.24 Exophytic meningioma of the anterior clinoid process extending into the cavernous sinus and around the optic canal (**a**, **b**). Small residuals of the tumor were left (**c**), and at the first sign of progressive growth (bottom right), fractionated stereotactic surgery was indicated

postponed for a long time. There are reports about radiosurgery, and these show that in the majority of cases, stable disease can be secured, although long-term results over several decades are not available yet [5]. Whatever therapy is selected, care should be taken that it is administered only to patients with progressive disease because the course can be stable without treatment for many years [25]. For these reasons, it is advocated to intervene early with exploratory surgery in medial sphenoid wing meningiomas as tumor may extend into the optic canal before that is detectable on MRI, and direct surgical inspection is the most sensitive technique to detect such extensions, and resection eliminates the need for radiation, at least until recurrence can be documented.

Radiosurgery as a *primary* modality is reserved to cases in which surgical manipulation

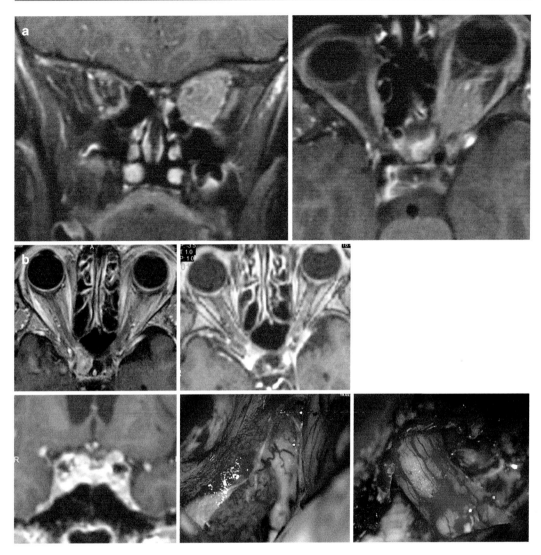

Fig. 8.25 (**a**) Biopsy proven meningioma of the optic nerve in a young boy, which upon inspection proved to be unseparable from the nerve and thus cannot be removed without risking blindness which in this case was not yet present. The optic canal was decompressed, and an intracranial extension was removed to prevent spread to the other side; eventually after years of progression and loss of vision, the whole orbit was decompressed and cosmeti-cally reconstructed with an epithesis. (**b**) Two cases of encased optic nerves where in the top row, the canal was opened, and all exophytic tumor removed but a remnant had to be left on the infiltrated nerve (left pre- and right postsurgery). The case in the bottom row presented with an engulfed optic nerve (intraoperative micrograph middle panel) which however was only overlapping allowing for complete removal and decompression (bottom right panel)

is associated with presently unacceptable morbidity and the likelihood of only subradical resection. As with the meningiomas which have a radiosurgical component in the interdisciplinary strategy, the locations are mostly at the skull base with true intracavernous meningiomas being the largest group but also locations in the cerebello-pontine angle and the perisellar region. In addition to location, age, comorbidities, and general status of health have to be included into the decision-making. The results of larger series show that disease control can be achieved in the majority of cases with acceptable morbidity which, however, is not negligible [31]. Total remissions, however, are rare which is expected when the induction of fibrous changes and stable disease is the major goal in these rather slowly proliferating lesions [41]. The issue of radiation as such, be it RT or SRS, is heavily debated and extensively reviewed [53, 70], and while a clear benefit shown in many series is acknowledged, the uniform application is still seen controversial, and the rates for tumor control, regression, and side effects vary widely most likely reflecting discordant histological gradings due to retrospective series and changing WHO guidelines. The inclusion of RT and SRS or the use of SRS instead of resection has to follow an individual evaluation of histology, grade of resection, risk of radiation damage, and risk of recurrence/progression.

Chemotherapy has never played a major role in the treatment of meningiomas. Even in anaplastic meningiomas, there is only limited experience and limited efficacy for the classical chemotherapeutic agents [13, 14, 43]. Hope has for a long time rested with the discoveries about the cell biology of meningiomas and the possibility to develop targeted approaches which in the context of meningioma hold only limited promise [59]. The intriguing presence of progesterone receptors has eventually been explored in a phase III clinical trial for non-resectable meningiomas, but no efficacy was seen for the synthetic antiprogestin mifepristone [36]. Also the detection of dopamine receptors [12] has not translated into therapeutic opportunities despite phase II clinical trials [30]. Because of their abundant vasculature, anti-angiogenic therapy has been explored, and there are early clinical indications that the small molecule tyrosine kinase inhibitor sunitinib may be active in atypical and anaplastic meningiomas when the vascular endothelial growth factor receptor 2 was present in the tumors [38]. The most widely used chemotherapeutic option with some limited efficacy comes from drawing an analogy to chronic lymphatic leukemia which also is a slowly proliferating disorder. Hydroxyurea which is effective in that disorder has shown a therapeutic effect also in some patients [50, 52], but a large randomized prospective phase III trial is still unavailable.

Also when used in combination with imatinib, a tyrosine kinase inhibitor, the efficacy is described as modest in a phase II trial [68].

Immunotherapy has become a major component in oncology but is still under evaluation for intrinsic brain tumors and not established for meningiomas. The analysis of components of the immune system which seem to be prerequisite for effective immune checkpoint inhibition has shown that potentially that approach is worth exploring but mainly for anaplastic meningiomas and clinical trials are outstanding [8].

8.9   Prognosis

The prognosis of meningiomas depends on their grade and their location. It can only be determined in the individual patient from regular follow-up. It has been difficult to find prognostic parameters based on histological markers except for grade and subtype. All other markers do not seem to have prognostic relevance. Based on the resection, the completeness of removal has been classified and basically distinguishes between a radical resection including the origin (Simpson grade 1), resection with coagulation of the origin (Simpson grade 2), partial resection (Simpson grade 3), and a mere biopsy (Simpson grade 4) [80].

Evidently there is better prognosis with more radical resection, but that may need to be revisited with the now widespread use of radiotherapeutic techniques for residual tumors. As a rule of thumb, one can expect permanent cure of a convexity meningioma grade WHO I or II which is fully resected in over 90% of the cases. Skull base meningiomas even when completely reduced to their site of origin will recur in 50% of the cases.

Anaplastic meningiomas have a poor prognosis and will eventually even metastasize.

To quote any numbers for average survival when facing patients is meaningless for the most part as there is no uniformity in the diagnosis of meningioma as such and the term "benign" is counterproductive in large unresectable skull base tumors (Fig. 8.8).

8.10   Follow-Up

Patients with resected meningiomas need to be followed regularly after treatment, and the scheduling includes WHO grade and degree of resection. After complete resection (Simpson grade 1) and WHO grade 1, first follow-up by MRI after the immediate post-op imaging should be at 1 year and, when that scan is clear, in intervals increasing from 2 to 3 years thereafter. In atypical meningiomas WHO grade II, the schedule should be 6 months for the first follow-up and then yearly for 3 years increasing to 2 years thereafter. For anaplastic meningiomas WHO grade III, the follow-up will be as for high-grade gliomas. Recurrent meningiomas when recapitulating the original tumor underlie the same considerations about resection, partial safe resection, and additional treatment with radiation or re-irradiation [87].

For resection Simpson grade 2 and above, the schedule depends on the dynamics of the residual. In some cases regrowth or increase in size cannot be detected for years even without treatment, and in some, growth detectible at 6 months will determine what kind of additional therapy is recommended. MRI is generally the best modality, but in cases of bone involvement at the skull base, CT may need to be done as well. Because imaging changes may be subtle in some patients, other interdisciplinary monitoring modalities may need to be included like regular ophthalmological assessment or audiograms when the tumor was in the area of the respective compromised cranial nerves and recurrence/progression impairing their function is feared. As it has been reported that patients with radiosurgical treatment for residual tumor may experience sudden aggressive growth with years of delay, special attention must be given to patients with such combined treatments.

Only when after 10 years there is no evidence for any activity of the disease, patients can be dismissed from regular follow-up. Bearing in mind that tumors may alter their growth characteristics over the years, patients can be advised that not each indication of a new tumor activity needs to be treated right away because it may not cause any symptoms and might be safely watched for some time. On the other hand, it must be pointed out that exactly because of the usually slow-growing nature, regular follow-up is important because symptoms from a recurrent or progressing lesion may arise only late and then optimal therapeutic opportunities may have been missed. There are no blood tests yet which would allow monitoring of tumor activity, but the development of detection techniques for tumor constituents in plasma such as extracellular vesicles may revolutionize the whole follow-up regimens.

8.11   Future Perspectives

Optimal definition of the treatment modalities in an interdisciplinary setting and evaluation of that concept in larger series with meticulous follow-up will make treatment of meningiomas safer and more efficacious on a much more individualized basis. Given the absence of any pharmacological treatment option and lack of perspective of such in the near future, therapy will for a long time rest on surgery and radiation. It is to be hoped that refined and meticulously clinically correlated gene expression analyses will lead to the definition of candidate genes for truly targeted therapies.

8.12   Other Meningeal Tumors

The 2016 WHO contains now a chapter of mesenchymal, non-meningothelial tumors [4]. According to this, *Haemangiopericytoma* which comprises about 2% of meningeal tumors [34] is now used synonymously with solitary fibrous tumor (SFT) which is the preferred terminology in the WHO classification. These tumors tend to occur at a younger age than the meningiomas with a peak incidence in the fourth and fifth decade. Also, there appears to be a slight prevalence for the male sex. By WHO grading they are allocated to the grades II and III, but the parameters distinguishing the two still need to be fully validated. The genetic alterations are different from meningioma with alterations of the chromosome 22 absent. Most alterations are found on chromosome 12q13 and 6p21.

As for clinical signs and symptoms, there is no difference between meningiomas and hemangiopericytomas. The neuroradiological features may be identical to meningioma (Fig. 8.26) but are somewhat different from meningiomas in respect to bone. The tumors tend to cause lytic lesions in bone and do not grow through the bone like the meningiomas which with rare exceptions either cause hyperostosis or just distend the bone without completely destroying it. The tumors are highly vascularized and upon angiography show a wealth of pathological vessels (Fig. 8.26), [51]. In contrast to meningiomas, calcifications are rare.

Treatment of hemangiopericytoma is more complex than that of the average meningioma. The tumors should be removed as completely as possible, and then there is a consensus that the region needs to be irradiated [3] because otherwise the rate of recurrence is 91% [89]. Especially with anaplastic tumors, the prognosis is bad without radical removal and radiation, but when achieved and completed, 5-year overall survival may be 90% [93]. Also, these tumors have a tendency to metastasize, primarily into bone [83]. No chemotherapeutic regimen has emerged as an effective standard [24]. Corresponding to the

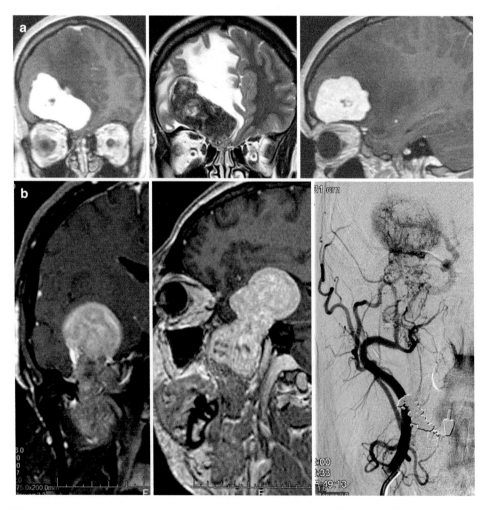

Fig. 8.26 Solitary fibrous tumor/hemangiopericytoma. (**a**) Frontobasal solitary fibrous tumor with massive edema but no infiltration to the brain and a very clean plane of dissection. The origin was a very small area of dural and bony infiltration at the orbital roof. (**b**) Large highly vascularized tumor growing destructively trough the temporal skull base which after partial embolization could be removed completely and is free from recurrence after 6 years

aggressiveness of the disease, patients need to be followed closely, especially to detect metastases. The high rate of recurrence and metastases is the cause for mortality, and despite aggressive treatment, up to 60% of the patients may have succumbed to the disease by 15 years [89].

8.12.1 Dural Lymphoma

Dural lymphomas present as contrast-enhancing lesions with an extension like a subdural hematoma, like a nodular meningioma with a dural tail, like an en plaque meningioma, or just as dural hypertrophy. Particularly suspicious is an extension deep into the arachnoid spaces and sulci (Fig. 8.26). Primary dural lymphomas are rare and not to be mistaken for primary CNS lymphoma (see Schlegel, this volume). They are mostly of the MALT type [28, 72] although other kinds and regular Hodgkin's disease have been reported [37]. They seem to have a better prognosis than PCNSL and respond well to cranial radiation [7]. Many of the reported dural lymphomas were unexpected, and therefore, some were resected like en plaque meningiomas. Cranial

radiation is to be recommended even after resection but certainly after biopsy.

8.12.2 Dural Metastases

Metastatic disease to the brain is seen with increasing frequency, but in comparison with the parenchymal or leptomeningeal variants, purely dural involvement is rare and is detected most frequently in the context of suspected meningioma [44, 86]. Whereas in intracranial disease, a metastasis is more readily suspected because of imaging characteristics and has a known primary in about 80% [92]; the diagnosis of a dural metastasis is made much more frequently when the primary tumor is still unknown [86]. This can be partially explained by the fact that dural metastases may occur in any type of cancer but show a spectrum which is different from intracranial disease. A large combined surgical and autoptic series showed a surprisingly broad spectrum including the expected high numbers of breast cancer as primary but an even higher number of underlying prostate cancer which can have extensive manifestation (Fig. 8.27) and also

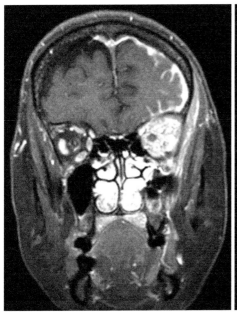
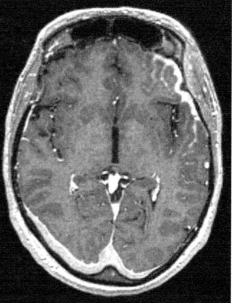

Fig. 8.27 Gd-enhanced MRI of a left frontal lesion which was observed for 5 years with deteriorating vision where the patient decidedly declined all offers for a biopsy. Because of an increasing exophthalmos, the lesion was biopsied, and it turned out to be the metastasis of a slowly growing lymphoma of which a cervical manifestation had been treated 7 years ago

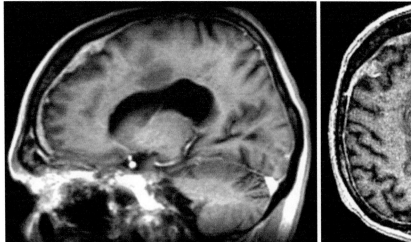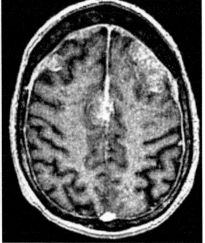

Fig. 8.28 Bihemispheric, mostly frontal en plaque, and nodular manifestation of a prostate carcinoma known for 6 years treated only with endocrine therapy. The patient presented with beginning signs of disorientation. No treatment was given because of rapid deterioration

such primaries as the larynx, gall bladder, and stomach, which otherwise rarely metastasize to brain [40].

When purely dural and an appearance like meningioma, the differential diagnosis is close to impossible without a tissue diagnosis because the neuroradiological techniques may not provide sufficient parameters for differentiation [42]. The tumors may be dural with a flat spread, be nodular, or show a combination of subdural-dural-skull extension. Depending on the context of the overall status of the patient, there may be an indication for resection, especially when the differential diagnosis toward meningioma cannot be made without histology and there is no known primary. As the spectrum of histological origins is very heterogeneous, there are no published series about the role of radiotherapy or chemotherapy as there are for leptomeningeal metastatic disease. How to proceed after histological verification of a dural metastasis will depend on the established treatment paradigms for the primary tumor and has to be determined in an interdisciplinary tumor board (Fig. 8.28).

References

1. Al-Mefti O (1991) Meningiomas. Raven Press, New York
2. Al-Mefti O (1998) Operative Atlas of Meningioma. Lippincott-Raven, Philadelphia
3. Alen JF, Lobato RD, Gomez PA, Boto GR, Lagares A, Ramos A, Ricoy JR (2001) Intracranial hemangiopericytoma: study of 12 cases. Acta Neurochir (Wien) 143:575–586
4. Antonescu CR, Paulus W, Perry A, Rushing EJ, Hainfellner JA, Bouvier C, Figarella-Branger D, von Deimling A, Wesseling P (2016) Mesenchymal, non-meningothelial tumours. In: Louis DN, Ohgaki H, Wiestler OD, Cavanee WK, Ellison DW, Figarella-Branger D, Perry A, Reifenberger G, von Deimling A (eds) WHO classification of tumours of the central nervous system. IARC Press, Lyon, pp 248–257
5. Becker G, Jeremic B, Pitz S, Buchgeister M, Wilhelm H, Schiefer U, Paulsen F, Zrenner E, Bamberg M (2002) Stereotactic fractionated radiotherapy in patients with optic nerve sheath meningioma. Int J Radiat Oncol Biol Phys 54:1422–1429
6. Bendszus M, Rao G, Burger R, Schaller C, Scheinemann K, Warmuth-Metz M, Hofmann E, Schramm J, Roosen K, Solymosi L (2000) Is there a benefit of preoperative meningioma embolization. Neurosurgery 47:1306–1311. ; discussion 1311–1302
7. Beriwal S, Hou JS, Miyamoto C, Garcia-Young JA (2003) Primary dural low grade BCL-2 negative

follicular lymphoma: a case report. J Neuro-Oncol 61:23–25

8. Bi WL, Wu WW, Santagata S, Reardon DA, Dunn IF (2016) Checkpoint inhibition in meningiomas. Immunotherapy 8:721–731

9. Borg A, Ekanayake J, Mair R, Smedley T, Brew S, Kitchen N, Samandouras G, Robertson F (2013) Preoperative particle and glue embolization of meningiomas: indications, results, and lessons learned from 117 consecutive patients. In: Neurosurgery, vol 73, pp ons244–ons251. ; discussion ons252

10. Buhl R, Hugo HH, Mehdorn HM (2001) Brain oedema in secretory meningiomas. J Clin Neurosci 8(Suppl 1):19–21

11. Bull WJ, Vandevender D, Cimino VG (2003) Reconstruction of defects of the cranial base. Tech Neurosurg 9:106–112

12. Carroll RS, Schrell UM, Zhang J, Dashner K, Nomikos P, Fahlbusch R, Black PM (1996) Dopamine D1, dopamine D2, and prolactin receptor messenger ribonucleic acid expression by the polymerase chain reaction in human meningiomas. Neurosurgery 38:367–375

13. Chamberlain MC (2001) Meningiomas. Curr Treat Options Neurol 3:67–76

14. Chamberlain MC, Tsao-Wei DD, Groshen S (2004) Temozolomide for treatment-resistant recurrent meningioma. Neurology 62:1210–1212

15. Chen WC, Magill ST, Englot DJ, Baal JD, Wagle S, Rick JW, McDermott MW (2017) Factors associated with pre- and postoperative seizures in 1033 patients undergoing supratentorial meningioma resection. Neurosurgery 81:297–306

16. Christensen HC, Kosteljanetz M, Johansen C (2003) Incidences of gliomas and meningiomas in Denmark, 1943 to 1997. Neurosurgery 52:1327–1333. ; discussion 1333–1324

17. Clark VE, Erson-Omay EZ, Serin A, Yin J, Cotney J, Ozduman K, Avsar T, Li J, Murray PB, Henegariu O, Yilmaz S, Gunel JM, Carrion-Grant G, Yilmaz B, Grady C, Tanrikulu B, Bakircioglu M, Kaymakcalan H, Caglayan AO, Sencar L, Ceyhun E, Atik AF, Bayri Y, Bai H, Kolb LE, Hebert RM, Omay SB, Mishra-Gorur K, Choi M, Overton JD, Holland EC, Mane S, State MW, Bilguvar K, Baehring JM, Gutin PH, Piepmeier JM, Vortmeyer A, Brennan CW, Pamir MN, Kilic T, Lifton RP, Noonan JP, Yasuno K, Gunel M (2013) Genomic analysis of non-NF2 meningiomas reveals mutations in TRAF7, KLF4, AKT1, and SMO. Science 339:1077–1080

18. Claus EB, Black PM, Bondy ML, Calvocoressi L, Schildkraut JM, Wiemels JL, Wrensch M (2007) Exogenous hormone use and meningioma risk: what do we tell our patients? Cancer 110:471–476

19. Claus EB, Calvocoressi L, Bondy ML, Schildkraut JM, Wiemels JL, Wrensch M (2011) Family and personal medical history and risk of meningioma. J Neurosurg 115:1072–1077

20. Claus EB, Calvocoressi L, Bondy ML, Wrensch M, Wiemels JL, Schildkraut JM (2013) Exogenous hormone use, reproductive factors, and risk of intracranial meningioma in females. J Neurosurg 118:649–656

21. Cossu G, Levivier M, Daniel RT, Messerer M (2015) The role of mifepristone in meningiomas management: a systematic review of the literature. Biomed Res Int 2015:267831

22. Couldwell WT, Cole CD, Al-Mefty O (2007) Patterns of skull base meningioma progression after failed radiosurgery. J Neurosurg 106:30–35

23. Dutour A, Kumar U, Panetta R, Ouafik L, Fina F, Sasi R, Patel YC (1998) Expression of somatostatin receptor subtypes in human brain tumors. Int J Cancer 76:620–627

24. Ecker RD, Marsh WR, Pollock BE, Kurtkaya-Yapicier O, McClelland R, Scheithauer BW, Buckner JC (2003) Hemangiopericytoma in the central nervous system: treatment, pathological features, and long-term follow up in 38 patients. J Neurosurg 98:1182–1187

25. Egan RA, Lessell S (2002) A contribution to the natural history of optic nerve sheath meningiomas. Arch Ophthalmol 120:1505–1508

26. Fountas KN, Kapsalaki EZ, Gotsis SD, Kapsalakis JZ, Smisson HF 3rd, Johnston KW, Robinson JS Jr, Papadakis N (2000) In vivo proton magnetic resonance spectroscopy of brain tumors. Stereotact Funct Neurosurg 74:83–94

27. Galldiks N, Albert NL, Sommerauer M, Grosu AL, Ganswindt U, Law I, Preusser M, Rhun EL, Vogelbaum MA, Zadeh G, Dhermain F, Weller M, Langen KJ, Tonn JC (2017) PET imaging in patients with meningioma-report of the RANO/PET gGroup. Neuro Oncol 19:1576–1587

28. Goetz P, Lafuente J, Revesz T, Galloway M, Dogan A, Kitchen N (2002) Primary low-grade B-cell lymphoma of mucosa-associated lymphoid tissue of the dura mimicking the presentation of an acute subdural hematoma. Case report and review of the literature. J Neurosurg 96:611–614

29. Goldbrunner R, Minniti G, Preusser M, Jenkinson MD, Sallabanda K, Houdart E, von Deimling A, Stavrinou P, Lefranc F, Lund-Johansen M, Moyal EC, Brandsma D, Henriksson R, Soffietti R, Weller M (2016) EANO guidelines for the diagnosis and treatment of meningiomas. Lancet Oncol 17:e383–e391

30. Grunberg SM (1994) Role of antiprogestational therapy for meningiomas. Hum Reprod 9(Suppl 1):202–207

31. Han JH, Kim DG, Chung HT, Park CK, Paek SH, Kim CY, Jung HW (2008) Gamma knife radiosurgery for skull base meningiomas: long-term radiologic and clinical outcome. Int J Radiat Oncol Biol Phys 72(5):1324–1332

32. Hart DJ, Gianotta SL (2003) Complex cranial base meningioma : combined management. Tech Neurosurg 9:86–92

33. Hsu DW, Efird JT, Hedley-Whyte ET (1997) Progesterone and estrogen receptors in meningiomas: prognostic considerations. J Neurosurg 86:113–120

34. Jääskeläinen J, Louis DN, Paulus W, Haltia M (2000) Haemangiopericytoma. In: Kleihues P, Cavanee WK (eds) Tumors of the central nervous system : pathology and genetics. IARC Press, Lyon

35. Jhawar BS, Fuchs CS, Colditz GA, Stampfer MJ (2003) Sex steroid hormone exposures and risk for meningioma. J Neurosurg 99:848–853

36. Ji Y, Rankin C, Grunberg S, Sherrod AE, Ahmadi J, Townsend JJ, Feun LG, Fredericks RK, Russell CA, Kabbinavar FF, Stelzer KJ, Schott A, Verschraegen C (2015) Double-blind phase III randomized trial of the antiprogestin agent mifepristone in the treatment of unresectable meningioma: SWOG S9005. J Clin Oncol 33:4093–4098

37. Johnson MD, Kinney MC, Scheithauer BW, Briley RJ, Hamilton K, McPherson WF, Barton JH Jr (2000) Primary intracerebral Hodgkin's disease mimicking meningioma: case report. Neurosurgery 47:454–456. ; discussion 456–457

38. Kaley TJ, Wen P, Schiff D, Ligon K, Haidar S, Karimi S, Lassman AB, Nolan CP, DeAngelis LM, Gavrilovic I, Norden A, Drappatz J, Lee EQ, Purow B, Plotkin SR, Batchelor T, Abrey LE, Omuro A (2015) Phase II trial of sunitinib for recurrent and progressive atypical and anaplastic meningioma. Neuro Oncol 17:116–121

39. Kaminski JM, Movsas B, King E, Yang C, Kronz JD, Alli PM, Williams J, Brem H (2001) Metastatic meningioma to the lung with multiple pleural metastases. Am J Clin Oncol 24:579–582

40. Kleinschmidt-DeMasters BK (2001) Dural metastases. A retrospective surgical and autopsy series. Arch Pathol Lab Med 125:880–887

41. Kondziolka D, Nathoo N, Flickinger JC, Niranjan A, Maitz AH, Lunsford LD (2003) Long-term results after radiosurgery for benign intracranial tumors. Neurosurgery 53:815–821. ; discussion 821–812

42. Kremer S, Grand S, Remy C, Pasquier B, Benabid AL, Bracard S, Le Bas JF (2004) Contribution of dynamic contrast MR imaging to the differentiation between dural metastasis and meningioma. Neuroradiology 46:642–648

43. Kyritsis AP (1996) Chemotherapy for meningiomas. J Neurooncol 29:269–272

44. Laidlaw JD, Kumar A, Chan A (2004) Dural metastases mimicking meningioma. Case report and review of the literature. J Clin Neurosci 11:780–783

45. Lamszus K (2004) Meningioma pathology, genetics, and biology. J Neuropathol Exp Neurol 63:275–286

46. Lamszus K, Kluwe L, Matschke J, Meissner H, Laas R, Westphal M (1999) Allelic losses at 1p, 9q, 10q, 14q, and 22q in the progression of aggressive meningiomas and undifferentiated meningeal sarcomas. Cancer Genet Cytogenet 110:103–110

47. Lamszus K, Lengler U, Schmidt NO, Stavrou D, Ergun S, Westphal M (2000) Vascular endothelial growth factor, hepatocyte growth factor/scatter factor, basic fibroblast growth factor, and placenta growth factor in human meningiomas and their relation to angiogenesis and malignancy. Neurosurgery 46:938–947. ; discussion 947–938

48. Lamszus K, Vahldiek F, Mautner VF, Schichor C, Tonn J, Stavrou D, Fillbrandt R, Westphal M, Kluwe L (2000) Allelic losses in neurofibromatosis 2-associated meningiomas. J Neuropathol Exp Neurol 59:504–512

49. Longstreth WT Jr, Phillips LE, Drangsholt M, Koepsell TD, Custer BS, Gehrels JA, van Belle G (2004) Dental X-rays and the risk of intracranial meningioma: a population-based case-control study. Cancer 100:1026–1034

50. Loven D, Hardoff R, Sever ZB, Steinmetz AP, Gornish M, Rappaport ZH, Fenig E, Ram Z, Sulkes A (2004) Non-resectable slow-growing meningiomas treated by hydroxyurea. J Neurooncol 67:221–226

51. Marc JA, Takei Y, Schechter MM, Hoffman JC (1975) Intracranial hemangiopericytomas. Angiography, pathology and differential diagnosis. Am J Roentgenol Radium Ther Nucl Med 125:823–832

52. Mason WP, Gentili F, Macdonald DR, Hariharan S, Cruz CR, Abrey LE (2002) Stabilization of disease progression by hydroxyurea in patients with recurrent or unresectable meningioma. J Neurosurg 97:341–346

53. Minniti G, Sacaringi F, F B (2017) Radiation therapy for intracranial meningiomas : current results and controversial issues. WFNOS Magazine 2:55–65

54. Mohammad MH, Chavredakis E, Zakaria R, Brodbelt A, Jenkinson MD (2017) A national survey of the management of patients with incidental meningioma in the United Kingdom. Br J Neurosurg 31:459–463

55. Mohme M, Emami P, Matschke J, Regelsberger J, Westphal M, Eicker SO (2016) Secretory meningiomas: characteristic features and clinical management of a unique subgroup. Neurosurg Clin N Am 27:181–187

56. Muracciole X, Regis J (2008) Radiosurgery and carcinogenesis risk. Prog Neurol Surg 21:207–213

57. Nakajima N, Fukuda H, Adachi H, Sasaki N, Yamaguchi M, Mitsuno Y, Kitagawa M, Horikawa F, Murao K, Yamada K (2017) Long-term volume reduction effects of endovascular embolization for intracranial meningioma: preliminary experience of 5 cases. World Neurosurg 105:591–598

58. Newman SA (2003) Optic nerve sheath meningiomas. Tech Neurosurg 9:64–77

59. Norden AD, Drappatz J, Wen PY (2007) Targeted drug therapy for meningiomas. Neurosurg Focus 23:E12

60. Ostrom QT, Gittleman H, Liao P, Vecchione-Koval T, Wolinsky Y, Kruchko C, Barnholtz-Sloan JS (2017) CBTRUS statistical report: primary brain and other central nervous system tumors diagnosed in the United States in 2010-2014. Neuro Oncol 19:v1–v88

61. Perry A, Banerjee R, Lohse CM, Kleinschmidt-DeMasters BK, Scheithauer BW (2002) A role for chromosome 9p21 deletions in the malignant progression of meningiomas and the prognosis of anaplastic meningiomas. Brain Pathol 12:183–190

62. Perry A, Dehner LP (2003) Meningeal tumors of childhood and infancy. An update and literature review. Brain Pathol 13:386–408

63. Perry A, Louis DN, Scheithauer BW, Budka H, von Deimling A (2007) Meningiomas. In: Louis DN, Ohgaki H, Wiestler OD, Cavanee WK (eds) WHO classification of tumors of the central nervous system. IARC Press, Lyon, pp 164–172

64. Perry A., Louis DN, Budka H., von Deimling A., Rushing E.J., Mawrin C., Claus E.B., Loeffler J, Sadetzki S Meningioma, in Louis D.N., Ohgaki H., Wiestler O.D., Cavanee W.K., Ellison D.W., Figarella-Branger D., Perry A., Reifenberger G., von Deimling A. (ed): WHO classification of tumors of the central nervous system. Lyon, IARC Press, 2016, pp 232–245

65. Preston DL, Ron E, Yonehara S, Kobuke T, Fujii H, Kishikawa M, Tokunaga M, Tokuoka S, Mabuchi K (2002) Tumors of the nervous system and pituitary gland associated with atomic bomb radiation exposure. J Natl Cancer Inst 94:1555–1563

66. Probst EN, Grzyska U, Westphal M, Zeumer H (1999) Preoperative embolization of intracranial meningiomas with a fibrin glue preparation. AJNR Am J Neuroradiol 20:1695–1702

67. Rachinger W, Stoecklein VM, Terpolilli NA, Haug AR, Ertl L, Poschl J, Schuller U, Schichor C, Thon N, Tonn JC (2015) Increased 68Ga-DOTATATE uptake in PET imaging discriminates meningioma and tumor-free tissue. J Nucl Med 56:347–353

68. Reardon DA, Norden AD, Desjardins A, Vredenburgh JJ, Herndon JE II, Coan A, Sampson JH, Gururangan S, Peters KB, McLendon RE, Norfleet JA, Lipp ES, Drappatz J, Wen PY, Friedman HS (2012) Phase II study of Gleevec(R) plus hydroxyurea (HU) in adults with progressive or recurrent meningioma. J Neurooncol 106:409–415

69. Richter B, Harinath L, Pu C, Stabingas K (2017) Metastatic spread of systemic neoplasms to central nervous system tumors: review of the literature and case presentation of esophageal carcinoma metastatic to meningioma. Clin Neuropathol 36:60–65, 2017

70. Rogers L, Barani I, Chamberlain M, Kaley TJ, McDermott M, Raizer J, Schiff D, Weber DC, Wen PY, Vogelbaum MA (2015) Meningiomas: knowledge base, treatment outcomes, and uncertainties. A RANO review. J Neurosurg 122:4–23

71. Rosen CL, Ammerman JM, Sekhar LN, Bank WO (2002) Outcome analysis of preoperative embolization in cranial base surgery. Acta Neurochir (Wien) 144:1157–1164

72. Rottnek M, Strauchen J, Moore F, Morgello S (2004) Primary dural mucosa-associated lymphoid tissue-type lymphoma: case report and review of the literature. J Neurooncol 68:19–23

73. Ruttledge MH, Sarrazin J, Rangaratnam S, Phelan CM, Twist E, Merel P, Delattre O, Thomas G, Nordenskjold M, Collins VP et al (1994) Evidence for the complete inactivation of the NF2 gene in the majority of sporadic meningiomas. Nat Genet 6:180–184

74. Sadetzki S, Modan B, Chetrit A, Freedman L (2000) An iatrogenic epidemic of benign meningioma. Am J Epidemiol 151:266–272

75. Sahm F, Schrimpf D, Olar A, Koelsche C, Reuss D, Bissel J, Kratz A, Capper D, Schefzyk S, Hielscher T, Wang Q, Sulman EP, Adeberg S, Koch A, Okuducu AF, Brehmer S, Schittenhelm J, Becker A, Brokinkel B, Schmidt M, Ull T, Gousias K, Kessler AF, Lamszus K, Debus J, Mawrin C, Kim YJ, Simon M, Ketter R, Paulus W, Aldape KD, Herold-Mende C, von Deimling A (2016) TERT promoter mutations and risk of recurrence in meningioma. J Natl Cancer Inst 108

76. Sayagues JM, Tabernero MD, Maillo A, Trelles O, Espinosa AB, Sarasquete ME, Merino M, Rasillo A, Vera JF, Santos-Briz A, de Alava E, Garcia-Macias MC, Orfao A (2006) Microarray-based analysis of spinal versus intracranial meningiomas: different clinical, biological, and genetic characteristics associated with distinct patterns of gene expression. J Neuropathol Exp Neurol 65:445–454

77. Sayegh ET, Burch EA, Henderson GA, Oh T, Bloch O, Parsa AT (2015) Tumor-to-tumor metastasis: breast carcinoma to meningioma. J Clin Neurosci 22:268–274

78. Schildkraut JM, Calvocoressi L, Wang F, Wrensch M, Bondy ML, Wiemels JL, Claus EB (2014) Endogenous and exogenous hormone exposure and the risk of meningioma in men. J Neurosurg 120:820–826

79. Seystahl K, Stoecklein V, Schuller U, Rushing E, Nicolas G, Schafer N, Ilhan H, Pangalu A, Weller M, Tonn JC, Sommerauer M, Albert NL (2016) Somatostatin receptor-targeted radionuclide therapy for progressive meningioma: benefit linked to 68Ga-DOTATATE/-TOC uptake. Neuro Oncol 18:1538–1547

80. Simpson D (1957) The recurrence of intracranial meningiomas after surgical treatment. J Neurol Neurosurg Psychiatry 20:22–29

81. Sindou M (2001) Meningiomas invading the sagittal or transverse sinuses, resection with venous reconstruction. J Clin Neurosci 8(Suppl 1):8–11

82. Sindou MP, Alvernia JE (2006) Results of attempted radical tumor removal and venous repair in 100 consecutive meningiomas involving the major dural sinuses. J Neurosurg 105:514–525

83. Soyuer S, Chang EL, Selek U, McCutcheon IE, Maor MH (2004) Intracranial meningeal hemangiopericytoma: the role of radiotherapy: report of 29 cases and review of the literature. Cancer 100:1491–1497

84. Strojan P, Popovic M, Jereb B (2000) Secondary intracranial meningiomas after high-dose cranial irradiation: report of five cases and review of the literature. Int J Radiat Oncol Biol Phys 48:65–73

85. Swensen R, Kirsch W (2002) Brain neoplasms in women: a review. Clin Obstet Gynecol 45:904–927

86. Tagle P, Villanueva P, Torrealba G, Huete I (2002) Intracranial metastasis or meningioma? An uncommon clinical diagnostic dilemma. Surg Neurol 58:241–245

87. Talacchi A, Muggiolu F, De Carlo A, Nicolato A, Locatelli F, Meglio M (2016) Recurrent atypical meningiomas: combining surgery and radiosurgery in

one effective multimodal treatment. World Neurosurg 87:565–572

88. Terpolilli NA, Rachinger W, Kunz M, Thon N, Flatz WH, Tonn JC, Schichor C (2016) Orbit-associated tumors: navigation and control of resection using intraoperative computed tomography. J Neurosurg 124:1319–1327

89. Vuorinen V, Sallinen P, Haapasalo H, Visakorpi T, Kallio M, Jaaskelainen J (1996) Outcome of 31 intracranial haemangiopericytomas: poor predictive value of cell proliferation indices. Acta Neurochir (Wien) 138:1399–1408

90. Wan WL, Geller JL, Feldon SE, Sadun AA (1990) Visual loss caused by rapidly progressive intracra-nial meningiomas during pregnancy. Ophthalmology 97:18–21

91. Weber RG, Bostrom J, Wolter M, Baudis M, Collins VP, Reifenberger G, Lichter P (1997) Analysis of genomic alterations in benign, atypical, and anaplastic menin-giomas: toward a genetic model of meningioma pro-gression. Proc Natl Acad Sci U S A 94:14719–14724

92. Westphal M, Heese O, de Wit M (2003) Intracranial metastases: therapeutic options. Ann Oncol 14(Suppl 3):iii4–ii10

93. Zhang GJ, Zhang LW, Li D, Wu Z, Zhang JT (2017) Analysis of prognostic factors, survival rates, and treatment in anaplastic Hemangiopericytoma. World Neurosurg 104:795–801

WHO II and III Gliomas

Shawn L. Hervey-Jumper, M. J. van de Bent,
Minesh P. Mehta, and Mitchel S. Berger

9.1 Epidemiology

Gliomas, as the most common primary intracranial tumor, have an increased prevalence among older individuals and those with European ethnicitiy [1]. WHO II and III gliomas are most common in patients 30–55 years of age. Populations with the highest incidence include individuals of Europe (5.5 per 100,000), North America (5.3 per 100,000), Australia (5.3 per 100,000), Western Asia (5.2 per 100,000), and North Africa decent (5 per 100,000) [1]. Following the introduction of computed tomography (CT) and magnetic resonance imaging (MRI) in the 1970s–1980s, there has been an increased prevalence of gliomas due to better imaging for radiographic detection.

Monogenetic Mendelian disorders represent 5% of overall glioma incidence as the vast majority of cases are sporadic. Optic nerve gliomas are found in 20% of children with neurofibromatosis type 1.

Neurofibromatosis type 2 is associated with intracranial and spinal ependymoma. Subependymal giant cell astrocytoma is found commonly in individuals with tuberous sclerosis. Li-Fraumeni and Lynch syndromes also have an increased prevalence of low-grade gliomas. Familial clusters in which first-degree relatives develop glioma represent 4% of cases; however there are no known risk variants with high penetrance [2]. Large genetic epidemiology population studies have identified seven genetic variants associated with increased risk of developing glioma [3–7]. These genes include epidermal growth factor receptor (EGFR), telomerase reverse transcriptase (TERT), coiled-coil domain containing 26 (CCDC26), cyclin-dependent kinase inhibitor 2B (CDKN2B), pleckstrin homology-like domain family B member 1 (PHLDB1), tumor protein p53 (TP53), and RTEL1 (a regulator of telomere elongation).

A history of prior brain or scalp exposure is the most securely established environmental risk factor associated with lifetime risk of glioma [8–10]. A study of patients treated for tinea capitis with scalp irradiation in Israel found the incidence of glioma doubled with a relative risk of 2.6 [11]. Additionally, allergic and immunological conditions such as allergic rhinitis, eczema, psoriasis, and asthma are thought to be protective against the risk of developing a glioma [12]. A recent meta-analysis involving over 60,000 patients illustrated the protective effects associated with allergic conditions [13]. Though long-term epide-

S. L. Hervey-Jumper · M. S. Berger (✉)
Department of Neurosurgery, University of California San Francisco, San Francisco, CA, USA
e-mail: Shawn.Hervey-Jumper@ucsf.edu; Mitchel.berger@ucsf.edu

M. J. van de Bent
Brain Tumor Center at Erasmus MC Cancer Institute, Rotterdam, the Netherlands
e-mail: m.vandenbent@erasmusmc.nl

M. P. Mehta
Miami Cancer Institute, Baptist Hospital, Miami, FL, USA

© Springer Nature Switzerland AG 2019
J.-C. Tonn et al. (eds.), *Oncology of CNS Tumors*, https://doi.org/10.1007/978-3-030-04152-6_9

miology studies have yet to be completed, one's risk of being diagnosed with a glioma does not appear to have an association with cellular phone use. This issue has been extensively studied over the past two decades. An initial report from the International Agency for Research on Cancer classified cellular phones as possible carcinogens; however all subsequent studies have failed to find any increased risk of glioma formation with increased cell phone exposure and use [1, 14].

9.2   Clinical Presentation

The constellation of physical signs and symptoms associated with WHO II and III gliomas can be highly variable depending on tumor size and location. The most common presenting symptom is seizures, and gliomas are highly epileptogenic nature. Many recent reports show seizures at presentation in as many as 81–85% of WHO II and III glioma patients [15, 16]. Additionally, both astrocytomas and oligodendrogliomas infiltrate into surrounding brain parenchyma; therefore proximity to the corticospinal tracts may result in impaired gait or hemiparesis. Similarly, gliomas located within the frontal pole may result in depression, abulia, or personality changes. Receptive or expressive aphasia may occur with gliomas involving the dominant hemisphere perisylvian language network. Parietal-lobe gliomas involving the primary somatosensory cortex may present with impaired balance, proprioception, distractibility, inferior quadrantanopia, aphasia, or anosognosia. Patients with temporal lobe gliomas are most likely to present with seizures, memory loss, or superior quadrantanopia, though no specific headaches occurring in up to 25% of patients [16]. Gliomas are found incidentally in rare circumstances (3.8% of patients); however incidental finding denotes a favorable prognosis [17].

9.3   Histology and Molecular Diagnosis: WHO 2016 Glioma Classification

The World Health Organization (WHO) central nervous system (CNS) tumor classification sys-

tem was updated in 2016 and provides a common nomenclature and platform for discussing primary CNS tumors. Recent molecular characterization studies have correlated genetic, gene expression, and DNA methylation profiles with overall and progression-free survival. This has led to reclassification of gliomas based on both histological and genetic subtypes and has enhanced our understanding of prognosis [18, 19]. Gliomas are therefore classified using a layered diagnosis according to histological as well as molecular criteria into astrocytomas and oligodendrogliomas. In this context, molecular and genetic data supplements rather than displaces histological classification. Layer 1 represents the final integrated diagnosis, layer 2 histological classification, layer 3 designates WHO grade, and layer 4 allows for integration of molecular information (Fig. 9.1). Layers 2 and 3 are assigned using microscopy and are therefore readily available; however layer 4 includes molecular data such as 1p19q codeletion status and IDH1/IDH2 which requires additional analysis. Integration of all four layers results in a single diagnostic entity, describing the tumor with sufficient clarity to permit prognostication (Fig. 9.1).

Grading of WHO II and III gliomas is influenced heavily on isocitrate dehydrogenase (IDH) 1 and 2 mutations in addition to balanced translocation of the p arm of chromosome 1 with the q arm of chromosome 19 (1p/19q codeletion). Oligodendrogliomas carry both IDH mutation and 1p19q codeletions. Infiltrating astrocytomas on the other hand never contain 1p19q codeletions and are subdivided based on the presence of IDH1 or IDH2 mutations. The previously popular oligoastrocytoma is now discouraged; therefore the diagnosis of oligoastrocytomas not otherwise specified (NOS) is only used when IDH mutation and 1p/19q codeletion testing has either failed or is not possible. The distinction between astrocytomas and oligodendrogliomas (which harbor IDH1 or 2 mutations and 1p19q codeletion) is clinically important particularly because WHO II and III oligodendrogliomas treated with radiation therapy followed by procarbazine, lomustine, and vincristine have significantly improved survival compared with astrocytomas [20].

Fig. 9.1 Diagnostic diagram for WHO II and III adult glioma

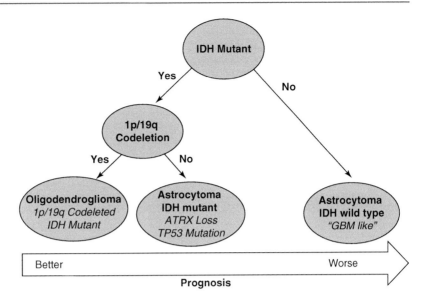

9.4 Neuroimaging

MRI with a gadolinium (Gd)-containing contrast agent is the imaging modality of choice. Computed tomography (CT) is generally reserved for those situations in which MRI is contraindicated, such as implanted pacemaker, metal fragment, or paramagnetic surgical clips, or where there is a need to image the extent of calcification or hemorrhage.

One of the most useful imaging studies is T1-weighted sagittal, Gd-enhanced (usually obtained in high-resolution modes such as SPGR or MP-RAGE) and unenhanced T1 axial images, T2-weighted axial images, and FLAIR (fluid-attenuated inversion recovery) sequences [21]. As is the case with CT contrast agents, Gd-based contrast leaks into parenchyma in areas with BBB breakdown, and the paramagnetic properties of Gd generate hyperintense signal on T1 scans. T1 images usually are better at demonstrating anatomy and areas of contrast enhancement. T2 and FLAIR images are more sensitive for detecting edema and infiltrative tumor. For G II tumors, enhancement is uncommon and the FLAIR abnormality represents the tumor. Tumor appearance on T1-weighted MRI is similar to that on CT, although tumor volumes are better delineated on MRI, particularly with low-grade neoplasms that do not demonstrate contrast enhancement. With the increasing incidence of posttreatment "pseudoprogression," additional specialized diffusion, perfusion, and spectroscopic sequences are being increasingly utilized to distinguish tumor from necrosis or pseudoprogression, and PET imaging may also have some role in this; in the United States, only FDG-PET is approved, but amino acid, FLT, and F-DOPA PET imaging is being evaluated. Diffusion-weighted and functional MR also has utility in guiding resection [22].

The characteristic radiographic features of grade II gliomas include an isodense lesion on CT, and on MRI, this lesion is isointense on T1 and hyperintense on T2 sequences [21]. Oligodendroglial tumors often contain calcifications, best visualized on CT. While WHO III gliomas may enhance with contrast, most low-grade gliomas demonstrate minimal to no enhancement with gadolinium, but new enhancement in a previously non-enhancing lesion is suggestive of malignant transformation, and, if clinically necessary, this area should be preferentially biopsied (Fig. 9.2) [23].

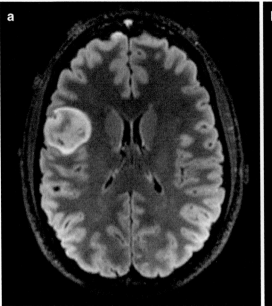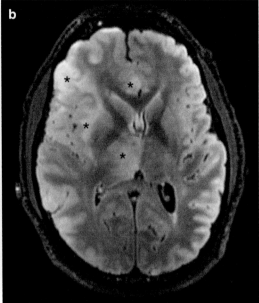

Fig. 9.2 Focal vs. WHO II gliomas. Low-grade gliomas may present either as focal tumors as illustrated by FLAIR signal limited to the right frontal lobe (**a**) or in a diffuse manner with FLAIR signal (denoted by asterisk) encompasses the right frontal operculum, insular cortex, thalamus, and cingulate gyrus (**b**)

9.5 Patient Outcome and Prognosis

The introduction of this revised WHO 2016 classification requires a reassessment of the survival of grade II and III glioma patients along molecular definitions. Table 9.1 summarizes the OS and PFS reported in molecular subtypes observed in prospective trials on diffuse grade II and III gliomas. Taken together, the reported median OS in *IDH*mt astrocytoma is in the 9- to 10-year range and in *IDH*mt 1p/19q-codeleted tumors more than 14 years [24]. *IDH*wt (anaplastic) glioma is no single entity, and OS in *IDH*wt astrocytoma with molecular characteristics of glioblastoma (with trisomy chromosome 7 and LOH 10q or with *TERT* promoter mutations) is significantly less [24–27]. Well-established clinical factors that affect outcome in diffuse grade II and III glioma include age, extent of resection, and performance status. Preliminary data suggest near total resection may be more important for IDHmt astrocytoma compared to oligodendroglioma, perhaps related to the increased sensitivity of

oligodendroglioma to adjuvant treatment [28, 29]. The grading of diffuse glioma is based on certain rather subjective characteristics such as the presence or absence of nuclear atypia, high cellularity, mitosis, endothelial proliferation, and necrosis. The clinical significance of grading of the diffuse gliomas within the WHO 2016 needs re-evaluation: the histological grade of *IDHmt* tumors is clinically less important compared to that grade of *IDHwt* tumors [24, 26, 30, 31]. Finding a molecular mutation alteration with clear impact on outcome within the molecular subgroups would be the molecular equivalent of histological grading. There is evidence from genome-wide methylation study prognosis that CIMP status (high versus low), homozygous loss of *CDKNA2A/B*, methylation of specific genes, and total copy number variation may correlate with survival [19, 32–34]. Combined analyses of methylation patterns and histological features suggested that necrosis on histological examination also affects outcome, but significantly less in the absence of homozygous loss of *CDKN2A/B*. Reports on the results on the clinical relevance of

Table 9.1 Median survival regardless of assigned treatment in the three major groups (*IDHwt*, *IDHmut*, *IDHmt* and 1p/19q codeleted) in historical prospective trials with retrospective molecular analysis

Histology/molecular subgroup	Treatment	*n*	Median PFS	Median OS
Low-grade glioma [26]				
IDH R132Hmt	RT ± PCV	71		13.1 years
IDHwt		42		5.1 years
Low-grade glioma [31]				
IDHmt 1p/19q codeleted	RT or TMZ	104	5.2 years	
IDHmt		165	4 years	NS
IDHwt		49	1.7 years	
Anaplastic astrocytoma [38]				
IDH R132H-mutated	RT/TMZ, BCNU of CCNU	49		7.9 years
IDHwt		54		2.8 years
Anaplastic oligodendroglioma[a] [16]				
IDHmt 1p/19q codeleted	RT ± PCV	49		9.5 years
IDH mt		20		3.1 years
IDHwt		55		1.1 years
Anaplastic oligodendroglioma[a] [28]				
IDHmt 1p/19q codeleted	RT/PCV	42		14.7 years
IDH mt		37		5.5 years
IDHwt		26		1.3 years
Anaplastic glioma [30, 64]				
IDHmt, 1p/19q codeleted	RT, PCV, or TMZ	69	7.5–8.7 years	NR
IDHmt		83	2.1–3.0 years	7.0–7.3 years
IDHwt		58	0.8 years	3.1–4.7 years

[a]NGS data on a subset of patients. *RT* radiotherapy, *TMZ* temozolomide, *BCNU* carmustine, CCNU (lomustine); *PCV* procarbazine, CCNA, and vincristine

other single markers are conflicting [26, 35–39]. Studies have shown a correlation between age, tumor grade, and total copy number alteration, which intuitively makes sense [26, 40]. Clearly, on a molecular level, both oligodendroglioma and astrocytoma *IDHmt* are heterogeneous tumors, and an integrated analysis of histological and molecular features may help to better predict outcome [34, 39].

9.6 Treatment Options

9.6.1 Surgical Resection

Given the natural history of gliomas, clinical observation of surgically treatable gliomas is rarely encouraged. The ultimate goal of surgical resection is to provide specimen used to establish the diagnosis, distinguishing between oligodendroglioma and astrocytoma, and provide cytoreduction [41–43]. Several studies have examined the role of surgical resection on progression-free survival and overall survival in patients with WHO II and III gliomas [16, 42, 44, 45]. Greater extent of resection affects the natural history of gliomas including time to malignant transformation. Time to malignant transformation from WHO grade II to WHO grades III or IV ranges from 4 to 29 months, depending on WHO grade, molecular characteristics, and extent of tumor resection [16, 42, 44, 46]. The decision to offer surgical resection versus tumor biopsy varies based on tumor location, tumor size, patient age, and baseline functional status. Treatment decisions must balance the natural history of the disease with perioperative morbidity.

Surgical resection plays a principal role in management. Cumulative evidence suggests that more extensive surgical resection of T1 post gadolinium-enhanced and FLAIR tissue on MRI is associated with longer survival and improved quality of life for patients with both low- and high-grade gliomas. Twenty-two studies since

1990 have examined the effect of extent of resection on patient survival and tumor progression for WHO grade II and III gliomas [16, 47–66]. Building on this body of work, a large population analysis of Norwegian patients [67] studied patients treated in two hospitals serving adjacent geographic regions. The treatment strategy differed between providers in these two hospitals, and there was little crossover between hospitals during the study period. Neurosurgeons from Hospital A favored glioma biopsy followed by watchful waiting, while Hospital B offered upfront tumor maximal resection at the time of diagnosis. After a median follow-up of 7 years, overall survival was superior for those individuals treated with early resection. Median survival in this study was 5.9 years for patients receiving tumor biopsy, while the group receiving early resection did not reach median survival by the end of the study period. Furthermore, 5-year survival was 60% for biopsy patients and 74% for those receiving early surgery [67]. For this reason incidentally found gliomas, which have yet to produce symptoms or demonstrate growth over time [17], are often treated with early resection which offers favorable outcome when compared with individuals presenting with symptoms [17].

In the era of novel molecular markers and 2016 WHO diagnostic criteria, there has been a new focus directed toward elucidating the impact of EOR among different molecular subtypes of both low- and high-grade gliomas. The center in this debate is the question of whether maximal resection is of greater benefit for molecularly unfavorable or molecularly favorable gliomas. Within the context of WHO II and III gliomas, initial evidence suggests that such differences do indeed exist. Kawaguchi et al. examined the impact of GTR versus non-GTR on clinical outcomes within three molecular subtypes of WHO grade III gliomas: IDH1/IDH2 mutation with 1p/19q codeletion, IDH1/IDH2 mutation without 1p/19q codeletion, and IDH1/IDH2 wild type. GTR led to a longer median OS and PFS than non-GTR; however focusing on outcomes between all three molecular groups, GTR only had a significant impact on overall survival in

patients with IDH1/IDH2 mutations without 1p/19q codeletion. No significant differences in survival were observed between GTR and non-GTR in patients with IDH1/IDH2 wild type or IDH1/IDH2 mutation with 1p/19q codeletion [29]. Cahill et al. similarly found that the prognostic significance of extent of resection differed in malignant astrocytomas based on their IDH1 status. After examining EOR in 157 patients with anaplastic astrocytomas and 250 patients with GBM, the authors reported that volume of residual enhancing tissue was associated with shorter overall survival in IDH1 wild-type tumors, thereby providing contradictory evidence compared to results from Kawaguchi et al. However, for IDH1 mutant tumors, both residual enhancing and non-enhancing tumor tissue were significantly associated with worse survival. Wijnenga et al. focused on extent of resection across molecular subtype for WHO II gliomas. Univariate analysis suggested that postoperative tumor volume was associated with overall survival in astrocytoma IDH-mutant patients but only demonstrated a trend toward significance within oligodendroglioma patients. In patients with IDH-mutant astrocytomas, a postoperative tumor volume of less than 25 cm^3 was associated with longer overall compared to residual volumes >25 cm^3 [28]. Taken together, the published literature highlights the fact that there are differences in clinical outcomes independently based on extent of glioma resection based and molecular subtype.

Prior to surgery each patient should have a detailed history, physical examination. Based on tumor location, a surgical approach should be considered which spares presumed functional areas while maximizing extent of resection. Glioma patients with tumors within or in close proximity to regions with language, sensorimotor, or neurocognitive significance should be considered for an awake or asleep brain mapping resection. A detailed motor examination, neuropsychological and language examination, may be indicated for dominant hemisphere lesions [68]. Management of seizures is particularly important before surgery, and corticosteroids such as dexamethasone should be administered to control periglioma edema, with doses ranging between 2 and 24 mg daily.

Direct cortical stimulation brain mapping is the gold standard approach for the identification and preservation of cortical and subcortical regions of functional significance during surgical resection of WHO II and III gliomas. Intraoperative brain mapping was introduced by Horsley and later by Penfield for the identification and preservation of functional sites [69, 70]. Cortical and subcortical stimulation depolarizes a focal area of the cortex which in turn evokes a functional response, depending on the stimulated region. There is significant variability of cortical and subcortical language organization [71]. Additionally, cortical and subcortical structures may be distorted by the tumor, resulting in localized mass effect. Multiple studies have found great individual variability in language sites responsible for motor planning and speech arrest between patients [72]. While typically the classic boundaries of Broca's area for motor speech are adjacent to face motor cortex, some studies have found that it is several centimeters from the sylvian fissure [72]. Even in patients with few neurologic symptoms preoperatively, it cannot be assumed that a glioma is well circumscribed and separate from functional pathways. The use of intraoperative stimulation is necessary to avoid neurologic deficits. The challenge in many cases is to maximize tumor resection while simultaneously minimizing risk of injury to vital cortical and subcortical structures.

Additional techniques such as intraoperative MRI (iMRI) and fluorescence-guided surgery are useful adjuvants to maximize extent of resection while minimizing perioperative morbidity. iMRI was first introduced in mid-1980s using 0.5 Tesla (T) magnets. Higher field-strength systems, such as 1.5 to 3 T magnets, now image with greater resolution. Intraoperative MRI is able to provide dynamic anatomic imaging during surgery to mitigate the changing environment during surgery due to loss of cerebrospinal fluid and cerebral edema. Intraoperative brain shift makes the interpretation and comparison of neuronavigation using preoperative images changing. Several studies have reported on the added benefit of iMRI-guided surgery to improve EOR for gliomas [73, 74]. A prospective randomized trial was performed that allocated 58 glioma patients to receive surgery with iMRI or conventional neurosurgical resection with neuronavigation. Gross total resection was achieved in 23 of 24 patients (96%) compared to the conventional treatment group (17 of 25 patients, 68%) [74]. This study provides level 1 evidence for the use of iMRI; however the median remaining enhancing tumor volume on postoperative imaging was 0.0 cm^3 in the iMRI group compared to 0.03 cm^3 in the conventional treatment group, and it remains to be determined whether a small volume of residual less than 0.1 cm^3 impacts outcome and justifies the added expense and operative time [74]. Fluorescence-guided surgery uses selective intracellular fluorescence to maximize EOR. 5-Aminolevulinic acid (5-ALA) is the most commonly used fluorescence agent in glioma surgery. 5-ALA is a natural biochemical precursor of hemoglobin that can be administered as a nonfluorescent prodrug [75]. When given at sufficient quantities, 5-ALA elicits synthesis and accumulation of intracellular fluorescent porphyrins in epithelial cells as well as rapidly dividing cancer cells including glioma tissue [75]. Porphyrin fluorescence can be visualized with an appropriate short wavelength filter. In a study of 531 patients with intracranial tumors treated by 5-ALA-guided resection or biopsy, the highest percentage of 5-ALA-positive fluorescence was detected in 96% of glioblastomas, 88% of anaplastic gliomas, 40% of LGG, and no WHO grade I gliomas [76, 77]. The utility of 5-ALA to aid in the visualization of residual tumor cells during resection of non-enhancing WHO II and III glioma is under investigation.

9.6.2 Chemotherapy

The efficacy of PCV (procarbazine, CCNU or lomustine, and vincristine) and temozolomide chemotherapy in grade II and III gliomas were initially shown in trials on recurrent tumors, with higher response rates and of longer duration in oligodendroglioma (in particular those

Table 9.2 Hazard ratio (HR) and 95% confidence intervals (CI) reported in trials on adjuvant chemotherapy in grade II and III glioma

Histology	Trial question	n	HR [95% CI] for OS
Anaplastic oligodendroglioma [25]	RT/PCV vs. RT	368	0.75 [0.60, 0.95]
Anaplastic oligodendroglioma [24]	RT/PCV-i vs. RT	291	0.79 [0.60, 1.04]
Low-grade glioma [26]	RT/PCV vs. RT	251	0.59 [0.42, 0.83]
Anaplastic astrocytoma [65]	RT/carmustine + DBD vs. RT	193	0.77 [0.56, 1.06]
Anaplastic glioma, 1p/19q intact [27]	RT vs. RT/TMZ	745	0.65[a] (0.45, 0.93)
Anaplastic glioma [30]	TMZ or PCV vs. RT	318	1.11 [0.8, 1.55]
Low-grade glioma [31]	RT vs. TMZ	447	1.16 [0.9, 1.5]
Anaplastic astrocytoma [38]	RT/TMZ vs. RT/lomustine or carmustine	197	0.94 [0.67, 1.32]

[a]99.145% confidence interval; primary endpoint PFS; *TMZ* temozolomide; *PCV* procarbazine, CCNU (lomustine), and vincristine; DBD dibromodulciterol; RT radiotherapy

with combined 1p/19q loss) compared to astrocytoma [78–82]. Randomized controlled trials have now shown that survival in newly diagnosed grade II and III glioma is improved if chemotherapy is added to radiotherapy (Table 9.2). Of the four trials that are now available, three used classical histological patient selection criteria and investigated the PCV regimen: two in anaplastic oligodendroglioma [83, 84] and one in low-grade glioma [20]. The last trial investigated temozolomide in 1p/19 non-codeleted anaplastic glioma [85]. In all these trials, increased survival was demonstrated with the addition of chemotherapy to radiotherapy, despite high crossover rates (56–79%) to salvage chemotherapy in the radiotherapy-only arm once patients developed tumor progression [20, 83–85]. Although initial reports of the trials on PCV chemotherapy in anaplastic oligodendroglioma suggested in particular survival benefit in patients with 1p/19q-codeleted tumors, subsequent studies suggested three related candidate markers predicting benefit to adjuvant PCV: *IDH* mutational status, CpG island methylator phenotype (CIMP), and *MGMT* promoter methylation [86, 87]. In the European study, *MGMT* promoter methylation assessed with a genomic-wide methylation assay was found to be the best predictor for benefit to chemotherapy; the US study identified IDH mutational status as a predictive factor.

Two European trials compared treatment with chemotherapy only to radiotherapy only: either PCV or temozolomide was compared to radiotherapy in a trial on anaplastic glioma, whereas temozolomide was compared to radiotherapy in a trial on low-grade glioma [88, 89]. Both studies failed to show improved outcome in patients initially treated with chemotherapy alone, with the suggestion of a worse outcome after initial chemotherapy-only in some analyses in the astrocytoma *IDHmt* strata [88, 89]. It needs to be realized that with temozolomide alone, even in the favorable 1p/19q-codeleted group, the median PFS with temozolomide alone is limited, and, in most reports around 5 years, for astrocytoma *IDHmt* PFS is in the 2.5–3.5 years [88–91]. Date on upfront PCV in molecularly defined oligodendroglioma is more limited; reports suggest a PFS of 5.5–8 years [88, 92]. A relatively small trial (n = 41) explored temozolomide induction therapy followed by thiotepa and busulfan myeloablative treatment with stem cell rescue. Among all 1p/19q-codeleted patients (n = 33), 5-year PFS was 50% and 5-year OS 93%; this PFS does not seem superior to results reported after temozolomide or PCV alone. That questions the contribution of the dose intensification on outcome; more follow-up is needed to fully understand OS [93]. The uncontrolled UCSF study on initial treatment with temozolomide alone reported a PFS of 3.6 years in IDH mt tumors and 4.9 years in 1p/19q-codeleted tumors, with a median OS of 11.2 and to 9.7 years, respectively [90]. This compares unfavorably with the 13–14 years reported in RTOG 9804 in IDH-mutant low-grade gliomas and 1p/19q-codeleted anaplastic oligodendroglioma in the adjuvant PCV trials [20, 83, 84]. As of today, a head-to-head trial of initial treatment with chemotherapy alone to initial treatment with both chemotherapy with radiotherapy is still lacking, but with the currently available data it appears justified to assume that combining radiotherapy with chemotherapy in newly diagnosed glioma patients will increase survival compared to single modality treatment (either radiotherapy alone or chemotherapy alone). A key argument in favor of chemotherapy alone is that this may avoid or delay radiotherapy-induced delayed cognitive effects, but the data from available studies suggest this is likely to jeopardize overall survival. Although better tolerated than PCV, the use of temozolomide has been associated with the development of a hypermutated tumor phenotype at progression through TMZ-induced mutations of mismatch repair pathway genes [94]. Although this indicates resistance to temozolomide, from a clinical perspective, the DNA mutational pattern at progression is less relevant than the total duration of treatment response and overall survival. A subgroup of *IDH* wild-type grade II and III glioma resemble at the molecular-level glioblastoma (presence of *TERT* promoter mutations, with or without 7+/10q LOH) with similar poor outcome [25, 26]. Combined chemo-irradiation with temozolomide should be considered in for these patients in view of their poor outcome [25, 27].

The Rationale for Nitrosourea-Based Chemotherapy Regimens Versus Temozolomide. The improved outcome after adjuvant chemotherapy in newly diagnosed grade II and III tumors was initially demonstrated in the studies that investigated *PCV chemotherapy. The more recent results of the CATNON trial show that adjuvant temozolomide results in prolonged survival in patients with anaplastic 1p/19q non-codeleted tumors; it seems reasonable to assume this will also hold true for grade II 1p/19q non-codeleted tumors. A study in anaplastic astrocytoma comparing adjuvant temozolomide to adjuvant BCNU or CCNU following radiotherapy observed no survival difference between these regimens but more myelosuppression in the nitrosourea-treated patients leading to more frequent early treatment discontinuation [95]. Temozolomide was also clearly better tolerated in comparison to PCV in the German trial

on anaplastic glioma [88]. Importantly, several retrospective analyses suggested a better outcome after PCV compared to temozolomide in 1p/19q-codeleted tumors [88, 96, 97]. The ongoing CODEL study (NCT00887146) compares adjuvant PCV to combined chemo-irradiation with temozolomide in codeleted grade II and III tumors, which will take many years to conclude.

Bevacizumab. Initial uncontrolled studies suggested efficacy of treatment with bevacizumab in relapsing grade II and III tumors, with results comparable to those in recurrent glioblastoma [98–101]. Response rates in these studies on non-glioblastoma tumors varied between 50 and 70%, with a PFS6 varying between 40 and 70% and OS between 9 and 15 months. Since those early days, controlled trials have failed to show an impact of bevacizumab on OS in glioblastoma despite an impact on PFS. This was documented both in first-line treatment and at progression with bevacizumab given as single agent or in combination with lomustine. Even more sobering, the TAVAREC randomized phase II trial in relapsing 1p/19q intact grade II and III glioma with enhancing disease showed that the addition of bevacizumab to temozolomide does not improve neither PFS nor OS in comparison to treatment with temozolomide alone [102]. In view of this, the role of bevacizumab in recurrent grade II and III tumors is limited to the palliative care setting (edema reduction, symptom improvement) without a real antitumor effect in glioma.

Salvage Chemotherapy. Past trials on recurrent grade II and III glioma have reported activity of the agents that are now used in first line following radiotherapy: PCV and temozolomide [79, 82, 103, 104]. The treatment of recurrent tumors after prior chemotherapy (either given adjuvant or after first progression) continues to represent a clinically unmet need. Data on second-line treatment with nitrosourea or temozolomide are limited and suggest only limited activity. Studies on second-line treatment in oligodendroglial tumors showed modest activity of PCV after prior temozolomide and vice versa; outcome was however no longer clearly associated with 1p/19q loss [105–107]. Single-agent lomustine showed some activity after prior radiotherapy and temozolomide, with a 40% 6 months PFS rate [108]. The interpretation of a small prospective but uncontrolled trial on sirolimus in progressive low-grade astrocytoma is cumbersome, due to the rather heterogeneous patient population and the lack of a control arm.

9.6.3 Radiotherapy

Understanding Who to Treat with Radiotherapy. WHO grade II LGGs with higher-risk features for tumor progression are presumed to receive the greatest benefit from therapeutic intervention; this specific hypothesis has not been prospectively tested. In 2002, Pignatti et al. performed a multivariate analysis from the EORTC 22844 and 22845 trials reporting five unfavorable prognostic factors for survival: age ≥ 40 years, astrocytoma histology, maximum diameter ≥ 6 cm, tumor crossing midline, and presence of neurologic deficits before surgery [109]. Low-risk patients, defined by the presence of up to two risk factors, displayed a median survival of 7.7 years versus 3.2 years for high-risk patients having three or more risk factors. The presence of mutations in either *IDH*1 or 2 is associated with significantly longer overall survival, leading the 2016 WHO classification to utilize this as a key variable [20, 110]. In RTOG 9802, a phase III trial for adult high-risk LGGs (here defined as patients <40 years old with an incomplete resection or >40 years old with any extent of resection), patients were randomized to RT versus RT plus procarbazine, lomustine, and vincristine (PCV) chemoradiotherapy (CRT). Compared with median survival of 7.8 years with RT and 13.3 years with CRT among all patients, IDH-mutated patients displayed a median survival of 10.1 years with RT, while median survival with chemoradiotherapy (CRT) was not reached [20]. Combined chromosomal 1p and 19q codeletion and 1;19 translocation are also associated with superior overall and progression-free survival in lower-grade glioma [111]. A secondary analysis of the NCCTG/RTOG/ECOG trial, which randomized LGG patients to 50.4 vs. 64.8 Gy, reported a median survival of 11.9 years for patients with 1;19 translocation versus 8.1

years without this alteration [57]. Specifically for oligodendroglioma, the median survival was 13.0 years for patients with a 1;19 translocation versus 9.1 years without [112]. In contrast, all grade III patients are considered high risk and treated with combinatorial radiochemotherapy, based on results from three large randomized trials [83–85].

Radiotherapy for WHO II Gliomas. The goals of RT for grade II LGG are to improve tumor control and survival while preventing/delaying malignant transformation and limiting the acute and late effects of treatment that may degrade quality of life. Randomized clinical trials have explored the roles of and dose for RT in LGG. The NCCTG/RTOG/ECOG trial randomized 203 adult G 2 LGG patients to 50.4 versus 64.8 Gy [57]. No statistically significant 5-year overall survival difference was observed between the arms. A secondary analysis on the cognitive effects of RT found that only 5.3% of patients deteriorated by 5 years, while most remained stable [113]. EORTC 22844 randomized 343 patients to 45 versus 59.4 Gy; 5-year overall survival rates were 58% in the 45 Gy arm versus 59% in the 59.4 Gy arm [51]. In the United States, it is generally accepted that a reasonable RT dose for GII LGG is 50–54 Gy.

EORTC 22845 examined the timing of RT for G II LGG, randomizing 314 LGG patients to early RT (54 Gy) versus deferred RT until progression [114]. Median progression-free survival was 5.3 years in the early RT arm versus 3.4 years in the deferred RT arm ($p < 0.0001$). However, because the majority of "observed" patients (65%) received RT, median overall survival was similar between the early and deferred RT arms (7.4 vs. 7.2 years, respectively). The proportion of patients with seizures at 1 year was significantly lower in the early RT group (25% vs. 41%, $p = 0.0329$), implying that tumor control has significant clinical benefit.

The lack of overall survival benefit has been used by some to justify deferring RT until progression for some patients with G II tumors. This can be considered for LGG patients with highly favorable prognostic features and no residual disease (e.g., younger than 40, MR-confirmed gross totally resected *IDH*-mutated WHO G II oligodendroglioma), provided they are carefully observed. RTOG 9802 included an observation cohort of so-called "low-risk" patients, who underwent resection without adjuvant therapy. One hundred and eleven patients, younger than 40, and had achieved a surgeon-determined gross total resection, were entered into the study; the overall survival rates at 2 and 5 years were 99 and 93%. The PFS rates at 2 and 5 years were 82 and 48% [115].

The recent publication of the mature results for higher-risk G II LGG patients in RTOG 9802 showed that patients selected for postoperative RT should also receive adjuvant chemotherapy, as discussed elsewhere in this chapter [20]. Median overall survival was also significantly improved for the CRT arm vs. RT arm (13.3 vs. 7.8 years). The added survival benefit from PCV was observed in all LGG histologies, with the greatest effect size in oligodendroglioma.

Because RT alone has not been shown to improve OS, the results of that arm could be viewed as equivalent to "observation"; however, RT in combination with PCV produces the longest OS described in a clinical trial, and therefore it is "fair" to ask whether chemotherapy alone (with delayed RT) could produce similar results. The EORTC 22033-26033 study randomized 477 LGG patients to receive 50.4 Gy RT versus dose-intense temozolomide (TMZ) [89]. Median progression-free survival was 39 months in the TMZ arm versus 46 months in the RT arm ($p = 0.22$). Patients with IDH mutation and non-1p19q-codeleted tumors had longer progression-free survival in the RT arm (55 months) vs. TMZ arm (36 months), but there were no differences in PFS for the IDH-mutated, IDH-codeleted, or IDH wild-type tumors. Mature OS data from this trial are still pending. A separate preliminary analysis of health-related quality of life and global cognitive functioning found no differences, belying the oft-quoted rationale for delaying radiotherapy, i.e., the assumed cognitive and QOL decline associated with its use, which in this randomized trial was no better or worse than TMZ alone [116]. While these preliminary results shed some light regarding the question of TMZ versus RT as monotherapy, overall survival

and quality of life results are pending longer follow-up. In the meantime, non-randomized data emerging from institutions where the "TMZ-first" principle had supplanted the upfront use of RT provide some interesting insights. Recently, Wahl et al. presented the findings of a single-arm phase II trial on 120 patients with WHO grade II gliomas treated with TMZ first [90]. Median progression-free and overall survival was 4.2 and 9.7 years. In RTOG 9802, median progression-free survival was 4.0 years in the RT arm versus 10.4 years in the CRT arm (significantly superior to TMZ first) [20]. Median overall survival with TMZ first in NCT 00313729 was 9.7 years, significantly lower than the 13.3 years achieved with RT plus PCV in RTOG 9802.

Radiotherapy for WHO III Gliomas. The current standard of care for patients with anaplastic oligodendrogliomas is maximal resection followed by postoperative radiotherapy and chemotherapy. The radiotherapy target volume includes both the postoperative cavity and any residual enhancing disease but also the FLAIR or T2 abnormality; unlike GBM, the postoperative FLAIR abnormality from anaplastic oligodendroglioma (and for that matter grade II gliomas) most likely represents residual tumor with minimal contribution from tumor-associated edema and therefore has to be included in the target volume. Indirect support for this comes from the small but growing body of data regarding supra-radical resection of lower-grade gliomas, where complete resection of all MR abnormality is associated with longer survival. Although the commonly used radiotherapy dose on prospective trials of anaplastic oligodendroglioma is 59.4 Gy, this never took into account molecular variability, and some have proposed that consideration could be made to lower the RT dose to 54 Gy for tumors with favorable prognostic features (e.g., 1p19q codeleted) to minimize long-term toxicity.

Two large randomized trials have investigated sequential chemoradiotherapy compared to radiotherapy alone in patients with anaplastic oligodendroglioma and oligoastrocytoma [83, 84]. With 11 years follow-up on RTOG 9402, the addition of PCV chemotherapy for radiotherapy did not impact overall survival for the overall cohort but did prolong overall survival for patients with loss of both 1p and 19q (from 7.7 to 14.7 years) [83]. Among patients without loss of 1p and 19q, PCV prior to radiotherapy prolonged survival for patients with IDH1-mutated tumors from 3.3 to 5.5 years. The EORTC trial reported similar findings [84]. Therefore, both the 1p19q codeleted and any IDH-mutated (with or without 1p19q codeletion) patient should receive chemoradiotherapy, but the role of combinatorial therapy for the 1p19q non-codeleted and IDH wild-type tumors is questionable.

The current standard of care for patients with anaplastic astrocytomas is maximal resection followed by radiotherapy and chemotherapy. The radiotherapy target volume and dose are similar to those for anaplastic oligodendroglioma. The effectiveness of adding temozolomide was tested in a phase III trial of non-1p19q-codeleted anaplastic glioma patients (the CATNON Intergroup trial). Preliminary results demonstrated prolongation of overall survival [85]. The NOA-04 trial compared radiation with two chemotherapy regimens for anaplastic gliomas, the majority of whom carried a diagnosis of anaplastic astrocytoma [88]. Patients were assigned to radiotherapy alone versus PCV versus temozolomide with time to treatment failure as the primary endpoint. Chemotherapy failures were salvaged with radiotherapy, and vice versa, and further, temozolomide failures were salvaged with PCV and vice versa, almost ensuring that every patient received every therapy at some point. Time to treatment failure was similar between each of the arms, as was overall survival, imputing that the sequence of radiotherapy, temozolomide, or PCV might not actually matter.

Technological Advances: Intensity Modulated Radiotherapy, Proton Therapy, and Carbon Therapy. As LGG patients may live for many years, it is important not only to improve survival but also to minimize RT-related late effects. Advances in RT delivery systems allow for more conformal radiation treatment planning to maximize RT doses to target volumes while minimizing dose to surrounding normal structures. Intensity-modulated radiation therapy (IMRT)

has been frequently utilized for the treatment of brain tumors and in many studies reported to offer improved conformity over traditional three-dimensional conformal radiotherapy (3DCRT) techniques [117–120]. Importantly, IMRT has the ability to reduce dose to surrounding critical structures such as the cochlea and hippocampus and is associated with decreased ototoxicity and neurotoxicity rates [121, 122].

The advantages of proton and carbon therapy are being investigated. One of the earliest experiences of proton therapy for LGG was a small series of 19 patients treated with protons in Germany, demonstrating low toxicity rates comparable to photon-based radiotherapy [123]. A pooled analysis of several proton centers found no grade III or greater side effects in LGG patients [124]. Sherman et al. reported a small cohort of 20 LGG patients treated with proton therapy who were prospectively evaluated with comprehensive neuropsychological testing [125]. At a median follow-up of 5 years, all patients exhibited stable cognitive functioning. A separate analysis from Shih et al. found that 20 LGG patients who underwent proton therapy experienced 3- and 5-year progression-free survival of 85 and 40% [126]. These results suggest that proton therapy may provide neurocognitive advantages over photons but may not confer overall or progression-free survival advantages. In Fig. 9.3, we demonstrate a left temporal lobe grade II oligodendroglioma case planned with protons and photons, demonstrating significant dosimetric superiority of proton therapy.

Ongoing Radiotherapy Trials for Low-Grade Glioma. NRG-BN005 is a phase II randomized trial of proton versus photon therapy for IDH-mutant low- and intermediate-grade gliomas using 54 Gy. The primary endpoint is to assess whether proton therapy preserves cognitive outcomes over time. A phase III trial in China (NCT01649830) is randomizing LGG patients to 54 Gy RT with or without adjuvant TMZ. A North American Intergroup trial (CODEL) is currently enrolling patients in order to compare chemoradiotherapy with either temozolomide or PCV for both grades III and II gliomas.

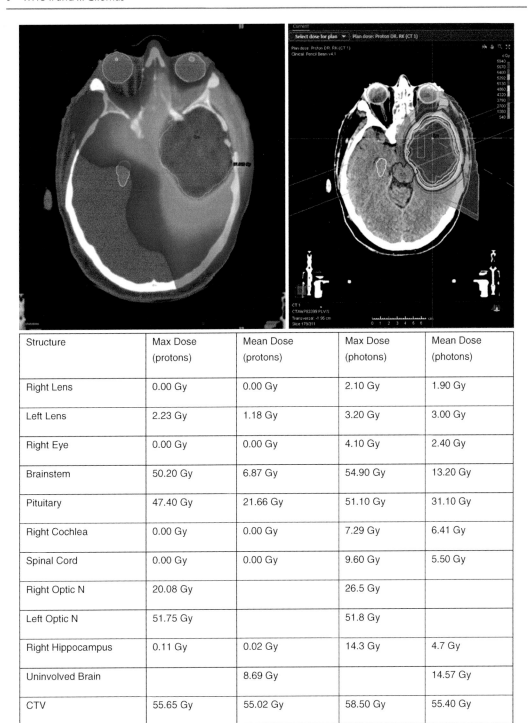

Structure	Max Dose (protons)	Mean Dose (protons)	Max Dose (photons)	Mean Dose (photons)
Right Lens	0.00 Gy	0.00 Gy	2.10 Gy	1.90 Gy
Left Lens	2.23 Gy	1.18 Gy	3.20 Gy	3.00 Gy
Right Eye	0.00 Gy	0.00 Gy	4.10 Gy	2.40 Gy
Brainstem	50.20 Gy	6.87 Gy	54.90 Gy	13.20 Gy
Pituitary	47.40 Gy	21.66 Gy	51.10 Gy	31.10 Gy
Right Cochlea	0.00 Gy	0.00 Gy	7.29 Gy	6.41 Gy
Spinal Cord	0.00 Gy	0.00 Gy	9.60 Gy	5.50 Gy
Right Optic N	20.08 Gy		26.5 Gy	
Left Optic N	51.75 Gy		51.8 Gy	
Right Hippocampus	0.11 Gy	0.02 Gy	14.3 Gy	4.7 Gy
Uninvolved Brain		8.69 Gy		14.57 Gy
CTV	55.65 Gy	55.02 Gy	58.50 Gy	55.40 Gy
PTV	55.68 Gy	54.99 Gy	58.50 Gy	55.20 Gy

Fig. 9.3 Radiation treatment planning for a 42-year-old man with a left temporal lobe oligodendroglioma, WHO grade II, who underwent subtotal resection with residual disease. He received radiotherapy to 5400 cGy in 180 cGy daily fractions. The T2 FLAIR MRI sequence with hyper-intensity. Clinical target volume is shown in red, and the prescription isodoses in color for photon IMRT plan on the left and proton planning on the right, demonstrating significant dose reduction to normal structures in favor of proton therapy; these data are tabulated below

9.6.4 Emerging Oncological Therapies for Low-Grade Glioma

Immunotherapy. In the United States, pembrolizumab and nivolumab have been registered for use in hypermutated, microsatellite instability (MSI)-high tumors. Data suggest that some IDH- mutated tumors that relapse after temozolomide also show microsatellite instability and a hypermutated phenotype, due to temozolomide-induced mutations in mismatch repair genes, but the frequency of this event is still poorly understood and requires more systematic studies in relapsing temozolomide-pretreated glioma [94, 127, 128]. Also, systematic studies on anti-PD1 and anti-PDL1 in MSI-high recurrent grade II and III glioma are still lacking. Several clinical projects aiming to induce an immune response against the IDH-mutated protein are ongoing, early studies have shown that indeed a cellular or humoral immune response can be elicited, but the clinical impact on outcome needs to be established [129].

IDH-Mutant Protein Inhibitors. An altered substrate affinity of the mutated IDH protein resulting in an increased production of 2-hydroxylutarate and a lowered concentration of α-ketoglutarate appears to be a key event in IDH-mutant glioma [130]. This results in a cascade of metabolic events, including the loss of functional activity of α-ketoglutarate-dependent enzymes, epigenetic changes (widespread DNA methylation or "CIMP"), and disruption of DNA repair mechanisms. Paradoxically, this may contribute to the sensitivity of IDH-mutant glioma to alkylating chemotherapy and radiotherapy [131, 132]. It is unclear whether IDH mutations alone are enough to induce a glioma, or whether other mutations are needed, and whether the mutation is still essential at the time of further tumor progression [133]. In some tumors the IDH mutation is actually lost at the time for further progression, probably due to chromosomal loss. Attempts to inhibit the mutant protein and restore intracellular 2-hydroxyglutarate levels have been effective in treatment-resistant IDHmt AML, resulting in a 20% complete response rate through differentiation of IDH-mutant precursor cells (and not by cytotoxicity) [134]. Similar attempts to treat glioma patients with IDHmt protein inhibitors have until now shown far from straightforward results. One hypothesis is that this treatment may be effective very early on in the course of the disease but perhaps not at a later stage. Much of this reasoning remains however speculative, and differences in response of IDHmt AML and glioma may very well reflect the histological context of the disease or differences between the organs and cells of origin. Others have emphasized the metabolic alterations that are induced by IDH mutations which may offer treatment options, such as a disturbed DNA single and double strand repair mechanisms [135–137]. Potentially, these make IDH-mutant cells sensitive for PARP inhibitors and trials are ongoing.

References

1. Ostrom QT, Bauchet L, Davis FG, Deltour I, Fisher JL, Langer CE et al (2014) The epidemiology of glioma in adults: a "state of the science" review. Neuro Oncol 16(7):896–913. https://doi.org/10.1093/neuonc/nou087
2. Osorio JA, Hervey-Jumper SL, Walsh KM, Clarke JL, Butowski NA, Prados MD et al (2015) Familial gliomas: cases in two pairs of brothers. J Neurooncol 121(1):135–140. https://doi.org/10.1007/s11060-014-1611-2
3. Shete S, Hosking FJ, Robertson LB, Dobbins SE, Sanson M, Malmer B et al (2009) Genome-wide association study identifies five susceptibility loci for glioma. Nat Genet 41(8):899–904. https://doi.org/10.1038/ng.407
4. Wrensch M, Jenkins RB, Chang JS, Yeh RF, Xiao Y, Decker PA et al (2009) Variants in the CDKN2B and RTEL1 regions are associated with high-grade glioma susceptibility. Nat Genet 41(8):905–908. https://doi.org/10.1038/ng.408
5. Sanson M, Hosking FJ, Shete S, Zelenika D, Dobbins SE, Ma Y et al (2011) Chromosome 7p11.2 (EGFR) variation influences glioma risk. Hum Mol Genet 20(14):2897–2904. https://doi.org/10.1093/hmg/ddr192
6. Stacey SN, Sulem P, Jonasdottir A, Masson G, Gudmundsson J, Gudbjartsson DF et al (2011) A germline variant in the TP53 polyadenylation signal confers cancer susceptibility. Nat Genet 43(11):1098–1103. https://doi.org/10.1038/ng.926
7. Rajaraman P, Melin BS, Wang Z, McKean-Cowdin R, Michaud DS, Wang SS et al (2012) Genome-wide

association study of glioma and meta-analysis. Hum Genet 131(12):1877–1888. https://doi.org/10.1007/s00439-012-1212-0

8. Preston DL, Ron E, Yonehara S, Kobuke T, Fujii H, Kishikawa M et al (2002) Tumors of the nervous system and pituitary gland associated with atomic bomb radiation exposure. J Natl Cancer Inst 94(20):1555–1563

9. Schwartzbaum JA, Fisher JL, Aldape KD, Wrensch M (2006) Epidemiology and molecular pathology of glioma. Nat Clin Pract Neurol 2:494. https://doi.org/10.1038/ncpneuro0289

10. Bondy ML, Scheurer ME, Malmer B, Barnholtz-Sloan JS, Davis FG, Il'yasova D et al (2008) Brain tumor epidemiology: consensus from the Brain Tumor Epidemiology Consortium. Cancer 113(7 Suppl):1953–1968. https://doi.org/10.1002/cncr.23741

11. Sadetzki S, Chetrit A, Freedman L, Stovall M, Modan B, Novikov I (2005) Long-term follow-up for brain tumor development after childhood exposure to ionizing radiation for tinea capitis. Radiat Res 163(4):424–432. https://doi.org/10.1667/rr3329

12. Turner MC, Krewski D, Armstrong BK, Chetrit A, Giles GG, Hours M et al (2013) Allergy and brain tumors in the INTERPHONE study: pooled results from Australia, Canada, France, Israel, and New Zealand. Cancer Causes Control 24(5):949–960. https://doi.org/10.1007/s10552-013-0171-7

13. Chen C, Xu T, Chen J, Zhou J, Yan Y, Lu Y et al (2011) Allergy and risk of glioma: a meta-analysis. Eur J Neurol 18(3):387–395. https://doi.org/10.1111/j.1468-1331.2010.03187.x

14. Baan R, Grosse Y, Lauby-Secretan B, El Ghissassi F, Bouvard V, Benbrahim-Tallaa L et al (2011) Carcinogenicity of radiofrequency electromagnetic fields. Lancet Oncol 12(7):624–626. https://doi.org/10.1016/s1470-2045(11)70147-4

15. Chang EF, Potts MB, Keles GE, Lamborn KR, Chang SM, Barbaro NM et al (2008) Seizure characteristics and control following resection in 332 patients with low-grade gliomas. J Neurosurg 108(2):227–235. https://doi.org/10.3171/JNS/2008/108/2/0227

16. Smith JS, Chang EF, Lamborn KR, Chang SM, Prados MD, Cha S et al (2008) Role of extent of resection in the long-term outcome of low-grade hemispheric gliomas. J Clin Oncol 26(8):1338–1345. https://doi.org/10.1200/JCO.2007.13.9337

17. Pallud J, Fontaine D, Duffau H, Mandonnet E, Sanai N, Taillandier L et al (2010) Natural history of incidental World Health Organization grade II gliomas. Ann Neurol 68(5):727–733. https://doi.org/10.1002/ana.22106

18. Cancer Genome Atlas Research Network, Brat DJ, Verhaak RG, Aldape KD, Yung WK, Salama SR et al (2015) Comprehensive, integrative genomic analysis of diffuse lower-grade gliomas. N Engl J Med 372(26):2481–2498. https://doi.org/10.1056/NEJMoa1402121

19. Ceccarelli M, Barthel FP, Malta TM, Sabedot TS, Salama SR, Murray BA et al (2016) Molecular profiling reveals biologically discrete subsets and pathways of progression in diffuse glioma. Cell 164(3):550–563. https://doi.org/10.1016/j.cell.2015.12.028

20. Buckner JC, Shaw EG, Pugh SL, Chakravarti A, Gilbert MR, Barger GR et al (2016) Radiation plus procarbazine, CCNU, and vincristine in low-grade glioma. N Engl J Med 374(14):1344–1355. https://doi.org/10.1056/NEJMoa1500925

21. Lote K, Egeland T, Hager B, Skullerud K, Hirschberg H (1998) Prognostic significance of CT contrast enhancement within histological subgroups of intracranial glioma. J Neurooncol 40(2):161–170

22. Roberts HC, Roberts TP, Brasch RC, Dillon WP (2000) Quantitative measurement of microvascular permeability in human brain tumors achieved using dynamic contrast-enhanced MR imaging: correlation with histologic grade. AJNR Am J Neuroradiol 21(5):891–899

23. Smits M (2016) Imaging of oligodendroglioma. Br J Radiol 89(1060):20150857. https://doi.org/10.1259/bjr.20150857

24. Pekmezci M, Rice T, Molinaro AM, Walsh KM, Decker PA, Hansen H et al (2017) Adult infiltrating gliomas with WHO 2016 integrated diagnosis: additional prognostic roles of ATRX and TERT. Acta Neuropathol 133(6):1001–1016. https://doi.org/10.1007/s00401-017-1690-1

25. Wijnenga MMJ, Dubbink HJ, French PJ, Synhaeve NE, Dinjens WNM, Atmodimedjo PN et al (2017) Molecular and clinical heterogeneity of adult diffuse low-grade IDH wild-type gliomas: assessment of TERT promoter mutation and chromosome 7 and 10 copy number status allows superior prognostic stratification. Acta Neuropathol 134(6):957–959. https://doi.org/10.1007/s00401-017-1781-z

26. Aoki K, Nakamura H, Suzuki H, Matsuo K, Kataoka K, Shimamura T et al (2018) Prognostic relevance of genetic alterations in diffuse lower-grade gliomas. Neuro Oncol 20(1):66–77. https://doi.org/10.1093/neuonc/nox132

27. Aibaidula A, Chan AK, Shi Z, Li Y, Zhang R, Yang R et al (2017) Adult IDH wild-type lower-grade gliomas should be further stratified. Neuro Oncol 19(10):1327–1337. https://doi.org/10.1093/neuonc/nox078

28. Wijnenga MMJ, French PJ, Dubbink HJ, Dinjens WNM, Atmodimedjo PN, Kros JM et al (2018) The impact of surgery in molecularly defined low-grade glioma: an integrated clinical, radiological, and molecular analysis. Neuro Oncol 20(1):103–112. https://doi.org/10.1093/neuonc/nox176

29. Kawaguchi T, Sonoda Y, Shibahara I, Saito R, Kanamori M, Kumabe T et al (2016) Impact of gross total resection in patients with WHO grade III glioma harboring the IDH 1/2 mutation without the 1p/19q co-deletion. J Neurooncol 129(3):505–514. https://doi.org/10.1007/s11060-016-2201-2

30. Reuss DE, Mamatjan Y, Schrimpf D, Capper D, Hovestadt V, Kratz A et al (2015) IDH mutant diffuse and anaplastic astrocytomas have similar age at presentation and little difference in survival: a grading problem for WHO. Acta Neuropathol 129(6):867–873. https://doi.org/10.1007/s00401-015-1438-8

31. Olar A, Wani KM, Alfaro-Munoz KD, Heathcock LE, van Thuijl HF, Gilbert MR et al (2015) IDH mutation status and role of WHO grade and mitotic index in overall survival in grade II-III diffuse gliomas. Acta Neuropathol 129(4):585–596. https://doi.org/10.1007/s00401-015-1398-z

32. Noushmehr H, Weisenberger DJ, Diefes K, Phillips HS, Pujara K, Berman BP et al (2010) Identification of a CpG island methylator phenotype that defines a distinct subgroup of glioma. Cancer Cell 17(5):510–522. https://doi.org/10.1016/j.ccr.2010.03.017

33. de Souza CF, Sabedot TS, Malta TM, Stetson L, Morozova O, Sokolov A et al (2018) A distinct DNA methylation shift in a subset of glioma CpG island methylator phenotype during tumor recurrence. Cell Rep 23(2):637–651. https://doi.org/10.1016/j.celrep.2018.03.107

34. Shirahata M, Ono T, Stichel D, Schrimpf D, Reuss DE, Sahm F et al (2018) Novel, improved grading system(s) for IDH-mutant astrocytic gliomas. Acta Neuropathol 136(1):153–166. https://doi.org/10.1007/s00401-018-1849-4

35. Alentorn A, Dehais C, Ducray F, Carpentier C, Mokhtari K, Figarella-Branger D et al (2015) Allelic loss of 9p21.3 is a prognostic factor in 1p/19q codeleted anaplastic gliomas. Neurology 85(15):1325–1331. https://doi.org/10.1212/wnl.0000000000002014

36. Wijnenga MMJ, French PJ, Dubbink HJ, Dinjens WNM, Atmodimedjo PN, Kros JM et al (2018) Prognostic relevance of mutations and copy number alterations assessed with targeted next generation sequencing in IDH mutant grade II glioma. J Neurooncol 139(2):349–357. https://doi.org/10.1007/s11060-018-2867-8

37. Gleize V, Alentorn A, Connen de Kerillis L, Labussiere M, Nadaradjane AA, Mundwiller E et al (2015) CIC inactivating mutations identify aggressive subset of 1p19q codeleted gliomas. Ann Neurol 78(3):355–374. https://doi.org/10.1002/ana.24443

38. Dubbink HJ, Atmodimedjo PN, Kros JM, French PJ, Sanson M, Idbaih A et al (2016) Molecular classification of anaplastic oligodendroglioma using next-generation sequencing: a report of the prospective randomized EORTC Brain Tumor Group 26951 phase III trial. Neuro Oncol 18(3):388–400. https://doi.org/10.1093/neuonc/nov182

39. Kamoun A, Idbaih A, Dehais C, Elarouci N, Carpentier C, Letouze E et al (2016) Integrated multi-omics analysis of oligodendroglial tumours identifies three subgroups of 1p/19q co-deleted gliomas. Nat Commun 7:11263. https://doi.org/10.1038/ncomms11263

40. Draaisma K, Wijnenga MM, Weenink B, Gao Y, Smid M, Robe P et al (2015) PI3 kinase mutations and mutational load as poor prognostic markers in diffuse glioma patients. Acta Neuropathol Commun 3:88. https://doi.org/10.1186/s40478-015-0265-4

41. Claus EB, Walsh KM, Wiencke JK, Molinaro AM, Wiemels JL, Schildkraut JM et al (2015) Survival and low-grade glioma: the emergence of genetic information. Neurosurg Focus 38(1):E6. https://doi.org/10.3171/2014.10.FOCUS12367

42. Eckel-Passow JE, Lachance DH, Molinaro AM, Walsh KM, Decker PA, Sicotte H et al (2015) Glioma groups based on 1p/19q, IDH, and TERT promoter mutations in tumors. N Engl J Med 372(26):2499–2508. https://doi.org/10.1056/NEJMoa1407279

43. Walsh KM, Wiencke JK, Lachance DH, Wiemels JL, Molinaro AM, Eckel-Passow JE et al (2015) Telomere maintenance and the etiology of adult glioma. Neuro Oncol 17(11):1445–1452. https://doi.org/10.1093/neuonc/nov082

44. Snyder LA, Wolf AB, Oppenlander ME, Bina R, Wilson JR, Ashby L et al (2014) The impact of extent of resection on malignant transformation of pure oligodendrogliomas. J Neurosurg 120(2):309–314. https://doi.org/10.3171/2013.10.JNS13368

45. Hervey-Jumper SL, Berger MS (2014) Role of surgical resection in low- and high-grade gliomas. Curr Treat Options Neurol 16(4):284

46. Frazier JL, Johnson MW, Burger PC, Weingart JD, Quinones-Hinojosa A (2010) Rapid malignant transformation of low-grade astrocytomas: report of 2 cases and review of the literature. World Neurosurg 73(1):53–62; discussion e5. https://doi.org/10.1016/j.surneu.2009.05.010

47. North CA, North RB, Epstein JA, Piantadosi S, Wharam MD (1990) Low-grade cerebral astrocytomas. Survival and quality of life after radiation therapy. Cancer 66(1):6–14

48. Whitton AC, Bloom HJ (1990) Low grade glioma of the cerebral hemispheres in adults: a retrospective analysis of 88 cases. Int J Radiat Oncol Biol Phys 18(4):783–786

49. Rajan B, Pickuth D, Ashley S, Traish D, Monro P, Elyan S et al (1994) The management of histologically unverified presumed cerebral gliomas with radiotherapy. Int J Radiat Oncol Biol Phys 28(2):405–413

50. Nicolato A, Gerosa MA, Fina P, Iuzzolino P, Giorgiutti F, Bricolo A (1995) Prognostic factors in low-grade supratentorial astrocytomas: a uni-multivariate statistical analysis in 76 surgically treated adult patients. Surg Neurol 44(3):208–221; discussion 21–3

51. Karim AB, Maat B, Hatlevoll R, Menten J, Rutten EH, Thomas DG et al (1996) A randomized trial on dose-response in radiation therapy of low-grade cerebral glioma: European Organization for Research and Treatment of Cancer (EORTC) Study 22844. Int J Radiat Oncol Biol Phys 36(3):549–556

52. Leighton C, Fisher B, Bauman G, Depiero S, Stitt L, MacDonald D et al (1997) Supratentorial low-grade glioma in adults: an analysis of prognostic factors and timing of radiation. J Clin Oncol 15(4):1294–1301. https://doi.org/10.1200/jco.1997.15.4.1294

53. Lote K, Egeland T, Hager B, Stenwig B, Skullerud K, Berg-Johnsen J et al (1997) Survival, prognostic factors, and therapeutic efficacy in low-grade glioma: a retrospective study in 379 patients. J Clin Oncol 15(9):3129–3140. https://doi.org/10.1200/jco.1997.15.9.3129

54. Peraud A, Ansari H, Bise K, Reulen H (1998) Clinical outcome of supratentorial astrocytoma WHO grade II. Acta Neurochir 140(12):1213–1222

55. van Veelen ML, Avezaat CJ, Kros JM, van Putten W, Vecht C (1998) Supratentorial low grade astrocytoma: prognostic factors, dedifferentiation, and the issue of early versus late surgery. J Neurol Neurosurg Psychiatry 64(5):581–587

56. Nakamura M, Konishi N, Tsunoda S, Nakase H, Tsuzuki T, Aoki H et al (2000) Analysis of prognostic and survival factors related to treatment of low-grade astrocytomas in adults. Oncology 58(2):108–116. https://doi.org/10.1159/000012087

57. Shaw E, Arusell R, Scheithauer B, O'Fallon J, O'Neill B, Dinapoli R et al (2002) Prospective randomized trial of low- versus high-dose radiation therapy in adults with supratentorial low-grade glioma: initial report of a North Central Cancer Treatment Group/Radiation Therapy Oncology Group/Eastern Cooperative Oncology Group study. J Clin Oncol 20(9):2267–2276. https://doi.org/10.1200/JCO.2002.09.126

58. Johannesen TB, Langmark F, Lote K (2003) Progress in long-term survival in adult patients with supratentorial low-grade gliomas: a population-based study of 993 patients in whom tumors were diagnosed between 1970 and 1993. J Neurosurg 99(5):854–862. https://doi.org/10.3171/jns.2003.99.5.0854

59. Scerrati M, Roselli R, Iacoangeli M, Pompucci A, Rossi GF (1996) Prognostic factors in low grade (WHO grade II) gliomas of the cerebral hemispheres: the role of surgery. J Neurol Neurosurg Psychiatry 61(3):291–296

60. Ito S, Chandler KL, Prados MD, Lamborn K, Wynne J, Malec MK et al (1994) Proliferative potential and prognostic evaluation of low-grade astrocytomas. J Neurooncol 19(1):1–9

61. Claus EB, Horlacher A, Hsu L, Schwartz RB, Dello-Iacono D, Talos F et al (2005) Survival rates in patients with low-grade glioma after intraoperative magnetic resonance image guidance. Cancer 103(6):1227–1233. https://doi.org/10.1002/cncr.20867

62. Yeh SA, Ho JT, Lui CC, Huang YJ, Hsiung CY, Huang EY (2005) Treatment outcomes and prognostic factors in patients with supratentorial low-grade gliomas. Br J Radiol 78(927):230–235. https://doi.org/10.1259/bjr/28534346

63. Shibamoto Y, Kitakabu Y, Takahashi M, Yamashita J, Oda Y, Kikuchi H et al (1993) Supratentorial low-grade astrocytoma. Correlation of computed tomography findings with effect of radiation therapy and prognostic variables. Cancer 72(1):190–195

64. Sanai N, Berger MS (2008) Glioma extent of resection and its impact on patient outcome. Neurosurgery 62(4):753–764.; ; discussion 264–6. https://doi.org/10.1227/01.neu.0000318159.21731.cf

65. Bauman G, Fisher B, Watling C, Cairncross JG, Macdonald D (2009) Adult supratentorial low-grade glioma: long-term experience at a single institution. Int J Radiat Oncol Biol Phys 75(5):1401–1407. https://doi.org/10.1016/j.ijrobp.2009.01.010

66. Incekara F, Olubiyi O, Ozdemir A, Lee T, Rigolo L, Golby A (2016) The value of pre- and intraoperative adjuncts on the extent of resection of hemispheric low-grade gliomas: a retrospective analysis. J Neurol Surg A Cent Eur Neurosurg 77(2):79–87. https://doi.org/10.1055/s-0035-1551830

67. Jakola AS, Myrmel KS, Kloster R, Torp SH, Lindal S, Unsgard G et al (2012) Comparison of a strategy favoring early surgical resection vs a strategy favoring watchful waiting in low-grade gliomas. JAMA 308(18):1881–1888. https://doi.org/10.1001/jama.2012.12807

68. Hervey-Jumper SL, Li J, Lau D, Molinaro AM, Perry DW, Meng L et al (2015) Awake craniotomy to maximize glioma resection: methods and technical nuances over a 27-year period. J Neurosurg 123(2):325–339. https://doi.org/10.3171/2014.10.JNS141520

69. Penfield W, Boldrey E (1937) Somatic motor and sensory representation in the cerebral cortex of man as studied by electrical stimulation. Brain 60(4):389–443. https://doi.org/10.1093/brain/60.4.389

70. Foerster O (1931) The cerebral cortex in man. Lancet 221:309–312

71. Herholz K, Thiel A, Wienhard K, Pietrzyk U, von Stockhausen HM, Karbe H et al (1996) Individual functional anatomy of verb generation. Neuroimage 3(3 Pt 1):185–194. https://doi.org/10.1006/nimg.1996.0020

72. Sanai N, Berger MS (2009) Operative techniques for gliomas and the value of extent of resection. Neurotherapeutics 6(3):478–486. https://doi.org/10.1016/j.nurt.2009.04.005

73. Schneider JP, Trantakis C, Rubach M, Schulz T, Dietrich J, Winkler D et al (2005) Intraoperative MRI to guide the resection of primary supratentorial glioblastoma multiforme—a quantitative radiological analysis. Neuroradiology 47(7):489–500. https://doi.org/10.1007/s00234-005-1397-1

74. Senft C, Bink A, Franz K, Vatter H, Gasser T, Seifert V (2011) Intraoperative MRI guidance and extent of resection in glioma surgery: a randomised, controlled trial. Lancet Oncol 12(11):997–1003. https://doi.org/10.1016/s1470-2045(11)70196-6

75. Stummer W, Stocker S, Wagner S, Stepp H, Fritsch C, Goetz C et al (1998) Intraoperative detection

of malignant gliomas by 5-aminolevulinic acid-induced porphyrin fluorescence. Neurosurgery 42(3):518–525; discussion 25-6

76. Marbacher S, Klinger E, Schwyzer L, Fischer I, Nevzati E, Diepers M et al (2014) Use of fluorescence to guide resection or biopsy of primary brain tumors and brain metastases. Neurosurg Focus 36(2):E10. https://doi.org/10.3171/2013.12.FOCUS13464

77. Stummer W, Pichlmeier U, Meinel T, Wiestler OD, Zanella F, Reulen H-J (2006) Fluorescence-guided surgery with 5-aminolevulinic acid for resection of malignant glioma: a randomised controlled multicentre phase III trial. Lancet Oncol 7(5):392–401. https://doi.org/10.1016/s1470-2045(06)70665-9

78. Cairncross G, Macdonald D, Ludwin S, Lee D, Cascino T, Buckner J et al (1994) Chemotherapy for anaplastic oligodendroglioma. National Cancer Institute of Canada Clinical Trials Group. J Clin Oncol 12(10):2013–2021. https://doi.org/10.1200/jco.1994.12.10.2013

79. Yung WK, Prados MD, Yaya-Tur R, Rosenfeld SS, Brada M, Friedman HS et al (1999) Multicenter phase II trial of temozolomide in patients with anaplastic astrocytoma or anaplastic oligoastrocytoma at first relapse. Temodal Brain Tumor Group J Clin Oncol 17(9):2762–2771. https://doi.org/10.1200/jco.1999.17.9.2762

80. van den Bent MJ, Taphoorn MJ, Brandes AA, Menten J, Stupp R, Frenay M et al (2003) Phase II study of first-line chemotherapy with temozolomide in recurrent oligodendroglial tumors: the European Organization for Research and Treatment of Cancer Brain Tumor Group Study 26971. J Clin Oncol 21(13):2525–2528. https://doi.org/10.1200/jco.2003.12.015

81. Cairncross JG, Ueki K, Zlatescu MC, Lisle DK, Finkelstein DM, Hammond RR et al (1998) Specific genetic predictors of chemotherapeutic response and survival in patients with anaplastic oligodendrogliomas. J Natl Cancer Inst 90(19):1473–1479

82. Taal W, Dubbink HJ, Zonnenberg CB, Zonnenberg BA, Postma TJ, Gijtenbeek JM et al (2011) First-line temozolomide chemotherapy in progressive low-grade astrocytomas after radiotherapy: molecular characteristics in relation to response. Neuro Oncol 13(2):235–241. https://doi.org/10.1093/neuonc/noq177

83. Cairncross G, Wang M, Shaw E, Jenkins R, Brachman D, Buckner J et al (2013) Phase III trial of chemoradiotherapy for anaplastic oligodendroglioma: long-term results of RTOG 9402. J Clin Oncol 31(3):337–343. https://doi.org/10.1200/jco.2012.43.2674

84. van den Bent MJ, Brandes AA, Taphoorn MJ, Kros JM, Kouwenhoven MC, Delattre JY et al (2013) Adjuvant procarbazine, lomustine, and vincristine chemotherapy in newly diagnosed anaplastic oligodendroglioma: long-term follow-up of EORTC brain tumor group study 26951. J Clin Oncol 31(3):344–350. https://doi.org/10.1200/jco.2012.43.2229

85. van den Bent MJ, Baumert B, Erridge SC, Vogelbaum MA, Nowak AK, Sanson M et al (2017) Interim results from the CATNON trial (EORTC study 26053-22054) of treatment with concurrent and adjuvant temozolomide for 1p/19q non-co-deleted anaplastic glioma: a phase 3, randomised, open-label intergroup study. Lancet 390(10103):1645–1653. https://doi.org/10.1016/s0140-6736(17)31442-3

86. Cairncross JG, Wang M, Jenkins RB, Shaw EG, Giannini C, Brachman DG et al (2014) Benefit from procarbazine, lomustine, and vincristine in oligodendroglial tumors is associated with mutation of IDH. J Clin Oncol 32(8):783–790. https://doi.org/10.1200/jco.2013.49.3726

87. van den Bent MJ, Erdem-Eraslan L, Idbaih A, de Rooi J, Eilers PH, Spliet WG et al (2013) MGMT-STP27 methylation status as predictive marker for response to PCV in anaplastic oligodendrogliomas and oligoastrocytomas. A report from EORTC study 26951. Clin Cancer Res 19(19):5513–5522. https://doi.org/10.1158/1078-0432.Ccr-13-1157

88. Wick W, Roth P, Hartmann C, Hau P, Nakamura M, Stockhammer F et al (2016) Long-term analysis of the NOA-04 randomized phase III trial of sequential radiochemotherapy of anaplastic glioma with PCV or temozolomide. Neuro Oncol 18(11):1529–1537. https://doi.org/10.1093/neuonc/now133

89. Baumert BG, Hegi ME, van den Bent MJ, von Deimling A, Gorlia T, Hoang-Xuan K et al (2016) Temozolomide chemotherapy versus radiotherapy in high-risk low-grade glioma (EORTC 22033-26033): a randomised, open-label, phase 3 intergroup study. Lancet Oncol 17(11):1521–1532. https://doi.org/10.1016/s1470-2045(16)30313-8

90. Wahl M, Phillips JJ, Molinaro AM, Lin Y, Perry A, Haas-Kogan DA et al (2017) Chemotherapy for adult low-grade gliomas: clinical outcomes by molecular subtype in a phase II study of adjuvant temozolomide. Neuro Oncol 19(2):242–251. https://doi.org/10.1093/neuonc/now176

91. Izquierdo C, Alentorn A, Idbaih A, Simo M, Kaloshi G, Ricard D et al (2018) Long-term impact of temozolomide on 1p/19q-codeleted low-grade glioma growth kinetics. J Neurooncol 136(3):533–539. https://doi.org/10.1007/s11060-017-2677-4

92. Taal W, van der Rijt CC, Dinjens WN, Sillevis Smitt PA, Wertenbroek AA, Bromberg JE et al (2015) Treatment of large low-grade oligodendroglial tumors with upfront procarbazine, lomustine, and vincristine chemotherapy with long follow-up: a retrospective cohort study with growth kinetics. J Neurooncol 121(2):365–372. https://doi.org/10.1007/s11060-014-1641-9

93. Thomas AA, Abrey LE, Terziev R, Raizer J, Martinez NL, Forsyth P et al (2017) Multicenter phase II study of temozolomide and myeloablative chemotherapy with autologous stem cell transplant for newly diagnosed anaplastic oligodendroglioma. Neuro Oncol 19(10):1380–1390. https://doi.org/10.1093/neuonc/nox086

94. Johnson BE, Mazor T, Hong C, Barnes M, Aihara K, CY ML et al (2014) Mutational analysis reveals the origin and therapy-driven evolution of recurrent glioma. Science 343(6167):189–193. https://doi.org/10.1126/science.1239947

95. Chang S, Zhang P, Cairncross JG, Gilbert MR, Bahary JP, Dolinskas CA et al (2017) Phase III randomized study of radiation and temozolomide versus radiation and nitrosourea therapy for anaplastic astrocytoma: results of NRG Oncology RTOG 9813. Neuro Oncol 19(2):252–258. https://doi.org/10.1093/neuonc/now236

96. Lassman AB, Iwamoto FM, Cloughesy TF, Aldape KD, Rivera AL, Eichler AF et al (2011) International retrospective study of over 1000 adults with anaplastic oligodendroglial tumors. Neuro Oncol 13(6):649–659. https://doi.org/10.1093/neuonc/nor040

97. Figarella-Branger D, Mokhtari K, Dehais C, Jouvet A, Uro-Coste E, Colin C et al (2014) Mitotic index, microvascular proliferation, and necrosis define 3 groups of 1p/19q codeleted anaplastic oligodendrogliomas associated with different genomic alterations. Neuro Oncol 16(9):1244–1254. https://doi.org/10.1093/neuonc/nou047

98. Desjardins A, Reardon DA, Herndon JE 2nd, Marcello J, Quinn JA, Rich JN et al (2008) Bevacizumab plus irinotecan in recurrent WHO grade 3 malignant gliomas. Clin Cancer Res 14(21):7068–7073. https://doi.org/10.1158/1078-0432.Ccr-08-0260

99. Chamberlain MC, Johnston S (2009) Bevacizumab for recurrent alkylator-refractory anaplastic oligodendroglioma. Cancer 115(8):1734–1743. https://doi.org/10.1002/cncr.24179

100. Chamberlain MC, Johnston S (2009) Salvage chemotherapy with bevacizumab for recurrent alkylator-refractory anaplastic astrocytoma. J Neurooncol 91(3):359–367. https://doi.org/10.1007/s11060-008-9722-2

101. Taillibert S, Vincent LA, Granger B, Marie Y, Carpentier C, Guillevin R et al (2009) Bevacizumab and irinotecan for recurrent oligodendroglial tumors. Neurology 72(18):1601–1606. https://doi.org/10.1212/WNL.0b013e3181a413be

102. Van Den Bent MJ, Klein M, Smits M, Reijneveld JC, Idbaih A, Clement P et al (2017) Final results of the EORTC Brain Tumor Group randomized phase II TAVAREC trial on temozolomide with or without bevacizumab in 1st recurrence grade II/III glioma without 1p/19q co-deletion. J Clin Oncol 35(15):2009

103. Cairncross JG, Macdonald DR (1988) Successful chemotherapy for recurrent malignant oligodendroglioma. Ann Neurol 23(4):360–364. https://doi.org/10.1002/ana.410230408

104. van den Bent M, Kros J, Schellens J, Krouwer H, Zonnenberg BA, Heimans J et al (1996) PCV-chemotherapy in anaplastic oligodendroglioma: time for a prospective, randomised study. J Neurooncol 30:130

105. van den Bent MJ, Chinot O, Boogerd W, Bravo Marques J, Taphoorn MJ, Kros JM et al (2003) Second-line chemotherapy with temozolomide in recurrent oligodendroglioma after PCV (procarbazine, lomustine and vincristine) chemotherapy: EORTC Brain Tumor Group phase II study 26972. Ann Oncol 14(4):599–602

106. Triebels VH, Taphoorn MJ, Brandes AA, Menten J, Frenay M, Tosoni A et al (2004) Salvage PCV chemotherapy for temozolomide-resistant oligodendrogliomas. Neurology 63(5):904–906

107. Kouwenhoven MC, Kros JM, French PJ, Biemond-ter Stege EM, Graveland WJ, Taphoorn MJ et al (2006) 1p/19q loss within oligodendroglioma is predictive for response to first line temozolomide but not to salvage treatment. Eur J Cancer 42(15):2499–2503. https://doi.org/10.1016/j.ejca.2006.05.021

108. Chamberlain MC (2015) Salvage therapy with lomustine for temozolomide refractory recurrent anaplastic astrocytoma: a retrospective study. J Neurooncol 122(2):329–338. https://doi.org/10.1007/s11060-014-1714-9

109. Pignatti F, van den Bent M, Curran D, Debruyne C, Sylvester R, Therasse P et al (2002) Prognostic factors for survival in adult patients with cerebral low-grade glioma. J Clin Oncol 20(8):2076–2084. https://doi.org/10.1200/jco.2002.08.121

110. Sun H, Yin L, Li S, Han S, Song G, Liu N et al (2013) Prognostic significance of IDH mutation in adult low-grade gliomas: a meta-analysis. J Neurooncol 113(2):277–284. https://doi.org/10.1007/s11060-013-1107-5

111. Reuss DE, Kratz A, Sahm F, Capper D, Schrimpf D, Koelsche C et al (2015) Adult IDH wild type astrocytomas biologically and clinically resolve into other tumor entities. Acta Neuropathol 130(3):407–417. https://doi.org/10.1007/s00401-015-1454-8

112. Jenkins RB, Blair H, Ballman KV, Giannini C, Arusell RM, Law M et al (2006) A t(1;19)(q10;p10) mediates the combined deletions of 1p and 19q and predicts a better prognosis of patients with oligodendroglioma. Cancer Res 66(20):9852–9861. https://doi.org/10.1158/0008-5472.Can-06-1796

113. Brown PD, Buckner JC, O'Fallon JR, Iturria NL, Brown CA, O'Neill BP et al (2003) Effects of radiotherapy on cognitive function in patients with low-grade glioma measured by the folstein mini-mental state examination. J Clin Oncol 21(13):2519–2524. https://doi.org/10.1200/jco.2003.04.172

114. van den Bent MJ, Afra D, de Witte O, Ben Hassel M, Schraub S, Hoang-Xuan K et al (2005) Long-term efficacy of early versus delayed radiotherapy for low-grade astrocytoma and oligodendroglioma in adults: the EORTC 22845 randomised trial. Lancet 366(9490):985–990. https://doi.org/10.1016/s0140-6736(05)67070-5

115. Shaw EG, Berkey B, Coons SW, Bullard D, Brachman D, Buckner JC et al (2008) Recurrence following neurosurgeon-determined gross-total resection of adult supratentorial low-grade glioma: results of a prospective clinical trial. J Neurosurg 109(5):835–841. https://doi.org/10.3171/jns/2008/109/11/0835

116. Reijneveld JC, Taphoorn MJ, Coens C, Bromberg JE, Mason WP, Hoang-Xuan K et al (2016) Health-related quality of life in patients with high-risk low-grade glioma (EORTC 22033-26033): a randomised, open-label, phase 3 intergroup study. Lancet

Oncol 17(11):1533–1542. https://doi.org/10.1016/s1470-2045(16)30305-9

117. Burnet NG, Jena R, Burton KE, Tudor GS, Scaife JE, Harris F et al (2014) Clinical and practical considerations for the use of intensity-modulated radiotherapy and image guidance in neuro-oncology. Clin Oncol (R Coll Radiol) 26(7):395–406. https://doi.org/10.1016/j.clon.2014.04.024

118. Hermanto U, Frija EK, Lii MJ, Chang EL, Mahajan A, Woo SY (2007) Intensity-modulated radiotherapy (IMRT) and conventional three-dimensional conformal radiotherapy for high-grade gliomas: does IMRT increase the integral dose to normal brain? Int J Radiat Oncol Biol Phys 67(4):1135–1144. https://doi.org/10.1016/j.ijrobp.2006.10.032

119. Navarria P, Pessina F, Cozzi L, Ascolese AM, Lobefalo F, Stravato A et al (2016) Can advanced new radiation therapy technologies improve outcome of high grade glioma (HGG) patients? analysis of 3D-conformal radiotherapy (3DCRT) versus volumetric-modulated arc therapy (VMAT) in patients treated with surgery, concomitant and adjuvant chemo-radiotherapy. BMC Cancer 16:362. https://doi.org/10.1186/s12885-016-2399-6

120. Yang Z, Zhang Z, Wang X, Hu Y, Lyu Z, Huo L et al (2016) Intensity-modulated radiotherapy for gliomas: dosimetric effects of changes in gross tumor volume on organs at risk and healthy brain tissue. OncoTargets and therapy 9:3545–3554. https://doi.org/10.2147/ott.S100455

121. Gondi V, Pugh SL, Tome WA, Caine C, Corn B, Kanner A et al (2014) Preservation of memory with conformal avoidance of the hippocampal neural stem-cell compartment during whole-brain radiotherapy for brain metastases (RTOG 0933): a phase II multi-institutional trial. J Clin Oncol 32(34):3810–3816. https://doi.org/10.1200/jco.2014.57.2909

122. Vieira WA, Weltman E, Chen MJ, da Silva NS, Cappellano AM, Pereira LD et al (2014) Ototoxicity evaluation in medulloblastoma patients treated with involved field boost using intensity-modulated radiation therapy (IMRT): a retrospective review. Radiat Oncol 9:158. https://doi.org/10.1186/1748-717x-9-158

123. Hauswald H, Rieken S, Ecker S, Kessel KA, Herfarth K, Debus J et al (2012) First experiences in treatment of low-grade glioma grade I and II with proton therapy. Radiat Oncol 7:189. https://doi.org/10.1186/1748-717x-7-189

124. Wilkinson B, Morgan H, Gondi V, Larson GL, Hartsell WF, Laramore GE et al (2016) Low levels of acute toxicity associated with proton therapy for low-grade glioma: a Proton Collaborative Group Study. Int J Radiat Oncol Biol Phys 96(2s):E135. https://doi.org/10.1016/j.ijrobp.2016.06.930

125. Sherman JC, Colvin MK, Mancuso SM, Batchelor TT, Oh KS, Loeffler JS et al (2016) Neurocognitive effects of proton radiation therapy in adults with low-grade glioma. J Neurooncol 126(1):157–164. https://doi.org/10.1007/s11060-015-1952-5

126. Shih HA, Sherman JC, Nachtigall LB, Colvin MK, Fullerton BC, Daartz J et al (2015) Proton therapy for low-grade gliomas: results from a prospective trial. Cancer 121(10):1712–1719. https://doi.org/10.1002/cncr.29237

127. van Thuijl HF, Mazor T, Johnson BE, Fouse SD, Aihara K, Hong C et al (2015) Evolution of DNA repair defects during malignant progression of low-grade gliomas after temozolomide treatment. Acta Neuropathol 129(4):597–607. https://doi.org/10.1007/s00401-015-1403-6

128. Choi S, Yu Y, Grimmer MR, Wahl M, Chang SM, Costello JF (2018) Temozolomide-associated hypermutation in gliomas. Neuro Oncol 20(10):1300–1309. https://doi.org/10.1093/neuonc/noy016

129. Platten M, Bunse L, Riehl D, Bunse T, Ochs K, Wick W (2018) Vaccine strategies in gliomas. Curr Treat Options Neurol 20(5):11. https://doi.org/10.1007/s11940-018-0498-1

130. Clark O, Yen K, Mellinghoff IK (2016) Molecular pathways: isocitrate dehydrogenase mutations in cancer. Clin Cancer Res 22(8):1837–1842. https://doi.org/10.1158/1078-0432.Ccr-13-1333

131. Molenaar RJ, Botman D, Smits MA, Hira VV, van Lith SA, Stap J et al (2015) Radioprotection of IDH1-mutated cancer cells by the IDH1-mutant inhibitor AGI-5198. Cancer Res 75(22):4790–4802. https://doi.org/10.1158/0008-5472.Can-14-3603

132. Wang P, Wu J, Ma S, Zhang L, Yao J, Hoadley KA et al (2015) Oncometabolite D-2-hydroxyglutarate inhibits ALKBH DNA repair enzymes and sensitizes IDH mutant cells to alkylating agents. Cell Rep 13(11):2353–2361. https://doi.org/10.1016/j.celrep.2015.11.029

133. Mazor T, Chesnelong C, Pankov A, Jalbert LE, Hong C, Hayes J et al (2017) Clonal expansion and epigenetic reprogramming following deletion or amplification of mutant IDH1. Proc Natl Acad Sci U S A 114(40):10743–10748. https://doi.org/10.1073/pnas.1708914114

134. Stein EM, DiNardo CD, Pollyea DA, Fathi AT, Roboz GJ, Altman JK et al (2017) Enasidenib in mutant IDH2 relapsed or refractory acute myeloid leukemia. Blood 130(6):722–731. https://doi.org/10.1182/blood-2017-04-779405

135. Lu Y, Kwintkiewicz J, Liu Y, Tech K, Frady LN, Su YT et al (2017) Chemosensitivity of IDH1-mutated gliomas due to an impairment in PARP1-mediated DNA repair. Cancer Res 77(7):1709–1718. https://doi.org/10.1158/0008-5472.Can-16-2773

136. Sulkowski PL, Corso CD, Robinson ND, Scanlon SE, Purshouse KR, Bai H et al (2017) 2-Hydroxyglutarate produced by neomorphic IDH mutations suppresses homologous recombination and induces PARP inhibitor sensitivity. Sci Transl Med 9(375). https://doi.org/10.1126/scitranslmed.aal2463.

137. Tateishi K, Higuchi F, Miller JJ, Koerner MVA, Lelic N, Shankar GM et al (2017) The alkylating chemotherapeutic temozolomide induces metabolic stress in IDH1-mutant cancers and potentiates NAD(+) depletion-mediated cytotoxicity. Cancer Res 77(15):4102–4115. https://doi.org/10.1158/0008-5472.Can-16-2263

Glioblastoma

10

Michael Weller, Colin Watts, David A. Reardon, and Minesh P. Mehta

10.1 Introduction

This chapter on glioblastoma is based on its definition in the revision of the fourth edition of the World Health Organization (WHO) Classification of Tumors of the Central Nervous System [1]. Glioblastoma is a tumor presumed to be of neuroglial origin and characterized by neovascularization and areas of focal necrosis commonly attributed to hypoxia [2]. It has been assigned the WHO grade IV, signifying an overall poor prognosis.

M. Weller (✉)
Department of Neurology, University Hospital and University of Zurich, Zurich, Switzerland
e-mail: michael.weller@usz.ch

C. Watts
Institute of Cancer and Genomic Sciences, University of Birmingham, Birmingham, UK
e-mail: C.Watts.2@bham.ac.uk

D. A. Reardon
Department of Medical Oncology, Center for Neuro-Oncology, Dana-Farber Cancer Institute, Boston, MA, USA
e-mail: david_reardon@dfci.harvard.edu

M. P. Mehta
Miami Cancer Institute, Baptist Health of South Florida and Florida International University, Baptist Hospital, Miami, FL, USA

10.2 Epidemiology

The annual incidence of glioblastoma is approximately 3 per 100,000 with probably similar risk throughout the world [3]. Glioblastoma has been diagnosed very rarely even in newborns, but the risk appears to increase steadily with age, resulting in a gradual increase of median age in the aging Western countries toward the mid- to late 1960s. In addition to age, genetic predisposition syndromes, e.g., affecting the p53 or DNA mismatch repair genes, or exposure of the cranium to irradiation have been identified as risk factors [4]. Studies on an association of glioblastoma risk with the use of mobile phones have remained largely inconclusive, although doubts on their safety continue to be expressed [5]. In contrast, there may be a small risk reduction in individuals affected by allergies [6]. No general cost-effective screening strategies are available; therefore, screening is limited to individuals at high genetic risk, on an individual case basis. Prevention strategies are not established, although first principle extrapolation would suggest minimization of exposure of the cranium to unnecessary radiation as one possible controllable approach; in this context, as an indirect example, reduction of exposure to radiation during dental procedures has been shown to reduce the risk of development of meningioma.

© Springer Nature Switzerland AG 2019
J.-C. Tonn et al. (eds.), *Oncology of CNS Tumors*, https://doi.org/10.1007/978-3-030-04152-6_10

10.3 Diagnosis

Glioblastomas are commonly diagnosed in patients with clinical features suggestive of a space-occupying lesion, mostly new onset seizures or gradual onset of focal neurological signs, personality changes, and evidence of increased intracranial pressure. The neurological workup of all brain tumor patients should ideally not only include a Mini Mental State Examination (MMSE) or a Montreal Cognitive Assessment (MOCA) but also a neuropsychological evaluation as a baseline for assessment in the further course of disease. The latter can be challenging for glioblastoma patients who present acutely to the Emergency Department, with rapidly progressive neurologic and cognitive decline.

Neuroimaging, in particular magnetic resonance imaging (MRI), remains the gold standard of diagnostic assessment in patients suspected of harboring a brain tumor [7]. MRI is also the preferred assessment modality in the course of disease, in particular to determine the activity of therapeutic interventions [8]. Spinal MRI is usually unnecessary except for patients with clinical symptoms or signs of spinal disease, or those presenting with a pattern of spread described as *gliomatosis cerebri*, or for those at recurrence who have subventricular spread of disease. Amino acid tracer-based positron emission tomography (PET) is increasingly used at specialized sites to identify the metabolically most active tumor region as a guidance for biopsy, to delineate the extension of tumor spread, and to distinguish between tumor progression and therapy-induced imaging changes [9], as well as, in an experimental context, to identify regions of the tumor that could be targeted for radiotherapy dose escalation. Serum or cerebrospinal fluid tests play no role as a screening or diagnostic tool for the detection of glioblastoma. The definitive diagnosis of glioblastoma is tissue-based and requires a surgical procedure. The diagnostic, therapeutic, and supportive care management plan for patients with glioblastoma should be developed ideally early on in a multidisciplinary setting according to institutional guidelines and should involve dedicated neuroradiologists and neuro-

pathologists as well as neurosurgeons, radiation oncologists, and neuro-oncologists.

10.4 Surgery

Surgery is an essential part of the multidisciplinary management of glioblastoma. The main objective of surgery is to obtain tissue for a molecular and histopathological diagnosis. The decision to operate should be based on clinical examination of the patient coupled with a detailed evaluation of MR imaging data. The functional status of the patient at presentation is critical in the surgical decision-making process [10]. Surgery may involve an open procedure via a craniotomy or a stereotactic biopsy. A stereotactic approach will allow precision biopsies with very low morbidity and mortality in experienced centers. In such situations, cytological specimens or frozen sections should be examined for quality and quantity before surgery is terminated.

A second objective of surgery is to remove as much of the tumor as possible without compromising neurological function. This is achieved via an open craniotomy, and the extent of cytoreduction is dependent on the proximity of eloquent functional brain tissue. Cytoreduction will facilitate radiotherapy by minimizing side effects caused by tumor swelling after the radiation.

Many studies have assessed the association of extent of resection with outcomes in glioblastoma patients over the past 20 years [11]. The European Organization for Research and Treatment of Cancer (EORTC) 26,981-22,981/ National Institute of Canada Clinical Trials Groups (NCIC) CE3 randomized phase III trial showed that those patients undergoing complete resection had a longer survival than those that underwent partial resection [12]. Further studies suggest similar survival advantage in patients who underwent complete resection versus partial resection, providing level 2b evidence of the benefit of surgery in glioblastoma. A recent meta-analysis of 12,607 patients from 34 studies concluded that there is an improvement in survival times, functional recovery, and tumor recurrence rate with increasing extents of safe resection [13]. However, there is an important but inherent bias in all studies that suggest a survival advantage; patients who undergo total resection are usually younger, with a good performance status, and have a glioma in a non-eloquent location. These data and informed guidelines provide a consensus that maximal resection likely provides a survival benefit. More recently research has focused on methods to maximize glioma resection using novel surgical approaches.

Advances in neurosurgical techniques allow safer, more aggressive surgery to maximize tumor resection while minimizing neurological deficit [11]. Surgical adjuncts including advanced neuronavigation, intraoperative magnetic resonance imaging, high-frequency ultrasonography, fluorescence-guided microsurgery using intraoperative fluorescence [14], functional mapping of motor and language pathways, and locally delivered therapies are extending the armamentarium of the neurosurgeon to provide patients with the best outcome (Fig. 10.1). Operating on elderly patients and those with recurrent disease, although controversial, is becoming more common due to emerging neurosurgical approaches.

Critically, these advances are based on the fact that preserving neurological function remains of higher priority than extent of resection, because no treatment approach to glioblastoma can be considered curative [15]. The extent of resection and potential complications from surgery should be documented by MRI within 24–72 h after surgery. Occasionally patients with large residual tumors that could have been resected without major risk are referred for a second opinion. A second look operation might be considered in such situations before further treatment is initiated.

The blood brain barrier is an obstacle that impairs selective delivery of systemic treatments to the local brain tumor area. Craniotomy and tumor resection provide an accessible cavity for local treatment of disease. BCNU (carmustine) wafers are an option of local delivery of chemotherapy that directly diffuses into the residual tumor cavity without causing systemic toxicity. Early studies in both the primary and recurrent setting provided evidence that the use of carmustine wafers in malignant glioma therapy was both safe and potentially efficacious. However,

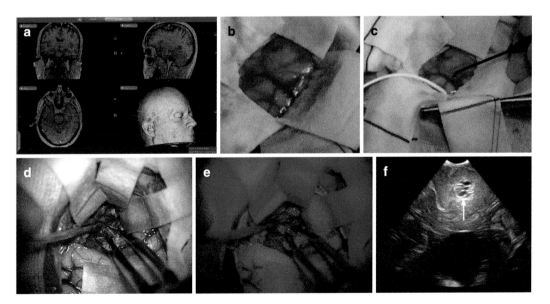

Fig. 10.1 Surgical approaches to glioblastoma. Modern surgical practice involves a multimodal approach: preoperative planning is coupled with intraoperative neuronavigation (**a**). Potentially eloquent but normal looking brain (**b**) can be further evaluated using intraoperative stimulation (**c**). These techniques can be used throughout the operation and can be augmented by intraoperative 5-aminolevulinic acid (**e**) and ultrasound (**f**) in selected patients

Table 10.1 Standards of care for glioblastoma per WHO classification

Tumor type	First-line treatment[a]	Salvage therapies[b,c]	Comments/references
Glioblastoma, IDH wild type, including giant cell glioblastoma, gliosarcoma, and epithelioid glioblastoma	TMZ/RT→TMZ, >70 years or reduced KPS RT (MGMT unmethylated), or TMZ/RT→TMZ or TMZ (MGMT methylated), ± tumor-treating fields[c]	Nitrosourea or TMZ rechallenge or bevacizumab[c], RT for RT-naïve patients	Stupp et al. [12] Stupp et al. [36] Wick et al. [43] Perry et al. [31]
Glioblastoma, IDH-mutant	(TMZ)/RT→TMZ	Nitrosourea (or TMZ rechallenge) or bevacizumab	Per extrapolation from IDH-mutant anaplastic astrocytoma [19]
Glioblastoma, NOS	TMZ/RT→TMZ, > 70 years or reduced KPS RT (MGMT unmethylated), or TMZ or TMZ/RT→TMZ (MGMT methylated), ± tumor-treating fields[c]	Nitrosourea or TMZ rechallenge or bevacizumab[c], RT for RT-naïve patients	See glioblastoma, IDH wild type

[a]Maximum safe surgery as feasible should be attempted in all patients with glioblastoma
[b]Second surgery should always be considered, but clinical benefit is probably limited to patients with tumors that can be gross totally resected
[c]Depending on local availability and reimbursement

subsequent clinical trial data confirmed that BCNU wafers do not confer a survival advantage in glioblastoma [16, 17]. There continues to be controversy on the safety and efficacy of BCNU wafers, and they are not recommended in current guidelines [15].

10.5 Histopathology and Molecular Diagnostics

The classification of glioblastoma should be based on the current WHO classification [1]. The majority of histological glioblastomas are IDH wild type, including the morphological variants of giant cell glioblastoma, gliosarcoma, and epitheloid glioblastoma. There are to date no clinical management implications of these glioblastoma variants. About 50% of the rare epitheloid glioblastomas carry a potentially "druggable" BRAF^{V600E} mutation. Molecular studies should include assessment of the IDH status first by immunohistochemistry for IDH1^{R132H} which represents the vast majority of mutations. If mutant IDH1^{R132H} protein is not detected, then sequencing to detect rare, other IDH1 mutations as well as IDH2 mutations should follow. This recommendation is valid only for patients younger than 55–60 years since IDH mutations are exceed-

ingly rare in the elderly [18]. "Not otherwise specified" (NOS) categories have been included in the WHO classification to label gliomas that were not tested for the relevant markers or that had inconclusive test results [1]. The following recommendations apply primarily to IDH wild-type glioblastoma. IDH-mutant glioblastomas are no longer uniformly treated the same way as IDH wild-type glioblastomas in many centers but may also be treated like IDH-mutant anaplastic astrocytoma [15], e.g., according to the results of the CATNON trial with maintenance temozolomide following resection and radiotherapy [19] (Table 10.1). Of note, to determine the potential impact of concurrent radiochemotherapy on outcome in patients with anaplastic astrocytoma in the CATNON trial requires longer follow-up.

10.6 Newly Diagnosed Glioblastoma

Further treatment beyond surgery is selected based on major prognostic factors. Outcome is overall significantly better for younger patients and patients in good general and neurological condition. Extent of resection has been confirmed as a favorable prognostic factor in essentially all major clinical trials, but it remains open to what extent this reflects benefit from reduced tumor burden versus less malignant biological behavior of lesions considered to be gross totally resectable.

Radiotherapy is part of the standard of care for glioblastoma since roughly a doubling of median survival was demonstrated 40 years ago [20] (Fig. 10.2). The superiority of radiotherapy over best supportive care was confirmed in an elderly glioblastoma patient population three decades later [21]. The target volume of radiotherapy usually comprises the resection cavity, any residual contrast-enhancing tumor, and a margin to cover microscopic disease, adapted to consider anatomical barriers to tumor cell spread; the FLAIR signal from the postoperative MRI is often used to guide this decision [22]. The optimal extent of this margin remains one of the unresolved radiotherapy questions, and a 2 cm margin is common, though not universally chosen. The standard dose for glioblastoma is 60 Gy delivered in fractions of 1.8–2 Gy fractions. An accelerated regimen of 40 Gy given in 15 fractions is commonly chosen for patients with reduced performance status or in the elderly [23]. Alternative hyper- or hypofrac-

tionated radiotherapy schedules, brachytherapy, and radiosurgery approaches have been explored in patients with newly diagnosed glioblastoma, but have not been shown to be superior to standard radiotherapy in randomized trials. Although focal radiotherapy dose-escalation techniques have not improved overall survival, it must be borne in mind that these trials and efforts were almost exclusively conducted in the pre-temozolomide era. The implication herein is that if microscopic disease remains inadequately addressed by radiotherapy—likely a very common phenomenon, as the true extent of microscopic spread is impossible to define and has been demonstrated to substantially exceed the conventional 2 cm margins used in radiotherapy—and dose escalation is attempted to a focal area without addressing the microscopic disease, no disease control benefit can be achieved. This has been validated in various dose escalation studies where high radiotherapy doses essentially necrotize the tumor within the high dose range, but peripheral recurrences still occur in more than 80% of the patients. The advent of temozolomide, with its potential ability to control microscopic disease, has therefore

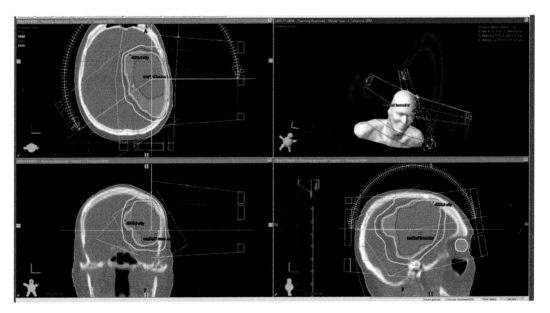

Fig. 10.2 Radiotherapy of glioblastoma. Volumetrically modulated arc therapy (VMAT) plan for a patient with left temporal glioblastoma. The volumes in purple and teal identify postoperative MR T1 contrast enhancement and

FLAIR abnormalities, which are encompassed by the radiotherapy prescription isodose lines in pink and yellow, using the arced field arrangement illustrated in the figure on the top right

resurrected the interest in focal dose escalation in radiotherapy, with a number of clinical trials underway.

Concomitant and six cycles of maintenance temozolomide chemotherapy plus radiotherapy (TMZ/RT→TMZ) became the standard of care for newly diagnosed adult glioblastoma patients in good general and neurological condition and aged up to 70 years in 2005 [12, 24]. Post hoc subgroup analysis revealed that the survival benefit afforded by the addition of temozolomide was essentially limited to patients with tumors which exhibited methylation of the promoter region of the MGMT gene [25]. The MGMT protein can repair the methylating DNA lesion induced by temozolomide. Accordingly, loss of MGMT gene expression renders cells sensitive to temozolomide. Despite considerable efforts to demonstrate that more intense temozolomide exposure up-front might improve outcome, neither increasing the dose of temozolomide in the first six cycles in a randomized trial [26] nor prolonging standard dose temozolomide beyond six cycles in two retrospective studies were associated with improved survival [27, 28].

Given the concern of limited tolerability of combined modality treatment and the large proportion of elderly patients who were not adequately represented in the first phase III trial demonstrating the efficacy of temozolomide [24], two ensuing trials compared radiotherapy alone with temozolomide alone in the elderly, NOA-08 and the Nordic trial [29, 30]. Both trials confirmed the superiority of temozolomide over radiotherapy in patients with tumors with MGMT promoter methylation but at the same time demonstrated that radiotherapy alone was superior to temozolomide alone in patients with tumors without MGMT promoter methylation. These studies thus defined standards of care for patients depending on MGMT promoter methylation status who are not considered eligible for combined modality treatment. More recently, the NCIC CE.6/EORTC 26062 trial revisited the comparison of TMZ/RT→TMZ versus RT alone [24], using a hypofractionated radiotherapy regimen [23], for newly diagnosed glioblastoma

patients aged 65 years or more. The efficacy of temozolomide was confirmed but again largely restricted to patients with tumors with MGMT promoter methylation [31]. The clinical benefit afforded by temozolomide in patients with MGMT promoter-unmethylated tumors did not reach statistical significance and therefore remains doubtful and must be weighed against the hematological toxicity and risk of infection. In the absence of a direct comparison between temozolomide alone and temozolomide chemoradiotherapy, elderly patients with MGMT promoter methylation who are candidates for combination therapy should be offered TMZ/RT→TMZ, whereas for patients with tumors without MGMT promoter methylation, a hypofractionated course of radiotherapy is a reasonable choice.

Best supportive care may be the preferred option in patients with extensive tumors and a Karnofsky performance score below 50, notably if they cannot provide informed consent for therapeutic interventions.

Numerous efforts at improving overall survival over that achieved by standard TMZ/RT→TMZ have failed. This includes phase III trials on the vascular endothelial growth factor receptor antibody bevacizumab [32, 33], the integrin antagonist cilengitide [34], and the epidermal growth factor receptor variant III-targeted vaccine rindopepimut [35]. In contrast, improved survival was seen with the addition of tumor-treating fields (TTFields), a novel treatment modality based on the exposure of the affected brain region to alternating electrical fields [36]. Several issues concerning the mode of action of this treatment, the interpretation of data and impact on quality of life remain a matter of debate [37]. That the results should not be considered meaningful because of the absence of a placebo arm in the randomized trial is a weak point of criticism because no previously approved therapy for glioblastoma been compared to a placebo except BCNU WAFERS [16]. The future expansion of the utilization of TTFields in the standard of care of newly diagnosed glioblastoma remains difficult to predict at present.

10.7   Recurrent Glioblastoma

All glioblastomas will eventually progress, either during or after first-line treatment. The therapeutic approach to recurrent glioblastoma is less uniform because several factors have to be taken into consideration which make a standardized management less feasible. A large number of patients appear not to be eligible for salvage treatment because of rapid neurological decline [38]. Tumor location and size determine whether second surgery or re-irradiation are options. Type, efficacy, and tolerability of prior treatment have to be considered for clinical decision-making, too [39].

Second surgery is an option for patients with local recurrence who have experienced stable disease from completion of postsurgical therapy for several months. By these criteria not more than one in four recurrent glioblastoma patients may be candidates for salvage surgery. Prospective randomized data to support this strategy are lacking, and careful retrospective analyses using prospectively collected imaging data from the DIRECTOR trial [40] suggest that patients may only benefit if a gross total resection of the enhancing tumor is achieved [41].

Although re-irradiation is commonly used in many centers, randomized data to support its activity are lacking, too. Favorable outcomes in retrospective single center studies are probably largely a result of patient selection. Many different fractionation regimens are being used, determined mainly by the tumor size, e.g., doses of 30–36 in 2–3 Gy fractions, and more recently higher single doses because of potential synergy with anti-angiogenic agents or checkpoint inhibition. None of these approaches can be considered standard of care as of today.

Among pharmacological treatment options, lomustine, re-exposure to temozolomide, sometimes in alternative dosing regimens, and bevacizumab are most commonly used. CCNU is now considered standard of care at least for clinical trials, although the 6-month progression-free survival rates remain low at around 20% [42, 43] and activity is particularly low if tumors lack MGMT promoter methylation. The efficacy of temozolomide rechallenge in any dosing regimen is prob-

ably in a similar range and equally dependent on MGMT promoter methylation [40, 44].

Bevacizumab is approved for the treatment of recurrent glioblastoma in the USA and various other countries, but not in the European Union. The initial approval was granted based on two prospective, but uncontrolled phase II trials which reported radiological response rates of 30% or more, higher than previously observed with other agents, and also progression-free survival times thought to be superior when compared with historical controls [45, 46]. The gain in progression-free survival was confirmed in the EORTC trial 26–101 which also served to confirm the approval of bevacizumab in the USA although no superiority of the combination of bevacizumab and lomustine over lomustine alone for overall survival was seen [43]. The failure of the PFS gain to result in improved survival was probably in part due to the "pseudoresponse" phenomenon associated with bevacizumab, i.e., decreasing mass effect and apparent tumor size assessed by contrast enhancement, without changing the progressive nature of the disease. Nevertheless, a role for bevacizumab in clinical practice is still considered by many neuro-oncologists because of the improved symptom control afforded by the agent and its potential for steroid-sparing. It has also been assumed that those patients who benefit most from bevacizumab were not adequately represented in the clinical trials that failed to demonstrate an overall survival effect of bevacizumab. However, an epidemiological study conducted in the Canton of Zurich, Switzerland, also failed to identify a change in overall survival since the introduction of bevacizumab at the population level [47], largely disassembling the above position. Tumor-treating fields were not superior to best physician's choice in a randomized phase III trial for patients with recurrent glioblastoma [48].

10.8   Follow-Up

Contrast-enhanced MRI according to a standard protocol is the method of choice for monitoring during therapy and follow-up. It is commonly conducted in 2–3-month intervals. There are no data to support that a shorter or longer imaging interval has a clinically meaningful impact. Longer intervals may be considered for the minority of patients who survive beyond 3 years. Neuropsychological, vision, and endocrine assessments are done as deemed necessary clinically. Neurorehabilitative measures should also be considered in the course of disease. In this context, it must be borne in mind that both steroids and antiseizure medications have numerous and considerable side effects, often leading to dramatic decline in quality of life, and the use of these should be closely monitored and minimized to the extent clinically possible. Every effort should be made to prepare patients and caregivers early enough for both the home care and the end-of-life phase [49]. Simple home modification approaches such as wheelchairs, ramps, vehicular access, alert alarms, support bars, accessible showers, shower benches, and safe kitchens go a very long way toward improving quality of life but are probably too often neglected. In this context, visiting nurses can prove to be a tremendously beneficial resource.

10.9   Outlook

Current areas of clinical research mainly concern new concepts of targeted therapy and immunotherapy as well as combinations thereof without and with radiotherapy. The most advanced targeted approach explores an antibody drug conjugate, ABT-414, which is directed against activated EGFR exposed at the cell surface. This activated conformation of EGFR is commonly found in tumors with EGFR gene amplification, including those with the EGFRvIII mutation. ABT-414 in combination with temozolomide showed promising activity in recurrent glioblastoma [19], and a randomized phase III trial of ABT-414 added to standard of care chemoradiotherapy in the first-line setting has completed enrolment.

New clinical trial concepts such as AGILE [50] have been designed to allow for rapid evaluation of novel targeted agents. After two negative phase III trials, of rindopepimut in the first-line setting and of nivolumab in the recurrent set-

ting, there is need for new concepts in the field of immunotherapy, including strategies for initial patient enrichment based on candidate biomarkers and their careful evaluation in well-designed phase I and II trials [51].

References

1. Louis DN, Perry A, Reifenberger G, von Deimling A, Figarella-Branger D, Cavenee WK, Ohgaki H, Wiestler OD, Kleihues P, Ellison DW (2016) The 2016 World Health Organization classification of tumors of the central nervous system: a summary. Acta Neuropathol 131:803–820
2. Weller M, Wick W, Aldape K, Brada M, Berger M, Pfister S, Nishikawa R, Rosenthal M, Wen PY, Stupp R, Reifenberger G (2015) Glioma. Nat Rev Dis Primers 1:15017
3. Ostrom QT, Gittleman H, Liao P, Vecchione-Koval T, Wolinsky Y, Kruchko C, Barnholtz-Sloan JS (2017) CBTRUS statistical report: primary brain and other central nervous system tumors diagnosed in the United States in 2010–2014. Neuro Oncol 19(Suppl_5):v1–v88
4. Rice T, Lachance DH, Molinaro AM, Eckel-Passow JE, Walsh KM, Barnholtz-Sloan J, Ostrom QT, Francis SS, Wiemels J, Jenkins RB, Wiencke JK, Wrensch MR (2016) Understanding inherited genetic risk of adult glioma—a review. Neurooncol Pract 3:10–16
5. Momoli F, Siemiatycki J, McBride ML, Parent MÉ, Richardson L, Bedard D, Platt R, Vrijheid M, Cardis E, Krewski D (2017) Probabilistic multiple-bias modeling applied to the Canadian data from the interphone study of mobile phone use and risk of glioma, meningioma, acoustic neuroma, and parotid gland tumors. Am J Epidemiol 186:885–889
6. Disney-Hogg L, Cornish AJ, Sud A, Law PJ, Kinnersley B, Jacobs DI, Ostrom QT, Labreche K, Eckel-Passow JE, Armstrong GN, Claus EB, Il'yasova D, Schildkraut J, Barnholtz-Sloan JS, Olson SH, Bernstein JL, Lai RK, Schoemaker MJ, Simon M, Hoffmann P, Nöthen MM, Jöckel KH, Chanock S, Rajaraman P, Johansen C, Jenkins RB, Melin BS, Wrensch MR, Sanson M, Bondy ML, Houlston RS (2018) Impact of atopy on risk of glioma: a Mendelian randomisation study. BMC Med 16:42
7. Ellingson BM, Bendszus M, Boxerman J, Barboriak D, Erickson BJ, Smits M, Nelson SJ, Gerstner E, Alexander B, Goldmacher G, Wick W, Vogelbaum M, Weller M, Galanis E, Kalpathy-Cramer J, Shankar L, Jacobs P, Pope WB, Yang D, Chung C, Knopp MV, Cha S, Van den Bent MJ, Chang S, Yung WKA, Cloughesy TF, Wen PY, Gilbert MR, The Jumpstarting Brain Tumor Drug Development Coalition Imaging Standardization Steering Committee (2015) Consensus recommendations for a standardized brain

tumor imaging protocol in clinical trials. Neuro Oncol 17:1188–1198

8. Wen PY, Macdonald DR, Reardon DA, Cloughesy TF, Sorensen AG, Galanis E, Degroot J, Wick W, Gilbert MR, Lassman AB, Tsien C, Mikkelsen T, Wong ET, Chamberlain MC, Stupp R, Lamborn KR, Vogelbaum MA, van den Bent MJ, Chang SM (2010) Updated response assessment criteria for high-grade gliomas: response assessment in neuro-oncology working group. J Clin Oncol 28:1963–1972

9. Albert NL, Weller M, Suchorska B, Galldiks N, Soffietti R, Kim MM, La Fougère C, Pope W, Law I, Arbizu J, Chamberlain M, Vogelbaum MA, Ellingson BM, Tonn JC (2016) Response Assessment in Neuro-Oncology Working Group and European Association for Neuro-Oncology recommendations for the clinical use of PET imaging in gliomas. Neuro Oncol 18:1199–1208

10. Watts C, Price SJ, Santarius T (2014) Current concepts in the surgical management of glioma patients. Clin Oncol 26:385–394

11. Watts C, Sanai N (2016) Surgical approaches for the gliomas. Handb Clin Neurol 134:51–69

12. Stupp R, Hegi ME, Mason WP, Van den Bent MJ, Taphoorn MJB, Janzer RC, Ludwin SK, Allgeier A, Fisher B, Belanger K, Hau P, Brandes AA, Gijtenbeek J, Marosi C, Vecht CJ, Mokhtari K, Wesseling P, Villa S, Eisenhauer E, Gorlia T, Weller M, Lacombe D, Cairncross JG, Mirimanoff RO; on behalf of the European Organisation for Research and Treatment of Cancer Brain Tumour and Radiation Oncology Groups and the National Cancer Institute of Canada Clinical Trials Group (2009) Effects of radiotherapy with concomitant and adjuvant temozolomide versus radiotherapy alone on survival in glioblastoma in a randomised phase III study: 5-year analysis of the EORTC-NCIC trial. Lancet Oncol 10:459–466

13. Almenawer SA, Badhiwala JH, Alhazzani W, Greenspoon J, Farrokhyar F, Yarascavitch B, Algird A, Kachur E, Cenic A, Sharieff W, Klurfan P, Gunnarsson T, Ajani O, Reddy K, Singh SK, Murty NK (2015) Biopsy versus partial versus gross total resection in older patients with high-grade glioma: a systematic review and meta-analysis. Neuro Oncol 17:868–881

14. Stummer W, Pichlmeier U, Meinel T, Wiestler OD, Zanella F, Reulen HJ, ALA-Glioma Study Group (2006) Fluorescence-guided surgery with 5-aminolevulinic acid for resection of malignant glioma: a randomised controlled multicentre phase III trial. Lancet Oncol 7:392–401

15. Weller M, van den Bent M, Tonn JC, Stupp R, Preusser M, Cohen-Jonathan-Moyal E, Henriksson R, Le Rhun E, Balana C, Chinot O, Bendszus M, Reijneveld JC, Dhermain F, French P, Marosi M, Watts C, Oberg I, Pilkington G, Baumert BG, Taphoorn MJB, Hegi M, Westphal M, Reifenberger R, Soffietti S, Wick W, for the European Association for Neuro-Oncology (EANO) Task Force on Gliomas (2017) EANO guideline on the diagnosis and treatment of adult astro-cytic and oligodendroglial gliomas. Lancet Oncol 18:e315–e329

16. Westphal M, Hilt DC, Bortey E, Delavault P, Olivares R, Warnke PC, Whittle IR, Jääskeläinen J, Ram Z (2003) A phase 3 trial of local chemotherapy with biodegradable carmustine (BCNU) wafers (Gliadel wafers) in patients with primary malignant glioma. Neuro Oncol 5:79–88

17. Westphal M, Ram Z, Riddle V, Hilt D, Bortey E, Executive Committee of the Gliadel Study Group (2006) Gliadel wafer in initial surgery for malignant glioma: long-term follow-up of a multicenter controlled trial. Acta Neurochir (Wien) 148:269–275

18. Hartmann C, Hentschel B, Wick W, Capper D, Felsberg J, Simon M, Westphal M, Schackert G, Meyermann R, Pietsch T, Reifenberger G, Weller M, Löffler M, von Deimling A (2010) Patients with IDH1 wild type anaplastic astroctytomas exhibit worse prognosis than IDH1-mutated glioblastomas, and IDH1 mutation status accounts for the unfavourable prognostic effect of higher age: implications for classification of gliomas. Acta Neuropathol 120:707–718

19. van den Bent MJ, Baumert B, Erridge SC, Vogelbaum MA, Nowak AK, Sanson M, Brandes AA, Clement PM, Baurain JF, Mason WP, Wheeler H, Chinot OL, Gill S, Griffin M, Brachman DG, Taal W, Rudà R, Weller M, McBain C, Reijneveld J, Enting RH, Weber DC, Lesimple T, Clenton S, Gijtenbeek A, Pascoe S, Herrlinger U, Hau P, Dhermain F, van Heuvel I, Stupp R, Aldape K, Jenkins RB, Dubbink HJ, Dinjens WNM, Wesseling P, Nuyens S, Golfinopoulos V, Gorlia T, Wick W, Kros JM (2017) Interim results from the CATNON trial (EORTC study 26053-22054) of treatment with concurrent and adjuvant temozolomide for 1p/19q non-co-deleted anaplastic glioma: a phase 3, randomised, open-label intergroup study. Lancet 390:1645–1653

20. Walker MD, Alexander E Jr, Hunt WE, MacCarty CS, Mahaley MS Jr, Mealey J Jr, Norrell HA, Owens G, Ransohoff J, Wilson CB, Gehan EA, Strike TA (1978) Evaluation of BCNU and/or radiotherapy in the treatment of anaplastic gliomas. A cooperative clinical trial. J Neurosurg 49:333–343

21. Keime-Guibert F, Chinot O, Taillandier L, Cartalat-Carel S, Frenay M, Kantor G, Guillamo JS, Jadaud E, Colin P, Bondiau PY, Meneï P, Loiseau H, Bernier V, Honnorat J, Barrié M, Mokhtari K, Mazeron JJ, Bissery A, Delattre JY, Association of French-Speaking Neuro-Oncologists (2007) Radiotherapy for glioblastoma in the elderly. N Engl J Med 356:1527–1535

22. Niyazi M, Brada M, Chalmers AJ, Combs SE, Erridge SC, Fiorentino A, Grosu AL, Lagerwaard FJ, Minniti G, Mirimanoff RO, Ricardi U, Short SC, Weber DC, Belka C (2016) ESTRO-ACROP guideline "target delineation of glioblastomas". Radiother Oncol 118:35–42

23. Roa W, Brasher PM, Bauman G, Anthes M, Bruera E, Chan A, Fisher B, Fulton D, Gulavita S, Hao C, Husain S, Murtha A, Petruk K, Stewart D, Tai P, Urtasun R,

Cairncross JG, Forsyth P (2004) Abbreviated course of radiation therapy in older patients with glioblastoma multiforme: a prospective randomized clinical trial. J Clin Oncol 22:1583–1588

24. Stupp R, Mason WP, van den Bent MJ, Weller M, Fisher B, Taphoorn MJB, Belanger K, Brandes AA, Cairncross JG, Marosi C, Bogdahn U, Curschmann J, Janzer RC, Ludwin S, Gorlia T, Allgeier A, Lacombe D, Eisenhauer E, Mirimanoff RO, on behalf of the European Organisation for Research and Treatment of Cancer (EORTC) Brain Tumor and Radiotherapy Groups and National Cancer Institute of Canada Clinical Trials Group (NCIC CTG) (2005) Radiotherapy plus concomitant and adjuvant temozolomide for patients with newly diagnosed glioblastoma. N Engl J Med 352:987–996

25. Hegi ME, Diserens AC, Gorlia T, Hamou MF, de Tribolet N, Weller M, Kros JM, Hainfellner JA, Mason WP, Mariani L, Bromberg JEC, Hau P, Mirimanoff RO, Cairncross G, Janzer R, Stupp R (2005) MGMT gene silencing and response to temozolomide in glioblastoma. N Engl J Med 352:997–1003

26. Gilbert MR, Wang M, Aldape KD, Stupp R, Hegi ME, Jaeckle KA, Armstrong TS, Wefel JS, Won M, Blumenthal DT, Mahajan A, Schultz CJ, Erridge S, Baumert B, Hopkins KI, Tzuk-Shina T, Brown PD, Chakravarti A, Curran WJ Jr, Mehta MP (2013) Dose-dense temozolomide for newly diagnosed glioblastoma: a randomized phase III clinical trial. J Clin Oncol 31:4085–4091

27. Blumenthal DT, Gorlia T, Gilbert MR, Kim MM, Nabors LB, Mason WP, Hegi ME, Zhang P, Golfinopoulos V, Perry JR, Nam DH, Erridge SC, Corn BW, Mirimanoff RO, Brown PD, Baumert BG, Mehta MP, Van den Bent MJ, Reardon DA, Weller M, Stupp R (2017) Is more better? The impact of extended adjuvant temozolomide in newly-diagnosed glioblastoma: a secondary analysis of EORTC and NRG oncology/RTOG. Neuro Oncol 19:1119–1126

28. Gramatzki D, Kickingereder P, Hentschel B, Felsberg J, Herrlinger U, Schackert G, Tonn JC, Westphal M, Sabel M, Schlegel U, Wick W, Pietsch T, Reifenberger G, Loeffler M, Bendszus M, Weller M (2017) Limited role for extended maintenance temozolomide for newly diagnosed glioblastoma. Neurology 88:1422–1430

29. Malmstrom A, Gronberg BH, Marosi C, Stupp R, Frappaz D, Schultz H, Abacioglu U, Tavelin B, Lhermitte B, Hegi ME, Rosell J, Henriksson R, Nordic Clinical Brain Tumour Study Group (NCBTSG) (2012) Temozolomide versus standard 6-week radiotherapy versus hypofractionated radiotherapy in patients older than 60 years with glioblastoma: the Nordic randomised, phase 3 trial. Lancet Oncol 13:916–926

30. Wick W, Platten M, Meisner C, Felsberg J, Tabatabai G, Simon M, Nikkhah G, Papsdorf K, Steinbach JP, Sabel M, Combs SE, Vesper J, Braun C, Meixensberger J, Ketter R, Mayer-Steinacker R, Reifenberger G, Weller M, for the Neurooncology Working Group (NOA) of the German Cancer Society (2012) Temozolomide chemotherapy alone versus radiotherapy alone for malignant astrocytoma in the elderly: the NOA-08 randomised, phase 3 trial. Lancet Oncol 13:707–715

31. Perry JR, Laperriere N, O'Callaghan CJ, Brandes AA, Menten J, Phillips C, Fay M, Nishikawa R, Cairncross JG, Roa W, Osoba D, Rossiter JP, Sahgal A, Hirte H, Laigle-Donadey F, Franceschi E, Chinot O, Golfinopoulos V, Fariselli L, Wick A, Feuvret L, Back M, Tills M, Winch C, Baumert BG, Wick W, Ding K, Mason WP, Trial Investigators (2017) Short-course radiation plus temozolomide in elderly patients with glioblastoma. N Engl J Med 376:1027–1037

32. Chinot OL, Wick W, Mason W, Henriksson R, Saran F, Nishikawa R, Carpentier AF, Hoang-Xuan K, Kavan P, Cernea D, Brandes AA, Hilton M, Abrey L, Cloughesy T (2014) Bevacizumab plus radiotherapy-temozolomide for newly diagnosed glioblastoma. N Engl J Med 370:709–722

33. Gilbert MR, Dignam JJ, Armstrong TS, Wefel JS, Blumenthal DT, Vogelbaum MA, Colman H, Chakravarti A, Pugh S, Won M, Jeraj R, Brown PD, Jaeckle KA, Schiff D, Stieber VW, Brachman DG, Werner-Wasik M, Tremont-Lukats IW, Sulman EP, Aldape KD, Curran WJ Jr, Mehta MP (2014) A randomized trial of bevacizumab for newly diagnosed glioblastoma. N Engl J Med 370:699–708

34. Stupp R, Hegi ME, Gorlia T, Erridge S, Perry J, Hong YK, Aldape KD, Lhermitte B, Pietsch T, Grujicic D, Steinbach JP, Wick W, Tarnawski R, Nam DH, Hau P, Weyerbrock A, Taphoorn MJB, Shen CC, Rao N, Thurzo L, Herrlinger U, Gupta T, Kortmann RD, Adamska K, McBain C, Brandes AA, Tonn JC, Schnell O, Wiegel T, Kim CK, Nabors LB, Reardon DA, Van den Bent MJ, Hicking C, Markivskyy A, Picard M, Weller M, on behalf of European Organisation for Research and Treatment of Cancer (EORTC), the Canadian Brain Tumor Consortium, and the CENTRIC Study Team (2014) Cilengitide combined with standard treatment for patients with newly diagnosed glioblastoma with methylated O6-methylguanine-DNA methyltransferase (MGMT) promoter: final results of the multicentre, randomised, open-label, controlled, phase 3 CENTRIC (EORTC 26071-22072) study. Lancet Oncol 15:1100–1108

35. Weller M, Butowski N, Tran DD, Recht LD, Lim M, Hirte H, Ashby L, Mechtler L, Goldlust SA, Iwamoto F, Drappatz J, O'Rourke DM, Wong M, Hamilton MG, Finocchiaro G, Perry J, Wick W, Green J, He Y, Turner CD, Yellin MJ, Keler T, Davis TA, Stupp R, Sampson JH, for the ACT IV Trial Investigators (2017) Rindopepimut with temozolomide for patients with newly diagnosed, EGFRvIII-expressing glioblastoma (ACT IV): results of a randomized, double-blind, international phase 3 trial. Lancet Oncol 18:1373–1385

36. Stupp R, Taillibert S, Kanner A, Read W, Steinberg DM, Lhermitte B, Toms S, Idbaih A, Ahluwalia MS, Fink K, Di Meco F, Lieberman F, Zhu JJ, Stragliotto

G, Tran DD, Brem S, Hottinger AF, Kirson ED, Lavy-Shahaf G, Weinberg U, Kim CY, Paek SH, Nicholas G, Bruna J, Hirte H, Weller M, Palti Y, Hegi ME, Ram Z (2017) Effect of tumor-treating fields plus maintenance temozolomide vs maintenance temozolomide alone on survival in patients with glioblastoma. A randomized clinical trial. J Am Med Assoc 318:2306–2316

37. Wick W (2016) TTFields: where does all the skepticism come from? Neuro Oncol 18:303–305
38. Gramatzki D, Dehler S, Rushing EJ, Zaugg K, Hofer S, Yonekawa Y, Bertalanffy H, Valavanis A, Korol D, Rohrmann S, Pless M, Oberle J, Roth P, Ohgaki H, Weller M (2016) Glioblastoma in the Canton of Zurich, Switzerland, revisited (2005–2009). Cancer 122:2206–2215
39. Weller M, Cloughesy T, Perry JR, Wick W (2013) Standards of care for treatment of recurrent glioblastoma—are we there yet? Neuro Oncol 15:4–27
40. Weller M, Tabatabai G, Kästner B, Felsberg J, Steinbach JP, Wick A, Schnell O, Hau P, Herrlinger U, Sabel MC, Wirsching HG, Ketter R, Bähr O, Platten M, Tonn JC, Schlegel U, Marosi C, Goldbrunner R, Stupp R, Homicsko K, Pichler J, Nikkhah G, Meixensberger J, Vajkoczy P, Kollias S, Hüsing J, Reifenberger R, Wick W, for the DIRECTOR Study Group (2015) MGMT promoter methylation is a strong prognostic biomarker for benefit from dose-intensified temozolomide rechallenge in progressive glioblastoma: the DIRECTOR trial. Clin Cancer Res 21:2057–2064
41. Suchorska B, Weller M, Tabatabai G, Senft C, Hau P, Sabel MC, Herrlinger U, Ketter R, Schlegel U, Marosi C, Reifenberger G, Wick W, Tonn JC, Wirsching HW (2016) Complete resection of contrast enhancing tumor volume is associated with improved survival in recurrent glioblastoma—results from the DIRECTOR trial. Neuro Oncol 18:549–566
42. Batchelor TT, Mulholland P, Neyns B, Nabors LB, Campone M, Wick A, Mason W, Mikkelsen T, Phuphanich S, Ashby LS, Degroot J, Gattamaneni R, Cher L, Rosenthal M, Payer F, Jürgensmeier JM, Jain RK, Sorensen AG, Xu J, Liu Q, van den Bent M (2013) Phase III randomized trial comparing the efficacy of cediranib as monotherapy, and in combination with lomustine, versus lomustine alone in patients with recurrent glioblastoma. J Clin Oncol 31:3212–3218
43. Wick W, Gorlia T, Bendszus M, Taphoorn M, Sahm F, Harting I, Brandes AA, Taal W, Domont J, Idbaih A, Campone M, Clement PM, Stupp R, Fabbro M, Le Rhun E, Dubois F, Weller M, von Deimling A, Golfinopoulos V, Bromberg JC, Platten M, Klein M, Van den Bent MJ (2017) Lomustine and bevacizumab in progressive glioblastoma. N Engl J Med 377:1954–1963

44. Perry JR, Belanger K, Mason WP, Fulton D, Kavan P, Easaw J, Shields C, Kirby S, Macdonald DR, Eisenstat DD, Thiessen B, Forsyth P, Pouliot JF (2010) Phase II trial of continuous dose-intense temozolomide in recurrent malignant glioma: RESCUE study. J Clin Oncol 28:2051–2057
45. Friedman HS, Prados MD, Wen PY, Mikkelsen T, Schiff D, Abrey LE, Yung WK, Paleologos N, Nicholas MK, Jensen R, Vredenburgh J, Huang J, Zheng M, Cloughesy T (2009) Bevacizumab alone and in combination with irinotecan in recurrent glioblastoma. J Clin Oncol 27:4733–4740
46. Kreisl TN, Kim L, Moore K, Duic P, Royce C, Stroud I, Garren N, Mackey M, Butman JA, Camphausen K, Park J, Albert PS, Fine HA (2009) Phase II trial of single-agent bevacizumab followed by bevacizumab plus irinotecan at tumor progression in recurrent glioblastoma. J Clin Oncol 27:740–745
47. Gramatzki D, Roth P, Rushing EJ, Weller J, Andratschke N, Hofer S, Korol D, Regli L, Pangalu A, Pless M, Oberle J, Bernays R, Moch H, Rohrmann S, Weller M (2018) Bevacizumab may improve quality of life, but not overall survival in glioblastoma: an epidemiological study. Ann Oncol 29:1431–1436
48. Stupp R, Wong ET, Kanner AA, Steinberg D, Engelhard H, Heidecke V, Kirson ED, Taillibert S, Liebermann F, Dbalý V, Ram Z, Villano JL, Rainov N, Weinberg U, Schiff D, Kunschner L, Raizer J, Honnorat J, Sloan A, Malkin M, Landolfi JC, Payer F, Mehdorn M, Weil RJ, Pannullo SC, Westphal M, Smrcka M, Chin L, Kostron H, Hofer S, Bruce J, Cosgrove R, Paleologous N, Palti Y, Gutin PH (2012) NovoTTF-100A versus physician's choice chemotherapy in recurrent glioblastoma: a randomised phase III trial of a novel treatment modality. Eur J Cancer 48(14):2192–2202
49. Pace A, Dirven L, Koekkoek JAF, Golla H, Fleming J, Rudà R, Marosi C, Le Rhun E, Grant R, Oliver K, Oberg I, Bulbeck HJ, Rooney AG, Henriksson R, Pasman HRW, Oberndorfer S, Weller M, Taphoorn MJB, on behalf of the European Association of Neuro-Oncology palliative care task force (2017) EANO guidelines for palliative care in adult glioma patients. Lancet Oncol 18:e330–e340
50. Alexander BM, Ba S, Berger MS, Berry DA, Cavenee WK, Chang SM, Cloughesy TF, Jiang T, Khasraw M, Li W, Mittman R, Poste GH, Wen PY, WKA Y, Barker AD, for the GBM AGILE Network (2018) Adaptive global innovative learning environment for glioblastoma: GBM AGILE. Clin Cancer Res 24:737–747
51. Lim M, Xia Y, Bettegowda C, Weller M (2018) Current state of immunotherapy for glioblastoma. Nat Rev Clin Oncol 15:422–442

Ependymomas and Tumors of the Ventricular System

11

Manfred Westphal

11.1 Definition

Ependymomas arise from the ventricular surface which is made up of ependymal cells. They occur throughout the whole central nervous system including the filum terminale. They may occur outside the ventricular structures, representing the rare ectopic ependymoma.

Neurocytoma describes a tumor occurring preferentially inside the ventricles which is a kind of neuroglial stem cell-like tumor with mostly minimal extension beyond the subependyma.

In addition to ependymomas and neurocytoma, tumors of the ventricular system include subependymomas which arise from the subependyma which is the cellular stratum underneath the ependymal layer. Another intrinsic tumor of the ventricular system arises from the choroid plexus, either as plexus papilloma or plexus carcinoma.

Ectopic tumors in that location are intraventricular meningiomas or metastases in the choroid plexus, the most frequent being from renal cell carcinoma and melanoma because they seem to have a certain tropism for this kind of highly vascularized tissue matrix [1]. Hemangioblastomas can also be found in the choroid plexus and are either sporadic or associated with von Hippel-Lindau disease.

In addition all glial tumors can exophytically extend into and compromise the ventricles and can have any glial histology from pilocytic astrocytoma to glioblastoma. The only specific astrocytoma of the ventricular system is the subependymal giant cell astrocytoma (SEGA) which is associated with tuberous sclerosis and arises from the subventricular zone.

11.2 Epidemiology

A comprehensive source for the epidemiology of tumors is the *Central Brain Tumor Registry of the United States* (*CBTRUS*), of which the latest 2017 edition covers the data collection time of 2010–2014 [2]. Adjusted to the US 2000 standard population ICD O-3 code, C71.5 (ventricular tumors) came out with an adjusted rate of 0.27 (per 100,000 person years). This was different for adults and children, which for *malignant* tumors came to a rate of 0.24 in children vs. 0.05 *nonmalignant* in contrast to adults which was rather constant with respective rates of 0.28 and 0.24. Looking for *ependymoma*, which includes many sites outside the ventricle, a total rate of 0.43 was found and for plexus tumors, 0.05. In the most recent survey, a total of 832 cases of tumors with ventricular location were reported among 75,970 cases of primary CNS tumors, translating into 1.1%.

M. Westphal (✉)
Department of Neurosurgery, University of Hamburg,
University Hospital Eppendorf, Hamburg,
Hamburg, Germany
e-mail: westphal@uke.de

© Springer Nature Switzerland AG 2019
J.-C. Tonn et al. (eds.), *Oncology of CNS Tumors*, https://doi.org/10.1007/978-3-030-04152-6_11

Ependymomas are a heterogeneous group of tumors with several subtypes and clear rules for grading, which however is uncertain in its clinical meaning so that molecular subclassifications will become the major correlate to clinical studies [3–5]. Epidemiological numbers for ependymomas frequently do not contain subdivisions between intraparenchymal, intraventricular, intramedullary, and cauda equina and therefore have to be viewed with caution. In the spinal cord, they are the most frequent neuroepithelial neoplasm [6]. The numbers vary between 3 and 9% of all neuroepithelial tumors in different reports, most of which have another primary focus. In children, ependymomas are the third most common tumor and account for 10% of all posterior fossa tumors in this population [7].

Choroid plexus tumors are rare and occur as WHO grade I tumors preferentially in children and young adults and WHO grade II (atypical) and grade III (plexus carcinoma) which occur at younger age with a mean age at diagnosis of 2.3 years [8]. In a recent survey, the prevalence of choroid plexus tumors was given as 0.3 cases per one million people [9]. This translates into 0.4–0.6% of all reported intracranial tumors. The tumors are more frequent in children [10] with a mean age at diagnosis of 3.5 years and no clear gender preference either in children or adults. Choroid plexus carcinomas are only a small subgroup of these tumors of which 80% occur in children [11].

Neurocytomas make up 0.25–0.5% of intracranial tumors [12]. They are given the WHO grade II but can have anaplastic features of which the clinical relevance is still uncertain [13]. They occur in all ages but mainly in young adulthood so that 75% of the cases are diagnosed between the age of 20 and 40 years [14]. They affect women and men equally. The most common site of occurrence is the anterior part of the lateral ventricle.

Ventricular meningiomas. In larger series of unselected meningiomas, a ventricular location was seen in only 1.3–1.5% but in a much higher incidence of 9.4% in the pediatric age group (reviewed in [15]). They are mostly located in the lateral ventricles with locations in the third or fourth ventricle being very rare. They originate from the choroid plexus.

Metastases become more frequent with extended life span of patients with cancer. Ventricular metastases are still rare and make up 6% of all ventricular tumors and less than 1% of intracranial metastases [16]. The choroid plexus seems to be a preferred site for metastases from renal cell carcinoma [17].

11.3 Molecular Genetics

For ependymomas, the most relevant finding over the past years has been the thorough molecular classification across all CNS compartments, histological grades, and age groups [5]. Ependymomas appear to have a distinct genetic phenotype which is different from other glial tumors. The otherwise characteristic mutations of p53, deletions or mutations of CDKN2A and CDKN2B and PTEN, or amplification of the EGF-R were reported to be absent [18], and this was confirmed except for supratentorial ependymomas of the RELA-subgroup where CDKN2A was lost, sometimes due to loss of chromosome 9 or 9p in 16% [5]. The only association of ependymomas is with NF-2 correlating to the epidemiological finding that in these patients, there is an increased frequency of intramedullary ependymomas (see Chap. 34). The molecular analysis of ependymomas showed that the DNA methylation pattern allows for a sharper distinction between groups than histopathology. Thus, nine groups were identified for three compartments, spinal (SP-EPN), posterior fossa (PF-EPN), and supratentorial (ST-EPN), with one type in each compartment corresponding to subependymoma. Focusing on the cranial tumors, the infratentorial tumors could be subdivided into two distinct groups, the PF-EPN-A and PF-EPN-B with distinct patterns. In the supratentorial group, a fusion gene involving the RELA-gene was predominantly found and is considered an oncogenic driver, and alternatively fusion genes involving the YAP-1 gene were found, thus resulting in the ST-EPN-RELA and ST-EPN-YAP-1 subgroups. These distinctions are now the basis for the formation of cohorts for clinical trials. None of the much improved molecular analyses have led to the development of targeted therapeutics neither for adults nor for children [19].

Plexus papillomas have provided even less cytogenetic or molecular genetic findings. Some anomalies were found in the 9p region, but no further specific characterization has been done. Like with meningiomas, comparative genomic hybridization provides a long list of sporadically altered chromosomal regions, but of pathophysiological distinction is possibly only an alteration in the Notch pathway [11]. Plexus carcinomas harbor mutations in the p53 gene but only in patients with the Li-Fraumeni phenotype [20].

There are no extensive investigations on molecular genetics of neurocytomas. The limited available data indicate only a gain of chromosome 7 in some cases, but no specific regions or genes have been implied [10, 12].

No specific genetic alterations have been reported for ventricular meningiomas which would distinguish them genetically from the majority of the other meningiomas.

11.4   Etiology and Prevention

No specific causes are known for ependymomas or other ventricular tumors. Thus there is no specific strategy for prevention. Except for the association with NF-2 [18], there are not even environmental or epidemiological predictors for these tumors. In known NF-2 cases, careful observation knowing about the possibility to develop such tumors may lead to earlier detection and an optimal timing for therapy.

Likewise, there is one other genetic syndrome associated with a pediatric ventricular tumor which is the subependymal giant cell astrocytoma which is associated with tuberous sclerosis [21].

Neurocytomas are considered neuroglial progenitor tumors [22, 23], and as such may be attributable to a deficit in definitive differentiation. There is no consistent coincidence with genetic syndromes or any kind of environmental exposure or ethnic preference.

11.5   Signs and Symptoms

Intracranial ependymomas occur mainly in children and especially in the posterior fossa (see also Chap. 29). But also adults may have tumors in this location and have the same imaging characteristics. When confined to the fourth ventricle, they may cause obstructive hydrocephalus with sudden headache of undulating intensity, nausea, vomiting (projectile), diplopia, and papilledema (Fig. 11.1). When they invade the floor of the fourth ventricle, they may cause also cranial nerve disorders, mostly again diplopia but also facial weakness. A preferred site is the foramen of Luschka where the tumors extend partly into the fourth ventricle and partly into the cerebellopontine angle. This causes similar symptoms but frequently also unilateral problems with the caudal cranial nerves and in cases of major compression of the medulla also hemiparesis or hemidystaxia because of loss of sensation. When extending across the foramen

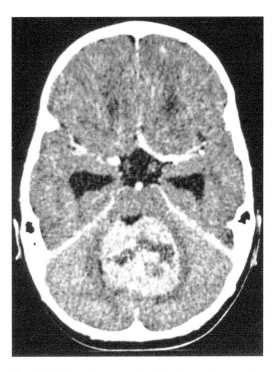

Fig. 11.1 Ependymoma in the fourth ventricle causing acute obstructive hydrocephalus. An immediate direct approach is desirable to avoid any complications from shunting-associated relief of supratentorial pressure

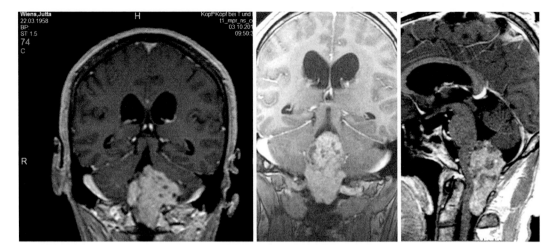

Fig. 11.2 Three different adult cases of ependymomas at the craniocervical junction. When located asymmetrically to one side (left panel), the tumor originates most likely from the inside border of the fourth ventricle at the foramen of Luschka. When located centrally with extension well up into the fourth ventricle, the attachments are often broad at the floor of the fourth ventricle (middle panel), and when located at the foramen of Magendie, the attachments are to be expected at the level of the obex (right panel) which was the case for all these three tumors which could all be totally removed

magnum, they may cause neck pain upon movement (Fig. 11.2). Spinal intramedullary ependymomas have different symptoms and will be discussed there (see Chap. 34).

The less frequent supratentorial intraventricular/periventricular ependymomas occur preferably in adults and will cause some kind of hydrocephalus. In a location within the lateral ventricle, it could be a trapped compartment or a monoventricular hydrocephalus. When located around the foramen of Monro, hydrocephalus can be biventricular (Fig. 11.3) with intermittent crises of severe headache like in the colloid cysts of the third ventricle. Ependymomas in the third ventricle can cause severe endocrinological problems when involving the hypothalamus or memory disorders when involving the fornices. The more dorsal locations lead to compression of the Sylvian aqueduct and cause triventricular hydrocephalus.

Ependymomas in adults have a tendency to also occur ectopically intraparenchymally, somewhere in the hemispheres (Fig. 11.4). There they will lead to the local symptoms identical to any other glioma including paresis, speech disorders, visual field impairment, as well as seizures.

The histology is usually unexpected, and there are no specific neuroradiological clues despite the high incidence of anaplastic tumors in this group. A dysembryogenic component of faulted migration pattern possibly in association with inadequate apoptotic potential must be suspected as part of their development.

In contrast to the ependymomas, plexus papillomas usually do not infiltrate their surroundings and respect the ependymal layer. Therefore the symptoms are those of local compression and of hydrocephalus which ranges between partial hydrocephalus from a trapped compartment to complete internal, non-communicating, obstructive hydrocephalus due to a lesion in the caudal part of the fourth ventricle. The same symptomatology pattern is true for the ventricular meningiomas and metastases. Meningiomas by virtue of their capacity to secrete large amounts of vascular endothelial growth factor may cause edema and metastases even more often do so as they may originate from the subependymal layer or when originating from the plexus have less respect for the ependyma than meningiomas or plexus papillomas.

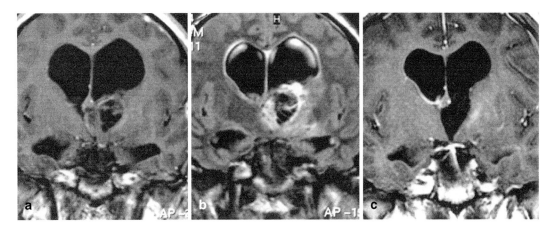

Fig. 11.3 Ependymoma arising from the ventricular wall around the area of the foramen of Monro (**a**, **b**). The lesion is inhomogeneously enhancing and has a cystic component and causes biventricular hydrocephalus. Via a frontal transcortical approach, this tumor can be removed (**c**), but because of the broad base, there is an extreme likelihood for recurrence warranting regular follow-up intervals. Because of the immediate vicinity of the hypothalamus and the yet undefined role of radiation for ependymoma, radiation is delayed until the activity of these tumors will reveal itself

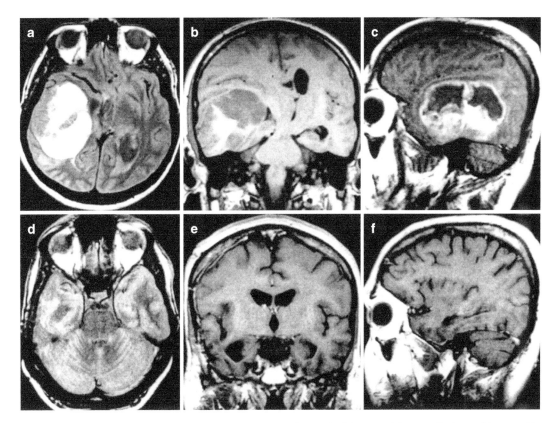

Fig. 11.4 Intraparenchymal ependymoma in a 46-year-old adult male patient (**a**–**c**) which was not suspected when the lesion was approached. The patient was treated afterward with external beam radiation and has a stable follow-up of 4 years (**d**–**f**)

11.6 Staging and Classification

There is an extensive appreciation of the histopathological and grading features in Chap. 1 by Reifenberger. According to the new WHO classification, subependymomas and the myxopapillary ependymomas of the filum terminale are considered to be grade WHO I tumors [4, 24]. There are four variants of grade II ependymoma: cellular, papillary, clear cell, and tanycytic [4]. Anaplastic ependymoma is considered to be grade III [3].

Tumors of the choroid plexus are either classified as grade I corresponding to choroid plexus papilloma or grade II when mitotic activity is present or histopathological signs of atypia which is to be expected in 15% of the cases. Grade III corresponds to the choroid plexus carcinoma [8].

Astrocytomas and oligodendrogliomas which extend exophytically into the ventricular system are also graded according to the WHO grading system and represent the whole spectrum.

Neurocytoma is considered to be grade II in the latest edition of the WHO [10, 12, 13]. There is much discussion about anaplasia in neurocytomas [25, 26], but at present it is preferred to speak about neurocytomas with atypical features when necrosis or a high mitotic labelling index is present and recommend an intensified clinical follow-up. The concept of malignancy has been used for the extraventricular location [27] even if it's not introduced in the WHO classification [12]. Aggressive neurocytomas are very rare, and only single cases in childhood have been reported [28].

11.7 Diagnostic Procedures

Clinical Signs. As most of these tumors occur in children (see there), the experienced neuropediatrician will suspect a posterior fossa tumor or another intracranial lesion causing hydrocephalus due to obstruction of the CSF pathways from some of the typical symptoms described above. Drowsiness, nausea, vomiting, papilledema, and singultus will be a grave warning sign. The "stiff neck," when children try to avoid neck pain from descended tonsils by holding their head upright

and almost fixed, is a pathognomonic sign which must not be missed.

Cerebrospinal Fluid (CSF). Ventricular tumors cause obstruction of the CSF pathways and thus create a pressure gradient which results in a vector of forces which can be aggravated by inadvertently selectively decompressing one distal compartment by puncture, i.e., lumbar. This can create downward or in rare cases upward herniation (when supratentorial relief by external ventricular drainage is associated with posterior fossa pressure), and therefore lumbar puncture may only be performed when this possibility is excluded and should not precede imaging. If obstruction of the CSF pathways warrants relief, an endoscopic third ventriculostomy (3VS) is preferable to external ventricular drainage with the risk of infection or a shunting procedure which may cause further dissemination in case of anaplastic tumors. Also, using an endoscope many ventricular tumors can be biopsied in the same setting. In any case, when obtaining CSF it should be analyzed for markers and cytology.

Neuroradiology. Overall, imaging is the most important diagnostic modality. CT allows the detection of calcifications in tumors and the assessment of the type and severity of hydrocephalus. Much more information is obtained in the MRI which allows to detect or at least speculate about the area of origin of the tumor. Furthermore, the three planes of representation are crucial for the planning of the surgical approach.

Supratentorial ependymomas (EPN-ST) are mostly in the ventricles and are difficult to distinguish from subependymoma which are more inert and sometimes even isointense. They can have a broad base of ependymal attachment and appear like an exophytic lesion of the brain (Fig. 11.3). On the other hand, they may arise from the septum pellucidum or any other area including the roof of the ventricles and then are sometimes undistinguishable from neurocytoma by imaging (Fig. 11.5). EPN-ST can also occur ectopically in the hemispheres and will cause local symptoms as any glial tumor. Cysts are more frequent with extraventricular location. Although they may completely fill a ventricle, CSF finds a

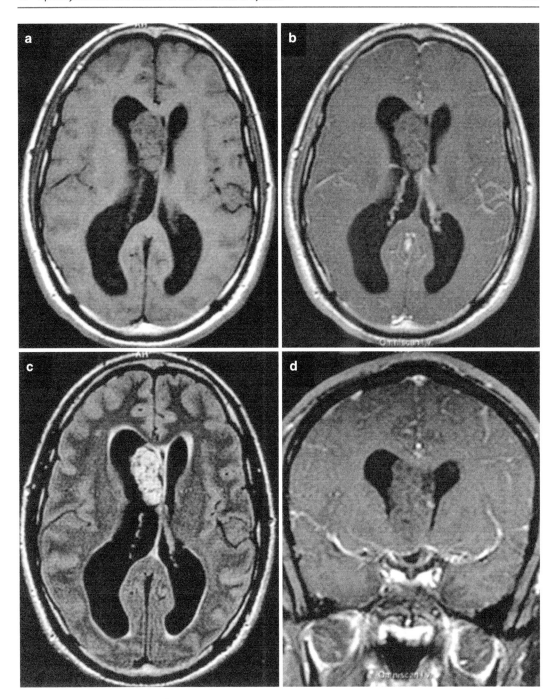

Fig. 11.5 Ependymoma of the region of the foramen of Monro (**a–d**) which was suspected to be neurocytoma but has clearly not that histology and a different immunohistochemical marker profile typical of a differentiated ependymoma (WHO II)

way to get past what indicates the small area of origin. EPN-PF is located infratentorially. They frequently show extension into the cerebellopontine angle (Figs. 11.2 and 11.6) or are located exclusively in the fourth ventricle (Fig. 11.1). In children the main differential diagnosis is medulloblastoma, and the diagnosis will only be made by intraoperative frozen section or definitive histology. As medulloblastoma, EPN-PF can have cystic components, show signs of prior hemorrhage, and vary between minimal and intensive enhancement after contrast, sometimes within the same tumor.

Choroid plexus papillomas tend to show a heterogeneous internal structure, frequently calcifications and very little reaction of the surrounding brain. They show intense staining due to their vascularization from the choroid plexus. They are usually central in the ventricles and occur anywhere where choroid plexus can be found. In children they are more frequent than in adults and are found usually in the lateral ventricles. In adults they tend to be more frequent in the fourth ventricle (Fig. 11.7).

Ventricular meningiomas have little calcification in CT, are homogeneously enhancing, and show very little reaction of the surrounding brain when only moderately distending the ventricles. As they slowly grow expansively in their "empty" compartment, they may grow to considerable size before becoming detected (Fig. 11.8). When they are large and lead to compression of the veins in the ventricles, they can cause congestive edema. The best imaging is obtained by MRI which is also needed for the planning of the surgical approach. In the case of a suspected meningioma, angiography is still sometimes performed, but it does not provide much useful information and is an unnecessarily added procedural risk to the patient. The blood supply is usually from the vessels of the choroid plexus and nothing more, but a faint blush can be seen. Because of this very peripheral vascularization, no high capacity feeding vessels can be distinguished, and as much as there is no option for embolization, there is no reason for it.

Neurocytomas are usually located in the lateral ventricles, have a broad attachment to the ependyma, are homogeneous in texture even when large, and show moderate enhancement after application of contrast media (Fig. 11.9). They tend to occur more frequently in the area around the foramen of Monro.

The major differential diagnosis for all intraventricular tumors is metastasis. The diagnosis of a metastasis is usually made in the context of a known primary. For intracranial metastases in general, one finds 20% in the absence of a known

primary, but this does not apply for the types which preferentially metastasize into the choroid plexus which are renal cell carcinoma and melanoma. They may have any of the appearances mentioned above. Interestingly, metastases seem to have an increased angiogenic activity which is known to be associated with an increased production of VEGF, and therefore edema is much more frequent and intense than with plexus papilloma, meningioma, or ependymoma.

Hemangioblastoma of the choroid plexus is another rare entity and may be very similar to a renal cell carcinoma but usually has more prominent (venous) blood vessels which can be seen as flow voids in its surroundings. As in other locations of hemangioblastomas, there may be cysts or signs of prior hemorrhage. In many cases a von Hippel-Lindau disease is known. This entity will be discussed separately (Chap. 16).

Another rare differential diagnosis can be cavernous hemangioma which is rare [29] but can be a surprise during surgery of when obtaining the final histological report (Fig. 11.10).

11.8   Treatment

Nearly all patients with ventricular tumors require a surgical intervention. Only rarely a tumor in the anterior part of the third ventricle (infundibulum) or posterior part (pineal region) will turn out to be a pure germinoma (see there), be diagnosed purely by CSF cytology and marker analysis in CSF and serum, and will be treated by radiation as the main component with optional chemotherapy [30].

Hydrocephalus is frequently a presenting sign and needs special consideration in respect to the timing of surgery. During the removal of a ventricular tumor, it may be very helpful to have distended ventricles to work in, and therefore definitive surgery is usually scheduled within a short period after diagnosis or even as an emergency. It is undesirable to have a ventriculoperitoneal shunt placed as a first measure in a center which cannot definitively deal with the lesion and then see the patient referred weeks later when the ventricular system has become normal or even slim. Also, placing a shunt prematurely

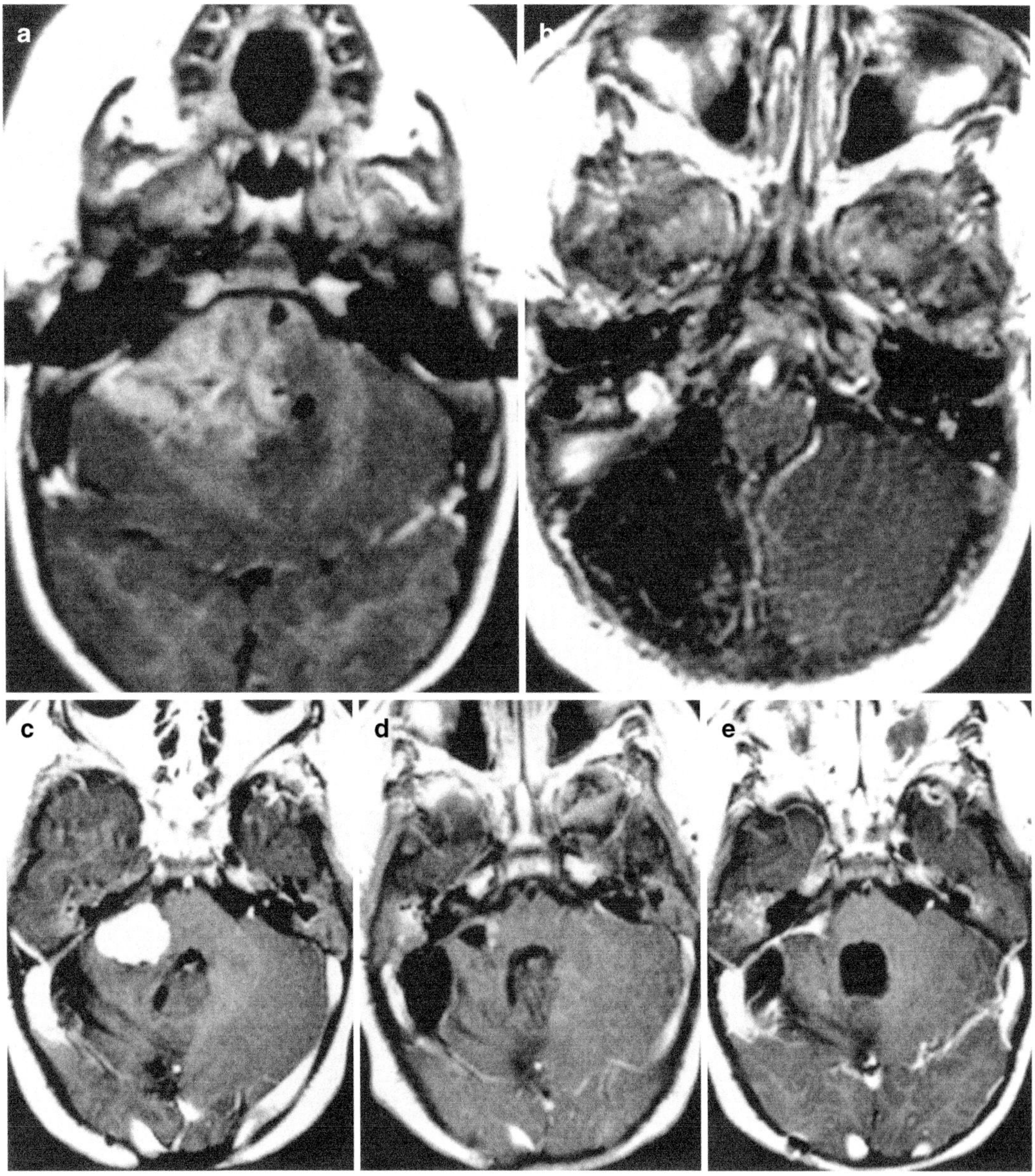

Fig. 11.6 Ependymoma of the foramen of Luschka of a 9-month-old child with extension around the brain stem and into the fourth ventricle (**a**). After near total resection (**b**) and radiation, the condition was stable for 2.5 years, and then a recurrence developed (**c**) which was again resected (**d**) with radiation of residuals which were tightly adherent to the nerve root exits of the caudal nerves and the facial nerve (**e**)

before the definitive diagnosis can be dangerous. There is a danger for peritoneal seeding although in one of the larger series which analyzed this phenomenon, this was more frequent for germinomas and medulloblastoma than ependymoma or plexus papilloma [31]. In a series of patients with extraneural metastasis of ependymoma, two patients with peritoneal seeding had shunts [32]. If surgery and relief of hydrocephalus cannot be in close timely association, a third ventriculostomy (3VS) is indicated because it is a small procedure, will leave no external drains which potentially could become infected, and provides also a biopsy opportunity so that a histology can

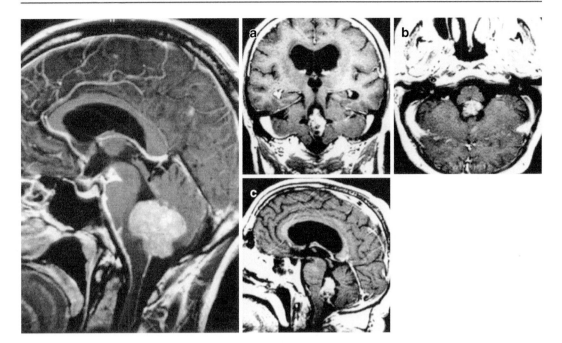

Fig. 11.7 Two examples of adult patients with plexus papillomas of the fourth ventricle. MRI with contrast of a large tumor in the fourth ventricle which was suspected to be adult medulloblastoma in a 38-year-old male patient but turned out to be a plexus papilloma which has been removed left panel [18]. (**b**) Plexus papilloma at the exit of the fourth ventricle in a 60-year-old man (**a–c**)

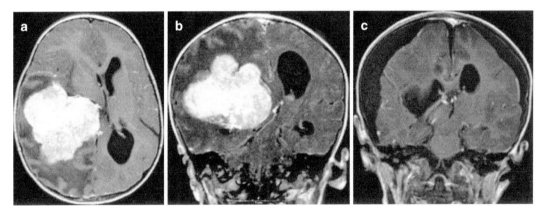

Fig. 11.8 Homogeneously enhancing tumor in the right trigonal area in a 4-year-old boy which turned out to be a ventricular meningioma (**a**, **b**) which could be removed without sequelae. (**c**) Ventricular meningiomas tend to be more frequent in boys which is in contrast to that disease elsewhere and later in life

be obtained [33]. The ventricular collapse after 3VS is also less compared to ventriculoperitoneal shunting or external drainage so that the situation for surgery does not deteriorate as much.

The approaches to the ventricular system are standardized for every location and are plentiful [34]. The approaches to the lateral ventricle depend on the location of the tumor, the extent of hydrocephalus, and the hemispheric dominance. With distended ventricles, the approaches are preferentially transcortical in the frontal area and are symmetrical for the hemispheres except for the trigonal area, where special consideration has to be taken on the dominant side and a more

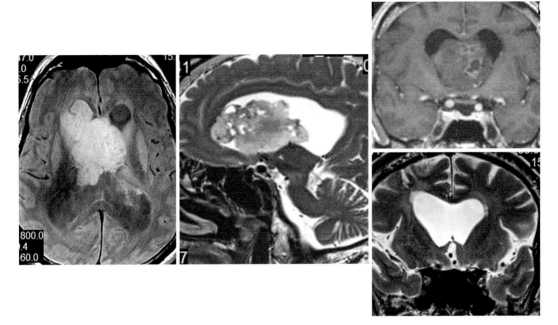

Fig. 11.9 Histologically confirmed neurocytoma arising in a 68-year-old patient with severe cognitive disorder and beginning drowsiness arising from a surprisingly small area of the septum pellucidum on the right side. There is no sign of edema in the FLAIR sequences (left panel) already indicating a respect for the ependyma and com- pletely exophytic growth. The septum was mostly dis- placed with some spontaneous perforations, and due to the soft nature of the tumor, it could be removed com- pletely through a small right frontal transcortical access. Without any adjuvant therapy, the result (right bottom T2-weighted panel) is stable since 3 years

basal or dorsal approach taken which leaves the angular gyrus area undisturbed. The third ven- tricle can be approached from the subfrontal region by the translaminar route or the transcorti- cal, transforaminal route in cases of a distended foramen of Monro. The interhemispheric, inter- forniceal approach is used for all processes in the central part of the third ventricle, but here a subchoroidal approach is a valid alternative [35, 36] (Fig. 11.10). The posterior part can easily be reached via a supracerebellar, infratentorial approach [37, 38] which gives easy access to all processes originating around the pineal region (Fig. 11.11). Should the venous system be placed inferiorly or is there only limited extension into the pineal region, transcallosal or transtentorial approaches may be more opportune [39]. Most infratentorial processes are approached by sub- occipital craniotomy and direct midline approach from the foramen of Magendie into the fourth ventricle, the so-called telovelar approach [40]. The further the head is anteflected, the more it is possible to work underneath the vermis without splitting it, thus avoiding the posterior fossa syn- drome mainly associated with prolonged mutism [41, 42]. Recent studies question the role of ver- mian splitting and see direct brain stem infiltra- tion as the main cause for mutism [43] but that may be more related to medulloblastoma.

Ependymomas. Few therapies for intracra- nial tumors are discussed as controversially, and inconclusively as those for ependymoma, but a recent survey concluded that the incorporation of biological understanding is of utmost impor- tance for further improvement [44]. With the new molecular classification system, there is at least a chance for better correlation of clinical stud- ies to homogeneous patient groups in the future [5]. There is almost no dissense that they should usually be resected as radically as possible and a wealth of information exists, predominantly in the pediatric literature, that the extent of resec- tion is the most important prognostic variable, correlating positively with survival (reviewed in

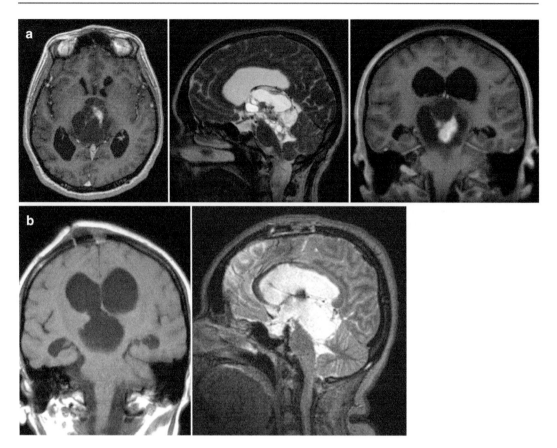

Fig. 11.10 (**a**) Large lesion in the third ventricle causing complex oculomotor disturbances with many heterogeneous cysts and signs of prior hemorrhage which was found to be consistent with a slowly developing pilocytic astrocytoma but turned out to be cavernous hemangioma. (**b**) This lesion was approached by subchoroidal approach allowing a good overview of the whole third ventricle way down to the fourth ventricle where a perforated gliotic velum with no impairment to CSF passage was left behind

[45]). What is to be a standard therapy has been controversial for a long time [7], but there is an emerging opinion that chemotherapy is to be used primarily in children under 12 years of age and adults with anaplastic recurrent tumors when all surgical and radiotherapeutic options have been exhausted (EANO guidelines) [46]. The role of surgery is firmly established. In the microsurgical age, mortality has dropped dramatically, and morbidity is related mainly to the involvement of the brain stem and cranial nerves. The numbers of patients surviving 5 years after complete (surgical microscope) resection versus subtotal/ partial resection show a statistically high significant difference (reviewed in [7]). In addition to extending survival, complete resection apparently leads to a significant reduction of spinal seeding. As spread of tumor beyond the site of origin can already be seen on preoperative imaging, it is not surprising that the neuroradiological evidence of spread is a negative prognostic sign [47]. The pattern for adults is somewhat different, because they arise more often in the supratentorial compartment and thus have a different surgical morbidity pattern when arising in the fourth ventricle [48]. Another poor sign seen in adults is the more frequent intraparenchymal localization because these tumors are nearly always anaplastic and correlated with poor survival [49].

The role of adjuvant chemotherapy is defined in the pediatric population and extrapolated to adults. It is still not firmly established, and no highly efficient regimen evaluated by a large study has been reported to date. The efficacy of chemotherapy is about that of radiation, sparing the children the radiation-induced sequelae which are a well-researched complication [50]. There is promise from a study alternating between a combination of carboplatin with vincristine and ifosfamide with etoposide [51]. The main goal of all chemotherapies in children is the delay of radiation which can be successfully achieved [52].

The role of radiation is controversial in many aspects. It has even been stated that in cases of MR-confirmed complete resection of grade II ependymoma, radiation maybe deferred until recurrence on an individual basis [53]. It has also been found that it may be beneficial for incompletely resected low-grade tumors but counterintuitively not for anaplastic lesions which have been completely removed [54]. As for the indication for craniospinal irradiation versus local radiation to the posterior fossa where most cases occur, there is apparently no difference in the rate of distant failures between groups receiving local radiation only compared to craniospinal regimens. When recurrences occur, they are almost always earlier in the posterior fossa before going to the spinal compartment. The doses delivered to the tumor area are between 45 and 50 Gy, and areas of macroscopic disease are given an extra 10 Gy. In the pediatric age group, there is now sufficient evidence that intensity of radiation, involved field, and age at the time of treatment will cause significant neuropsychological sequelae [55]. On the other hand, these are experiences from the past, and with the modern radiation techniques allowing for extreme limitation of the target volumes and minimization of collateral damage, the outcomes may be much better when present-day treatment series are evaluated. There is already a small study that radiosurgery for focal residual or recurrent disease may extend survival time [56].

Prognostic factors for tumors of the choroid plexus are mostly derived from small series and the limitation of conclusions from small numbers. For treatment, plexus papillomas are resected and then followed at regular intervals. As they can be easily resected, there is no use for adjuvant therapies when gross total resection is achieved [57, 58], and that is an accepted regimen for children as well as for adults. Even local recurrences of well-differentiated plexus papillomas in the adult are rather reoperated [59]. Complete resection appears to be an independent favorable prognostic parameter with a very high rate of 10-year progression-free survival in papillomas [60], and the negative prognostic parameter was the presence of carcinoma. Carcinomas of the plexus are much more difficult, occur mostly in small children, and carry a poor prognosis. They are treated with combination of surgery radiation and chemotherapy [60], but the true impact of adjuvant therapies is still debated. Prognosis is significantly worse than for papilloma [58].

Plexus meningiomas are resected like papillomas and then followed [15]. Radiosurgery may be considered in selected cases, but the high incidence of increased radiation toxicity and unsatisfactory tumor control in the long term leaves this modality for patients who for any reason cannot be given surgical treatment [15].

Neurocytomas, although a potentially benign, well-differentiated tumor entity, still raise controversial therapeutic issue. Whenever possible, gross total resection should be achieved and when completed offers excellent long-term tumor control [61]. This is usually possible in the anterior part of the lateral ventricles when not encasing the fornices. When they extend too far into the third ventricle and involve the fornices, a subradical approach must be taken. The same is true when the tumors arise with a broad ventricular base in the middle part of the ventricles or the trigonal area. In these instances, the issue of additional radiation is raised, and the remaining most controversial issue for neurocytomas is the indication for and the timing of radiation. There is clearly a benefit for patients after incomplete resection, tumors in inoperable location and for recurrent, well-differentiated lesions, and a strong recommendation to give radiation to patients with tumors carrying anaplastic features [61–63]. Radiation after gross total resection is not beneficial because while prolonging the event-free survival, it does not extend overall survival [62]. When during follow-up rapid regrowth is seen, the patients should undergo radiation which will lead to long-term control or complete cures, respectively [64]. There seems to be a slight advantage for stereotactic radiosurgery over conventional fractionated radiotherapy [65]. The role of radiation or radiosurgery as primary therapy is not clear, and there is no systematic evaluation because of the primate of surgery. There are only few reports about chemotherapy which was mostly given to patients with recurrence despite resection and radiation [66, 67] or very aggressive cases in children [28]. The most relevant prognostic parameters are the completeness of resection and for the likelihood of recurrence the KI67 labelling index [61].

Neuro-endoscopy has an important role in the treatment of ventricular tumors, mostly for the relief of hydrocephalus and biopsy [33]. In particular lesions in the posterior part of the third ventricle which are related to the complex pathology of the pineal region (see there) need a ventriculostomy rather than external ventricular drainage or shunt (Fig. 11.12) unless the patient has a combination of obstructive and malresorptive hydrocephalus. During ventriculostomy it is possible to take an endoscopic biopsy so that chemotherapy or radiation may be started before a surgical option is considered.

There are tumors which do not arise from the proper ventricular tissue matrix but nevertheless have exophytic growth into the ventricles, leading to partial hydrocephalus. These are frequently best approached by direct transventricular route to get to the exophytic part which in some cases may be the only part which can be resected (Figs. 11.13–11.15). Craniopharyngiomas and optic nerve gliomas, which also frequently affect the third ventricle and can be mistaken for intraventricular tumors, can sometimes easily be decompressed via the translaminar approach (Fig. 11.16) but may not be approachable when recurrent and no dissection plane is present to the hypothalamic boundaries (Fig. 11.17). Aggressive surgical approaches to the third ventricle and its surroundings have unwanted sequelae, in particular eating and weight disorders [68, 69]. Therefore radiation is indicated when tumors are infiltrative or recurrent [70].

11.9   Follow-Up and Prognosis

In all patients with ependymomas, the extent of resection is documented by postoperative MRI, preferably within 2 days after surgery. In the more aggressive tumors (WHO III), a spinal MRI is always performed to obtain staging information.

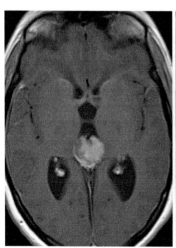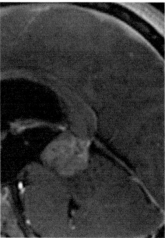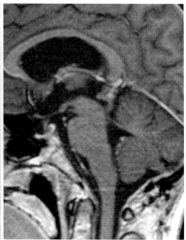

Fig. 11.11 Tumor in the posterior part of the third ventricle/pineal region (left and middle panel) which was removed via the supracerebellar approach and turned out to be pineocytoma with proportions of pineoblastoma which otherwise could have easily been missed by stereotactic biopsy. Complete resolution after surgery followed by local radiation (right panel)

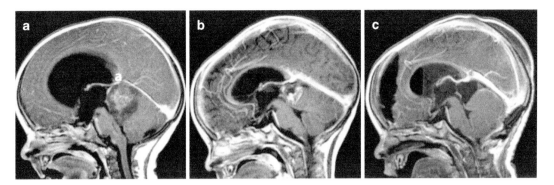

Fig. 11.12 Histologically confirmed atypical teratoid/ rhabdoid tumor (ATRT) in an 8-month-old boy which was biopsied on the occasion of a ventriculostomy (**a**). The diagnosis led to chemotherapy after which the tumor shrank significantly (**b**) and was then removed completely (**c**). A malresorptive component of the hydrocephalus required shunting after the ventriculostomy

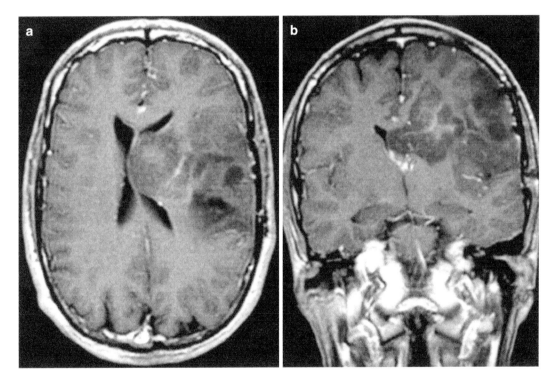

Fig. 11.13 A case of a hemispheric glioma in a 40-year-old male patient which extends into the lateral ventricles with a large exophytic component. In this case this was a histologically proven oligodendroglioma of the left insular region which had remained stable over several years without treatment but then developed a nodular satellite obliterating parts of the lateral ventricle. This was removed by direct transcortical approach

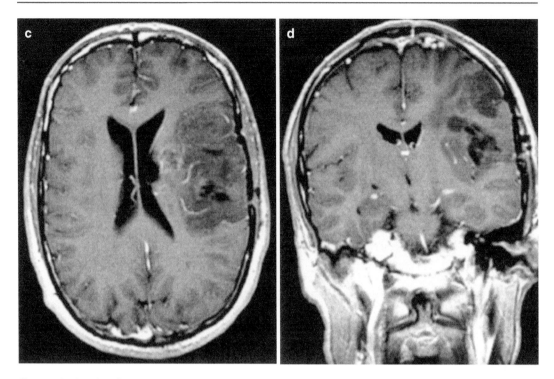

Fig. 11.13 (continued)

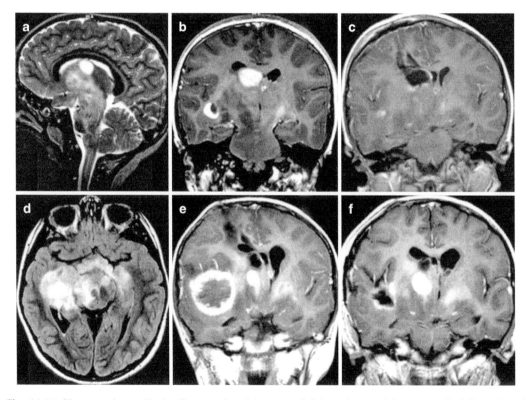

Fig. 11.14 Very complex pediatric (5 years, female) pilocytic astrocytoma of the optic nerve involving basal ganglia and brain stem which intermittently forms contrast-enhancing rapidly growing foci, one of which protruded into the ventricle, was well delineated, and could be removed completely by direct transcortical approach as other foci which were removed at later stages

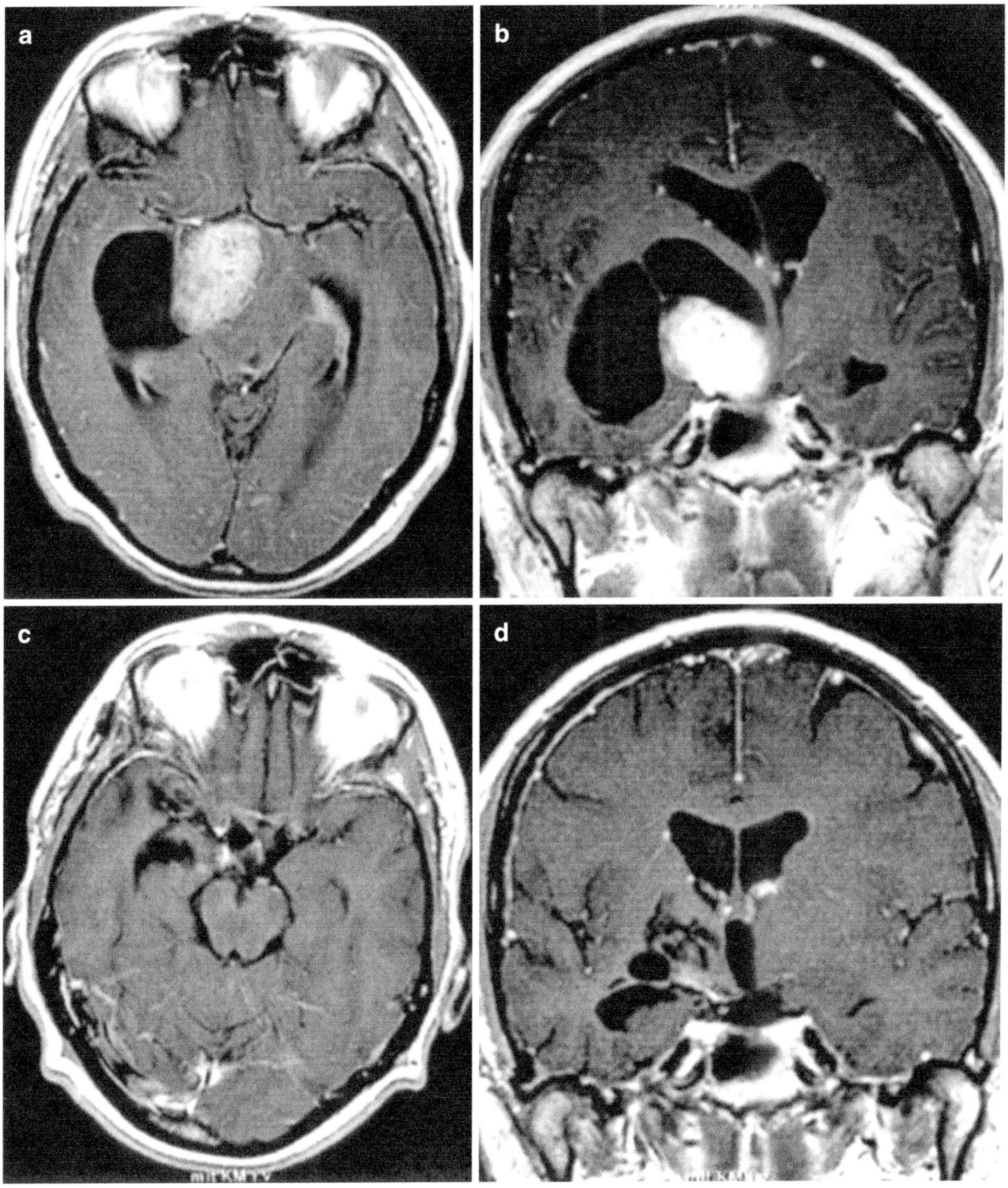

Fig. 11.15 Large tumor of the temporal horn (**a, b**) which after near-complete microsurgical removal (**c, d**) turned out to be an exophytically grown pilocytic astrocytoma of the optic tract in a 40-year-old woman

Depending on the treatment protocol chosen, patients are observed without any further treatment and followed at regular intervals or treated with radiation and/or chemotherapy after which they are also followed. The intervals for imaging are initially every 6 months but can be shorter when the tumors are WHO III and the treatment protocols call for shorter intervals. When the situation is stable, the periods between the follow-up visits can be extended to yearly to eventually biannual visits. There is much controversy as to what are prognostic parameters because histology is not

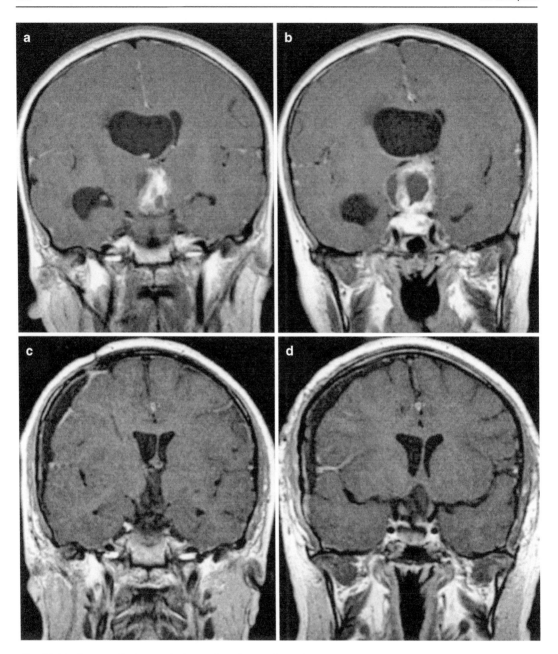

Fig. 11.16 Gross total microsurgical resection of a mostly cystic, recurrent craniopharyngioma of the third ventricle which is presently stable for 3 years after adjuvant radiotherapy

predictive of outcome, and even the occurrence of extraneural metastases occurs to the same degree with grade II and grade III lesions [32].

Plexus papillomas and meningiomas and hemangioblastomas are followed with initially 6-month intervals, then yearly visits after 2 years, and then biannual follow-up after 5 years. Neurocytomas may require radiation already after the first operation when they possess anaplastic feature. Thereafter they are followed with 6-month intervals. Also for the grade II lesions, close observation for regrowth is required for 3 years with 6-month intervals.

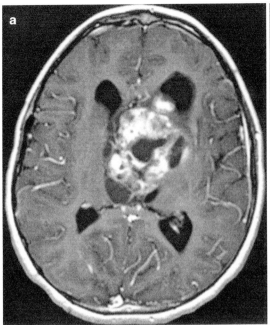
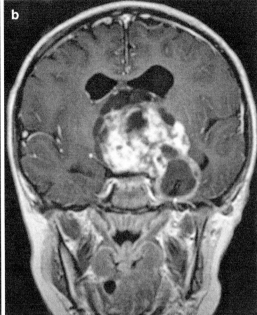

Fig. 11.17 Progressive development of an optic nerve glioma (pilocytic) which had been subradically approached already a few years earlier. As the cysts turned out to be part of the tumor all around, a dissection plane could not be expected so that in the absence of major neurological deficits, shunting and adjuvant therapies were preferred to a resective attempt

Metastases are treated and followed according to the histology of the primary tumor and the development of the disease outside the brain. With neurological deterioration in the absence of solid tumor and no local recurrence, the development of meningeal carcinomatosis has to be considered, but there are no reports of an association with metastasis to the choroid plexus.

References

1. Vecil GG, Lang FF (2003) Surgical resection of metastatic intraventricular tumors. Neurosurg Clin N Am 14:593–606
2. Ostrom QT, Gittleman H, Liao P, Vecchione-Koval T, Wolinsky Y, Kruchko C, Barnholtz-Sloan JS (2017) CBTRUS statistical report: primary brain and other central nervous system tumors diagnosed in the United States in 2010–2014. Neuro Oncol 19:v1–v88
3. Ellison DW, McLendon R, Wiestler OD, Kros JM, Korshunov A, Ng H-K, Witt H, Hirose T (2016) Anaplastic ependymoma. In: Louis DN, Ohgaki H, Wiestler OD, Cavanee WK, Ellison DW, Figarella-Branger D, Perry A, Reifenberger G, von Deimling A (eds) WHO classification of tumors of the central nervous system. IARC Press, Lyon, pp 113–114
4. Ellison DW, McLendon R, Wiestler OD, Kros JM, Korshunov A, Ng H-K, Witt H, Hirose T (2016) Ependymoma. In: Louis DN, Ohgaki H, Wiestler OD, Cavanee WK, Ellison DW, Figarella-Branger D, Perry A, Reifenberger G, von Deimling A (eds) WHO classification of tumors of the central nervous system. IARC Press, Lyon, pp 106–111
5. Pajtler KW, Witt H, Sill M, Jones DT, Hovestadt V, Kratochwil F, Wani K, Tatevossian R, Punchihewa C, Johann P, Reimand J, Warnatz HJ, Ryzhova M, Mack S, Ramaswamy V, Capper D, Schweizer L, Sieber L, Wittmann A, Huang Z, van Sluis P, Volckmann R, Koster J, Versteeg R, Fults D, Toledano H, Avigad S, Hoffman LM, Donson AM, Foreman N, Hewer E, Zitterbart K, Gilbert M, Armstrong TS, Gupta N, Allen JC, Karajannis MA, Zagzag D, Hasselblatt M, Kulozik AE, Witt O, Collins VP, von Hoff K, Rutkowski S, Pietsch T, Bader G, Yaspo ML, von Deimling A, Lichter P, Taylor MD, Gilbertson R, Ellison DW, Aldape K, Korshunov A, Kool M, Pfister SM (2015) Molecular classification of ependymal tumors across all CNS compartments, histopathological grades, and age groups. Cancer Cell 27:728–743
6. McLendon RE, Wiestler OD, Kros JM, Korshunov A, Ng H-K (2007) Ependymoma. In: Louis DN, Ohgaki H, Wiestler OD, Cavanee W (eds) WHO classification

of tumors of the central nervous system. IARC, Lyon, pp 74–78

7. Teo C, Nakaji P, Symons P, Tobias V, Cohn R, Smee R (2003) Ependymoma. Childs Nerv Syst 19:270–285

8. Paulus W, Brandner S, Hawkins C, Tihan TT (2016) Choroid plexus papilloma. In: Louis DN, Ohgaki H, Wiestler OD, Cavanee WK, Ellison DW, Figarella-Branger D, Perry A, Reifenberger G, von Deimling A (eds) WHO classification of tumors of the central nervous system. IARC Press, Lyon, pp 124–129

9. Waldron JS, Tihan T (2003) Epidemiology and pathology of intraventricular tumors. Neurosurg Clin N Am 14:469–482

10. Aguzzi A, Brandner S, Paulus W (2000) Choroid plexus tumors. In: Kleihues P, Cavanee W (eds) Tumours of the nervous system: pathology and genetics. IARC Press, Lyon

11. Paulus W, Brandner S (2007) Choroid plexus tumors. In: Louis DN, Ohgaki H, Wiestler OD, Cavanee W (eds) WHO classification of tumors of the central nervous system. IARC, Lyon, pp 82–85

12. Figarella-Branger D, Söylemezoglu F, Burger PC (2007) Central neurocytoma. In: Louis D, Ohgaki H, Wiestler OD, Cavanee W (eds) WHO classification of tumors of the central nervous system. IARC, Lyon, pp 106–109

13. Figarella-Branger D, Söyemezoglu F, Burger P, Park S-H, Honavar MT (2016) Central neurocytoma. In: Louis DN, Ohgaki H, Wiestler OD, Cavanee WK, Ellison DW, Figarella-Branger D, Perry A, Reifenberger G, von Deimling A (eds) WHO classification of tumors of the central nervous system. IARC Press, Lyon, pp 113–114

14. Lee J, Chang SM, McDermott MW, Parsa AT (2003) Intraventricular neurocytomas. Neurosurg Clin N Am 14:483–508

15. McDermott MW (2003) Intraventricular meningiomas. Neurosurg Clin N Am 14:559–569

16. Kohno M, Matsutani M, Sasaki T, Takakura K (1996) Solitary metastasis to the choroid plexus of the lateral ventricle. Report of three cases and a review of the literature. J Neurooncol 27:47–52

17. Shapira Y, Hadelsberg UP, Kanner AA, Ram Z, Roth J (2014) The ventricular system and choroid plexus as a primary site for renal cell carcinoma metastasis. Acta Neurochir (Wien) 156:1469–1474

18. Ebert C, von Haken M, Meyer-Puttlitz B, Wiestler OD, Reifenberger G, Pietsch T, von Deimling A (1999) Molecular genetic analysis of ependymal tumors. NF2 mutations and chromosome 22q loss occur preferentially in intramedullary spinal ependymomas. Am J Pathol 155:627–632

19. Khatua S, Ramaswamy V, Bouffet E (2017) Current therapy and the evolving molecular landscape of paediatric ependymoma. Eur J Cancer 70:34–41

20. Tabori U, Shlien A, Baskin B, Levitt S, Ray P, Alon N, Hawkins C, Bouffet E, Pienkowska M, Lafay-Cousin L, Gozali A, Zhukova N, Shane L, Gonzalez I, Finlay J, Malkin D (2010) TP53 alterations determine clinical subgroups and survival of patients with choroid plexus tumors. J Clin Oncol 28:1995–2001

21. Wiestler OD, Lopes BS, Green AJ, Vinters HV (2000) Tuberous sclerosis complex and subependymal giant cell astrocytoma. In: Kleihues P, Cavanee W (eds) Tumours of the nervous system: pathology and genetics. IARC, Lyon

22. Westphal M, Meissner H, Matschke J, Herrmann HD (1998) Tissue culture of human neurocytomas induces the expression of glial fibrillary acidic protein. J Neurocytol 27:805–816

23. Westphal M, Stavrou D, Nausch H, Valdueza JM, Herrmann HD (1994) Human neurocytoma cells in culture show characteristics of astroglial differentiation. J Neurosci Res 38:698–704

24. McLendon R, Schiffer D, Rosenblum M, Wiestler OD, Rushing EJ, Hirose T, Santi M (2016) Subependymoma. In: Louis DN, Ohgaki H, Wiestler OD, Cavanee WK, Ellison DW, Figarella-Branger D, Perry A, Reifenberger G, von Deimling A (eds) WHO classification of tumors of the central nervous system. IARC Press, Lyon, pp 106–111

25. Kuchiki H, Kayama T, Sakurada K, Saino M, Kawakami K, Sato S (2002) Two cases of atypical central neurocytomas. Brain Tumor Pathol 19:105–110

26. Mackenzie IR (1999) Central neurocytoma: histologic atypia, proliferation potential, and clinical outcome. Cancer 85:1606–1610

27. Vallat-Decouvelaere AV, Gauchez P, Varlet P, Delisle MB, Popovic M, Boissonnet H, Gigaud M, Mikol J, Hassoun J (2000) So-called malignant and extraventricular neurocytomas: reality or wrong diagnosis? A critical review about two overdiagnosed cases. J Neurooncol 48:161–172

28. Buchbinder D, Danielpour M, Yong WH, Salamon N, Lasky J (2010) Treatment of atypical central neurocytoma in a child with high dose chemotherapy and autologous stem cell rescue. J Neurooncol 97:429–437

29. Chadduck WM, Binet EF, Farrell FW Jr, Araoz CA, Reding DL (1985) Intraventricular cavernous hemangioma: report of three cases and review of the literature. Neurosurgery 16:189–197

30. Osuka S, Tsuboi K, Takano S, Ishikawa E, Matsushita A, Tokuuye K, Akine Y, Matsumura A (2007) Long-term outcome of patients with intracranial germinoma. J Neurooncol 83:71–79

31. Rickert CH (1998) Abdominal metastases of pediatric brain tumors via ventriculo-peritoneal shunts. Childs Nerv Syst 14:10–14

32. Newton HB, Henson J, Walker RW (1992) Extraneural metastases in ependymoma. J Neurooncol 14:135–142

33. Kunwar S (2003) Endoscopic adjuncts to intraventricular surgery. Neurosurg Clin N Am 14:547–557

34. Anderson RC, Ghatan S, Feldstein NA (2003) Surgical approaches to tumors of the lateral ventricle. Neurosurg Clin N Am 14:509–525

35. Wen HT, Rhoton AL Jr, de Oliveira E (1998) Transchoroidal approach to the third ventricle: an anatomic study of the choroidal fissure and its clinical application. Neurosurgery 42:1205–1217; discussion 1217–1209

36. Winkler PA, Ilmberger J, Krishnan KG, Reulen HJ (2000) Transcallosal interforniceal-transforaminal approach for removing lesions occupying the third ventricular space: clinical and neuropsychological results. Neurosurgery 46:879–888; discussion 888–890

37. Herrmann HD, Winkler D, Westphal M (1992) Treatment of tumours of the pineal region and posterior part of the third ventricle. Acta Neurochir (Wien) 116:137–146

38. Stein BM (1971) The infratentorial supracerebellar approach to pineal lesions. J Neurosurg 35:197–202

39. Lozier AP, Bruce JN (2003) Surgical approaches to posterior third ventricular tumors. Neurosurg Clin N Am 14:527–545

40. Winkler EA, Birk H, Safaee M, Yue JK, Burke JF, Viner JA, Pekmezci M, Perry A, Aghi MK, Berger MS, McDermott MW (2016) Surgical resection of fourth ventricular ependymomas: case series and technical nuances. J Neurooncol 130:341–349

41. Ersahin Y, Mutluer S, Cagli S, Duman Y (1996) Cerebellar mutism: report of seven cases and review of the literature. Neurosurgery 38:60–65; discussion 66

42. Pollack IF (1997) Posterior fossa syndrome. Int Rev Neurobiol 41:411–432

43. Tamburrini G, Frassanito P, Chieffo D, Massimi L, Caldarelli M, Di Rocco C (2015) Cerebellar mutism. Childs Nerv Syst 31:1841–1851

44. Wu J, Armstrong TS, Gilbert MR (2016) Biology and management of ependymomas. Neuro Oncol 18:902–913

45. Hamilton RL, Pollack IF (1997) The molecular biology of ependymomas. Brain Pathol 7:807–822

46. Ruda R, Reifenberger G, Frappaz D, Pfister SM, Laprie A, Santarius T, Roth P, Tonn JC, Soffietti R, Weller M, Moyal EC (2018) EANO guidelines for the diagnosis and treatment of ependymal tumors. Neuro Oncol 20:445–456

47. Chen CJ, Tseng YC, Hsu HL, Jung SM (2004) Imaging predictors of intracranial ependymomas. J Comput Assist Tomogr 28:407–413

48. Schwartz TH, Kim S, Glick RS, Bagiella E, Balmaceda C, Fetell MR, Stein BM, Sisti MB, Bruce JN (1999) Supratentorial ependymomas in adult patients. Neurosurgery 44:721–731

49. Guyotat J, Signorelli F, Desme S, Frappaz D, Madarassy G, Montange MF, Jouvet A, Bret P (2002) Intracranial ependymomas in adult patients: analyses of prognostic factors. J Neurooncol 60:255–268

50. von Hoff K, Kieffer V, Habrand JL, Kalifa C, Dellatolas G, Grill J (2008) Impairment of intellectual functions after surgery and posterior fossa irradiation in children with ependymoma is related to age and neurologic complications. BMC Cancer 8:15

51. Needle MN, Goldwein JW, Grass J, Cnaan A, Bergman I, Molloy P, Sutton L, Zhao H, Garvin JH Jr, Phillips PC (1997) Adjuvant chemotherapy for the treatment of intracranial ependymoma of childhood. Cancer 80:341–347

52. Grill J, Le Deley MC, Gambarelli D, Raquin MA, Couanet D, Pierre-Kahn A, Habrand JL, Doz F, Frappaz D, Gentet JC, Edan C, Chastagner P, Kalifa C (2001) Postoperative chemotherapy without irradiation for ependymoma in children under 5 years of age: a multicenter trial of the French Society of Pediatric Oncology. J Clin Oncol 19:1288–1296

53. Reni M, Gatta G, Mazza E, Vecht C (2007) Ependymoma. Crit Rev Oncol Hematol 63:81–89

54. Metellus P, Barrie M, Figarella-Branger D, Chinot O, Giorgi R, Gouvernet J, Jouvet A, Guyotat J (2007) Multicentric French study on adult intracranial ependymomas: prognostic factors analysis and therapeutic considerations from a cohort of 152 patients. Brain 130:1338–1349

55. Mulhern RK, Merchant TE, Gajjar A, Reddick WE, Kun LE (2004) Late neurocognitive sequelae in survivors of brain tumours in childhood. Lancet Oncol 5:399–408

56. Mansur DB, Drzymala RE, Rich KM, Klein EE, Simpson JR (2004) The efficacy of stereotactic radiosurgery in the management of intracranial ependymoma. J Neurooncol 66:187–190

57. Krishnan S, Brown PD, Scheithauer BW, Ebersold MJ, Hammack JE, Buckner JC (2004) Choroid plexus papillomas: a single institutional experience. J Neurooncol 68:49–55

58. Wolff JE, Sajedi M, Brant R, Coppes MJ, Egeler RM (2002) Choroid plexus tumours. Br J Cancer 87:1086–1091

59. Heese O, Lamszus K, Grzyska U, Westphal M (2002) Diffuse arachnoidal enhancement of a well differentiated choroid plexus papilloma. Acta Neurochir (Wien) 144:723–728

60. Bettegowda C, Adogwa O, Mehta V, Chaichana KL, Weingart J, Carson BS, Jallo GI, Ahn ES (2012) Treatment of choroid plexus tumors: a 20-year single institutional experience. J Neurosurg Pediatr 10:398–405

61. Lee SJ, Bui TT, Chen CH, Lagman C, Chung LK, Sidhu S, Seo DJ, Yong WH, Siegal TL, Kim M, Yang I (2016) Central neurocytoma: a review of clinical management and histopathologic features. Brain Tumor Res Treat 4:49–57

62. Leenstra JL, Rodriguez FJ, Frechette CM, Giannini C, Stafford SL, Pollock BE, Schild SE, Scheithauer BW, Jenkins RB, Buckner JC, Brown PD (2007) Central neurocytoma: management recommendations based on a 35-year experience. Int J Radiat Oncol Biol Phys 67:1145–1154

63. Rades D, Schild SE (2006) Treatment recommendations for the various subgroups of neurocytomas. J Neurooncol 77:305–309

64. Rades D, Fehlauer F, Schild SE (2004) Treatment of atypical neurocytomas. Cancer 100:814–817

65. Garcia RM, Ivan ME, Oh T, Barani I, Parsa AT (2014) Intraventricular neurocytomas: a systematic review of stereotactic radiosurgery and fractionated conventional radiotherapy for residual or recurrent tumors. Clin Neurol Neurosurg 117:55–64

66. Brandes AA, Amist P, Gardiman M, Volpin L, Danieli D, Guglielmi B, Carollo C, Pinna G, Turazzi S, Monfardini S (2000) Chemotherapy in patients with recurrent and progressive central neurocytoma. Cancer 88:169–174

67. Brandes AA, Amista P, Gardiman M, Volpin L, Danieli D, Guglielmi B, Carollo C, Pinna G, Turazzi S, Monfardini S (2000) Chemotherapy in patients with recurrent and progressive central neurocytoma. Cancer 88:169–174

68. Pinto G, Bussieres L, Recasens C, Souberbielle JC, Zerah M, Brauner R (2000) Hormonal factors influencing weight and growth pattern in craniopharyngioma. Horm Res 53:163–169

69. Skorzewska A, Lal S, Waserman J, Guyda H (1989) Abnormal food-seeking behavior after surgery for craniopharyngioma. Neuropsychobiology 21:17–20

70. Kalapurakal JA, Goldman S, Hsieh YC, Tomita T, Marymont MH (2003) Clinical outcome in children with craniopharyngioma treated with primary surgery and radiotherapy deferred until relapse. Med Pediatr Oncol 40:214–218

Pituitary Adenomas

12

Jörg Flitsch, Davis G. Taylor, and John A. Jane Jr

12.1 Introduction

The pituitary gland lies within the sella turcica and is connected to the hypothalamus by the pituitary stalk. As in any other gland, benign tumors occur frequently. Pituitary adenomas develop from anterior pituitary cells and are divided into hormone-secreting and nonfunctioning adenomas. Additionally, tumors are characterized according to their size into micro- (<10 mm) and macroadenomas (≥10 mm). Older data from the brain tumor register of the USA report an average incidence of 0.9 per 100,000 people per year [1]. More recent studies assume a 3–5 times higher incidence [2]. From autopsy studies, it is reported that in about 10%, mostly small adenomas were found in the pituitary gland [3].

Pituitary adenomas can be diagnosed as an incidental finding during imaging studies of the brain ("incidentaloma") or because of clinical symptoms. Symptoms may be secondary to the tumor size, e.g., headaches, visual disturbances, and pituitary insufficiencies, or due to hormone secretion of the tumor. According to the current WHO classification, tumors are classified as "regular" adenomas, aggressive adenomas with increased mitotic and proliferative activity, and pituitary carcinomas. Pituitary carcinomas are rare, and the diagnosis requires proven metastases [4]. The hormone status of the adenomas can be classified by immunohistochemistry. However, the identification of hormone expression in adenomas does not necessarily correlate with hormone secretion.

Except for prolactinomas, surgical resection is the treatment of choice for nonfunctioning and hormone-secreting adenomas, with high remission rates in microadenomas and decent results in macroadenomas. In the era of MR imaging, several classification systems have been proposed to predict resection likelihood. The most frequently used classification system is the Knosp grading, focusing on the extension of the tumor into the cavernous sinus with respect to the carotid artery [5]. Although biologically benign, invasive adenomas can result in therapeutic challenges.

Despite progress in knowledge, the pathogenesis of most adenomas remains unclear. About 5% of all pituitary adenomas are caused by germline mutations [6]. Known causes for increased adenoma occurrence are MEN 1, MEN 4, Carney

J. Flitsch (✉)
Hypophysenchirurgie/Klinik für Neurochirurgie, Universitätskrankenhaus Hamburg-Eppendorf, Hamburg, Germany
e-mail: flitsch@uke.de

D. G. Taylor · J. A. Jane Jr
Department of Neurosurgery, University of Virginia Health System, Charlottesville, VA, USA
e-mail: DT4AA@virginia.edu;
jaj2k@hscmail.mcc.virginia.edu

© Springer Nature Switzerland AG 2019
J.-C. Tonn et al. (eds.), *Oncology of CNS Tumors*, https://doi.org/10.1007/978-3-030-04152-6_12

complex, and McCune-Albright syndrome. More recently, AIP mutations were identified for the familial occurrence of isolated pituitary adenomas (FIPA), especially in acromegaly [2]. Other known mutations include Gs alpha activating mutation of the alpha-subunit of the adenylate cyclase-stimulating protein, found in acromegaly; PTTG overexpression of the pituitary tumor transforming gene; truncated form of the fibroblast growth factor 4; and somatic mutation of USP8 deubiquitinase gene in Cushing's disease through EGF-receptor signaling activation [7–11]. So far, no specific somatic mutations have been found in sporadic nonfunctioning adenomas by exome sequencing [12].

With rare exception, most pituitary adenomas can be approached using the transsphenoidal technique under microscopic or endoscopic guidance. In microadenomas, resection rates of up to 95% are reported, dropping to about 60% in macroadenomas. The surgical complication rate is considered low; the overall rate is about 7% and mainly consisting of CSF fistulas, meningitis, and pituitary insufficiencies [13]. Approved pharmacotherapy is available for prolactinomas (dopamine agonists), as second-line therapy for acromegaly (somatostatin analogues, GH-receptor antagonist), and Cushing's disease (somatostatin analogue, steroid genesis inhibitors (EMA), and steroid receptor antagonist (FDA)). Radiotherapy is associated with a high success rate in controlling tumor growth, and hormone secretion control may be achieved in about 50% over a period of 5–10 years. In the following, each subtype of adenoma will be discussed.

12.2 Nonfunctioning or Clinically Inactive Pituitary Adenoma

Nonfunctioning pituitary adenomas refer to a diverse group of tumors whose common feature is a lack of clinical hormone activity. Either no or nearly no hormone is secreted or the secreted hormone shows no biological activity. By histological means, these tumors are classified as FSH/LH adenomas (gonadotropinomas), null cell adenomas, or silent ACTH/GH/PRL/TSH adenomas, the latter with positive immunostaining for the respective hormone but no secretion into circulation.

About 25% of all adenomas are nonsecreting adenomas; the prevalence is assumed to be 22 per 100,000, making it the second most common adenoma type after prolactinomas and the most frequently surgically treated adenoma type [14]. Most nonsecreting adenomas are clinically diagnosed as macroadenomas, since a significant size is required to cause compression symptoms. Visual acuity loss and visual field disturbances are common symptoms, the occurrence reported in several studies from 18 to 78% [15]. Eye movement disorders caused by third, fourth, or sixth nerve palsy are less frequent (4–16%) and usually found after acute tumor hemorrhage or apoplexy, which can simulate symptoms of acute SAH with devastating headaches. Patients with pituitary adenomas frequently report headaches (17–75%) [15]. Some authors advocate a surgical resection even of microadenomas in case of intractable headaches, assuming a causal connection [16].

Pituitary insufficiencies presenting with symptoms such as fatigue, loss of libido/erection, weight loss or weight gain, hypotension, or amenorrhea can also be the leading clinical symptom, usually with an at least several months ongoing history. The pituitary axes are affected in a different speed and timing: somatotropic and gonadotropic insufficiencies occur prior to thyrotropic and corticotropic insufficiencies in most patients [15].

Incidental findings of pituitary adenomas are more frequent with the widespread use of imaging studies for other reasons ("incidentalomas"). In these cases and after an endocrinological work-up to rule out hormone secretion and pituitary insufficiencies, a follow-up by MR imaging is justified [17].

12.2.1 Diagnostic Work-Up

Unlike in hormone-secreting adenomas, there is no known tumor marker. The diagnosis as well as follow-up is mostly based on imaging studies.

Thin-sliced MR imaging of the sellar region with and without contrast enhancement (1.5 or 3 T) is the diagnostic tool of choice, showing the tumor size and extension including invasiveness. As mentioned above, the Knosp grading system is useful to predict surgical resection chances [5]. If an MRI is not an option, CT imaging should be obtained, allowing sagittal and coronal reconstructions (Fig. 12.1).

Endocrine work-up is mandatory to rule out hormone secretion of the tumor as well as to evaluate pituitary function. It is of main impor-

tance to rule out prolactinomas, since pituitary stalk deviation (stalk effect) can cause moderate hyperprolactinemia. In general, prolactin levels in the setting of stalk effect are below 100 µg/L, whereas prolactin levels >200 µg/L (10 × ULN) in a macroadenoma are indicative of a prolactinoma [18]. Other causes of hyperprolactinemia (pharmacotherapy) have to be ruled out; in giant adenomas a high-dose hook effect has to be considered and excluded by dilution of the blood sample. Anterior lobe function is altered in up to 85% of nonfunctioning adenomas requiring surgery [19].

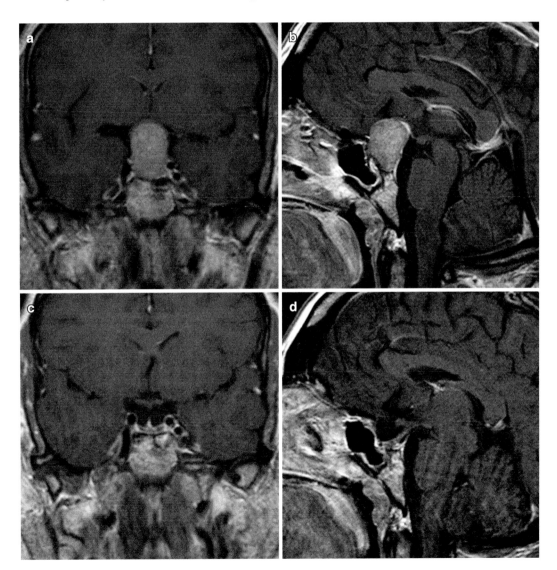

Fig. 12.1 Contrast-enhanced MRI of the pituitary region before (**a**, **b**) and after (**c**, **d**) removal of a nonfunctioning pituitary macroadenoma with optic chiasm compression

In most patients, a basal early morning hormone panel allows sufficient information; sometimes stimulation test may be necessary [20]. Diabetes insipidus is not a common symptom of nonfunctioning adenomas at presentation.

12.2.2 Therapy

In case of chiasm syndrome, eye movement alterations, and acute symptomatic hemorrhage, intervention is recommended [21]. Treatment can furthermore be considered in case of proven tumor growth during follow-up, intractable headaches, planned pregnancy, or occurrence of pituitary insufficiencies.

Treatment of choice is transsphenoidal surgery, either microscopic or endoscopic [22]. Nowadays, there are different intraoperative guidance and support systems available; however, current literature does not show superiority compared to traditional techniques. Tumor decompression is immediately achieved by surgery. However, incomplete resection is frequent in up to 36%. Therefore, relief of chiasm compression syndrome is reported in the majority (75–91%) of patients [23]. Even pituitary insufficiency can improve. Complications of transsphenoidal surgery are considered low; a more recent meta-analysis reported a morbidity of 7% and a mortality under 1% [24]. New pituitary insufficiencies occur in about 5% of treated patients [25].

Surgery is indicated in most patients with chiasmal compression. Those without chiasmal compression may be considered for surgery depending on their expected risk of becoming symptomatic from tumor growth depending on their age, life expectancy, and comorbidities [21]. Although pituitary apoplexy has been considered an indication for surgical intervention, select patients can be successfully treated conservatively.

Treatment of choice is transsphenoidal surgery, either microscopic or endoscopic [22]. In modern practice there are different intraoperative guidance and support systems available; however, current literature does not show superiority compared to traditional techniques. Tumor

decompression is immediately achieved by surgery; however, incomplete resection is frequent in up to 36%. Therefore, relief of chiasm compression syndrome is reported in the majority (75–91%) of patients [23]. Preoperative pituitary insufficiency improves in a minority of patients. Complications of transsphenoidal surgery are considered low; a more recent meta-analysis reported a morbidity of 7% and a mortality under 1% [24]. New pituitary insufficiencies occur in about 5% of treated patients [25].

There is no approved pharmacotherapy for the treatment of nonfunctioning adenomas. Since membrane-bound dopamine-2 and somatostatin receptors (mostly subtypes 1, 2, and 3) have been found in these tumors as well, dopamine agonists and somatostatin analogues have been tried, unfortunately with limited success.

Radiotherapy is considered in case of residual or recurrent disease. Growth control rates of about 90% are reported [15]. Stereotactic methods are state of the art, either fractionated or as single dose (radiosurgery). Side effects of radiotherapy include pituitary insufficiency (50% in 5–10 years), optic neuropathy (1–5%), an increase of cerebrovascular events, and a risk increase for benign as well as malignant intracranial tumors (1.6–2.4 times).

12.3 Hormone-Secreting Adenomas

12.3.1 ACTH-Secreting Adenomas (Cushing's Disease)

Endogenous hypercortisolism (Cushing's syndrome) is rare with an estimated annual incidence of 0.7–2.4 per one million and connected with an increased morbidity and mortality risk [26]. In about 70% of patients, the origin is an ACTH-secreting pituitary adenoma (Cushing's disease), overstimulating the adrenals with consecutive elevation of cortisol. The female to male ratio is 3 to 1, and most patients are diagnosed in the third to fifth decade of life. The time from initial symptoms to diagnosis usually takes about 5 years [27]. Clinically, the disease is characterized by many changes; the most prominent changes to discriminate from other conditions are petechial/easy bruising, facial plethora, proximal myopathy, and striae distensae. In childhood, weight gain in combination with growth arrest is typical [28]. Regarding the pathogenesis, the recent detection of USP-8 mutations in a number of ACTH adenomas has been a hallmark, showing an activation of EGF-receptor signaling [8].

12.3.1.1 Diagnostic Work-Up

Even in experienced hands, the diagnostic work-up of Cushing's disease can be challenging. The first step in suspected Cushing's syndrome is the detection of hypercortisolism, which can be done by repeated sampling of urine-free cortisol (UFC) and late-night salivary cortisol or a 1 mg dexamethasone suppression test [28].

In cases of detectable or elevated ACTH in hypercortisolism, ACTH-dependent Cushing's syndrome is diagnosed, requiring further separation of pituitary and ectopic disease. The high-dose dexamethasone test (8 mg) and CRH-stimulation test in combination best discriminate both conditions. In dubious cases, inferior petrosal sinus sampling (IPSS) is considered the gold standard to diagnose pituitary vs. ectopic disease and is particularly useful in the setting of MRI negative Cushing's.

If all tests lead to pituitary origin, thin-sliced MR imaging of the pituitary (3 T with and without contrast enhancement) is the study of choice. Unlike in other adenoma types, microadenomas are common (~90%). Even with sophisticated imaging protocols, not all adenomas are visualized [29]. Therefore, additional diagnostic tests and studies have been developed to help localize small adenomas, like central venous sampling or PET-MRI studies, enriching the armory [30, 31].

12.3.1.2 Therapy

After diagnosis, therapy is recommended in all patients, and transsphenoidal surgery is the treatment of choice, ideally resulting in early hypo-cortisolemia as a marker for complete resection [28]. In most patients, cortisol and ACTH levels drop within 16–24 h, but in some it may take up to 72 h. Early morning cortisol and ACTH

determination without prior replacement help the clinician to distinguish between remission and persistent disease in most cases. Cortisol levels below 18 µg/L (50 nmol/L) are considered the best result regarding long-term remission. Levels below 57 µg/L (140 nmol/L) or 72 µg/L (200 nmol/L) are reported to be adequate as early signs of remission. Furthermore, ACTH levels below 10 pg/mL predict long-term remission [32–35].

The patients experience a phase of secondary adrenal insufficiency as a sign of successful treatment. The restitution of the hypothalamic-pituitary-adrenal axis takes on average about 18 months, in children on average 12 months [36]. Especially in the beginning, patients require increased cortisol substitution doses above the recommended 10–25 mg/die hydrocortisone (~10 mg/m^2 body surface) for adrenal insufficiency. Insufficient substitution leads to signs of steroid withdrawal like bone and joint aches, loss of appetite, and adynamia. Surgery in experienced hands can lead to remission rates of ~90% in microadenomas and ~65% in macroadenomas. Recurrence rates of 10–65% are reported in literature [37]. Surgery has to be reconsidered first in case of recurrence.

Complications after surgery mostly comprise of anterior lobe insufficiencies, especially after re-surgery, transient diabetes insipidus or SIADH, CSF fistulas, and rarely neurological deficits. Patients with Cushing's disease are in a state of hypercoagulability and therefore are at risk for thromboembolic events, especially during the perioperative phase [38]. The authors support the preventive administration of low-dose heparin perioperatively.

Pharmacotherapy has been long used for the treatment of hypercortisolism, but only recently several drugs have been approved as second-line treatment options. Pasireotide, a multi-ligand somatostatin analogue, is approved by the FDA and EMA for Cushing's disease, lowering ACTH secretion and achieving normal UFC in about 20% of treated patients after 6 months. Ketoconazole (50% drop of UFC in 75% of patients) and metyrapone (75% normalization of UFC), steroid genesis inhibitors, have been approved by the EMA for treatment of hypercortisolism. For the treatment of glucose intolerance and diabetes mellitus in Cushing's syndrome, mifepristone, a glucocorticoid receptor antagonist, has been approved by the FDA. All substances have considerable high rates of side effects, making a long-term treatment difficult and therefore are second choice. In clinical use but not approved are cabergoline, fluconazole, etomidate, aminoglutethimide, and mitotane.

Radiotherapy is recommended in patients after failed surgery or in case of recurrent disease. Because of the time span between radiotherapy and biochemical effect, patients should additionally receive medical therapy. Stereotactic radiotherapy is state of the art; there is no clear-cut advantage when comparing fractionated or radiosurgical methods. Whereas tumor control is achieved in nearly all patients, biochemical control varies between published series from 28 to 86% [37]. Risks apply as described in the section nonfunctioning adenomas.

Bilateral adrenalectomy is reserved for severe cases in whom hypercortisolemia cannot be controlled by other means, resulting in lifelong adrenal insufficiency. In these patients, the risk of Nelson's syndrome development is present, requiring careful monitoring of ACTH and regular MRIs.

12.3.2 TSH-Secreting Adenomas (TSHomas)

TSH-secreting adenomas account for only 1–2% of all pituitary adenomas and have a prevalence of 2.8 per one million [39, 40]. These adenomas are a potential misdiagnosed cause of hyperthyroidism. Before the correct diagnosis is made, many patients have undergone thyroid surgery or symptomatic pharmacotherapy. Also, since TSH determination is used as a screening parameter for hypothyroidism without additional determination of peripheral thyroid hormones, patients may even falsely receive thyroid hormone replacement therapy, worsening the symptoms.

12.3.2.1 Diagnostic Work-Up
Clinically, signs of hyperthyroidism should lead to an endocrinological work-up, showing elevated

peripheral thyroid hormones with detectable TSH (normal or elevated). The main differential diagnosis of this hormone constellation is resistance to thyroid hormone action (Refetoff syndrome), which usually does not present with clinical signs of hyperthyroidism. To differentiate between both conditions, the determination of alpha-subunit, which is increased in most TSHomas, can be helpful [39]. In today's clinical practice, the thyroid hormone receptor mutations can be confirmed by molecular-biological means; several mutations have been described. In case of true TSH-dependent hyperthyroidism, MR imaging is the final step to confirm the diagnosis.

12.3.2.2 Therapy
The treatment of choice is transsphenoidal surgery [39, 41]. Surgical results show a high remission rate and low complication rates [41, 42]. Invasion is frequently reported [43]. Second-line treatment consists of first-generation somatostatin analogues (octreotide or lanreotide). So far, there are no reports on the use of second-generation somatostatin analogues. In some cases, dopamine agonist therapy may be considered prior to somatostatin analogue therapy. Presurgical somatostatin analogue therapy may be used to improve clinical symptoms as well as to reduce tumor size. For some patients, radiotherapy may be considered for residual, non-resectable tumor tissue.

12.3.3 Growth Hormone-Secreting Adenomas (Acromegaly)

Growth hormone (GH)-secreting adenomas account for about 30% of functioning pituitary tumors with a prevalence of 40 per one million [44]. The presentation of acromegaly patients is typical for a protracted course of changes in physical appearance, including facial coarseness, macroglossia, and enlargement of the hands and feet [45]. Cardiovascular comorbidities are common (a consequence of GH hypersecretion), and the associations with heart disease, diabetes, hypertension, and chronic pain lead to reduced quality of life and increased mortality among these patients, with GH levels directly correlating with mortality rate [45, 46]. Due to the prolonged time to diagnosis, these patients often present with macroadenomas and associated findings of cavernous sinus invasion or clinical symptoms of optic chiasm compression [47].

12.3.3.1 Diagnostic Work-Up

Initial laboratory evaluation of acromegaly or suspicion of GH-secreting adenomas should include a serum insulin growth factor (IGF-1) level. IGF-1, a measure of systemic response to elevated GH, is almost always elevated in GH-secreting adenomas, but confirmation should be performed with an oral glucose tolerance test, whereby the patient is given an oral dose of 75 g of glucose, and growth hormone concentration is measured at time 0 and then every 30 min for 2 h. Patients with GH > 0.4 ng/mL at 2 h following administration of oral glucose are diagnosed with acromegaly and should undergo full endocrine evaluation to rule out hypopituitarism and MRI to assess for a pituitary adenoma [48, 49].

12.3.3.2 Therapy

Following diagnosis, a multidisciplinary team including endocrinologists and neurosurgeons is utilized to medically optimize the patient's care. Due to the significant comorbidities associated with continued elevation of GH, surgery can be considered as initial treatment, but some authors recommend medical therapy as a first-line treatment, particularly in patients with significant comorbidities, the elderly, or those patients where surgical resection is unlikely to provide a biochemical cure (cavernous sinus or dural invasion). Initial treatment with somatostatin analogues can result in normalization of IGF-1 in as many as 68% of patients achieving normalization of IGF-1 at 18 weeks, with significant improvement in prevalence of hypertension, hyperlipidemia, and cardiac dysfunction [50–52]. Pre-treatment GH levels are predictive of post-operative success, and so the positive effects of medical treatment and the ability to reduce tumor size and reduce GH levels have led some authors to advocate for neoadjuvant treatment of acromegalic patients prior to elective surgery to reduce

the tumor burden and improve normalization of GH and IGF-1 [53]. Surgery offers the most rapid and definitive opportunity for biochemical cure of microadenomas and noninvasive macroadenomas and can result in a 65% reduction in preoperative GH levels within 2 days of surgery [54, 55]. Aggressive resection should be performed as IGF levels will remain persistently elevated until the GH is less than 10 ng/mL, and persistent elevations in IGF-1 are directly related to patient mortality [56, 57].

In many cases, such as with cavernous sinus invasion, a long-term surgical remission is unlikely. Three medications are used as adjuvant or neoadjuvant treatment in the management of acromegaly with proven efficacy: somatostatin analogues, GH-receptor antagonists, and dopamine agonists. Somatostatin analogues have been shown to reduce GH levels and normalize IGF-1 in as many as 61% of patients and a radiographic tumor response in 20% of tumors [47, 58].

For patients with cavernous sinus invasion, residual tumor, recurrent acromegaly, or medical failure, radiosurgery has a proven benefit in the treatment of patients with persistent acromegaly, demonstrating remission in as many as 82.6% of patients at 8 years and with a median time to remission of 26 months [59, 60].

12.3.4 Prolactin-Secreting Adenomas (Prolactinoma)

Prolactinomas are the most common pituitary adenoma, representing 40% of all pituitary adenomas [61]. Patients typically present based on sex with symptoms of amenorrhea (90%) and galactorrhea (80%) among women and impotence among men [61]. Unlike the other adenomas previously mentioned, these tumors are frequently responsive to medication and, generally, should undergo medical treatment.

12.3.4.1 Diagnostic Work-Up

Laboratory assessment of prolactinoma should involve endocrine assessment of prolactin function. Normal levels are less than 25 μg/L in women. Initial evaluation should involve review of current medications for any dopamine antagonist medications. If no offending agent is appreciated, MRI should be obtained. Prolactin level correlates directly with adenoma size. Macroadenomas with prolactinemia less than 150 µg/L are unlikely to be true prolactinomas, and are more likely representative of stalk effect and reduced dopamine inhibition due a nonfunctioning macroadenoma's compressive effects or may be artificially low in prolactinomas due to the "hook" effect, which is an artifact that occurs with oversaturation of the immunoassay for prolactin [61, 62]. More typically, prolactin macroadenomas will demonstrate levels well over 200 µg/L [61, 62].

12.3.4.2 Therapy

Once the diagnosis of hyperprolactinemia is made and the presence of a pituitary adenoma confirmed, the treatment team must weigh the appropriate course of management. Even among untreated microadenomas, some tumors will undergo spontaneous involution with improvement of clinical symptoms [63]. If intervention is pursued, most cases of prolactinoma can be safely treated with medical therapy, primarily with dopamine agonists bromocriptine or cabergoline [61, 64–66]. In general, cabergoline is the initial treatment of choice due to greater patient tolerance and tumor response and normalization of prolactin levels compared to bromocriptine [67, 68].

Occasionally, however, surgery may be indicated in patients with medication intolerance or tumor resistance to dopamine agonist therapy, as well as in some patients with microadenomas or noninvasive intrasellar macroadenomas [61, 65, 69, 70]. Some studies have demonstrated improved medication responsiveness and normalization of prolactin levels following transsphenoidal resection of previously resistant prolactinomas [61, 69, 71].

For those patients resistant to medical and surgical treatment, radiosurgery can also be considered. Radiotherapy has been demonstrated to have tumor growth control in up to 89% of patients with 26% of patients achieving endocrine remission at 24.5 months and 50% by 42.3 months [72–74].

12.4 Follow-Up

In all patients, a follow-up is recommended. Even after surgical resection with no visual tumor remnant on MR imaging, recurrences in about 12% are reported; in cases of visible residual disease, recurrences occur in up to 50% of nonfunctioning adenomas [75]. Follow-up timing of imaging studies varies between patients and depends on treatment mode, and usually after therapy initiation, a 3- to 6-month follow-up scan is advisable. In hormone-secreting adenomas, endocrinological follow-up allows determination of the respective hormone function; therefore there is a tendency to reduce imaging studies in case of clear remission. Especially the recently discussed potential harmfulness of gadolinium should limit its use until more data is available [76]. After proof of a stable situation, the time span can be extended from an annual MRI to several years. The development of new clinical symptoms may lead to short-term MR imaging.

Endocrinological follow-up is mandatory to control treatment effects as well as to rule out new pituitary insufficiencies. After initial treatment, a follow-up is recommended within 6–12 weeks and afterward under stable clinical conditions every 6–12 months. Tumor recurrence or previous radiotherapy can alter the pituitary function even years after initial therapy [77]. Additionally, ophthalomological examinations should be considered if appropriate, especially after radiotherapy.

References

1. Surawicz TS, McCarthy BJ, Kupelian V, Jukich PJ, Bruner JM, Davis FG (1999) Descriptive epidemiology of primary brain and CNS tumors: results from the central brain tumor registry of the United States, 1990–1994. Neuro Oncol 1:14–25
2. Daly AF, Tichomirowa MA, Beckers A (2009) The epidemiology and genetics of pituitary adenomas. Best Pract Res Clin Endocrinol Metab 23:543–554
3. Buurman H, Saeger W (2006) Subclinical adenomas in postmortem pituitaries: classification and correlations to clinical data. Eur J Endocrinol 154:753–758
4. Saeger W, Ludecke DK, Buchfelder M, Fahlbusch R, Quabbe HJ, Petersenn S (2007) Pathohistological classification of pituitary tumors: 10 years of experience with the German pituitary tumor registry. Eur J Endocrinol 156:203–216

5. Knosp E, Steiner E, Kitz K, Matula C (1993) Pituitary adenomas with invasion of the cavernous sinus space: a magnetic resonance imaging classification compared with surgical findings. Neurosurgery 33:610–617; discussion 7–8

6. Caimari F, Korbonits M (2016) Novel genetic causes of pituitary adenomas. Clin Cancer Res 22:5030–5042

7. Ezzat S, Zheng L, Zhu XF, Wu GE, Asa SL (2002) Targeted expression of a human pituitary tumor-derived isoform of FGF receptor-4 recapitulates pituitary tumorigenesis. J Clin Invest 109:69–78

8. Reincke M, Sbiera S, Hayakawa A et al (2015) Mutations in the deubiquitinase gene USP8 cause Cushing's disease. Nat Genet 47:31–38

9. Ronchi CL, Peverelli E, Herterich S et al (2016) Landscape of somatic mutations in sporadic GH-secreting pituitary adenomas. Eur J Endocrinol 174:363–372

10. Vallar L, Spada A, Giannattasio G (1987) Altered Gs and adenylate cyclase activity in human GH-secreting pituitary adenomas. Nature 330:566–568

11. Vlotides G, Eigler T, Melmed S (2007) Pituitary tumor-transforming gene: physiology and implications for tumorigenesis. Endocr Rev 28:165–186

12. Newey PJ, Nesbit MA, Rimmer AJ et al (2013) Whole-exome sequencing studies of nonfunctioning pituitary adenomas. J Clin Endocrinol Metab 98:E796–E800

13. Halvorsen H, Ramm-Pettersen J, Josefsen R et al (2014) Surgical complications after transsphenoidal microscopic and endoscopic surgery for pituitary adenoma: a consecutive series of 506 procedures. Acta Neurochir 156:441–449

14. Fernandez A, Karavitaki N, Wass JA (2010) Prevalence of pituitary adenomas: a community-based, cross-sectional study in Banbury (Oxfordshire, UK). Clin Endocrinol 72:377–382

15. Molitch ME (2014) Nonfunctioning pituitary tumors. Handb Clin Neurol 124:167–184

16. Fleseriu M, Yedinak C, Campbell C, Delashaw JB (2009) Significant headache improvement after transsphenoidal surgery in patients with small sellar lesions. J Neurosurg 110:354–358

17. Ludecke DK (2003) [Management of patients with non-functioning pituitary adenomas. Summary of results of an expert conference of the Hypophysis Work Group of the German Society of Endocrinology, Friedewald, 15–17 February 2002]. Med Klin (Munich) 98:616–627

18. Melmed S, Casanueva FF, Hoffman AR et al (2011) Diagnosis and treatment of hyperprolactinemia: an Endocrine Society Clinical Practice Guideline. J Clin Endocrinol Metab 96:273–288

19. Nomikos P, Ladar C, Fahlbusch R, Buchfelder M (2004) Impact of primary surgery on pituitary function in patients with non-functioning pituitary adenomas—a study on 721 patients. Acta Neurochir 146:27–35

20. Fleseriu M, Bodach ME, Tumialan LM et al (2016) Congress of Neurological Surgeons systematic review and evidence-based guideline for Pretreatment endocrine evaluation of patients with nonfunctioning pituitary adenomas. Neurosurgery 79:E527–E529

21. Freda PU, Beckers AM, Katznelson L et al (2011) Pituitary incidentaloma: an endocrine society clinical practice guideline. J Clin Endocrinol Metab 96:894–904

22. Kuo JS, Barkhoudarian G, Farrell CJ et al (2016) Congress of Neurological Surgeons systematic review and evidence-based guideline on surgical techniques and technologies for the management of patients with nonfunctioning pituitary adenomas. Neurosurgery 79:E536–E538

23. Lucas JW, Bodach ME, Tumialan LM et al (2016) Congress of Neurological Surgeons systematic review and evidence-based guideline on primary management of patients with nonfunctioning pituitary adenomas. Neurosurgery 79:E533–E535

24. Murad MH, Fernandez-Balsells MM, Barwise A et al (2010) Outcomes of surgical treatment for nonfunctioning pituitary adenomas: a systematic review and meta-analysis. Clin Endocrinol 73:777–791

25. Webb SM, Rigla M, Wagner A, Oliver B, Bartumeus F (1999) Recovery of hypopituitarism after neurosurgical treatment of pituitary adenomas. J Clin Endocrinol Metab 84:3696–3700

26. Sharma ST, Nieman LK, Feelders RA (2015) Cushing's syndrome: epidemiology and developments in disease management. Clin Epidemiol 7:281–293

27. Flitsch J, Spitzner S, Ludecke DK (2000) Emotional disorders in patients with different types of pituitary adenomas and factors affecting the diagnostic process. Exp Clin Endocrinol Diabetes 108:480–485

28. Nieman LK, Biller BM, Findling JW et al (2008) The diagnosis of Cushing's syndrome: an Endocrine Society Clinical Practice Guideline. J Clin Endocrinol Metab 93:1526–1540

29. Grober Y, Grober H, Wintermark M, Jane JA Jr, Oldfield EH (2018) Comparison of MRI techniques for detecting microadenomas in Cushing's disease. J Neurosurg 128:1051–1057

30. Burkhardt T, Flitsch J, van Leyen P et al (2015) Cavernous sinus sampling in patients with Cushing's disease. Neurosurg Focus 38:E6

31. Ikeda H, Abe T, Watanabe K (2010) Usefulness of composite methionine-positron emission tomography/3.0-tesla magnetic resonance imaging to detect the localization and extent of early-stage Cushing adenoma. J Neurosurg 112:750–755

32. Alwani RA, de Herder WW, van Aken MO et al (2010) Biochemical predictors of outcome of pituitary surgery for Cushing's disease. Neuroendocrinology 91:169–178

33. Flitsch J, Knappe UJ, Ludecke DK (2003) The use of postoperative ACTH levels as a marker for successful transsphenoidal microsurgery in Cushing's disease. Zentralbl Neurochir 64:6–11

34. Starke RM, Reames DL, Chen CJ, Laws ER, Jane JA Jr (2013) Endoscopic transsphenoidal surgery for Cushing disease: techniques, outcomes, and predictors of remission. Neurosurgery 72:240–247; discussion 7

35. Trainer PJ, Lawrie HS, Verhelst J et al (1993) Transsphenoidal resection in Cushing's disease: undetectable serum cortisol as the definition of successful treatment. Clin Endocrinol 38:73–78

36. Flitsch J, Ludecke DK, Knappe UJ, Saeger W (1999) Correlates of long-term hypocortisolism after transsphenoidal microsurgery for Cushing's disease. Exp Clin Endocrinol Diabetes 107:183–189

37. Nieman LK, Biller BM, Findling JW et al (2015) Treatment of Cushing's syndrome: an Endocrine Society Clinical Practice Guideline. J Clin Endocrinol Metab 100:2807–2831

38. Boscaro M, Sonino N, Scarda A et al (2002) Anticoagulant prophylaxis markedly reduces thromboembolic complications in Cushing's syndrome. J Clin Endocrinol Metab 87:3662–3666

39. Beck-Peccoz P, Persani L, Mannavola D, Campi I (2009) Pituitary tumours: TSH-secreting adenomas. Best Pract Res Clin Endocrinol Metab 23:597–606

40. Onnestam L, Berinder K, Burman P et al (2013) National incidence and prevalence of TSH-secreting pituitary adenomas in Sweden. J Clin Endocrinol Metab 98:626–635

41. Rotermund R, Riedel N, Burkhardt T et al (2017) Surgical treatment and outcome of TSH-producing pituitary adenomas. Acta Neurochir 159:1219–1226

42. Malchiodi E, Profka E, Ferrante E et al (2014) Thyrotropin-secreting pituitary adenomas: outcome of pituitary surgery and irradiation. J Clin Endocrinol Metab 99:2069–2076

43. Laws ER, Vance ML, Jane JA Jr (2006) TSH adenomas. Pituitary 9:313–315

44. Jane JA Jr, Thapar K, Laws ER Jr (2001) Acromegaly: historical perspectives and current therapy. J Neurooncol 54:129–137

45. Colao A, Ferone D, Marzullo P, Lombardi G (2004) Systemic complications of acromegaly: epidemiology, pathogenesis, and management. Endocr Rev 25:102–152

46. Abosch A, Tyrrell JB, Lamborn KR, Hannegan LT, Applebury CB, Wilson CB (1998) Transsphenoidal microsurgery for growth hormone-secreting pituitary adenomas: initial outcome and long-term results. J Clin Endocrinol Metab 83:3411–3418

47. Bush ZM, Vance ML (2008) Management of acromegaly: is there a role for primary medical therapy? Rev Endocr Metab Disord 9:83–94

48. Carmichael JD, Bonert VS, Mirocha JM, Melmed S (2009) The utility of oral glucose tolerance testing for diagnosis and assessment of treatment outcomes in 166 patients with acromegaly. J Clin Endocrinol Metab 94:523–527

49. Clemmons DR, Van Wyk JJ, Ridgway EC, Kliman B, Kjellberg RN, Underwood LE (1979) Evaluation of acromegaly by radioimmunoassay of somatomedin-C. N Engl J Med 301:1138–1142

50. Colao A, Auriemma RS, Galdiero M, Lombardi G, Pivonello R (2009) Effects of initial therapy for five years with somatostatin analogs for acromegaly on growth hormone and insulin-like growth factor-I levels, tumor shrinkage, and cardiovascular disease: a prospective study. J Clin Endocrinol Metab 94:3746–3756

51. Higham CE, Atkinson AB, Aylwin S et al (2012) Effective combination treatment with cabergoline and low-dose pegvisomant in active acromegaly: a prospective clinical trial. J Clin Endocrinol Metab 97:1187–1193

52. Lim DS, Fleseriu M (2017) The role of combination medical therapy in the treatment of acromegaly. Pituitary 20:136–148

53. Colao A, Ferone D, Cappabianca P et al (1997) Effect of octreotide pretreatment on surgical outcome in acromegaly. J Clin Endocrinol Metab 82:3308–3314

54. Nomikos P, Buchfelder M, Fahlbusch R (2005) The outcome of surgery in 668 patients with acromegaly using current criteria of biochemical 'cure'. Eur J Endocrinol 152:379–387

55. Yu M, Bruns DE, Jane JA Jr et al (2017) Decrease of serum IGF-I following transsphenoidal pituitary surgery for acromegaly. Clin Chem 63:486–494

56. Holdaway IM, Rajasoorya RC, Gamble GD (2004) Factors influencing mortality in acromegaly. J Clin Endocrinol Metab 89:667–674

57. Oldfield EH, Jane JA Jr, Thorner MO, Pledger CL, Sheehan JP, Vance ML (2017) Correlation between GH and IGF-1 during treatment for acromegaly. J Neurosurg 126:1959–1966

58. Colao A, Ferone D, Marzullo P et al (2001) Long-term effects of depot long-acting somatostatin analog octreotide on hormone levels and tumor mass in acromegaly. J Clin Endocrinol Metab 86:2779–2786

59. Lee CC, Vance ML, Lopes MB, Xu Z, Chen CJ, Sheehan J (2015) Stereotactic radiosurgery for acromegaly: outcomes by adenoma subtype. Pituitary 18:326–334

60. Lee CC, Vance ML, Xu Z et al (2014) Stereotactic radiosurgery for acromegaly. J Clin Endocrinol Metab 99:1273–1281

61. Casanueva FF, Molitch ME, Schlechte JA et al (2006) Guidelines of the pituitary society for the diagnosis and management of prolactinomas. Clin Endocrinol 65:265–273

62. Schlechte JA (2003) Clinical practice. Prolactinoma. N Engl J Med 349:2035–2041

63. Schlechte J, Dolan K, Sherman B, Chapler F, Luciano A (1989) The natural history of untreated hyperprolactinemia: a prospective analysis. J Clin Endocrinol Metab 68:412–418

64. Ferrari CI, Abs R, Bevan JS et al (1997) Treatment of macroprolactinoma with cabergoline: a study of 85 patients. Clin Endocrinol 46:409–413

65. Molitch ME (2002) Medical management of prolactin-secreting pituitary adenomas. Pituitary 5:55–65

66. Molitch ME, Elton RL, Blackwell RE et al (1985) Bromocriptine as primary therapy for prolactin-secreting macroadenomas: results of a prospective multicenter study. J Clin Endocrinol Metab 60:698–705

67. Verhelst J, Abs R, Maiter D et al (1999) Cabergoline in the treatment of hyperprolactinemia: a study in 455 patients. J Clin Endocrinol Metab 84:2518–2522

68. Webster J, Piscitelli G, Polli A, Ferrari CI, Ismail I, Scanlon MF (1994) A comparison of cabergoline and bromocriptine in the treatment of hyperprolactinemic amenorrhea. Cabergoline Comparative Study Group. N Engl J Med 331:904–909

69. Hamilton DK, Vance ML, Boulos PT, Laws ER (2005) Surgical outcomes in hyporesponsive prolactinomas: analysis of patients with resistance or intolerance to dopamine agonists. Pituitary 8:53–60

70. Ogiwara T, Horiuchi T, Nagm A, Goto T, Hongo K (2017) Significance of surgical management for cystic prolactinoma. Pituitary 20:225–230

71. Andereggen L, Frey J, Andres RH et al (2017) 10-year follow-up study comparing primary medical vs. surgical therapy in women with prolactinomas. Endocrine 55:223–230

72. Cohen-Inbar O, Xu Z, Schlesinger D, Vance ML, Sheehan JP (2015) Gamma knife radiosurgery for medically and surgically refractory prolactinomas: long-term results. Pituitary 18:820–830

73. Molitch ME (2014) Management of medically refractory prolactinoma. J Neurooncol 117:421–428

74. Pouratian N, Sheehan J, Jagannathan J, Laws ER Jr, Steiner L, Vance ML (2006) Gamma knife radiosurgery for medically and surgically refractory prolactinomas. Neurosurgery 59:255–266; discussion 255–266

75. Chen Y, Wang CD, Su ZP et al (2012) Natural history of postoperative nonfunctioning pituitary adenomas: a systematic review and meta-analysis. Neuroendocrinology 96:333–342

76. Tedeschi E, Caranci F, Giordano F, Angelini V, Cocozza S, Brunetti A (2017) Gadolinium retention in the body: what we know and what we can do. Radiol Med 122:589–600

77. Ziu M, Dunn IF, Hess C et al (2016) Congress of Neurological Surgeons systematic review and evidence-based guideline on posttreatment follow-up evaluation of patients with nonfunctioning pituitary adenomas. Neurosurgery 79:E541–E543

Tumors of the Pineal Region

13

Manfred Westphal

13.1 Definition

Pineal region tumors (PRTs) are not homogeneous as can be guessed already by the name which describes a region rather than a histological relationship. PRTs are located in the niche of the pineal gland in the posterior part of the third ventricle underneath the splenium and above or arising from the quadrigeminal plate. Basically, any kind of tumor can be found in this region because of the presence of brain parenchyma (quadrigeminal plate), pineal gland, choroid plexus, and dural folds of the anterior rim of the tentorial/falcine junction (Fig. 13.1). Therefore ubiquitous tumors like gliomas, meningiomas, and metastases are seen here as well as tumors intrinsic to the region like pineal parenchymal tumors but also lesions occurring here preferentially like germ cell tumors and non-germinomatous germ cell tumors (NGGCT) including teratomas. In addition the pineal gland has a tendency to form intrinsic cysts which can be very difficult to distinguish from cystic tumors (Fig. 13.2).

Therefore, upon diagnosis, pineal region lesions need to be very carefully assessed considering all parameters like epidemiology (age, sex, geographic region), morphology, case history, concurrent symptoms, and neuroradiologi-

M. Westphal (✉)
Department of Neurosurgery, University of Hamburg,
Hamburg, Germany
e-mail: westphal@uke.de

cal appearance. Unsurprisingly there is no unique treatment approach to pineal lesions but rather an individual, lesion-specific approach, considering age and histology leading to differentiated multidisciplinary therapeutic approaches including surgery, radiation oncology, chemotherapy, and endocrinology.

13.1.1 Epidemiology

PRTs are rare with an annual rate of 0.04 per 100,000, and germ cell tumors and cysts in that same report [1] account for an annual rate of 0.1, but this is only partially accounting for the pineal region (germ cell tumors) or neoplasia (cysts), respectively. In the pediatric population, the rate is 0.05. Thus there is an almost constant rate throughout life but with distinct lesion spectra in the pediatric and adult population [1]. Specifically germ cell tumors have a remarkable distribution with an incidence of 0.4 per 1,000,000 for both males and females up to 9 years of age and then a very different annual rate of 3.4 vs 0.08 for males and females, resp., between 10 and 29 years [2]. Beyond the pediatric and young adult population, germ cell tumors are extremely rare and lack the male predominance [3]. For true germinomas there is pronounced male prevalence [4]. Interestingly, these tumors have an interesting ethnic distribution and make up 70% of PRT in Japanese registries [5].

© Springer Nature Switzerland AG 2019
J.-C. Tonn et al. (eds.), *Oncology of CNS Tumors*, https://doi.org/10.1007/978-3-030-04152-6_13

Fig. 13.1 Sagittal MRI of
a normal pineal region
showing the pineal gland,
the tectal plate (lamina
quadrigemina), the vein of
Galen, and the Sylvian
aqueduct as borders of the
location

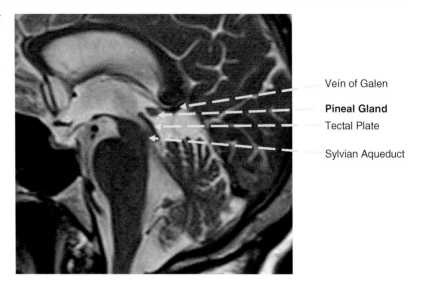

Veín of Galen

Pineal Gland

Tectal Plate

Sylvian Aqueduct

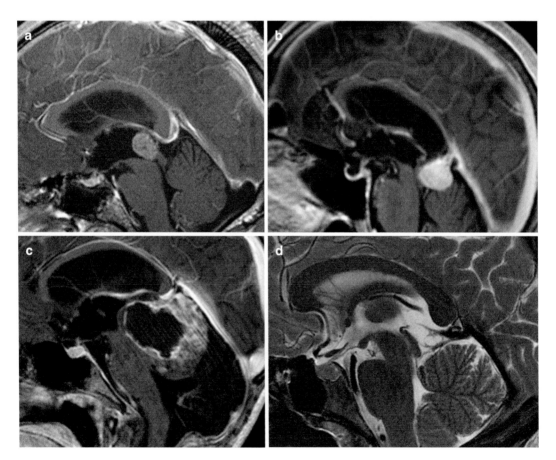

Fig. 13.2 Spectrum of MRI appearances of lesion in the pineal region: (**a**): Pineal parenchymal tumor, pineocytoma.
(**b**): Meningioma. (**c**) Pilocytic astrocytoma. (**d**) Pineal cyst

Pineal parenchymal tumors occur in child- and adulthood but are also rare beyond age 50. Large epidemiological studies are missing, so one has to resolve to the individual series finding an average age at diagnosis of 28 years [6] or to compilations, where in a recent study of 29 publications including 127 patients, an average age of 33 years and a male/female ratio of 1:1.6 was found [7]. In the higher age groups, metastases become more prevalent, and that number is increasing with the longer survival of cancer patients, but except for the location, there are no specifics for these tumors which are treated under the same specific algorithms used for brain metastases of the respective entity.

Pineal cysts are common in children, and in a systematic study, they were found in routine 3 T MRI in 57% of children. Unless specific symptoms can be related to the cyst which is usually related to large size and hydrocephalus, no further follow-up is required [8, 9]. In adults there may be specific and bothersome symptoms, for the most part, intermittent tension headaches (hydrocephalus related), and when operated after careful consideration of the risk/benefit ratio, the majority experience improved symptom burden, and almost 50% become symptom-free [9].

13.1.2 Pathology

The intrinsic PRTs are basically the pineal parenchymal tumors. The specific histopathological and molecular genetic aspects of these tumors are dealt with in this book in Part I, Chap. 1, by Reifenberger et al. Most importantly it is to be borne in mind that these tumors may be heterogeneous and that between the purely WHO grade I tumors and the pineoblastoma (WHO grade IV), there are tumors with the so-called intermediate differentiation (grade II or III) which have to be treated more aggressively as they can progress to pineoblastoma; therefore a resection in toto to obtain a full histological analysis is desirable (Figs. 13.3 and 13.4).

Every now and then, a new entity is defined such as the papillary tumors of the pineal region which are the most recent addition to PRTs, and each entity carries its own prognosis [10]. With the introduction of molecular genetics, the definition of entities has become sharper, and specific mutation like the INI-1 mutation defines the atypical teratoid rhabdoid tumors (ATRT) which in detail are described in the pathology chapter mentioned above. Clinically relevant is the common fact that the tumors may be mixed with germinomatous and teratomatous components and that a biopsy may miss a component, so it is preferable to obtain a representative portion of any tumor (Fig. 13.5a, b).

13.1.3 Symptomatology

Because of their vicinity to the Sylvian aqueduct, pineal region tumors will cause obstructive hydrocephalus which can develop chronically in slowly expanding lesions but can also develop

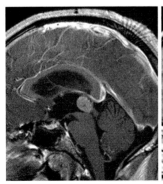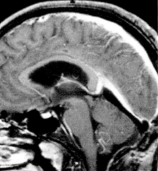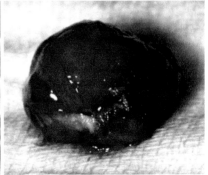

Fig. 13.3 In toto removal of a pineocytoma allowing for complete histological analysis

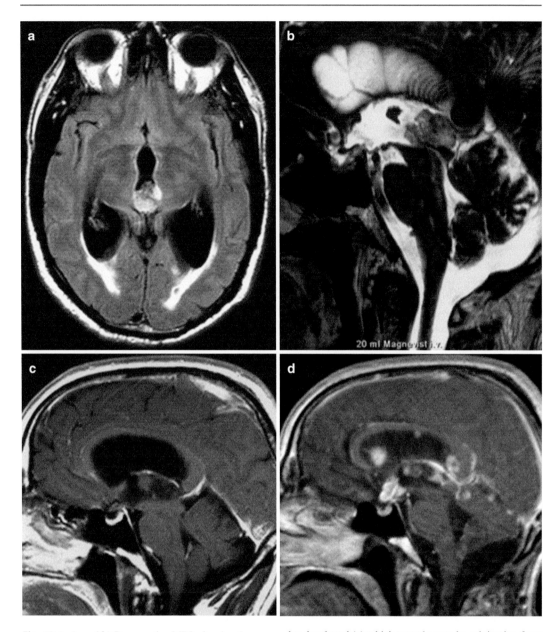

Fig. 13.4 (**a** and **b**) Preoperative MRI of a pineal parenchymal tumor considered to be a pineocytoma, in which
within 1 year postoperatively a malresorptive hydrocephalus developed (**c**) which turned out to be originating from
disseminated pineoblastoma of which the patient succumbed (**d**)

acutely or come to a situation of acute decompen-
sation of a long-standing hydrocephalus resulting in raised intracranial pressure (ICP). This
goes along with headache, nausea, unsteady gait
and diffusely blurred vision (papilledema), and
maybe diplopia. Oculomotor symptoms are also
frequent from pressure on the quadrigeminal plate
sometimes resulting in upward gaze paralysis
(Parinaud's syndrome) or diffuse diplopia, meaning a difficulty to fuse images which is different
from the distinct oculomotor deficits attributed to
cranial nerve palsies. These signs are, however,
much rarer as a presenting sign than as transient
postoperative sequelae.

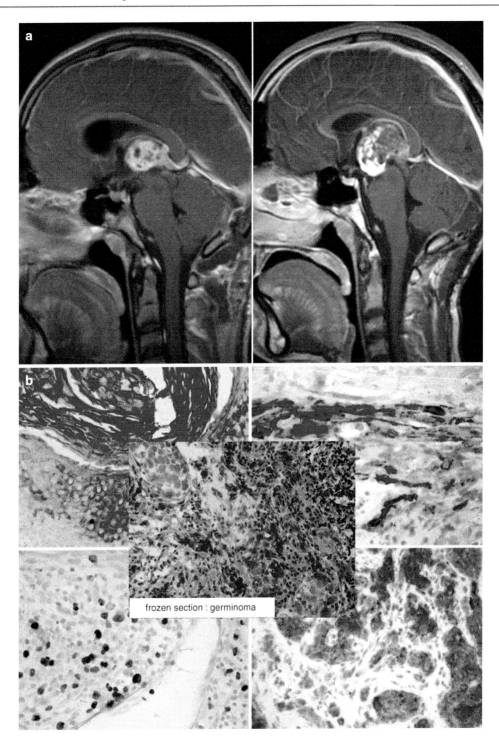

frozen section : germinoma

Fig. 13.5 (**a**) Initial presentation of a slowly growing mature teratoma in a young patient (left) for whom further therapy after initial extended biopsy (**b**) was refused, and after a 2-year follow-up and an expanding lesion after radiation and chemotherapy, the patient was withdrawn from further observation by his caregivers. (**b**) Frozen section of the lesion shown in (**a**) which was thought to be a germinoma but larger additional specimens taken from a different region showed the mixed composition of a teratoma with high proliferation shown by Ki67 stain. After radiation and chemotherapy, the lesion continued to grow but very slowly (**a**, right panel)

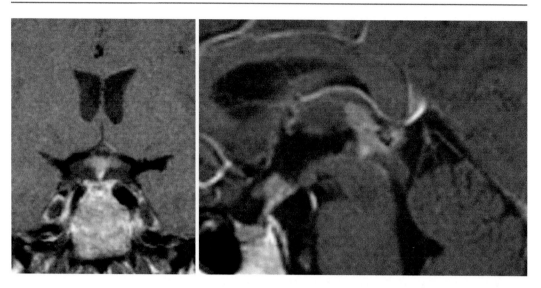

Fig. 13.6 Typical multifocal pure germinoma with deposits in the pineal region and the suprasellar area

Endocrine syndromes such as precocious puberty are indicative of hormone-producing tumors, most likely a non-germinomatous germ cell tumor (NGGCT, see below).

As the main producer of melatonin [11], the pineal gland is long known to be involved in the regulation of the circadian rhythm [12], but only very few people notice that they may have a related disturbance, as they got gradually used to it and consider it an idiosyncrasy. In these cases the environment needs to be asked specifically. When occurring as a postoperative sequelae, the patients tend to notice and require specific medication [13].

13.1.4 Diagnostic Procedures

Imaging is the backbone of diagnosis of PRT (Fig. 13.2). Usually because of emergency diagnosis in the case of raised ICP, a computerized tomography (CT) scan will show triventricular hydrocephalus and a mass in the pineal region which can be solid, cystic, calcified, and surrounded by edema. This is followed by a magnetic resonance tomography (MRI) which clarifies the anatomic situation [14], the relationship to the neighboring structures, and the texture of the lesion in respect to homogeneity and characteristics of contrast enhancement. Often this allows already to suspect a certain category of lesions or exclude some entities. A very het-

erogeneous lesion with cysts, fat, and calcifications is highly suspicious of a teratoma, whereas a homogeneously enhancing lesion with fuzzy edges in the presence of a secondary lesion in the hypothalamic area or in the ventricles is highly suspicious of a germinoma (Fig. 13.6).

As for further imaging modalities, positron emission tomography has been used in individual cases to monitor therapy [15, 16], but there are no specific clues from MRI spectroscopy to define pineal region lesions.

In addition to imaging which for most intracranial tumors is the only presurgical diagnostic measure, pineal lesions may show distinct markers in serum or cerebrospinal fluid (CSF, Table 13.1). Whereas serum markers are unproblematic, obtaining CSF is to be seen with great caution in case of obstructive hydrocephalus where lumbar puncture is problematic. CSF is best obtained when an endoscopic procedure is performed either for biopsy or third ventriculostomy (3VS, see below) or when in an emergency situation in the absence of endoscopic expertise an external ventricular drain is inserted.

The interpretation of markers is not easy, and only few have proven to be indicative of the mostly rare underlying pathology. There are secretory NGGCT which are positive for alpha-fetoprotein or beta-HCG or both. NGGCT may on the other hand also be nonsecretory (Table 13.1). If the markers in serum and/or CSF are very high,

Table 13.1 Markers for distinct pineal lesions in serum or cerebrospinal fluid

Histology	Alpha-fetoprotein	Beta-chorionic gonadotrophin	Human placental alkaline phosphatase
Germinoma	–	+/–	+
Mature teratoma	–	–	+/–
Malignant teratoma	+/–	+/–	+/–
Undifferentiated germ cell tumor	+/–	+/–	+/–
Choriocarcinoma	–	+	+/–
Endodermal sinus tumor syn.: yolk sac tumor	+	–	+/–
Embryonal carcinoma	+	+	+/–
Pineocytoma	–	–	–
Pineoblastoma	–	–	–

This table is modified after [73, 74]

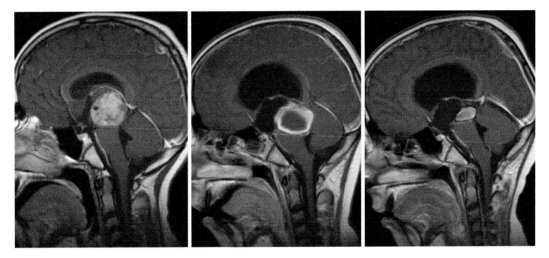

Fig. 13.7 Marker "proven" embryonal carcinoma which was treated with high-dose chemotherapy which after induction led to massive hemorrhagic transformation with severe neurological impairment and no option to relieve the immediate brain stem compression due to severe bone marrow toxicity. The tumor regressed over 4 years but the patient remained vegetative

histological diagnosis may be foregone to start with a chemotherapy regimen right away, although detrimental intratumoral hemorrhage may occur as a consequence to dramatic tumor response (Fig. 13.7). Human placental alkaline phosphatase (HPLAP) was for a long time considered to be a useful marker for any kind of pineal lesion, but it is mostly ambiguous and basically only supports the diagnosis of pure germinoma (Table 13.1).

13.1.5 Cytology

Analysis of cells in the CSF may be a part of the initial diagnostics, provided that CSF can be obtained in the absence of obstructive hydro-cephalus. It is mandatory for aggressive tumors to allow staging as that determines the extent of therapy and prognosis [17, 18].

13.1.6 Therapy

There are several useful treatment algorithms in the literature [19–21], and the initial consideration always concerns the presence or absence of hydrocephalus and when present its immediate management. With hydrocephalus as the leading symptom, establishing adequate CSF flow is mandatory. This can be achieved optimally by the immediate, safe resection of the lesion. In cases where the necessary expertise for such neurosurgical procedure is not available, 3VS, an endoscopic ventriculostomy of the floor of the third ventricle to the prepontine cistern will be the most frequent and best validated procedure introduced decades ago [22]. In that context, it is mandatory to obtain CSF for the analysis of markers and cytology. It may also be possible during 3VS to gain access to the anterior aspect of a PRT in the third ventricle and get a biopsy [23, 24] so that in cases of very chemosensitive tumors, a presurgical, neo-adjuvant therapy can be implemented (see below). If the lesion looks as if it has to be approached surgically anyway, an attempt for biopsy may be forgone. Both techniques, resection and 3VS, require some specialized expertise, but it is absolutely desirable to proceed in this way as an external ventricular drainage only adds the risk of infectious complications. However, it is still preferable to an a priori ventriculoperitoneal shunt, which in case of a malignant tumor may cause dissemination [25]. If a lesion looks a priori nonsurgical and tissue diagnosis is needed in the absence of hydrocephalus, stereotactic biopsy (STX) has an accuracy of 98% vs 78% for endoscopic biopsy and in addition is burdened with a much lower complication rate [26], so a carefully planned STX is advocated. There is some evidence that PET may help in selecting an area of interest for a biopsy in heterogeneous lesions [27].

The detection of some markers in serum or CSF allows the selection of therapy without tissue when clinical parameters are also typical. Several entities of PRT are primarily treated by radiation and/or chemotherapy. When, for example, the diagnosis of germinoma is established (pediatric male, multicentric, positive HPLAP, positive CSF cytology), standard therapy is radiation with or without chemotherapy. The doses and fields vary greatly according to disease localization, either being the whole brain or whole ventricle plus local boost or craniospinal radiation with local boost with or without chemotherapy. A constant feature of the multicenter as well as institutional studies is the goal to reduce the radiation dose because of the neuroendocrine and neuropsychological sequelae especially for young children [28–33]. The control rate of all regimens is about 90% or higher, but to eventually define the minimally effective dose with maximally maintained neuropsychological performance is still

an ongoing effort due to the rarity of the disease and the very long follow-up times for each new regimen. Germinoma may, however, be only a component of otherwise complex mixed tumors like mature or immature teratoma (Fig. 13.5b). In these cases, the germinomatous component will respond to radiation and chemotherapy but may result only in the transition of an immature teratoma into a mature, slowly progressing lesion (Fig. 13.5a).

Treatment of NGGCT is more complex. When confirmed by an unequivocal marker profile or ideally histology to rule out mixed histologies, intense chemotherapy regimens are the first measure which usually lead to disappearance or shrinkage of the tumors (Fig. 13.8). It has to be borne in mind that the first dosing of chemotherapy may cause severely symptomatic hemorrhage, so careful monitoring at that stage is recommend to be able to rapidly react to such situation (Fig. 13.7). After successful shrinkage of the tumor after the first block of chemotherapy, some regimens pursue resection of the remnant followed by further chemotherapy [34]. Even after complete resolution, it is common practice to perform a "second-look" surgery [35, 36]. Large series looking at neo-adjuvant therapies with and without second-look surgery found a benefit in second-look surgery and even a 100% event-free 5-year survival when the lesion was completely resected before the chemotherapy regimens [37]. When widespread dissemination is present already at diagnosis, craniospinal radiation is mandatory (Fig. 13.9).

Likewise, biopsy-proven atypical teratoid rhabdoid tumors (ATRT) of the pineal region are treated by adjuvant measures and then resected should there be a residual.

13.2 Surgery

For many lesions in the pineal region, the most efficacious, definitive therapy is resection as it also addresses hydrocephalus [38]. However, depending on the available neurosurgical expertise, the locally established therapeutic regimens, or the expected histology, a PRT may get biopsied as the first measure. There is little justification

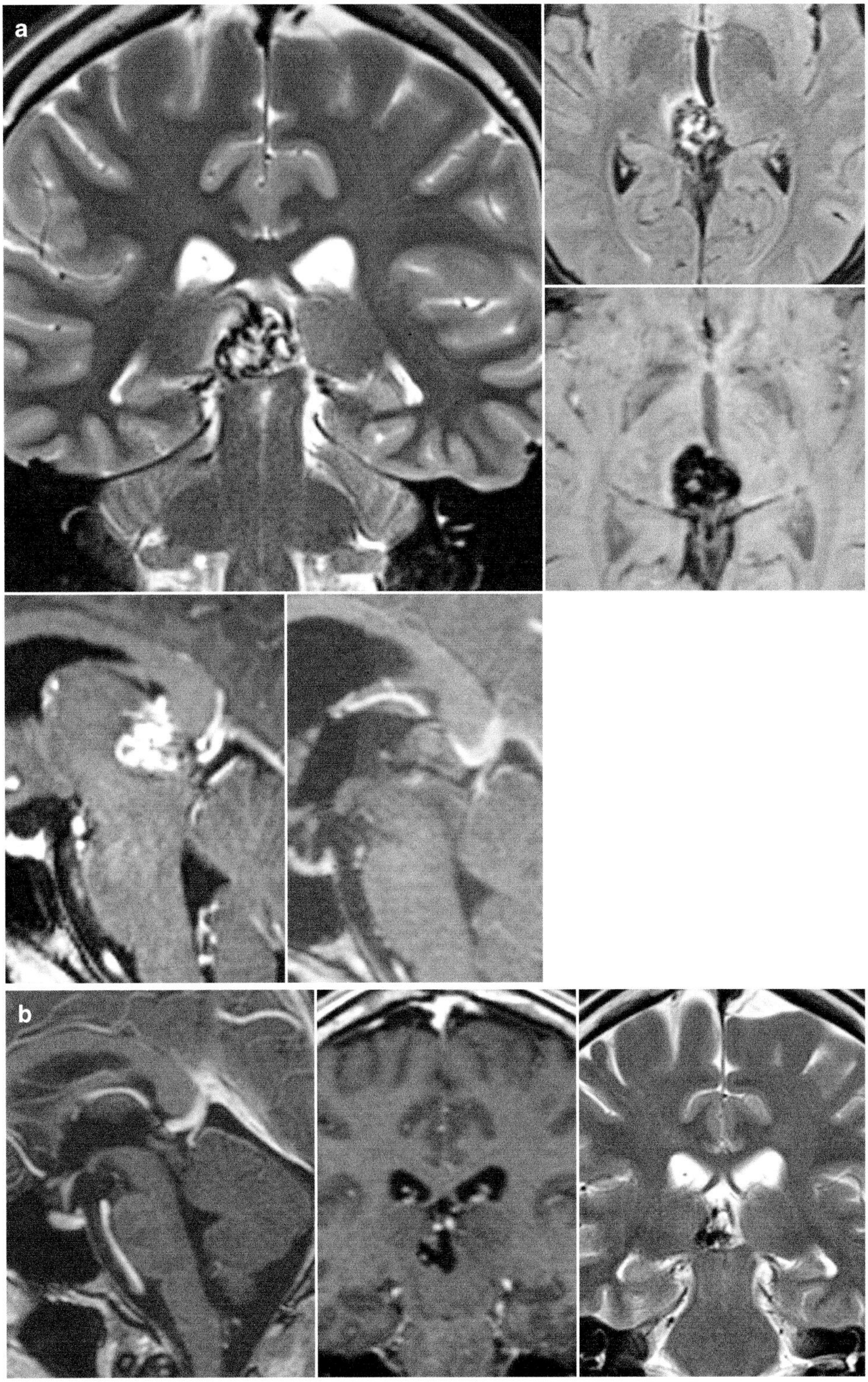

Fig. 13.8 (a) ß-HCG-positive embryonal carcinoma appearing like a cavernous hemangioma with a strong hemosiderin signal which was partially resected and basically devascularized (b) to avoid hemorrhagic complica-tions during high-dose chemotherapy. (b) Same embryonal carcinoma after partial removal and reconstitution of direct CSF passage (left) and after intense chemotherapy for 2 months, T1 with gadolinium

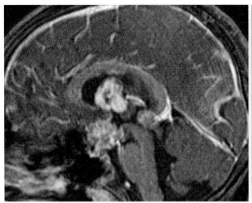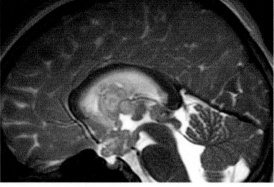

Fig. 13.9 Newly diagnosed NGGCT positive for AFP and ß-HCG in CSF obtained on the occasion of placement of a Rickham reservoir. Dissemination in the whole ven-tricular system constitutes a high-risk situation; initial treatment is chemotherapy

for an endoscopic procedure for biopsy only, but when performing a 3VS, an endoscopic biopsy may be attempted. In cases where the tumor is pushing a layer of ependyma in front or is covered by the posterior commissure, biopsy may be negative, but that can be resolved with another attempt or with resection. Neuro-endoscopic biopsies may not only be negative but may also have the pitfall of missing a major component in mixed histologies [39] which may be less of an issue in well-planned STX.

Surgical approaches for resection developed gradually, given the infrequency of the lesions which prolongs refinement of technique to which repetitive adaptation is key but over many decades, the basic approaches have been refined and are well established and time tested. The most frequently used approach is supracerebellar infratentorial in the midline [40, 41], but transtentorial or transcallosal and endoscopic approaches are also described [42, 43]. They are mostly selected because of venous considerations of the deep venous system which before MRI was assessed by angiography to diagnose and assess PRTs [44].

The most common complications of pineal surgery relate to the irritation of the quadrigeminal plate like diplopia or upward gaze paralysis (Parinaud's syndrome) [40, 45]. Depending on the positioning, immediate postoperative pneumocephalus is frequently seen in the sitting position [46] but

apart from transient headache is not a problem, and when a perioperative ventricular drain is inserted, no pressure builds up. Reported complications from pneumocephalus are rare. When planning patients for surgery in the sitting position, cardiac ultrasound to detect a patent foramen ovale is mandatory to assess the risk of a paradoxical air embolism in case of air entry into the venous system.

Resection is the most definitive treatment for pineocytoma (WHO grade 1) as they are well-differentiated lesions and when completely resected will not recur. It may be impossible in some cases to differentiate between a cystic pineocytoma and a pineal cyst [21]. If a cystic pineocytoma is suspected, the attempt should be to completely remove the lesion, preferable in one piece. If the lesion is suspected to be a benign pineal cyst, a remnant should be left after confirmation by intraoperative frozen section to retain some endocrine pineal function. There are reports of incompletely resected PPTs or recurrence, and in such cases, one might consider re-resection or stereotactic radiation (see below). For PPT a complete as possible histopathological analysis is very important as these tumors may present with an intermediate WHO grade which may rapidly deteriorate, so that the detection of anaplastic features should result in additive therapies [47]. For a primarily aggressive tumor like the pineoblastoma, no surgical risks should be taken at complete resection as these tumors infiltrate the surround-

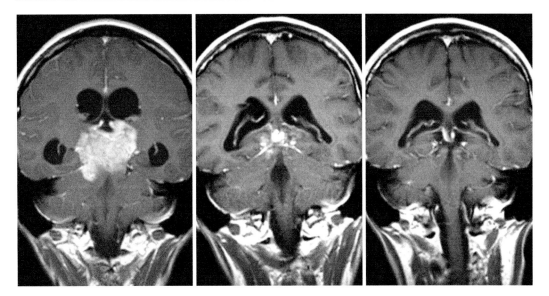

Fig. 13.10 Initial presentation of a large and irregular pineoblastoma (left) with extensive decompression reconstituting normal CSF passage but clearly residual tumor in the anticipated infiltrative edges (middle). After 10 years follow-up, stable complete remission after chemotherapy and whole-brain radiation but marked cognitive decline (right)

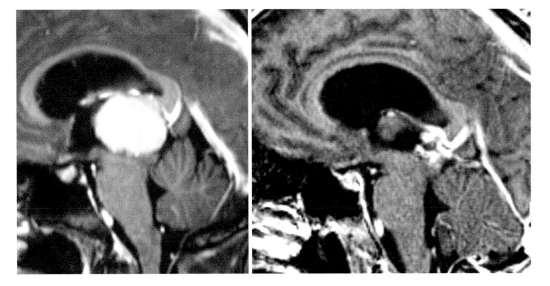

Fig. 13.11 NGGCT with almost complete response to chemotherapy and radiation. Second-look surgery indicated but refused by patient

ings and will need to be treated aggressively with radiation and chemotherapy anyway (Fig. 13.10). In case there is a residual (Fig. 13.11), a "second look" is recommended. In a large prospective series of 26 patients, the rate of complete resection was only 6/26, but in a multivariate analysis, incomplete resection had no influence on survival [48], likewise in a series of papillary tumors of the pineal region for which only the proliferative activity seemed to be prognostic [49].

Other PRTs which are amenable for cure by resection are mature teratomas or residuals after neo-adjuvant therapy of NGGCT [34] or "foreign" lesions like meningioma. There is no structured analysis of the role of surgery for any kind of recurrent PRTs.

Endoscopic techniques are explored as an alternative to open microsurgical resection, and small series report results similar to open procedure [43] in a very mixed spectrum of histologies including cysts so the applicability to general tumor situations is limited. For cysts it appears to be an alternative method, although the difference of technical involvement is not extensive [50].

13.2.1 Chemotherapy

As mentioned above, typical marker-positive tumors, mostly NGGCT, can be treated with up-front chemotherapy as a kind of sandwich regimen in which the first block of chemotherapy is given to consolidate and shrink the tumor, mostly aiming at immature undifferentiated components which is then followed by resection or a "second-look surgery" and another postsurgical boost [51]. Chemotherapy is also a mandatory component for pineoblastoma. The chemotherapeutics used are based on consortional clinical trials which are adapted over decades and include platinum-based compounds, etoposide, bleomycin, and irinotecan among others.

13.2.2 Radiation

There are reports that pineal parenchymal tumors can be stabilized with external beam radiotherapy alone without chemotherapy and that this may be indicated where radical surgery cannot be achieved because of the difficult location of these tumors [52]. Such statements originate from the rarity of the disease and the lack of experience for most neurosurgeons who will be confronted with these tumors only very infrequently. However, there is now sufficient documentation that any pineal lesion can be safely approached by surgery [40] and especially PPTs removed completely with minimal complication and no late side effects

from radiation which is to be expected with external beam field irradiation in the vicinity of both fornices. If there is any role for radiation in PPTs, it is for growing remnants which had to be left behind for rare adverse anatomical situations or intermediate differentiation with uncertain prognosis, and for these radiosurgery has been shown to be a very effective method [53].

Side effects from radiation have to be differentiated between different regimens. In pineoblastoma same as in high-risk medulloblastoma (incomplete resection, leptomeningeal spread), whole-brain radiation is applied, and for medulloblastoma and disseminated ependymoma, late sequelae and neurocognitive deficits are well known [54, 55] leading to radiation concepts avoiding dose and volume [56]. By extrapolation and unpublished experiences of individual cases for pineoblastoma and absence of large series as in medulloblastoma, this will apply as well. The sequelae seen, for example, in whole-brain radiation for germinomas are also substantial but somewhat different as a smaller dose is given and these two entities should not be cross-referenced [32].

13.2.3 Radiosurgery

Radiosurgery is reported to be an effective method for long-term control of residual pineocytomas [53], but as there are sequelae to be expected from radiosurgery, appropriate techniques should be employed to resect these tumors completely which is possible in most cases [21]. There is a debate, however, whether radiosurgery despite the wide spectrum of histological entities and possible sequelae deserves early consideration in the management of PRTs because of surgical morbidity in small-volume centers and the reduced cost and hospital stay [57, 58]. There is ample evidence that radiosurgery can be effective over a wide spectrum of lesions [59]. However, its role has to be defined individually for each patient, and in contrast to past reports, histology must be obtained to assess where it is most efficacious so it can be considered as part of a multimodal treatment [60]. In case of failure of radiosurgery, surgery is still an option [61].

A role for brachytherapy has not been established and is reportedly used only in rare cases [16].

13.2.4 Prognosis

As the group of pineal region tumors is so heterogeneous, there cannot be a general statement except for the already mentioned procedural sequelae of surgery which in modern times has a mortality below 1% [40, 45] and depending on the series, the entities treated, and approaches chosen, a very acceptable morbidity with transient or persistent oculomotor disturbances being the main concern. As for most patients the acute/subacute hydrocephalus is the immediate concern, adequate treatment resolves that issue permanently in 80–90% of patients. Nevertheless it has been reported that in up to 20% of patients, hydrocephalus fails to resolve, so the patients become shunt dependent [62].

Series looking at prognosis of PRT are rare and mostly limited by the complexity of diagnoses. In a series of primary pineal parenchymal tumors (PPTs) combining pineocytomas and pineoblastomas, relapse is rare in pineocytomas but 60% for pineoblastoma in the observation period [63] with 20% development of dementia, leukoencephalopathy, or memory loss attributed to radiation [63]. On the other hand, when PPTs are completely resected or treated with radiosurgery for a rare remnant, or treated adequately when carefully assessed for risk factors [64], the prognosis is excellent without the sequelae from cranial radiation. For germinomas, the prognosis is generally excellent [4]. Survival reported on one representative series is 95% 5-year survival and long-term cures [65]. Also NGGCT when treated adequately have a much improved prognosis over the last decades with 72% progression-free 5-year survival [36] with high-dose chemotherapy and reduction of radiation whenever possible, but due to frequently necessary craniospinal radiation, neurocognitive sequelae are to be expected and will be reported in the next years. Other late sequelae include failure in the spinal compartment despite control of the intracranial situation (Fig. 13.12).

13.2.5 Pineal Cysts and Tectal Gliomas

In the context of PRT, there are two more entities which need to be considered, pineal cysts and tectal gliomas.

As for pineal cysts, the only issue is the differentiation to cystic pineocytoma which on some cases with thick walls is almost impossible and is a histological task, requiring surgery. It will therefore be unavoidable that cysts which impose as tumor get removed and tumors which impose as cysts will only be treated adequately after a long time of being taken for a cyst. As mentioned above, cysts are common and in the absence of related symptoms do not need surgery. Symptoms are mostly unspecific like intermittent headache (possibly from aqueductal stenosis) or ocular disturbances but almost never a marked hydrocephalus. With resection via the supratentorial approach, symptom relief can be achieved in more than 90% of the patients with no morbidity in a large series although other smaller series using other approaches report complication rates of up to 20% (reviewed in [66]). Leaving some pineal tissue behind allows for residual pineal secretory function [66].

Tectal gliomas on the other hand are true tumors of the pineal region albeit not of the gland. They are rare and occur mostly in the pediatric population and make up only 5% of the already rare pediatric brain stem tumors [67]. Mostly they are symptomatic with hydrocephalus because of aqueductal compression. The reported series are small and treatment as well as histologies is heterogeneous. An emerging theme is the foremost treatment of hydrocephalus and the neurocognitive decline related to these lesions independent of management [68]. The need for treatment is seen controversial. While one series treated 11 children with CSF diversion only and observed no progression in lesions less than 1.5 cm in diameter [69], other series reporting neuropsychological impairment in all patients based intervention on enhancement or progression and treated with biopsy only, partial resection, or radiosurgery, depending on histology [68]. Similarly another series reported a differential approach based on presenting imag-

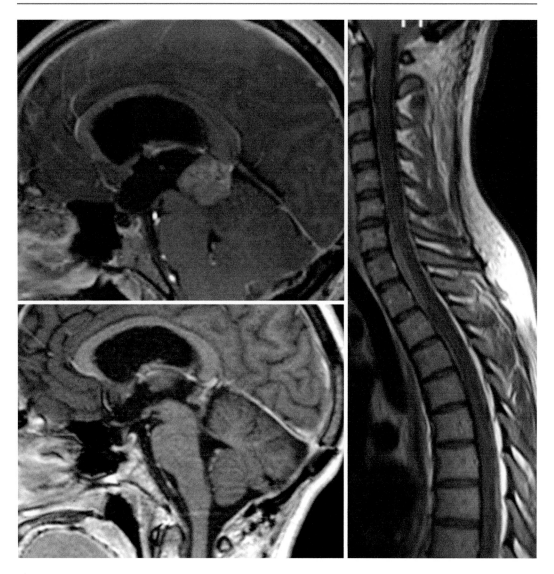

Fig. 13.12 Complete radiological response in a case of pineoblastoma to chemotherapy and cranial radiation but failure in the spinal subdural compartment with late metastatic spread along the whole spinal cord

ing, imaging progression, or clinical progression and supports hydrocephalus associated with neuropsychological impairment [70]. In another series of 11 patients, all were treated with radiosurgery with excellent results as for tumor control but lack of histology in half of the series and no neuropsychological data [71]. Pediatric tectal tumors are considered as indolent lesions [72], as progression seems to occur only in a low percentage of cases, maximally 25% in the reported series. Nevertheless, the notion that biopsy or surgical intervention, especially in children, is too dangerous [71] is untenable especially as all series

unequivocally document an extremely heterogeneous spectrum of histologies; and thus a uniform management is inappropriate, and therapy selection at progression requires tissue confirmation.

Tectal tumors seen in the adult population are naturally different as the hydrocephalus associated with the pediatric tumors leads to early diagnosis. The spectrum is more that of malignant gliomas (Fig. 13.13), which may have a history of a small indolent "low-grade" precursor lesion, but also metastases and "tumefactive" vascular lesions like cavernous hemangiomas are found. In addition to either transient or permanent

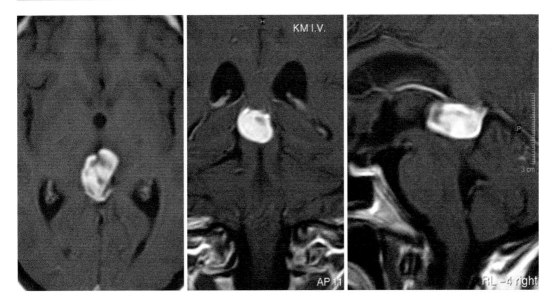

Fig. 13.13 Tectal tumor which upon biopsy and partial removal turned out to be an oligodendroglioma NOS

CSF diversion, adult lesions will generally be approached surgically either for attempted resection or at least a therapy guiding biopsy.

References

1. Ostrom QT, Gittleman H, Xu J, Kromer C, Wolinsky Y, Kruchko C et al (2016) CBTRUS statistical report: primary brain and other central nervous system tumors diagnosed in the United States in 2009-2013. Neuro Oncol 18(Suppl 5):v1–v75
2. Poynter JN, Fonstad R, Tolar J, Spector LG, Ross JA (2014) Incidence of intracranial germ cell tumors by race in the United States, 1992-2010. J Neurooncol 120(2):381–388
3. Villano JL, Propp JM, Porter KR, Stewart AK, Valyi-Nagy T, Li X et al (2008) Malignant pineal germ-cell tumors: an analysis of cases from three tumor registries. Neuro Oncol 10(2):121–130
4. Calaminus G, Bamberg M, Baranzelli MC, Benoit Y, di Montezemolo LC, Fossati-Bellani F et al (1994) Intracranial germ cell tumors: a comprehensive update of the European data. Neuropediatrics 25(1):26–32
5. Kang JK, Jeun SS, Hong YK, Park CK, Son BC, Lee IW et al (1998) Experience with pineal region tumors. Childs Nerv Syst 14(1–2):63–68
6. Chatterjee D, Lath K, Singla N, Kumar N, Radotra BD (2017) Pathologic prognostic factors of pineal parenchymal tumor of intermediate differentiation. Appl Immunohistochem Mol Morphol. https://doi.org/10.1097/PAI.0000000000000565
7. Mallick S, Benson R, Rath GK (2016) Patterns of care and survival outcomes in patients with pineal parenchymal tumor of intermediate differentiation: an individual patient data analysis. Radiother Oncol 121(2):204–208
8. Whitehead MT, Oh CC, Choudhri AF (2013) Incidental pineal cysts in children who undergo 3-T MRI. Pediatr Radiol 43(12):1577–1583
9. Majovsky M, Netuka D, Benes V (2017) Conservative and surgical treatment of patients with pineal cysts: prospective case series of 110 patients. World Neurosurg 105:199–205
10. Edson MA, Fuller GN, Allen PK, Levine NB, Ghia AJ, Mahajan A et al (2015) Outcomes after surgery and radiotherapy for papillary tumor of the pineal region. World Neurosurg 84(1):76–81
11. Brzezinski A (1997) Melatonin in humans. N Engl J Med 336(3):186–195
12. Wiederanders RE, Evans GW (1967) Circadian rhythms and the pineal gland. J Lancet 87(8):277–280
13. Hardeland R (2012) Neurobiology, pathophysiology, and treatment of melatonin deficiency and dysfunction. ScientificWorldJournal 2012:640389
14. Satoh H, Uozumi T, Kiya K, Kurisu K, Arita K, Sumida M et al (1995) MRI of pineal region tumours: relationship between tumours and adjacent structures. Neuroradiology 37(8):624–630
15. Panagiotidis E, Shankar A, Afaq A, Bomanji J (2014) Assessing therapy response of secreting pineal germ cell tumor on simultaneous 18F-choline PET/MRI. Clin Nucl Med 39(9):e387–e388
16. Julow J, Viola A, Major T (2006) Review of radiosurgery of pineal parenchymal tumors. Long survival following 125-iodine brachytherapy of pineoblastomas in 2 cases. Minim Invasive Neurosurg 49(5):276–281
17. Baumgartner JE, Edwards MS (1992) Pineal tumors. Neurosurg Clin N Am 3(4):853–862

18. Chang SM, Lillis-Hearne PK, Larson DA, Wara WM, Bollen AW, Prados MD (1995) Pineoblastoma in adults. Neurosurgery 37(3):383–390; discussion 90–1

19. Zaazoue MA, Goumnerova LC (2016) Pineal region tumors: a simplified management scheme. Childs Nerv Syst 32(11):2041–2045

20. Sonabend AM, Bowden S, Bruce JN (2016) Microsurgical resection of pineal region tumors. J Neurooncol 130(2):351–366

21. Westphal M, Emami P (2015) Pineal lesions: a multidisciplinary challenge. Adv Tech Stand Neurosurg 42:79–102

22. Jones RF, Stening WA, Brydon M (1990) Endoscopic third ventriculostomy. Neurosurgery 26(1):86–91; discussion-2

23. Yurtseven T, Ersahin Y, Demirtas E, Mutluer S (2003) Neuroendoscopic biopsy for intraventricular tumors. Minim Invasive Neurosurg 46(5):293–299

24. Ahmed AI, Zaben MJ, Mathad NV, Sparrow OC (2015) Endoscopic biopsy and third ventriculostomy for the management of pineal region tumors. World Neurosurg 83(4):543–547

25. Cranston PE, Hatten MT, Smith EE (1992) Metastatic pineoblastoma via a ventriculoperitoneal shunt: CT demonstration. Comput Med Imaging Graph 16(5):349–351

26. Balossier A, Blond S, Reyns N (2016) Endoscopic versus stereotactic procedure for pineal tumor biopsies: focus on overall efficacy rate. World Neurosurg 92:223–228

27. Pirotte BJ, Lubansu A, Massager N, Wikler D, Van Bogaert P, Levivier M et al (2010) Clinical impact of integrating positron emission tomography during surgery in 85 children with brain tumors. J Neurosurg Pediatr 5(5):486–499

28. Bouffet E, Baranzelli MC, Patte C, Portas M, Edan C, Chastagner P et al (1999) Combined treatment modality for intracranial germinomas: results of a multicentre SFOP experience. Societe Francaise d'Oncologie Pediatrique. Br J Cancer 79(7–8):1199–1204

29. Calaminus G, Kortmann R, Worch J, Nicholson JC, Alapetite C, Garre ML et al (2013) SIOP CNS GCT 96: final report of outcome of a prospective, multinational nonrandomized trial for children and adults with intracranial germinoma, comparing craniospinal irradiation alone with chemotherapy followed by focal primary site irradiation for patients with localized disease. Neuro Oncol 15(6):788–796

30. Cheng S, Kilday JP, Laperriere N, Janzen L, Drake J, Bouffet E et al (2016) Outcomes of children with central nervous system germinoma treated with multiagent chemotherapy followed by reduced radiation. J Neurooncol 127(1):173–180

31. Haas-Kogan DA, Missett BT, Wara WM, Donaldson SS, Lamborn KR, Prados MD et al (2003) Radiation therapy for intracranial germ cell tumors. Int J Radiat Oncol Biol Phys 56(2):511–518

32. Liang SY, Yang TF, Chen YW, Liang ML, Chen HH, Chang KP et al (2013) Neuropsychological functions and quality of life in survived patients with intracranial germ cell tumors after treatment. Neuro Oncol 15(11):1543–1551

33. Odagiri K, Omura M, Hata M, Aida N, Niwa T, Ogino I et al (2012) Treatment outcomes, growth height, and neuroendocrine functions in patients with intracranial germ cell tumors treated with chemoradiation therapy. Int J Radiat Oncol Biol Phys 84(3):632–638

34. Herrmann HD, Westphal M, Winkler K, Laas RW, Schulte FJ (1994) Treatment of nongerminomatous germ-cell tumors of the pineal region. Neurosurgery 34(3):524–529; discussion 9

35. Nakamura H, Takeshima H, Makino K, Kuratsu J (2007) Evaluation of residual tissues after adjuvant therapy in germ cell tumors. Pediatr Neurosurg 43(2):82–91

36. Calaminus G, Frappaz D, Kortmann RD, Krefeld B, Saran F, Pietsch T et al (2017) Outcome of patients with intracranial non-germinomatous germ cell tumors-lessons from the SIOP-CNS-GCT-96 trial. Neuro Oncol 19(12):1661–1672

37. Goldman S, Bouffet E, Fisher PG, Allen JC, Robertson PL, Chuba PJ et al (2015) Phase II trial assessing the ability of neoadjuvant chemotherapy with or without second-look surgery to eliminate measurable disease for nongerminomatous germ cell tumors: a Children's Oncology Group Study. J Clin Oncol 33(22):2464–2471

38. Stein BM, Fetell MR (1985) Therapeutic modalities for pineal region tumors. Clin Neurosurg 32:445–455

39. Kinoshita Y, Yamasaki F, Tominaga A, Saito T, Sakoguchi T, Takayasu T et al (2017) Pitfalls of a neuroendoscopic biopsy of intraventricular germ cell tumors. World Neurosurg 106:430–434

40. Hernesniemi J, Romani R, Albayrak BS, Lehto H, Dashti R, Ramsey C 3rd et al (2008) Microsurgical management of pineal region lesions: personal experience with 119 patients. Surg Neurol 70(6):576–583

41. Stein BM (1971) The infratentorial supracerebellar approach to pineal lesions. J Neurosurg 35(2):197–202

42. Liu JK (2016) Endoscopic-assisted interhemispheric parieto-occipital transtentorial approach for microsurgical resection of a pineal region tumor: operative video and technical nuances. Neurosurg Focus 40 Video Suppl 1:2016.1.FocusVid.15450

43. Thaher F, Kurucz P, Fuellbier L, Bittl M, Hopf NJ (2014) Endoscopic surgery for tumors of the pineal region via a paramedian infratentorial supracerebellar keyhole approach (PISKA). Neurosurg Rev 37(4):677–684

44. Raimondi AJ, Tomita T (1982) Pineal tumors in childhood. Epidemiology, pathophysiology, and surgical approaches. Childs Brain 9(3–4):239–266

45. Qi S, Fan J, Zhang XA, Zhang H, Qiu B, Fang L (2014) Radical resection of nongerminomatous pineal region tumors via the occipital transtentorial approach based on arachnoidal consideration: experience on a series of 143 patients. Acta Neurochir (Wien) 156(12):2253–2262

46. Dallier F, Di Roio C (2015) Sitting position for pineal surgery: some anaesthetic considerations. Neurochirurgie 61(2–3):164–167

47. Pusztaszeri M, Pica A, Janzer R (2006) Pineal parenchymal tumors of intermediate differentiation in adults: case report and literature review. Neuropathology 26(2):153–157

48. Gerber NU, von Hoff K, Resch A, Ottensmeier H, Kwiecien R, Faldum A et al (2014) Treatment of children with central nervous system primitive neuroectodermal tumors/pinealoblastomas in the prospective multicentric trial HIT 2000 using hyperfractionated radiation therapy followed by maintenance chemotherapy. Int J Radiat Oncol Biol Phys 89(4):863–871

49. Heim S, Beschorner R, Mittelbronn M, Keyvani K, Riemenschneider MJ, Vajtai I et al (2014) Increased mitotic and proliferative activity are associated with worse prognosis in papillary tumors of the pineal region. Am J Surg Pathol 38(1):106–110

50. Gui S, Bai J, Wang X, Zong X, Li C, Cao L et al (2016) Assessment of endoscopic treatment for quadrigeminal cistern arachnoid cysts: a 7-year experience with 28 cases. Childs Nerv Syst 32(4):647–654

51. Herrmann HD, Winkler D, Westphal M (1992) Treatment of tumours of the pineal region and posterior part of the third ventricle. Acta Neurochir (Wien) 116(2–4):137–146

52. Das P, McKinstry S, Devadass A, Herron B, Conkey DS (2016) Are we over treating Pineal Parenchymal tumour with intermediate differentiation? Assessing the role of localised radiation therapy and literature review. Springerplus 5:26

53. Wilson DA, Awad AW, Brachman D, Coons SW, McBride H, Youssef E et al (2012) Long-term radiosurgical control of subtotally resected adult pineocytomas. J Neurosurg 117(2):212–217

54. Mulhern RK, Palmer SL, Merchant TE, Wallace D, Kocak M, Brouwers P et al (2005) Neurocognitive consequences of risk-adapted therapy for childhood medulloblastoma. J Clin Oncol 23(24):5511–5519

55. Camara-Costa H, Resch A, Kieffer V, Lalande C, Poggi G, Kennedy C et al (2015) Neuropsychological outcome of children treated for standard risk medulloblastoma in the PNET4 European randomized controlled trial of hyperfractionated versus standard radiation therapy and maintenance chemotherapy. Int J Radiat Oncol Biol Phys 92(5):978–985

56. Lafay-Cousin L, Bouffet E, Hawkins C, Amid A, Huang A, Mabbott DJ (2009) Impact of radiation avoidance on survival and neurocognitive outcome in infant medulloblastoma. Curr Oncol 16(6):21–28

57. Li W, Zhang B, Kang W, Dong B, Ma X, Song J et al (2015) Gamma knife radiosurgery (GKRS) for pineal region tumors: a study of 147 cases. World J Surg Oncol 13:304

58. Hanft SJ, Isaacson SR, Bruce JN (2011) Stereotactic radiosurgery for pineal region tumors. Neurosurg Clin N Am 22(3):413–420, ix

59. Yianni J, Rowe J, Khandanpour N, Nagy G, Hoggard N, Radatz M et al (2012) Stereotactic radiosurgery for pineal tumours. Br J Neurosurg 26(3):361–366

60. Balossier A, Blond S, Touzet G, Sarrazin T, Lartigau E, Reyns N (2015) Role of radiosurgery in the management of pineal region tumours: indications, method, outcome. Neurochirurgie 61(2–3):216–222

61. Nanda A, Kalakoti P, Patra DP, Maiti T, Sun H (2017) Microsurgical resection after failed gamma knife radiosurgery of papillary tumor of the pineal gland. World Neurosurg 105:1031.e1

62. Zhang Z, Wang H, Cheng H, Fan Y, Hang C, Sun K et al (2013) Management of hydrocephalus secondary to pineal region tumors. Clin Neurol Neurosurg 115(9):1809–1813

63. Villa S, Miller RC, Krengli M, Abusaris H, Baumert BG, Servagi-Vernat S et al (2012) Primary pineal tumors: outcome and prognostic factors—a study from the Rare Cancer Network (RCN). Clin Transl Oncol 14(11):827–834

64. Yu T, Sun X, Wang J, Ren X, Lin N, Lin S (2016) Twenty-seven cases of pineal parenchymal tumours of intermediate differentiation: mitotic count, Ki-67 labelling index and extent of resection predict prognosis. J Neurol Neurosurg Psychiatry 87(4):386–395

65. Lee SH, Jung KW, Ha J, Oh CM, Kim H, Park HJ et al (2017) Nationwide population-based incidence and survival rates of malignant central nervous system germ cell tumors in Korea, 2005-2012. Cancer Res Treat 49(2):494–501

66. Majovsky M, Netuka D, Benes V (2018) Is surgery for pineal cysts safe and effective? Short review. Neurosurg Rev 41(1):119–124

67. Igboechi C, Vaddiparti A, Sorenson EP, Rozzelle CJ, Tubbs RS, Loukas M (2013) Tectal plate gliomas: a review. Childs Nerv Syst 29(10):1827–1833

68. Aarsen FK, Arts WF, Van Veelen-Vincent ML, Lequin MH, Catsman-Berrevoets CE (2014) Long-term outcome in children with low grade tectal tumours and obstructive hydrocephalus. Eur J Paediatr Neurol 18(4):469–474

69. Grant GA, Avellino AM, Loeser JD, Ellenbogen RG, Berger MS, Roberts TS (1999) Management of intrinsic gliomas of the tectal plate in children. A ten-year review. Pediatr Neurosurg 31(4):170–176

70. Gass D, Dewire M, Chow L, Rose SR, Lawson S, Stevenson C et al (2015) Pediatric tectal plate gliomas: a review of clinical outcomes, endocrinopathies, and neuropsychological sequelae. J Neurooncol 122(1):169–177

71. El-Shehaby AM, Reda WA, Abdel Karim KM, Emad Eldin RM, Esene IN (2015) Gamma Knife radiosurgery for low-grade tectal gliomas. Acta Neurochir (Wien) 157(2):247–256

72. Bowers DC, Georgiades C, Aronson LJ, Carson BS, Weingart JD, Wharam MD et al (2000) Tectal gliomas: natural history of an indolent lesion in pediatric patients. Pediatr Neurosurg 32(1):24–29

73. Janss AJ, Mapstone TB (2010) Pineal region tumors in children. In: Tonn JC, Westphal M, Rutka JT (eds) Oncology of CNS tumors. Springer, Heidelberg, pp 545–552

74. Sawamura Y, Radovanovic I, de Tribolet N (2010) Tumors of the pineal region. In: Tonn JC, Westphal M, Rutka JT (eds) Oncology of CNS tumors. Springer, Heidelberg, pp 239–249

Tumors of the Cranial Nerves

14

Jörg-Christian Tonn, Alexander Muacevic,
and Roland Goldbrunner

14.1 Epidemiology

The most frequent tumors of the cranial nerves are referred to as schwannomas (formerly neuromas). They may develop in most cranial nerves, except I and II, which do not have Schwann cells, except for very rare cases of ectopic pediatric olfactory schwannomas. Cranial nerve tumors (CNT) account for 8.4% of intracranial tumors [1]. The incidence is rising since the distribution of MRI became widespread. The incidence of the most common CNT, the vestibular schwannoma (VS), is estimated to be 1.3 per 100,000 inhabitants per year nowadays compared with 0.8 in the period between 1976 and 1983 [2]. Furthermore, the incidence of CNT is higher in patients with neurofibromatosis type 2 (NF2).

Another group of tumors with a frequent relation to cranial nerves is the meningiomas. However, they originate from the arachnoidal cell layer and not directly from neural structures. Therefore, it seems appropriate to focus this contribution on those meningiomas that have a similar close relation to cranial nerves, such as the schwannomas. These are the optic nerve sheath meningioma (ONSM) and the meningiomas extending into the optic canal. Meningiomas like the fronto-orbital tumors compressing the olfactory nerve are not dealt with. Meningiomas of the cavernous sinus or the petroclival meningiomas that may compress optic pathway structures are also excluded. ONSM and the meningiomas extending into the optic canal account for 1–2% of all meningiomas [3].

There are further very rare cranial nerve tumors. Optic pathway gliomas (optic nerve glioma, ONG) emerge in NF1 children below the age of 7 years and as a separate entity in non-NF1 patients also in older children and in adults [4, 5]. ONGs are increasingly considered as markers of enhanced risk in patients and their families for subsequent development of central nervous system tumors [6]. The incidence of ONG is about 1:10,000.

Malignant peripheral nerve sheath tumors (MPNSTs) account for about 5% of malignant soft tissue tumors. The involvement of cranial nerves is very seldom [7], and if it occurs, the trigeminal nerve or the vestibulocochlear nerve is affected predominantly [8, 9]. The prevalence of neurofibromatosis type 1 (NF1) is around 1:4000, and NF1 patients have an

J.-C. Tonn (✉)
Department of Neurosurgery, LMU München,
München, Germany
e-mail: joerg.christian.tonn@med.uni-muenchen.de

A. Muacevic (✉)
CyberKnife Zentrum München, München, Germany
e-mail: alexander.muacevic@cyber-knife.net

R. Goldbrunner (✉)
Department of General Neurosurgery, Center for
Neurosurgery, University of Cologne,
Cologne, Germany
e-mail: roland.goldbrunner@uk-koeln.de

© Springer Nature Switzerland AG 2019
J.-C. Tonn et al. (eds.), *Oncology of CNS Tumors*, https://doi.org/10.1007/978-3-030-04152-6_14

approximately 10% lifetime risk of developing MPNST. Esthesioneuroblastoma (synonym: olfactory neuroblastoma) is a small round cell tumor type originating from the olfactory epithelium. About a thousand examples of this very rare tumor have been described so far [10].

14.2 Symptoms and Clinical Signs

Clinical symptoms of the CNT depend on three factors: the cranial nerve that is associated with the tumor; the tumor's growth velocity, which is slow in most benign lesions; and the size of the tumor. Larger tumors may compromise other cranial nerves and functional areas of the brain in the vicinity of the lesion (Fig. 14.1). In general, the first clinical symptoms are specific deficits of the cranial nerve involved by the tumor.

Optic gliomas and meningiomas of the optic nerve sheath may cause progressive loss of vision, bulbar protrusion, and congestion of sclera vessels. The malignant esthesioneuroblastoma is frequently associated with recurrent epistaxis.

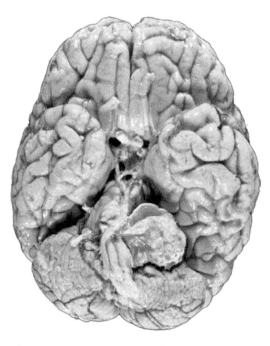

Fig. 14.1 Autopsy specimen of a patient who died because of a large vestibular schwannoma (VS) displacing the brain stem

Facial neuropathy is frequent in trigeminal schwannomas. Vertigo, tinnitus, and hearing loss are key symptoms of VS. Peripheral facial nerve palsies indicate schwannomas of the ganglion geniculi. Swallowing difficulties and the sensation of having a lump in the throat are signs of schwannomas of the jugular foramen and the caudal cranial nerves. With increasing tumor size, further symptoms may develop: trigeminal deficits in VS, ataxia, and cardiac arrhythmia in schwannomas of the caudal cranial nerves. If the craniospinal fluid (CSF) passage is compromised by larger schwannomas, the symptomatology of obstructive hydrocephalus may develop.

14.3 Diagnostics

Diagnostic workup includes clinical examination (with the specialties of neurology, ophthalmology, and audiology), neurophysiology, and neuroimaging. Neurophysiology helps to analyze the specific function of a cranial nerve compromised by a tumor. Imaging basically consists of high-resolution MRI, rarely CT. Nowadays, sophisticated MRI techniques and contrast media are used to characterize a tumorous lesion noninvasively and to support the therapeutic decision-making. PET imaging, especially using ^{68}Ga-DOTATATE/DOTATOC, might help to differentiate meningiomas from schwannomas and other tumors [11].

Differential diagnostic considerations for a mass of the optic nerve within the orbit include ONG or ONSM, schwannoma, and granulomatous disease, specifically neurosarcoidosis, cavernous hemangioma, dermoid, and metastases. The circumferential, homogenously enhancing appearance of the lesion with a thin residual segment of the optic nerve centrally strongly suggests a meningioma. However, ONG and ONSM are sometimes difficult to differentiate even with elaborate imaging [12, 13]. In cases of canalicular optic nerve meningioma, the diagnosis may be missed for a longer time period. Clinical features can lead to a misdiagnosis of optic neuritis or ischemic optic neuropathy, and the diagnosis can sometimes be made only by high-spatial-resolution contrast-enhanced MR findings, including native and contrast-enhanced scanning and fat suppression sequences [14]. ^{68}Ga-DOTATATE-PET imaging has been shown to discriminate ONSM from other lesions [15, 16]. Hence, surgery just to obtain a biopsy to validate ONSM is no longer necessary.

The differentiation in tumors of the cavernous sinus and Meckel's cave between schwannoma of the trigeminal nerve and meningioma can be made without difficulty in most cases. Here, the clinical symptoms may be of help, because meningiomas are frequently associated with mild oculomotor deficits, whereas schwannomas are associated with trigeminal neuralgia or neuropathy. Furthermore, the topographic extension is quite specific for each of the two entities. This can be evaluated reasonably well by MRI. Again, PET imaging, especially using ^{68}Ga-DOTATATE/ DOTATOC, might help to differentiate meningiomas from schwannomas and other tumors [17]. The rare cases of cavernous sinus cavernomas may require digital angiography for diagnosis before resection.

Difficulties in the differential diagnosis between meningioma and schwannoma frequently arise in lesions of the cerebellopontine angle. Since the presenting symptoms are not specific, a refined MRI analysis revealing the matrix structure of the tumor under study will predict the histology with high probability in most instances. The differential diagnosis of lesions in the cerebellopontine angle furthermore comprises inflammatory or vascular lesions and metastases including CNS dissemination/meningeal carcinomatosis (Fig. 14.2) [18]. The lat-

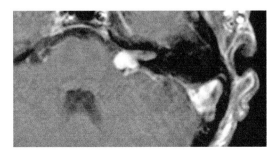

Fig. 14.2 A fast-growing lesion in the left cerebellopontine angle mimicking a VS. The tumor turned out to be a malignant lymphoma

ter may imitate bilateral VS as in NF2 patients. Further lesions of the cerebellopontine angle to be taken into account in the differential diagnosis are glomus tympanicum tumors and cholesteatoma (epidermoid cysts).

The differential diagnosis of lesions associated with the caudal cranial nerves and with the area of the jugular foramen comprises schwannomas, meningiomas, metastases, and a few very rare lesions like the chloroma. Of clinical significance are the tumors of the glomus jugulare (formerly also referred to as paraganglioma). However, these tumors originate from specialized neural crest cells and affect the cranial nerves only by compression or displacement, and thus they are not cranial nerve tumors in the strict sense of the word. Jugular glomus tumors usually present with pulsatile tinnitus, hearing loss, hoarseness, and dysphagia. The chromaffin tumor type may be associated with hypertension. In such tumors, radionuclide imaging may support the diagnosis. Angiography shows highly vascularized tumors that therefore lend themselves to embolization (see below).

14.4 Staging and Classification

Most nerve tumors are benign (according to WHO grade I) [19]. Optic nerve gliomas are the principal CNS neoplasm in NF1 [20]. Although the histology of these tumors typically reveals pilocytic astrocytoma (WHO grade I) [21], they can present within the entire spectrum of astrocytic neoplasias, including glioblastoma (WHO grade IV) [22]. Still, malignant optic gliomas are rare tumors. They are usually found in adults. Meningiomas in close contact to cranial nerves and schwannomas are normally benign. Although schwannomas associated with NF2 may have a higher proliferative activity, this does not indicate malignant behavior [23]. Apparently, loss of merlin expression constitutes a genetic alteration shared by all schwannomas [24].

In contrast, malignant peripheral nerve sheath tumors (MPNSTs) correspond to WHO grade III or IV [20]. These tumors are also referred to as malignant schwannomas and as malignant triton tumor if they show rhabdomyosarcomatous differentiation [7, 23]. They are associated with NF1 [23], and as a basic principle, they arise de novo [25]. Several variants of MPNST have been identified. A minority of MPNSTs show epithelioid or perineurial cell differentiation. These tumors carry a more favorable prognosis than anaplastic or glandular MPNST or malignant triton tumor [23, 26].

Esthesioneuroblastomas (synonym, neuroblastomas of the olfactory nerve) are malignant neuroectodermal tumors of WHO grade IV that tend to metastasize. Their matrix consists of the olfactory receptor cells in the upper nasal cavity [23].

Clinical classification is normally done for the purpose of assigning an appropriate therapy to any individual cranial nerve tumor. For ONSM, the crucial question is whether there is an extension into the intracranial space or not. In pure intraorbital meningiomas, the tumor is amenable to complete excision if necessary. In case of intracranial extension of an ONSM, surgical therapy is not useful. However, if intracranial meningiomas (not ONSM) extend into the optic canal, the surgical approach depends on the localization of the meningioma in relation to the optic nerve and on the origin of the tumor [27].

Several classifications have been proposed for VS. They all categorize according to tumor size, which is the most decisive outcome predictor. A summary of the classification systems is given in Table 14.1 [30, 31].

A surgical classification of trigeminal schwannomas (TNS) was published by Samii and co-workers in 1995 [32] (Table 14.2). This classification uses the topographic extension of trigeminal schwannomas as a guideline to determine the best surgical approach in order to achieve complete resection.

In a very similar way, Samii also classified the surgical approaches to the tumors of the jugular foramen, including schwannomas of the caudal cranial nerves (Table 14.3) [33].

Kadish and co-workers developed a staging system of esthesioneuroblastoma that suggests a treatment policy correlated to the anatomical extension of these tumors [34]. The Kadish classification is given in Table 14.4.

Table 14.1 Classification of vestibular schwannoma (VS)

Size (Tos)	Grade (Koos)	Class (Samii)	Definition of tumor size
	Grade I	T1	Purely intracanalicular lesion
	Grade II	T2	VS protruding into the cerebellopontine angle without brain stem contact
<1 cm	IIA	T2	Tumor diameter < 1 cm
1–1.8 cm	IIB	T2	Tumor diameter 1–1.8 cm
	Grade III	T3a	Filling cerebellopontine angle cistern
		T3b	Reaching the brain stem
	Grade IV	T4a	Brain stem compression
		T4b	Severely dislocating the brain stem and compressing the fourth ventricle

Synopsis according to Tos [28], Koos [29], and Samii [30]

Table 14.2 Surgical classification of trigeminal schwannomas (TNS) according to Samii [33]

Type	Definition of tumor extension
Type A	Intracranial predominantly in the middle fossa
Type B	Intracranial predominantly in the posterior fossa
Type C	Intracranial dumbbell-shaped in the middle and posterior fossa
Type D	Extracranial with intracranial extension

14.5 Treatment

Treatment options for benign tumors comprise watchful waiting, microsurgery, radiosurgery, and the variants of modern fractionated radiation therapy. In the era of MRI, slowly growing tumors no longer implicate a vital risk (Fig. 14.1). They mainly constitute a functional problem for the patient concerning a specific neural deficit. Since many of them are diagnosed in patients in their most active period of professional and social life, the benign behavior of these lesions has to be taken into account when deciding on therapy. In this respect, radiosurgery has been established as an alternative to microsurgery for schwannomas

Table 14.3 Surgical classification of jugular foramen schwannomas according to Samii [33]

Type	Definition of tumor extension
Type A	Primarily at the cerebellopontine angle with minimal enlargement of the FJ
Type B	Tumors primarily in the FJ with intracranial extension
Type C	Primarily extracranial tumor with extension into the FJ
Type D	Dumbbell-shaped tumors with both intra- and extracranial components

FJ foramen jugulare

Table 14.4 Staging of esthesioneuroblastoma according to Kadish [34]

Group	Definition
Group A	Tumor is limited to the nasal cavity
Group B	Tumor is localized to the nasal cavity and paranasal sinuses
Group C	Tumor extends beyond the nasal cavity and paranasal sinuses

and meningiomas. For large tumors, radiosurgery may be used as an adjunct to microsurgery if a lesion cannot be completely removed without significant risk. Stereotactic radiotherapy (and intensity-modulated conformal radiotherapy) is specifically indicated in large schwannomas and meningiomas diagnosed in inoperable patients and in patients with optic nerve gliomas and optic nerve sheath meningiomas if the vision is spared. Classic whole-brain radiation therapy no longer plays a role in the treatment of benign tumors of the cranial nerves.

Malignant tumors as a rule deserve resection and adjunct fractionated radiation therapy and/or chemotherapy with a therapeutic strategy being set up by multidisciplinary tumor boards.

14.5.1 Meningioma Associated with Cranial Nerves

Meningiomas associated with the optic nerve may be either ONSM or sinus cavernous meningiomas extending into the optic canal or suprasellar meningiomas displacing the optic chiasm. Except for ONSM, in all other meningiomas compressing or displacing segments of the optic nerve, surgery is generally the first-line treatment in order to relieve compression of the optic nerve and to achieve at least partial tumor resection. Some of these meningiomas cannot be removed completely. In such cases, either radiosurgery or fractionated stereotactic radiation therapy is indicated as a second-line treatment [17].

The natural course of ONSM is slow progression leading to progressive optic neuropathy, impairment of visual acuity until blindness, and proptosis. Because ONSMs are typically circumferential to the optic nerve and adhere tightly to the perineural microvessels, it is impossible to avoid trauma to the optic nerve during surgery and, therefore, not to compromise the patient's vision. Thus, surgical resection is no therapeutic option. As ^{68}Ga-DOTATATE-PET imaging has been shown to discriminate ONSM from other lesions, surgery just to obtain a biopsy to validate ONSM is no longer necessary [11, 15, 16].

In patients already being blind on the affected eye, excision of the tumor, including the optic nerve and its meningeal sheath, is possible whenever growth of a tumor extension posteriorly beyond the optic canal into the intracranial side is documented. Standard treatment of ONSM is stereotactic fractionated radiation and conformal radiotherapy [4, 35–42]. Favorable results have been published at least in the short term, and primary stereotactic fractionated radiation therapy has been advocated to preserve vision in patients with ONSM better than observation alone [4, 37, 41, 43]. However, recently, radiation retinopathy and loss of vision after fractionated stereotactic radiotherapy for ONSM were reported [44]. Because of this observation, only symptomatic patients should be treated, and caution in not overestimating the potential of fractionated stereotactic and three-dimensional conformal radiotherapy is warranted due to the well-known long latency of radiation damage to sensitive structures other than the optic nerve itself. Radiosurgery does not play a role in patients with ONSM and preserved vision, but in blind patients and small tumors, it can substitute for any other type of therapy very elegantly.

For meningiomas extending into the optic canal from the inside of the skull, surgical unroofing is the preferred treatment. The surgical approach in this situation depends on the localization of the meningioma in relation to the optic nerve [27, 45].

Meningiomas in association with other cranial nerves are found among the meningiomas of the middle or posterior fossa cerebri. In general, such lesions are primary candidates for resection if they are progressive, symptomatic, or of considerable size at diagnosis. If complete resection turns out to be too risky in an individual case, adjunct radiosurgery is recommended for small tumor remnants. In residual meningiomas too large for radiosurgery and in progressive meningiomas en plaque, fractionated radiation therapy is used. Today these lesions are indications for stereotactic radiotherapy or intensity-modulated (highly conformal) radiation therapy. For small skull base meningiomas with progressive growth proven by appropriate sequential MRI, primary radiosurgery is an effective and only minimally invasive treatment.

14.5.2 Optic Nerve Glioma

The role of surgical intervention in intraorbital optic nerve gliomas (ONGs) is still a subject of debate [46, 47]. Surgery must be in any case be embedded in a personalized treatment concept with watchful waiting, chemotherapy, and radiotherapy as potential combinations [6, 48]. In some patients the radiological assessment of therapeutic response can be difficult. For this purpose a proptosis index has been created that correlates with a therapeutic response and/or with progressive disease [49]. Progressive chiasmatic tumors are best treated by either chemotherapy or, especially in progressive disease after previous chemotherapy, fractionated radiotherapy. Modern variants of radiotherapy (stereotactic fractionated radiotherapy, proton therapy) allow effective treatment of ONG. In contrast to conventional radiotherapy, it provides the potential of sparing the pituitary gland in chiasmatic lesions. In some instances, vision may even improve after this type of radiotherapy [50]. Exophytic chiasmatic tumors may be treated by chiasm-preserv-

ing surgery and subsequent radiotherapy [51]. Radiosurgery can also be used as an effective adjuvant therapy in selected cases [52].

Rare cases of adult malignant optic nerve glioma have been published. These tumors may mimic optic neuritis in their initial presentation. On MRI, malignant glioma cannot be distinguished from optic nerve enlargement due to other causes.

14.5.3 Schwannomas

14.5.3.1 Orbital Cavity Schwannoma

Intraorbital schwannoma accounts for about 1–2% of all neoplasms of the orbit. Orbital schwannoma on MRI usually appears as hypointense on T1WI and hyperintense on T2WI, with homogeneous or heterogeneous enhancement [53]. Among the tumors of the orbit, patients with intraorbital schwannoma have the most favorable prognosis in terms of both visual function and long-term quality of life. Therefore, removal of orbital cavity schwannomas should not be postponed since the surgical outcome is very good provided a meticulous dissection to preserve function of the intraorbital muscles [54].

14.5.4 Vestibular Schwannoma

14.5.4.1 General Aspects

The most common tumor of the cerebellopontine angle are vestibular schwannomas (VS). Formerly, they have been termed "acoustic neuroma," but in fact the majority of tumors arise from the vestibular nerves, and the term "schwannoma" reflects the cellular heritage more precisely. There has been much discussion about mobile phones as potential risk factors for development of VS. However, despite telephone use might increase the risk of developing ipsilateral brain tumors in general, there has not been found any reliable interrelation for mobile phone use and VS yet [55]. They are benign tumors and unless very large, not life-threatening. Mean annual growth rate according to recent meta-analysis is 1 mm/year. Presenting symptoms are vertigo, tinnitus, and/or hearing loss, which compromise the patients' quality of life. After longer periods of growth, VS may additionally cause hydrocephalus, facial nerve palsy, trigeminal neuropathy, and ataxia by brain stem compression. The degree of hearing loss depends on the width of the internal auditory canal (in relation to the tumor size) and the extension of the VS into the depth of the internal auditory canal. The incidence of both facial and trigeminal nerve deficits is correlated to the extension of the tumor at diagnosis and found in 6% and 9%, respectively [56]. Typically, VS grows slowly but not continuously [57]. The proliferative activity of VS seems to be higher in younger patients and with NF2. However, in many patients, there are longer periods of very slow growth or growth arrest [58–60]. Even spontaneous regression has been described in 6–13% of VS [58, 60]. Taking into account this naturally heterogeneous behavior of VS, the appropriate timing of any therapeutic intervention is an important issue [61]. Apart from a strategy of "watchful waiting," surgery and radiation therapy are available. There is no specific chemotherapy for VS.

There are different surgical approaches, and there are several types of radiation therapy, including radiosurgery. All types of therapy have been proven to be highly effective in VS, although tumor recurrences are always possible, even in up to 10% in the long term after complete resection [62]. The historical evolution of surgery and radiosurgery has developed rather in parallel for the last three decades.

Microsurgery. Surgery for acoustic neuroma has a long history. Sir Charles Balance is known to have performed the first resection of one acoustic neuroma in 1894 and to have published the initial results in 1907. In his series, the mortality was around 80%. In 1917, Harvey Cushing, one of the early pioneers of neurosurgery, reported a reduced mortality rate of 11%. Just two decades later, Walter E. Dandy, another pioneer of neurosurgery, succeeded in reducing the lethal outcomes in his surgical series of acoustic neuroma below 5%. Today, the surgical mortality rate is below 1% [63]. MRI became available in the middle of the 1980s, and since then, increasing

numbers of small tumors have been detected. Microsurgical approaches in conjunction with the evolution of intraoperative facial nerve monitoring improved the chance to preserve facial nerve function during surgery [64, 65]. However, the possibility of sparing facial nerve function after surgery is dependent also on the anatomical extension of the tumor in relation to the facial nerve [66]. The majority of patients with postoperative facial nerve palsy showed at least partial functional recovery in a long-term follow-up; in these patients tumor size was detected to be a factor associated with the postoperative prognosis [30, 67–69]. Furthermore, facial nerve preservation is significantly reduced in recurrent tumors [70]. By analogy, the chance to preserve hearing increased also due to both the advent of microsurgery and the development of intraoperative neuromonitoring [65, 71]. In small- and medium-sized VS (classes T1 to T3; Fig. 14.3), a useful level of hearing can be preserved in about 60% of the patients. However, the real chance of hearing preservation depends on the presurgical hearing level, the anatomical extension (intra- vs extra-canalicular), the size of the tumor, the length of tumor-cochlear nerve contact [72], and the surgical approach. Furthermore, it continues to remain difficult to compare hearing results of different series due to the lack of a generally accepted standard of reporting hearing preservation results.

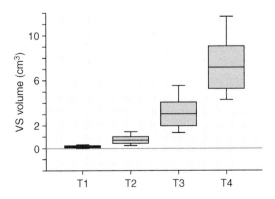

Fig. 14.3 Correlation between tumor volume (y-$axis$, cm³) and T-classification (x-$axis$, T1, T2, T3, T4) in 300 patients treated for VS by Gamma Knife surgery. T-classification according to Tos [28], Samii [64], and Koos [29]

Neurosurgeons and ENT surgeons have developed different avenues to access VS. In small intracanalicular tumors with ipsilateral deafness, a translabyrinthine approach can be used. In small intracanalicular tumors with ipsilateral hearing, the subtemporal approach is recommended. Larger tumors are resected via a suboccipital-retromastoid craniotomy. There are also combined surgical approaches, for example, the translabyrinthine-transtentorial access. Planned partial resection can be used in large VS with tumors tightly adhering to the facial nerve or the brain stem in order to minimize functional trauma [73, 74].

Evolution of Radiosurgery. Radiosurgery as a therapeutic concept has a history of more than half a century. Lars Leksell conceived the radiosurgical treatment principle in 1951, developed the prototype of the Gamma Knife, and was the first to apply it to an acoustic neuroma in 1968. His initial treatment report was published in 1971 [75]. Subsequently, radiosurgery for VS evolved into an evidence-based treatment standard. Technical progress in radiosurgery for VS translating into improved clinical outcome was achieved by the introduction of MRI for use in treatment planning and follow-up [76]. An important step forward was the introduction of the multiple isocenter treatments in the Gamma Knife method in 1990. Biological risk parameters of radiosurgery were identified as well as the tolerance doses of the cranial nerves associated with VS. Leveling off the marginal dose to an optimum of 12–13 Gy was shown to be effective in suppressing tumor growth while better preserving neurological function [56, 77]. Tumor volumetry was shown to be adequate to quantify the treatment outcome following radiosurgery. There is now broad awareness that radiosurgically treated schwannomas are subjected to a chronic and dynamic process that includes a transient increase of size due to tissue swelling (interstitial edema). Several centers have documented unequivocally the favorable long-term outcomes of radiosurgery for acoustic neuromas [31, 78–82]. The Gamma Knife indication has also been established for VS recurring after surgery [21, 83, 84] and for NF2 schwannomas [85, 86].

Gamma Knife radiosurgery as an alternative to microsurgery was postulated by Lunsford in 1992 [87]. In 1994, Hudgins and co-workers published a decision analysis comparing microsurgery and radiosurgery. They concluded that when patients prefer the preservation of facial nerve function even if that requires leaving a tumor remnant, then Gamma Knife radiosurgery is a better treatment strategy than microsurgical resection [88]. A very newsworthy evidence-based comparison of stereotactic radiosurgery and microsurgical resection showed that the best quality of evidence (levels 2 and 3) shows superior outcomes for VS patients having stereotactic radiosurgery compared to surgical resection, allowing a grade B recommendation for this approach [89]. This has been confirmed by a very recent meta-analysis [90]. Microsurgery for vestibular schwannoma after failed radiosurgery may present some technical difficulties. In such cases subtotal resection without dissection of the facial nerve and tumor has been advocated, because growth of the residual tumor is rare [70, 91]. However, the results do not support a change in the possibility of first intention radiosurgical treatment of small- to medium-sized vestibular schwannomas [92, 93]. Basically, radiosurgery is also effective for patients with recurrent tumors after the first radiosurgery although little information is available to evaluate this approach further [94]. Regarding cost-effectiveness and from a societal perspective, radiosurgery has been verified to be less expensive than microsurgical resection provided that the rate of tumor progression after radiosurgery remains low with long-term follow-up [9]. In bilateral VS associated with NF2, the results of radiosurgery do not seem to be as good as for patients with sporadic unilateral tumors. But in selected patients, radiosurgery may be considered for primary tumor management [95].

Gamma Knife radiosurgery has been performed in ambulatory patients in Munich, Germany, since 1994. The results are in agreement with other current published data. Primary Gamma Knife radiosurgery was applied to 169 (71%) patients, while 70 (29%) were treated by radiosurgery for residual or recurrent tumor after surgery. At 6 years, the tumor control rate in unilateral VS was 97% with a minimum follow-up time of 2 years after Gamma Knife radiosurgery (Figs. 14.4 and 14.5). Including salvage radiosurgery, the tumor control rate was 99%. The interval between the first and the salvage radiosurgeries was 2.4 years. In patients with complete facial nerve function, this was preserved after Gamma Knife surgery in all instances. In patients treated twice with the Gamma Knife, no facial deficit occurred. In the subpopulation of patients with some degree of facial neuropathy before radiosurgery, the risk of additional facial neuropathy was 10%. These symptoms were mild to moderate and transient. Trigeminal neuropathy was observed for larger tumors (class T3 and T4) and pertained also to two patients treated twice. Trigeminal neuropathy was transient, required no medication, and correlated to transient tumor swelling. In 17 patients treated for NF2 schwannomas, the recurrence rate was higher due to a reduced dose level accepted in order to spare hearing better (Fig. 14.5).

In 2005 the CyberKnife [67] replaced the Gamma Knife in our outpatient RS service. Within the first 3 years, more than 230 patients with vestibular schwannomas were treated. This figure is indicative of an increased rate of acoustic neuroma treatments and supports the parity of microsurgery and radiosurgery for VS today [89]. Preliminary experience shows improved clinical outcome when compared to our previous radiosurgical experience.

The quality of the physical dose parameters obtained with the CyberKnife is equal or somewhat superior to that obtained with the Gamma Knife and because vestibular schwannomas today are treated at earlier stages than in former years

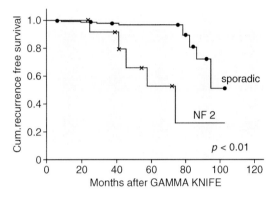

Fig. 14.5 Tumor control after outpatient Gamma Knife radiosurgery (225 sporadic VS; 14 NF2 tumors). The recurrence rate for NF2 schwannomas is significantly ($p < 0.01$) higher due to a reduced dose level intentionally given to preserve hearing better. The maximum dose to the tumor was 25.0 (range 15.3–31.1) Gy in sporadic tumors and 23.0 (range 15.7–27.0) Gy in NF2 tumors

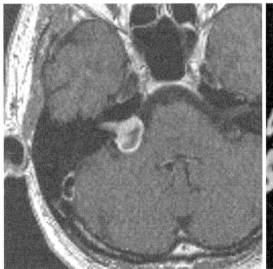

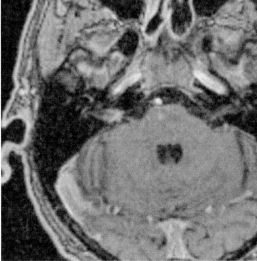

Fig. 14.4 VS on the right side treated by Gamma Knife surgery (*left image*). Follow-up examination after 6 years reveals subtotal regression (*right image*)

when the pretreatment hearing level is higher and the tumors are smaller [78, 96].

Linear Accelerator Radiosurgery. The principle of radiosurgery can also be performed by other radiation delivery devices, e.g., linear accelerators. These are either adapted for stereotactic irradiation or are dedicated systems. There are several reports on linear accelerator radiosurgery for VS [97–99]. In general, linear accelerator radiosurgery yielded a high tumor control rate equivalent to the Gamma Knife results.

Stereotactic Fractionated Radiation Therapy. Fractionated stereotactic radiotherapy offers an additional therapeutic approach for VS. The rationale for the strategy is that fractionation will allow complications to be reduced while maintaining the same degree of long-term tumor control achieved by radiosurgery [100]. In a single institution trial in particular, a higher rate of serviceable hearing preservation was claimed for fractionated stereotactic radiotherapy than with Gamma Knife radiosurgery [4]. However, there are also reports of hearing loss after fractionated stereotactic radiotherapy [101]. Single institution trials as well as pooled data showed that both radiosurgery and fractionated stereotactic radiotherapy can be considered equally effective [102]. Proton beam irradiation is another type of fractionated stereotactic radiotherapy. A tumor control rate reported for proton therapy of VS was similar to the results of Gamma Knife radiosurgery. However, the facial nerve toxicity was higher [103].

Most studies on fractionated stereotactic radiotherapy are handicapped by a rather short follow-up time. This aspect is especially noteworthy because fractionation delays the tissue response significantly in comparison to radiosurgery. The time interval for the manifestation of radiation toxicity is less than 1 year in radiosurgery, but it may take several years in fractionated stereotactic radiotherapy. This makes valid comparisons of both treatment methods difficult. Furthermore, in fractionated stereotactic radiotherapy, a higher total dose of radiation has to be applied to compensate for a fractionation effect compromising tumor control. In contrast to radiosurgery, the structures of the inner ear are in the range of fractionated stereotactic radiotherapy. This may cause hearing loss due to radiation toxicity affecting the hair cells in the inner ear [104].

Taking into consideration the argument of radiation protection, it seems rational to restrict fractionated stereotactic radiotherapy to selected patients with large tumors and risk factors for surgery.

Medical Therapy. Based on preclinical data, different drugs have been proposed for "targeted therapy" in selected NF2 cases. Bevacizumab, a monoclonal antibody against VEGF, has been reported to induce hearing improvement and tumor shrinkage in progressive vestibular schwannomas (VS) in NF2. The need for intravenous injections, continuous treatment, and long-term adverse events (hypertension, proteinuria, hemorrhage) are the main drawbacks.

Lapatinib seemed promising in a single phase II trial but is not currently used in clinical practice. Erlotinib has not been associated with radiographic or hearing responses. Everolimus has been evaluated in phase II trials and did not induce tumor shrinkage, but seems to prolong time to tumor progression in selected cases. By now, bevacizumab is the only drug proposed for medical treatment in very selected NF2 patients [105–110].

Key Issues of Decision-Making in VS. In order to identify in a practical manner the best type of treatment in an individual patient, the following key issues and answers to the major questions may be used:

1. There are differences in the invasiveness and risk profile of the treatment modalities.
2. Concerning the variants of radiation therapy (mainly radiosurgery or fractionated radiotherapy), there are considerable distinctions in dose burden to normal tissue.
3. Radiation therapy kills the tumor cells but leaves the tumor mass at the disposal of the biological capacity of the body to resolve it. With surgery, the tumor mass is removed but at the expense of the invasiveness of trephination and tissue dissection.
4. In case of surgery, the choice of the surgical approach depends on the residual hearing level, the size of the tumor, and the surgeon's experience and preferences.

Further questions determining the surgical indication are the following:

(a) Is it a sporadic VS or is it a case of NF2?
(b) Is the hearing preserved in the contralateral ear or not?
(c) Is it a native tumor, or is it tumor recurrence:
  • after surgery or
  • after radiation therapy
(d) Are there conditions indicating an elevated surgical risk for the patient?

Questions with impact on the radiosurgical (or radiotherapeutic) indication are:

(a) Is the diagnosis of the tumor histology certain enough to allow noninvasive therapy?
(b) How active is the tumor concerning clinical symptoms, and how fast growing is the tumor as documented by follow-up imaging?
(c) Is the size (volume) small enough for radiosurgery?
(d) Are there conditions associated with increased radiosensitivity (diabetes mellitus)?
(e) What is the psychological condition of the patient concerning radiation therapy?
(f) What is the comparative profile of other treatment options?
(g) Concerning the issue of radiation protection, which type of radiotherapy is effective by delivering the lowest dose?

In many clinical situations, several treatment strategies are conceivable, indicating a possibility for patients to select the therapy according to their own needs or preferences [111, 112].

Bearing in mind the various treatment alternatives, it is not surprising that there is no general agreement regarding therapeutic decisions. There is no prospective randomized trial comparing microsurgery (including the various surgical approaches), radiation therapy (including radiosurgery, stereotactic radiation therapy, proton beam therapy), and the "watchful waiting" strategy [112]. It is clear that both surgery and radiation therapy have experienced a consider-

able synchronous progress during the last four decades. It is further clear that tumor size remains a decisive prognostic factor in terms of functional outcome for any type of therapy. In case of primary radiosurgical treatment, the differential diagnosis of the lesions in the cerebellopontine angle has to be regarded. It includes inflammatory, vascular, and neoplastic lesions [18]. Because also metastatic lesions (Fig. 14.2) may seed in the cerebellopontine angle, mimicking a VS, it is not recommended to treat VS-like lesions by radiosurgery in patients with a settled diagnosis of cancer. Although it is an important issue of concern, the risk of carcinogenesis or malignant transformation due to radiosurgery of VS is exceptionally low (0.3%) [24, 35, 113, 114].

Primary Treatment of Sporadic VS. Large tumors with significant brain stem compression usually require surgical resection. Large tumors in inoperable patients can be treated by stereotactic fractionated radiotherapy. However, nowadays more and more smaller-sized tumors are being identified. For such VS, microsurgery and radiosurgery are equivalent therapeutic methods, and, in non-symptomatic lesions, even watchful waiting is an option [112]. Radiosurgery is associated with a lower rate of immediate and long-term development of facial and trigeminal neuropathy, postoperative complications, and hospital stay. Radiosurgery yields better measurable hearing preservation than microsurgery and an equivalent serviceable hearing preservation rate and tumor growth control [49]. For preservation of function, near-total resection (with intentionally left small remnants at the facial and cochlear nerve) has shown to be a valid concept with very good functional results and low risk of further tumor progression [87, 115–117]. Concerning radiosurgery as a management option, a statement of Kondziolka published in 2003 reads as follows: "Patients must be able to accept the concept of tumor control rather than tumor removal. Physicians should strive to educate their patients with information from the peer-reviewed literature. Confusion exists among patients because the information from Internet sources, newsletters, support groups, and physicians has not always been validated and supported by outcomes data.

Although we are asked to provide our opinions, our comments should not be based on myth, conjecture, training bias, or socioeconomic concerns" [118]. This, however, should serve as a general rule in counseling patients.

Neurofibromatosis Type 2. Patients with NF2 pose specific challenges, particularly in regard to preservation of hearing and other cranial nerve functions. In NF2 patients with bilateral tumors, the questions arise: which side should be treated first, and which type of therapy is preferable? If useful hearing is preserved on both sides, it can be recommended to start treatment directed to the more active tumor (in clinical and radiological terms). If radiosurgery is used for this first approach, one should wait for at least 2 and, even better, 3 years thereafter to see how well the hearing is preserved on the treated side and how the therapeutic effect (tumor control, tumor shrinkage) manifests. In such situations, we tend to reduce the radiosurgical dose by about 10% in order to spare the hearing better. This is basically at the expense of a reduced tumor control rate, however, and therefore it seems important to know the individual radiosensitivity of the patient's VS before treatment of the other side is performed. If the bilateral tumors are too large for radiosurgery, either a surgical resection (preferentially approaching the larger tumor) or a stereotactic radiotherapy with a classic fractionation scheme (30 times 1.8 Gy) is indicated. Surgery should be conservative in order to minimize the risk of deafness, and in case of tumor remnants, they could be treated by second-line radiosurgery. Our own experience with VS patients with preserved useful hearing after partial tumor resection, including opening of the internal auditory canal, shows that the risk of radiation-induced hearing loss is quite low in this situation. Stereotactic radiosurgery appears to be a safe and effective alternative to surgery for NF2-VS with high rates of local control and significantly lower facial nerve complications [85].

Recurrent or Residual VS: Combined Treatment. After intentionally near-total or subtotal resection, a watch-and-scan policy is warranted as only a minority of remnants do progress; however, the risk is correlated to the size of the remnant.

In cases of recurrences after radiosurgery, both radiosurgical retreatment and surgery are possible. In contrast to earlier experiences when higher doses were used in radiosurgery and when the dose planning was not as precise as today, there is nowadays no increased surgical difficulty due to the delivered radiosurgery dose. However, the functional risk for the facial nerve is slightly higher, and a very meticulous, conservative dissection technique is required [119, 120]. Furthermore, it has to be considered that recurrent VS treated with radiosurgery has a lower proliferation potential compared with recurrences following microsurgery. Radiation-induced apoptosis is thought to contribute to the lower tumor cell proliferation of radiosurgically treated tumors. In VS recurring after surgery, radiosurgery may be used preferentially because the risk of (additional) damage to the facial nerve is lower than with a second operation.

VS Associated with the Only Hearing Ear. A further issue of importance is the situation in patients with a VS associated with the only hearing ear. This situation is more common in NF2 patients. There is no method available to compare objectively and prospectively the outcome of hearing concerning surgery, radiosurgery, and fractionated stereotactic radiotherapy in such situations. However, there are guidelines common to these treatment options. Firstly, the better the higher the pretreatment level of hearing is, the better is the chance of hearing preservation. Secondly, the chance of hearing preservation depends strongly on the size of the tumor. Both issues would speak in favor of early proactive treatment. However, for all treatment options, including surgery, there is some risk of delayed hearing loss, even in the absence of residual tumor. The time course of hearing loss may be different in regard of the type of therapy. In general, hearing decreases within a few days after surgery, within a few months after radiosurgery, and within a few years after stereotactic fractionated radiotherapy. However, there are considerable individual variations [101, 121]. It is therefore advisable to present this situation to the individual patient and to identify the treatment of choice together with the patient.

Non-vestibular Schwannoma. Surgery has been the first-line treatment for non-vestibular schwannoma (NVS) for five decades. The results of surgery have considerably improved during this time period [32, 33, 89]. The risks of microsurgery are characterized by a low percentage of general morbidity (CSF leakage, hemorrhage, etc.) and between 30 and 60% specific morbidity, e.g., new or increased cranial nerve deficits. The latter are mostly transient and/or mild. There are specific treatment reports dealing with selected CNT treated by surgery [32, 89], radiosurgery [122], or stereotactic fractionated radiotherapy [123]. Radiosurgery and radiation therapy avoid the risks of the invasive surgical approaches. However, radiosurgery is useful for small tumors only but with very good results concerning tumor control and functional integrity [123–125]. The drawback of fractionated radiation therapy is the higher dose load (an issue of radiation protection) and the much longer time needed compared with radiosurgery. Therefore, fractionated stereotactic radiation therapy should be restricted to NVSs that are both inoperable and too large for Gamma Knife surgery. In many instances, a combined approach of microsurgery and radiosurgery is preferable. According to the literature, this strategy has been applied in about half of the radiosurgically treated NVS. Regarding the specific risk of radiation toxicity to the cranial nerve, radiosurgery and stereotactic fractionated radiation therapy are not inferior to the specific risks of surgery.

Although microsurgical resection in general remains the method of choice for NVS, radiosurgery can be used as an additional or alternative method in suitable patients. The therapeutic profile of radiosurgery is characterized by a very high tumor control rate (over 95%), mostly associated with significant tumor shrinkage. As a rule, specific side effects are mild and transient [124].

14.5.5 Malignant Peripheral Nerve Sheath Tumors

Malignant peripheral nerve sheath tumors (MPNSTs) derive from Schwann cells or pluripotent cells of the neural crest. Delay of diagnosis is common, especially in lesions affecting proximal parts of the peripheral nervous system. Patients with centrally located tumors have a poorer prognosis than those with peripheral tumors [126]. The management of patients with MPNST involves a multimodality approach. The goal of surgery is complete resection with negative margins. Adjuvant irradiation with doses up to 60 Gy and more and other means of local dose escalation are associated with improved local control of disease [127]. Tumor diameter of <5 cm, gross total resection of the tumor, and younger age are favorable prognostic variables [128].

14.5.6 Esthesioneuroblastoma

Olfactory neuroblastomas (or esthesioneuroblastomas) are most frequently staged using a system proposed by Kadish et al. in 1976 and adjusted by Chao 2001 [34, 129]:

- Group A: Limited to the nasal cavity
- Group B: Limited to the nasal cavity and paranasal sinuses
- Group C: Extends beyond the nasal cavity and paranasal sinuses:
  - Base of skull
  - Intracranial compartment
  - Orbit
- Group D (added by Chao): Cervical nodal metastases

Imaging plays a key role in the accurate staging including both computed tomography (CT) and magnetic resonance imaging (MRI). CT should be performed with thin slices (1 mm thick) and in both coronal and sagittal planes as it is essential for evaluation of the osseous involvement. The most important information gained from MRI is defining the soft tissue extent and assessment of suspected intracranial, orbital, or skull base invasion of tumor. MRI is also excellent at distinguishing dural involvement from parenchymal involvement [130].

Esthesioneuroblastoma is potentially curable by surgical resection and radiation therapy. Surgical treatment alone is effective for low-grade tumors if tumor-free margins can be obtained (Kadish stage A) [131]. Nowadays, with modern imaging used for diagnostic workup, esthesioneuroblastoma should be either endoscopically or via an endoscopic-assisted microsurgical approach [132, 133]. Kadish stage B ought to be treated by surgical tumor resection in combination with radiotherapy [131]. Large tumors (Kadish stage C) should be considered for preoperative chemotherapy and postoperative radiotherapy [133, 134]. Preoperative tumor extension with skull base penetration, intraorbital growth, and Kadish C stage compromise the disease-free survival significantly [135]. Multimodality treatment (surgery plus pre- or postoperative chemotherapy plus postoperative radiation therapy) appears to be highly efficient in preventing local and systemic relapse in patients with such advanced esthesioneuroblastomas [135]. Nevertheless, tumor recurrence is not uncommon. Neck metastases, when present, should be excised using a modified neck dissection. Distant metastases may present at any time during the course of the disease and may respond to local radiotherapy or systemic chemotherapy [136]. Five-year survival currently appears to be optimized by neoadjuvant chemotherapy, surgery followed by postoperative radiotherapy, and additional chemotherapy, depending on the state of disease [132, 134, 137–139]. Because recurrence can appear after 5 or even 10 years, long-term follow-up is mandatory [133, 136].

14.6 Prognosis/Quality of Life

The prognosis and the quality of life have synchronously improved during the last decades for patients with benign tumors of the cranial nerves. The reason for this favorable development is the progress achieved in diagnostic imaging and simultaneously the technical advances of microsurgery and radiation therapy, including the success of radiosurgery. Early diagnosis leads to superior treatment results. Lifetime tumor control is routine for benign tumors. Nowadays, preservation of neurological function is no longer a claim but reality in many aspects. Much of the

success can be attributed to the fact that in many clinical settings, treatment alternatives are available, offering the choice of less invasive and less risky therapeutic strategies. Further considerable progress has become possible by combined treatment. The treatment of large VS by conservative microsurgery and adjunct radiosurgery to spare the facial nerve function may serve as a suitable example.

14.7 Follow-Up/Specific Problems and Measures

Considerable knowledge has accumulated to show that a lifelong follow-up is mandatory in all cases of cranial nerve tumors, even in patients with complete resection. Tumor recurrences may develop in the long term because of a manifestation of biological tumor heterogeneity. MRI is the method of choice to perform sequential imaging over the years. The timing of the follow-up examinations depends on the individual treatment applied and on the histology of the tumor. In completely resected schwannomas, the follow-up interval may be 1 or 2 years in the first period after surgery. It can be extended to 3–5 years later. In cases with radiation therapy or radiosurgery, the first follow-up examination should be after 6 months and then once a year. In tumors showing a regular response to radiosurgery, after 5 years the examination intervals may be expanded to 3–5 years for the remaining lifetime. In cases with tumor swelling or in cases showing questionable tumor progression or recurrence, a reexamination should be performed earlier, e.g., after 6 months. In irregular cases, the examination intervals should be scheduled individually according to the further development of the treated tumor. It has to be kept in mind that there is a dynamic response of benign cranial nerve tumors to radiation therapy and to radiosurgery. After single-dose irradiation, there may be a continuous shrinkage of the treated tumor over the years. However, there are also cases with transient tumor increase before shrinking. Other tumors remain stable, indicating growth arrest, while other tumors show a tumor increase in the first period after radiosurgery and then remain stable. Because of these different reactions of benign cranial nerve tumors to radiation therapy/radiosurgery, it seems impossible to define a treatment failure or tumor recurrence before 2 years have elapsed after radiosurgery. This peculiarity demands a sophisticated follow-up regimen under the responsibility of the radiosurgical team.

For malignant tumors of the cranial nerves, a tighter follow-up time schedule is necessary, which is again based on MRI. In this setting, not only the local tumor control but also the issue of distant metastases is evaluated. This requires a more extensive examination protocol that is dependent on the type of the tumor under question.

References

1. Ostrom QT, Gittleman H, Xu J, Kromer C, Wolinsky Y, Kruchko C, Barnholtz-Sloan JS (2016) CBTRUS statistical report: primary brain and other central nervous system tumors diagnosed in the United States in 2009-2013. Neuro Oncol 18(Suppl 5):v1–v75
2. Too M, Stangerup SE, Caye-Thomasen P, Tos T, Thomsen J (2004) What is the real incidence of vestibular schwannoma? Arch Otolaryngol Head Neck Surg 130:216–220
3. Dutton JJ (1992) Optic nerve sheath meningiomas. Surv Ophthalmol 37:167–183
4. Andrews DW, Faroozan R, Yang BP, Hudes RS, Werner-Wasik M, Kim SM, Sergott RC, Savino PJ, Shields J, Shields C, Downes MB, Simeone FA, Goldman HW, Curran WJ Jr (2002) Fractionated stereotactic radiotherapy for the treatment of optic nerve sheath meningiomas: preliminary observations of 33 optic nerves in 30 patients with historical comparison to observation with or without prior surgery. Neurosurgery 51:890–902; discussion 903–894
5. Mornet E, Kania R, Sauvaget E, Herman P, Tran Ba Huy P (2013) Vestibular schwannoma and cellphones. Results, limits and perspectives of clinical studies. Eur Ann Otorhinolaryngol Head Neck Dis 130(5):275–282
6. Walker D (2003) Recent advances in optic nerve glioma with a focus on the young patient. Curr Opin Neurol 16:657–664
7. Best PV (1987) Malignant triton tumour in the cerebellopontine angle. Report of a case. Acta Neuropathol (Berl) 74:92–96
8. Akimoto J, Ito H, Kudo M (2000) Primary intracranial malignant schwannoma of trigeminal nerve. A case report with review of the literature. Acta Neurochir (Wien) 142:591–595
9. Banerjee R, Moriarty JP, Foote RL, Pollock BE (2008) Comparison of the surgical and follow-up costs associated with microsurgical resection and stereotactic radiosurgery for vestibular schwannoma. J Neurosurg 108(6):1220–1224
10. Kumar M, Fallon RJ, Hill JS, Davis MM (2002) Esthesioneuroblastoma in children. J Pediatr Hematol Oncol 24:482–487
11. Galldiks N, Albert NL, Sommerauer M, Grosu AL, Ganswindt U, Law I, Preusser M, Rhun EL, Vogelbaum MA, Zadeh G, Dhermain F, Weller M, Langen KJ, Tonn JC (2017) PET imaging in patients with meningioma-report of the RANO/PET Group. Neuro Oncol 19(12):1576–1587
12. Liauw L, Vielvoye GJ, de Keizer RJ, van Duinen SG (1996) Optic nerve glioma mimicking an optic nerve meningioma. Clin Neurol Neurosurg 98:258–261
13. Ortiz O, Schochet SS, Kotzan JM, Kostick D (1996) Radiologic-pathologic correlation: meningioma of the optic nerve sheath. AJNR Am J Neuroradiol 17:901–906
14. Jackson A, Patankar T, Laitt RD (2003) Intracanalicular optic nerve meningioma: a serious diagnostic pitfall. AJNR Am J Neuroradiol 24:1167–1170
15. Klingenstein A, Haug AR, Miller C, Hintschich C (2015) Ga-68-DOTA-TATE PET/CT for discrimination of tumors of the optic pathway. Orbit 34(1):16–22
16. Purohit BS, Vargas MI, Ailianou A, Merlini L, Poletti PA, Platon A, Delattre BM, Rager O, Burkhardt K, Becker M (2016) Orbital tumours and tumour-like lesions: exploring the armamentarium of multiparametric imaging. Insights Imaging 7(1):43–68
17. Goldbrunner R, Minniti G, Preusser M, Jenkinson MD, Sallabanda K, Houdart E, von Deimling A, Stavrinou P, Lefranc F, Lund-Johansen M, Moyal EC, Brandsma D, Henriksson R, Soffietti R, Weller M (2016) EANO guidelines for the diagnosis and treatment of meningiomas. Lancet Oncol 17(9):e383–e391
18. Slooff JL (1984) Pathological anatomical findings in the cerebellopontine angle. A review. In: Pfaltz CR (ed) Advances in oto-rhino-laryngology, vol 34. S. Karger, Basel-München-Paris-London, pp 89–103
19. Louis DN, Perry A, Reifenberger G, von Deimling A, Figarella-Branger D, Cavenee WK, Ohgaki H, Wiestler OD, Kleihues P, Ellison DW (2016) The 2016 World Health Organization Classification of Tumors of the Central Nervous System: a summary. Acta Neuropathol 131(6):803–820
20. Kalamarides M, Acosta MT, Babovic-Vuksanovic D, Carpen O, Cichowski K, Evans DG, Giancotti F, Hanemann CO, Ingram D, Lloyd AC, Mayes DA, Messiaen L, Morrison H, North K, Packer R, Pan D, Stemmer-Rachamimov A, Upadhyaya M, Viskochil D, Wallace MR, Hunter-Schaedle K, Ratner N (2012) Neurofibromatosis 2011: a report of the

Children's Tumor Foundation annual meeting. Acta Neuropathol 123(3):369–380

21. Pollock BE, Lunsford LD, Flickinger JC, Clyde BL, Kondziolka D (1998) Vestibular schwannoma management. Part I. Failed microsurgery and the role of delayed stereotactic radiosurgery. J Neurosurg 89:944–948

22. Cirak B (2003) Optic nerve glioma. J Neurosurg 99:246; author reply 246

23. Kleihues P, Cavenee WK (1997) Pathology and genetics of tumours of the nervous system. International Agency for Research on Cancer, Lyon

24. Woordruff JM, Kourea HP, Louis DN (1997) Schwannoma. In: Kleihues P, Cavenee WK (eds) Pathology and genetics of tumours of the nervous system. International Agency for Research on Cancer, Lyon, pp 126–132

25. Nair AG, Pathak RS, Iyer VR, Gandhi RA (2014) Optic nerve glioma: an update. Int Ophthalmol 34(4):999–1005

26. Hirose T, Scheithauer BW, Sano T (1998) Perineurial malignant peripheral nerve sheath tumor (MPNST): a clinicopathologic, immunohistochemical, and ultrastructural study of seven cases. Am J Surg Pathol 22:1368–1378

27. Shimano H, Nagasawa S, Kawabata S, Ogawa R, Ohta T (2000) Surgical strategy for meningioma extension into the optic canal. Neurol Med Chir (Tokyo) 40:447–451; discussion 451–442

28. Tos M, Thomsen J (1992) Proposal of classification of tumor size in acoustic neuroma surgery. In: Tos M, Thomsen J (eds) Proceedings of the first international conference on acoustic neuroma Copenhagen, Denmark, August 25–29, 1991. Kugler Publications, Amsterdam/New York, pp 133–137

29. Koos WT, Day JD, Matula C, Levy DI (1998) Neurotopographic considerations in the microsurgical treatment of small acoustic neurinomas. J Neurosurg 88:506–512

30. Samii M, Matthies C (1997) Management of 1,000 vestibular schwannomas (acoustic neuromas): surgical management and results with an emphasis on complications and how to avoid them. Neurosurgery 40:11–21; discussion 21–13

31. Kondziolka D, Lunsford LD, McLaughlin MR, Fl ickinger JC (1998) Long-term outcomes after radiosurgery for acoustic neuromas [see comments]. N Engl J Med 339:1426–1433

32. Samii M, Migliori MM, Tatagiba M, Babu R (1995) Surgical treatment of trigeminal schwannomas. J Neurosurg 82:711–718

33. Samii M, Babu RP, Tatagiba M, Sepehrnia A (1995) Surgical treatment of jugular foramen schwannomas. J Neurosurg 82:924–932

34. Kadish S, Goodman M, Wang CC (1976) Olfactory neuroblastoma. A clinical analysis of 17 cases. Cancer 37:1571–1576

35. Romanelli P, Wowra B, Muacevic A (2007) Multisession CyberKnife radiosurgery for optic nerve sheath meningiomas. Neurosurg Focus 23(6):E11

36. Jeremic B, Pitz S (2007) Primary optic nerve sheath meningioma: stereotactic fractionated radiation therapy as an emerging treatment of choice. Cancer 110(4):714–722

37. Becker G, Jeremic B, Pitz S, Buchgeister M, Wilhelm H, Schiefer U, Paulsen F, Zrenner E, Bamberg M (2002) Stereotactic fractionated radiotherapy in patients with optic nerve sheath meningioma. Int J Radiat Oncol Biol Phys 54:1422–1429

38. Eddleman CS, Liu JK (2007) Optic nerve sheath meningioma: current diagnosis and treatment. Neurosurg Focus 23(5):E4

39. Litre CF, Noudel R, Colin P, Sherpereel B, Peruzzi P, Rousseaux P (2007) [Fractionated stereotactic radiotherapy for optic nerve sheath meningioma: eight cases]. Neurochirurgie 53(5):333–338

40. Llorente-Gonzalez S, Arbizu-Duralde A, Pastora-Salvador N (2008) [Fractionated stereotactic radiotherapy in optic nerve sheath meningioma]. Arch Soc Esp Oftalmol 83(7):441–444

41. Pitz S, Becker G, Schiefer U, Wilhelm H, Jeremic B, Bamberg M, Zrenner E (2002) Stereotactic fractionated irradiation of optic nerve sheath meningioma: a new treatment alternative. Br J Ophthalmol 86:1265–1268

42. Vagefi MR, Larson DA, Horton JC (2006) Optic nerve sheath meningioma: visual improvement during radiation treatment. Am J Ophthalmol 142(2):343–344

43. Turbin RE, Thompson CR, Kennerdell JS, Cockerham KP, Kupersmith MJ (2002) A long-term visual outcome comparison in patients with optic nerve sheath meningioma managed with observation, surgery, radiotherapy, or surgery and radiotherapy. Ophthalmology 109:890–899; discussion 899–900

44. Subramanian PS, Bressler NM, Miller NR (2004) Radiation retinopathy after fractionated stereotactic radiotherapy for optic nerve sheath meningioma. Ophthalmology 111:565–567

45. Combs SE, Ganswindt U, Foote RL, Kondziolka D, Tonn JC (2012) State-of-the-art treatment alternatives for base of skull meningiomas: complementing and controversial indications for neurosurgery, stereotactic and robotic based radiosurgery or modern fractionated radiation techniques. Radiat Oncol 7:226

46. Goodden J, Pizer B, Pettorini B, Williams D, Blair J, Didi M, Thorp N, Mallucci C (2014) The role of surgery in optic pathway/hypothalamic gliomas in children. J Neurosurg Pediatr 13(1):1–12

47. Sawamura Y, Kamada K, Kamoshima Y, Yamaguchi S, Tajima T, Tsubaki J, Fujimaki T (2008) Role of surgery for optic pathway/hypothalamic astrocytomas in children. Neuro Oncol 10(5):725–733

48. Fried I, Tabori U, Tihan T, Reginald A, Bouffet E (2013) Optic pathway gliomas: a review. CNS Oncol 2(2):143–159

49. Diaz RJ, Laughlin S, Nicolin G, Buncic JR, Bouffet E, Bartels U (2008) Assessment of chemotherapeutic response in children with proptosis due to optic nerve glioma. Childs Nerv Syst 24(6):707–712

50. Debus J, Kocagoncu KO, Hoss A, Wenz F, Wannenmacher M (1999) Fractionated stereotactic radiotherapy (FSRT) for optic glioma. Int J Radiat Oncol Biol Phys 44:243–248

51. Astrup J (2003) Natural history and clinical management of optic pathway glioma. Br J Neurosurg 17:327–335

52. Lim YJ, Leem W (1996) Two cases of gamma knife radiosurgery for low-grade optic chiasm glioma. Stereotact Funct Neurosurg 66(1):174–183

53. Wang Y, Xiao LH (2008) Orbital schwannomas: findings from magnetic resonance imaging in 62 cases. Eye (Lond) 22(8):1034–1039

54. Iida Y, Sakata K, Kobayashi N, Tatezuki J, Manaka H, Kawasaki T (2016) Orbital Abducens Nerve Schwannoma: a case report and review of the literature. NMC Case Rep J 3(4):107–109

55. Bortkiewicz A, Gadzicka E, Szymczak W (2017) Mobile phone use and risk for intracranial tumors and salivary gland tumors—a meta-analysis. Int J Occup Med Environ Health 30(1):27–43

56. Hirato M, Inoue H, Zama A, Ohye C, Shibazaki T, Andou Y (1996) Gamma Knife radiosurgery for acoustic schwannoma: effects of low radiation dose and functional prognosis. Stereotact Funct Neurosurg 66:134–141

57. Nikolopoulos TP, Fortnum H, O'Donoghue G, Baguley D (2010) Acoustic neuroma growth: a systematic review of the evidence. Otol Neurotol 31(3):478–485

58. Charabi S, Tos M, Thomsen J, Charabi B, Mantoni M (2000) Vestibular schwannoma growth–long-term results. Acta Otolaryngol Suppl 543:7–10

59. Miller T, Lau T, Vasan R, Danner C, Youssef AS, van Loveren H, Agazzi S (2014) Reporting success rates in the treatment of vestibular schwannomas: are we accounting for the natural history? J Clin Neurosci 21(6):914–918

60. Walsh RM, Bath AP, Bance ML, Keller A, Tator CH, Rutka JA (2000) The natural history of untreated vestibular schwannomas. Is there a role for conservative management? Rev Laryngol Otol Rhinol 121:21–26

61. Hajioff D, Raut VV, Walsh RM, Bath AP, Bance ML, Guha A, Tator CH, Rutka JA (2008) Conservative management of vestibular schwannomas: third review of a 10-year prospective study. Clin Otolaryngol 33(3):255–259

62. Thomassin JM, Pellet W, Epron JP, Braccini F, Roche PH (2001) [Recurrent acoustic neurinoma after complete surgical resection]. Ann Otolaryngol Chir Cervicofac 118:3–10

63. McClelland S 3rd, Kim E, Murphy JD, Jaboin JJ (2017) Operative mortality rates of acoustic neuroma surgery: a national cancer database analysis. Otol Neurotol 38(5):751–753

64. Samii M, Tatagiba M, Matthies C (2001) Vestibular schwannomas: surgical approach. J Neurosurg 94(1):144–146

65. Tonn JC, Schlake HP, Goldbrunner R, Milewski C, Helms J, Roosen K (2000) Acoustic neuroma surgery as an interdisciplinary approach: a neurosurgical series of 508 patients. J Neurol Neurosurg Psychiatry 69:161–166

66. Strauss C (2002) The facial nerve in medial acoustic neuromas. J Neurosurg 97:1083–1090

67. Acioly MA, Gharabaghi A, Liebsch M, Carvalho CH, Aguiar PH, Tatagiba M (2011) Quantitative parameters of facial motor evoked potential during vestibular schwannoma surgery predict postoperative facial nerve function. Acta Neurochir (Wien) 153(6):1169–1179

68. Goldbrunner RH, Schlake HP, Milewski C, Tonn JC, Helms J, Roosen K (2000) Quantitative parameters of intraoperative electromyography predict facial nerve outcomes for vestibular schwannoma surgery. Neurosurgery 46(5):1140–1146

69. Veronezi RJ, Fernandes YB, Borges G, Ramina R (2008) Long-term facial nerve clinical evaluation following vestibular schwannoma surgery. Arq Neuropsiquiatr 66(2A):194–198

70. Slattery WH 3rd (2009) Microsurgery after radiosurgery or radiotherapy for vestibular schwannomas. Otolaryngol Clin North Am 42(4):707–715

71. Yang J, Grayeli AB, Barylyak R, Elgarem H (2008) Functional outcome of retrosigmoid approach in vestibular schwannoma surgery. Acta Otolaryngol 128(8):881–886

72. Ahsan SF, Huq F, Seidman M, Taylor A (2017) Long-term hearing preservation after resection of vestibular schwannoma: a systematic review and meta-analysis. Otol Neurotol 38(10):1505–1511

73. Daniel RT, Tuleasca C, George M, Pralong E, Schiappacasse L, Zeverino M, Maire R, Levivier M (2017) Preserving normal facial nerve function and improving hearing outcome in large vestibular schwannomas with a combined approach: planned subtotal resection followed by gamma knife radiosurgery. Acta Neurochir (Wien) 159(7):1197–1211

74. Syed MI, Wolf A, Ilan O, Hughes CO, Chung J, Tymianski M, Pothier DD, Rutka JA (2017) The behaviour of residual tumour after the intentional incomplete excision of a vestibular schwannoma: is it such a bad thing to leave some behind? Clin Otolaryngol 42(1):92–99

75. Leksell L (1971) A note on the treatment of acoustic tumours. Acta Chir Scand 137:763–765

76. Too SY, Lufkin RB, Rand R, Robinson JD, Hanafee W (1990) Volume growth rate of acoustic neuromas on MRI post-stereotactic radiosurgery. Comput Med Imaging Graph 14:53–59

77. Flickinger JC, Kondziolka D, Niranjan A, Voynov G, Maitz A, Lunsford LD (2003) Acoustic neuroma radiosurgery with marginal tumor doses of 12 to 13/Gy. Int J Radiat Oncol Biol Phys 57:S325

78. Mahboubi H, Sahyouni R, Moshtaghi O, Tadokoro K, Ghavami Y, Ziai K, Lin HW, Djalilian HR (2017) CyberKnife for treatment of vestibular schwannoma: a meta-analysis. Otolaryngol Head Neck Surg 157(1):7–15

79. Noren G, Arndt J, Hindmarsh T, Hirsch A (1988) Stereotactic radiosurgical treatment of acoustic neurinomas. In: Lunsford DL (ed) Modern stereotactic neurosurgery. Martinus Nijhoff, Boston, pp 481–489

80. Pan SY, Liu SA, Sun MH, Tsou HK, Lee SD, Chen YJ, Sheehan J, Sheu ML, Pan HC (2017) Outcome of hearing preservation related to tumor morphologic analysis in acoustic neuromas treated by gamma knife radiosurgery. Radiat Oncol 12(1):134

81. Pellet W, Regis J, Roche PH, Delsanti C (2003) Relative indications for radiosurgery and microsurgery for acoustic schwannoma. Adv Tech Stand Neurosurg 28:227–282; discussion 282–224

82. Unger F, Walch C, Papaefthymiou G, Eustacchio S, Feichtinger K, Quehenberger F, Pendl G (2002) Long term results of radiosurgery for vestibular schwannomas. Zentralbl Neurochir 63:52–58

83. Fu VX, Verheul JB, Beute GN, Leenstra S, Kunst HPM, Mulder JJS, Hanssens PEJ (2017) Retreatment of vestibular schwannoma with Gamma Knife radiosurgery: clinical outcome, tumor control, and review of literature. J Neurosurg 6:1–9

84. Lin RH, Wang TC, Lin CD, Lin HL, Chung HK, Wang CY, Tsou YA, Tsai MH (2017) Predictors of hearing outcomes following low-dose stereotactic radiosurgery in patients with vestibular schwannomas: a retrospective cohort review. Clin Neurol Neurosurg 162:16–21

85. Chung LK, Nguyen TP, Sheppard JP, Lagman C, Tenn S, Lee P, Kaprealian T, Chin R, Gopen Q, Yang I (2018) A systematic review of radiosurgery versus surgery for neurofibromatosis type 2 vestibular schwannomas. World Neurosurg 109:47–58

86. Subach BR, Kondziolka D, Lunsford LD, Bissonette DJ, Flickinger JC, Maitz AH (1999) Stereotactic radiosurgery in the management of acoustic neuromas associated with neurofibromatosis type 2 [see comments]. J Neurosurg 90:815–822

87. Gurgel RK, Dogru S, Amdur RL, Monfared A (2012) Facial nerve outcomes after surgery for large vestibular schwannomas: do surgical approach and extent of resection matter? Neurosurg Focus 33(3):E16

88. Hudgins WR (1994) Patients' attitude about outcomes and the role of gamma knife radiosurgery in the treatment of vestibular schwannomas. Neurosurgery 34:459–463; discussion 463–455

89. Kim CS, Chang SO, Oh SH, Ahn SH, Hwang CH, Lee HJ (2003) Management of intratemporal facial nerve schwannoma. Otol Neurotol 24:312–316

90. Tsao MN, Sahgal A, Xu W, De Salles A, Hayashi M, Levivier M, Ma L, Martinez R, Régis J, Ryu S, Slotman BJ, Paddick I (2017) Stereotactic radiosurgery for vestibular schwannoma: International Stereotactic Radiosurgery Society (ISRS) Practice Guideline. J Radiosurg SBRT 5(1):5–24

91. Shuto T, Inomori S, Matsunaga S, Fujino H (2008) Microsurgery for vestibular schwannoma after gamma knife radiosurgery. Acta Neurochir (Wien) 150(3):229–234; discussion 34

92. Pollock BE, Driscoll CL, Foote RL, Link MJ, Gorman DA, Bauch CD et al (2006) Patient outcomes after vestibular schwannoma management: a prospective comparison of microsurgical resection and stereotactic radiosurgery. Neurosurgery 59(1):77–85; discussion 77–85

93. Roche PH, Khalil M, Thomassin JM, Delsanti C, Regis J (2008) Surgical removal of vestibular schwannoma after failed gamma knife radiosurgery. Prog Neurol Surg 21:152–157

94. Pollock BE, Link MJ (2008) Vestibular schwannoma radiosurgery after previous surgical resection or stereotactic radiosurgery. Prog Neurol Surg 21:163–168

95. Mathieu D, Kondziolka D, Flickinger JC, Niranjan A, Williamson R, Martin JJ et al (2007) Stereotactic radiosurgery for vestibular schwannomas in patients with neurofibromatosis type 2: an analysis of tumor control, complications, and hearing preservation rates. Neurosurgery 60(3):460–468; discussion 8–70

96. Wowra B, Muacevic A, Fürweger C, Schichor C, Tonn JC (2012) Therapeutic profile of single-fraction radiosurgery of vestibular schwannoma: unrelated malignancy predicts tumor control. Neuro Oncol 14(7):902–909. https://doi.org/10.1093/neu-onc/nos085. Epub 2012 May 3

97. Bendel M, Kocher M, Müller R-P, Sturm V, Voges J (1998) Stereotaktische Einzeldosiskonvergenzbestrahlung am Linearbeschleuniger bei Akustikusneurinomen. Strahlenther Onkol 174(Sondernr 1):35

98. Martens F, Verbeke L, Piessens M, Van Vyve M (1994) Stereotactic radiosurgery of vestibular schwannomas with a linear accelerator. Acta Neurochir Suppl 62:88–92

99. Suh JH, Barnett GH, Sohn JW, Kupelian PA, Cohen BH (2000) Results of linear accelerator-based stereotactic radiosurgery for recurrent and newly diagnosed acoustic neuromas. Int J Cancer 90:145–151

100. Szumacher E, Schwartz ML, Tsao M, Jaywant S, Franssen E, Wong CS, Ramaseshan R, Lightstone AW, Michaels H, Hayter C, Laperriere NJ (2002) Fractionated stereotactic radiotherapy for the treatment of vestibular schwannomas: combined experience of the Toronto-Sunnybrook Regional Cancer Centre and the Princess Margaret Hospital. Int J Radiat Oncol Biol Phys 53:987–991

101. Sakamoto T, Shirato H, Takeichi N, Aoyama H, Kagei K, Nishioka T, Fukuda S (2001) Medication for hearing loss after fractionated stereotactic radiotherapy (SRT) for vestibular schwannoma. Int J Radiat Oncol Biol Phys 50:1295–1298

102. Combs SE, Engelhard C, Kopp C, Wiedenmann N, Schramm O, Prokic V, Debus J, Molls M, Grosu AL (2015) Long-term outcome after highly advanced single-dose or fractionated radiotherapy in patients

with vestibular schwannomas—pooled results from 3 large German centers. Radiother Oncol 114(3):378–383

103. Harsh GR, Thornton AF, Chapman PH, Bussiere MR, Rabinov JD, Loeffler JS (2002) Proton beam stereotactic radiosurgery of vestibular schwannomas. Int J Radiat Oncol Biol Phys 54:35–44

104. Talmi YP, Finkelstein Y, Zohar Y (1989) Postirradiation hearing loss. Audiology 28:121–126

105. Blakeley JO, Ye X, Duda DG, Halpin CF, Bergner AL, Muzikansky A, Merker VL, Gerstner ER, Fayad LM, Ahlawat S, Jacobs MA, Jain RK, Zalewski C, Dombi E, Widemann BC, Plotkin SR (2016) Efficacy and biomarker study of bevacizumab for hearing loss resulting from neurofibromatosis type 2-associated vestibular schwannomas. J Clin Oncol 34(14):1669–1667

106. Goutagny S, Kalamarides M (2018) Medical treatment in neurofibromatosis type 2. Review of the literature and presentation of clinical reports. Neurochirurgie 64(5):370–374

107. Karajannis MA, Legault G, Hagiwara M, Ballas MS, Brown K, Nusbaum AO, Hochman T, Goldberg JD, Koch KM, Golfinos JG, Roland JT, Allen JC (2012) Phase II trial of lapatinib in adult and pediatric patients with neurofibromatosis type 2 and progressive vestibular schwannomas. Neuro Oncol 14(9):1163–1170

108. Karajannis MA, Legault G, Hagiwara M, Giancotti FG, Filatov A, Derman A, Hochman T, Goldberg JD, Vega E, Wisoff JH, Golfinos JG, Merkelson A, Roland JT, Allen JC (2014) Phase II study of everolimus in children and adults with neurofibromatosis type 2 and progressive vestibular schwannomas. Neuro Oncol 16(2):292–297

109. Morris KA, Golding JF, Blesing C, Evans DG, Ferner RE, Foweraker K, Halliday D, Jena R, McBain C, McCabe MG, Swampillai A, Warner N, Wilson S, Parry A, Afridi SK, UK NF2 Research Group (2017) Toxicity profile of bevacizumab in the UK Neurofibromatosis type 2 cohort. J Neurooncol 131(1):117–124

110. Plotkin SR, Halpin C, McKenna MJ, Loeffler JS, Batchelor TT, Barker FG 2nd (2010) Erlotinib for progressive vestibular schwannoma in neurofibromatosis 2 patients. Otol Neurotol 31(7):1135–1143

111. Berkowitz O, Han YY, Talbott EO, Iyer AK, Kano H, Kondziolka D, Brown MA, Lunsford LD (2017) Gamma knife radiosurgery for vestibular schwannomas and quality of life evaluation. Stereotact Funct Neurosurg 95(3):166–173

112. Soulier G, van Leeuwen BM, Putter H, Jansen JC, Malessy MJA, van Benthem PPG, van der Mey AGL, Stiggelbout AM (2017) Quality of life in 807 patients with vestibular schwannoma: comparing treatment modalities. Otolaryngol Head Neck Surg 157(1):92–98

113. Maducdoc MM, Ghavami Y, Linskey ME, Djalilian HR (2015) Evaluation of reported malignant transformation of vestibular schwannoma: de novo and

after stereotactic radiosurgery or surgery. Otol Neurotol 36(8):1301

114. Pollock BE, Link MJ, Stafford SL, Parney IF, Garces YI, Foote RL (2017) The risk of radiation-induced tumors or malignant transformation after single-fraction intracranial radiosurgery: results based on a 25-year experience. Int J Radiat Oncol Biol Phys 97(5):919–923

115. Gurgel RK, Theodosopoulos PV, Jackler RK (2012) Subtotal/near-total treatment of vestibular schwannomas. Curr Opin Otolaryngol Head Neck Surg 20(5):380–384

116. Monfared A, Corrales CE, Theodosopoulos PV, Blevins NH, Oghalai JS, Selesnick SH, Lee H, Gurgel RK, Hansen MR, Nelson RF, Gantz BJ, Kutz JW Jr, Isaacson B, Roland PS, Amdur R, Jackler RK (2016) Facial nerve outcome and tumor control rate as a function of degree of resection in treatment of large acoustic neuromas: preliminary report of the Acoustic Neuroma Subtotal Resection Study (ANSRS). Neurosurgery 79(2):194–203

117. Roche PH, Ribeiro T, Khalil M, Soumare O, Thomassin JM, Pellet W (2008) Recurrence of vestibular schwannomas after surgery. Prog Neurol Surg 21:89–89

118. Kondziolka D, Lunsford LD, Flickinger JC (2003) Acoustic tumors: operation versus radiation–making sense of opposing viewpoints. Part II. Acoustic neuromas: sorting out management options. Clin Neurosurg 50:313–328

119. Husseini ST, Piccirillo E, Taibah A, Almutair T, Sequino G, Sanna M (2013) Salvage surgery of vestibular schwannoma after failed radiotherapy: the Gruppo Otologico experience and review of the literature. Am J Otolaryngol 34(2):107–114

120. Wise SC, Carlson ML, Tveiten ØV, Driscoll CL, Myrseth E, Lund-Johansen M, Link MJ (2016) Surgical salvage of recurrent vestibular schwannoma following prior stereotactic radiosurgery. Laryngoscope 126(11):2580–2586

121. Chang SD, Poen J, Hancock SL, Martin DP, Adler JR Jr (1998) Acute hearing loss following fractionated stereotactic radiosurgery for acoustic neuroma. Report of two cases. J Neurosurg 89:321–325

122. Muthukumar N, Kondziolka D, Lunsford LD, Fl ickinger JC (1999) Stereotactic radiosurgery for jugular foramen schwannomas. Surg Neurol 52:172–179

123. Xu F, Pan S, Alonso F, Dekker SE, Bambakidis NC (2017) Intracranial facial nerve schwannomas: current management and review of literature. World Neurosurg 100:444–449

124. Langlois AM, Iorio-Morin C, Masson-Côté L, Mathieu D (2018) Gamma knife stereotactic radiosurgery for nonvestibular cranial nerve schwannomas. World Neurosurg 110:e1031–e1039, pii: S1878-8750(17)32096-X

125. Peciu-Florianu I, Tuleasca C, Comps JN, Schiappacasse L, Zeverino M, Daniel RT, Levivier M (2017) Radiosurgery in trochlear

and abducens nerve schwannomas: case series and systematic review. Acta Neurochir (Wien) 159(12):2409–2418

126. Kunisada T, Kawai A, Ozaki T, Sugihara S, Taguchi K, Inoue H (1997) A clinical analysis of malignant schwannoma. Acta Med Okayama 51:87–92

127. Wong WW, Hirose T, Scheithauer BW, Schild SE, Gunderson LL (1998) Malignant peripheral nerve sheath tumor: analysis of treatment outcome. Int J Radiat Oncol Biol Phys 42:351–360

128. Baehring JM, Betensky RA, Batchelor TT (2003) Malignant peripheral nerve sheath tumor: the clinical spectrum and outcome of treatment. Neurology 61:696–698

129. Chao KS, Kaplan C, Simpson JR, Haughey B, Spector GJ, Sessions DG, Arquette M (2001) Esthesioneuroblastoma: the impact of treatment modality. Head Neck 23(9):749–757

130. Dublin AB, Bobinski M (2016) Imaging characteristics of olfactory neuroblastoma (esthesioneuroblastoma). J Neurol Surg B Skull Base 77(1):1–5

131. Lunsford LD, Kondziolka D, Fl ickinger JC (1992) Radiosurgery as an alternative to microsurgery of acoustic tumors. Clin Neurosurg 38:619–634

132. Schwartz JS, Palmer JN, Adappa ND (2016) Contemporary management of esthesioneuroblastoma. Curr Opin Otolaryngol Head Neck Surg 24(1):63–69

133. Theilgaard SA, Buchwald C, Ingeholm P, Kornum Larsen S, Eriksen JG, Sand Hansen H (2003) Esthesioneuroblastoma: a Danish demographic study of 40 patients registered between 1978 and 2000. Acta Otolaryngol 123:433–439

134. Lapierre A, Selmaji I, Samlali H, Brahmi T, Yossi S (2016) Neoadjuvant chemotherapy could be an effective treatment for tumor reduction, improving surgical resection and reducing its complications. Cancer Radiother 20(8):783–789

135. Gruber G, Laedrach K, Baumert B, Caversaccio M, Raveh J, Greiner R (2002) Esthesioneuroblastoma: irradiation alone and surgery alone are not enough. Int J Radiat Oncol Biol Phys 54:486–491

136. Morita A, Ebersold MJ, Olsen KD, Foote RL, Lewis JE, Quast LM (1993) Esthesioneuroblastoma: prognosis and management. Neurosurgery 32:706–714; discussion 714–705

137. Bartel R, Gonzalez-Compta X, Cisa E, Cruellas F, Torres A, Rovira A, Manos M (2018) Importance of neoadjuvant chemotherapy in olfactory neuroblastoma treatment: series report and literature review. Acta Otorrinolaringol Esp 69(4):208–213

138. Bradley PJ, Jones NS, Robertson I (2003) Diagnosis and management of esthesioneuroblastoma. Curr Opin Otolaryngol Head Neck Surg 11:112–118

139. Turri-Zanoni M, Maragliano R, Battaglia P, Giovannardi M, Antognoni P, Lombardi D, Morassi ML, Pasquini E, Tarchini P, Asioli S, Foschini MP, Sessa F, Nicolai P, Castelnuovo P, La Rosa S (2017) The clinicopathological spectrum of olfactory neuroblastoma and sinonasal neuroendocrine neoplasms: refinements in diagnostic criteria and impact of multimodal treatments on survival. Oral Oncol 74:21–29

Hemangioblastoma and von Hippel-Lindau Disease

15

Ranjit Ganguly, David Dornbos III,
Jonathan L. Finlay, and Russell R. Lonser

15.1 Hemangioblastoma

15.1.1 Overview

Hemangioblastomas are pathologically benign (WHO grade I), vascular neoplasms found almost exclusively within the central nervous system (CNS). These tumors account for 10% of all posterior fossa tumors (2% of all intracranial tumors) and are the most common primary posterior fossa tumor in adults. While two-thirds of hemangioblastomas occur sporadically, one-third of cases arise in the context of the familial neoplasia syndrome, von Hippel-Lindau disease (VHL). Whether they occur sporadically or in the context of VHL, 99% of hemangioblastomas occur below the tentorium, in the brainstem, cerebellum, and spinal cord. Over 80% of VHL patients will develop a CNS hemangioblastoma during their lifetime, and 95% of these patients will develop multiple hemangioblastomas [1].

R. Ganguly · D. Dornbos III · R. R. Lonser (✉)
Department of Neurological Surgery, The Ohio State University Wexner Medical Center,
Columbus, OH, USA
e-mail: Ranjit.Ganguly@osumc.edu;
David.Dornbos@osumc.edu;
russell.lonser@osumc.edu

J. L. Finlay
Division of Hematology, Oncology and Bone Marrow Transplant, Nationwide Children's Hospital,
Columbus, OH, USA
e-mail: Jonathan.Finlay@nationwidechildrens.org

Hemangioblastoma-associated signs and symptoms are based on location and size of the tumor and/or the presence of a peritumoral cyst or syrinx. While the indications can differ for treatment of sporadic and VHL-associated hemangioblastomas, surgical resection remains the treatment of choice.

15.1.2 Clinical Presentation

The initial manifestation of sporadic hemangioblastomas tends to be headache (85%) [2]. In the VHL population, 90% of hemangioblastomas are asymptomatic and identified on surveillance imaging [3]. Symptom formation is caused by tumor mass effect and/or associated peritumoral edema/cyst. Seventy percent of symptomatic cerebellar hemangioblastomas and 90% of symptomatic spinal hemangioblastomas had an associated peritumoral cyst or syrinx [4]. Cyst growth tends to be tenfold greater than tumor growth and is largely responsible for symptom formation [1]. In fact, 41% of asymptomatic hemangioblastomas with an associated peritumoral cyst progress to become symptomatic, requiring surgical resection [5].

In those patients that are symptomatic, anatomic location is the main determinant of signs and symptoms. Patients with symptomatic cerebellar lesions typically reported headache (77%) and gait ataxia (57%), along with nausea/vomiting, vertigo,

© Springer Nature Switzerland AG 2019
J.-C. Tonn et al. (eds.), *Oncology of CNS Tumors*, https://doi.org/10.1007/978-3-030-04152-6_15

speech difficulties, and dysmetria [6]. Patients with symptomatic brainstem lesions often reported headaches (83%), nausea/vomiting (50%), and hyperesthesias (55%) [7]. Patients with spinal cord hemangioblastomas can experience hyperesthesia (83%), weakness (65%), gait ataxia (65%), and pain (17%) [8, 9]. Symptomatic cauda equina or nerve root lesions often cause pain (67%), numbness (50%), or urinary complaints (33%) [10].

15.1.3 Diagnosis

Hemangioblastomas are typically diagnosed through radiographic imaging, and contrast-enhanced magnetic resonance (MR) imaging is the most sensitive and specific imaging modality to identify hemangioblastomas (Fig. 15.1). As hemangioblastomas are highly vascular, they enhance vividly and discretely on contrast-enhanced T1-weighted MR imaging. Peritumoral edema

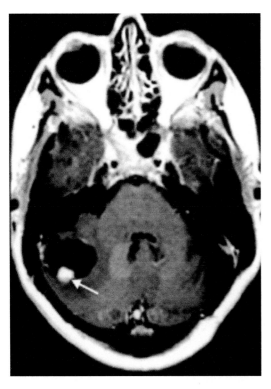

Fig. 15.1 Axial post-contrast T1-weighted MRI showing an enhancing lesion (arrows) with a peritumoral cyst

and cysts are best visualized with T2-weighted and fluid-attenuated inversion-recovery (FLAIR) sequences (Fig. 15.2). Occasionally, digital subtraction angiography may be used to evaluate tumor vascularity, particularly in larger lesions. On angiography, hemangioblastomas demonstrate enlarged feeding arteries, early draining veins, and a dense tumor blush that persists into the venous phase.

15.1.4 Clinical Management of Hemangioblastoma

Assessment. Given the strong association between hemangioblastomas and VHL, patients with a newly diagnosed hemangioblastoma should be screened for VHL. Once a CNS hemangioblastoma has been identified, brain and total spine imaging should be obtained to screen for lesions elsewhere in the CNS. Given the systemic lesions associated with VHL, abdominal imaging and a retinal fundoscopic examination should be performed as part of the initial screening [11].

Management. In patients presenting with a single CNS hemangioblastoma, no family history of VHL disease and no evidence of systemic VHL manifestations, only 4% of patients will be found to have a detectable VHL mutation. Such individuals are typically less than 40 years of age [12]. For patients with an isolated hemangioblastoma, VHL mutation analysis is recommended, in addition to abdominal imaging, 24-h urine catecholamines and ophthalmologic examination. Long-term surveillance for patients with a solitary CNS hemangioblastoma largely depends on age and genetic analysis. Patients harboring a germline VHL mutation require lifelong surveillance, in addition to screening of at-risk relatives [12]. Given the association between younger age at presentation and VHL disease, younger patients should be kept under close surveillance, even in the setting of negative mutation analysis as genetic mosaicism may lead to false-negative testing [12, 13]. Furthermore, the risk of familial VHL disease in a patient presenting with a solitary hemangioblastoma over 50 years of age is quite low [12].

Fig. 15.2 Sagittal (**a**) and axial (**c**) post-contrast T1-weighted MRI showing an enhancing spinal cord lesion at C5 (arrows). Sagittal (**b**) and axial (**d**) T2-weighted images revealing the extent of edema and syrinx formation (arrows)

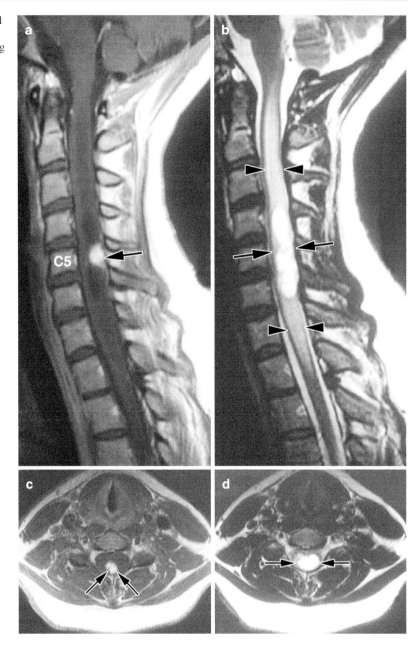

In the VHL population, the multiplicity of tumors and classic saltatory growth pattern generates unpredictable tumor growth. As such, radiographic progression alone is not an indication for treatment, and surgical resection is generally reserved for symptomatic lesions [3, 14]. While nearly 50% of tumors will demonstrate growth on surveillance imaging, only 6% will progress to become symptomatic requiring operative intervention [3], and avoiding surgery on these asymptomatic enlarging tumors eliminates approximately four unnecessary surgeries per patient per decade [1, 15, 16]. Excellent neurologic function with minimal morbidity can be obtained in the VHL population with this treatment paradigm.

15.2   Treatment

15.2.1 Surgical Resection

The treatment of choice for symptomatic hemangioblastoma is complete resection. Biopsies and subtotal resections are avoided due to high risk for intraoperative and postoperative hemorrhage, and complete resection is curative. The tumor mass is removed using circumferential coagulation and sharp transection of the associated vessels. Although surgeon preference ultimately determines the surgical approach, the majority of cerebellar tumors are resected with a midline suboccipital craniotomy. Similarly, 75% of brainstem lesions arise at the obex, requiring a similar approach [17]. Two-thirds of spinal cord tumors are found within the dorsal root entry zone, typically appropriate for a simple posterior, midline approach [8]. While short-term transient deficits may arise after surgery, these typically resolve within 2 weeks to 6 months, and greater than 90% and 98% of patients exhibit long-term neurologic stability or improvement following resection of spinal cord and cerebellar lesions, respectively [8, 18].

Peritumoral edema and subsequent cyst formation are often the underlying source of symptom development as the cyst volume tends to be substantially larger than the associated tumor. Vascular permeability of CNS hemangioblastomas leads to extravasation of fluid into the interstitial spaces of the tumor and surrounding parenchyma [19, 20]. As such, resection of the cyst wall is not needed, as tumor resection removes the underlying driver of cyst formation.

15.2.2 Stereotactic Radiosurgery

Stereotactic radiosurgery has been used for CNS hemangioblastomas as a primary and adjunctive treatment. A prospective analysis of VHL patients undergoing stereotactic radiosurgery as a primary treatment for cerebellar and brainstem hemangioblastomas found that lesions that underwent stereotactic radiosurgery had similar long-term (7 years or more) clinical and radiographic outcomes as untreated tumors [21]. While previous studies revealed a possible benefit of radiosurgery [22, 23], this likely represents normal periods of quiescent tumor growth. For this reason, stereotactic radiosurgery is typically reserved for treatment of hemangioblastomas that are not surgically resectable and/or in patients who cannot tolerate surgery. Moreover, stereotactic radiosurgery has limited efficacy on peritumoral cysts and can even increase vascular permeability, exacerbating edema, and peritumoral cyst progression.

15.2.3 Arteriography and Embolization

Preoperative embolization has been previously advocated as a means to reduce tumor vascularity prior to resection. However, a recent analysis demonstrated that embolization does not improve resection, decrease blood loss, or reduce operative complications [24]. Furthermore, preoperative particle embolization of cerebellar hemangioblastomas has been associated with a heightened risk of intratumoral hemorrhage, in addition to standard procedural risks [24, 25].

15.2.4 Pathologic Findings

On gross examination, hemangioblastomas appear as highly vascular, red lesions with a nodular surface. They have prominent dilated and tortuous vessels. Hemangioblastomas are histologically characterized by a proliferative capillary network and large, neoplastic, vacuolated stromal cells (Fig. 15.3) [26]. Hyperchromatic nuclei, cyst wall gliosis, and Rosenthal fibers are also commonly seen. These WHO grade I lesions lack fibrillary cells, necrosis, and atypical or mitotic figures. Immunohistochemical staining of stroma is positive for neuron-specific enolase (NSE), reticulin, CD34, vascular endothelial growth factor (VEGF), and inhibin alpha.

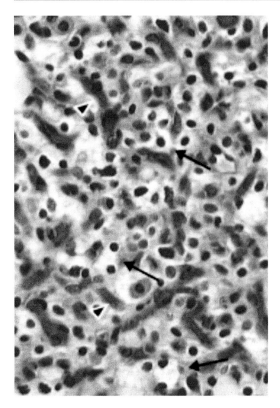

Fig. 15.3 Hematoxylin and eosin staining of a hemangioblastoma showing lipid-laden stromal cells (arrows) distributed within a capillary network (arrowheads)

15.3 von Hippel-Lindau Disease

15.3.1 Overview

VHL is an inherited disease caused by a germline mutation of the VHL tumor suppressor gene on the short arm of chromosome 3 (3p25-26) [27]. It is transmitted in an autosomal dominant manner with 90% penetrance by 65 years of age [28] and an incidence of approximately 1 in 36,000 live births [7]. Loss of heterozygosity predisposes these individuals to a distinct set of CNS and visceral lesions. CNS lesions include hemangioblastomas and endolymphatic sac tumors (ELSTs), while visceral lesions include renal cell carcinoma and renal cysts, adrenal gland tumors, pancreatic neuroendocrine tumors and cysts, pheochromocytomas, and adnexal cystadenomas. The VHL phenotype is highly variable. Familial VHL can

Table 15.1 Genotype-phenotype classifications in familial von Hippel-Lindau disease

VHL classification	Clinical characteristics
Type 1	CNS hemangioblastomas
	Retinal hemangioblastomas
	Pancreatic neoplasms/cysts
	Renal cell carcinoma
Type 2A	CNS hemangioblastomas
	Retinal hemangioblastomas
	Pheochromocytoma
Type 2B	CNS hemangioblastomas
	Retinal hemangioblastomas
	Pheochromocytoma
	Renal cell carcinoma
	Pancreatic neoplasms/cysts
Type 2C	Pheochromocytoma only

be categorized into Type 1 or Type 2, based on the absence or presence of pheochromocytoma, respectively (Table 15.1) [15]. Type 2 families are subdivided based on their risk of developing renal cell carcinoma (RCC). Type 2A and Type 2B families have a low and high incidence of RCC, respectively, whereas Type 2C exists for those only afflicted by pheochromocytoma [7].

The average life expectancy has improved considerably for VHL patients. Although CNS hemangioblastomas are the main cause of mortality in this patient population, male and female life expectancy is now 67 and 60 years, respectively, given proper treatment [14, 29]. While 80% of VHL patients will develop a hemangioblastoma in their lifetime, the majority arise in the third to fourth decades of life [1]. Systemically, 25–45% of patients develop RCC by age 40, and 10–20% develop pheochromocytoma by age 30 [7]. While CNS disease is the most common cause of mortality, RCC is also a common cause of death in patients with VHL [30]. Management of patients who develop RCC may include nephrectomy, renal ablation, dialysis, and renal transplantation as indicated by the severity of renal involvement and dysfunction [31].

15.3.2 VHL Protein

Inactivation of the VHL tumor suppressor gene underlies VHL disease pathogenesis. The VHL protein is known to be involved in maintenance of primary cilia and microtubule function [32], regulation of cytokinesis, regulation of angiogenesis, extracellular matrix integrity [33], and cell cycle regulation [34]. On the molecular level, the VHL protein forms a stable complex with elongin B, elongin C, and cullin 2. This proteolytic complex functions as an E3 ubiquitin ligase for proteasomal degradation for target molecules [35–37]. The VHL protein also has important interactions with hypoxia-inducible factor-1 alpha (HIF-1a). In normal cells, VHL protein ubiquinates HIF-1a, targeting it for degradation. In VHL, HIF-1a accumulates, increasing transcription of a variety of HIF-controlled genes, including vascular endothelial growth factor (VEGF), a major mechanism underlying the vascular nature of these tumors.

15.3.3 Clinical Presentation

CNS hemangioblastomas are certainly the most common tumor affecting VHL patients (60–80%), presenting at an average age of 33 years [7]. Overall, approximately 50% of CNS hemangioblastomas in patients with VHL are in the spinal cord, 40% in the cerebellum, and 10% in the brainstem. Less than 1% of CNS hemangioblastomas are located supratentorially [7]. Fifty percent of VHL patients present with retinal hemangioblastomas, often earlier than other CNS manifestations, at an average age of 25 years [38]. VHL patients are also predisposed to develop multiple cysts throughout the kidneys, pancreas, and liver, and these patients also carry an increased risk of malignancy, such as RCC and pheochromocytoma [39, 40]. In addition to CNS hemangioblastomas, other common manifestations of VHL disease include endolymphatic sac tumors, paragangliomas, glomus tumors, and neuroendocrine neoplasms.

15.3.4 Diagnosis

The diagnosis of VHL can be made if an individual has one of the following combinations of clinical factors: a family history of VHL and one CNS hemangioblastoma, endolymphatic sac tumor, RCC, or pheochromocytoma; at least two CNS hemangioblastomas; or one CNS hemangioblastoma and a VHL-associated visceral tumor [7, 41–43]. Diagnosis may also be made through genetic testing [44], although disease mosaicism has been reported in up to 5% of patients, which may lead to false-negative genetic testing [12, 13]. Phenotypic expressivity is highly variable among VHL patients and families. It is not possible to reliably predict the severity of VHL manifestations based on genetic testing.

15.3.5 Treatment Considerations in VHL

In VHL patients, hemangioblastoma recurrence after complete surgical resection is rare [4, 15]. However, new tumor formation is common, and these patients require regular surveillance. Given the degree of new tumor formation, treatment is reserved for symptomatic tumors or those that show clear evidence of significant growth. In unresectable spinal cord or brainstem lesions, or for patients that are poor surgical candidates, stereotactic radiosurgery may represent an alternative treatment modality.

Patients with known VHL should be evaluated annually by a team of specialists, including neurosurgery, ophthalmology, nephrology, urology, and endocrinology (Table 15.2) [45, 46].

Table 15.2 Recommended intervals for screening of at-risk individuals

Test	Starting age (frequency)
Ophthalmoscopy	Infancy (annual)
Plasma or 24-h urine catecholamines and metanephrines	2 years (annual and when blood pressure is raised)
MRI of craniospinal axis	11 years (annual)
CT and MRI of internal auditory canal	Onset of symptoms (hearing loss, tinnitus, vertigo, or balance difficulties)
Abdominal ultrasound	8 years (annual)
CT of the abdomen	18 years (annual)
Audiology examination	When clinically indicated

Actual practices may vary based on individual patient presentation, characteristics, and manifestations of disease

Annual evaluations include ophthalmologic evaluation, nephrology evaluation with urine or plasma catecholamines and metanephrines, MRI of the brain and spinal cord, and abdominal imaging [7]. Psychiatric and neuropsychological evaluations should also be available, as patients are at significant risk of developing psychiatric disorders [46]. Lastly, first-degree relatives of VHL patients should undergo screening with genetic counseling and mutation analysis if the specific mutation has been identified.

15.3.6 Chemotherapy

Many patients with VHL or sporadic inoperable hemangioblastomas may potentially benefit from systemic targeted therapies, although to date, no reproducible proven drug therapy against hemangioblastoma has been identified. Recent case reports and research have drawn attention to inhibition of growth factors or tyrosine kinase [47], VEGF [48], or somatostatin [49]. Researchers have also investigated octreotide (an octapeptide that mimics and thereby inhibits naturally produced somatostatin) [49], pazopanib (a tyrosine kinase and VEGF inhibitor) [50], bevacizumab [51], thalidomide, interferon alfa-2a [52], and other potential therapeutic agents to target hemangioblastomas, although none have yet yielded meaningful clinical benefits.

References

1. Wanebo JE, Lonser RR, Glenn GM, Oldfield EH (2003) The natural history of hemangioblastomas of the central nervous system in patients with von Hippel-Lindau disease. J Neurosurg 98(1):82–94
2. Liao CC, Huang YH (2014) Clinical features and surgical outcomes of sporadic cerebellar hemangioblastomas. Clin Neurol Neurosurg 125:160–165
3. Lonser RR, Butman JA, Huntoon K, Asthagiri AR, Wu T, Bakhtian KD et al (2014) Prospective natural history study of central nervous system hemangioblastomas in von Hippel-Lindau disease. J Neurosurg 120(5):1055–1062
4. Lonser RR (2014) Surgical management of sporadic spinal cord hemangioblastomas. World Neurosurg 82(5):632–633
5. Huntoon K, Wu T, Elder JB, Butman JA, Chew EY, Linehan WM et al (2016) Biological and clinical impact of hemangioblastoma-associated peritumoral cysts in von Hippel-Lindau disease. J Neurosurg 124(4):971–976
6. Butman JA, Linehan WM, Lonser RR (2008) Neurologic manifestations of von Hippel-Lindau disease. JAMA 300(11):1334–1342
7. Lonser RR, Glenn GM, Walther M, Chew EY, Libutti SK, Linehan WM et al (2003) von Hippel-Lindau disease. Lancet 361(9374):2059–2067
8. Lonser RR, Weil RJ, Wanebo JE, DeVroom HL, Oldfield EH (2003) Surgical management of spinal cord hemangioblastomas in patients with von Hippel-Lindau disease. J Neurosurg 98(1):106–116
9. Wind JJ, Lonser RR (2011) Management of von Hippel-Lindau disease-associated CNS lesions. Expert Rev Neurother 11(10):1433–1441
10. Mehta GU, Montgomery BK, Maggio DM, Chittiboina P, Oldfield EH, Lonser RR (2017) Functional outcome after resection of Von Hippel-Lindau disease-associated cauda equina hemangioblastomas: an observational cohort study. Oper Neurosurg (Hagerstown) 13(4):435–440
11. Singh AD, Nouri M, Shields CL, Shields JA, Smith AF (2001) Retinal capillary hemangioma: a comparison of sporadic cases and cases associated with von Hippel-Lindau disease. Ophthalmology 108(10):1907–1911
12. Woodward ER, Wall K, Forsyth J, Macdonald F, Maher ER (2007) VHL mutation analysis in patients with isolated central nervous system haemangioblastoma. Brain 130(Pt 3):836–842
13. Ding X, Zhang C, Frerich JM, Germanwala A, Yang C, Lonser RR et al (2014) De novo VHL germline mutation detected in a patient with mild clinical phenotype of von Hippel-Lindau disease. J Neurosurg 121(2):384–386
14. Feletti A, Anglani M, Scarpa B, Schiavi F, Boaretto F, Zovato S et al (2016) Von Hippel-Lindau disease: an evaluation of natural history and functional disability. Neuro Oncol 18(7):1011–1020
15. Ammerman JM, Lonser RR, Dambrosia J, Butman JA, Oldfield EH (2006) Long-term natural history of hemangioblastomas in patients with von Hippel-Lindau disease: implications for treatment. J Neurosurg 105(2):248–255
16. Lonser RR, Vortmeyer AO, Butman JA, Glasker S, Finn MA, Ammerman JM et al (2005) Edema is a precursor to central nervous system peritumoral cyst formation. Ann Neurol 58(3):392–399
17. Wind JJ, Bakhtian KD, Sweet JA, Mehta GU, Thawani JP, Asthagiri AR et al (2011) Long-term outcome after resection of brainstem hemangioblastomas in von Hippel-Lindau disease. J Neurosurg 114(5):1312–1318
18. Jagannathan J, Lonser RR, Smith R, DeVroom HL, Oldfield EH (2008) Surgical management of cerebellar hemangioblastomas in patients with von Hippel-Lindau disease. J Neurosurg 108(2):210–222

19. Lonser RR, Butman JA, Oldfield EH (2006) Pathogenesis of tumor-associated syringomyelia demonstrated by peritumoral contrast material leakage. Case illustration. J Neurosurg Spine 4(5):426

20. Lohle PN, van Mameren H, Zwinderman KH, Teepen HL, Go KG, Wilmink JT (2000) On the pathogenesis of brain tumour cysts: a volumetric study of tumour, oedema and cyst. Neuroradiology 42(9):639–642

21. Asthagiri AR, Mehta GU, Zach L, Li X, Butman JA, Camphausen KA et al (2010) Prospective evaluation of radiosurgery for hemangioblastomas in von Hippel-Lindau disease. Neuro Oncol 12(1):80–86

22. Simone CB 2nd, Lonser RR, Ondos J, Oldfield EH, Camphausen K, Simone NL (2011) Infratentorial craniospinal irradiation for von Hippel-Lindau: a retrospective study supporting a new treatment for patients with CNS hemangioblastomas. Neuro Oncol 13(9):1030–1036

23. Kano H, Shuto T, Iwai Y, Sheehan J, Yamamoto M, McBride HL et al (2015) Stereotactic radiosurgery for intracranial hemangioblastomas: a retrospective international outcome study. J Neurosurg 122(6):1469–1478

24. Ampie L, Choy W, Lamano JB, Kesavabhotla K, Kaur R, Parsa AT et al (2016) Safety and outcomes of preoperative embolization of intracranial hemangioblastomas: a systematic review. Clin Neurol Neurosurg 150:143–151

25. Cornelius JF, Saint-Maurice JP, Bresson D, George B, Houdart E (2007) Hemorrhage after particle embolization of hemangioblastomas: comparison of outcomes in spinal and cerebellar lesions. J Neurosurg 106(6):994–998

26. Vortmeyer AO, Gnarra JR, Emmert-Buck MR, Katz D, Linehan WM, Oldfield EH et al (1997) von Hippel-Lindau gene deletion detected in the stromal cell component of a cerebellar hemangioblastoma associated with von Hippel-Lindau disease. Hum Pathol 28(5):540–543

27. Maher ER, Neumann HP, Richard S (2011) von Hippel-Lindau disease: a clinical and scientific review. Eur J Hum Genet 19(6):617–623

28. Maher ER, Iselius L, Yates JR, Littler M, Benjamin C, Harris R et al (1991) Von Hippel-Lindau disease: a genetic study. J Med Genet 28(7):443–447

29. Binderup ML, Jensen AM, Budtz-Jorgensen E, Bisgaard ML (2017) Survival and causes of death in patients with von Hippel-Lindau disease. J Med Genet 54(1):11–18

30. Maher ER, Yates JR, Harries R, Benjamin C, Harris R, Moore AT et al (1990) Clinical features and natural history of von Hippel-Lindau disease. Q J Med 77(283):1151–1163

31. Ploussard G, Droupy S, Ferlicot S, Ples R, Rocher L, Richard S et al (2007) Local recurrence after nephron-sparing surgery in von Hippel-Lindau disease. Urology 70(3):435–439

32. Thoma CR, Frew IJ, Hoerner CR, Montani M, Moch H, Krek W (2007) pVHL and GSK3beta are components of a primary cilium-maintenance signalling network. Nat Cell Biol 9(5):588–595

33. Lolkema MP, Gervais ML, Snijckers CM, Hill RP, Giles RH, Voest EE et al (2005) Tumor suppression by the von Hippel-Lindau protein requires phosphorylation of the acidic domain. J Biol Chem 280(23):22205–22211

34. Roe JS, Kim H, Lee SM, Kim ST, Cho EJ, Youn HD (2006) p53 stabilization and transactivation by a von Hippel-Lindau protein. Mol Cell 22(3):395–405

35. Sufan RI, Jewett MA, Ohh M (2004) The role of von Hippel-Lindau tumor suppressor protein and hypoxia in renal clear cell carcinoma. Am J Physiol Renal Physiol 287(1):F1–F6

36. Kaelin WG Jr (2002) Molecular basis of the VHL hereditary cancer syndrome. Nat Rev Cancer 2(9):673–682

37. Barry RE, Krek W (2004) The von Hippel-Lindau tumour suppressor: a multi-faceted inhibitor of tumourigenesis. Trends Mol Med 10(9):466–472

38. Niemela M, Lemeta S, Sainio M, Rauma S, Pukkala E, Kere J et al (2000) Hemangioblastomas of the retina: impact of von Hippel-Lindau disease. Invest Ophthalmol Vis Sci 41(7):1909–1915

39. Wong WT, Agron E, Coleman HR, Tran T, Reed GF, Csaky K et al (2008) Clinical characterization of retinal capillary hemangioblastomas in a large population of patients with von Hippel-Lindau disease. Ophthalmology 115(1):181–188

40. Weil RJ, Lonser RR, DeVroom HL, Wanebo JE, Oldfield EH (2003) Surgical management of brainstem hemangioblastomas in patients with von Hippel-Lindau disease. J Neurosurg 98(1):95–105

41. Chittiboina P, Lonser RR (2015) Von Hippel-Lindau disease. Handb Clin Neurol 132:139–156

42. Lamiell JM, Salazar FG, Hsia YE (1989) von Hippel-Lindau disease affecting 43 members of a single kindred. Medicine (Baltimore) 68(1):1–29

43. Melmon KL, Rosen SW (1964) Lindau's disease. Review of the literature and study of a large kindred. Am J Med 36:595–617

44. Stolle C, Glenn G, Zbar B, Humphrey JS, Choyke P, Walther M et al (1998) Improved detection of germline mutations in the von Hippel-Lindau disease tumor suppressor gene. Hum Mutat 12(6):417–423

45. Choyke PL, Glenn GM, Walther MM, Patronas NJ, Linehan WM, Zbar B (1995) von Hippel-Lindau disease: genetic, clinical, and imaging features. Radiology 194(3):629–642

46. Schmid S, Gillessen S, Binet I, Brandle M, Engeler D, Greiner J et al (2014) Management of von Hippel-Lindau disease: an interdisciplinary review. Oncol Res Treat 37(12):761–771

47. Kim BY, Jonasch E, McCutcheon IE (2012) Pazopanib therapy for cerebellar hemangioblastomas in von Hippel-Lindau disease: case report. Target Oncol 7(2):145–149

48. Pierscianek D, Wolf S, Keyvani K, El Hindy N, Stein KP, Sandalcioglu IE et al (2017) Study of angiogenic signaling pathways in hemangioblastoma. Neuropathology 37(1):3–11

49. Sizdahkhani S, Feldman MJ, Piazza MG, Ksendzovsky A, Edwards NA, Ray-Chaudhury A et al (2017) Somatostatin receptor expression on von Hippel-Lindau-associated hemangioblastomas offers novel therapeutic target. Sci Rep 7:40822

50. Migliorini D, Haller S, Merkler D, Pugliesi-Rinaldi A, Koka A, Schaller K et al (2015) Recurrent multiple CNS hemangioblastomas with VHL disease treated with pazopanib: a case report and literature review. CNS Oncol 4(6):387–392

51. Slim E, Antoun J, Kourie HR, Schakkal A, Cherfan G (2014) Intravitreal bevacizumab for retinal capillary hemangioblastoma: a case series and literature review. Can J Ophthalmol 49(5):450–457

52. Capitanio JF, Mazza E, Motta M, Mortini P, Reni M (2013) Mechanisms, indications and results of salvage systemic therapy for sporadic and von Hippel-Lindau related hemangioblastomas of the central nervous system. Crit Rev Oncol Hematol 86(1):69–84

Orbital Tumors

16

Christoph Hintschich, Ullrich Müller-Lisse,
and Geoffrey E. Rose

16.1 Introduction

Orbital tumors can either be developmental, such as dermoid cysts, or acquired lesions (inflammatory masses, vascular anomalies, and benign or malignant neoplasms). Only the diagnosis and management of discrete structural lesions of the orbit will be presented in this chapter, and we will not address vascular or inflammatory disease.

16.2 Epidemiology

As orbital tumors are rare, the exact incidence of orbital tumors is difficult to obtain, but based on the tumor register of the former German Democratic Republic and the American Cancer Society, the estimated incidence is less than 1 per 100,000 population. Better estimates are available for sex- and age-related incidences for orbital conditions: A relatively high incidence in the first decade of life

is followed by the lowest risk during the second decade. The frequency of orbital tumors gradually increases from 25 to 75 years of age, after which a fairly sharp decrease occurs, and this results in more than 50% of all orbital tumors occurring between the fifth and seventh decades. There is no significant male or female preponderance.

Although Graves' orbitopathy is the commonest orbital disease, when excluding cystic and vascular lesions, orbital neoplasms comprise about 20% of all orbital conditions, and their diversity reflects the wide spectrum of orbital tissues. The five most common primary tumors in adults are cavernous hemangioma, lymphoma, orbital inflammatory masses, meningiomas, and optic nerve glioma. The most common secondary tumors are very different: sinus mucocele, squamous cell carcinoma, cranial meningioma, vascular malformations, and malignant melanoma. Children show a different spectrum of orbital tumors, the commonest being dermoid cysts, capillary hemangiomas, lymphangiomas, rhabdomyosarcomas, neuroblastomas, and optic nerve tumors.

16.3 Orbital Anatomy

16.3.1 Dimensions

The bony orbit is a confined space in the skull that contains and protects the eyeball and its accessory organs with the orbital soft tissues. It

C. Hintschich (✉)
Augenklinik der Universität München,
München, Germany
e-mail: christoph.hintschich@med.uni-muenchen.de

U. Müller-Lisse
Oberarzt CT, Medizinische Klinik,
München, Germany
e-mail: ullrich.mueller-lisse@med.uni-muenchen.de

G. E. Rose
Moorfields Eye Hospital, London, UK
e-mail: geoff.rose@breathemail.net

© Springer Nature Switzerland AG 2019
J.-C. Tonn et al. (eds.), *Oncology of CNS Tumors*, https://doi.org/10.1007/978-3-030-04152-6_16

is pyramidal with four walls narrowing posteriorly toward the apex, at which site many nerves and vessels pass to the cranial cavity. The bony orbital volume averages about 27 mL, with the globe taking up about 7–8 mL volume, the extraocular muscles about 5 mL, and the fat about 10–13 mL. The optic canal is usually 40–45 mm behind the medial orbital rim, and a simple "24–12–6" rule helps to memorize some key orbital distances: 24 mm from the medial orbital margin to the anterior ethmoidal neurovascular bundle, 12 mm further to the posterior ethmoidal bundle, and 6 mm from the latter to the optic canal. The anterior and posterior ethmoidal bundles also serve to define the upper limit of the medial orbital wall at the skull base.

16.3.2 Bony Walls

Each orbital wall has a particular relation to neighboring structures: The orbital *roof*, formed by the frontal and sphenoid bones, lies beneath the frontal sinus and the anterior cranial fossa. The *medial wall*—formed from the ethmoid, lacrimal, sphenoid, and maxillary bones—has the ethmoid and part of the sphenoid sinuses lying medially. The *orbital floor*, formed by the maxillary, zygomatic, and palatine bones, lies above the maxillary antrum. Finally, the *lateral wall*—comprising part of the zygoma, sphenoid, and frontal bones—has the temporalis fossa (with the temporalis muscle) lying laterally and posterolaterally abuts the middle cranial fossa. Anteriorly, the orbit is defined by the globe and the eyelid complex, the latter with its medial and lateral canthal tendons and orbital septum, and the septum, a thin and elastic membrane acting as an important barrier between the intra- and extraorbital spaces. The bony orbital entrance is the strongest part of the orbit, the weakest part being the orbital floor and medial wall.

16.3.3 Orbital Foramina and Fissures

A number of fissures and foramina in the bony walls accommodate neurovascular structures,

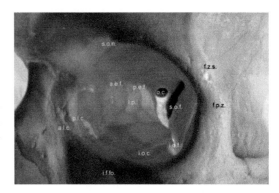

Fig. 16.1 Osteology and foramina of the left orbit: The orbit is bounded anteriorly by the anterior (*a.l.c*) and posterior lacrimal crests (*p.l.c*) and the frontal process of the zygoma (*f.p.z*), limited superiorly by the frontozygomatic suture (*f.z.s*). The supraorbital ridge is indented on its inner one third by the supraorbital notch (*s.o.n*). The medial wall comprises the thin lamina papyracea (*l.p*) of the ethmoid air cells, the upper limit of which is marked by the anterior (*a.e.f*) and posterior ethmoidal foramina (*p.e.f*); the floor is traversed by the infraorbital canal (*i.o.c*) passing from the inferior orbital fissure (*i.o.f*) anteromedially to exit on the cheek as the infraorbital foramen (*i.f.fo*). The superior orbital fissure (*s.o.f*) and optic canal (*o.c*) are also clearly seen

which are essential for normal ocular function and also provide valuable landmarks during orbital surgery (Fig. 16.1). The supraorbital neurovascular bundle may pass through a canal or notch in the superior orbital rim, the nerves being the frontal and lacrimal branches of the ophthalmic division of the trigeminal nerve. The infraorbital neurovascular bundle—passing from the inferior orbital fissure, along the infraorbital canal, and reaching the cheek through the *infraorbital foramen*—contains fibers from the maxillary division of the trigeminal nerve and subserves sensation for the cheek, upper lid, and anterior upper teeth.

The *inferior orbital fissure*, which is 20 mm long, separates the orbital floor from the lateral wall and contains fat, the infraorbital nerve, and veins leaving the orbit for the pterygopalatine fossa. Further posteriorly and superiorly, at the junction of the lateral wall and the roof, lies the shorter *superior orbital fissure*, through which several important structures pass: the superior and inferior divisions of the oculomotor nerve, the trochlear nerve, the abducens nerve, the first division of the trigeminal nerve, and the venous connections between the orbit and the cavernous sinus. The superior orbital fissure is divided into a lateral and a medial part by the fibrous annulus of Zinn, the origin of the recti. The lateral part transmits the lacrimal, frontal, and trochlear nerves, the superior ophthalmic vein, and the anastomosis of the recurrent lacrimal and middle meningeal arteries, while the medial part of the fissure transmits the superior and inferior divisions of the oculomotor nerve, the nasociliary nerve, the abducens nerve, and the sympathetic nerves. Finally, in the orbital apex, medial to the superior orbital fissure, lies the optic foramen through which passes the optic nerve in its meninges and the ophthalmic artery. The optic nerve, about 4 mm in diameter, takes an "S"-shaped course for its 30-mm orbital portion and has a 9-mm-long intracanalicular section and about 10 mm of intracranial length before joining the optic chiasm. The intraorbital nerve is surrounded by dura, arachnoid, and pia mater from the optic canal to the globe. The intracanalicular part is immobile as its dural sheath is fused to the periosteum of the optic canal – the latter making the intracanalicular nerve particularly vulnerable to blunt trauma and edema.

The zygomatic neurovascular bundle passes inferolaterally through the orbital wall just behind the orbital rim, and division during surgery only rarely causes a clinically significant sensory deficit. In its very anterior part, between the anterior and posterior lacrimal crest, the medial wall forms the nasolacrimal fossa with the opening of the nasolacrimal duct, and this area should generally be avoided during orbital exploration to avoid damage to the lacrimal drainage apparatus.

16.3.4 Periorbita and Surgical Spaces

The periorbita covers all bones of the orbit and is only loosely attached to the underlying bone (except at the orbital rim and at suture lines), giving readily available extraperiosteal spaces that can be used to surgical advantage, or in which an abscess can develop.

Multiple connective tissue septa have been described between all orbital structures, these maintaining the spatial separation of structures—such as the extraocular muscles—and also defining the so-called surgical spaces, which are relevant for the description of orbital pathology and for planning surgery. The orbit can be divided into four surgical spaces: the subperiosteal (extraperiosteal) space, the intraperiosteal extraconal space, the intraconal space, and the sub-Tenon's space.

The Subperiosteal (Extraperiosteal) Space. The subperiosteal space, existing only when created surgically or when filled by a pathological process, lies between the periorbita and the bony orbital walls and is crossed by a number of structures. The subperiosteal space can be reached through several approaches, such as transcutaneous or transconjunctival incisions, and the periosteum should be incised outside the orbit and then elevated over the rim.

Extraconal Space. Lying behind the orbital rim in the superotemporal quadrant, the lacrimal gland is the dominant extraconal structure, and it is readily approached through an upper lid skin crease incision; lateral orbitotomy is readily performed through a lateral extension of this incision if required for intact excision of the gland—as with suspected pleomorphic adenomas. Other structures in the extraconal space are the oblique muscles, trochlea, orbital fat, sensory nerves, trochlear (motor) nerve, and some vessels.

Intraconal Space. The intraconal space lies within the recti and their interconnecting septa and contains the optic nerve, intraconal orbital fat, motor nerves, and some blood vessels. The ophthalmic artery enters through the optic foramen and divides to form the central retinal artery (most importantly), which arises near the apex, passes forward beneath the optic nerve, and loops laterally over the optic nerve in three-quarters of people, to finally pierce the optic nerve dura in a variable position—usually in the inferomedial aspect about 1 cm behind the globe.

Optic nerve tumors lying within the intraconal space may be accessed by several routes such as a superomedial upper lid incision, through a medial conjunctival incision (with disinsertion of the medial rectus muscle in some cases) or laterally via a lateral canthotomy with or without bone removal. During a lateral orbitotomy approach with bone resection, the intraconal space is usually entered by passing below the lateral rectus muscle.

Sub-tenon's Space. This potential space, located between the globe and the anterior surface of Tenon's capsule, can be enlarged by inflammatory fluid—as in posterior scleritis—or infiltrated by extraocular growth of intraocular tumors (e.g., with choroidal melanoma).

16.4   Symptoms and Signs

Orbital symptoms include lid swelling, globe displacement, a feeling of "pressure," ocular discomfort due to corneal exposure and drying, or epiphora. Abnormal ocular motility can cause double vision (diplopia), and a patient may notice visual failure due to direct nerve compression or raised intraorbital pressure, visual failure being manifest as loss of acuity, loss of color perception, impaired stereoscopic functions, poor distance judgment, field loss, or premature presbyopic symptoms. Pain—generally due to inflammation—may be a rare, but important, symptom of orbital malignancy (Tables 16.1 and 16.2).

Tumor growth inside the orbital confines causes an expansion of orbital soft tissues and, in some cases, a rise in orbital pressure. Proptosis—an axial protrusion of the globe—is a significant sign often caused by a retrobulbar mass, such as intraconal cavernous hemangiomas (Fig. 16.2a) or optic nerve tumors. The globe may, in addition, be displaced vertically or horizontally, inferomedial displacement, for example, being due to a lacrimal gland mass (Fig. 16.3a) or intraorbital dermoid cyst. Inferolateral displacement is typically due to frontoethmoidal mucoceles (Fig. 16.4f), vascular lesion, neural tumors, or dermoid cysts. Common masses in the inferonasal quadrant are lymphoma, vascular lesions, or mesenchymal tumors, and the inferotemporal quadrant is the location of lymphoma, arteriosclerotic hemorrhage, and rare tumors.

Other signs of orbital disease include disturbance of ocular motility, eyelid asymmetry (Figs. 16.4a and 16.5a), conjunctival inflammation and swelling (chemosis) (Figs. 16.6a and 16.7a), optic nerve head swelling (Fig. 16.5c), choroidal folds (Fig. 16.2b), and periocular sensory loss.

16.5   Clinical History and Orbital Examination

16.5.1 History

A thorough history will characterize the disease and its progression and, in most cases, provides the likely diagnosis. As well as the current state of general health, enquiry should be made about previous sinus disease or surgery, endocrine (especially thyroid) dysfunction, immunological disease, malignancies, infections, injuries, and any abnormal skin pigmentations, with café-au-lait spots being almost pathognomonic for neurofibromatosis (Fig. 16.8b, c). Systemic medication, in particular anticoagulants, should also be recorded and any prior orbital surgery noted.

The temporal sequence of symptoms will often indicate the nature of the disease: The onset of proptosis, taken with age, is a valuable criterion for the differential diagnosis, and we distinguish

Table 16.1 Signs of orbital tumors

Exophthalmos
Horizontal or vertical displacement of the eyeball
Motility disorder
Visual acuity/visual field reduction
Optic nerve head edema and choroidal folds
Ptosis and eyelid distortion or swelling

Table 16.2 Symptoms of orbital tumors

Double vision (diplopia)
Visual acuity/visual field reduction
Pressure feeling
Foreign body sensation
Pain
Hypesthesia
Eyelid swelling and bulging eye

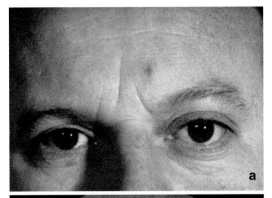

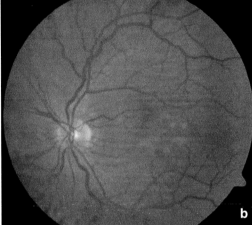

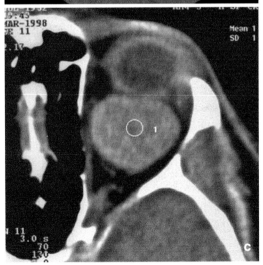

Fig. 16.2 (**a–c**) Adult onset proptosis of slow progression: (**a**) Slowly progressive left proptosis with reduced visual acuity and hypermetropic refractive shift due to choroidal folds (**b**), these changes being caused by the slow growth of a well-defined, round, intraconal mass (**c**), most commonly a cavernous hemangioma

onsets that are acute, subacute, chronic, or acute on chronic (see below). If disease progression is slow, a patient might not notice the changes, and in most cases, it is invaluable to compare their actual appearance with old portrait photographs. The order in which symptoms occur can also suggest the position of an orbital mass. Anterior masses often cause globe displacement and diplopia before affecting visual acuity, whereas apical tumors often cause visual loss with only minimal diplopia or proptosis.

Accurate symptoms from an observant patient are valuable in making a preliminary diagnosis. With optic neuropathy, the patient might notice a different color balance in each eye, mention a reduction in color "brightness," or have difficulty with depth perception and coordination. Obscurations of vision on extremes of gaze or on suddenly standing occur with compromised optic nerve circulation, as seen with optic nerve meningiomas, large retrobulbar masses, or severe thyroid eye disease. The nature of the pain gives a clue to the cause of the orbital disease: Dull retro-ocular "pressure" or ache is generally due to a deep intraorbital mass, whereas sharp pain is due to corneal exposure problems. Orbital myositis causes a background periorbital ache with severe lancinating pain on looking out of the field of action of the affected muscle. Severe persistent pain, most common with inflammation, may be a rare symptom of orbital malignancy, with periocular sensory loss being present in some patients.

16.5.2 Examination

Examination should start with a general examination of the patient, ideally under daylight, looking for facial asymmetry, for displacement of the globe, or for orbital or periorbital masses. Skin changes, such as discoloration, may indicate an underlying vascular anomaly or neurofibroma (Fig. 16.8b, c), whereas skin infiltration and induration may occur with systemic lymphoma or sarcoid.

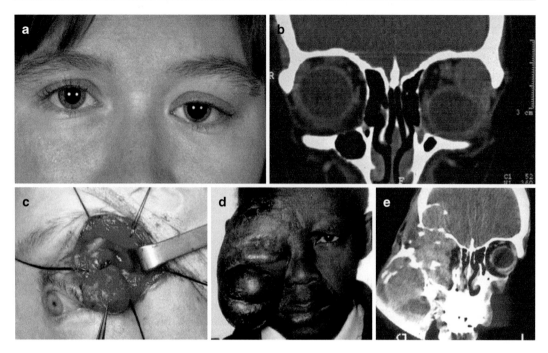

Fig. 16.3 (**a**) Pleomorphic adenoma of the left lacrimal gland, presenting as slowly progressive painless proptosis with diplopia on extreme left gaze; the left globe is also displaced inferiorly by the well-defined mass in the lacrimal gland (**b**), which is also causing some flattening of the globe. Pleomorphic adenomas should be excised intact (**c**), as they carry a risk of later malignant transformation (so-called malignant mixed tumor), when the patient will present with an accelerated history (**d**), and imaging may then show bone invasion and destruction (**e**)

Asymmetry or changes of the eyelids—such as swelling, erythema, ptosis, loss of the eyelid sulcus, or skin crease (Figs. 16.2a, 16.4c, 16.5a, and 16.6a)—should be sought. A record should be made of an eyelid's relationship to the corneal limbus: If the upper lid does not cover the upper limbus by 2 mm (or if there is upper scleral show), upper eyelid retraction is present, and this is the most common and most sensitive clinical sign of thyroid eye disease (Graves' disease), with lid retraction and hang-up on downgaze being rarely due to orbital malignancy. Lower lid scleral show is less specific, since this is mainly due to involutional lower lid laxity or significant proptosis. Upper lid movements (levator excursion), position on downgaze (lid hang-up), and failure of eyelid closure (lagophthalmos) are important clinical details. Levator function is measured as difference (mm) in lid position between maximal up- and downgaze, with the frontalis action blocked by pressing the thumb against the forehead. Facial weakness and lagophthalmos should be recorded, with particular attention being paid to the presence of frontalis sparing—this indicating an upper motor neuron (central) facial nerve palsy. Hearing should always be checked with facial nerve lesions, this being easily tested clinically by rustling two fingertips together near the patient's ear. The eyelids should be everted and fornices examined for masses, such as fat prolapse, lacrimal gland enlargement or prolapse, or a subconjunctival "salmon patch" (typical for lymphoma) (Fig. 16.7b).

Palpation. The orbital margin should be examined for palpable discontinuity, notches, or foreign body, and the shape, size, surface texture, and attachment of any mass should be assessed. A lesion can be well or ill-defined, with a round or irregular shape, soft or hard, and non-tender or painful. Some masses will be palpable only on posterior ballottement of the globe or—if attached near the globe—on certain positions of gaze. Variation in the size of a mass with Valsalva maneuver or a "filling-and-emptying" sign with

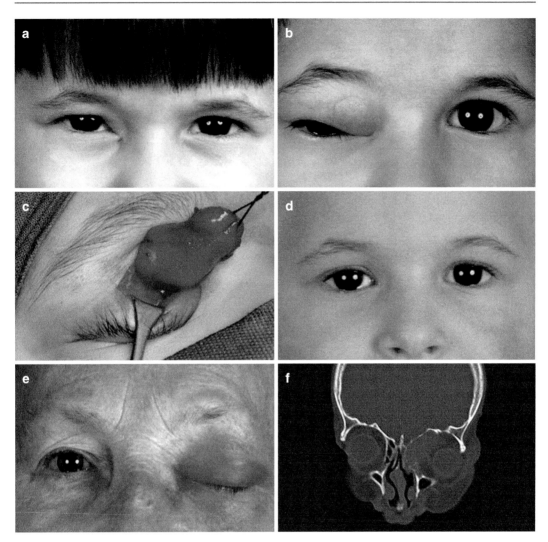

Fig. 16.4 (**a–f**) Orbital lesion of subacute onset. (**a**) Slight painless swelling of a child's right upper lid, which developed into a significant superonasal quadrant mass within a month of onset (**b**). The mass, an embryonal rhabdomyosarcoma, was excised intact (**c**), and after adjuvant chemotherapy, the child was still disease-free 5 years later (**d**). (**e**) Within days, increasing left upper lid redness and swelling due to a chronic frontoethmoidal mucocele erupting into the left orbit; the mass, originating within the sinuses, is shown on coronal CT (**f**)

pressure may indicate a low-pressure vascular malformation or a meningocele.

Palpation of the preauricular, submandibular, and clavicular lymph node regions is important in the clinical evaluation of orbital masses, especially malignancy.

Examination of Globe Position. The globe may be displaced in any dimension and thereby indicates the location of a mass: In most cases the eyeball is displaced away from a tumor (Figs. 16.2c, 16.3a, b, and 16.4f), although fibrosis due to scirrhous carcinomas (e.g., breast metastases) or inflammation may cause enophthalmos. Proptosis, axial anterior displacement of the globe, is readily assessed when unilateral by an "up-the-nose" view but is formally measured by exophthalmometry. The exophthalmometer is placed firmly on the lateral orbital rims and, with the examined eye in the primary position, the corneal position is noted on the instrument scale; parallax errors should be avoided, and the distance between both orbital rims is noted for

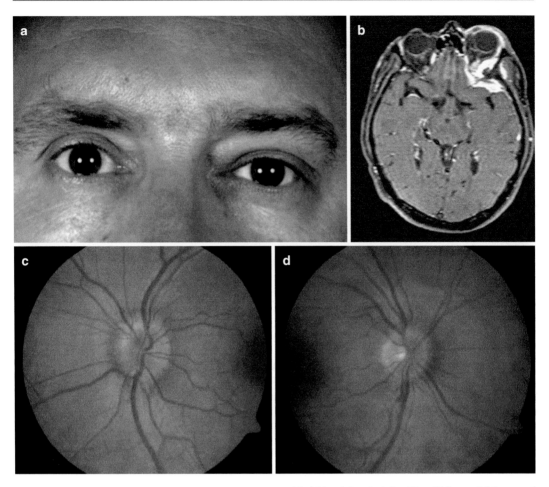

Fig. 16.5 (**a–c**) Slowly progressive displacement of the left eye due to sphenoidal wing meningioma. (**a**) The left globe shows hypoglobus and exophthalmos, with some "fullness" of the upper lid sulcus. (**b**) MRI shows a high-signal lesion "en-plaque" to the greater wing of the sphe-noid and involving the left orbit, middle cranial fossa, and temporalis fossa. Compression of the left optic nerve, manifest as mild disc swelling (**c**, **d**), is associated with some impairment of function

reproducibility. There is variation in exophthal-mometer readings between different examiners or instruments, but any readings greater than 22 mm are probably abnormal. Of greater impor-tance, however, is an interocular difference of more than 2 mm or a changing value. Non-axial globe displacement may be assessed clinically by placing a ruler horizontally across the nasal bridge and estimating the position of the pupil-lary center in the horizontal and vertical axes.

Proptosis is mainly due to retrobulbar masses, but it is important to differentiate between real proptosis and "pseudo-proptosis," where a condi-tion mimics a proptotic eye. Upper eyelid retrac-tion with widening of the palpebral aperture and upper scleral show can easily be mistaken for proptosis. The elongated myopic globe leads to abnormally high exophthalmometer readings and is a cause of pseudo-proptosis. Unilateral enoph-thalmos due, for example, to breast metastases can give the appearance of a relative protrusion of the other globe. An abnormal orbital rim or the shallow orbits of cranial anomalies may mimic proptosis.

Extraocular Muscle and Periorbital Sensory Functions. Extraocular muscle func-tion is assessed by asking the patient to follow a fingertip, for example, and any restriction is

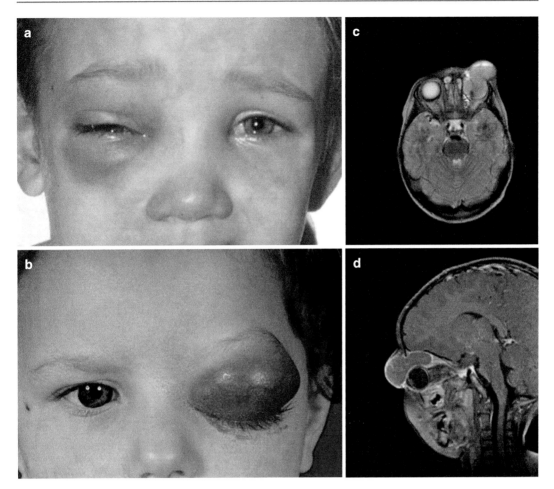

Fig. 16.6 (a–d) Childhood orbital lesions of acute onset. (a) Acute orbital cellulitis in an unwell child due to spread of bacterial infection from the right ethmoid sinus. (b) Overnight onset of massive left orbital hemorrhage from a lymphangiomas/varix; MRI demonstrates a lobulated mass (c) throughout the upper part of the orbit, with evidence of a fluid level with the characteristics of layering blood (d). Clinical photographs from the Moorfields Eye Hospital, London

recorded. Double vision may be present in primary position or in extreme gaze, most commonly due to mechanical restriction and more rarely to neurological deficit. Any limitation, if present, needs quantification by a detailed orthoptic examination.

The sensory function of the ophthalmic and maxillary branches of the trigeminal nerve should be assessed, as it can be impaired by orbital masses and tends to indicate the site, rather than the nature, of orbital disease.

Assessment of Visual Functions. Visual assessment is of paramount importance. Although a normal acuity does not exclude orbital disease, the best acuity for distance and near must be recorded. Color testing, particularly a difference between two eyes (tested with the "hue panel D-15" test), often gives an early indication of optic neuropathy.

The test for a relative afferent pupillary defect (RAPD) is the least subjective method and a very sensitive test for optic neuropathy. It is performed using a bright torch light, with the patient gazing into distance in a semi-dark room. The light is directed into one pupil from just off the visual axis and swung, alternately, from one to the

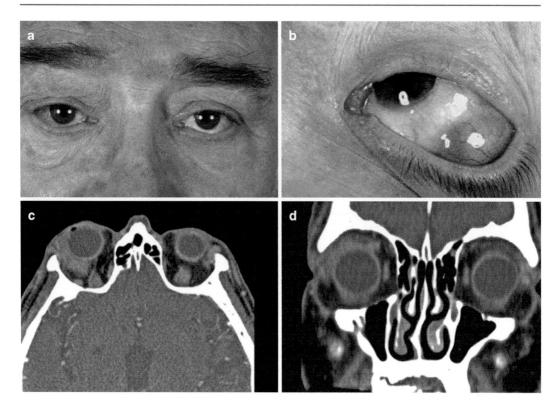

Fig. 16.7 Slowly progressive proptosis in adulthood, due to orbital lymphoma. (**a**) Subtle, right, painless proptosis due to a pink subconjunctival mass of lymphomatous tissue ((**b**) viewed from above). CT shows the mass arising from the right lacrimal gland and cloaking the globe both posteriorly (**c**) and superiorly (**d**)

other pupil, remaining for 2–3 s at each pupil. As both pupils should remain small, a positive RAPD is indicated by an anomalous dilatation of the pupil on the side with loss of afferent stimulus—this generally being due to optic nerve or extensive retinal disease (distinguished by fundal examination).

16.5.3 Additional Examinations

Visual Field Assessment. Confrontational visual field testing will reveal major defects, such as hemianopia or sensory inattention, but field examination with Goldmann or automated perimetry provides a more accurate permanent record. Goldmann perimetry is particularly useful when the visual acuity is reduced or with loss of the far-temporal visual field, whereas automated perimetry can better distinguish the depth of a field defect (Fig. 16.9d). Visual field testing should be repeated to check for reproducibility.

Tumors of the orbit, optic canal, or chiasm frequently impair visual function and cause visual field defects, which may be typical for certain locations: Field defects due to apical orbital disease are predominately centrocecal scotomas; scotomas due to intraorbital optic nerve lesions are typically central, centrocecal, or enlargement of the blind spot; a generalized constriction of the peripheral field may be a nonspecific sign of optic neuropathy. Compression of the intracranial optic nerve causes a "junctional scotoma," in which an ipsilateral central scotoma is associated with a contralateral superotemporal scotoma, the latter being due to involvement of contralateral inferonasal optic nerve fibers at the knee of von Willebrand.

Disease progression or improvement of optic nerve function may be monitored with ongoing visual fields, for example, with review or treatment of orbital meningiomas.

Visual Evoked Potentials. Normal pattern visual evoked potentials (VEP) help to distinguish

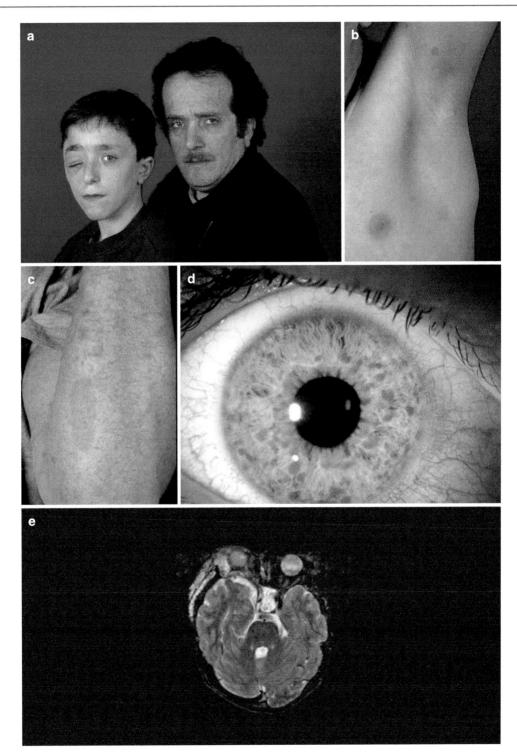

Fig. 16.8 (**a–e**) Systemic involvement in chronically progressive orbital disease, neurofibromatosis. (**a**) Father and son with type I neurofibromatosis, the son having a large plexiform neurofibroma of the right orbit and the father having widespread cutaneous neurofibromas. Other stigmata of neurofibromatosis include axillary freckles (**b**), café-au-lait spots (**c**), and Lisch nodules of the iris stroma (**d**). MRI (**e**) demonstrates marked dysplasia and widespread involvement of the right orbit, together with parenchymal anomalies of the cerebral tissues

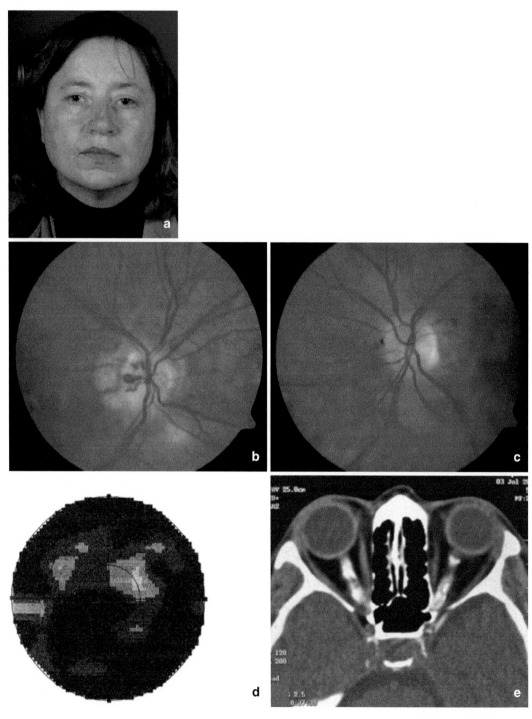

Fig. 16.9 (**a–e**) Gradual onset of progressive, painless visual failure in adulthood without significant proptosis (**a**) due to bilateral optic nerve sheath meningioma. The right optic disc (**b**) is atrophic, with marked optociliary shunt vessels, and the left disc (**c**) shows temporal atrophy; visual field testing was possible only on the left eye (**d**) and shows gross impairment. Bilateral calcified optic nerves, pathognomonic of optic nerve sheath meningioma, are clearly shown on CT (**e**); a slight flattening of the posterior pole of both globes (especially the left) is also evident due to a "splinting" effect of the optic nerve tumors

the cause of a decreased visual capacity. A prolonged delay, reduced voltage, and a change of the configuration indicate optic neuropathy, and VEP is a sensitive and objective method for detecting, quantifying, and monitoring optic neuropathy.

16.5.4 Imaging

Orbital Ultrasonography. Orbital ultrasonography provides useful information about the location, size, shape, tissue characteristics, and vascular features of orbital tumors; as it is a noninvasive technique, it is very helpful for long-term follow-up assessments. Ultrasound examination is especially useful for intraocular pathology involving the orbit, such as extrascleral extension of choroidal melanoma, for confirming the cystic nature of a mass and in the sizing of orbital lesions and (with Doppler flow studies) the vascular flow within orbital tumors. Because of the bony confinement and the ultrasound frequency

used, echography is poor for masses within the posterior half of the orbit.

Computed Tomography. The natural difference in X-ray attenuation between the orbital structures and fat provides the excellent soft-tissue resolution of CT; it also provides superb bone detail and is very sensitive for tissue calcification or radio-opaque foreign bodies. With its high resolution, thin-slice (0.6–1 mm) CT with contrast is still the single most instructive imaging technique and should be the first choice for imaging adult orbital disease; in most cases CT will indicate the site and probable nature of the lesion, and no other imaging will be required (Figs. 16.3b, 16.7c, d, 16.9e, and 16.10c).

Like conventional radiography (CR), computed tomography (CT) applies the respective absorption and transmission of X-ray electromagnetic waves to obtain a signal. However, unlike CR, both the X-ray source and the detector row opposite to it circle around the subject under

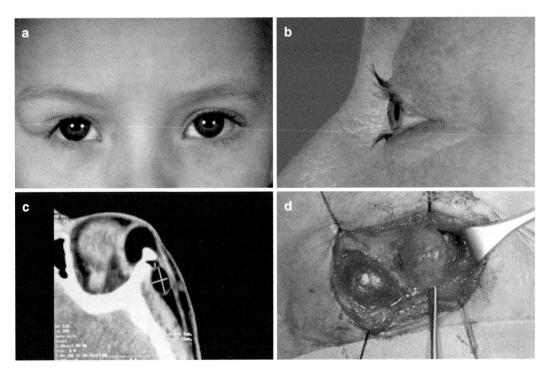

Fig. 16.10 (**a–d**) Dermoid cysts of the orbit, with history of slow progression. (**a**) A typical mobile cyst at the superotemporal rim of the child's right orbit. (**b**) A more complex, dumbbell dermoid straddling the orbital rim with both an orbital and a temporalis fossa component, shown well on imaging (**c**) and at surgery (**d**)

investigation, gathering signals from each angular position along the way. In incremental CT, the respective courses of the X-ray source and the detector row truly describe a circle around the subject, who is lying still in the center of that circle. However, in spiral (or helical) CT, the subject moves through that circle while the X-ray source and the detector row are on their way. Therefore, the course of the CT signals describes a helix rather than a circle. The resulting image data set is three-dimensional. This specific property in principle allows for the reconstruction of CT images in any desired plane. Reconstruction of CT images in any other than the axial (or transversal) plane of images has only become meaningful since the advent of multi-detector-row CT (MDCT, also known as multi-slice CT, or MSCT). Instead of just one detector row opposite to the X-ray source, MDCT has several, which gain signal simultaneously. The MDCT approach is more dose-efficient and time-efficient and provides more image data points along the long axis of the subject than the single-detector row approach. The spatial resolution of MDCT scans along the long axis of the subject (through-plane resolution) is approximately 0.6 mm in current clinical whole-body MDCT scanners. The in-plane resolution of MDCT images, which usually have an imaging matrix of 512×512 points, depends on the field of view (FoV) of the reconstructed images. While the FoV could be 40–50 cm in width in a wide-shouldered individual undergoing a whole-body MDCT scan, it could be 12–15 cm in an orbital MDCT reconstruction, with an edge length of 0.25–0.30 mm per image point. Therefore, CT provides superb anatomical detail in orbital structures. CT images are the results of complex mathematical calculations carried out by a computer. Each image point within the matrix of a CT image is assigned a numerical value (which translates into a grayscale value in the visible image), depending on the calculated average X-ray attenuation within the subject at that point. X-ray attenuation, in turn, is linearly correlated with physical density of the subject in any point. Therefore, CT distinguishes soft-tissue structures within the orbit, e.g., the eye bulb, optic nerve, muscles, and blood vessels, from both orbital fat and periorbital bone structures and their respective canals and fissures. Air within the paranasal sinuses (but also air within the orbit that results from some pathologic process) discerns as clearly from the soft tissue, fat, and bone as metallic objects, whether from osteosynthesis or from other foreign bodies. Natural physical density is similar in different soft tissues within the human body. Therefore, pathological processes affecting soft tissue or tumors of soft tissue density will not distinguish in density from normal soft tissue. However, after intravenous injection of X-ray contrast media, CT density increases rapidly in tissue with increased (neo-) vascularization, e.g., inflammatory tissue and many malignant tumors. The physiological principle behind soft-tissue contrast enhancement in CT imaging is like in magnetic resonance imaging (MRI, see below). Since it precisely locates the site of pathological change, CT will therefore be the method of first choice, at least in adults, and suffice for orbital imaging in most instances. MRI may be considered as an alternative cross-sectional imaging method, particularly in children. The need for intravenous administration of contrast media will depend on the specific indication for CT scanning and should be discussed with or left at the discretion of the radiologist. Modern MDCT scanners are widely available. MDCT scans are fast, with image data acquisition times in the range of seconds, and generally less expensive than MRI scans of the same range. Radiation exposure is a trade-off to be weighed against the advantages of MDCT imaging.

Magnetic Resonance Imaging. MRI, free of ionizing radiation and able to provide soft-tissue differentiation, can provide images in several planes, but it is expensive, time-consuming, and extremely liable to acts due to motion during image acquisition. MRI is, however, rarely specific for a diagnosis and is not routinely required for orbital patients. Specific indications include the evaluation of optic nerve lesions (especially in the region of the optic canal and chiasm), of suspected radiolucent orbital foreign bodies, where coexistent central nervous system disease is suspected (such as demyelination), and the extent of sphenoid wing meningiomas (Fig. 16.5c).

Magnetic resonance imaging (MRI) uses the specific electromagnetic properties of hydrogen nuclei to obtain cross-sectional images. The respective ranges of electromagnetic wavelengths applied in MRI and in X-ray-based imaging methods differ considerably. Therefore, there is no useful or harmful radiation exposure associated with MRI examinations. However, MRI requires a strong, static external magnetic field to align the magnetic moments of hydrogen nuclei inside the subject under investigation either parallel or antiparallel to one another. The most common clinical MRI scanners are based on superconducting magnets and operate at magnetic field strengths of either 1.5 or 3.0 T. Electromagnetic coils inside the scanner induce energy into the subject under investigation by means of radiofrequency pulses. That energy changes the direction of the magnetic moments of hydrogen nuclei. When the radiofrequency pulse ends, the magnetic moments of the hydrogen nuclei return to their previous positions, either parallel or antiparallel to the external magnetic field. While returning, the magnetic moments give off their added energy by emitting electromagnetic radiofrequency waves. This phenomenon is called magnetic resonance. The release of energy in radiofrequency waves provides the signal for MRI. Both the strength and the time course of the signal depend on the respective binding properties of hydrogen in the tissues under scrutiny. A technical program that manipulates the course of events within a magnetic resonance experiment is called a "sequence." Sequences may emphasize signal emanating from hydrogen nuclei in specific bindings and suppress or eliminate signal from hydrogen nuclei in other bindings. Other technical manipulations, e.g., phase encoding or frequency encoding, allow for localization of the source of magnetic resonance within the scanner. Thereby, MRI provides complex information on physical and chemical tissue properties that can be localized to specific points in an image matrix. Usually, sequence-dependent signal strength at each point is expressed as a gray-scale value in the MR image. MRI data can be gathered for three-dimensional volumes, with subsequent calculation of two-dimensional, cross-sectional images, by means of a "3D sequence." However, a "2D sequence," which creates individual images, may take less time, show a higher signal-to-noise ratio, and provide higher spatial resolution in its pre-defined plane of imaging than a 3D sequence. Combinations of different sequences are usually applied for MRI of the orbit. T2-weighted MR images, which show water with high-signal intensity, fat with intermediate signal intensity, and muscle with low signal intensity, distinguish, e.g., cerebrospinal fluid in the optic nerve sheath from soft tissue. T1-weighted MR images are susceptible to contrast change after intravenous administration of gadolinium-based contrast media. Soft tissue shows intermediate to low signal intensity in unenhanced T1-weighted MR images. However, after intravenous injection of contrast media, signal intensity increases rapidly in tissue with increased (neo-)vascularization, e.g., inflammatory tissue and many malignant tumors. Since adipose tissue shows with bright contrast at T1-weighted imaging, fat signal suppression may improve the delineation of inflammatory or tumor tissue. Different variants and derivatives of T1- and T2-weighted MR sequences are widely applied in MRI of the orbit. Diffusion-weighted imaging, which depicts restrictions to free Brownian motion of water molecules in tissues under investigation, has been the subject of research in orbital imaging but is not (yet) routinely used. Depending on the respective combination of sequences, MRI examinations may be time-consuming and, therefore, expensive. While MRI is highly sensitive for orbital disease, its findings are often not specific to any disease or pathological process. Specific indications for MRI of the orbit include known or suspected disease of the optic nerve, optic chiasm, meningeal membranes (Fig. 16.5c), or the central nervous system and the search for non-metallic foreign bodies which are not delineated by computed tomography.

Positron-Emission Tomography and Combined Computed Tomography. 68Ga-DOTA-TATE PET/CT combines morphological and metabolic information in a single examination

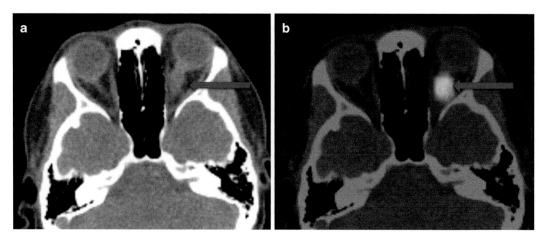

Fig. 16.11 (**a**) CT showing perineural orbital lesion. (**b**) DOTA-TATE PET/CT signalling optic nerve sheath meningioma

with excellent sensitivity and specificity. It has become a valuable tool for meningioma detection and has an essential influence on therapy decisions (Fig. 16.11).

Positron-emission tomography and combined computed tomography (PET-CT) has recently shown its value in the investigation of orbital diseases. Specific biochemical tissue properties can be studied by means of radioactively labelled tracers which are injected intravenously, accumulate in the target tissue, and emit positrons. Emitted positrons are annihilated upon meeting with electrons. Each annihilation of one positron and one electron sends off a pair of photons which simultaneously tissue albeit in opposite directions. Coincidental registration of photons with exactly opposite flight directions provides the signal in positron-emission tomography (PET). Reference to the PET-scanning matrix localizes the origin of positron emission. Accumulation of tracers to specific sites increases the number of photon counts emanating from the respective points of origin. Number of counts per point of origin can be expressed in cross-sectional PET images as a specific gray-scale or color-scale level. However, correction for different tissue attenuation of signal emission is necessary for the correct visualization and interpretation of PET images. Modern combined PET-CT applies computed-tomography (CT) images for both attenuation correction and attribution of PET sig-

nals to specific morphologic sites within the body. Interpretation of combined image information from both PET and CT improves diagnostic accuracy, whether by reviewing PET images and CT images side-by-side or by looking at gray-scale CT images with super-imposed, color-coded PET images. Two different PET tracers with very different properties have been successfully applied to specific orbital diseases. Radioactively labelled glucose (18F-fluorodeoxyglucose, or FDG) accumulates in tissue with increased cell energy metabolism. Although increased energy metabolism is not specific to any disease, FDG accumulation is particularly strong in malignant tumors, e.g., lymphoma, or squamous cell carcinoma. Besides localizing sites of disease inside and around the orbit, FDG localizes concomitant primary or metastatic foci elsewhere in the body. Specific binding to somatostatin receptors (SSR) is the biochemical principle in PET examinations with gallium-labelled DOTA-TATE (68Ga-DOTA-TATE, also known as DOTA-octreotate, oxodotreotide, and DOTA-(Tyr3)-octreotate or DOTA-0-Tyr3-Octreotate). SSR are expressed by neuroendocrine cells and their tumors. However, meningiomas demonstrate high uptake of DOTA-TATE. Therefore, DOTA-TATE PET-CT detects, localizes, and determines the extent of meningiomas affecting the orbit and helps to distinguish between meningiomas and gliomas if necessary.

16.6 An Approach to Differential Diagnosis

An accurate history and examination are the basis for any diagnosis, with imaging providing further definition of the extent of the mass, or extra evidence in favor or against the provisional diagnosis.

Proptosis, the most common clinical sign of an orbital tumor, can be used as an approach to diagnosis when considered in relation to the patient's age. The rate of onset can be considered as acute (minutes to hours), subacute (days to weeks), chronic (over months), or acute on chronic, the latter being a chronic condition with recent dramatic acceleration.

16.6.1 Acute Onset

1. Orbital hemorrhage, often of overnight onset, resolves only slowly, and bruising may appear a few days later (Fig. 16.6). Children generally have an underlying vascular anomaly, whereas adults are often arteriopathic and taking antiplatelet drugs. Children may suffer vagally induced vomiting. The management consists of CT (if there is diagnostic doubt) and visual monitoring, with drainage indicated if there is major visual impairment, significant progression, or persistent proptosis.
2. Acute infective orbital cellulitis shows a progression over hours, generally after a prodromal illness with headache, nasal discharge, and fever. The orbit is painful, tense, and active, and passive ocular motility shows marked impairment. Eventually there may be visual loss. Orbital infection is an ophthalmological emergency and needs *immediate* treatment with intravenous antibiotics (prior to imaging), close monitoring of vision, and then orbital CT to confirm the diagnosis. Drainage is indicated for acute compressive optic neuropathy or persistent orbital abscess.
3. Arteriovenous shunts, generally in patients with arterial disease, develop within minutes to hours and are characterized by a painless

protrusion, acute "red eye" with chemosis, and a global reduction of orbital functions. CT and ultrasound echography should be performed, visual acuity and intraocular pressure monitored, and where ocular complications occur, interventional radiology should be considered.

16.6.2 Subacute Onset

1. Childhood malignancies are characterized by subacute onset, often in an otherwise well child, and the tumor may present with a tense, inflamed, and painful orbit (Fig. 16.4). Open incisional biopsy is always indicated, and the appropriate therapy depends on the histological diagnosis. Rhabdomyosarcomas typically are well defined and do *not* occur in extraocular muscles.
2. Childhood capillary hemangiomas develop over months, the lesions being soft and causing only mild impairment of orbital functions. Often there is an expansion of the hemangioma when the child cries or catches a cold.
3. Adult inflammation may show variable progression over weeks, with pain, tenderness, lid swelling, and redness, and may be associated with a marked loss of orbital functions. Biopsy is necessary and may reveal granulomatous, xanthogranulomatous, or lymphocytic inflammations. Biopsy is not required where the history and course of the disease are appropriate, as with thyroid eye disease, idiopathic orbital myositis, or orbital apex inflammation. The last is characterized by an acute, rapid onset of painful, complete ophthalmoplegia, a numb forehead, mild proptosis, and often significant optic neuropathy.
4. Orbital infections in adults may progress over weeks if due to low-grade or unusual organisms—such as fungi, parasites as in hydatid disease, or tuberculosis—and these infections are often painless with only mild inflammatory signs.
5. Adult metastatic disease may show a subacute, relentless progression over weeks, and

about 75% of patients will have a known systemic malignancy. The clinical picture is typically one of painful proptosis, sometimes with inflammatory signs, and a marked reduction of orbital functions. CT scan and systemic tests are obligatory, open biopsy indicated in most cases, and treatment will often involve orbital radiotherapy and systemic chemotherapy or hormonal therapy.

16.6.3 Chronic Onset

1. Childhood benign tumors, such as retrobulbar dermoid or optic nerve tumors, present as slowly progressive proptosis with mild changes in orbital function. Some may be found by chance while imaging for other conditions, such as neurofibromatosis. Imaging may be advisable in some cases, and monitoring of visual development is compulsory.
2. Sinus mucoceles or tumors may progress slowly and present late, and there may be a history of sinus surgery or facial trauma. Inferior displacement of the globe is common, with some limitation of globe movements.
3. Osseous disease, such as fibrous dysplasia, osteoma, or sphenoid wing meningioma, develops slowly at any age, being manifest as facial asymmetry or optic neuropathy (Fig. 16.5).
4. Adult benign tumors show a chronic progression over years, with globe displacement that may be axial or non-axial (Figs. 16.2 and 16.8). Generally, these tumors are painless, and often there is only a mild change in orbital functions. Observation may be appropriate if orbital function is normal, and CT shows a well-defined mass, but otherwise the mass should be excised.
5. Some adult malignant tumors, such as low-grade lymphomas or some sarcomas, may show a painless, slow progression without significant loss of orbital function (Fig. 16.7). All ill-defined, infiltrative orbital masses should be biopsied.
6. Adult low-grade inflammation is usually a chronic disease with swelling, proptosis, and globe displacement. It may be painless, non-erythematous, and possibly organ-specific, as with dacryoadenitis. Treatment usually consists of incisional or excision biopsy followed by immunosuppression and, in some cases, low-dose orbital radiotherapy.
7. Most adult vascular lesions, arising from an "evolution" of venous anomalies or enlargement of arterial anomalies, are of chronic nature and may cause chronic pain and a moderate loss of function. CT scan and Doppler ultrasonography are of diagnostic help, and sometimes an MRI angiogram may be indicated. Venous anomalies should be observed where possible, and arteriovenous malformations usually need treatment by interventional radiology.

16.6.4 Acute-on-Chronic Onset

1. A sudden acceleration of a previously very slowly progressive proptosis suggests the malignant transformation of a formerly benign tumor, such as carcinoma in pleomorphic adenoma (Fig. 16.3), sarcoma in fibrous dysplasia, or lymphoma in Sjögren's syndrome.
2. Occasionally, a low-grade malignancy will transform into a higher-grade lesion as, for example, with lymphomas or in the dedifferentiation of sarcomas.
3. In both adults and children, venous anomalies may undergo spontaneous thrombosis, causing acute pain, signs of inflammation, and a dramatic increase in proptosis with a marked loss of function. Either a surgical intervention or, in some cases, anticoagulants and medical therapy may be required if orbital functions are severely impaired.

16.7 Common Orbital Tumors

The prevalence of various orbital tumors varies with age, with structural anomalies and benign tumors being more common in childhood and acquired benign or malignant neoplasms being typical of adulthood.

16.7.1 Benign Orbital Tumors

The likely diagnosis for many benign orbital tumors can be based on a typical history and examination, with confirmation by CT if necessary. Childhood benign lesions are relatively common, the most frequent being dermoid or epidermoid cysts (up to about one third of referrals) and capillary hemangiomas in up to about 15% of cases. In contrast, dermoid cysts very rarely remain occult until adulthood, and benign tumors in adults tend to be acquired lesions, such as cavernous hemangiomas, benign peripheral nerve sheath tumors, optic nerve tumors, and various, distinctly rare, lacrimal gland and mesenchymal tumors.

16.7.1.1 Orbital Cystic Tumors

Orbital cysts generally arise from developmental sequestration of epithelium within the orbit, by traumatic implantation, or from orbital encroachment by epithelial-lined sinus lesions.

Congenital dermoid and epidermoid cysts, often noted shortly after birth, are most commonly located near the orbital rim at the zygomaticofrontal suture and may present with firm, smooth preseptal masses that may be mobile over the bone or fixed deeply (Fig. 16.10a); in some cases the dermoid passes through a hole or notch in the orbital rim (Fig. 16.10b–d), and very rarely, a dermoid cyst is open to the skin surface and presents as an intermittently discharging sinus. These cysts slowly enlarge from the continued accumulation of epithelial debris, and leakage of the lipid contents may cause intermittent marked inflammation. Retrobulbar dermoid cysts, which may occasionally have a conjunctival epithelial lining, tend to present late in life with progressive proptosis or orbital inflammation.

Mobile, anteriorly situated, and characteristic lesions do not require radiological investigation and should be excised through an upper lid skin crease incision or through an incision hidden on the brow hairs; likewise, fixed dermoid cysts do not necessitate imaging if the surgeon is adequately experienced to follow the lesion to its limits. The tissues should be divided right down to the surface of the cyst (there being a tendency to dissect tissues remote from the lesion) and this plane followed by blunt dissection; in some cases it is necessary to remove the underlying periosteum or follow the lesion into or through the orbital wall. Deep orbital dermoids, as with any tumor presenting with proptosis, require thin-slice CT with bone windows to show associated osseous clefts or canals. CT will often show a smooth, "scalloped" erosion of the neighboring bone as a result of pressure from the mass, although this is a nonspecific sign suggesting a long-standing benign orbital lesion. Intraoperative rupture of a dermoid cyst may lead to a marked postoperative inflammation, and any spilt contents should be removed and residual oily debris "floated out" from the operative field by copious saline irrigation. Incomplete excision of the epithelial lining will lead to recurrent inflammation with formation of a discharging cutaneous fistula through the operative incision.

Dermolipomas are allied to dermoid cysts, in that they comprise cutaneous epithelium and fat sequestered on the ocular surface and typically overlie the lateral and superolateral sclera. The abnormal epithelium, often hair-bearing, causes a chronic ocular irritation and discharge and may be removed by microdissection, with care being taken to avoid damage to the neighboring lacrimal gland ductules.

Paranasal sinus mucoceles most commonly arise in the ethmoid and frontal sinuses, and their enlargement with mucus retention leads to a slow encroachment on the neighboring orbit and globe displacement; orbital cellulitis may occur with secondary infection of the retained sinus secretions (Fig. 16.4e, f). CT scan shows a cystic cavity expanding the paranasal sinus cavity, with patchy thinning or loss of the bone, and MR images can show a wide variation in signal intensities within the lesions. Once any infection has been controlled with systemic antibiotics, the mucocele and other sinus disease should receive definitive treatment from an otorhinolaryngologist, this treatment typically being drainage of retained secretions, reestablishment of new drainage pathways for the affected sinuses, and possibly removal of the mucocele lining.

16.7.1.2 Orbital Vascular Tumors

Many vascular anomalies, such as varices, lymphangiomas, and arteriovenous anomalies, are rather diffuse within the orbit and do not form discrete, tumorlike masses. Childhood capillary hemangiomas and cavernous hemangiomas in adults do, however, present as well-defined tumors with appropriate orbital signs.

Capillary hemangiomas occur in up to 2% of infants and typically appear soon after birth, enlarge, and then undergo a spontaneous involution, with most having resolved by 7 years of age. Unlike rapidly growing malignancies of infancy (such as rhabdomyosarcoma), capillary hemangiomas show multiple vessels with very high flow rates—generally above 50 cm/s—and arterial waveform. Unless the rare necessity for surgical resection is being considered, CT or MRI is only rarely needed for the diagnosis but generally shows a rather irregular lesion with marked contrast enhancement. Affected children should be monitored and treated for their visual development, and if the visual impairment is due to tumor bulk, these hemangiomas are usually treated with systemic or topical β-blockers (e.g., systemic propranolol) or, more rarely, with intralesional steroids or resection.

The most common adult benign orbital tumor, cavernous hemangiomas, usually arise in retrobulbar tissues and present as painless, very slowly progressive proptosis in the fourth or fifth decades; vision may be reduced due to induced presbyopia, choroidal folds, or optic nerve compression (Fig. 16.2). CT scanning reveals a well-defined, round intraconal tumor, with only very slow and patchy contrast enhancement, which commonly displaces the optic nerve medially. Some hemangiomas are wedged in the orbital apex and tend to present early due to optic neuropathy. Asymptomatic tumors—discovered on imaging for other reasons—should be monitored for orbital signs and the lesion removed through an anterior or lateral orbitotomy if there is optic neuropathy, significant proptosis, or diplopia.

16.7.1.3 Benign Lacrimal Gland Lesions

Lacrimal gland masses can be due to chronic dacryoadenitis or benign neoplasms, but the tendency for these conditions to present in a similar fashion to malignancy complicates the management of these patients. Mismanagement of benign conditions can lead to serious consequences as with, for example, malignant recurrence after biopsy of a benign pleomorphic adenoma.

Pleomorphic adenomas are a rare, benign, epithelial neoplasm of the lacrimal gland, typically arising in the orbital lobe and presenting in the fourth or fifth decades as a slow onset of painless proptosis and inferomedial displacement of the globe. To prevent inadvertent biopsy, it is imperative to diagnose the tumor based on clinical history and CT scanning. The ovoid orbital lobe tumors typically lie entirely within the orbit, show a smooth expansion of the lacrimal gland fossa, calcify rarely, and displace and flatten the globe (Fig. 16.3a–c). In contrast, the rare palpebral lobe tumors show a normal gland with an enlarged, rounded, anterior surface extending outside the orbital rim. The key to treatment of pleomorphic adenomas is preoperative recognition, with avoidance of biopsy. Because of the risk of late malignant transformation, tumors of the orbital lobe should be excised intact—sometimes requiring lateral orbitotomy—and breach of the "pseudocapsule" of compressed tissues avoided; to this end, the tumor is handled at all times with a malleable retractor and not with any sharp-edged instruments.

Incisional biopsy should be considered wherever a persistent lacrimal gland mass is accompanied by a history and signs suggestive of chronic inflammation as lacrimal gland carcinoma will be present in some cases. Acute inflammation presents as a painful, swollen, tender upper eyelid, often with an "S"-shaped ptosis, whereas chronic dacryoadenitis more typically presents as a bilateral painless mass. CT or MR images show diffuse lacrimal gland enlargement with "spillover" into the neighboring preseptal and orbital tissues—a radiological appearance that cannot be differentiated from infiltrative malignancies, such as lymphoma.

16.7.1.4 Benign Optic Nerve Tumors

Primary optic nerve meningiomas or gliomas (juvenile pilocytic astrocytoma) are usually benign and present in children or young adults.

Glioma is the most common optic nerve tumor but comprises only 3% of orbital tumors. One third of gliomas are related to type I neurofibromatosis, these having a better visual prognosis than those in patients without NF1. Gliomas generally cause painless proptosis and visual loss ranging from mild to severe. In the early stages, fundus examination may show a swollen optic disc, which later may become pale with the appearance of a retinochoroidal shunt vessel on the margin of the disc. Imaging shows a fusiform enlargement of the optic nerve, often with a characteristic intraorbital kink, and MRI is especially useful for detailing the intracanalicular and intracranial portions of the nerve. Gliomas show a variable clinical course. Most orbital gliomas remain stable for a long time, but some—although benign—may show infiltrative growth and systemic spread. Asymptomatic tumors should be followed clinically and radiologically. Chemotherapy, radiotherapy, and neurosurgical resection should be considered if an optic nerve glioma is showing progression with a threat to the chiasm, whereas a transcanthal resection of the orbital tumor—sparing the eye—may be considered for gross proptosis. Microscopic control of the resection margins may be helpful as the extent of tumor is ill-defined radiologically. The prognosis is generally good for solely orbital glioma and the mortality, other than with intracerebral disease, less than 5%.

Orbital meningiomas are benign neoplasms arising from the meninges, and there are two distinct forms—optic nerve sheath meningioma (Fig. 16.9) and sphenoid wing meningiomas (Fig. 16.5)—which are both frequent in middle-aged women. Optic nerve meningiomas cause minimal proptosis but profoundly affect vision due to impairment of optic nerve perfusion. The affected eye presents with a swollen or atrophic optic disc, occasionally with retinochoroidal shunt vessels. When the tumor is confined to the optic canal, it can mimic optic neuritis, and the diagnosis may be more difficult. CT scan typically shows a diffuse expansion of the optic nerve and, in some cases, a "train-track" parallel calcification of the optic nerve sheath. MRI may demonstrate a normal or small optic nerve passing through an enlarged sheath. Early meningioma should be suspected in any young patient with unusual visual symptoms, such as obscurations, and needs careful radiological examination.

The therapy of optic nerve sheath meningioma is conservative, since surgical excision invariably leads to blindness. High-dose radiotherapy should be considered for optic nerve meningiomas with clinical progression and, in most patients, will slow tumor growth and stabilize or improve vision. Optic nerve meningiomas in younger people should be considered for neurosurgical resection, as the disease appears to have a more active course in this group and probably carries a higher risk of chiasmal involvement.

16.7.1.5 Benign Tumors of the Peripheral Nerve, Bone, or Mesenchyme

Solitary benign nerve sheath tumors, such as neurilemmoma (schwannoma) and neurofibroma, arise from peripheral nerves, comprising about 4% of orbital neoplasms. They present either in the intraconal space (with an imaging appearance like cavernous hemangiomas) or as a sausage-like mass along the orbital roof, causing slowly progressive proptosis and hypoglobus. Orbital neurilemmoma, derived from Schwann cells, usually occurs in middle-aged adults and causes painless proptosis with symptoms similar to those of cavernous hemangioma; they are readily cured by surgery. Neurofibromas are composed of a combination of Schwann, perineural, and fibroblastoid cells, and often axons are present in localized, diffuse, or plexiform types of lesion. Localized neurofibromas are generally not related to NF1, whereas the plexiform type has a very strong association (Fig. 16.8). Although both NF1 and NF2 have ophthalmic manifestations, type 1 has the greatest ophthalmic significance as it is ten times more common than type 2 (the former with an incidence of 1:3000) and has a number of ophthalmic manifestations, including Lisch nodules, neurofibromas, dysplasia of the sphenoid wing, and optic nerve glioma.

Plexiform neurofibromas, the most common and complex of orbital peripheral nerve tumors, grow along the nerves and form a characteristic "bag of worms." They are very vascular and diffusely interconnected with normal tissues, the overlying skin being thickened, and typically affect the upper eyelid and lacrimal gland. Although orbital plexiform neurofibromas are benign, they cause significant problems with continuous growth to sometimes grotesque dimensions, visual impairment or blindness, and, rarely, even death due to impairment of vital intracranial structures. Surgical resection presents considerable difficulty and consists of—often repeated—tumor debulking, which is never curative.

There are many rare tumors that affect the orbital bone, but the most common in adulthood is sphenoid wing meningioma and, in children, osteomas. Sphenoid wing meningioma—unrelated to optic nerve meningioma—tends to present in middle age with chronic variable lid swelling, chemosis, and mild proptosis. CT scan shows hyperostosis of the greater wing of the sphenoid with en-plaque soft tissue on the lateral wall of the orbit, the temporalis fossa, or the middle cranial fossa (Fig. 16.5b). Although metastases may very rarely present with a similar radiological appearance, the clinical behavior is different—with sphenoid wing meningioma progressing very slowly and usually not requiring any active treatment; a rapidly progressing tumor should probably undergo biopsy to exclude metastatic disease with a view to radiotherapy or neurosurgical resection if shown to be meningioma. As progestogens may act as a stimulus to the growth of sphenoid wing meningiomas, it is prudent to discourage the use of hormone replacement therapy in postmenopausal women with this condition.

Benign mesenchymal tumors of the orbit, such as solitary fibrous tumors or hemangiopericytomas, are very rare and typically present as painless proptosis with diplopia. The masses, generally well defined but cloaking normal orbital structures, are often located in the superonasal quadrant of the orbit and may be en-plaque with the orbital periosteum. These tumors should, where possible, be excised intact, as they carry a significant risk of pervasive tumor recurrence with piecemeal primary excision.

16.7.2 Malignant Orbital Tumors

Primary or secondary orbital malignancy can affect all ages and should be considered wherever there is rapidly or relentlessly progressive disease, an inflammatory picture, or where a condition—presumed to be benign—fails to show appropriate clinical behavior (Table 16.3).

16.7.2.1 Malignant Orbital Tumors of Childhood

Rhabdomyosarcoma is the most common primary orbital malignancy of childhood and arises from pluripotent mesenchyme that normally differentiates into striated muscle cells. Showing a peak incidence at about 7 years of age, rhabdomyosarcoma often presents with signs of acute orbital inflammation, and a suspicion of underlying malignancy should be entertained with any unilateral orbital disease in childhood. The tumor mass may be located anywhere in the orbital soft tissues, most commonly in the superomedial quadrant, and typically does *not* arise in the extraocular muscles (Fig. 16.4a–c). Imaging will usually demonstrate a fairly well-defined, round mass with moderate contrast enhancement, arising within the orbital fat and flattening the globe; expansion of the thin bone of the childhood orbit is quite common. Doppler ultrasonography

Table 16.3 The five most common primary and secondary orbital tumors (according to Henderson)

Primary orbital tumors	Secondary orbital tumors
Hemangioma	Mucocele
Malignant lymphoma	Squamous cell carcinoma
Orbital inflammation (pseudotumor)	Meningioma
Meningioma	Vascular malformation
Optic nerve glioma	Malignant melanoma

Table 16.4 Most common orbital tumors in childhood (according to Henderson)

Dermoid cyst
Hemangioma
Rhabdomyosarcoma
Neuroblastoma
Glioma

assists in differentiating rhabdomyosarcoma from capillary hemangioma, the latter showing marked vascularity. Urgent incisional biopsy will provide the diagnosis—although macroscopic excision may be possible for well-defined tumors—and a systemic evaluation (including whole-body CT and a bone marrow biopsy) is required to look for metastatic disease prior to systemic and local tumor therapy. Long-term side effects of orbital radiotherapy include cataract, dry eye with secondary corneal scarring, loss of skin appendages (lashes and brow hair), atrophy of orbital fat, and, if performed in infancy, retardation of orbital bone growth. There is also a risk of late radiation-induced periorbital malignancies, such as fibrosarcoma and osteosarcoma, and there may be an increased propensity to certain other primary tumors in adulthood (Table 16.4).

Both neuroblastoma and acute myeloid leukemias may present as metastases within the orbital soft tissues or bone, the clinical presentation being very similar to rhabdomyosarcoma, with rapidly progressive proptosis and orbital inflammatory signs. The Langerhans cell histiocytoses are a group of malignant diseases affecting this cell lineage, although the variant found most commonly in children (eosinophilic granuloma) verges on a benign proliferation and is readily treated—after biopsy—with intralesional or systemic steroids.

All of these childhood tumors require urgent biopsy, systemic investigation, and chemotherapy with, in some cases, radiotherapy. Although the prognosis for vision with most of the hematological malignancies is generally good, there is a significant mortality, depending on prechemotherapy disease staging.

16.7.2.2 Orbital Lymphoma in Adults

Orbital lymphocytic lesions display a spectrum from benign morphology, showing a well-organized follicular pattern (so-called reactive lymphoid hyperplasia), through the rare "atypical lymphoid hyperplasia" with poorly organized or disrupted follicles, to frankly malignant lymphoma. Improved tissue diagnosis has shown that many lesions previously labelled "atypical lymphoid hyperplasia" are, in fact, lymphomas displaying various degrees of follicular destruc-

tion. Primary lymphomas of the orbit are effectively all of the non-Hodgkin's B-cell type, and the extremely rare orbital T-cell lymphomas occur only in patients with systemic disease. Depending on the grade of lymphoma, up to about one half of patients presenting with orbital disease will be found to have systemic involvement within 6 months of presentation.

Orbital lymphomas typically present in those over 50 with a slowly progressive, painless, pink subconjunctival mass or—if deeper in the orbit—with eyelid swelling, globe displacement, or diplopia (Fig. 16.7). CT scan commonly shows a moderately well-defined soft-tissue mass, which may be bilateral, cloaking the globe and other orbital structures; tumor calcification and bone destruction are distinctly rare. Biopsy is mandatory, as the CT and MRI characteristics of lymphomas are indistinguishable from orbital inflammation. As the contemporary diagnosis of lymphoma depends on structural analysis, open biopsy is recommended because, in contrast to fine-needle aspiration biopsy, it provides a structured sample with minimal disruption. All patients with lymphoid lesions should undergo investigation for systemic disease, including whole-body PET-CT scan and bone marrow biopsy if the lymphoma is of higher grades.

Although some conjunctival lymphomas progress only very slowly and may be kept under observation, most such low-grade orbital lymphomas respond very well to about 2400 cGy fractionated radiotherapy or to oral chemotherapy. Patients with high-grade lymphomas have, however, a much higher chance of systemic disease and usually require multiple cycles of more aggressive chemotherapy, and adjunctive orbital radiotherapy (often to 3500 cGy) may be used to accelerate resolution of the orbital disease. When the disease is confined to the orbit, the visual prognosis is excellent and complications unusual. The overall mortality varies according to the histological grade and staging, and at least 10 years' review is required after primary therapy.

16.7.2.3 Lacrimal Gland Carcinomas

With a peak incidence in the fourth decade, adenoid cystic carcinoma is the most common epithelial malignancy of the lacrimal gland, and other carcinomas (primary adenocarcinoma, mucoepidermoid carcinoma, squamous carcinoma, or malignant mixed tumors; Fig. 16.3d, e) are much rarer; malignant mixed tumors arise within a long-standing pleomorphic adenoma or in recurrent tumor after incomplete resection of a benign pleomorphic adenoma. The diagnosis of lacrimal carcinoma is suggested by persistent periocular ache, ocular displacement, and upper lid swelling progressing over a few months and a non-tender lacrimal gland mass. CT scan shows an enlarged gland molding to the globe, flecks of calcification in about one third of tumors, extension along the lateral orbital wall with medial displacement of lateral rectus (the "lateral wedge sign"), and—in more advanced cases—erosion of the cortical bone in the lacrimal gland fossa.

Biopsy of suspected lacrimal gland malignancy should be through an upper lid skin crease incision, and adenoid cystic carcinoma is composed of cords of malignant epithelial cells, often with cystic spaces giving a "Swiss cheese" pattern. Adenoid cystic carcinoma has a tendency to perineural spread (into the cavernous sinus and pterygopalatine fossa) and also tends to infiltrate beyond the macroscopic boundaries evident at surgery or radiologically. As recurrent lacrimal carcinoma may not present for more than a decade after primary therapy, treatment cannot realistically be considered a "cure" until at least 20 years have elapsed without disease. The optimum treatment for lacrimal carcinoma appears to be local macroscopic debulking—without resection of the bone—followed by high-dose radiotherapy (55–60 Gy) to the lateral part of the orbit, the orbital roof, the superior orbital fissure, and the anterior part of the ipsilateral cavernous sinus; major cranio-orbital resection ("super-exenteration") appears to worsen the prognosis for this disease. Deliberate surgical breach of an intact lateral orbital wall should be avoided, as this may encourage tumor seeding into the cranial diploe and a relentless, fatal recurrence of local disease. Implantation brachytherapy has been used to deliver a high radiation dosage to the tumor bed while relatively sparing the globe,

but it does not treat the cavernous sinus or pterygopalatine fossa, areas in which tumor recurrence occurs after perineural invasion. Intracarotid chemotherapy may have a role as an adjunct to radiotherapy in advanced disease.

The long-term prognosis is probably one of the worst of all orbital tumors with a 10-year survival rate of approximately 50%.

16.7.2.4 Secondary Orbital Malignancy from the Eyelids, Paranasal Sinuses, or Globe

Orbital exenteration, with craniofacial resection in some cases, is generally required where there is extensive orbital involvement by secondary spread of tumors from the globe or from sites around the orbit.

Extensive meibomian gland carcinoma and neglected basal cell or squamous carcinomas tend to invade the orbit and conjunctival fornices, causing diplopia, and tumor fixation to underlying bone suggests advanced disease. Painful perineural invasion, usually from forehead tumors with infiltration along the frontal nerve, is most common with squamous cell carcinoma and may not be associated with a significant orbital mass. Likewise, sebaceous (meibomian gland) carcinoma may show intraepithelial pagetoid invasion across the conjunctiva or skin remote from an apparently localized eyelid mass.

Squamous carcinoma from the paranasal sinuses or pharynx is the most common secondary epithelial neoplasm of the orbit, either with direct bone destruction or microscopic perineural spread through, for example, the ethmoid foramina or the inferior orbital fissure. Management involves diagnostic biopsy, wide surgical clearance, and later radiotherapy and chemotherapy.

Other rare tumors of the paranasal sinuses that may involve the orbit include adenoid cystic carcinoma, adenocarcinoma, esthesioneuroblastoma, and melanoma.

Uveal malignant melanoma is the most common primary intraocular tumor of adulthood, and orbital extension probably occurs through the emissary veins, although aggressive tumors may reach the orbit by direct scleral invasion or through the optic nerve head. As there is often coexistent systemic disease, orbital extension of uveal melanoma carries a poor prognosis, although future advances in tumor-directed chemotherapy may improve this outlook. Extraocular extension of retinoblastoma—the most common childhood ocular malignancy—occurs in about 8% of cases and carries a poor prognosis, despite systemic chemotherapy and local radiotherapy.

16.7.2.5 Orbital Metastases in Adults

Although adulthood metastases occur more commonly in the uveal tract, orbital metastases (which occur by hematological spread in the absence of orbital lymphatics) form 2–3% of all orbital tumors and may arise from an occult primary tumor. The most common primary sites are the breast, prostate, lung, kidney, and the gastrointestinal tract, and such lesions typically present with painful proptosis and diplopia, in some cases resembling orbital inflammation. Malignancy should be considered whenever an orbital disease progresses despite treatment. An exception with regard to the most typical clinical sign of an orbital tumor, proptosis, is the spontaneous enophthalmos in the case of a metastatic scirrhous breast cancer. The mechanism is contraction of fibroblasts in the diffuse scirrhous breast cancer metastases, leading to a retraction of the globe.

A multidisciplinary approach involving the ophthalmologist, family physician, pathologist, and oncologist is essential for an adequate management of these patients. Treatment from an ophthalmologic standpoint includes preservation of vision and relief of pain. Radiotherapy, chemotherapy, and hormonal therapy can often achieve these goals. After possibly debulking the tumor, the mainstay of therapy is local treatment with about 5500 cGy fractionated radiotherapy. Radical surgery is contraindicated except in rare cases, when exenteration may be considered if the orbit is the sole metastasis (e.g., carcinoid, renal carcinoma). Most treatments are palliative, with avoidance of discomfort and preservation of vision (if possible), but dry eye and troublesome diplopia are major problems, particularly after radiation.

16.7.2.6 Rare Adulthood Malignancies of Mesenchymal or Neural Origin

Sarcomas of the orbit are extremely rare. The highly malignant osteosarcoma is often secondary to childhood orbital radiotherapy in genetically predisposed individuals (with prior retinoblastoma), and even with radical clearance, the tumor is almost uniformly fatal within 2 years. Children may present with metastatic Ewing's sarcoma or Wilms' tumor within the orbit and will require systemic therapy after diagnosis.

Fibrosarcomas arise as a primary orbital tumor or as a secondary tumor from adjacent sinuses or the site of prior radiotherapy. Exenteration is often necessary for wide clearance or palliation with radiotherapy and chemotherapy. The prognosis for vision and life is variable, but it is best for primary juvenile fibrosarcomas.

Several rare orbital tumors present with a spectrum of disease from benign to malignant. With a poor prognosis, malignant fibrous histiocytomas generally present with a well-defined mass in the superonasal quadrant, and even after wide excision, recurrence of these radioresistant and chemoresistant tumors is common. Hemangiopericytoma, likewise, has a spectrum of malignancy and should be treated by wide and, if possible, intact resection.

Leiomyosarcoma, a tumor of smooth muscle, and liposarcomas of various degrees of differentiation present considerable diagnostic difficulties and have been reported to involve the orbit very rarely.

Of Schwann cell origin, the extremely rare malignant neurilemmoma may arise spontaneously or in association with neurofibromatosis. It presents as a slowly progressive lid mass or proptosis. CT scan shows an ill-defined mass, and management involves wide surgical clearance with adjunctive radiotherapy or chemotherapy. The prognosis is poor, as these tumors tend to invade the middle cranial fossa and develop pulmonary metastases.

16.8 Principles of Surgical Management

Orbital tumors generally require excision, either intact if well-defined or as an incisional biopsy or piecemeal excision if ill-defined or pervasive. Pleomorphic adenomas of the lacrimal gland must be excised intact and are the only absolute contraindication to incisional biopsy or piecemeal excision; disruption of the pseudocapsule predisposes to a late and infiltrative recurrence of these neoplasms, with these recurrences often being malignant.

It is possible for the experienced orbital surgeon to approach all areas of the orbit through cosmetically "hidden" incisions, and there is almost no indication for using transcranial approaches for solely orbital disease. Cranioorbitotomy should be reserved for cases where there is a need to remove both an intracranial and an orbital mass, such as intracanalicular optic nerve gliomas, masses straddling the superior orbital fissure, and large craniofacial osseous lesions (such as meningiomas). Likewise, the various craniofacial approaches—such as lateral rhinostomy, trans-frontal mid-face resection, or trans-oral mid-face "degloving"—should be reserved for cases of sinus disease involving the orbit or skull base.

16.8.1 Principles of Anterior Orbitotomy

A skin incision of about 3 cm is placed in a suitably hidden position, generally the upper eyelid skin crease or lower eyelid "tear trough," and the underlying orbicularis oculi muscle cauterized and divided at the midpoint of the skin incision. The points of a pair of scissors are inserted through the defect, opened widely along the line of the muscle to separate the fibers by blunt dissection, and any remaining bridging tissue diathermied and divided to reveal the underlying orbital septum. The septum is likewise divided along the line of incision to expose the orbital fat, and the direction of the orbital mass ascertained by analysis of the imaging and by palpation.

A closed pair of blunt-tipped scissors is gently directed through the orbital fat toward the site to be biopsied, the scissors opened widely to reveal the depths of the tissues, and—before withdrawing the scissors—a 12–16-mm malleable retractor is inserted alongside the opened scissors to maintain the plane and depth of exploration. This maneuver is repeated until the abnormal tissue is reached (the surgical assistant maintaining the access with a pair of malleable retractors), and meticulous hemostasis is essential as it can otherwise be almost impossible to recognize subtly abnormal orbital tissues, such as edematous or infiltrated fat.

When the abnormal tissue is located, a relatively large biopsy should be taken using a number 11 blade or noncrushing biopsy forceps. The tissue should preferably be gripped once only, to avoid crush artifact, with a single larger piece being more diagnostic than multiple fragments. Complete hemostasis should be established with bipolar cautery, a vacuum drain placed if there is a concern about tissue fluid collection at the orbital apex, and the orbicularis muscle and skin closed with a running 6/0 nylon suture.

16.8.2 Principles of Lateral Orbitotomy

An upper lid skin crease incision is extended laterally to about 1 cm below the lateral canthus, the tissues opened to the superolateral orbital rim, and the periosteum incised 6 mm outside the rim from the lateral one third of the supraorbital ridge to the level of the zygomatic arch. The periosteum is raised across the rim into the orbit and separated from the inner aspect of the lateral wall, with cautery and division of any bridging vessels. Two axial-plane saw cuts are made at the upper and lower ends of the osteotomy, drill holes placed on either side of each cut and—using a burr—the inner aspect of the lateral wall fragment weakened about 1 cm behind the rim; the fragment is then out-fractured and trimmed, swung laterally on temporalis, and the periosteum opened to provide access for the intraorbital procedure.

After achieving intraorbital hemostasis, a vacuum drain is placed within the intraconal space and passed out through the skin overlying the temporalis fossa. The bone is swung medially into the correct position; fixed in place with a 4/0 absorbable suture passed through the drill holes, the deep subcutaneous tissues over the outer canthus; and further laterally repaired with a 5/0 absorbable suture and the skin closed with a running 6/0 nylon suture. The patient should be nursed half-recumbent after surgery and excessive drainage reported. If the patient develops severe and increasing pain, the vision in the affected eye and the state of the orbit should be checked—a very tense orbit with markedly decreased vision, a relative afferent pupillary defect, and loss of eye movements suggesting significant accumulation of orbital hemorrhage that might lead to irreversible visual loss. Should this emergency occur, the drain should be moved slightly to see if fluid drainage can be reestablished, and if this does not succeed, the operative site should be reopened at the "bedside" and any accumulation of blood allowed to drain. The vacuum drain is removed when active fluid drainage has ceased (usually 8–12 h after surgery), and postoperative systemic anti-inflammatory medications at high dosage are useful—particularly where there has been manipulation in the region of the superior orbital fissure or optic nerve. The patient should refrain from vigorous exercise for 10 days after surgery, normal ocular ductions should be encouraged, and the skin suture removed at 1 week.

Complications after lateral orbitotomy are mainly related to the nature of the intraorbital procedure rather than the approach. It is common to develop diplopia due to mechanical weakness of ocular ductions (particularly abduction), and this typically improves over several weeks, but motor neuropraxias, fairly common with surgery near the orbital apex and superior orbital fissure, may take some months to recover. Postoperative mydriasis—probably due to denervation at the ciliary ganglion—is relatively common and may be permanent, and total loss of vision is a distinct risk with any surgery involving the posterior half of the orbit.

16.8.3 Principles of Orbital Exenteration

Exenteration, necessary for the treatment of various pervasive malignant or benign orbital diseases, involves the complete removal of the eyeball, retrobulbar soft tissues, and, in some cases, the eyelids. Skin-sparing exenteration provides a very rapid rehabilitation and is particularly useful for benign disease, post-septal intraorbital malignancy, and the palliation of fungating terminal orbital malignancy.

The skin incision should be placed well clear of the malignancy, either near the orbital rim if dealing with extensive eyelid malignancy invading the orbit or alongside the lash line for a skin-sparing exenteration when the skin and orbicularis oculi muscle is undermined to the orbital rim. The periosteum is incised just outside the rim, raised intact over the rim and posteriorly into the orbit, with areas of adherence being found at the arcus marginalis, the trochlear fossa, the interosseous suture lines, and the lacrimal crest. The anterior and posterior ethmoidal vessels should be cauterized and divided, along with the nasolacrimal duct and any vessels crossing between the orbit and the lateral orbital wall or floor. Care should be taken to avoid damage to the lamina papyracea, as ethmoidal sinus damage can lead to a chronic sino-orbital fistula. Once the orbital contents have been mobilized within the periosteum, the posterior tissues are divided about 7–10 mm from the apex, this being best achieved from the lateral side, using a monopolar diathermy in a blended cutting and coagulation mode. The ophthalmic artery should also be cauterized with bipolar diathermy, and any persistent bleeding from the bones should be plugged with bone wax. With skin-sparing exenteration, the orbicularis of the residual upper and lower lid flaps are sutured using buried 5/0 absorbable sutures, and the skin closed with continuous 6/0 nylon to create an air-tight closure to encourage retraction of the surface. Where complete exenteration of the eyelids and orbit has been performed, the socket can be left to granulate or lined with split-thickness skin grafts. Exenteration can be complicated by postoperative infection, necrosis of flaps and grafts, or delayed socket granulation. Disruption of the lamina papyracea leads to communication between the ethmoid sinuses and the exenteration cavity (a sino-orbital fistula), and failure of closure of the nasolacrimal duct may cause a lacrimal "blowhole" (**a** and Fig. 16.3d, e), and Augenklinik der Universität München (**b–d**, Figs. 16.2, 16.3a–c, 16.4, 16.5, 16.7, 16.8, 16.9, and 16.10).

Suggested Reading

1. Harris GJ, Logani SC (1999) Eyelid crease incision for lateral orbitotomy. Ophthalmic Plast Reconstr Surg 15:9–16
2. Henderson JW (1994) Orbital tumors, 3rd edn. Raven Press, New York
3. Klingenstein A, Haug AR, Miller C, Hintschich C (2015) Ga-68-DOTA-TATE PET/CT for discrimination of tumors of the optic pathway. Orbit 34(1):16–22
4. Lacey B, Chang W, Rootman J (1999) Nonthyroid causes of extraocular muscle disease. Surv Ophthalmol 44:187–213
5. Lacey B, Rootman J, Marotta TR (1999) Distensible venous malformations of the orbit: clinical and hemodynamic features and a new technique for management. Ophthalmology 106:1197–1209
6. McNab AA, Wright JE (1990) Lateral orbitotomy—a review. Aust N Z J Ophthalmol 18:281–286
7. Moreiras JVP, Prada MC, Coloma J, Beverra EP (2004) Orbit: examination, diagnosis, microsurgery and pathology, 1st edn. Highlights of Ophthalmology International, Panama
8. Rootman J (1999) Diseases of the orbit. A multidisciplinary approach, 2nd edn. J.B. Lippincott, Philadelphia
9. Rootman J, Kao SC, Graeb DA (1992) Multidisciplinary approaches to complicated vascular lesions of the orbit. Ophthalmology 99:1440–1446
10. Rootman J, Stewart B, Goldberg RA (1995) Orbital surgery. A conceptual approach, 1st edn. Lippincott-Raven, Philadelphia
11. Rose GE (1996) Clinical examination in orbital disease. In: Bosniak S (ed) Principals and practice of ophthalmic plastic and reconstructive surgery, 1st edn. W.B. Saunders, Philadelphia, pp 860–873
12. Rose GE, Wright JE (1992) Pleomorphic adenomas of the lacrimal gland. Br J Ophthalmol 76:395–400
13. Rose GE, Wright JE (1994) Trigeminal sensory loss and orbital disease. Br J Ophthalmol 78:427–429
14. Wright JE, McNab AA, McDonald WI (1989) Primary optic nerve sheath meningioma. Br J Ophthalmol 73:960–966
15. Wright JE, McNab AA, McDonald WI (1989) Optic nerve glioma and the management of optic nerve tumors of the young. Br J Ophthalmol 73:967–974
16. Wright JE, Rose GE, Garner A (1992) Primary malignant neoplasms of the lacrimal gland. Br J Ophthalmol 76:401–407

Primary CNS Lymphoma

17

Lakshmi Nayak and Uwe Schlegel

17.1 Epidemiology, Incidence and Prognostic Factors

Primary CNS lymphomas are rare highly aggressive brain tumours. They belong to the group of extra nodal NHL and affect exclusively the brain parenchyma, meninges and rarely the spinal cord [1, 2]. In about 10 to 15% of PCNSL, patients are affected by a vitreoretinal lymphoma, either prior to appearance of the CNS lymphoma, at presentation or during the course of the disease [3–5]. Leptomeningeal involvement may be detectable by CNS analysis in about 15% of cases. Highly proliferative diffuse large B-cell lymphomas (DLBCL) comprise more than 95% of lymphomas with CNS manifestation; these are PCNSL according to the WHO classification system [6]. Low-grade malignant B-cell lymphomas and T-cell lymphomas are extremely rare [2]. PCNSL comprise 2–4% of all primary intracranial tumours; their annual incidence is 0.5 per 100,000 [1, 2]. While in past decades patients with HIV infection were frequently affected by PCNSL, this number has dropped dramatically due to the induction of highly active antiretroviral therapy (HAART) [7]. On the other hand, the incidence of PCNSL is increasing in medically immunocompromised patients such as post-transplant lymphoproliferative disorder (PTLD), which is often associated with Epstein-Barr virus (EBV) reactivation. Prognostic factors, such as age, clinical performance state, involvement of deep brain structures, certain laboratory and cerebral spinal fluid (CSF) findings, have been associated with prognosis [8]. In clinical practice, however, only older age and low clinical performance status play a role as factors undoubtedly associated with worse prognosis.

17.2 Diagnostic Procedures

The **clinical symptoms** in PCNSL are unspecific and generally evolve within a few weeks due to rapid tumour growth. More than 50% of patients present with a psycho-organic syndrome including psychomotor slowing, disorientation and other symptoms. About 50% of patients are affected by neurological symptoms, depending on tumour localisation. Signs of raised intracranial pressure, epileptic seizures and cranial nerve palsies are rare [1, 2]. In case of vitreoretinal ocular involvement, blurred vision and mouches volantes (ocular floaters) may occur [3, 4, 9].

L. Nayak (✉)
Center for CNS Lymphoma, Center for Neuro-Oncology, Dana-Farber Cancer Institute, Harvard Medical School, Boston, MA, USA
e-mail: Lakshmi_Nayak@dfci.harvard.edu

U. Schlegel
Department of Neurology, University Hospital Bochum Knappschaftskrankenhaus, Bochum, Germany
e-mail: Uwe.schlegel@kk-bochum.de

Leptomeningeal involvement usually is clinically asymptomatic.

The most important diagnostic measure is cranial **magnetic resonance imaging (MRI)** without and with contrast media application. Lesions are characteristically unifocal and intensively and homogenously contrast enhancing and typically localise adjacent to the lateral ventricles. Multifocal lesions can occur in about a third of cases [10, 11]. Due to a high density of tumour cells, diffusion restriction is high, such that PCNSL present as bright hyperintense lesions in diffusion-weighted images (DWI) [12]. DWI may be used to separate PCNSL from atypical glioblastoma [13]. Their differential diagnosis on MRI, however, comprises not only other primary intracranial tumours and metastases but also inflammatory space occupying lesions as, for example, tumefactive multiple sclerosis, sarcoidosis, other granulomas, vasculitis and infectious lesions as abscesses, opportunistic infections like toxoplasmosis, progressive multifocal leukoencephalopathy (PML) and others [11, 12]. Nearly all PCNSL lesions enhance and this is typically homogenous; about 10–15% of the lesions may enhance heterogeneously [12]. Necrosis and peripheral, ring-like enhancement are uncommon in the immunocompetent but may be found in the immunocompromised. While all these imaging findings are characteristic of PCNSL, there are no pathognomonic imaging findings for this tumour. Advanced imaging techniques may be helpful in some cases as described for DWI [13, 14]. Intratumoural susceptibility signals from SWI, likely related to microhaemorrhage, are more common and extensive in GBM than in PCNSL [12].

Cerebrospinal fluid (CSF) analysis is part of the recommended work-up in all patients with suspected brain lymphoma, unless contraindicated for raised intracranial pressure [2, 15, 16]. Its analysis comprises conventional cytomorphology, flow cytometry and monoclonality assessment by polymerase chain reaction (PCR). These tests are positive only in patients with leptomeningeal involvement leading to mobilisation of tumour cells into the CSF space and are present in only a minority of cases. In a large prospective study comprising more than 400 patients, lymphoma was detected in the CSF by cytomorphology in 12%, by PCR in 10% and by imaging in 4% [17]. These findings are more frequent in patients with CSF pleocytosis. Several **CSF markers** have been investigated for their diagnostic value, including microRNA (miRNA) patterns [18], CXC chemokine ligand 13 (CXCL-13) [19], interleukin 10 [20], neopterin [21] and others [12]. Proteome analysis recently has identified proteins in the CSF of PCNSL patients involved in ectodermal shedding [22]. Neither of these interesting CSF markers has been validated in independent patient cohorts, and their use for definitive diagnosis in PCNSL is not yet recommended. In rare instances the definitive diagnosis of PCNSL can be made by CSF analysis alone. In all other cases, histopathologic verification of CNS lymphoma is mandatory.

Tumour tissue for **pathological examination** (see below) can be achieved by surgical resection, open biopsy or most frequently stereotactic biopsy. It is recommended to withhold treatment with steroids, since this may lead to shrinkage of the tumour and to apoptotic cell death of B-cell lymphomas, leaving the pathologist with a specimen that shows unspecific (often T-cell-dominated) inflammatory changes, which reflects a possible corticosteroid-mitigated-lymphoma [10]. In case of such a non-diagnostic pathology, which is otherwise unexpected in PCNSL [23], it is advisable to reduce/omit steroids, to carry out a control MRI after 4–6 weeks or earlier in case of clinical deterioration and to go for a second biopsy in case of tumour growth. After histopathologic conformation of brain lymphoma (see below), a systematic standardised **staging** is recommended by the international PCNSL collaborative group (IPCG) [24] (listed in Table 17.1): This comprises computer tomography (CT) without and with contrast media of the neck, thorax and abdomen. Alternatively ^{18}F-glucose positron emission tomography (PET)-CT of the whole body can be used for detecting occult systemic tumour. Recommended staging also includes bone marrow aspirate for cytology and histology. Admittedly, systemic occult lymphoma confined to the bone marrow and not detectable in

Table 17.1 Recommended staging in CNS lymphoma; adapted to the IPCG recommendations [24]

- Taking history with special consideration of possible immunosuppression
- Clinical neurological examination; signs of intracranial pressure
- MRI of the brain without and with gadolinium
- CSF analysis including cytopathology (also in samples with normal cell count), flow cytometry using antibodies against B-cell surface (CD19, CD20, kappa/lambda light chains) and against T-cell surface markers, in particular in samples with pleocytosis. PCR-based detection of B-cell clonality is suggested. Lumbar puncture is contraindicated in cases of raised intracranial pressure
- Ophthalmological examination including slit-lamp investigation.
- Systemic staging with:
  - Palpation of peripheral lymph nodes
  - CT neck, thorax, abdomen (may be substituted by whole body ^{18}F-Glucose-PET-CT)
  - Bone marrow aspirate (cytology, histology and immunophenotyping)
  - Palpation and ultrasound of testes
- HIV testing

other organs is exceptional in the case of brain lymphoma. Ultrasound of testes and palpation of lymph nodes are to be carried out in case ^{18}F-glucose PET-CT is not available. Careful ophthalmological examination including slit-lamp examination is part of standard staging to exclude or detect vitreoretinal lymphoma accompanying PCNSL. HIV testing is mandatory, and additional opportunistic (latent) infections should be ruled out prior to administration of rituximab and aggressive chemotherapy. This comprises testing for EBV infection, CMV infection and hepatitis.

17.3 Histopathology and Molecular Pathogenesis

Microscopically, PCNSL is a highly cellular neoplasm composed of large lymphoid cells [6]. At the periphery, an angiocentric growth pattern of tumour cells is typical, and vascular walls with lymphoid cell infiltration show concentric lamellae of reticulin fibres, pathognomonic for PCNSL. Small T-lymphocytes are often intermingled with large lymphoma cells

and may dominate the picture in case of steroid pretreatment [6, 25]. Neoplastic cells are large and possess atypical, round nuclei with a single or multiple nucleoli, resembling centroblasts or immunoblasts. Mitotic figures and apoptotic bodies are frequently seen. PCNSL are mature B-cell lymphomas expressing Pan-B-cell-markers, as CD20 and CD79a [25]. Other markers frequently expressed in DLBCL are BCL6 (60–80%), MUM1/IRF4 (90%), CD10 (10–20%) and BCL2 [25]. Cell surface immunoglobulins are IgM and IgD with light chain restriction. The proliferation index KI67 frequently is between 70 and 90% of all tumour cells [25].

Molecular genetic analysis shows that PCNSL is a distinct lymphoma entity, in which neoplastic cells correspond to the late germinal centre exit B-cell expressing BCL6 and IRF4 [25, 26]. Translocation of BCL6 gene with promotor substitution, observed in about one third of PCNSL, induces constitutive BCL6 activity, which has oncogenic properties and contributes to keeping lymphoma cells in the germinal centre stage [25]. Activation of pathways for B-cell signalling also fosters lymphoma survival. Toll-like receptor (TLR) pathway is activated by mutations of MYD88, which was demonstrated in 1/3 of PCNSL [27]. MYD88 plays a key role as an adapter molecule to transducing signals from Toll-like receptors. B-cell receptor (BCR) signalling cascade is also altered by mutations of CD79B and CARD11 [28]. The activation of these signalling pathways, alone or in synergy, produces constitutive activation of the nuclear factor (NK)-kappa B pathway and then contributes to proliferation and survival of lymphoma cells [29]. PCNSL show frequently an ongoing mutation in the variable immunoglobulin heavy chain [30–32], and post-translationally modified CNS driver auto-antigens have been proposed to attract systemic B-lymphoma cells (or pre-lymphoma cells) [33] through the vasculature. In the brain as an immunoprivileged site, they may expand through clonal evolution by, for example, acquiring additional mutations in the variable region of the immunoglobulin heavy chain [31]. This mechanism is supported by the pathological feature, since most PCNSL show a perivascular growth pattern. Most recently candidates for such post-translationally modified CNS driver auto-antigens have been found in 8/12 PCNSL specimens with hyper N-glycosylated SAMD14 and neurabin-1 [34]. These findings may support the role of chronic antigen stimulation by post-translationally modified CNS driver auto-antigens in the genesis of PCNSL, and they may serve as an explanation for the CNS tropism [34].

17.4 First-Line Treatment

As is true in general for lymphomas, PCNSL are sensitive to radiotherapy and chemotherapy. **Surgical resection** was supposed to play no therapeutic role. This issue has been addressed by an unplanned post hoc analysis of a large series of patients having been included in a randomised phase 3 trial [35]. An analysis of patients with single lesions found a longer progression-free survival (PFS) and a trend to a longer overall survival (OS) for those with total or subtotal resection as compared to those with biopsy alone [36]. However, only 318 of 551 patients included in this trial had been treated per protocol, and those were undertreated with regard to current treatment standard [35, 37]. Prognosis is much better today due to efficient immunochemotherapy (see below), and outcome mainly is determined by complete response to efficient systemic therapy [2, 38]. It also needs to be considered that PCNSL is a "whole brain disease" [39] and that surgical resection could be harmful given the risk of irreversible neurological deficits from resection based on the tumour location. Therefore, an attempt of resection may not be justified for a tumour entity that rapidly shrinks and eventually disappears as a consequence of efficient systemic therapy. In conclusion, biopsy is the procedure of choice to gain tissue when an MRI suggests a brain lymphoma [1, 2].

In the past, **whole brain radiotherapy** (WBRT) had been applied as the sole treatment modality of PCNSL with median survival of no more than 1 to 1.5 years [40, 41]. Since high-dose intravenous MTX had been identified as the most important treatment-related factor independently correlated with longer survival [42], in the past two decades, MTX-based chemotherapy, followed by WBRT as consolidation, has been exploited in many single-arm phase 2 trials (see Table 17.2), in one randomised phase 2 trial [52] and in one large randomised phase 3 trial [35, 37]. Notwithstanding the heterogeneity of clinical data, the addition of WBRT to intensified MTX-based polychemotherapy has never been proven to add significantly to overall survival [61], neither in retrospective analysis [62] nor in prospective clinical trials [35, 37]. On the other hand, the deleterious late neurotoxic side effects of WBRT in addition to MTX-based chemotherapy need to be considered. Delayed neurotoxicity in PCNSL became evident in the 1990s with prolonged patients' survival as a result of HDMTX-based chemotherapy, followed by WBRT. In patients over 60 years treated with HDMTX i.v. and MTX i.c.v., followed by WBRT and systemic HDaraC, a 100% rate of severe cognitive dysfunction, presenting as a dementing disease, was reported, while younger patients less frequently suffered from this side effect and with more delay [15]. Late neurotoxicity can be recognised by radiographic findings such as diffuse white matter disease and cortical, subcortical atrophy [63]; see Fig. 17.1. The true prevalence of late neurotoxicity is likely underestimated, since clinical follow-up in most trials did not comprise formal neurocognitive testing [64]. The risk of delayed neurotoxicity increases with age but is also present in younger patients. There is a whole body of literature strongly suggesting that WBRT rather than chemotherapy is the primary mediator of neurotoxicity. In a retrospective analysis of 185 patients, WBRT was the only factor associated with clinically manifest delayed neurotoxicity in the multivariate setting [65]. These results were confirmed by long-term evaluations using both neuropsychometric testing and MRI showing significantly higher scores from tests of selective attention and memory and less T2-abnormalities on MRI after HDMTX-based chemotherapy alone than after combined therapy [66]. Preservation of cognitive function was reported after chemotherapy alone

Table 17.2 Selection of prospective trials and first-line therapy of PCNSL

Reference	N	Med. age (ys)	Regimen (induction → intensification/consolidation)	Response (ORR/CR, in %)	Med. PFS (mo)	Med. OS (mo)
Conventional chemotherapy, all age groups, $n \geq 40$						
Pels et al., 2003 [43]	65	62	MTX, vincristine, ifosfamide, cyclophosphamide → araC/vindesine	71/61	21 (TTP)	54
Jurgens et al., 2010 [44]	30 (≤60 ys)	52	MTX, prednisolone + araC i.c.v.		64	>80
	35 (>60 ys)				30	34
Rubenstein et al., 2013 [45]	44	61	R, MTX, TMZ → etoposide, araC	77/66	29	>59
Pulczynski et al., 2015 [46]	39 (≤65 ys)	55	R, MTX, ifosfamide, cyclophosphamide → araC, vindesine liposomal araC intrathecally	70/59	10 (DoR)	>22
	27 (>66 ys)	70	R, MTX, TMZ → araC, vindesine, liposomal araC intrathecally maintenance with TMZ for 12 months	81/69	>22 (DoR)	>22
Conventional chemotherapy in elderly patients (>60 years), $n \geq 40$						
Hoang-Xuan et al., 2003 [47]	50	72	MTX, procarbazine, lomustine → MTX + araC i.t.	48/42	7	14
Omuro et al., 2015 [48]	95	72	MTX + TMZ	71/45	6	14
		73	MTX + procarbazine, vincristine → araC	82/62	10	31
Fritsch et al., 2017 [49]	107	73	R, MTX, procarbazine (lomustine) maintenance: procarbazine for 6 mo	49/36	10	21
Chemotherapyie + WBRT, $n \geq 40$						
DeAngelis et al., 2002 [16]	102	57	MTX, procarbazine, vincristine, MTX i.c.v. → RT	94	24	37
Poortmans et al., 2003 [50]	52	51	MTX, teniposide, BCNU MTX, araC + hydrocortisone i.t. → RT	81/69	NA	46
Korfel et al., 2005 [51]	56	60	MTX, BCNU, procarbazine → RT	61/54	10	12
Ferreri et al., 2009 [52]	79	58	MTX → RT	41/18	5 (FFS)	10
		59	MTX + araC → RT	69/46	9 (FFS)	31
Thiel et al., 2010 [35]	551 (318 per protocol)	61	MTX, (ifosfamide) → araC	54/35	12	37
			MTX, (ifosfamide) → RT		18	32
Morris et al., 2013 [53]	52	60	R, MTX, procarbazine, vincristine → araC + dose-reduced RT	95/79	92	>70
Glass et al., 2016 [54]	53	57	R, MTX, TMZ → dose-reduced RT Maintenance with TMZ for 11 mo	85/51	64	90
High-dose chemotherapy + autologous stem cell transplantation (HDC-ASCT) +/− RT, $n \geq 30$						
Illerhaus et al., 2006 [55] Kasenda et al., 2012 [56]	30	54	MTX, araC, TT → HD-AST (BCNU, TT) + RT	92/38	>64 104	
Omuro et al., 2015 [57]	32	57	MTX, procarbazine, vincristine → HDC-ASCT (busulfan, TT, cyclophosphamide)	96/45	>84	>84

(continued)

Table 17.2 (continued)

Reference	N	Med. age (ys)	Regimen (induction → intensification/ consolidation)	Response (ORR/CR, in %)	Med. PFS (mo)	Med. OS (mo)
Illerhaus et al., 2016 [58]	79	56	R, MTX → ara-C,TT → HDC-ASCT (BCNU,TT), RT (in n = 10 with no CR after HDC-ASCT)	80/23	74	>84
Ferreri et al., 2016 [59] Ferreri et al., 2017 [60]	75	58	MTX, araC → HDC-ASCT (BCNU, TT) or WBRT	53/23	6, PFS-2: 80% WBRT, 69% HDC-ASCT	12
	69	57	R, MTX, araC → HDC-ASCT (BCNU, TT) or WBRT	74/30	20 PFS-2: 80% WBRT, 69% HDC-ASCT	30
	75	57	R, MTX, araC, TT (MATRix) → HDC-ASCT (BCNU, TT) or WBRT	86/49	>20 PFS-2: 80% WBRT, 69% HDC-ASCT	>30

N number of patients, *ORR* overall response rate, *CR* complete response rate, *PR* partial response rate, *ys* years, *mo* months, *i.c.v.* intracerebroventricular (via Ommaya reservoir), *i.t.* intrathecally, *MTX* methotrexate, *araC* cytarabine, *TT* thiotepa, *TMZ* temozolomide, *BCNU* carmustine, *(WB)RT* (whole brain) radiotherapy, *FFS* failure-free survival, *TTP* time to progression, *DoR* duration of response, *PFS-2* progression-free survival fraction at 2 years

[67]. In the "Bonn trial" after a median follow-up of 100 months, 21 patients out of 65 initially included were still alive, and 19 of those completed serial neuropsychologic and QOL examination showing no late neurotoxicity nor a decline of QOL [44]. Ongoing trials to exploit the role of low-dose radiotherapy (e.g. 23.4 Gy WBRT) [53] or methods to spare the hippocampus [68] should be considered experimental at this time. In conclusion, WBRT should no longer be considered part of first-line therapy for patients who can tolerate intensified HDMTX-based chemotherapy. Even experts reluctant to take the "risk" of omitting WBRT in PCNSL acknowledge the fact that this is a reasonable consolidation instead of WBRT for patients able to tolerate intensified chemotherapy [69, 70].

Despite ongoing clinical research to define the optimal treatment for PCNSL, there is a broad consensus that successful **systemic ther-apy**, as the sole first-line treatment, is based on **HDMTX-based induction**, followed by some **consolidation** chemotherapy ([1, 2]; see also Table 17.2). Figure 17.2 shows a typical example of a complete response to MTX-based induction (MTX/ifosfamide/rituximab X 3), followed by consolidation with intensified conventional chemotherapy and durable remission for >2.5 years. Irrespective of the lack of class 1 evidence, the following therapeutic recommendations can be given for first-line therapy in PCNSL:

High-dose MTX (HD-MTX ≥ 3 g/m^2 infused over 4 h under vigorous hyperhydration and urine alkalisation) is the most effective single therapy and backbone of every successful combination therapy. HDMTX must be dose-reduced in renal insufficiency. Specifically, glomerular filtration rate (GFR) needs to be determined prior to HDMTX application, and HDMTX should not be administered at a GFR < 50 mL/min. Several cycles of HDMTX need to be administered. HDMTX alone, however, in general does not lead to sustained responses [71, 72] and needs to be combined with other substances able to cross the blood-brain barrier [73], such as **HDaraC**

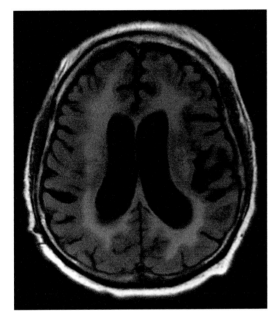

Fig. 17.1 Axial T2 FLAIR image demonstrating periventricular hyperintense T2 signal changes, cortical atrophy and hydrocephalus suggesting leukoencephalopathy in patient with PCNSL 3 years after treatment with HD-MTX followed by whole brain radiotherapy

[52], **thiotepa** [59, 60], **ifosfamide** [35, 37] or **temozolomide** [45]. Many of these substances have been shown to increase response rate while increasing systemic toxicity. The **CD20 antibody rituximab** has been analysed for additional therapeutic efficacy in a retrospective analysis and in several prospective randomised trials. In a prospective randomised trial, the addition of rituximab to HDMTX and HDaraC increased the response rate [59]. It is generally accepted that rituximab should be included in first-line therapy [1, 2].

Consolidation chemotherapy may be applied as intensive conventional chemotherapy as in the CALGB 50202 trial with etoposide and HDaraC [45] or with HDaraC, cyclophosphamide/ifosfamide and i.c.v. chemotherapy as in the Bonn trial [43, 44]. Details of these chemotherapy regimens are given in Table 17.2, which comprises also other regimens, most importantly those following the concept of HDC-ASCT [48, 55, 58–60, 74]. Among those high-dose concepts, most promising results have been achieved with the "Freiburg protocol" [58], which, after induction and stem cell mobilisation with low-dose thiotepa and araC, comprises high-dose chemotherapy with BCNU and thiotepa, both substances readily able to cross the intact blood-brain barrier. In a single-arm phase 2 trial, which comprised whole

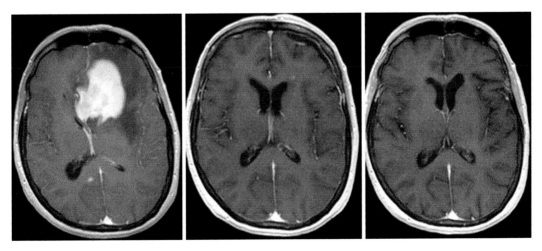

Fig. 17.2 Axial T1 post-gadolinium contrast images of a 64-year-old woman with PCNSL at presentation showing a contrast-enhancing lesion in the left frontal lobe, a complete response to treatment with HD-MTX, ifosfamide and rituximab that is sustained at 2.5 years after diagnosis

brain radiotherapy of only 10/79 non-CR patients, results in 79 patients were excellent with a PFS fraction of more than 50% after 5 years [58]. These results admittedly have been achieved in a selected group of patients, being 70 years old or younger and considered fit for HDC-ASCT, but were realised in a multicentre setting, comprising 15 different German centres. According to the concept of induction chemotherapy, followed by consolidation, the ELSG32 study was carried out, exploiting three different induction regimens after a first randomisation step, followed by either HDC-ASCT or WBRT (also in a randomised fashion). For details see Table 17.2. While the highest response rate was achieved with the most aggressive induction regimen HDMTX/ HDaraC/Thiotepa/rituximab (MATRix) X 4, this regimen turned out to be toxic, and only 64% of patients received consolidation [59]. If less than two thirds of young and fit patients considered to qualify for HDC-ASCT made it for consolidation within a clinical trial, it is most questionable that "MATRix" qualifies for routine clinical use. The progression-free survival rate of the whole group after consolidation was consequently disappointing ([59, 60]; see also Table 17.2). It seems more reasonable to achieve tumour response and clinical amelioration with a much less toxic induction regimen, e.g. based on HDMTX and rituximab as in the Freiburg trial [58], in order to put patients into a situation where they can tolerate either intensified conventional chemotherapy or HDC-ASCT for consolidation.

With respect to **intracerebroventricular (i.c.v.)** administration of chemotherapy, as applied in the Bonn protocol, no evidence exists for the additional benefit of such a regimen. However, leptomeningeal disease is frequent in PCNSL with tumour cells adjacent to the meninges and not detectable in the CSF compartment. The CSF may well be a sanctuary of survival for tumour cells due to failure to kill cells by cytotoxic drug concentrations after i.v. administration. Sustained drug cytotoxic concentrations, however, can be achieved by daily administration of low-dose MTX plus prednisolone, followed by araC via an Ommaya reservoir [43]. This theoretical consideration was supported by our obser-

vation that omitting i.c.v. therapy in the original Bonn protocol in a consecutive trial was associated with a high rate of early relapses, most frequently affecting the leptomeninges and the CSF compartment [75]. While there is no evidence for the additional efficacy of i.c.v. therapy, it is a reasonable approach to intensify treatment in elderly people, for which systemic therapy cannot be escalated for reasons of systemic toxicity.

17.5 First-Line Treatment for Elderly Patients

As mentioned earlier, older age is one of the most important prognostic factors, consistently found to be independently associated with poor prognosis in newly diagnosed PCNSL. Specifically, patients over 60 years of age at initial diagnosis are found to do poorly. Additionally, tolerance to therapy has also been found to be worse in older patients in the setting of clinical trials. Treatment-associated toxicities may be higher due to the presence of multiple medical comorbidities in the elderly population making them more susceptible to side effects. Not only is there a concern for acute toxicity from chemotherapy, the risk for delayed neurotoxicity from whole brain radiotherapy is much higher in patients over 60 years of age [76]. Although the Memorial Sloan Kettering Cancer Center prognostic model identified an age cut-off at 50 years, the cut-off based on IELSG scoring system was 60 years, and many other studies have demonstrated age over 60 as a negative prognostic factor. This is a significant concern as greater than 50% of the patients are above this age given the median age at diagnosis in this disease is 65 years. Although there has been a significant improvement in outcomes related to advances in treatment over the last 40 years, survival in elderly patients remains poor. In a population study using two national databases in the United States, the median OS survival improved from 12 months in the 1970s to 26 months in 2010. However, this survival benefit was not seen in patients >70 years of age, in whom median OS remained at 6–7 months over 40 years [77].

There have been fewer prospective clinical trials in the elderly with median progression-free survival ranging from 6 to 16 months and median overall survival, 14 to 31 months [46–49]. A multicentre, randomised, phase 2 study of HD-MTX and temozolomide versus HD-MTX (3.5 g/m^2), procarbazine, vincristine and HDaraC (3 g/m^3) in patients >60 years of age (median age, 73 years) with KPS >40 demonstrated no significant difference with regard to survival, toxicities, quality of life and neurocognitive status [48]. The authors noted that there was a trend towards improved outcomes in the HDaraC group. While toxicities and HD-MTX dose reductions were common, the majority of patients did not need to discontinue drugs. The PRIMAIN study evaluated the efficacy of three cycles of rituximab, HD-MTX (3 g/m^2; total nine doses over three cycles), procarbazine and lomustine (R-MPL) followed by maintenance treatment with procarbazine in 107 elderly patients (median age, 73 years) with newly diagnosed PCNSL [49]. Lomustine was dropped during the study due to infectious complications, and 38 of these patients received only R-MP. Approximately 40% of the patients did not reach end of treatment (three cycles) primarily due to death or toxicities. The 2-year PFS and OS were 37% and 47%, respectively. A recent meta-analysis of 783 patients with a median age of 68 years (range, 60–90 years) indicated that HD-MTX-based treatment was beneficial and associated with better survival [78]. Whole brain radiotherapy was delivered to 35% of patients as initial therapy and found to be associated with improved survival but also increased neurotoxicity. The majority of patients died from progressive disease; treatment-related deaths were seen in 12% of patients, although cause of death was unknown in 23% of patients. In a retrospective review of 24 very old patients ≥80 years of age, 92% were safely treated with a HD-MTX-based regimen and tolerated it well with reasonable results; 62.5% had an objective response and 2-year OS was 33% [79]. Although thiotepa-based HDC-ASCT has been increasingly employed for consolidation in younger patients, its use in the elderly population particularly given the concerns for transplant-associated mortal-

ity risk is met with trepidation. In a retrospective study of 52 selected patients ≥65 years of age (median age 68.5 years), there were only 2 transplant-related deaths, and 2-year PFS and OS were 62% and 71%, respectively [80]. Some of the recent prospective autologous transplant studies have included patients up to 70 or 72 years of age, and its safety and efficacy in this population remain to be demonstrated. In general, treatment in the elderly needs to be individualised. While many patients can likely tolerate HD-MTX-based chemotherapy, in those patients with medical comorbidities, the risk-benefit ratio needs to be weighed while making treatment decisions.

17.6 Considerations for the Immunosuppressed

Immunosuppression is a known risk factor for development of PCNSL. In the 1980s during the HIV/AIDS epidemic, there was an increase in incidence of PCNSL in young adults which dropped significantly after the introduction of antiretroviral therapy (ART) in the mid-1990s. An association with EBV has been seen in 75–100% of patients. PCNSL patients with HIV have been excluded from clinical trials, and current guidelines recommend treatment with HD-MTX-based chemotherapy with or without whole brain radiotherapy [81]. There are case reports of success with HDC-ASCT in these patients [82, 83]. While prognosis of these patients has been poor, many of the reported studies were from the pre-antiretroviral therapy (ART) era. ART can be safely given in conjunction with chemotherapy which has led to improved survival in these patient populations.

More recently, with the use of immunosuppressive drugs for autoimmune disorders, there has been an increase in the risk of development of PCNSL in these patients particularly those who are on chronic immunosuppressive agents for several years. CNS PTLD (post-transplant lymphoproliferative disorder) can be seen in patients on immunosuppressive drugs after organ transplant and accounts for 5–15% of all PTLD cases [84]. Unlike systemic PTLD which typically appears within the first year after transplantation, CNS PTLD has been known to develop much later and represents a distinct clinicopathologic entity [85]. The vast majority of PCNSL in immunocompromised patients are associated with EBV infections, although EBV positivity is not required for the diagnosis. It is important to distinguish CNS PTLD from immunocompetent PCNSL as prognosis and treatment strategies may differ. In a large multicentre retrospective study of 84 patients with CNS PTLD after solid organ transplantation, the most common organ transplantation was kidney (79%), and the majority (83%) of patients developed late-onset PTLD [86]. The common immunosuppressive agents used were mycophenolate, cyclosporine and tacrolimus. The majority of patients had reduction in immunosuppressive drug, and 48% received HD-MTX-based treatment, by itself or in combination with rituximab, HDaraC or other chemotherapy. Whole brain radiotherapy was delivered to 19 patients alone or after chemotherapy. The median PFS and OS were 8 and 17 months, respectively, with no treatment-related differences in survival.

17.7 Treatment for Vitreoretinal Lymphoma

Intraocular lymphoma can occur in conjunction with brain parenchymal or leptomeningeal lymphoma, precede it or occur by itself as primary vitreoretinal lymphoma (PVRL). The optimal treatment for intraocular lymphoma is not established as data from prospective studies are limited to studies of PCNSL that include a few patients with PVRL and mostly retrospective reviews. Systemic HD-MTX and HDaraC appear to adequately penetrate this space as observed by clinical responses, although recurrences may occur. Focal treatment with intraocular chemotherapy or radiation has also been tried. The exact risk of brain dissemination is unclear with varying numbers reported from different studies. There is no prospective data on how the treatment of PVRL impacts CNS involvement and overall survival.

The IPCG reported on 83 patients with PVRL of whom 27% received focal therapy and 63%

underwent extensive systemic chemotherapy and whole brain radiotherapy [4]. Relapses in the brain occurred in 62% of patients and did not depend on the type of initial treatment. Also, there was no difference in survival. In a more recent retrospective cohort of 78 patients with PVRL seen across 17 European ophthalmologic centres, CNS lymphoma developed in 36% of the patient at a median follow-up period of 49 months [87]. Here too, there was no statistically significant difference in the risk of developing CNS disease whether patients received focal/ocular therapy, systemic therapy or both. Based on these retrospective studies and the lack of reliable predictors for CNS relapse from PVRL, patients could receive focal therapy alone, although some argue that the treatment should not differ from PCNSL. The treatment decision ultimately depends on the individual patient characteristics, presentation, comorbidities and risk of treatment-associated toxicities.

Intraocular lymphoma in conjunction with brain lymphoma is not associated with a worse prognosis according to one study, and these patients are treated similarly to PCNSL without intraocular disease [9]. In this retrospective study of 221 patients of PCNSL with intraocular involvement, 46% of patients received ocular therapy in addition to treatment for their brain lymphoma. While there was improved disease control in those that received additional ocular therapy, there was no impact on overall survival. Whether focal therapy in the form of intraocular chemotherapy or ocular radiotherapy needs to be added to systemic therapy continues to remain a matter of debate, and dedicated trials are necessary to address this issue.

17.8 Treatment of Recurrent PCNSL

Approximately 50–60% of patients with PCNSL develop recurrence of disease, and in addition to that, one third are primary refractory to first-line therapy [15, 88, 89]. Recurrent and refractory PCNSL remains a challenge due to the aggressive course of the disease and lack of optimal salvage options. Without treatment, median OS in this setting is 2 months. The majority of recurrences occur in the first 2 years of initial diagnosis. However, late relapses up to 5 and 10 years from initial diagnosis have been seen [90]. While most recurrences are restricted to the central nervous system, systemic relapses have also been seen. Limited insight into the biology of recurrent and refractory disease, lack of uniform upfront treatment, heterogeneous sites of recurrence and advancing age pose challenges to the development of randomised clinical trials.

Several retrospective studies using chemotherapy and WBRT have shown varying efficacy and outcomes. Re-challenge with HD-MTX has been studied in the retrospective setting and has been found to be quite effective with high objective response rates of 85–91% and median OS of 41–62 months [91, 92]. WBRT in the salvage setting demonstrated response rates of up to 79% with a median OS of 11–16 months [93, 94]. Other agents such as procarbazine, vincristine and lomustine, temozolomide alone or in combination with rituximab, bendamustine, cytarabine and pemetrexed have been used with reasonable response rates for all agents.

Promising results from these retrospective studies led to prospective trials with some of these agents which have been fairly disappointing with poor responses and limited durability in the responders. Single-agent temozolomide in 37 patients with recurrent and refractory PCNSL led to objective response rates of 31%, but median PFS was 2.8 months. Single-agent rituximab was found to demonstrate objective responses in 42% of patients, but again median PFS was poor and below 2 months [95]. Combination of the two agents did not seem to add to efficacy or survival in a single-arm phase 2 study [96]. Single-agent pemetrexed in a prospective trial demonstrated modest activity at 55% response rate and median PFS of 6 months [97]. The most impressive results were from a French multicentre prospective study of HDaraC and etoposide followed by thiotepa-based ASCT with a median PFS of almost 1 year and a 2-year OS of 45% [98]. The same group also reported a retrospective series of 79 patients with a median age of 52 years (range 23–67 years) in whom HDC-

ASCT resulted in durable responses with a median PFS of 18 months and 2-year OS probability of 68% [99]. However, the analysis of these 79 patients included 11 with PVRL, 11 patients with partial response to first-line and 5 with no prior therapy [99]. Promising results have been achieved as well with the "Freiburg high-dose protocol" for relapsed and refractory PCNSL in a German series [100]. However, these studies were restricted to patients under 65 years of age. While HDC-ASCT is a viable option for younger patients, the elderly are not candidates for this approach. Additionally, given that many young patients currently undergo HDC-ASCT for consolidation in the upfront setting, their options are limited upon recurrence from transplant.

Both HD-MTX and WBRT have not been studied prospectively in the recurrent and refractory setting. HD-MTX re-challenge can be considered in those who previously responded to it and developed a late recurrence after a long period of remission [50, 92]. WBRT is reasonable in patients who have previously not received it, are young with good performance status and have reasonable cognitive function and if no other salvage options exist.

17.9 Novel Agents, Experimental Therapy and Ongoing Trials

Recent insights into the biology and molecular pathogenesis of PCNSL based on comprehensive genomic analysis [101] have led to identification of potential actionable molecular targets [102, 103]. This has led to the development of several phase 1 and 2 trials in patients with recurrent and refractory PCNSL.

The first reported study of a targeted agent, temsirolimus, an mTOR (mammalian target of rapamycin) inhibitor, in a phase 2 multicentre trial demonstrated a remarkable objective response rate of 54% [10]. Unfortunately, the responses were not durable and median PFS was 2.1 months. This certainly indicates activity of mTOR inhibition in this disease but also highlights the development of resistance as commonly seen in several targeted agents. In another study, the PI3K/AKT/mTOR pathway was targeted using panPI3K inhibitor, buparlisib, with a response seen in 1 out of 4 patients [104]. A multicentre phase 1/2 study of PQR309 which is a PI3K/mTOR inhibitor is currently ongoing (NCT02669511).

Targeting TLR and BCR signalling pathway via BTK inhibition with ibrutinib has demonstrated encouraging results. A phase 1 dose-escalation study of single-agent ibrutinib resulted in an objective response rate of 77% with a median PFS of 4.6 months [105]. Dose-dependent CSF concentrations of ibrutinib were seen in patients receiving higher doses of ibrutinib (up to 840 mg oral daily dose). Initial results from a multicentre phase 2 study of ibrutinib at 560 mg daily in recurrent and refractory PCNSL and primary intraocular lymphoma have shown similar promising results with objective responses in 50% of patients within 2 months of treatment [106]. In a phase 1 study of ibrutinib in combination with chemotherapy, 83% of patients were found to have objective radiographic responses during a 2-week window period when patients were treated with single-agent ibrutinib [107]. This study was associated with a high frequency of fungal infections with aspergillus in 39% of patients. The other two single-agent ibrutinib studies have reported a lower incidence of aspergillus infections at ≤5%. It is interesting to note that the activity of BTK inhibition with ibrutinib in PCNSL is much higher than in systemic DLBCL which is low at 25% and may be explained by the high frequency of observed MYD88 L265P mutations in PCNSL. There is preclinical evidence to support synergy of mTOR/PI3K inhibition and BTK inhibition [105]. While the responses with temsirolimus and ibrutinib have been short, the ORR in both was quite high. It is possible that combination therapy as seen from excellent preclinical evidence of synergy may demonstrate durable responses, and further combination studies will be informative.

Immunomodulatory agents or IMids like lenalidomide and pomalidomide have been investigated in PCNSL, and early results seem promising. IMids likely utilise multiple mechanisms including altering the tumour microenvironment as well as stimulating NK cells and leading to T-cell expansion, in addition to inhibition of IRF4 and MYC pro-survival pathways. Rubenstein and colleagues conducted a phase 1 study of lenalidomide monotherapy and lenalidomide in combination with intraventricular and intravenous rituximab in recurrent CNS lymphoma [108]. The maximum tolerated dose of lenalidomide in this study was 15 mg/day. Additionally, the highest CSF concentrations were achieved at this dose, and dose-dependent increase in CSF drug penetration was noted. Objective responses were seen in 64% of patients receiving lenalidomide monotherapy. Elevated CSF kynurenine (metabolite via degradation of indoleamine-2,3 dioxygenase (IDO)) concentration was found to correlate with progressive disease and resistance to lenalidomide as was elevated CSF lactate, both of which could be used as biomarkers in future studies. The combination of lenalidomide and rituximab was evaluated in a French multicentre phase 2 study in 50 patients, and an objective response rate of 67% was reported with a median PFS of 8.1 months [109]. Lenalidomide maintenance is currently being evaluated as a consolidative approach in the context of randomised studies and may be a good option for consolidation particularly for elderly patients who are unable to undergo autologous transplant or whole brain radiotherapy.

Checkpoint inhibitors are also being investigated in PCNSL based on the preclinical evidence and presence of chromosomal 9p24.1/PDL1/PDL2 copy number alterations (copy gain, amplification and additional translocations) which may be the genetic basis of immune evasion in this disease. A case series of five patients with recurrent and refractory CNS lymphoma demonstrated objective responses to treatment with nivolumab [110]. There are currently ongoing clinical trials investigating the use of nivolumab (NCT02857426) and pembrolizumab (NCT02779101) in PCNSL.

The above-mentioned targeted agents seem to have evidence of clinical activity in addition to a biologic rationale in PCNSL, although mechanisms of resistance to these agents exist and combination therapies may be necessary.

17.10 Follow-Up

The International Primary Central Nervous System Lymphoma Collaborative Study Group (IPCG) recommends monitoring and follow-up of patients after completing therapy every 3 months for 2 years, every 6 months for the following 3 years and then yearly for 5 years [24]. Given that late relapses do occur beyond 5 years and can impact neurologic function, up to 10 years of follow-up is reasonable. While most patients with a recurrence will develop neurologic symptoms, asymptomatic relapses have been seen in approximately 25% of patients detected on routine imaging. Detection of asymptomatic recurrence is of great value in PCNSL so as to institute treatment before the development of neurologic deterioration. Additionally, in patients that remain progression-free and alive, there is a significant risk of delayed neurotoxicity and associated morbidity and mortality. For that reason, it is important to follow patients clinically and with imaging.

17.11 Conclusions

PCNSL is an aggressive disease with unique biologic features requiring a multidisciplinary approach. Recent progress has led to improvement in outcomes, but this is not reflected in the elderly population. Current trials are focused on optimisation of frontline treatment to improve long-term disease control reducing the risk of long-term treatment-associated neurotoxicity as well as treatment of recurrent and refractory disease. Targeted agents and immunotherapy hold promise and demand further investigation.

References

1. Hoang-Xuan K, Bessell E, Bromberg J et al (2015) Diagnosis and treatment of primary CNS lymphoma in immunocompetent patients: guidelines from the European association for neuro-oncology. Lancet Oncol 16:e322–e332
2. Korfel A, Schlegel U (2013) Diagnosis and treatment of primary CNS lymphoma. Nat Rev Neurol 9:317–327
3. Fend F, Ferreri AJ, Coupland SE (2016) How we diagnose and treat vitreoretinal lymphoma. Br J Haematol 173:680–692
4. Grimm SA, Pulido JS, Jahnke K et al (2007) Primary intraocular lymphoma: an international primary central nervous system lymphoma collaborative group report. Ann Oncol 18:1851–1855
5. Kakkassery V, Schroers R, Coupland SE et al (2017) Vitreous microRNA levels as diagnostic biomarkers for vitreoretinal lymphoma. Blood 129:3130–3133
6. Deckert M, Paulus W, Kluin PM, Ferry JA (2016) Lymphomas. In: Louis DN, Ohgaki H, Wiestler OD, Cavenee WK et al (eds) World Health Organization histological classification of tumours of the central Nervous System. IARC, Lyon, pp 272–277
7. Skiest DJ, Crosby C (2003) Survival is prolonged by highly active antiretroviral therapy in aids patients with primary central nervous system lymphoma. AIDS 17:1787–1793
8. Ferreri AJ, Blay JY, Reni M et al (2003) Prognostic scoring system for primary CNS lymphomas: the international extranodal lymphoma study group experience. J Clin Oncol 21:266–272
9. Grimm SA, McCannel CA, Omuro AM et al (2008) Primary CNS lymphoma with intraocular involvement: international PCNSL collaborative group report. Neurology 71:1355–1360
10. Korfel A, Schlegel U, Herrlinger U et al (2016) Phase II trial of temsirolimus for relapsed/refractory primary CNS lymphoma. J Clin Oncol 34:1757–1763
11. Kuker W, Nagele T, Korfel A et al (2005) Primary central nervous system lymphomas (PCNSL): MRI features at presentation in 100 patients. J Neuro-Oncol 72:169–177
12. Korfel A, Schlegel U, Johnson DR et al (2017) Case-based review: primary central nervous system lymphoma. Neuro-Oncol Pract 4:46–59
13. Kickingereder P, Wiestler B, Sahm F et al (2014) Primary central nervous system lymphoma and atypical glioblastoma: multiparametric differentiation by using diffusion-, perfusion-, and susceptibility-weighted MR imaging. Radiology 272:843–850
14. Hatzoglou V, Oh JH, Buck O et al (2018) Pretreatment dynamic contrast-enhanced MRI biomarkers correlate with progression-free survival in primary central nervous system lymphoma. J Neurooncol 140(2):351–358
15. Abrey LE, DeAngelis LM, Yahalom J (1998) Long-term survival in primary CNS lymphoma. J Clin Oncol 16:859–863
16. DeAngelis LM, Seiferheld W, Schold SC et al (2002) Combination chemotherapy radiotherapy for primary central nervous system lymphoma: Radiation Therapy Oncology Group Study 93-10. J Clin Oncol 20:4643–4648
17. Korfel A, Weller M, Martus P et al (2012) Prognostic impact of meningeal dissemination in primary CNS lymphoma (PCNSL): experience from the G-PCNSL-SG1 trial. Ann Oncol 23:2374–2380
18. Baraniskin A, Kuhnhenn J, Schlegel U et al (2011) Identification of microRNAs in the cerebrospinal

fluid as marker for primary diffuse large B-cell lymphoma of the central nervous system. Blood 117:3140–3146

19. Fischer L, Korfel A, Pfeiffer S et al (2009) CXCL13 and CXCL12 in central nervous system lymphoma patients. Clin Cancer Res 15:5968–5973

20. Rubenstein JL, Wong VS, Kadoch C et al (2013) CXCL13 plus interleukin 10 is highly specific for the diagnosis of CNS lymphoma. Blood 121:4740–4748

21. Viaccoz A, Ducray F, Tholance Y et al (2015) CSF neopterin level as a diagnostic marker in primary central nervous system lymphoma. Neuro Oncol 17:1497–1503

22. Waldera-Lupa DM, Etemad-Parishanzadeh O, Brocksieper M, Kirchgaessler N, Seidel S, Kowalski T, Montesinos-Rongen M, Deckert M, Schlegel U, Stühler K (2017) Proteomic changes in cerebrospinal fluid from primary central nervous system lymphoma patients are associated with protein ectodomain shedding. Oncotarget 8(66):110118–110132

23. Porter AB, Giannini C, Kaufmann T et al (2008) Primary central nervous system lymphoma can be histologically diagnosed after previous corticosteroid use: a pilot study to determine whether corticosteroids prevent the diagnosis of primary central nervous system lymphoma. Ann Neurol 63:662–667

24. Abrey LE, Batchelor TT, Ferreri AJ et al (2005) Report of an international workshop to standardize baseline evaluation and response criteria for primary CNS lymphoma. J Clin Oncol 23:5034–5043

25. Deckert M, Brunn A, Montesinos-Rongen M et al (2014) Primary lymphoma of the central nervous system—a diagnostic challenge. Hematol Oncol 32:57–67

26. Montesinos-Rongen M, Kuppers R, Schluter D et al (1999) Primary central nervous system lymphomas are derived from germinal-center B cells and show a preferential usage of the V4-34 gene segment. Am J Pathol 155:2077–2086

27. Montesinos-Rongen M, Godlewska E, Brunn A et al (2011) Activating L265P mutations of the MYD88 gene are common in primary central nervous system lymphoma. Acta Neuropathol 122:791–792

28. Montesinos-Rongen M, Schmitz R, Brunn A et al (2010) Mutations of CARD11 but not TNFAIP3 may activate the NF-kappaB pathway in primary CNS lymphoma. Acta Neuropathol 120:529–535

29. Montesinos-Rongen M, Schafer E, Siebert R et al (2012) Genes regulating the B cell receptor pathway are recurrently mutated in primary central nervous system lymphoma. Acta Neuropathol 124:905–906

30. Montesinos-Rongen M, Van Roost D, Schaller C et al (2004) Primary diffuse large b-cell lymphomas of the central nervous system are targeted by aberrant somatic hypermutation. Blood 103:1869–1875

31. Pels H, Montesinos-Rongen M, Schaller C et al (2004) Clonal evolution as pathogenetic mechanism in relapse of primary CNS lymphoma. Neurology 63:167–169

32. Pels H, Montesinos-Rongen M, Schaller C et al (2005) VH gene analysis of primary CNS lymphomas. J Neurol Sci 228:143–147

33. Brandt A, Matschke J, Fehrle W et al (2018) A significant proportion of patients with primary central nervous system lymphoma harbor clonal bone marrow B-cells. Leuk Lymphoma 1–7 [Epub ahead of print]

34. Thurner L, Preuss KD, Bewarder M et al (2018) Hyper N-glycosilated SAMD14 and neurabin-I as driver CNS autoantigens of PCNSL. Blood 132(26):2744–2753

35. Thiel E, Korfel A, Martus P et al (2010) High-dose methotrexate with or without whole brain radiotherapy for primary CNS lymphoma (G-PCNSL-SG-1): a phase 3, randomised, non-inferiority trial. Lancet Oncol 11:1036–1047

36. Weller M, Martus P, Roth P et al (2012) Surgery for primary CNS lymphoma? Challenging a paradigm. Neuro Oncol 14:1481–1484

37. Korfel A, Thiel E, Martus P et al (2015) Randomized phase III study of whole-brain radiotherapy for primary CNS lymphoma. Neurology 84:1242–1248

38. Pels H, Juergens A, Schirgens I et al (2010) Early complete response during chemotherapy predicts favorable outcome in patients with primary CNS lymphoma. Neuro Oncol 12:720–724

39. Lai R, Rosenblum MK, DeAngelis LM (2002) Primary CNS lymphoma: a whole-brain disease? Neurology 59:1557–1562

40. Kwak YK, Choi BO, Choi KH et al (2017) Radiotherapy as an alternative treatment option for primary central nervous system lymphoma patients who are noncandidates for chemotherapy. Oncotarget 8:106858–106865

41. Nelson DF, Martz KL, Bonner H et al (1992) Non-Hodgkin's lymphoma of the brain: can high dose, large volume radiation therapy improve survival? Report on a prospective trial by the Radiation Therapy Oncology Group (RTOG): RTOG 8315. Int J Radiat Oncol Biol Phys 23:9–17

42. Blay JY, Conroy T, Chevreau C et al (1998) High-dose methotrexate for the treatment of primary cerebral lymphomas: analysis of survival and late neurologic toxicity in a retrospective series. J Clin Oncol 16:864–871

43. Pels H, Schmidt-Wolf IG, Glasmacher A et al (2003) Primary central nervous system lymphoma: results of a pilot and phase II study of systemic and intraventricular chemotherapy with deferred radiotherapy. J Clin Oncol 21:4489–4495

44. Juergens A, Pels H, Rogowski S et al (2010) Long-term survival with favorable cognitive outcome after chemotherapy in primary central nervous system lymphoma. Ann Neurol 67:182–189

45. Rubenstein JL, Hsi ED, Johnson JL et al (2013) Intensive chemotherapy and immunotherapy in patients with newly diagnosed primary CNS lymphoma: CALGB 50202 (Alliance 50202). J Clin Oncol 3:3061–3068

46. Pulczynski EJ, Kuittinen O, Erlanson M et al (2015) Successful change of treatment strategy in elderly patients with primary central nervous system lymphoma by de-escalating induction and introducing temozolomide maintenance: results from a phase II study by the Nordic Lymphoma Group. Haematologica 100:534–540

47. Hoang-Xuan K, Taillandier L, Chinot O et al (2003) Chemotherapy alone as initial treatment for primary CNS lymphoma in patients older than 60 years: a multicenter phase II study (26952) of the European organization for research and treatment of cancer brain tumor group. J Clin Oncol 21:2726–2731

48. Omuro A, Chinot O, Taillandier L et al (2015) Methotrexate and temozolomide versus methotrexate, procarbazine, vincristine, and cytarabine for primary CNS lymphoma in an elderly population: an intergroup anocef-goelams randomised phase 2 trial. Lancet Haematol 2:e251–e259

49. Fritsch K, Kasenda B, Schorb E et al (2017) High-dose methotrexate-based immuno-chemotherapy for elderly primary CNS lymphoma patients (PRIMAIN study). Leukemia 31:846–852

50. Poortmans PM, Kluin-Nelemans HC, Haaxma-Reiche H et al (2003) High-dose methotrexate-based chemotherapy followed by consolidating radiotherapy in non-AIDS-related primary central nervous system lymphoma: European Organization for Research and Treatment of Cancer Lymphoma Group Phase II Trial 20962. J Clin Oncol 21:4483–4488

51. Korfel A, Martus P, Nowrousian MR, Hossfeld DK, Kirchen H, Brucher J et al (2005) Response to chemotherapy and treating institution predict survival in primary central nervous system lymphoma. Br J Haematol 128:177–183

52. Ferreri AJ, Reni M, Foppoli M et al (2009) High-dose cytarabine plus high-dose methotrexate versus high-dose methotrexate alone in patients with primary CNS lymphoma: a randomised phase 2 trial. Lancet 374:1512–1520

53. Morris PG, Correa DD, Yahalom J et al (2013) Rituximab, methotrexate, procarbazine, and vincristine followed by consolidation reduced-dose whole-brain radiotherapy and cytarabine in newly diagnosed primary CNS lymphoma: final results and long-term outcome. J Clin Oncol 31:3971–3979

54. Glass J, Won M, Schultz CJ et al (2016) Phase I and II study of induction chemotherapy with methotrexate, rituximab, and temozolomide, followed by whole-brain radiotherapy and postirradiation temozolomide for primary CNS lymphoma: NRG Oncology RTOG 0227. J Clin Oncol 34:1620–1625

55. Illerhaus G, Marks R, Ihorst G et al (2006) High-dose chemotherapy with autologous stem-cell transplantation and hyperfractionated radiotherapy as first-line treatment of primary CNS lymphoma. J Clin Oncol 24:3865–3870

56. Kasenda B, Schorb E, Fritsch K et al (2012) Prognosis after high-dose chemotherapy followed by autologous stem-cell transplantation as first-line treatment in primary CNS lymphoma—a long-term follow-up study. Ann Oncol 23:2670–2675

57. Omuro AM, Correa DD, DeAngelis LM et al (2015) R-MPV followed by high-dose chemotherapy with TBC and autologous stem-cell transplant for newly diagnosed primary CNS lymphoma. Blood 125:1403–1410

58. Illerhaus G, Kasenda B, Ihorst G et al (2016) High-dose chemotherapy with autologous haemopoietic stem cell transplantation for newly diagnosed primary CNS lymphoma: a prospective, single-arm, phase 2 trial. Lancet Haematol 3:e388–e397

59. Ferreri AJ, Cwynarski K, Pulczynski E et al (2016) Chemoimmunotherapy with methotrexate, cytarabine, thiotepa, and rituximab (matrix regimen) in patients with primary CNS lymphoma: results of the first randomisation of the international extranodal lymphoma study group-32 (IELSG32) phase 2 trial. Lancet Haematol 3:e217–e227

60. Ferreri AJ, Cwynarski K, Pulczynski E et al (2017) Whole-brain radiotherapy or autologous stem-cell transplantation as consolidation strategies after high-dose methotrexate-based chemoimmunotherapy in patients with primary CNS lymphoma: results of the second randomisation of the International Extranodal Lymphoma Study Group-32 phase 2 trial. Lancet Haematol 11:e510–e523

61. Schlegel U, Korfel A (2018) Is whole-brain radiotherapy (WBRT) still a standard treatment for primary central nervous system lymphomas (PCNSL)? Curr Treat Neurol

62. Ferreri AJ, Reni M, Pasini F et al (2002) A multicenter study of treatment of primary CNS lymphoma. Neurology 58:1513–1520

63. Lai R, Abrey LE, Rosenblum MK et al (2004) Treatment-induced leukoencephalopathy in primary CNS lymphoma. Neurology 62:451–456

64. Correa DD, Maron L, Harder H et al (2007) Cognitive functions in primary central nervous system lymphoma. Literature review and assessment guidelines. Ann Oncol 18:1145–1151

65. Omuro AM, Ben-Porat LS, Panageas KS et al (2005) Delayed neurotoxicity in primary central nervous system lymphoma. Arch Neurol 62:1595–1600

66. Doolittle ND, Korfel A, Lubow M et al (2013) Long-term cognitive function, neuroimaging and quality of life in primary CNS lymphoma. Neurology 81:84–92

67. Harder H, Holtel H, Bromberg JE et al (2004) Cognitive status and quality of life after treatment for primary CNS lymphoma. Neurology 62:544–547

68. Wagner H, Ali A, Glantz M et al (2017) Role of hippocampal-avoidance whole brain radiation therapy (HA-WBRT) in patients with primary CNS lymphoma (PCNSL). Int J Radiat Oncol Biol Phys 99(2 Suppl):E424

69. Ferreri AJ, Illerhaus G (2016) The role of autologous stem cell transplantation in primary central nervous system lymphoma. Blood 127:13

70. Kasenda B, Loeffler J, Illerhaus G et al (2016) The role of whole brain radiation in primary CNS lymphoma. Blood 128:32–36

71. Batchelor T, Carson K, O'Neill A et al (2003) Treatment of primary CNS lymphoma with methotrexate and deferred radiotherapy: a report of NABTT 96-07. J Clin Oncol 21:1044–1049

72. Herrlinger U, Küker W, Uhl M et al (2005) NOA-03 trial of high-dose methotrexate in primary central nervous system lymphoma: final report. Ann Neurol 57:843–884

73. Bergner N, Monsef I, Illerhaus G et al (2012) Role of chemotherapy additional to high-dose methotrexate for primary central nervous system lymphoma (PCNSL). Cochrane Database Syst Rev 11:CD009355

74. Houillier C, Taillandier L, Lamy T et al (2016) Whole Brain Radiotherapy (WBRT) versus intensive chemotherapy with haematopoietic stem cell rescue (IC + HCR) for primary central nervous system lymphoma (PCNSL) in young patients: an intergroup anocef-goelams randomized phase II trial (PRECIS). Blood 128:782

75. Pels H, Juergens A, Glasmacher A et al (2009) Early relapses in primary CNS lymphoma after response to polychemotherapy without intraventricular treatment: results of a phase II study. J Neuro-Oncol 91:299–305

76. Correa DD, Shi W, Abrey LE et al (2012) Cognitive functions in primary CNS lymphoma after single or combined modality regimens. Neuro Oncol 14:101–108

77. Mendez JS, Ostrom QT, Gittleman H et al (2018) The elderly left behind changes in survival trends of primary central nervous system lymphoma over the past 4 decades. Neuro Oncol 20:687–694

78. Kasenda B, Ferreri AJ, Marturano E et al (2015) First-line treatment and outcome of elderly patients with primary central nervous system lymphoma (PCNSL)—a systematic review and individual patient data meta-analysis. Ann Oncol 26(7):1305–1313

79. Welch MR, Omuro A, DeAngelis LM (2012) Outcomes of the oldest patients with primary CNS lymphoma treated at Memorial Sloan-Kettering Cancer Center. Neuro Oncol 14(10):1304–1311

80. Schorb E, Fox CP, Fritsch K et al (2017) High-dose thiotepa-based chemotherapy with autologous stem cell support in elderly patients with primary central nervous system lymphoma: a European retrospective study. Bone Marrow Transplant 52(8):1113–1119

81. Gonzalez-Aguilar A, Soto-Hernandez JL (2011) The management of primary central nervous system lymphoma related to AIDS in the HAART era. Curr Opin Oncol 23(6):648–653

82. O'Neill A, Mikesch A, Fritsch K et al (2015) Outcomes for HIV-positive patients with primary central nervous system lymphoma after high-dose chemotherapy and auto-SCT. Bone Marrow Transplant 50(7):999–1000

83. Wieters I, Atta J, Kann G et al (2014) Autologous stem cell transplantation in HIV-related lymphoma in the rituximab era—a feasibility study in a monocentric cohort. J Int AIDS Soc 17:19648

84. Castenello-Sanchez AA, Li S, Qian J et al (2004) Primary central nervous system posttransplant lymphoproliferative disorders. Am J Clin Pathol 121(2):246–253

85. Kempf C, Tinguely M, Rishing EJ (2013) Posttransplant lymphoproliferative disorder of the central nervous system. Pathobiology 80(6):310–318

86. Evens AM, Choquet S, Krol-Desrosiers AR et al (2013) Primary CNS posttransplant lymphoproliferative disease (PTLD): an international report of 84 cases in the modern era. Am J Transplant 13(6):1512–1522

87. Riemens A, Bromberg J, Touitou V et al (2015) Treatment strategies in primary vitreoretinal lymphoma: a 17-center European collaborative study. JAMA Ophthalmol 133:191–197

88. Jahnke K, Thiel E, Martus P et al (2006) Relapse of primary central nervous system lymphoma: clinical features, outcome and prognostic factors. J Neurooncol. 80(2):159–165

89. Langner-Lemercier S, Houillier C, Soussain C et al (2016) Primary CNS lymphoma at first relapse/progression: characteristics, management, and outcome of 256 patients from the French LOC network. Neuro Oncol [Internet] 18(9):1297–1303

90. Nayak L, Hedvat C, Rosenblum MK, Abrey LE, DeAngelis LM (2011) Late relapse in primary central nervous system lymphoma: clonal persistence. Neuro Oncol 13(5):525–529

91. Pentsova E, Deangelis LM, Omuro A (2014) Methotrexate re-challenge for recurrent primary central nervous system lymphoma. J Neuro-Oncol 117:161–165

92. Plotkin SR, Betensky RA, Hochberg FH et al (2004) Treatment of relapsed central nervous system lymphoma with high-dose methotrexate. Clin Cancer Res 10:5643–5646

93. Hottinger AF, DeAngelis LM, Yahalom J et al (2007) Salvage whole brain radiotherapy for recurrent or refractory primary CNS lymphoma. Neurology 69:1178–1182

94. Nguyen PL, Chakravarti A, Finkelstein DM et al (2005) Results of whole-brain radiation as salvage of methotrexate failure for immunocompetent patients with primary CNS lymphoma. J Clin Oncol 23:1507–1513

95. Batchelor TT, Grossman SA, Mikkelsen T et al (2011) Rituximab monotherapy for patients with recurrent primary CNS lymphoma. Neurology 76(10):929–930

96. Nayak L, Abrey LE, Drappatz J et al (2013) Multicenter phase II study of rituximab and temozolomide in recurrent primary central nervous system lymphoma. Leuk Lymphoma 54:58–61

97. Raizer JJ, Rademaker A, Evens AM et al (2012) Pemetrexed in the treatment of relapsed/refractory

primary central nervous system lymphoma. Cancer 118(15):3743–3748

98. Soussain C, Hoang-Xuan K, Taillandier L et al (2008) Intensive chemotherapy followed by hematopoietic stem-cell rescue for refractory and recurrent primary CNS and intraocular lymphoma: Societe Française de Greffe de Moelle Osseuse-Therapie Cellulaire. J Clin Oncol 26(15):2512–2518

99. Soussain C, Choquet S, Fourme E et al (2012) Intensive chemotherapy with thiotepa, busulfan and cyclophosphamide and hematopoietic stem cell rescue in relapsed or refractory primary central nervous system lymphoma and intraocular lymphoma: a retrospective study of 79 cases. Haematologica 97:1751–1756

100. Kasenda B, Ihorst G, Schroers R et al (2017) High-dose chemotherapy with autologous haematopoietic stem cell support for relapsed or refractory primary CNS lymphoma: a prospective multicentre trial by the German cooperative PCNSL study group. Leukemia 31:2623–2629

101. Vater I, Montesinos-Rongen M, Schlesner M et al (2015) The mutational pattern of primary lymphoma of the central nervous system determined by whole-exome sequencing. Leukemia 29:677–685

102. Illerhaus G, Schorb E, Kasenda B (2018) Novel agents for primary central nervous system lymphoma: evidence and perspectives. Blood 132:681–688

103. Mendez JS, Grommes C (2018) Treatment of primary central nervous system lymphoma: from chemotherapy to small molecules. Am Soc Clin Oncol Educ Book 38:604–615

104. Grommes C, Pentsova E, Nolan C et al (2016) Phase II study of single agent buparlisib in recurrent/refractory primary (PCNSL) and secondary CNS lymphoma (SCNSL). Ann Oncol 27; abstract

105. Grommes S, Pastore A, Palaskas N et al (2017) Ibrutinib unmasks critical role of bruton tyrosine kinase in primary CNS lymphoma. Cancer Discov 7:1018–1029

106. Choquet S, Bijou F, Houot R et al (2016) Ibrutinib monotherapy in relapse or refractory primary CNS lymphoma (PCNSL) and primary vitreo-retinal lymphoma (PVRL). Result of the interim analysis of the iLOC phase II study from the Lysa and the French LOC network. Blood 128:784; abstract.

107. Lionakis MS, Dunleavy K, Roschewski M et al (2017) Inhibition of B cell receptor signaling by ibrutinib in primary CNS lymphoma. Cancer Cell 31(6):833–843

108. Rubenstein JL, Geng H, Fraser EJ et al (2018) Phase 1 investigation of lenalidomide/rituximab and outcomes of lenalidomide as maintenance in relapsed CNS lymphoma. Blood Adv 2:1595–1607

109. Ghesquieres H, Houillier C, Chinot O et al (2016) Rituximab-lenalidomide (REVRI) in relapse or refractory primary central nervous system (PCNSL) or vitreo retinal lymphoma (PVRL): results of a "proof of concept" phase II study of the French LOC network. Blood 128:785; abstract.

110. Nayak L, Iwamoto FM, LaCasce A et al (2017) Pd-1 blockade with nivolumab in relapsed/refractory primary central nervous system and testicular lymphoma. Blood 129:3071–3073

Brain Metastases and Leptomeningeal Metastases

18

Lynn Mubita, Ian Lee, Mira Shah, Emilie Le Rhun, and Steven Kalkanis

18.1 Introduction

Cancer remains the second leading cause of death in the United States. Each year, 23,800 new cases of metastatic cancer to the central nervous system are diagnosed [1]. These numbers are expected to rise in part due to the aging population, earlier diagnoses, and more effective treatment strategies. Ten times more common than primary brain tumors, central nervous system metastases pose a serious and significant complication of cancer as they can impair quality of life by causing neurological dysfunction. Presenting symptoms range from headache to seizures to focal deficits such as hemiparesis, aphasia, or hemianopia. When brain metastases are not treated, they lead to progressive neurological decline and eventual death. Similar to evolution of metastases in other parts of the body, brain metastases share early cellular sequences of events that lead to their formation, such as mutations that facilitate cellular detachment from basement membranes, intravasation, and endothelial adhesion. Brain metastases are most frequently located in the cerebral hemispheres, followed by the cerebellum and, lastly, in the brain stem, likely due to differing proportions of blood flow. However, there are certain types of cancers which tend to metastasize to specific organs preferentially. This "seed and soil" theory was initially proposed by Stephen Paget in 1889. For example, malignancies such as melanoma and small cell lung cancer have a disproportionately high metastatic rate to the brain [2].

In adults, the most common sources of brain metastases in order of decreasing frequency include lung carcinoma, breast carcinoma, melanoma, renal carcinoma, gastrointestinal carcinoma, thyroid carcinoma, lymphoma, and unknown primary carcinoma [2] (Table 18.1). The optimal treatment for patients with metastatic cancer to the brain remains controversial. Treatment options are chosen based on prognostic factors such as number and presentation of metastases to the brain, performance status of the patient, molecular status of the primary disease, previous treatment, and clinical judgment. This chapter explores the current consensus on the management and treatment of brain metastases and of leptomeningeal metastases.

L. Mubita · I. Lee · S. Kalkanis (✉)
Department of Neurosurgery, Henry Ford Health System, Detroit, MI, USA
e-mail: ilee1@hfhs.org; skalkan1@hfhs.org

M. Shah
Department of Radiation Oncology, Henry Ford Health System, Detroit, MI, USA
e-mail: MSHAH6@hfhs.org

E. Le Rhun
Univ. Lille, U-1192, Lille, France

Inserm, U-1192, Lille, France

Neuro-oncology, Neurosurgery Department, CHU Lille, Lille, France

Neurology, Breast Cancer Department, Oscar Lambret Center, Lille, France

© Springer Nature Switzerland AG 2019
J.-C. Tonn et al. (eds.), *Oncology of CNS Tumors*, https://doi.org/10.1007/978-3-030-04152-6_18

Table 18.1 Primary sites of origin in brain metastases

Site of Origin (in %)	Barnholtz-Sloan et al. [3]	Schouten el al. [4]	Fabi et al. [5]	Stark et al. [6]	Lagerwaard et al. [7]
Lung	19.90	16.3	44	50	56
Melanoma	6.90	7.4	6	7	–
Renal	6.5	9.8	–	–	4
Breast	5.1	5	30	15	16
Colorectal	1.8	1.2	9	8	–

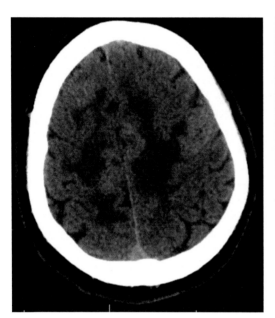

Fig. 18.1 Non-contrast CT scan of the brain showing cerebral edema associated with brain metastases

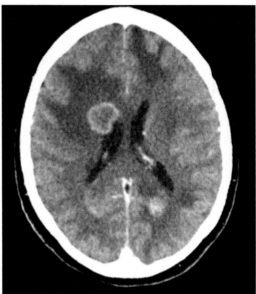

Fig. 18.2 Post-Contrast CT head of brain showing ring enhancing brain metastasis

18.2 Imaging Findings

Imaging is essential in the diagnosis and eventual treatment of patients with brain metastases. Patients who present with new neurological symptoms may be diagnosed initially with brain computed tomography (CT) or magnetic resonance imaging (MRI). CT is often the initial imaging modality used to identify brain metastases, but MRI is the imaging modality of choice to determine further treatment. Brain metastases on CT may appear as single or multiple lesions, surrounded by varying amounts of vasogenic edema (Fig. 18.1). These lesions may range in signal characteristics from hypodense to hyperdense and may have varying degrees of hemorrhage/hyperdensity within them. CT is often used as a screening tool in the diagnosis of brain metasta-

ses and can be followed by a gadolinium-enhanced magnetic resonance imaging (MRI) study, depending on the patient's clinical stability. CT with contrast may suffice for the patient that is not clinically stable to tolerate lying flat for an MRI, the imaging modality of choice, which typically takes between 30 min to an hour. It can demonstrate ring, nodular, or solid enhancement (Fig. 18.2). MRI usually demonstrates iso- to hypointense signal on T1-weighted imaging, as well as hyperintense signal on T2-weighted imaging, with contrast enhancement (Fig. 18.3). Once a diagnosis is solidified, advanced MRI techniques may be used for staging purposes as well as for surgical planning. Such techniques include MR spectroscopy, MR perfusion, diffusion tensor imaging, and functional MRI, among others. Then, treatment strategies are chosen.

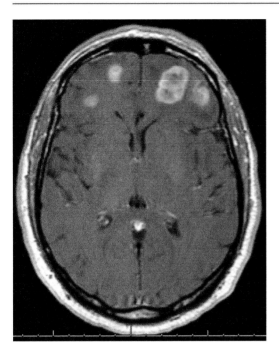

Fig. 18.3 Post-gadolinium T1 weighted MRI brain showing multiple metastatic tumors

18.3 Treatment Strategies

The development of brain metastasis in a patient with systemic cancer represents a poor prognosis. Decision for a particular treatment is based on prognostic factors such as number of metastases to the brain, location of the metastases, size and presentation of the metastases, performance status of the patient, molecular status of the primary disease previous treatment, and clinical judgment. They can broadly be divided into two categories—symptomatic or supportive care and therapeutic treatment.

18.3.1 Symptomatic/Supportive Care

Clinically, symptoms from brain metastases arise due to increased intracranial pressure or from mass effect in eloquent areas. These symptoms can be very generalized in the form of headaches and changes in mental status ranging from lethargy to coma or with focal signs such as hemiparesis or aphasias. The goal of symptomatic/supportive care is to ease the burden of symptoms in patients. Reasons for choosing symptomatic/supportive care may vary from disease burden, poor performance status, and poor prognosis to multifocal lesions involving eloquent brain, which would result in significant morbidity with other treatment strategies.

Control of edema and mass effect is commonly achieved with steroids. Steroids stabilize the tumor vasculature, which has increased permeability relative to normal brain parenchyma, thus decreasing the edema in the tumor and surrounding parenchyma. By doing so, symptoms related to mass effect, such as headache, nausea, and altered mental status, can be relieved. In addition, chemotherapeutic agents, which can be used palliatively, often rely on hydrostatic pressure to penetrate brain parenchyma and might be able to better penetrate areas with tumor infiltration. Dexamethasone, which has low mineralocorticoid activity, is frequently used. In periods over 6 weeks, patients may be subject to various side effects including decreased immune function and susceptibility to opportunistic infections, gastrointestinal dyspepsia or reflux, steroid myopathy, changes in mood, difficulty in sleeping/insomnia, and/or serum glucose derangements in patients with diabetes. Prophylaxis with Bactrim, use of proton pump inhibitors, and limiting steroid use duration and dosage may help curb these side effects. It is advisable to keep the dosage to the lowest possible amount that will treat the symptoms without causing too many side effects. Many physicians utilize a slow taper to achieve this, which also minimizes the possibility of rebound edema. In patients with acute rises in intracranial pressure and pending herniation, hypertonic saline and/or mannitol may be used in short courses [3].

Seizure control is achieved with antiepileptic drugs. Most physicians do not prophylactically prescribe antiepileptic drugs in patients who do not already have seizures, as the rates of seizures are not decreased and the side effects may cause more harm than benefit [4]. Some physicians will prescribe antiepileptics only in the perioperative period with a plan to taper the medication off after surgery. In the small subset of patients that do have seizures in the immediate postoperative period, seizures can be attributed to temporarily lowered seizure thresholds from cortical irritation during surgery, and most will recover. Of the patients diagnosed with brain metastases, 20% have seizures as their presenting symptom. Most commonly, physicians prescribe phenytoin as a first-line agent for treatment of their seizures. These have the unfortunate side effect of upregulating the hepatic cytochrome P450 system and may lead to adverse side effects with other medications. There are newer agents, such as levetiracetam and topiramate, which do not upregulate this hepatic microsomal system that may be used.

Symptomatic/supportive care also includes providing support and access for challenges posed by new neurological deficits. Patients may have severely decreased level of function with paresis or plegia requiring physical and/or occupational therapy. Assistive devices such as mechanical wheelchairs and walkers may be necessary. In patients who require straight catheterization, supplies must be provided and nursing care available.

18.3.2 Therapeutic Treatment

The main aim of therapeutic treatment is to decrease disease burden with a goal to control disease, increase survival and improve quality of life. Therapeutic treatment options include surgical resection, chemotherapy, and radiation (including whole brain and/or stereotactic radiosurgery). These options may be used alone or in combination. Various methods have been published in an effort to determine what the most optimal treatment strategy is for individual patients. One such method, which is frequently used, was established in 1997 by the Radiation Therapy Oncology Group, RTOG (Table 18.1). This method classifies patients with brain metastases into three groups according to prognostic factors such as age and Karnofsky Performance Status, identified by recursive partitioning analysis, RPA [5]. Another method, the Graded Prognostic Assessment (GPA), is a more objective measure in patients with brain metastases [6]

and has been developed using molecular markers for different primaries (mol-GPA) [7, 8].

18.4 Surgery

Surgical resection provides an opportunity to immediately improve neurological function due to removal of mass effect, thus potentially improving quality of life. In addition, surgery allows for histological tissue diagnosis when the diagnosis is unknown or for validation of molecular biomarkers. Due to advances in surgical technique, including image-guided resection with improved localization, surgical morbidity and mortality have improved significantly [3]. This is even more significant in large hospitals that have high volume in surgery, with one study quoting 1.8% mortality compared to 4.4% in smaller hospitals [9].

Generally, surgery is a reasonable first treatment option in a patient with good performance status who has a single metastasis. This comes from the results of two, groundbreaking, prospective randomized clinical trials. In these studies, patients with good functional status and a single brain metastasis were randomized to receive either needle biopsy of the metastasis followed by whole brain radiation or surgical resection followed by whole brain radiation. Patients in the surgery and whole brain radiation group had fewer local recurrences, improved survival, and improved Karnofsky Performance Status (KPS) than patients who received whole brain radiation alone [10, 11]. Surgery should therefore be undertaken with the goal of complete cytoreduction, which may improve survival when combined with other treatment strategies. In patients with active systemic disease and low performance status, surgery does not provide as much benefit as these results have not been duplicated when the criteria are expanded to include patients with lower Karnofsky Performance Status [12].

A meta-analysis published by the Cochrane Collaboration showed that surgical resection improved functionally independent survival, but did not statistically improve overall survival [13]. However, each included study had small numbers of participants and highly selected patient populations limiting the generalizability of these results.

In patients who have multiple brain metastases, the decision-making is more complex. Studies in the literature comparing the effects of surgery in patients with multiple metastases with or without whole brain radiation are conflicting [14]. More recent studies show that surgical resection may be a reasonable option in patients with multiple metastases who have good performance status [15, 16]. Broadly speaking, the role of surgery in patients with multiple metastasis is limited to resection of the largest lesion if it is life threatening and also to establish a histological tissue diagnosis.

18.5 Systemic Therapy

Chemotherapy is generally regarded as a last-line treatment choice for brain metastasis and is often used in patients who have failed other treatment strategies. Brain metastases often develop in patients in the later stages of their disease course. As such, various treatments of the primary tumor, including chemotherapy, have already been attempted, and the tumors may be resistant to chemotherapy. Unique to the central nervous system is the presence of the blood-brain barrier, although commonly disrupted in brain metastases, which provides a formidable barricade to the penetration of most chemotherapeutic agents into the brain, with the presence of endothelial tight junctions. In addition, active pumps such as the multidrug resistance protein actively remove drugs from within the blood-brain barrier.

In a select few patients with brain metastasis, diagnosis is made after screening imaging is performed for other reasons (except for small cell lung cancer, where screening for brain metastases is routinely performed). These patients may not be symptomatic from their metastasis, and chemotherapy, targeted therapy, or immunotherapy may be used primary to treat the primary cancer with the added benefit of treating the metastasis.

Some chemotherapy regimens have shown activity against a select few histopathologies,

with promise in crossing the blood-brain barrier. For example, brain metastases from non-small cell lung carcinoma have responded to platinum-based therapy with and/or without temozolomide and tyrosine kinase inhibitors, as these cross the blood-brain barrier in significant amounts. Brain metastases from breast cancer have response rates varying from 30 to 60%, particularly with chemotherapy regimens that include cyclophosphamide and methotrexate. Capecitabine and gemcitabine have shown activity as well. Germ cell tumors and non-Hodgkin's lymphoma when metastasized to the brain are preferentially treated with chemotherapy.

Research is currently being done to explore the relationship to certain drugs that, when given with radiation, act as radiation sensitizers [18]. Efaproxiral is a synthetic modifier of hemoglobin that, when given in combination with whole brain radiation therapy, significantly improves response rates for non-small cell lung carcinoma and breast cancer. It does not, however, improve survival [17]. Another compound, motexafin gadolinium, was studied in 401 patients. Despite not improving overall survival in patients when given in combination with whole brain radiation, in a subset of patients who had non-small cell lung carcinoma, neurological function was improved [18].

Another active area of research involves targeted molecular agents. For example, gefitinib, which is an oral tyrosine kinase inhibitor of the epidermal growth factor receptor, is effective against certain subtypes of non-small cell lung carcinoma. A prospective trial showed that gefitinib controlled brain metastases in 27% of patients by a median duration of 4 months [19]. In mice models of human breast tumors, genetically engineered oncolytic viruses are administered via carotid injection, with results showing survival benefit in those mice [20].

Up to half of melanomas contain a BRAF mutation, most commonly V600E (80%) and V600K (14%), which represent single point mutations replacing valine with glutamate or lysine, respectively [21]. Melanoma cells with these mutations have ongoing kinase activity and uncontrolled cell growth. Metastatic melanoma models showed that suppression of these mutations slowed tumor growth, making BRAF a logical target for potential chemotherapeutic treatment. One such drug, vemurafenib, was the first BRAF inhibitor to be approved by the FDA (Food and Drug Administration) and showed promise in a phase 3 randomized clinical trial in which 675 patients with untreated metastatic melanoma had improved response rates and 6-month overall survival compared to standard of care chemotherapy with dacarbazine [22]. Combinations of targeted agents and immunotherapy represent potential new inter-

esting therapeutic options, but only preliminary results are available Overall, due to these encouraging results, multiple clinical trials for a variety of histologies are ongoing (Table 18.2).

18.6 Radiation Therapy

18.6.1 Whole Brain Radiation

Whole brain radiation has been the favored treatment in patients who have multiple brain metasta-

Table 18.2 Active chemotherapy trials for brain metastases

Primary Site	Chemotherapy agent	Clinicaltrials.gov Identifier
All	Ceritinib	NCT02605746
All	Nivolumab	NCT02978404
All	Palbociclib	NCT02896335
All	Pembrolizumab	NCT02886585
All	Ropidoxuridine	NCT02993146
All	Sunitinib	NCT00981890
Breast	Atezolizumab	NCT03483012
Breast	Cabozantinib, Trastuzumab	NCT02260531
Breast	Cisplatin, Veliparib	NCT02595905
Breast	Eribulin Mesylate	NCT02581839, NCT03412955
Breast	Etirinotecan	NCT02915744
Breast	Irinotecan	NCT03328884
Breast	Lapatinib	NCT01622868
Breast	Palbociclib	NCT02774681
Breast	T-DM1, Temozolomide	NCT03190967
Breast	Tucatinib, Capecitabine, Trastuzumab	NCT02614794
Breast, NSCLC, Melanoma	Abemaciclib	NCT02308020
Lung, Breast	Afatinib	NCT02768337
Lung, Breast	Etirinotecan	NCT02312622
Lung, Neuroendocrine	VX-970	NCT02589522
Melanoma	Bevacizumab, Atezolizumab	NCT03175432
Melanoma	Buparlisib	NCT02452294
Melanoma	Dabrafenib, Trametinib	NCT02974803
Melanoma	Fotemustine, Ipilimumab, Nivolumab	NCT02460068
Melanoma	Nivolumab, Ipilimumab	NCT02621515
Melanoma	Vemurafenib, Cobimetinib	NCT03430947
Melanoma, NSCLC	Pembrolizumab, Bevacizumab	NCT02681549
NSCLC	Alectinib, Bevacizumab	NCT02521051
NSCLC	AZD9291	NCT02736513, NCT03257124
NSCLC	Bevacizumab, Erlotinib	NCT02655536
NSCLC	Cabozantinib	NCT02132598
NSCLC	EGFR-TKI	NCT02714010
NSCLC	Gefitinib, Pemetrexed/Cisplatin	NCT01951469
NSCLC	Nivolumab	NCT02696993
NSCLC	Osimertinib, Bevacizumab	NCT02971501
NSCLC	Pembrolizumab	NCT02858869
Solid Tumor	LY3381916	NCT03343613
Solid Tumor	Meclofenamate	NCT02429570

ses. It provides relief of symptoms in 75–80% of patients with brain metastases [23]. The treatment paradigm involves a total of dose of 30 Gy, usually given over ten fractions. Whole brain radiation therapy alone gives patients an overall median survival of 3–5 months, depending upon RPA class [24]. In the RPA classification scheme, class II and III patients (who have low Karnofsky Performance Status and poorly controlled systemic disease) would receive palliative whole brain radiation. Additionally, symptomatic leptomeningeal carcinomatosis is best treated with whole brain radiation. Yet, overall the role of WBRT is limited in leptomeningeal metastases, as no survival benefit has been demonstrated in retrospective cohorts of patients, and WBRT should be limited to extensive nodular disease or symptomatic linear leptomeningeal metastases [25].

There have been a few studies that compared WBRT with supportive care. In one study, median survival was reported as higher in the group that received whole brain radiation [23]. In a more contemporary multi-institutional trial comparing dexamethasone and supportive care with and without WBRT, little difference was seen in the two treatment groups, leading to the conclusion that the WBRT added little benefit [26]. However, when whole brain radiation was compared to surgery alone, the addition of whole brain radiation led to reduction in recurrence rate and death due to neurological reasons, but did not increase overall survival [27].

As mentioned previously, newer studies are in place to analyze the effect of radiosensitizing agents such as gemcitabine [28], but results have been conflicting. ENRICH (Enhancing Whole Brain Radiation Therapy In Patients With Breast Cancer and Hypoxic Brain Metastasis) is a phase III trial of efaproxiral which is ongoing. Celecoxib is currently being studied [29].

Side effects of whole brain radiation can be divided into short and long term. Short-term effects include hair loss, xerostomia, altered taste, nausea, and fatigue. Long-term effects include cognitive decline ranging from memory impairment to depression, hydrocephalus, and neuroendocrine dysfunction [30]. The standard dose paradigm which limits daily radiation to 3 Gy attempts to minimize these side effects.

Prophylactic whole brain radiation has been used in clinical trials, particularly in patients with non-small cell lung carcinoma, who have a very high incidence of brain metastatic recurrence [27]. Current therapy for small cell carcinoma involves chemotherapy, radiation, and surgery, which is not enough to treat brain metastatic recurrences. In patients who received prophylactic whole brain radiation, studies have shown a decreased incidence of metastatic recurrence [31, 32]. An ongoing phase III clinical trial comparing prophylactic whole brain radiation to observation, however, did not show any survival advantage [33].

18.6.2 Stereotactic Radiosurgery (SRS)

Stereotactic radiosurgery is a very accurate radiation therapy technique that uses multiple convergent beams of radiation to treat a discrete lesion in most often a single dose; these treatments are also fractionated at times depending on size and location to critical structures and local edema. Stereotactic radiosurgery techniques produce a steep dose fall around the target, thereby limiting radiation to normal tissue. Doses may vary from 15 to 24 Gy and more than one lesion may be treated at a time. The maximum tolerated dose is inversely proportionate to the size of the lesion. Therefore, as the tumor size increases, the maximum tolerated dose decreases. Thus, stereotactic radiosurgery is advised for lesions that are 3–4 cm or less. Stereotactic radiosurgery utilizes relatively higher doses of radiation in a single treatment compared to whole brain radiation. Thus, the risk of radiation necrosis is increased with radiosurgery when compared to whole brain radiation therapy. This risk increases in patients who have already received whole brain radiation prior to receiving stereotactic radiosurgery. Radiation necrosis can be difficult to distinguish from tumor recurrence and often requires long-term medical treatment, with steroids, for example. Various radiological studies, such as diffusion-weighted MRI or PET scans, can be used to differentiate between the two.

Although the various treatment modalities are complementary, stereotactic radiosurgery has the advantage, compared to surgical resection and chemotherapy, of being less invasive and being able to treat multiple lesions in one setting. It can therefore be done on an outpatient basis with minimal to no recovery time, making it ideal for patients.

In patients who have deep-seated lesions, or lesions in eloquent areas that may pose significant morbidity for surgical resection, stereotactic radiosurgery may be considered an alternative to surgery. Retrospective studies in the literature show that these two treatment modalities are similar; however, stereotactic radiosurgery has been shown to only increase survival when coupled with WBRT [34]; there is an advantage to SRS regarding cognitive decline. As with surgical resection, patient selection is critical, as those with poor performance status are less likely to have good outcomes.

A study performed at Mayo Clinic compared patients treated with surgery to those treated with stereotactic radiosurgery. One year survival was 56% in the stereotactic radiosurgery group and 62% in the surgery group, with local control being better in the stereotactic radiosurgery group compared to the surgery group as judged by lack of recurrence in the stereotactic radiosurgery compared to 58% in the surgery group [35].

Interstitial brachytherapy involves the placement of radioactive material into the wall of a surgical cavity to deliver doses of radiation to any residual tumor left after surgery. Currently, this is experimental treatment. GliaSite is one such delivery system that utilizes an inflatable balloon catheter [36].

Symptoms present as a result of obstruction of normal CSF flow or by direct tumor invasion. Typical symptoms and signs include headache, nausea, vomiting, cranial nerve deficits, gait disorders, sensorimotor deficits, cauda equina syndrome, and back pain. Whole neuraxis gadolinium-enhanced MRI is recommended for screening [25]. The identification of tumor cells in the cerebrospinal fluid confirms the diagnosis. Positive cytology is seen in 50–70% of specimens on the first lumbar puncture, with most diagnoses being made on the third attempt [38]. The prognosis of leptomeningeal metastasis is dire, with median survival of 4 months [39]. Therapeutic options include combination of systemic pharmacotherapy based on molecular profile, intra-cerebrospinal fluid therapy, and focal radiation. Intra-cerebrospinal fluid therapy can be administered via lumbar puncture or via a ventricular device. Most common therapeutic agents include methotrexate and cytarabine. Intra-cerebrospinal fluid trastuzumab may be an option for HER2-positive breast cancer [40]. Toxicity varies with the agents and includes seizures, arachnoiditis, headaches, nausea, emesis, and even delayed necrotizing leukoencephalopathy [39]. Focal radiotherapy should be considered for focal symptomatic lesions. The role of WBRT is limited in leptomeningeal metastases, as no survival benefit has been demonstrated in retrospective cohorts of patients, and WBRT should be limited to extensive nodular disease or symptomatic linear leptomeningeal metastases.

18.7 Leptomeningeal Metastases

Leptomeningeal metastasis, which is a rare complication of cancer, results in metastatic spread of disease to the meninges of the brain and spinal cord, by direct invasion [37], either through the bloodstream or the lymphatic system [38]. It can arise from either solid tumors or hematological malignancies. Common primaries include breast and lung cancer, melanoma, lymphomas, and leukemias. Leptomeningeal metastases can present with varied symptoms.

18.8 Conclusions

Brain metastases are a common and unfortunate complication of cancer, with significant impact on patients' quality of life and function. Once a diagnosis is made, treatment decision-making is based on patient functional status, extent and molecular characteristics of primary disease, and number and location of the metastatic lesions. Patients who have poor functional status, significantly advanced disease burden, and multiple metastases including leptomeningeal metastases may be considered for symptomatic/supportive care.

Patients who have good functional status and a single metastatic lesion should be considered for surgical resection or stereotactic radiosurgery depending on the location of the lesion. Multiple lesions can be treated with whole brain radiation. Chemotherapy should also be considered with targeted therapies and immunotherapy geared toward histological subtypes. Treatment options can be used in combination and must be tailored to the individual patient.

Leptomeningeal metastases present a complication of brain cancer with a dire prognosis. Treatment options include intrathecal chemotherapy and systemic pharmacotherapy with or without focal radiotherapy. Treatment strategies should be based on overall patient performance.

References

1. Cancer facts and figures. Statistics for 2017 [online resource] (2017) American Cancer Society, Atlanta. https://www.cancer.org/research/cancer-facts-statistics/all-cancer-facts-figures/cancer-facts-figures-2017.html
2. Zimm S, Wampler GL, Stablein D et al (1981) Intracerebral metastases in solid-tumor patients: natural history and results of treatment. Cancer 48(2):384–394
3. Shaffrey ME, Mut M, Asher AL et al (2004) Brain metastases. Curr Probl Surg 41:665–741
4. Glantz MJ, Cole BF, Forsyth PA et al (2000) Practice parameter: anticonvulsant prophylaxis in patients with newly diagnosed brain tumors. Report of the Quality Standards Subcommittee of the American Academy of Neurology. Neurology 54(10):1886–1893
5. Gaspar L, Scott C, Rotman M et al (1997) Recursive partitioning analysis (RPA) of prognostic factors in three Radiation Therapy Oncology Group (RTOG) brain metastases trials. Int J Radiat Oncol Biol Phys 37(4):745–751
6. Sperduto PW et al (2008) A new prognostic index and comparison to three other indices for patients with brain metastases: an analysis of 1960 patients in the RTOG database. Int J Radiat Oncol Biol Phys 70(2):510–514
7. Sperduto PW, Jiang W, Brown PD, Braunstein S, Sneed P, Wattson DA, Shih HA, Bangdiwala A, Shanley R, Lockney NA, Beal K, Lou E, Amatruda T, Sperduto WA, Kirkpatrick JP, Yeh N, Gaspar LE, Molitoris JK, Masucci L, Roberge D, Yu J, Chiang V, Mehta M (2017) Estimating survival in melanoma patients with brain metastases: an update of the graded prognostic assessment for melanoma using molecular markers (melanoma-molGPA). Int J Radiat Oncol Biol Phys 99(4):812–816
8. Sperduto PW, Yang TJ, Beal K, Pan H, Brown PD, Bangdiwala A, Shanley R, Yeh N, Gaspar LE, Braunstein S, Sneed P, Boyle J, Kirkpatrick JP, Mak KS, Shih HA, Engelman A, Roberge D, Arvold ND, Alexander B, Awad MM, Contessa J, Chiang V, Hardie J, Ma D, Lou E, Sperduto W, Mehta MP (2017) Estimating survival in patients with lung cancer and brain metastases: an update of the graded prognostic assessment for lung cancer using molecular markers (Lung-molGPA). JAMA Oncol 3(6):827–831
9. Barker FG 2nd (2004) Craniotomy for the resection of metastatic brain tumors in the U.S., 1988–2000: decreasing mortality and the effect of provider caseload. Cancer 100:999–1007
10. Patchell RA, Tibbs PA, Walsh JW et al (1990) A randomized trial of surgery in the treatment of single metastases to the brain. N Engl J Med 322(8):494–500
11. Vecht CJ, Haaxma-Reiche H, Noordijk EM et al (1993) Treatment of single brain metastasis: radiotherapy alone or combined with neurosurgery? Ann Neurol 33(6):583–590
12. Mintz AH, Kestle J, Rathbone MP et al (1996) A randomized trial to assess the efficacy of surgery in addition to radiotherapy in patients with a single cerebral metastasis. Cancer 78(7):1470–1476
13. Hart MG, Grant R, Walker M, Dickinson H (2005) Surgical resection and whole brain radiation therapy versus whole brain radiation therapy alone for single brain metastases. Cochrane Database Syst Rev (1):CD003292
14. Black PM, Johnson MD (2004) Surgical resection for patients with solid brain metastases: current status. J Neurooncol 69:119–124
15. Paek SH, Audu PB, Sperling MR et al (2005) Reevaluation of surgery for the treatment of brain metastases: review of 208 patients with single or multiple brain metastases treated at one institution with modern neurosurgical techniques. Neurosurgery 56:1021–1034
16. Stark AM, Tscheslog H, Buhl R et al (2005) Surgical treatment for brain metastases: prognostic factors and survival in 177 patients. Neurosurg Rev 28:115–119
17. Stea B, Suh JH, Boyd AP et al (2006) Whole-brain radiotherapy with or without efaproxiral for the treatment of brain metastases: determinants of response and its prognostic value for subsequent survival. Int J Radiat Oncol Biol Phys 64(4):1023–1030
18. Meyers CA, Smith JA, Bezjak A et al (2004) Neurocognitive function and progression in patients with brain metastases treated with whole-brain radiation and motexafin gadolinium: results of a randomized phase III trial. J Clin Oncol 22(1):157–165
19. Ceresoli GL, Cappuzzo F, Gregorc V et al (2004) Gefitinib in patients with brain metastases from non-

small-cell lung cancer: a prospective trial. Ann Oncol 15:1042–1047

20. Liu R, Martuza RL, Rabkin SD (2005) Intracarotid delivery of oncolytic HSV vector G47Delta to metastatic breast cancer in the brain. Gene Ther 12:647–654

21. Sampson JH, Carter JH Jr, Friedman AH, Seigler HF (1998) Demographics, prognosis, and therapy in 702 patients with brain metastases from malignant melanoma. J Neurosurg 88(1):11–20

22. Chapman PB, Hauschild A, Robert C et al (2011) BRIM-3 Study Group Improved survival with vemurafenib in melanoma with BRAF V600E mutation. N Engl J Med 364(26):2507–2516

23. Pease NJ, Edwards A, Moss LJ (2005) Effectiveness of whole brain radiotherapy in the treatment of brain metastases: a systematic review. Palliat Med 19(4):288–299

24. Plotkin SR, Wen PY (2003) Brain metastases. In: Samuels MA, Feske SK (eds) Office practice of neurology, 2nd edn. Churchill Livingstone, Philadelphia, pp 1101–1106

25. Le Rhun E, Weller M, Brandsma D, Van den Bent M, de Azambuja E, Henriksson R, Boulanger T, Peters S, Watts C, Wick W, Wesseling P, Rudà R, Preusser M, EANO Executive Board and ESMO Guidelines Committee (2017) EANO-ESMO Clinical Practice Guidelines for diagnosis, treatment and follow-up of patients with leptomeningeal metastasis from solid tumours. Ann Oncol 28(Suppl 4):iv84–iv99. https://doi.org/10.1093/annonc/mdx221

26. Mulvenna P, Nankivell M, Barton R, Faivre-Finn C, Wilson P, McColl E, Moore B, Brisbane I, Ardron D, Holt T, Morgan S, Lee C, Waite K, Bayman N, Pugh C, Sydes B, Stephens R, Parmar MK, Langley RE (2016) Dexamethasone and supportive care with or without whole brain radiotherapy in treating patients with non-small cell lung cancer with brain metastases unsuitable for resection or stereotactic radiotherapy (QUARTZ): results from a phase 3, non-inferiority, randomised trial. Lancet 388(10055):2004–2014

27. Patchell RA, Tibbs PA, Regine WF et al (1998) Postoperative radiotherapy in the treatment of single metastases to the brain: a randomized trial. JAMA 280:1485–1489

28. Maraveyas A, Sgouros J, Upadhyay S et al (2005) Gemcitabine twice weekly as a radiosensitiser for the treatment of brain metastases in patients with carcinoma: a phase I study. Br J Cancer 92:815–819

29. Cerchietti LC, Bonomi MR, Navigante AH et al (2005) Phase I/II study of selective cyclooxygenase-2 inhibitor celecoxib as a radiation sensitizer in patients with unresectable brain metastases. J Neurooncol 71:73–81

30. Kondziolka D, Niranjan A, Flickinger JC, Lunsford LD (2005) Radiosurgery with or without whole-brain radiotherapy for brain metastases: the patients' perspective regarding complications. Am J Clin Oncol 28:173–179

31. Tsao MN, Lloyd NS, Wong RK et al (2005) Radiotherapeutic management of brain metastases: a systematic review and meta-analysis. Cancer Treat Rev 31:256–273

32. Lester JF, Macbeth FR, Coles B (2005) Prophylactic cranial irradiation for preventing brain metastases in patients undergoing radical treatment for non-small-cell lung cancer: a Cochrane review. Int J Radiat Oncol Biol Phys 2005:23

33. Gore E, Choy H (2004) Non-small cell lung cancer and central nervous system metastases: should we be using prophylactic cranial irradiation? Semin Radiat Oncol 14:292–297

34. Andrews DW, Scott CB, Sperduto PW et al (2004) Whole brain radiation therapy with or without stereotactic radiosurgery boost for patients with one to three brain metastases: phase III results of the RTOG 9508 randomized trial. Lancet 363(9422):1665–1672

35. O'Neill BP, Iturria NJ, Link MJ et al (2003) A comparison of surgical resection and stereotactic radiosurgery in the treatment of solitary brain metastases. Int J Radiat Oncol Biol Phys 55:1169–1176

36. Chan TA, Weingart JD, Parisi M et al (2005) Treatment of recurrent glioblastoma multiforme with GliaSite brachytherapy. Int J Radiat Oncol Biol Phys 62:1133–1139

37. Kokkoris CP (1983) Leptomeningeal carcinomatosis. How does cancer reach the pia-arachnoid? Cancer 51:154–160

38. Glass JP, Melamed M, Chernik NL et al (1979) Malignant cells in cerebrospinal fluid (CSF): the meaning of a positive CSF cytology. Neurology 29:1369–1375

39. Boogerd W, Hart AAM, van der Sande JJ et al (1991) Meningeal carcinomatosis in breast cancer. Prognostic factors and influence of treatment. Cancer 67:1685–1695

40. Bonneau C, Paintaud G, Trédan O, Dubot C, Desvignes C, Dieras V, Taillibert S, Tresca P, Turbiez I, Li J, Passot C, Mefti F, Mouret-Fourme E, Le Rhun E, Gutierrez M (2018) Phase I feasibility study for intrathecal administration of trastuzumab in patients with HER2 positive breast carcinomatous meningitis. Eur J Cancer 95:75–84. https://doi.org/10.1016/j.ejca.2018.02.032. Epub 2018 Apr 7

Part III

Pediatric Neurooncology

James T. Rutka

Neurocutaneous Syndromes

Michael S. Taccone and James T. Rutka

19.1 Introduction

Neurocutaneous disorders are a heterogeneous group of genetic disorders characterized by abnormalities of the skin and nervous systems due to their common embryological origin. These disorders have inconsistent definitions, and therefore there is lack of consensus regarding which diseases belong to this category. In general, and for the purposes of this chapter, the neurofibromatoses, Sturge-Weber syndrome, von Hippel-Lindau syndrome, and Gorlin syndrome are accepted neurocutaneous disorders and will

M. S. Taccone
Division of Neurosurgery, The Ottawa Hospital, Ottawa, ON, Canada

Division of Neurosurgery, Department of Surgery, University of Ottawa, Ottawa, ON, Canada

Arthur & Sonia Labatt Brain Tumour Research Centre, The Hospital for Sick Children, Toronto, ON, Canada

Division of Neurosurgery, The Hospital for Sick Children, Toronto, ON, Canada
e-mail: michael.taccone@sickkids.ca

J. T. Rutka (✉)
Arthur & Sonia Labatt Brain Tumour Research Centre, The Hospital for Sick Children, Toronto, ON, Canada

Division of Neurosurgery, The Hospital for Sick Children, Toronto, ON, Canada

Department of Surgery, University of Toronto, Toronto, ON, Canada
e-mail: James.rutka@sickkids.ca

be discussed. Genetic aberrations in cell growth pathways are fundamental to all neurocutaneous syndromes which predispose these patients to developmental abnormalities and neoplasms of the central and peripheral nervous systems, skull, skin, and eyes. Therefore, these heterogeneous disorders are also known as tumor predisposition syndromes.

All neurocutaneous disorders, with the exception of Sturge-Weber syndrome, are genetically inherited, and their complications and predisposition risks persist lifelong. As well, due to the commonality of multiple organ involvement, cognitive difficulties, and developmental delay, these patients are best managed by multidisciplinary teams which include neurologists, neurosurgeons, neuropsychologists, neuro-oncologists, neuro-ophthalmologists and dermatologists to best maximize their productive potential and monitor complications.

19.2 The Neurofibromatoses

The neurofibromatoses encompass at least three distinct genetic disorders: neurofibromatosis 1 (NF1), neurofibromatosis 2 (NF2), and schwannomatosis (SCWS). Although each has a unique underlying genetic etiology, they share some common features including tumors of neuroectodermal origin [1]. Of these tumor predisposition syndromes, NF1 is the most common, followed by NF2 and schwannomatosis which are rarer.

© Springer Nature Switzerland AG 2019
J.-C. Tonn et al. (eds.), *Oncology of CNS Tumors*, https://doi.org/10.1007/978-3-030-04152-6_19

19.2.1 Neurofibromatosis Type 1

19.2.1.1 Epidemiology and Pathophysiology

NF1, which is more classically known as von Recklinghausen's disease, is a peripheral form of neurofibromatosis and accounts for up to 96% of all NF cases [2]. With an incidence of 1 in 3000 live births, it is one of the most commonly inherited neurological disorders and the most common neurocutaneous syndrome [3, 4]. Its pattern of inheritance is autosomal dominant, with high penetrance and variable expression leading to a heterogeneous phenotype even among patients with a family history. However, up to half of all patients with NF1 lack a discernable family history whose disease instead arises from de novo gene mutations the neurofibromin (NF-1) tumor suppressor gene. Loss-of-function mutations in *NF-1* are thought to cause the disease as about 80% of germline mutations lead to truncation of the gene product [5]. The *NF-1* gene has been mapped to chromosome 17q11.2. It functions by downregulating the activity of P21-RAS, a cellular proto-oncogene that affects various signaling pathways involved in tumorigenesis, including the mammalian target of rapamycin (mTOR), mitogen-activated protein (MAP) kinase, and stem cell factor/c-Kit signaling pathways [6, 7]. Therefore, NF1 also belongs to a group of disorders now known as the RASopathies [8].

19.2.1.2 Clinical Manifestations

Due to its neuroectodermal origin, symptoms and signs of NF1 are referable to systems and structures which develop from the neural plate (Table 19.1). Thus, clinical manifestations typically involve the dermatologic, ophthalmologic, musculoskeletal, peripheral, and central nervous systems. The appearance of specific clinical features is usually age-dependent [9].

Skin Manifestations

One common and pathognomonic cutaneous lesion in NF1 is the café au lait macule [4]. This often-darkened area of abnormal skin pigmentation with regular borders and even coloration can vary in size from a few millimeters up to several centimeters in diameter (Fig. 19.1). These lesions

Table 19.1 Tissues of neuroectodermal origin

Neuroectoderm	
Neural crest cells	Neural tube
Melanocytes	Rhombencephalon
Facial cartilage	Mesencephalon
Aorticopulmonary septum	Prosencephalon
Ciliary body of the eye	Spinal cord and motor neurons
Adrenal medulla	Retina
Parafollicular cells in the thyroid	Posterior pituitary
Skull base	
Dorsal root ganglia	
Ganglia of the autonomic nervous system	

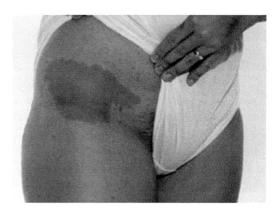

Fig. 19.1 Café au lait macule in patient with NF1. NF1 patient with characteristic café au lait macule of the inguinal region

are often evident at birth, usually before the child's first birthday. Up to 95% of adults with NF1 will display at least one café au lait macule, with 78% having six or more. A second cutaneous sign is skinfold freckling, seen in regions such as the submammary fold, axilla, or inguinal regions. These may be absent initially but will typically develop later as the child approaches puberty.

Ophthalmologic Manifestations

Iris hamartomas (Lisch nodules) are the most common ophthalmologic abnormality in NF1 patients. They are present in >74% of patients with NF1 but do not appear in NF2 [10]. These nodules consist of masses of melanocytes and appear as raised, pigmented lesions best seen by slit-lamp examination. Like skinfold freckling, iris hamartomas are often absent in early child-hood, showing increased prevalence with age.

Musculoskeletal Manifestations

Musculoskeletal abnormalities associated with NF1 include scalloping of the vertebral bodies, kyphoscoliosis, and idiopathic vertebral dyspla-sia [11]. Scoliosis typically becomes apparent between the ages of 6 and 10. Other bony abnor-malities include thinning of long-bone cortex, pseudoarthrosis, and dysplasia of the sphenoid wing. Osteoporosis is also common among this population. One study of 460 patients determined that NF1 patients over age 40 have an increased incidence of fractures [12]. Rarely, malignancies such as rhabdomyosarcoma may develop.

Peripheral Nervous System Manifestations

NF1 patients may harbor abnormalities in both the peripheral (PNS) and central nervous system (CNS). Within the PNS, a cardinal feature of NF1 is the presence of multiple cutaneous and subcutaneous neurofibromas, often found in the thoracoabdominal region or around the nipple-areolar complex. These can also be found along peripheral nerves, blood vessels, as well as the gastrointestinal viscera. It is not uncommon for NF1 patients to develop up to thousands of these benign lesions, making it the most common tumor associated with this disorder. Cutaneous neurofibromas typically develop during ado-lescence and pregnancy, suggesting a hormonal influence. They are usually small, rubbery lesions with a slight purple discoloration of the overlying skin. Despite their frequency, these lesions pose primarily a cosmetic problem for NF1 patients, with malignant transformation occurring rarely.

Neurofibromas also develop in the paraspinal region, arising from the dorsal roots in the cervi-cal or lumbar regions. If they extend through the intervertebral foramen, they may take on a char-acteristic "dumbbell" shape, with further growth into the spinal canal. If large enough, these lesions may produce symptoms of myelo-radiculopathy.

Plexiform neurofibromas are another lesion seen within the PNS in NF1 patients. These lesions are almost exclusively congenital in nature or appear during early childhood and dif-

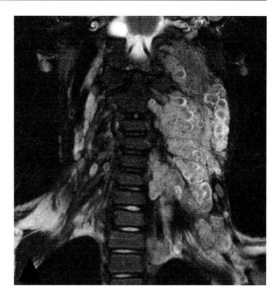

Fig. 19.2 Plexiform neurofibroma in patient with NF1. Coronal view T2-weighted MRI demonstrating a plexi-form neurofibroma of the cervical sympathetic chain in an adult NF1 patient who presented with neck mass

fusely involve larger peripheral nerves or the sympathetic chain (Fig. 19.2). Although not pathognomonic, the presence of a plexiform neu-rofibroma is highly suggestive of underlying NF1 [13]. Approximately 30% of NF1 patients have clinically detectable plexiform neurofibromas, with multiple lesions being present in 9–21% of cases [14–16]. Imaging studies reveal plexi-form neurofibromas in up to 50% of NF1 patients [17]. Although some remain asymptomatic, these lesions can present as a painful expanding mass and have the potential to cause overgrowth of an extremity or neurologic dysfunction of the involved area [18].

Plexiform neurofibromas possess the poten-tial for malignant transformation, forming a neu-rofibrosarcoma or malignant peripheral nerve sheath tumor (MPNST). These highly malignant Schwann cell tumors affect up to 10% of NF1 patients [19]. Conversely, approximately 50% of patients with MPNST have NF1. Compared to MPNSTs occurring in patients without NF1, those occurring in the context of this syndrome are diagnosed earlier and are associated with significantly shorter progression-free and over-all survival [20]. In one cohort which has had 60 patients followed-up or diagnosed with MPNST since 2009, 37 of 60 (61.6%) survived 5 years or more from the time of initial diagnosis [21]. The development of such tumors may be heralded by the onset of new neurologic deficits, pain, or rapid growth of a plexiform neurofibroma [18, 22]. One must have a high index of suspicion for MPNSTs under these circumstances, given their aggressive behavior and potential to metastasize.

Central Nervous System Manifestations

Within the CNS, the most common tumor seen in NF1 patients is the optic pathway glioma (OPG) (Fig. 19.3). OPGs account for 2–5% of all childhood brain tumors, and up to 15–20% of NF1 patients are affected by this lesion [23]. Although development of this tumor can occur at any age, the incidence peaks in childhood, usually prior to 6 years of age. Females appear to be at higher risk than males. Generally, OPGs are slow-growing, WHO grade I pilocytic astrocytomas. OPGs arising in the context of NF1 tend to exhibit a more benign clinical course than spontaneous tumors

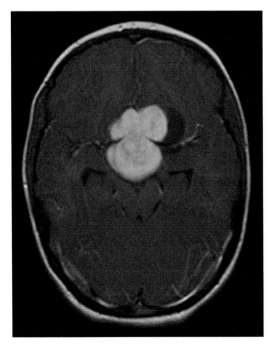

Fig. 19.3 Optic pathway glioma in patient with NF1. Axial view T1-weighted post-gadolinium-enhanced MRI demonstrating large optic pathway glioma in a child with NF1. Note non-enhancing cystic component

[24]. OPGs may arise anywhere along the optic pathway, although the prechiasmal optic nerve is the most common location in NF1 patients [25]. Rarely, these tumors develop further posteriorly, within the optic radiations themselves [26]. In the NF1 patient, OPGs may remain asymptomatic in up to half the patients [27]. When symptoms arise, patients may suffer from diplopia, proptosis, altered visual fields, or impaired acuity. Hypothalamic or endocrine dysfunction (such as precocious puberty) may also occur. Even among symptomatic patients, OPGs in NF1 patients may remain quite stable. As a result, presymptomatic radiologic screening is not required.

In addition to OPGs, NF1 patients are susceptible to developing supratentorial, infratentorial, and brain stem gliomas of various histological grades [28]. Hemispheric gliomas (Fig. 19.4) and posterior fossa gliomas occur in 0.5% and 1.0% of NF1 patients, respectively. As expected, the symptoms and signs of these lesions depend on their particular location but may include those of increased intracranial pressure, hydrocephalus, focal motor or sensory deficits, cerebellar dysfunction, or seizures. The spectrum of gliomas in the NF1 patient is susceptible to include pilocytic astrocytoma (WHO grade I) and all grades of diffuse gliomas (WHO grades II–IV) [29]. Perhaps not surprisingly, overall and progression-free survival for NF1 patients that develop gliomas is significantly better for those with pilocytic lesions versus diffusely infiltrating ones [29].

Nonneoplastic manifestations of NF1 within the CNS include cognitive impairment, attention-deficit hyperactivity disorder, aqueductal stenosis, Chiari malformation, hydrocephalus, epilepsy, and idiopathic macrocephaly [17, 30–34]. In addition, one may find the radiologic phenomenon of focal areas of increased T2-weighted signal on imaging studies—imaging correlates of possible spongiform myelinopathy and markers of poor cognitive and fine motor performance [35].

19.2.1.3 Diagnosis and Management

Diagnostic Criteria

The diagnosis of NF1 is essentially a clinical one and is purely based upon the presence of

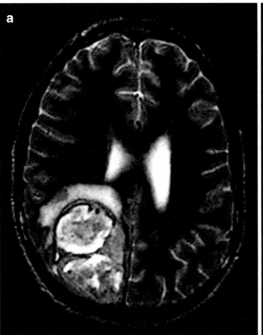
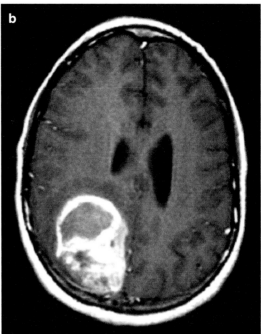

Fig. 19.4 Hemispheric high-grade glioma in patient with NF1. MRI of NF1 patient with high-grade glioma. (**a**) Axial view T2-weighted MRI of a large right parieto-occipital high-grade glioma demonstrating heterointen-sity and surrounding vasogenic edema with mass effect on the right lateral ventricle. (**b**) Axial view T1-weighted post-gadolinium-enhanced MRI of parieto-occipital high-grade glioma demonstrating avid ring enhancement

characteristic clinical features (Table 19.2). Only in cases of suspected children who do not fully meet the diagnostic criteria is genetic testing required. The diagnostic criteria released by the National Institutes of Health (NIH) are both highly sensitive and specific for the diagnosis of NF1 and are positive in all but the youngest patients [36]. In a study of over 1800 NF1 patients, by age 8, 97% meet these criteria, and by 20 years of age, virtually all patients meet the criteria [36].

The differential diagnosis in NF1 includes disorders associated with abnormal pigmentation, tumors that may be confused with neurofibromas, and other forms of neurofibromatosis [17, 30]. The most common to rule out are Legius syndrome, constitutional mismatch repair deficiency syndrome, neurofibromatosis type 2, and Noonan syndrome. Genetic tests have been developed to assess for mutations in the NF1 gene [37]. These tests are readily available and able to detect a mutation in the *NF1* gene in 95% of individuals who meet clinical diagnostic criteria [38]. The utility of genetic testing is in its ability to

Table 19.2 Diagnostic criteria for neurofibromatosis type 1 (NF1) (Gutmann et al. [82])

The patient should have two or more of the following
1. Six or more café au lait spots
   - 1.5 cm or larger in postpubertal individuals
   - 0.5 cm or larger in prepubertal individuals
2. Two or more neurofibromas of any type or one or more plexiform neurofibroma
3. Freckling in the axilla or groin
4. Optic pathway glioma
5. Two or more Lisch nodules (benign iris hamartomas)
6. A distinctive bony lesion
   - Dysplasia of the sphenoid bone
   - Dysplasia or thinning of long-bone cortex

confirm the diagnosis of NF1 in equivocal patients and to screen members of the same family for the identical mutation. Genetic testing is required for prenatal or preimplantation diagnosis. It is important to realize that a positive genetic test for the *NF1* gene does not correlate with the severity of the symptoms or complication rate however.

Diagnostic imaging is a critical component of not only the diagnostic workup but also the long-term follow-up of patients with NF1. For this, various imaging modalities can be useful depending on the workup in question. Plain film X-rays are of utility in the diagnosis of appendicular bony abnormalities. For spinal deformity such as kyphoscoliosis, CT scans with coronal and sagittal reformats as well as three-foot standing plain films can be useful. As with all tumor disposition syndromes however, due to the lifelong nature of NF1, cumulative exposure to ionizing radiation needs to be carefully considered in this population. Therefore, the neuroimaging modality of choice in the management of NF1 patients is MRI and should be used preferentially over X-ray or CT scan when possible. MRI scan of the craniospinal axis, with and without contrast, in addition to assessing spinal alignment pathology, is able to detect the presence of optic pathway, brain stem, and hemispheric and posterior fossa gliomas. In addition, paraspinal lesions may be identified with this modality. Another finding identified by MRI in NF1 patients is the presence of regions of increased signal involving the basal ganglia, thalamus, brain stem, and cerebellum on T2-weighted images, referred to as "unidentified bright objects" (UBOs) (Fig. 19.5) [39]. Although not pathognomonic, the presence of such lesions appears to be highly specific to NF1 and can be helpful in reaching the diagnosis in the presence of other suggestive clinical findings [39]. However, these lesions may spontaneously disappear as patients age, typically by adulthood [40].

Outside of the CNS, contrast-enhanced MRI may be of some utility in the diagnosis of MPNSTs as well, with these lesions appearing heterogeneous due to the presence of necrosis and intratumoral hemorrhage [41]. A case-control series examining tumor burden by whole-body MRI in NF1 patients with known MPNST versus those without found that among NF1 patients age 30 years or younger, those with MPNST had a significantly greater median neurofibroma volume and median number of plexiform neurofibromas, a large proportion of which were internal and not evident on clinical exam [42]. The

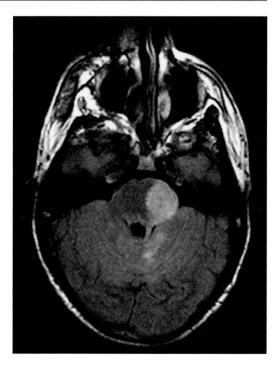

Fig. 19.5 Unidentified bright objects in patient with NF1. Axial view T2-weighted MRI of NF1 patient demonstrating characteristic high-signal intensity areas colloquially known as "unidentified bright objects." Note areas of high-signal intensity within the brainstem and cerebellum

authors concluded that whole-body imaging may identify a subset of NF1 patients at increased risk of developing MPNST and would allow for closer surveillance in this patient population [42]. Additional modalities, such as positron emission tomography (PET), can be useful in the determination of malignant transformation from plexiform neurofibroma to MPNST, although combination of PET imaging tracers may be required to determine tumor grade [43–45]. Therefore, this should only be reserved for cases with a high index of suspicion for transformation.

19.2.1.4 Clinical Management

Surveillance and Screening

Children suspected of having NF1 should be evaluated by a multidisciplinary team that includes pediatric neurology, genetics, and ophthalmology. This team should examine the child for diagnostic criteria and treatable complications, provide anticipatory guidance, and refer to specialists as needed. In particular, a complete ophthalmologic exam by either a pediatric or neuro-ophthalmologist is recommended on a yearly basis up to 10 years of age and every 2–3 years afterward or as symptoms arise [46]. Children with symptoms or abnormal clinical exams should go on to receive relevant diagnostic imaging.

Surgical Management

Surgery is often required for the treatment of the majority of benign and malignant tumors associated with NF1. Cutaneous and subcutaneous neurofibromas are easily excisable and can be resected if desired by the patient for cosmetic reasons. Plexiform neurofibromas, on the other hand, have high degrees of vascularity, are large, and typically occur within a neural plexus making them difficult to treat surgically. Rarely is a complete resection possible. In addition, the risk of incurring a postoperative sensory or motor deficit is not insignificant. Therefore, surgical treatment of this lesion should be approached cautiously and may not be indicated for the minimally symptomatic patient. Resection should be reserved only for the patient who experiences functional compromise as a result of continued tumor growth [18]. Conversely, when the malignant transformation of this tumor to a MPNST is suspected, prompt investigation and treatment is warranted which includes an initial biopsy to confirm the diagnosis of MPNST. Targeted biopsy may be attempted using FDG-PET to identify suspected regions of increased malignancy within the lesion [17]. This is followed at a second stage by either an attempt at gross total resection with tumor-free margins or by limb amputation. The patient then undergoes adjuvant radiation and occasionally chemotherapy [47, 48]. Despite this aggressive strategy, prognosis is poor, with a 5- and 10-year survival rate of 60 and 45%, respectively, according to a recent study [49].

As previously mentioned, OPGs are the most common CNS tumor in patients with NF1. Surgery however in these patients must be carefully considered. As is the case with most tumors affecting eloquent regions, the potential for surgical morbidity is not insignificant, and therefore treatment recommendations depend on the patient's symptoms, evidence of clinical progression, and the location of the tumor itself. Intraorbital or prechiasmatic lesions causing significant proptosis, visual loss, or exhibiting rapid growth may warrant treatment. Even in these cases, however, the role of surgical excision is limited to those scenarios in which visual impairment is significant making complete resection feasible or those in which significant mass effect exists, necessitating debulking. Additionally, numerous case reports exist of NF1-associated OPGs spontaneously regressing without intervention, [50–53] highlighting the importance of a watch-and-wait approach in minimally symptomatic patients.

The other intracranial gliomas (brainstem, posterior fossa, hemispheric) are often followed with serial imaging studies as these can behave more indolently in the NF1 population as compared to sporadic. However, occasionally these tumors can exhibit significant mass effect or accelerated growth in the posterior fossa or supratentorial compartment, leading to the need for surgical management if herniation or hydrocephalus develops.

Radiation Therapy

Where surgery fails to achieve tumor-free margins, radiation therapy serves a role as an adjunct in the treatment of MPNSTs. Additionally, it may also serve as a primary treatment modality for symptomatic, progressive OPGs. Up to 80% local control rates for OPGs following radiation therapy have been described, with either tumor shrinkage or stabilization seen on follow-up imaging studies. Recently, one group has attempted single-session stereotactic radiosurgery on 22 adult and pediatric patients with OPG with a 90% overall response rate [54]. Although the risk is much reduced with stereotactic radiosurgery, radiation therapy can incur significant morbidity, however, such as cognitive dysfunction, postradiation ischemic events, or endocrinologic disturbances [55]. Radiotherapy for OPGs has also been associated with increased risk of developing secondary malignancies in the NF1 population [56]. In addition to intracranial lesions, radiotherapy has been applied with some success to treat benign extramedullary spinal tumors in NF1, with long-term control demonstrated over a 3-year follow-up period [57]. At the moment, radiation therapy is used sparingly in patients with NF1 given its potential long-term complications.

Chemotherapy

In order to avoid iatrogenic complications secondary to radiation therapy, investigators have studied the role and efficacy of chemotherapy in treating gliomas associated with NF1. Single- and multi-agent chemotherapy regimens have been attempted with wide variability in success [58–66]. The most common strategy includes a regimen of cisplatin and vincristine. This combination [17] leads to a 89% 5-year overall and 61% 5-year radiation therapy-free survival [61]. Because of the surprisingly high response rate, chemotherapeutic regimens have been preferred over radiation as initial therapy—especially in those aged 5 years or younger.

19.2.1.5 Prognosis and Quality of Life

The overall prognosis and quality of life for NF1 patients are limited by their propensity for tumor development, which continues for life [67]. Between 3 to 15% of NF1 patients develop a malignancy during the course of their disease, [68] a major factor that contributes to an overall 15-year-shorter life expectancy compared to the general population [68, 69]. An analysis of American death certificates revealed that in patients with NF1 who died before age 30, a malignant neoplasm was more likely to be listed as their cause of death [69]. For those patients likely to have a shortened life expectancy, risk factors included the presence of a CNS tumor located outside of the optic pathway or the diagnosis of a symptomatic tumor in adulthood [55]. Unsurprisingly, a diagnosis of MPNST also contributes to a shortened life expectancy in this population.

19.2.1.6 Future Perspectives

Currently there is no cure or genetic therapy to reverse the effects of NF1. Future therapeutic strategies must take into account the often underappreciated genetic heterogeneity of this disorder. Multiple clinical trials with rational drug targeting at various points in the RAS pathway have been met with mediocre, negative, or even paradoxical results caused by compensatory cellular signaling mechanisms [70]. Therapeutic strategies employed thus far include MEK inhibition, VEGF inhibition, EGFR inhibition, mTOR inhibitors, or a combination of these two [70]. A phase I trial has been completed using MEK inhibitor selumetinib in pediatric patients with recurrent or refractory LGGs. Three of the five patients with NF1 completed 26, 20, and 4 cycles, respectively [71]. The results of the phase II study using the same agent have been published in an abstract form in 25 children with NF1. All had some degree of radiographic shrinkage, which exceeded 50% in nearly 40% of patients [70]. Further supporting the potential efficacy of MEK inhibition is its use in NF-associated plexiform neurofibromas, as greater than 70% of patients showed sustainable radiographic and or clinical benefit [70]. Future advances in the management of these patients may lie in the field of small-molecule, targeted chemotherapy. Preclinical and clinical data suggest that the receptor tyrosine kinase inhibitor imatinib, or other inhibitors of downstream targets in the RAS pathway, may prove to be of benefit in the treatment of NF1 patients [72, 73].

19.2.2 Neurofibromatosis Type 2

19.2.2.1 Epidemiology and Pathophysiology

NF2 is a rarer form of neurofibromatosis, with an annual incidence of approximately 1/25,000 [74]. As with NF1, NF2 is an autosomal dominant disorder, with no particular predilection for race or sex. The responsible gene (*NF-2*) is located on chromosome 22q11 and encodes the tumor suppressor protein called *merlin*, an acronym for moesin-ezrin-radixin-like protein.

Merlin (also known as schwannomin) belongs to the ERM family of proteins and is thought to play several roles, including negatively regulating RAC-dependent signaling, receptor tyrosine kinase signaling and trafficking, and possibly mediating contact-dependent inhibition of cell proliferation [9, 75]. This occurs through its involvement in multiple pathways such as phosphoinositide 3-kinase (PI3K)/AKT, RAF/MAPK, and mTOR. Merlin also controls the availability of cell membrane surface receptors VEGF, Notch, EGFR, and other members of the ErbB family [74, 76–78]. Loss of heterozygosity for the *NF-2* gene has been demonstrated in multiple NF2-associated tumors. In addition, the particular type of gene mutation may influence the severity of the expressed phenotype, as well as the spectrum of tumors a particular patient is at risk of developing [79]. For example, frameshift and nonsense mutations which result in truncated protein expression result in a more severe phenotype and poorer prognosis than missense or inframe deletions which carry the best prognosis [80]. Although NF2 exists in family cohorts, it is important to recognize that greater than one-half of cases represent de novo mutations and occur in the absence of a positive family history [81].

In distinction with NF1, NF2 patients typically become symptomatic during the second or third decades of life. Only 10% of patients are symptomatic before 10 years of age [82]. The majority, however, develop symptoms by the age of 40, often due to the presence of intracranial lesions such as vestibular schwannomas.

19.2.2.2 Clinical Manifestations

As with NF1, patients with NF2 are prone to develop abnormalities of the ophthalmologic system and multiple neoplasms involving the central and peripheral nervous systems. In contrast, however, is a lack of cutaneous findings which are not a prominent feature of NF2. The average age of onset of symptoms in NF2 is between 18 and 24 years of age [17].

Ophthalmologic Manifestations

Ophthalmologic manifestations in patients with NF2 include the development of juvenile posterior subcapsular lenticular opacities—occurring in up to 50% of affected individuals. Patients, when symptomatic, may present with visual impairment as a result. Other findings include retinal or iris hamartomas and epiretinal membranes.

Central Nervous System Manifestations

The hallmark lesions associated with NF2 are bilateral vestibular schwannomas (acoustic neuromas) (Fig. 19.6). Patients with unilateral vestibular schwannomas plus additional NF2-associated nervous system tumors have a significant risk of developing a contralateral vestibular tumor during their lifetime, especially if they present before 18 years of age [83]. By age 70, nearly all (90%) patients will develop bilateral vestibular schwannomas. Compared with sporadic cases, NF2 patients with vestibular schwannomas often become symptomatic at an earlier age. Presenting symptoms are similar and include sensorineural hearing loss, tinnitus, imbalance, headache, or facial nerve dysfunction.

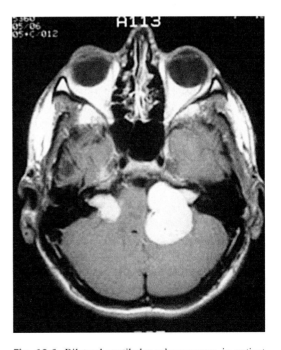

Fig. 19.6 Bilateral vestibular schwannomas in patient with NF2. Axial view T1-weighted post-gadolinium-enhanced MRI of NF2 patient demonstrating bilateral homogeneously enhancing vestibular masses consistent with vestibular schwannomas

The behavior of these lesions is quite variable, with growth rates between 1 and 10 mm per year reported.

NF2 patients are also at risk of developing additional tumors of the neuraxis. These include meningiomas, schwannomas (other than vestibular schwannomas), ependymomas, and rarely astrocytomas. Of these tumors, meningiomas are the most common and can occur intracranially or within the spine. They may be isolated or multiple in number. Their natural history and symptomatic presentation mirrors sporadic meningioma in the general population. In addition to schwannomas which arise from the superior division of the vestibular nerve, these tumors can arise elsewhere in NF2 patients, and not uncommonly involve the trigeminal and oculomotor nerves. Extracanially, schwannomas can also develop along sensory roots in the cervicothoracic region as well as outside of the spine along cutaneous nerves [84]. Such dermal schwannomas may be confused with cutaneous neurofibromas; however, histological examination reveals they are composed entirely of Schwann cells [9]. Extramedullary spinal tumors (schwannomas and meningiomas) can be detected radiologically in up to 90% of NF2 patients, although only approximately 30% become symptomatic [17]. Their associated symptomatology relates to the locations in which they arise.

Ependymomas are the most common intra-axial tumors in NF2 patients. Again, the behavior of these lesions (both intracranial and intramedullary within the spinal cord) parallels similar lesions found spontaneously in the general population.

19.2.2.3 Diagnosis

The diagnosis of NF2 remains a clinical one (Table 19.3). As with NF1, the diagnostic workup of suspected NF2 should involve the concerted efforts of a multidisciplinary team with interest and expertise in this disorder. Definitive diagnosis of NF2 may pose a challenge, especially in the young, owing to the fact that peripheral nerve schwannomas, meningiomas, spinal tumors, and ocular findings can often appear prior to vestibular schwannomas [17]. Additionally, the clinician must also distinguish NF2 from the related but

Table 19.3 Diagnostic criteria for neurofibromatosis type 2 (Gutmann et al. [82])

Patients with the following clinical features have confirmed (definite) NF2:	Patients with the following clinical features should be further evaluated for (presumptive or probable) NF2:
Bilateral vestibular schwannomas (VS) *Or* Family history of NF2 (first-degree family relative) *Plus* Unilateral VS <30 years *Or* Any two of the following: • Meningioma • Glioma • Schwannoma • Juvenile posterior subcapsular lenticular opacities/juvenile cortical cataract	Unilateral VS <30 years *Plus* Any of the following: • Meningioma • Glioma • Schwannoma • Juvenile posterior subcapsular lenticular opacities/ juvenile cortical cataract
	Multiple meningiomas (2 or more) *Plus* One of the following: • Unilateral VS <30 years • Glioma • Schwannoma • Juvenile posterior subcapsular lenticular opacities/ juvenile cortical cataract

clinically distinct syndrome, schwannomatosis, in which multiple schwannomas occur in the absence of vestibular tumors or germline mutations of the *NF-2* gene [17]. Annual examinations for patients between the ages of 15 and 45 years have been recommended [82]. In addition to a thorough clinical exam, further workup should include imaging of the craniospinal axis, audiometry, and possibly brainstem auditory-evoked response (BAER) testing. Contrast-enhanced MRI of the brain, including images centered on the internal auditory meatus, will disclose the presence of vestibular nerve tumors as well as other intracranial pathologies. MRI of the spine may reveal the presence of intramedullary ependymomas, spinal meningiomas, or schwannomas of sensory roots. In patients with positive findings of a vestibular schwannoma, audiometry helps assess and document the severity of high-tone sensorineural hearing loss typical for the NF2 patient. Detailed genetic testing is available for NF2 and will detect an abnormality in *NF-2* in about 93% of families who have multiple members affected [85]. Due to genetic heterogeneity and mosaicism however, genetic testing for this disease although specific is far from sensitive.

19.2.2.4 Clinical Management

Surveillance and Screening

In patients with NF2 and vestibular schwannomas, the clinical course is difficult to predict, owing to the variable growth rates described for these lesions. As such, the initial treatment strategy often consists of close observation, repeat clinical assessment, and serial neuroimaging. If progressive symptomatic deterioration, rapid growth rate, or evidence of neural compression due to tumor mass is noted, intervention may be required. The optimal treatment strategy for NF2 patients with bilateral vestibular schwannomas has received much attention over the years, with controversy continuing regarding which modality is most appropriate–surgery versus radiation therapy—and under what circumstances.

These patients require annual histories and physicals with ophthalmologic, audiology, and cutaneous evaluations. Imaging recommendations include annual brain MRI, beginning at 10 years of age. If negative, MRI frequency can be reduced to every 2 years. If, however, the study yields characteristic tumor findings, brain MRI should be repeated twice yearly in the first year and then annually if stable. MRI should include thin-slice (1–3 mm thickness) post-contrast imaging through the internal auditory meatus, in at least two views (usually axial and coronal).

Similarly, spinal MRI is recommended every 24–36 months beginning at the start of 10 years of age. Should the initial scan prove normal, the imaging interval can be increased to once every 3–5 years. However, once tumors are detected, imaging should be repeated in six months' time.

Staging and Classification

Pertaining specifically to those patients with vestibular schwannomas, two classification systems often used are the House-Brackmann and Gardner-Robertson scales. These grading systems evaluate facial and cochlear nerve function, respectively, and provide a means of quantifying the degree of injury to these nerves both before and after therapy.

Surgical Management

In all cases, the goal of therapy in the management of vestibular schwannomas is twofold: to preserve function and maintain or improve quality of life. Microsurgical resection has long been considered the gold standard treatment for vestibular schwannomas. Several authors view microsurgery as a superior treatment modality for achieving tumor control compared to radiation therapy strategies [86]. Surgery is generally preferred over radiation when symptoms due to mass effect are present, such as in the case of brainstem compression. In instances of hearing deterioration or facial nerve dysfunction, the choice of surgery over radiation is less obvious.

Multiple surgical strategies and approaches are used in the clinical setting for these lesions. These include the retrosigmoid-suboccipital, translabyrinthine, and subtemporal-middle fossa approaches. Factors which affect the most desirable surgical approach are (1) size of the lesion, (2) its location (intracanalicular vs. cerebellopontine angle), and (3) whether hearing preservation is a goal of the surgery. Those who advocate surgery for these lesions suggest that early surgery, when lesions are smallest, will provide for the best chance of both complete resection and preservation of hearing and facial nerve function [87]. Samii et al. reviewed their extensive surgical experience for 120 vestibular schwannomas in 82 NF2 patients treated during the period from 1978 to 1993 [88]. Among this group of patients, bilateral resections were accomplished in 38, while unilateral resections were done in 44 patients. Complete excision was possible in 105 of the tumors. Anatomic facial nerve preservation was achieved in 85% of cases. Attempts at hearing preservation were successful in approximately 36% of patients and were generally better for those with smaller lesions. In a more recent review of 145 consecutive NF2 patients who underwent resection of vestibular schwannoma, Samii et al. report an overall hearing preservation rate of 35% [87]. When only patients with useful preoperative hearing were included, the rate of hearing preservation was 65% [87]. Another group which used the middle fossa approach for vestibular tumor resection in a cohort of pediatric NF2 patients reported a bilateral hearing preservation rate of 75% among 12 children operated on for bilateral tumors [89]. This same study reported a facial nerve preservation rate (House-Brackmann grade I or II) of 81% among a total of 47 cases [89].

Due to the development of and treatment for bilateral vestibular tumors, NF2 patients are at high risk for hearing loss due to cochlear nerve damage. In those with hearing loss, these patients may benefit from auditory brain stem implants [90, 91]. When the anatomic and physiologic integrity of the cochlear nerve is preserved and promontory stimulation confirms that residual cochlear nerve function exists, cochlear nerve implantation offers another option with good success for the NF2 patient [92]. However, up to 8 weeks of postsurgical recovery time can be required before reliable testing of residual cochlear nerve function can be performed [92].

Patients with NF2 may require surgical treatment for other lesions, such as meningioma, schwannoma, or ependymoma. Treatment decisions and approach regarding these lesions generally parallel their spontaneously occurring counterparts in the non-NF2 population.

Radiation Therapy

Modalities for the treatment of vestibular schwannomas in the NF2 patient that have gained favor more recently include fractionated stereotactic radiotherapy and stereotactic radiosurgery. Tumor control rates up to 98–100% have been demonstrated with these modalities, along with rates of hearing preservation equal to those reported in surgical series [79, 93]. Rowe et al. reviewed their experience using stereotactic radiosurgery for the treatment of vestibular schwannomas in NF2 patients [94]. They observed that only 20% of treated patients went on to require surgical treatment of the same lesion during an 8-year follow-up period. In addition, they reported

complications of facial and trigeminal neuropathy in only 5% and 2% of patients, respectively. More recently, Rowe et al. reported a functional hearing preservation rate of approximately 40% 3 years following radiosurgery for vestibular schwannomas in NF2 [94]. Mathieu et al. recently reviewed their results using gamma-knife radiosurgery for 74 vestibular tumors in 62 NF2 patients [95]. They observed actuarial tumor control and hearing preservation rates of 85% and 48% at 5 years, respectively [95]. New facial neuropathy and new trigeminal neuropathy occurred in 8% and 4% of cases, respectively, with tumor size and radiosurgery dose being predictive of incurring treatment-related deficits [95]. Radiosurgery is becoming an increasingly more commonly utilized alternative to traditional microsurgical resection, providing tumor control, or at least a delay in need for subsequent resection, with acceptable treatment-related morbidity [96]. In a recent study examining radiosurgery in patients with bilateral vestibular schwannomas, Vachhani et al. demonstrated 5-year actuarial tumor control rates of 92% on the treated side compared with only 21% on the untreated side [97]. It is important to keep in mind however that for lesions which exert their symptoms due to mass effect and require debulking, reduction in tumor volume can take up to 1–2 years posttreatment with radiosurgery.

While surgical resection remains the primary treatment modality for benign extramedullary spinal tumors in NF2, radiosurgery has shown some efficacy at local tumor control over a 3-year follow-up period [57]. Longer follow-up is needed, however, to determine the long-term efficacy of this strategy.

19.2.2.5   Prognosis and Quality of Life

The overall prognosis and quality of life for NF2 patients are as variable as the phenotypic severity of this disorder. As mentioned, quality of life may be impaired significantly due to the development of hearing impairment. In addition, ophthalmologic abnormalities such as juvenile posterior subcapsular cataracts may add to their disability by impairing vision. One significant treatment-related morbidity, facial nerve paresis, can be extremely distressing and disfiguring for these patients as well, not to mention the increased ophthalmologic risks of corneal abrasion or exposure keratitis which are lifelong.

19.3 Schwannomatosis

19.3.1 Epidemiology and Pathophysiology

SCWS is another form of the neurofibromatosis which is most similar to NF2. However, this disorder lacks the cutaneous findings of both NF1 and NF2. In addition, SCWS is driven by genetically distinct germline mutations which lead to the development of multiple non-cutaneous schwannomas during adulthood, without the presence of bilateral vestibular schwannomas as in NF2. Patients with SCWS represent approximately 2–10% of individuals who undergo schwannoma surgery [98]. Its incidence is believed to be approximately 0.58 per 100,000 [99].

As mentioned, patients with SCWS present in adulthood, typically in their 40s, with multiple and often painful schwannomas [100]. Up to 20% of patients have a positive family history. There is no known predilection for race or sex. Loss-of-function mutations in genes *SMARCB1* and *LZTR1* which act as tumor suppressors are thought to be responsible for the majority of cases. *SMARCB1*, known also as *INI1*, is thought to act as tumor suppressor by regulating cell cycle function and thus inhibiting differentiation, proliferation, and growth. In *SMARCB1*-mutant tumors, a four-hit hypothesis is believed to occur, whereby hit 1 occurs in the germline affected allele, hit 2 occurs in the second wild-type *SMARCB1* allele, followed by hits 3 and 4 which occur in the *NF-2* gene merlin [101]. The result is unregulated Schwann cell growth leading to schwannoma development. This phenomenon is thought to occur in 40–50% of patients with SCWS. In those without a *SMARCB1* mutation, loss-of-function mutations in *LZTR1* have been identified in up to 80% [102].

19.3.2 Clinical Manifestations

As with NF1 and NF2, patients with SCWS have a lifelong risk of tumor development, and thus a risk factor for multiple tumors has been shown to be increasing age [103]. With regard to clinical presentation, one retrospective series of 87 patients determined that the most common presentation was pain unassociated with a mass (46%) [100]. Tumor burden in this group included peripheral schwannomas (89%), spinal schwannomas (74%), intracranial nonvestibular schwannomas (9%), and intracranial meningiomas (5%). However, the most common overall symptom in this population was pain (68%) and persisted despite aggressive intervention. Unfortunately, due to this, depression and anxiety have a higher prevalence in patients with SCWS.

In addition to schwannomas and meningiomas, some families with rhabdoid tumors have also been reported in the literature [104, 105].

19.3.3 Diagnosis

Due to its similarity to NF2, making a diagnosis of SCWS can be difficult. The diagnostic criteria of SCWS have been revised multiple times in recent years. Currently, patients who meet the criteria can be diagnosed with definite, possible, or segmental neurofibromatosis (Table 19.4) [106]. Those individuals who meet the criteria for definite or possible SCWS can be further divided into familial or sporadic SCWS based on whether first-degree relatives are affected or not [107].

19.3.4 Clinical Management

Patients should be managed in multidisciplinary clinics with expertise in neurofibromatosis whenever possible. Treatment for these patients is primarily symptomatic and aims to address pain. In the case of clinically apparent tumor which causes mass effect resulting in neurological compromise, surgery is typically employed to restore function and improve quality of life. Neuropathic

Table 19.4 Diagnostic criteria for schwannomatosis (Baser et al. [106])

Criteria for definite, possible, and segmental schwannomatosis		
Definite	Possible	Segmental
1. Age > 30 years and all of the following: • Two or more nonintradermal schwannomas, at least one with histologic confirmation • Diagnostic criteria for NF2 not fulfilled • No evidence of vestibular tumor on high-resolution MRI • No first-degree relative with NF2 • No known constitutional NF2 mutation OR 2. One pathologically confirmed nonvestibular schwannoma plus a first-degree relative who meets the above criteria	1. Age < 30 years and all of the following: • Two or more nonintradermal schwannomas, at least one with histologic confirmation • Diagnostic criteria for NF2 not fulfilled • No evidence of vestibular tumor on high-resolution MRI • No first-degree relative with NF2 • No known constitutional NF2 mutation OR 2. Age > 45 years and all of the following: • Two or more nonintradermal schwannomas, at least one with histologic confirmation • No symptoms of eighth cranial nerve dysfunction • No first-degree relative with NF2 • No known constitutional NF2 mutation OR 3. Radiographic evidence of a nonvestibular schwannoma and a first-degree relative meeting criteria for definite schwannomatosis	1. Meets criteria for either definite or possible schwannomatosis limited to one limb or ≤ 5 contiguous spine segments

pain is frequently treated with GABA-like agents such as pregabalin or gabapentin with some success. Unfortunately, surgery typically does little to relieve pain in these individuals and paradoxically may exacerbate it.

It is useful to regularly assess these patients for anxiety and depression given the higher than average presence of these disorders in this population.

19.3.5 Prognosis and Quality of Life

The clinical spectrum and natural history of SCWS as of yet are poorly defined making it difficult to determine accurate life expectancy and prognosis in this group. However, based on population studies to date, there does not appear to be a shortened lifespan. Quality of life is mostly impacted by pain which can result in depression and anxiety.

19.4 Tuberous Sclerosis Complex

19.4.1 Epidemiology and Pathophysiology

Tuberous sclerosis complex (TSC) is an autosomal dominant disorder, characterized by the presence of multiple, hamartomatous abnormalities affecting several organ systems, including the brain, eyes, heart, lung, liver, kidney, and skin. In addition, neoplasms can occur, in particular within the CNS and kidneys. TSC has an annual incidence of approximately 1 in 6000, making it the second most common of the neurocutaneous syndromes after NF1 [108]. It shows no preference for sex or race. Like NF1, up to half of cases are thought to be due to new mutations. Mutations in two separate genes, *TSC1* and *TSC2*, were first identified in genetic linkage analysis of families with TSC [109]. *TSC1* is located on chromosome 9q34 and encodes the protein product hamartin.

The *TSC2* gene is found on chromosome 16p13.3 and encodes the protein tuberin. Of sporadic cases of TSC, nearly three quarters are thought to be due to new mutations in the *TSC2* gene [110]. The protein products of these two genes – hamartin and tuberin – have been shown to function together as a heterodimeric complex, negatively regulating the insulin receptor/phosphoinositide 3-kinase/mTOR pathway, thereby helping to control cell growth and division [111–113].

19.4.2 Clinical Manifestations

Classically, the symptoms and signs of TSC as defined by Vogt's triad have included seizures, neurocognitive delay, and the presence of a facial angiofibroma (adenoma sebaceum). This triad, however, is only completely present in one-third of TSC patients. In contrast, nearly all patients have at least one or more of the skin manifestations seen in TSC. As with other neurocutaneous syndromes, the symptoms and signs of TSC are referable to the dermatologic, ophthalmologic, and nervous systems. In addition, these patients may suffer from cardiac, pulmonary, and renal abnormalities as detailed below.

19.4.2.1 Central Nervous System Manifestations

Neurologic symptoms are the most common cause of morbidity and mortality in TSC patients [108]. Within the CNS, TSC patients are prone to develop numerous lesions and cytoarchitectural abnormalities. Among these are the characteristic cortical tubers, subependymal nodules, subependymal giant cell astrocytoma (SEGA) (Fig. 19.7), cortical dysplasia, and radial migration abnormalities. Involvement of the spinal cord is uncommon in TSC. Although uncommon, an association with intracranial aneurysms has also been reported in TSC patients.

Cortical tubers are the most common CNS manifestation of the disease. These hamartomas are usually situated at the gray-white matter junction within the frontal lobes, although they may occur in other lobes as well. They range from 1

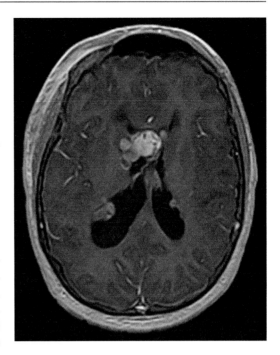

Fig. 19.7 Subependymal giant cell astrocytoma in a patient with TSC. Axial view T1-weighted post-gadolinium-enhanced MRI demonstrating a cystic inhomogeneously enhancing intraventricular subependymal giant cell astrocytoma obstructing Monroe's foramen with associated ventricular dilatation in a patient with tuberous sclerosis

to 2 cm in size and consist of firm, pale gliotic plaques pathologically. The normal laminar cortical architecture is disrupted around these tubers. Over time, these lesions may accumulate progressive calcification or undergo cystic degeneration.

In addition to cortical tubers, subependymal nodules around the lateral ventricles can develop. These characteristic lesions usually range in size from 1 to 10 mm and are distributed along the head of the caudate nucleus as well as the strio-thalamic zone of the lateral ventricle. Over time, they may increase in number and show evidence of calcification.

A third structural lesion thought to be unique to TSC patients is the SEGA. Up to 6% of TSC patients develop this tumor. Typically, they arise within the ventricle in the region of the foramen of Monro and are thought to arise from the transformation and overgrowth of a subependymal nodule. On occasion, one finds a SEGA within the parenchyma itself – thought to be secondary to degeneration of a cortical tuber [114]. Symptoms of increased intracranial pressure or a change in the patient's previous seizure pattern may signal the development of this lesion.

The presence of these cortical tubers has been linked to the development of both the seizure disorder and cognitive dysfunction seen in the TSC patients [115, 116]. Despite appearing neurologically normal at birth, up to 85% of TSC patients eventually suffer from a seizure disorder [108, 116, 117]. In fact, the onset of seizures may be the first symptom of this disorder in a child. The majority become symptomatic within the first 2–3 years of life. The initial pattern is usually one of flexion myoclonus, with EEG evidence of hypsarrhythmia. This pattern may evolve into psychomotor or generalized tonic-clonic epilepsy as the disease progresses.

Cognitive dysfunction is also common in TSC—seen in up to 50% of patients [108]. Additionally, patients with TSC are at increased risk of developing autism, behavioral disorders, and psychosocial difficulties. Collectively, these are termed TSC-associated neuropsychiatric disorders.

19.4.2.2 Cutaneous Manifestations

The cutaneous lesions of TSC are not pathognomonic but occur in more than 90% of patients with TSC. These lesions include hypomelanotic macules, shagreen patches, periungual fibromas, and facial angiofibromas [118]. Ash-leaf spots (hypomelanotic macules) are one of the earliest cutaneous findings. These lesions which are often present at birth appear as dull-white polygonal regions of hypopigmentation. They are not, however, pathognomonic for TSC and can be seen among the general population. Another cutaneous sign of TSC is the shagreen patch. This lesion consists of an orange peel-textured hamartoma of the skin, found most commonly in the lumbosacral region. Up to 20% of TSC patients may exhibit a shagreen patch, often during early childhood. In many TSC patients, facial angiofibromas may develop during childhood. This acneiform-like lesion usually is found in a malar distribution, can be disfiguring, and can reduce quality of life.

19.4.2.3 Ophthalmologic Manifestations

The ophthalmologic manifestations of TSC include retinal phakomas (astrocytomas), which occur in 50–75% of patients [119]. In addition, achromic retinal patches may be seen. Neither of these lesions produces visual impairment.

19.4.2.4 Cardiac Manifestations

Cardiac rhabdomyomas can be found in up to 50% of TSC patients. Most patients suffer little clinical impact from these lesions. Some, however, develop heart failure secondary to outflow obstruction or impaired cardiac contractility. Less frequently, these lesions may incite arrhythmias or thromboembolic events. Typically, rhabdomyomas decrease in size and may disappear altogether, with symptomatic patients requiring medical management alone.

19.4.2.5 Pulmonary Manifestations

Pulmonary complications in TSC are uncommon, affecting approximately 2–5% of females with TSC. A potentially fatal pulmonary manifestation of TSC is lymphangioleiomyomatosis, which typically develops during the fourth decade of life, causing symptoms of dyspnea, hemoptysis, or spontaneous pneumothorax.

19.4.2.6 Renal Manifestations

Multiple different renal lesions can develop in TSC patients. These often become symptomatic during the second decade of life. The most common among these lesions is the benign angiomyolipoma – seen in approximately 70–80% of TSC patients [120]. Renal cysts occur in approximately 20% of patients. Less common findings include angiomyoliposarcoma, oncocytoma, and renal cell carcinoma.

19.4.3 Diagnosis

The diagnostic criteria of TSC have been recently revised and updated (Table 19.5) [121, 122]. These include 11 major and 6 minor features. However, independent of clinical findings, detection of a pathogenic mutation in *TSC1* or *TSC2* in non-lesional

Table 19.5 Updated diagnostic criteria for tuberous sclerosis complex (Northrup and Krueger [121])

Genetic diagnostic criteria	Clinical diagnostic criteria
Genetic findings	*Major features*
A pathogenic mutation in *TSC1* or *TSC2*, defined as:	1. Hypomelanotic macules (≥3, at least 5 mm in diameter)
1. A mutation that clearly inactivates TSC1 or TSC2	2. Angiofibromas (≥3) or fibrous cephalic plaque
(a) An out-of-frame insertion	3. Ungal fibromas (≥2)
(b) An out-of-frame deletion	4. Shagreen patch
(c) Nonsense mutation	5. Multiple retinal hamartomas
2. A mutation that prevents protein synthesis	6. Cortical dysplasias[a]
(a) Large genomic deletion	7. Subependymal nodules
3. A missense mutation whose effect on protein function has been established by functional assessment	8. Subependymal giant cell astrocytoma
Notes:	9. Cardiac rhabdomyoma
Other *TSC1* or *TSC2* variants whose effects on function are less certain do not meet these criteria and are not sufficient to make a definite diagnosis of TSC	10. Lymphangioleiomyomatosis (LAM)[b]
10–25% of patients do not have an identifiable genetic mutation which is known	11. Angiomyolipomas (≥2)[b]
	Minor features
	1. "Confetti" skin lesions
	2. Dental enamel pits (≥3)
	3. Intraoral fibromas (≥2)
	4. Retinal achromic patch
	5. Multiple renal cysts
	6. Nonrenal hamartomas

Definite diagnosis: (1) Presence of a pathogenic mutation in normal tissue; (2) two major features or one major feature and ≥ 2 minor features

Possible diagnosis: Either one major feature or ≥ 2 minor features

[a]Includes tubers and cerebral white matter radial migration lines

[b]A combination of the two major clinical features (LAM and angiomyolipomas) without other features does not meet criteria for a definitive diagnosis

tissue is sufficient to make a diagnosis of TSC. As with all neurocutaneous syndromes, initial investigation of a patient suspected to have TSC should involve a multidisciplinary workup, including detailed ophthalmologic and fundoscopic exams, dermatologic screen, and a clinical neurologic and neurodevelopmental assessment. Also of importance are the inclusion of neuroimaging studies and echocardiography and renal ultrasound or CT.

CT scan usually demonstrates cortical tubers and subependymal nodules which appear as focal regions of increased attenuation. These lesions enhance very little with intravenous contrast agent. The subependymal nodules have been described as resembling "candle drippings" along the walls of the lateral ventricles. On MRI, however, these lesions are more heterogeneous in appearance and have minimal peripheral contrast enhancement. Significant enhancement of a subependymal nodule, nodules greater than 10 mm in diameter or exhibiting rapid growth between serial imaging studies, or nodules caus-

ing hydrocephalus are worrisome for the development of a SEGA [108]. TSC patients should undergo regular MRI every 1–3 years to monitor for SEGA [108]. This should be continued at least until 25 years of age but should be offered more frequently if a SEGA is identified or if patients are unable to reliably report subtle symptoms due to cognitive delay.

In patients with seizures, further workup, including EEG studies, video-EEG monitoring, magnetoencephalography, or invasive monitoring with electrocorticography, may facilitate identification of the epileptic focus. Advanced MRI techniques such as diffusion-weighted MRI may aid in identifying which tuber, among many, could be causative of the patient's seizures [123]. Tubers with elevated apparent diffusion coefficients and reduced fractional anisotropy are associated with increased epileptic potential [123, 124]. In addition, evidence of hypometabolism on FDG-PET imaging may assist in identifying epileptogenic tubers [125].

19.4.4 Clinical Management

19.4.4.1 Surgical Management

The neurosurgical management of TSC patients is performed for three main indications: the control of intractable seizures, the resection of SEGAs, and the treatment of hydrocephalus.

Up to 63% of patients with TSC may develop medication refractory seizures [126]. In these children epilepsy surgery can be challenging due to many reasons. Firstly, the presence of multiple cortical tubers can make identification of the epileptogenic focus difficult. Second, occasionally, more than one focus may be present. Better outcomes are expected when a single cortical tuber can be identified as the epicenter of a patient's seizure activity, showing a strong correlation between imaging and EEG studies [127]. Although challenging, the presence of multiple tubers, however, is not an absolute contraindication to surgery. In some cases, use of invasive intracranial EEG monitoring may allow the surgeon to pinpoint the primary seizure focus and assist with rational surgical planning [128].

In patients who lack a clear seizure focus, surgery can still be beneficial and offered with a more palliative goal in mind, such as reducing the severity or frequency of seizures. An example of this is a corpus callosotomy, which can be helpful in children who suffer from frequent drop attacks.

Surgery also serves a role in the treatment of TSC patients who develop SEGA. Be it via a interhemispheric transcallosal or transfrontal transcortical approach, complete surgical excision of this tumor remains the standard of care. Many advocate that early diagnosis followed by complete excision may minimize the morbidity and mortality associated with this complication of TSC [116, 129]. Due to either location, size, or patient factors, some patients may not tolerate surgical excision of these lesions however. In this group of patients, a palliative CSF diversion procedure may be warranted if and when the lesion causes obstructive hydrocephalus. Alternatively, nonsurgical alternatives may be tried including novel targeted drug therapies or stereotactic radiosurgery [130].

19.4.4.2 Nonsurgical Management

The medical management of epilepsy associated with TSC depends on the pattern of seizures observed. Children with infantile spasms may respond to adrenocorticotrophic hormone (ACTH) therapy [131]. The antiepileptic medication vigabatrin has also shown promise as an effective drug for treating infantile spasms in the context of TSC [132]. Patients with generalized seizures may benefit from treatment with benzodiazepines, with or without the addition of sodium valproate. Children with complex partial and focal motor seizures can be treated with various antiepileptic medications, including carbamazepine, phenytoin, lamotrigine, or primidone [133, 134].

Novel therapies for SEGA have recently been approved for use in the clinical setting and are particularly valuable for those tumors which are not amenable to surgical therapies. Everolimus is one such drug which is now frequently used after demonstrating remarkable tumor regression in multiple clinical trials [130]. In addition to targeted drug therapies, stereotactic radiosurgery has emerged as an increasingly popular treatment option when either recurrence or symptomatic residual tumor is present postsurgery. However, given its inability to reduce tumor size dramatically, it should not be offered in cases which demonstrate SEGA-associated hydrocephalus.

19.4.5 Prognosis and Quality of Life

As disease phenotypes can be heterogeneous even among affected families, the long-term prognosis and quality of life for TSC patients are variable. Patients with mild phenotypes can lead nearly normal lives without obvious impairment. Others may experience significant morbidity and a reduced life expectancy. The most worrisome complications relate to the CNS and renal systems. Young patients may suffer from serious morbidity or death due to the development of SEGA. Older patients are at risk of developing end-stage renal failure. Death occasionally can result from status epilepticus or pneumonia. Even in the absence of these feared complications, large facial angiofibromas can have a significant lifelong impact on quality of life and self-image.

19.4.6 Future Perspectives

Increased understanding regarding the molecular basis of TSC may lead to the development of new, targeted therapies in the near future. As mentioned previously, the *TSC1* and *TSC2* gene products work together to inhibit signaling via the insulin receptor/PI3K/mTOR pathway. Inhibitors of mTOR have been developed and have shown efficacy in causing regression of SEGAs [135]. Interestingly, mTOR inhibitors have shown promise as not only oncologic therapies but have also been effective as anti-seizure therapy in some patients [130]. These drugs, along with others such as the farnesyl transferase inhibitors, are already in use in the clinic and may serve an increasingly important role in the treatment of patients with TSC in the near future [136].

19.5 Von Hippel-Lindau Disease

19.5.1 Epidemiology and Pathophysiology

Von Hippel-Lindau disease (VHL) is an autosomal dominant, inherited disorder characterized by cystic or neoplastic changes in many organ systems, in addition to the development of benign hemangioblastomas of the CNS. It has also been referred to as retinocerebellar angiomatosis due to the vascular changes evident in both the ophthalmologic and nervous systems. The annual incidence of VHL is approximately 1 in 36,000 births [137].

The *VHL* tumor suppressor gene has been identified on chromosome 3p25. Its gene product normally plays a role in targeting the alpha subunit of hypoxia-inducible factor (*HIF*) for ubiquitination, and subsequent proteasomal degradation, thereby helping to limit angiogenic activity [138]. With *VHL* mutated, *HIF* activity rises leading to increased proliferation and subsequent tumor growth [139].

19.5.2 Clinical Manifestations

19.5.2.1 Central Nervous System Manifestations

The most common CNS manifestation of VHL is the characteristic cerebellar hemangioblastoma (Fig. 19.8). Approximately 60–80% of VHL patients ultimately develop a CNS hemangioblastoma [140]. Three-quarters of these lesions are cerebellar in location, with the majority of the remaining hemangioblastomas located within the spinal cord. Hemangioblastomas of the cerebral hemispheres account for only a small minority of lesions. The majority of symptomatic cerebellar and spinal hemangioblastomas are associated with a cyst, which typically is larger than the tumor nodule itself [140]. Patients with cerebellar lesions may present with complaints because of increased intracranial pressure, such as headache, nausea, vomiting, or visual disturbances. Less often, they may present suddenly with symptoms secondary to acute hemorrhage, including gross cerebellar dysfunction or a decreased level of consciousness. In a large review series of 80 VHL patients operated on for cerebellar hemangioblastoma, headache, ataxia, dysmetria, and hydrocephalus were observed in 75%, 55%, 29%, and 28%, respectively [141]. Interestingly, nervous system hemangioblastomas also represent an early and preferred site for tumor-to-tumor metastasis from systemic primary cancers (such as renal cell carcinoma) in the VHL patient [142]. Compared to hemangioblastomas arising in the general population, those occurring in VHL patients tend to become symptomatic at an earlier age, with a mean age at diagnosis in the third decade of life [114, 140]. In addition, among VHL patients who develop hemangioblastomas, approximately 90% develop multiple lesions [140]. In addition to hemangioblastomas, 10–15% of VHL patients develop endolymphatic sac tumors [140].

Spinal hemangioblastomas also occur in VHL patients (Fig. 19.9). These lesions are predominantly intramedullary in location and typically abut the pial surface of the cord. The cystic component seen in cerebellar hemangioblastomas is often absent in the spinal cord; however, an associated

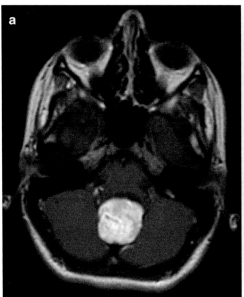 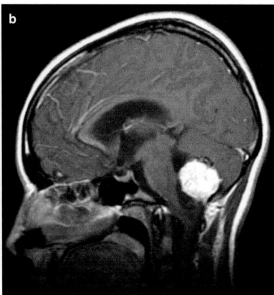

Fig. 19.8 Cerebellar hemangioblastoma in a patient with VHL. MRI of VHL patient with a cerebellar hemangioblastoma. Axial (**a**) and sagittal (**b**) view T1-weighted post-gadolinium-enhanced MRI of a midline cerebellar hemangioblastoma demonstrating almost homogenous enhancement. Note characteristic "popcorn-like" enhancement

syrinx may be evident. Patients with spinal hemangioblastomas may be asymptomatic or may develop pain or long tract findings.

19.5.2.2 Ophthalmologic Manifestations

A common ophthalmologic manifestation of VHL is the retinal hemangioblastoma. These lesions occur in over half of all VHL patients and become symptomatic in approximately 20% of them. They typically arise bilaterally and in multiple locations. Fluorescein retinal angiography aids in the early detection of these lesions. Early detection and treatment may minimize the risks of hemorrhage and retinal detachment.

19.5.2.3 Other Systemic Manifestations

Additional systemic findings associated with VHL include pancreatic cysts and islet cell tumors, renal cysts, and renal cell carcinoma, as well as pheochromocytoma.

19.5.3 Diagnosis

The diagnosis of VHL is no longer primarily a clinical one with the growing role of genetics in medicine [143]. Previously, a diagnosis of VHL was made confidently in the presence of one major manifestation of the disease in a patient with a positive family history or at least two major features (at least one being a hemangioblastoma) in a patient lacking this family history [144]. Although this still holds true, due to the advancement and ease of access to genetic testing and its high specificity and sensitivity in VHL, more and more patients with pathognomonic lesions are being sent for genetic diagnostics [143].

Despite the fact that the majority of patients diagnosed with a cerebellar hemangioblastoma do not suffer from VHL, one should maintain a high index of suspicion for this disease. Few patients ultimately diagnosed with VHL actually have a known positive family history for this disorder. Patients with multiple lesions, or those presenting at a young age, are in a high-risk group

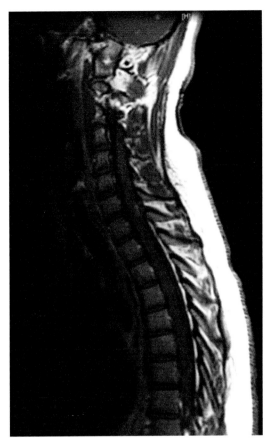

Fig. 19.9 Spinal hemangiomas in a patient with VHL. Sagittal view T1-weighted post-gadolinium-enhanced MRI of a patient with prominent enhancing intradural intramedullary hemangioma of the lower cervical spinal cord

for having VHL as the underlying etiology for their hemangioblastomas.

The most common diagnostic adjuncts for the diagnosis of the CNS manifestations of VHL are CT and MRI scans. On CT scan of the brain, hemangioblastomas typically appear as a cystic mass with an associated hyperdense mural nodule that enhances brightly with IV contrast. This nodule often abuts a pial surface. Most lesions are found within the cerebellar hemispheres. Contrast-enhanced MRI remains the most sensitive diagnostic modality for detecting CNS hemangioblastomas [140]. MRI of the brain reveals a hypo- to isointense nodule

on T1-weighted images and hyperintense on T2-weighted images, which enhances strongly with contrast administration. Angiography may be slightly more sensitive for the detection of smaller lesions, but is not commonly used as an initial investigation in this patient population.

Upon confirmation of the diagnosis of VHL, adequate follow-up and monitoring are required. Between the ages of 0 and 2 years, annual physical examination including an ophthalmologic assessment is warranted. Urine catecholamines should be measured every 1–2 years after this point. At approximately age 11, serial imaging of the craniospinal axis along with abdominal ultrasound is recommended on a biannual basis [145].

19.5.4 Clinical Management

19.5.4.1 Surgical Management

The treatment of cerebellar hemangioblastomas in VHL parallels the treatment used in the spontaneously arising variety. The management challenge posed by the VHL patient stems from the number of hemangioblastomas they may harbor. A recent review from the National Institutes of Health examined 19 VHL patients with a total of 143 lesions over a period of more than 10 years in order to identify factors predictive of symptomatic progression of these lesions [146]. They observed that the hemangioblastomas tended to grow in a stuttering pattern and that the lesions that ultimately became symptomatic may not have been those initially identified by neuroimaging [146]. While 97% of lesions demonstrated asymptomatic progression on serial imaging, only 50% ultimately required treatment for symptomatic progression [146]. In general, symptomatic progression was related to the rate of growth of the tumor or associated cyst and lesion location (cerebellum vs. brain stem vs. spinal cord) [146]. Based on their observations, they issued caution regarding recommending treatment for lesions based on asymptomatic growth demonstrated on imaging alone [146]. A larger review of 160 VHL patients with 655 CNS hemangioblastomas also observed variable growth rates for these lesions [147]. A threshold for symptomatic progression based on tumor size or rate of growth could not be clearly defined [147]. Others recommend resection of asymptomatic lesions showing radiographic progression alone in order to prevent the development of permanent deficits [148]. Surgical resection, however, has been shown to result in symptomatic improvement in the vast majority of patients [141]. When necessary, complete surgical excision is the goal of treatment, taking care to remove the mural nodule in order to prevent recurrence. The wall of the accompanying cyst does not need to be resected in its entirety. Patients presenting with preoperative hydrocephalus rarely will require permanent CSF diversion following resection of the lesion [141]. For asymptomatic spinal lesions, observation with serial imaging is one strategy often used. Once symptomatic, an attempt at surgical resection should be considered [119, 149, 150]. Some authors, however, suggest selective surgical resection for asymptomatic spinal hemangioblastomas [151]. After complete resection, the appearance of additional lesions is more likely to represent new primary lesions rather than a recurrence.

19.5.4.2   Radiation Therapy

Although not common, radiosurgery has been used as a modality in the treatment of hemangioblastomas associated with VHL. Chang et al. reviewed their experience treating 29 lesions in 13 patients with underlying VHL using linear accelerator-based radiosurgery [120]. Their mean follow-up was just under 4 years. Only one lesion (3%) showed evidence of progression during this period. Five lesions disappeared on subsequent imaging studies, 16 regressed, and 7 remained unchanged. Despite somewhat limited follow-up, they suggested that radiosurgery may be an alternative to microsurgical resection of hemangioblastomas. Due to the stuttering nature of tumor growth, however, the lack of radiographic progression following radiosurgery may simply reflect the natural history of the lesion and not a treatment effect. Longer follow-up is needed to determine the true value of this

treatment modality for hemangioblastoma [140]. This modality may prove useful in treating those lesions that are difficult to access or those in which the risks of surgical resection in an asymptomatic patient may be prohibitive as in the case of high spinal cord lesions.

19.5.5   Prognosis and Quality of Life

The main contributors to a poor prognosis or reduced quality of life in VHL patients are the presence of CNS hemangioblastomas or the development of renal cell carcinoma. Niemela et al. examined a series of 110 consecutive patients diagnosed with CNS hemangioblastoma during the period from 1953 to 1993, 14 of whom had underlying VHL [152]. Among the VHL patients, the mean age at diagnosis of their CNS hemangioblastoma was 33 years, and the mean age at which renal cell carcinoma developed was 43 years of age.

19.6   Sturge-Weber Syndrome

19.6.1   Epidemiology and Pathophysiology

Sturge-Weber syndrome (SWS) is a rare neurocutaneous syndrome involving the vasculature of the skin, eyes, meninges, and brain. SWS is a sporadic congenital neurocutaneous syndrome caused by somatic mutations in *GNAQ* on chromosome 9q21 and thus not a heritable disorder [153]. *GNAQ* mutation activates a set of signaling pathways that are thought to result in either nonsyndromic port-wine stains or SWS, depending upon what stage of embryonic development is affected [153]. Unlike other neurocutaneous syndromes in this chapter, tumorigenesis is not a feature of this disorder. The vascular anomalies seen in SWS are thought to stem from abnormal embryogenesis during weeks 5–8 of gestation. There appears to be no predilection for any particular race or sex in SWS. The incidence is thought to be approximately 1 in 20,000 to 1 in 50,000 [154]. A rare variant of this disorder is known as Klippel-Trenaunay-Weber syndrome or spinal cutaneous angiomatosis. This subgroup of patients exhibit dermatomally distributed cutaneous hemangiomas, with spinal hemangiomas involving the same dermatomal region of the cord.

19.6.2 Clinical Manifestations

The cardinal clinical features of SWS include a congenital, unilateral facial nevus, seizures, mental retardation, hemiparesis, and altered vision. The characteristic facial nevus (port-wine stain or salmon patch) is typically located along the first or second division of the trigeminal nerve. This nevus may persist transiently or permanently. On occasion, a bilateral nevus is present.

In the forme fruste of SWS, this cutaneous lesion may be entirely absent. In addition, the presence of such a nevus is not pathognomonic for SWS, as most children born with this lesion do not have underlying SWS.

19.6.2.1 Ophthalmologic Manifestations

The ophthalmologic manifestations of SWS include glaucoma, retinal detachment, retinal vascular tortuosity, strabismus, and buphthalmos. In addition, choroidal, conjunctival, or episcleral hemangiomas may be seen. Of these disorders, glaucoma is the most common, affecting between 30 and 50% of SWS patients. Glaucoma usually develops in the eye ipsilateral to the facial nevus and often during the first 2 years of life.

19.6.2.2 Central Nervous System Manifestations

Within the CNS, and ipsilateral to the facial nevus, patients with SWS may develop leptomeningeal venous angiomatosis. In up to 15%, this abnormality occurs bilaterally. Pathologically, this lesion consists of thin-walled venous malformations within the pia mater, causing the meninges to take on a thick, darkened purple appearance. The underlying brain often shows evidence of cortical atrophy, calcification, as well as associated enlargement of the choroid plexus. This leptomeningeal angiomatosis may produce symptoms including hemiparesis, visual disturbance (hemianopsia), seizures, and cognitive impairment. These findings are often present to some degree prior to 2 years of age. Seizures affect up to 85% of SWS patients [155]. Seizure onset occurs typically during the first year of life, prior to the development of hemiparesis [156, 157]. The seizure semiology is often that of either partial motor or generalized tonic-clonic epilepsy and may follow a remitting and relapsing course. In addition, hypoxia and microcirculatory stasis are thought to play a role in seizure etiology. In addition to seizures, some children may show a stepwise pattern of neurologic decline, thought to be secondary to ischemic events resulting from venous occlusion [158].

19.6.3 Diagnosis

The diagnosis of SWS is often possible based on the characteristic facial nevus, combined with findings at neuroimaging. On CT scan, the brain typically shows evidence of calcification of meningeal arteries, cortical and subcortical veins, and atrophy of the associated cortex (Fig. 19.10). MRI of the brain with IV contrast may disclose areas of meningeal angiomatosis. Since calcification may not be evident in the earliest stages of disease, MRI may be more appropriate in the initial workup of these patients. Perfusion abnormalities may be identified using modalities such as single-photon emission computed tomography or positron emission tomography. Abnormalities seen with these modalities may precede evidence of atrophy or calcification seen later on CT or MRI scans [159]. Recently, MR spectroscopy has shown utility in detecting intracranial abnormalities that elude conventional MRI scans [147]. Reduced frontal lobe N-acetylaspartate (NAA) was associated with earlier seizure onset and motor impairment [147]. Susceptibility-weighted MRI acquisition offers the potential to more clearly identify enlarged transmedullary veins, periventricular veins, cortical gyriform abnormalities, and abnormalities of the gray-white matter interface [160].

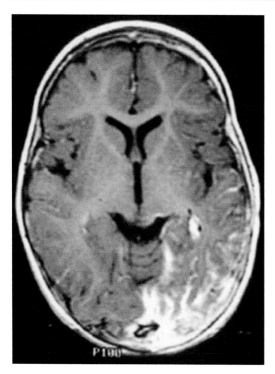

Fig. 19.10 Vascular calcification in patient with SWS. Axial view T1-weighted post-gadolinium-enhanced MRI of a patient with prominent meningeal arterial, cortical, and subcortical vein calcification of the left parieto-occipital lobe in a patient with Sturge-Weber syndrome

EEG is routine in the workup of SWS patients suffering from epilepsy. Video-EEG monitoring is useful in the preoperative planning stage. In addition, invasive cortical monitoring or magnetoencephalography may assist in defining the seizure focus in these patients.

19.6.4 Clinical Management

19.6.4.1 Surgical Management
The primary role for neurosurgery in SWS patients is for control of medically refractory epilepsy. Due to the rarity of this disorder, it is difficult to define the most appropriate treatment strategy for these patients. Early surgery has been proposed by some authors in order to prevent subsequent development of hemiparesis [161, 162]. Hoffman et al. reported on the relationship between seizure control and subsequent developmental outcome, comparing children with SWS treated surgically

versus those managed medically. They found a higher chance of maintaining normal or nearly normal function (as measured by intelligence quotient scores) using surgical therapy as opposed to continued medical management. Others suggest reserving surgery solely for patients with medically intractable seizures and progressive neurologic decline [163]. Many surgical strategies have been employed in the treatment of these patients, including focal cortical resection, peri-insular hemispherectomy, hemispherectomy, lobectomy, corpus callosotomy, posterior quadrant disconnection, and vagal nerve stimulation. Surgery may provide complete relief from seizure in up to 65–81% of patients, with additional patients experiencing some degree of reduction in seizure frequency or severity [164].

19.6.4.2 Medical Management
Medical management of seizures in SWS is usually the first-line treatment. Seizure control is possible in up to 40% of SWS patients using antiepileptic medications [164]. Multiple agents have been used [158].

19.6.5 Prognosis and Quality of Life

The prognosis and quality of life of patients with SWS relate in part to whether the disease affecting the CNS is focal or holo-hemispheric [158]. Up to 50–60% with holo-hemispheric SWS will have some degree of developmental delay. Profound delay is expected in cases of bilateral CNS SWS. Patients with focal SWS are expected to have a decent prognosis and quality of life provided that their seizures are well controlled either surgically or medically.

19.7 Gorlin Syndrome

19.7.1 Epidemiology and Pathophysiology

Gorlin syndrome, also known as Gorlin-Goltz syndrome, nevoid basal cell carcinoma syndrome, or basal cell nevus syndrome, is a rare cancer predisposition syndrome with an autosomal dominant pattern of inheritance without sex or race predilection and a typical incidence of 1 in 57,000 to 1 in 256,000, [165, 166] although in some populations the incidence is as high as 1 in 15,000 [167]. Approximately 75% of individuals have a first-degree relative with the syndrome, with the remainder representing de novo mutations in germline candidate genes. The disease was first described in 1960 by Gorlin and Goltz in patients who shared the features of multiple basal cell carcinomas (BCC), jaw cysts, and bifid ribs [168]. This multisystem disorder is caused by germline mutations in genes involved in the sonic hedgehog (*SHH*) signaling pathway; the most well-studied of which are the human homolog of the patched (*PTCH1*) gene found at 9q22.3 and suppressor of fused (*SUFU*) [169–173]. The *PTCH1* gene product is a receptor for *SHH* or other *SHH*-related ligands. *SHH* binding to mutant *PTCH1* results in an alteration in *Smo* (smoothened) activity which is normally repressed by *PTCH1* [174]. Mutant PTCH1 therefore results in *Smo* activation of the signaling complex of *Gli-1* (glioma-associated oncogene) and *SUFU* [175]. Germline mutations in both *SUFU* and *PTCH1* are associated with loss of heterozygosity of the remaining allele in the tumor and activation of the *SHH* pathway. In addition to *PTCH1* and *SUFU*, *PTCH2* which shares high homology with *PTCH1* has also been found to contribute to tumorigenesis in Gorlin syndrome [176]. The activation of *PTCH1*, *PTCH2*, and *SUFU* results in unregulated expression of pathways involved in proliferation and inhibition of apoptosis [176, 177].

19.7.2 Clinical Manifestations

Patients with Gorlin syndrome can experience an array of phenotypic abnormalities, even within an affected family [166]. More relevant to its diagnostic criteria are abnormalities of the skin, skeletal system, genitourinary system, and the central nervous system. Most individuals with the disorder exhibit clinical manifestations by early childhood, and therefore diagnosis in infancy can be difficult if no positive family history is present.

19.7.2.1 Craniofacial Manifestations

Characteristic facial features have been described in over 50% of affected individuals. These include coarse facial appearance, frontal bossing, macrocephaly, and hypertelorism [166, 178]. Keratocystic odontogenic tumors (KOT) are also commonly present in individuals and can range from asymptomatic to painful and may also cause of abnormal dentition. One study of 105 patients with Gorlin syndrome determined that by age 20, 75% of patients develop KOT [166]. Other less common head and neck abnormalities can include cleft palate and strabismus [166].

19.7.2.2 Skeletal and Limb Manifestations

Perhaps some of the most clinically interesting manifestations in Gorlin syndrome are those which affect the skeletal system. Abnormalities affecting the ribs occur in 38% of affected individuals [166]. These include bifid ribs, marked widening of the anterior ends of ribs, fusion defects, and modeling defects. Asides from rib deformities, patients with this syndrome have been known to develop various developmental anomalies such as polydactyly, syndactyly, and Sprengel deformity which is seen in 10–40% of patients [179]. Also, patients with Gorlin syndrome are more likely to develop spinal deformities such as kyphoscoliosis and when present is typically severe.

19.7.2.3 Skin Manifestations

The hallmark of Gorlin syndrome is the propensity for these patients to develop multiple BCCs [180]. In the span of a patient's lifetime, as many as 500 BCCs may develop and are more frequent in those with lighter skin pigmentation as well as individuals who live in geographic locations with higher indices of ultraviolet radiation exposure [178]. Compared to sporadic BCC, in Gorlin syndrome patients, these lesions are often more clinically aggressive and develop much earlier in life – typically in adolescence although reports exist as early as 2 years of age [181, 182]. BCCs are found most commonly on the face but are also frequently identified on the trunk and limbs, anywhere skin is exposed to sun. Other skin manifestations in Gorlin syndrome include palmar and plantar pits in as many as 65–87% of patients and develop early in life, with up to 80% presenting by 10 years of age.

19.7.2.4 Central Nervous System Manifestations

Medulloblastoma is more frequently observed in Gorlin syndrome than in the general population, likely due to germline mutations in *PTCH* and *SUFU* which activate the SHH signaling pathway [183]. The link between Gorlin syndrome and medulloblastoma was first reported by Kimonis et al. in 1997 [166]. As many as 5% of patients with Gorlin syndrome develop medulloblastoma, usually by 3 years of age although occurrences have been reported as late as age 7 or 8 [179]. These tumors are exclusively driven by SHH and typically appear desmoplastic on histology. Interestingly, although Gorlin syndrome has no sex predilection, the ratio of medulloblastoma in these patients is skewed toward females at a ratio of 3:1 in distinction to sporadic medullo-blastoma which is more common in males [179]. Perplexingly, medulloblastoma in Gorlin syndrome has a less aggressive clinical behavior than its sporadic counterpart [179]. Other CNS tumors are also seen in affected individuals with a higher frequency than the general population likely due to activation of *SUFU* and *Gli-1*.

Medulloblastomas most often originate in the cerebellar vermis (Fig. 19.11), although rarely, more so in older patients, they can also occur in the cerebellar hemisphere. Imaging typically reveals a midline cerebellar mass appearing hyperdense on noncontrast computed tomography, intermediate signal intensity on T2-weighted MRI due to high cellularity, shows intense and homogenous enhancement, and causes obstructive hydrocephalus by infiltration of the fourth ventricle and invasion of the brainstem, with CSF seeding to spinal cord and meninges seen in 30% of cases [184, 185].

Non-oncologic central nervous system manifestations seen in Gorlin syndrome are seizures as well as structural or developmental anomalies [179, 180, 186, 187]. A recent study revealed that the brains of affected patients have unique morphological characteristics including larger size of the cerebrum, cerebellum, and ventricular system compared to normal individuals [186]. A proportion of patients can also exhibit cysts or dysgenesis in virtually any intracranial compartment. These include colloid cysts of third ventricle, arachnoid cysts, intraparenchymal cysts, and cysts of the septum pellucidum and vermian dysgenesis [179]. In addition, calcifications of meningeal structures can occur, most commonly calcification of the falx cerebri followed by the tentorium cerebelli, the pectinate ligament, and the diaphragma sellae [166]. Historically, these calcifications were identified on plain film radiography of the child's skull. In present day, they are more likely to be noticed on the scout image of computed tomography.

Seizures in these individuals are mostly associated with tumors, cysts, and structural anomalies but may also result from focal neuronal heterotopia [188]. Intellectual disabilities are found in approximately 5% of individuals [179].

19.7.2.5 Abdominal, Genitourinary, and Renal Manifestations

One of the most common genitourinary manifestations of Gorlin syndrome are ovarian fibromas or cysts. Occurring in up to 25–50% of females, these are often bilateral and evade clinical detection unless large, calcified, or twisted [179, 189]. A much smaller proportion, 5–10%, of males have been reported to show signs of hypogonadotropic hypogonadism such as anosmia, cryptorchidism, female pubic escutcheon, gynecomastia, or scant pubic hair [178].

Various renal anomalies are reported in 5% of the individuals with Gorlin syndrome. These include horseshoe kidney, L-shaped kidney, unilateral renal agenesis, renal cysts, and duplication of renal pelvis or ureters [190]. Within the abdomen, thin-walled mesenteric chylous and lymphatic cysts have been reported [190].

19.7.3 Diagnosis

Similar to other neurocutaneous disorders, the diagnosis of Gorlin syndrome is based on clinical

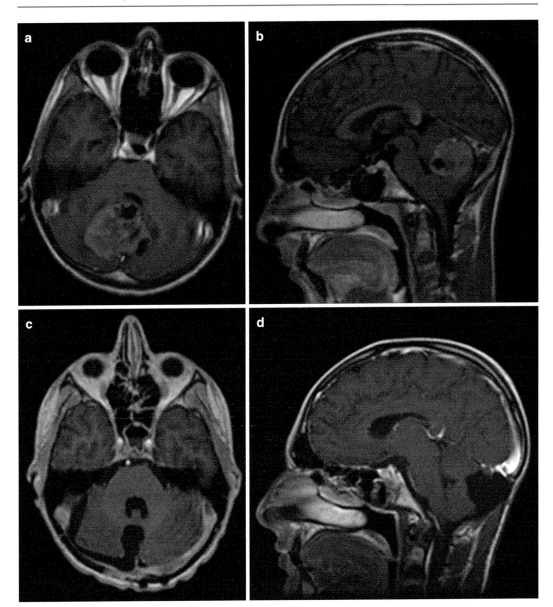

Fig. 19.11 Pre- and postoperative MRI of patient with medulloblastoma. Axial (**a**) and sagittal (**b**) view T1-weighted post-gadolinium-enhanced MRI of a midline medulloblastoma. Postoperative axial (**c**) and sagittal (**d**) view T1-weighted post-gadolinium-enhanced MRI demonstrating gross total resection

findings in the majority of cases. Initial diagnostic criteria were suggested by Evans et al. in 1993 [189]. This was revised 4 years later by Kimonis and colleagues [166]. In 2011, however, after the first meeting of the international colloquium of basal cell nevus syndrome, Bree and colleagues have proposed the most recent and widely accepted diagnostic criteria [191]. Under this consensus statement, a diagnosis of Gorlin syndrome can be made with near certainty if the patient has (1) one major criterion and molecular confirmation, (2) two major criteria, or (3) one major and two minor criteria (Table 19.6) [191].

In patients who meet criteria for clinical diagnosis, the detection rate of a *PTCH1* mutation is as high as 60–75% [187, 191]. However, genetic testing of

Table 19.6 Diagnostic criteria for Gorlin syndrome (Bree et al. [191])

Major criteria	Minor criteria
1. BCC prior to 20 years of age or excessive BCCs out of proportion to prior sun exposure and skin type	1. Rib anomalies
2. Odontogenic keratocyst of the jaw prior to 20 years of age	2. Other specific skeletal malformations and radiologic changes (i.e., vertebral anomalies, kyphoscoliosis, short fourth metacarpals, postaxial polydactyly)
3. Palmar or plantar pitting	3. Macrocephaly
4. Lamellar calcification of the falx cerebri	4. Cleft lip or cleft palate
5. Medulloblastoma (typically desmoplastic)	5. Ovarian fibroma or cardiac fibroma
6. First-degree relative with Gorlin syndrome	6. Lymphomesenteric cysts
	7. Ocular abnormalities (i.e., strabismus, hypertelorism, congenital cataracts, glaucoma, coloboma)

A suspected diagnosis of Gorlin syndrome could be made if:
1. Presence of one major criterion plus molecular confirmation (i.e., somatic PTCH1 mutation)
2. Two major criteria
3. One major and two minor criteria

the *PTCH1* mutation for the purpose of diagnosing Gorlin syndrome is controversial and reserved only for a small list of clinical scenarios. These typically include (1) prenatal testing if known familial mutation, (2) confirmatory diagnosis in patients with some clinical signs but not meeting criteria, and (3) predictive testing for patients with an affected family member who is at risk but does not meet clinical criteria [191]. Of course, this genetic testing does not take into account alternate driver mutations *PTCH2* and *SUFU* for which the diagnostic utility of genetic testing is less clear. Clinically, the consensus diagnostic workup for Gorlin syndrome has been recently proposed, beginning with a targeted medical history and physical exam followed by relevant imaging with or without genetic testing [191].

19.7.4 Management

19.7.4.1 Screening and Surveillance

All pediatric patients with Gorlin syndrome require annual contrasted brain MRI with epilepsy protocol until the age of 8, after which, it can be safely discontinued if findings are stable. If, however, patients become symptomatic of a suspected brain pathology, MRI imaging should be repeated sooner. All patients should also be seen annually by a medical geneticist, to ensure proper multidisciplinary issues are being adequately addressed with appropriate referrals being made. Annual full dermatologic evaluation is recommended until the discovery of an initial BCC at which point evaluations should be performed as frequent as every 6 months. Panoramic X-ray films should be performed as a baseline at 3 years of age or as soon as tolerated to detect possible jaw cysts. With respect to scoliosis, baseline radiographic films with scoliosis protocol should be obtained by 1 year of age or at time of diagnosis, whichever soonest. This should be repeated if abnormal every 6 months thereafter.

Developmental screening should include routine well-child visits. If children fail to meet developmental milestones, further investigation is warranted as appropriate. Regular vision, hearing, and speech screenings should be performed annually and continued into school age. One baseline ophthalmology assessment is warranted and is to be repeated only if symptomatic. All patients should undergo an initial psychological evaluation with follow-up arranged according to initial recommendations and findings.

Adult patients with Gorlin syndrome should undergo more frequent dermatologic evaluations, at least three times yearly. Digital panoramic X-ray should be performed yearly or more frequent if documented KOTs present. Prenatal or preconception genetic counseling should be offered to all couples determined to be high risk. Psychological evaluation should be performed on an as needed basis. In those patients with a history of medulloblastoma, annual neurological examinations are highly recommended.

As with all tumor predisposition syndromes, in both children and adults, care should be taken to limit exposure of ionizing radiation during diagnostic evaluations. Radiographs and computed tomography should be used sparsely, with the benefit versus risk to the patient's long-term health carefully considered. Whenever possible, diagnostic modalities which avoid the use of ionizing radiation should be used.

19.7.4.2 Radiation Therapy

Typically, all malignant tumors of the CNS are treated with a combination of surgery, radiation, and/or chemotherapy. However, in patients with Gorlin syndrome, this classic three-pronged approach poses a dilemma due to the increased risk for malignant tumor formation with ionizing radiation exposure and for spontaneous development of BCC both from existing basal cell nevi and apparently unaffected skin [192–196]. Because medulloblastoma in Gorlin syndrome has a peak incidence at 2 years of age, it is almost always the first oncologic manifestation in affected individuals [185]. In one recent study, three out of nine children received ionizing radiation as therapy for their medulloblastomas prior to a diagnosis of Gorlin syndrome; this radiation led to secondary cancers and ultimately proved fatal in two of the patients [197]. Therefore, in patients presenting with medulloblastoma, particularly those younger than age 5, Gorlin syndrome should first be ruled out to avoid untoward iatrogenic complications caused by radiation therapy—and is one such instance where genetic testing may be helpful in an otherwise asymptomatic child with medulloblastoma.

19.7.4.3 Surgery and Chemotherapy

As the histology of medulloblastoma is exclusively desmoplastic or with extensive nodularity,

patients with Gorlin syndrome typically have a favorable prognosis if diagnosed with medulloblastoma. This is an important consideration given that radiation therapy should be given sparingly or avoided altogether.

Gross total to near-total surgical resection is therefore fundamental to best achieve long-term survival. Ideally, a residual of less than or equal to 1.5 cm^3 is compatible with a favorable outcome and allows for initiation of standard-risk chemotherapy with or without stem cell rescue. Chemotherapeutic protocols vary according to center and practitioner preference but typically include a 3–4 drug combination of vincristine, cisplatin, topotecan, lomustine, and/or cyclophosphamide.

19.7.4.4 Targeted Biological Therapies

Sonidegib and vismodegib are two hedgehog-pathway inhibitors which are the first well-characterized targeted biological therapies to obtain approval for clinical use in North America for BCC. Both sonidegib and vismodegib function as SMO antagonists. These drugs and others are currently under investigation for use in children with medulloblastoma as well as other CNS and non-CNS tumors [198].

19.7.4.5 Other Considerations

Given that informed and health-aware patients with Gorlin syndrome take necessary precautions to avoid exposure to ultraviolet radiation, the incidence of Vitamin D deficiency in this population is elevated. Therefore, Vitamin D levels should be monitored closely and supplemented as appropriate.

19.7.5 Prognosis and Quality of Life

With much owed to modern developments in diagnostics, therapies and clinical knowledge, prompt identification, surveillance, and medical care of patients with Gorlin syndrome have resulted in expected survival that equals or approaches national averages. Development of BCCs and other malignancies can be minimal with avoidance of exposure to ultraviolet and ionizing radiation. Quality of life has been shown to be inversely related to number of BCCs [199]. Despite this and the small proportion who experience cognitive delay, most find meaning in life as evidenced by quality of life scores which are similar to the general population [199].

19.8 Conclusions

The neurocutaneous disorders described in this chapter comprise a fascinating array of conditions in which cutaneous lesions are typically found in conjunction with benign or malignant neoplasms of the peripheral or central nervous system. While the molecular genetics of these disorders are becoming well known and appreciated, the genotype-phenotype variability remains an important area of active investigation. With the advent of drug therapy for SEGAs in the context of tuberous sclerosis, there is hope that novel pharmacotherapeutics will be developed for some of the other neurocutaneous disorders.

References

1. Campian J, Gutmann DH (2017) CNS Tumors in Neurofibromatosis. J Clin Oncol 35:2378–2385
2. Karnes PS (1998) Neurofibromatosis: a common neurocutaneous disorder. Mayo Clin Proc 73:1071–1076
3. Huson SM, Compston DA, Clark P, Harper PS (1989) A genetic study of von Recklinghausen neurofibromatosis in south East Wales. I. Prevalence, fitness, mutation rate, and effect of parental transmission on severity. J Med Genet 26:704–711
4. Lammert M, Friedman JM, Kluwe L, Mautner VF (2005) Prevalence of neurofibromatosis 1 in German children at elementary school enrollment. Arch Dermatol 141:71–74
5. Jett K, Friedman JM (2010) Clinical and genetic aspects of neurofibromatosis 1. Genet Med 12:1–11
6. Dilworth JT et al (2006) Molecular targets for emerging anti-tumor therapies for neurofibromatosis type 1. Biochem Pharmacol 72:1485–1492
7. Khalaf WF et al (2007) K-ras is critical for modulating multiple c-kit-mediated cellular functions in wild-type and Nf1+/− mast cells. J Immunol 1950(178):2527–2534
8. Hand JL (2015) What's new with common genetic skin disorders? Curr Opin Pediatr 27:460–465
9. McClatchey AI (2007) Neurofibromatosis. Annu Rev Pathol 2:191–216
10. Kliegman R, Nelson WE (2011) Nelson textbook of pediatrics. Elsevier/Saunders, Philadelphia, PA
11. Gutmann DH et al (2017) Neurofibromatosis type 1. Nat Rev Dis Primer 3:17004
12. Heervä E et al (2012) A controlled register-based study of 460 neurofibromatosis 1 patients: increased fracture risk in children and adults over 41 years of age. J Bone Miner Res 27:2333–2337
13. Lin V, Daniel S, Forte V (2004) Is a plexiform neurofibroma pathognomonic of neurofibromatosis type I? Laryngoscope 114:1410–1414
14. Friedman JM, Birch PH (1997) Type 1 neurofibromatosis: a descriptive analysis of the disorder in 1,728 patients. Am J Med Genet 70:138–143
15. Huson SM, Harper PS, Compston DA (1988) Von Recklinghausen neurofibromatosis. A clinical and population study in south-East Wales. Brain J Neurol 111(Pt 6):1355–1381
16. Waggoner DJ, Towbin J, Gottesman G, Gutmann DH (2000) Clinic-based study of plexiform neurofibromas in neurofibromatosis 1. Am J Med Genet 92:132–135
17. Ferner RE (2007) Neurofibromatosis 1 and neurofibromatosis 2: a twenty first century perspective. Lancet Neurol 6:340–351
18. Serletis D et al (2007) Massive plexiform neurofibromas in childhood: natural history and management issues. J Neurosurg 106:363–367
19. Coffin CM, Davis JL, Borinstein SC (2014) Syndrome-associated soft tissue tumours. Histopathology 64:68–87
20. Hagel C et al (2007) Histopathology and clinical outcome of NF1-associated vs. sporadic malignant peripheral nerve sheath tumors. J Neuro-Oncol 82:187–192
21. Rauen KA et al (2015) Recent developments in neurofibromatoses and RASopathies: management, diagnosis and current and future therapeutic avenues. Am J Med Genet A 167:1–10
22. Friedrich RE, Hartmann M, Mautner VF (2007) Malignant peripheral nerve sheath tumors (MPNST) in NF1-affected children. Anticancer Res 27:1957–1960
23. de Blank PMK et al (2017) Optic pathway gliomas in neurofibromatosis type 1: an update: surveillance, treatment indications, and biomarkers of vision. J Neuroophthalmol 37(Suppl 1):S23–S32
24. Czyzyk E, Jóźwiak S, Roszkowski M, Schwartz RA (2003) Optic pathway gliomas in children with and without neurofibromatosis 1. J Child Neurol 18:471–478
25. Shamji MF, Benoit BG (2007) Syndromic and sporadic pediatric optic pathway gliomas: review of clinical and histopathological differences and treatment implications. Neurosurg Focus 23:E3

26. Liu GT et al (2004) Optic radiation involvement in optic pathway gliomas in neurofibromatosis. Am J Ophthalmol 137:407–414

27. Listernick R, Charrow J, Greenwald M, Mets M (1994) Natural history of optic pathway tumors in children with neurofibromatosis type 1: a longitudinal study. J Pediatr 125:63–66

28. Rosser T, Packer RJ (2002) Intracranial neoplasms in children with neurofibromatosis 1. J Child Neurol 17:630–637-651

29. Rodriguez FJ et al (2008) Gliomas in neurofibromatosis type 1: a clinicopathologic study of 100 patients. J Neuropathol Exp Neurol 67:240–249

30. Ferner RE et al (2007) Guidelines for the diagnosis and management of individuals with neurofibromatosis 1. J Med Genet 44:81–88

31. Burgio F et al (2017) Numerical activities of daily living in adults with neurofibromatosis type 1. J Intellect Disabil Res 61(11):1069–1077. https://doi.org/10.1111/jir.12408

32. Cipolletta S, Spina G, Spoto A (2018) Psychosocial functioning, self-image, and quality of life in children and adolescents with neurofibromatosis type 1. Child Care Health Dev 44(2):260–268. https://doi.org/10.1111/cch.12496

33. Pecoraro A et al (2017) Epilepsy in neurofibromatosis type 1. Epilepsy Behav 73:137–141

34. Vogel AC, Gutmann DH, Morris SM (2017) Neurodevelopmental disorders in children with neurofibromatosis type 1. Dev Med Child Neurol 59(11):1112–1116. https://doi.org/10.1111/dmcn.13526

35. Feldmann R, Denecke J, Grenzebach M, Schuierer G, Weglage J (2003) Neurofibromatosis type 1: motor and cognitive function and T2-weighted MRI hyperintensities. Neurology 61:1725–1728

36. DeBella K, Szudek J, Friedman JM (2000) Use of the national institutes of health criteria for diagnosis of neurofibromatosis 1 in children. Pediatrics 105:608–614

37. Heim RA, Silverman LM, Farber RA, Kam-Morgan LN, Luce MC (1994) Screening for truncated NF1 proteins. Nat Genet 8:218–219

38. Messiaen LM et al (2000) Exhaustive mutation analysis of the NF1 gene allows identification of 95% of mutations and reveals a high frequency of unusual splicing defects. Hum Mutat 15:541–555

39. Lopes Ferraz Filho JR et al (2008) Unidentified bright objects on brain MRI in children as a diagnostic criterion for neurofibromatosis type 1. Pediatr Radiol 38:305–310

40. Shen MH, Harper PS, Upadhyaya M (1996) Molecular genetics of neurofibromatosis type 1 (NF1). J Med Genet 33:2–17

41. Mautner VF et al (2003) Malignant peripheral nerve sheath tumours in neurofibromatosis type 1: MRI supports the diagnosis of malignant plexiform neurofibroma. Neuroradiology 45:618–625

42. Mautner V-F et al (2008) Assessment of benign tumor burden by whole-body MRI in patients with neurofibromatosis 1. NeuroOncol 10:593–598

43. Bredella MA et al (2007) Value of PET in the assessment of patients with neurofibromatosis type 1. AJR Am J Roentgenol 189:928–935

44. Ferner RE et al (2008) [18F]2-fluoro-2-deoxy-D-glucose positron emission tomography (FDG PET) as a diagnostic tool for neurofibromatosis 1 (NF1) associated malignant peripheral nerve sheath tumours (MPNSTs): a long-term clinical study. Ann Oncol 19:390–394

45. Ferner RE et al (2000) Evaluation of (18)fluorodeoxyglucose positron emission tomography ((18)FDG PET) in the detection of malignant peripheral nerve sheath tumours arising from within plexiform neurofibromas in neurofibromatosis 1. J Neurol Neurosurg Psychiatry 68:353–357

46. King A, Listernick R, Charrow J, Piersall L, Gutmann DH (2003) Optic pathway gliomas in neurofibromatosis type 1: the effect of presenting symptoms on outcome. Am J Med Genet A 122A:95–99

47. Gachiani J, Kim D, Nelson A, Kline D (2007) Surgical management of malignant peripheral nerve sheath tumors. Neurosurg Focus 22:E13

48. Perrin RG, Guha A (2004) Malignant peripheral nerve sheath tumors. Neurosurg Clin N Am 15:203–216

49. Stucky C-CH et al (2012) Malignant peripheral nerve sheath tumors (MPNST): the Mayo Clinic experience. Ann Surg Oncol 19:878–885

50. Piccirilli M et al (2006) Spontaneous regression of optic pathways gliomas in three patients with neurofibromatosis type I and critical review of the literature. Childs Nerv Syst 22:1332–1337

51. Pruzan NL, de Alba Campomanes A, Gorovoy IR, Hoyt C (2015) Spontaneous regression of a massive sporadic Chiasmal optic pathway glioma. J Child Neurol 30:1196–1198

52. Parsa CF et al (2001) Spontaneous regression of optic gliomas: thirteen cases documented by serial neuroimaging. Arch Ophthalmol 1960(119):516–529

53. Perilongo G et al (1999) Spontaneous partial regression of low-grade glioma in children with neurofibromatosis-1: a real possibility. J Child Neurol 14:352–356

54. El-Shehaby AMN, Reda WA, Abdel Karim KM, Emad Eldin RM, Nabeel AM (2016) Single-session gamma knife radiosurgery for optic pathway/hypothalamic gliomas. Spec Suppl 125:50–57

55. Guillamo J-S et al (2003) Prognostic factors of CNS tumours in Neurofibromatosis 1 (NF1): a retrospective study of 104 patients. Brain J Neurol 126:152–160

56. Sharif S et al (2006) Second primary tumors in neurofibromatosis 1 patients treated for optic glioma: substantial risks after radiotherapy. J Clin Oncol 24:2570–2575

57. Gerszten PC, Burton SA, Ozhasoglu C, McCue KJ, Quinn AE (2008) Radiosurgery for benign intradural spinal tumors. Neurosurgery 62:887–895-896

58. Chamberlain MC, Grafe MR (1995) Recurrent chiasmatic-hypothalamic glioma treated with oral etoposide. J Clin Oncol 13:2072–2076

59. Friedman HS et al (1992) Treatment of children with progressive or recurrent brain tumors with carboplatin

or iproplatin: a Pediatric oncology group randomized phase II study. J Clin Oncol 10:249–256

60. Gajjar A et al (1993) Response of pediatric low grade gliomas to chemotherapy. Pediatr Neurosurg 19:113–118-120

61. Laithier V et al (2003) Progression-free survival in children with optic pathway tumors: dependence on age and the quality of the response to chemotherapy--results of the first French prospective study for the French Society of Pediatric Oncology. J Clin Oncol 21:4572–4578

62. Mahoney DH et al (2000) Carboplatin is effective therapy for young children with progressive optic pathway tumors: a Pediatric oncology group phase II study. NeuroOncol 2:213–220

63. Massimino M et al (2002) High response rate to cisplatin/etoposide regimen in childhood low-grade glioma. J Clin Oncol 20:4209–4216

64. Packer RJ et al (1988) Treatment of chiasmatic/hypothalamic gliomas of childhood with chemotherapy: an update. Ann Neurol 23:79–85

65. Pons MA et al (1992) Chemotherapy with vincristine (VCR) and etoposide (VP-16) in children with low-grade astrocytoma. J Neuro-Oncol 14:151–158

66. Rosenstock JG et al (1985) Chiasmatic optic glioma treated with chemotherapy. A preliminary report. J Neurosurg 63:862–866

67. Gutmann DH et al (2003) Molecular analysis of astrocytomas presenting after age 10 in individuals with NF1. Neurology 61:1397–1400

68. Bader JL (1986) Neurofibromatosis and cancer. Ann N Y Acad Sci 486:57–65

69. Rasmussen SA, Yang Q, Friedman JM (2001) Mortality in neurofibromatosis 1: an analysis using U.S. death certificates. Am J Hum Genet 68:1110–1118

70. Khatua S, Gutmann DH, Packer RJ (2018) Neurofibromatosis type 1 and optic pathway glioma: molecular interplay and therapeutic insights. Pediatr Blood Cancer. https://doi.org/10.1002/pbc.26838

71. Banerjee A et al (2017) A phase I trial of the MEK inhibitor selumetinib (AZD6244) in pediatric patients with recurrent or refractory low-grade glioma: a Pediatric Brain Tumor Consortium (PBTC) study. NeuroOncol 19:1135–1144

72. Wei J et al (2014) Nilotinib is more potent than imatinib for treating plexiform neurofibroma in vitro and in vivo. PLoS One 9:e107760

73. Khelifa I, Saurat JH, Prins C (2015) Use of imatinib in a patient with cutaneous vasculopathy in the context of von Recklinghausen disease/neurofibromatosis. Br J Dermatol 172:253–256

74. Evans DG et al (2009) Consensus recommendations to accelerate clinical trials for neurofibromatosis type 2. Clin Cancer Res 15:5032–5039

75. Pećina-Šlaus N (2013) Merlin, the NF2 gene product. Pathol Oncol Res POR 19:365–373

76. Ammoun S, Hanemann CO (2011) Emerging therapeutic targets in schwannomas and other merlin-deficient tumors. Nat Rev Neurol 7:392–399

77. Scoles DR (2008) The merlin interacting proteins reveal multiple targets for NF2 therapy. Biochim Biophys Acta 1785:32–54

78. Uesaka T et al (2007) Expression of VEGF and its receptor genes in intracranial schwannomas. J Neuro-Oncol 83:259–266

79. Baser ME et al (2004) Genotype-phenotype correlations for nervous system tumors in neurofibromatosis 2: a population-based study. Am J Hum Genet 75:231–239

80. Cranial meningiomas in 411 neurofibromatosis type 2 (NF2) patients with proven gene mutations: clear positional effect of mutations, but absence of female severity effect on age at onset. J Med Genet. http://jmg.bmj.com.myaccess.library.utoronto.ca/content/48/4/261.long. Accessed 25 Oct 2017

81. Evans DGR (2009) Neurofibromatosis type 2 (NF2): a clinical and molecular review. Orphanet J Rare Dis 4:16

82. Gutmann DH et al (1997) The diagnostic evaluation and multidisciplinary management of neurofibromatosis 1 and neurofibromatosis 2. JAMA 278:51–57

83. Evans DGR et al (2008) What are the implications in individuals with unilateral vestibular schwannoma and other neurogenic tumors? J Neurosurg 108:92–96

84. Fisher LM, Doherty JK, Lev MH, Slattery WH (2007) Distribution of nonvestibular cranial nerve schwannomas in neurofibromatosis 2. Otol Neurotol 28:1083–1090

85. Evans DGR et al (2007) Mosaicism in neurofibromatosis type 2: an update of risk based on uni/bilaterality of vestibular schwannoma at presentation and sensitive mutation analysis including multiple ligation-dependent probe amplification. J Med Genet 44:424–428

86. Moffat DA, Quaranta N, Baguley DM, Hardy DG, Chang P (2003) Management strategies in neurofibromatosis type 2. Eur Arch Otorhinolaryngol 260:12–18

87. Samii M, Gerganov V, Samii A (2008) Microsurgery management of vestibular schwannomas in neurofibromatosis type 2: indications and results. Prog Neurol Surg 21:169–175

88. Samii M, Matthies C, Tatagiba M (1997) Management of vestibular schwannomas (acoustic neuromas): auditory and facial nerve function after resection of 120 vestibular schwannomas in patients with neurofibromatosis 2. Neurosurgery 40:696–705-706

89. Slattery WH, Fisher LM, Hitselberger W, Friedman RA, Brackmann DE (2007) Hearing preservation surgery for neurofibromatosis type 2-related vestibular schwannoma in pediatric patients. J Neurosurg 106:255–260

90. Schwartz MS, Otto SR, Brackmann DE, Hitselberger WE, Shannon RV (2003) Use of a multichannel auditory brainstem implant for neurofibromatosis type 2. Stereotact Funct Neurosurg 81:110–114

91. Schwartz MS, Otto SR, Shannon RV, Hitselberger WE, Brackmann DE (2008) Auditory brainstem implants. Neurother J Am Soc Exp Neurother 5:128–136

92. Neff BA et al (2007) Cochlear implantation in the neurofibromatosis type 2 patient: long-term follow-up. Laryngoscope 117:1069–1072

93. Subach BR et al (1999) Stereotactic radiosurgery in the management of acoustic neuromas associated with neurofibromatosis type 2. J Neurosurg 90:815–822

94. Rowe J, Radatz M, Kemeny A (2008) Radiosurgery for type II neurofibromatosis. Prog Neurol Surg 21:176–182

95. Mathieu D et al (2007) Stereotactic radiosurgery for vestibular schwannomas in patients with neurofibromatosis type 2: an analysis of tumor control, complications, and hearing preservation rates. Neurosurgery 60:460–468-470

96. Linskey ME, Lunsford LD, Flickinger JC (1992) Tumor control after stereotactic radiosurgery in neurofibromatosis patients with bilateral acoustic tumors. Neurosurgery 31:829-838-839

97. Vachhani JA, Friedman WA (2007) Radiosurgery in patients with bilateral vestibular schwannomas. Stereotact Funct Neurosurg 85:273–278

98. Gonzalvo A et al (2011) Schwannomatosis, sporadic schwannomatosis, and familial schwannomatosis: a surgical series with long-term follow-up. Clinical article. J Neurosurg 114:756–762

99. Antinheimo J et al (2000) Population-based analysis of sporadic and type 2 neurofibromatosis-associated meningiomas and schwannomas. Neurology 54:71–76

100. Merker VL, Esparza S, Smith MJ, Stemmer-Rachamimov A, Plotkin SR (2012) Clinical features of schwannomatosis: a retrospective analysis of 87 patients. Oncologist 17:1317–1322

101. Sestini R, Bacci C, Provenzano A, Genuardi M, Papi L (2008) Evidence of a four-hit mechanism involving SMARCB1 and NF2 in schwannomatosis-associated schwannomas. Hum Mutat 29:227–231

102. Piotrowski A et al (2014) Germline loss-of-function mutations in LZTR1 predispose to an inherited disorder of multiple schwannomas. Nat Genet 46:182–187

103. Plotkin SR et al (2012) Quantitative assessment of whole-body tumor burden in adult patients with neurofibromatosis. PLoS One 7:e35711

104. Carter JM et al (2012) Epithelioid malignant peripheral nerve sheath tumor arising in a schwannoma, in a patient with 'neuroblastoma-like' schwannomatosis and a novel germline SMARCB1 mutation. Am J Surg Pathol 36:154–160

105. Swensen JJ et al (2009) Familial occurrence of schwannomas and malignant rhabdoid tumour associated with a duplication in SMARCB1. J Med Genet 46:68–72

106. Baser ME, Friedman JM, Evans DGR (2006) Increasing the specificity of diagnostic criteria for schwannomatosis. Neurology 66:730–732

107. MacCollin M et al (2003) Familial schwannomatosis: exclusion of the NF2 locus as the germline event. Neurology 60:1968–1974

108. Baskin HJ (2008) The pathogenesis and imaging of the tuberous sclerosis complex. Pediatr Radiol 38:936–952

109. Sampson JR, Harris PC (1994) The molecular genetics of tuberous sclerosis. Hum Mol Genet 3 Spec No:1477–1480

110. Jones AC et al (1997) Molecular genetic and phenotypic analysis reveals differences between TSC1 and TSC2 associated familial and sporadic tuberous sclerosis. Hum Mol Genet 6:2155–2161

111. Kwiatkowski DJ (2003) Rhebbing up mTOR: new insights on TSC1 and TSC2, and the pathogenesis of tuberous sclerosis. Cancer Biol Ther 2:471–476

112. Manning BD, Cantley LC (2003) United at last: the tuberous sclerosis complex gene products connect the phosphoinositide 3-kinase/Akt pathway to mammalian target of rapamycin (mTOR) signalling. Biochem Soc Trans 31:573–578

113. Sampson JR (2003) TSC1 and TSC2: genes that are mutated in the human genetic disorder tuberous sclerosis. Biochem Soc Trans 31:592–596

114. Conway JE et al (2001) Hemangioblastomas of the central nervous system in von Hippel-Lindau syndrome and sporadic disease. Neurosurgery 48:55–62-63

115. O'Callaghan FJK et al (2004) The relation of infantile spasms, tubers, and intelligence in tuberous sclerosis complex. Arch Dis Child 89:530–533

116. Webb DW, Fryer AE, Osborne JP (1996) Morbidity associated with tuberous sclerosis: a population study. Dev Med Child Neurol 38:146–155

117. Sparagana SP, Roach ES (2000) Tuberous sclerosis complex. Curr Opin Neurol 13:115–119

118. Roach ES, Gomez MR, Northrup H (1998) Tuberous sclerosis complex consensus conference: revised clinical diagnostic criteria. J Child Neurol 13:624–628

119. Neumann HP et al (1989) Hemangioblastomas of the central nervous system. A 10-year study with special reference to von Hippel-Lindau syndrome. J Neurosurg 70:24–30

120. Chang SD et al (1998) Treatment of hemangioblastomas in von Hippel-Lindau disease with linear accelerator-based radiosurgery. Neurosurgery 43:28–34-35

121. Northrup H, Krueger DA (2013) Tuberous sclerosis complex diagnostic criteria update: recommendations of the 2012 international tuberous sclerosis complex consensus conference. Pediatr Neurol 49:243–254

122. Teng JMC et al (2014) Dermatologic and dental aspects of the 2012 international tuberous sclerosis complex consensus statements. JAMA Dermatol 150:1095–1101

123. Jansen FE et al (2003) Diffusion-weighted magnetic resonance imaging and identification of the epileptogenic tuber in patients with tuberous sclerosis. Arch Neurol 60:1580–1584

124. Luat AF, Makki M, Chugani HT (2007) Neuroimaging in tuberous sclerosis complex. Curr Opin Neurol 20:142–150

125. Chandra PS et al (2006) FDG-PET/MRI coregistration and diffusion-tensor imaging distinguish epileptogenic tubers and cortex in patients with tuberous sclerosis complex: a preliminary report. Epilepsia 47:1543–1549

126. Chu-Shore CJ, Major P, Camposano S, Muzykewicz D, Thiele EA (2010) The natural history of epilepsy in tuberous sclerosis complex. Epilepsia 51:1236–1241

127. Karenfort M, Kruse B, Freitag H, Pannek H, Tuxhorn I (2002) Epilepsy surgery outcome in children with focal epilepsy due to tuberous sclerosis complex. Neuropediatrics 33:255–261

128. Weiner HL (2004) Tuberous sclerosis and multiple tubers: localizing the epileptogenic zone. Epilepsia 45(Suppl 4):41–42

129. Roszkowski M, Drabik K, Barszcz S, Jozwiak S (1995) Surgical treatment of intraventricular tumors associated with tuberous sclerosis. Childs Nerv Syst 11:335–339

130. Beaumont TL, Limbrick DD, Smyth MD (2012) Advances in the management of subependymal giant cell astrocytoma. Childs Nerv Syst 28:963–968

131. Riikonen R, Simell O (1990) Tuberous sclerosis and infantile spasms. Dev Med Child Neurol 32:203–209

132. Curatolo P, Seri S, Verdecchia M, Bombardieri R (2001) Infantile spasms in tuberous sclerosis complex. Brain and Development 23:502–507

133. Franz DN et al (2001) Lamotrigine therapy of epilepsy in tuberous sclerosis. Epilepsia 42:935–940

134. Kotagal P, Rothner AD (1993) Epilepsy in the setting of neurocutaneous syndromes. Epilepsia 34(Suppl 3):S71–S78

135. Franz DN et al (2006) Rapamycin causes regression of astrocytomas in tuberous sclerosis complex. Ann Neurol 59:490–498

136. Pan D, Dong J, Zhang Y, Gao X (2004) Tuberous sclerosis complex: from drosophila to human disease. Trends Cell Biol 14:78–85

137. Lonser RR et al (2003) von Hippel-Lindau disease. Lancet Lond Engl 361:2059–2067

138. Kaelin WG (2002) Molecular basis of the VHL hereditary cancer syndrome. Nat Rev Cancer 2:673–682

139. Koh MY, Lemos R, Liu X, Powis G (2011) The hypoxia-associated factor switches cells from HIF-1α- to HIF-2α-dependent signaling promoting stem cell characteristics, aggressive tumor growth and invasion. Cancer Res 71:4015–4027

140. Butman JA, Linehan WM, Lonser RR (2008) Neurologic manifestations of von Hippel-Lindau disease. JAMA 300:1334–1342

141. Jagannathan J, Lonser RR, Smith R, DeVroom HL, Oldfield EH (2008) Surgical management of cerebellar hemangioblastomas in patients with von Hippel-Lindau disease. J Neurosurg 108:210–222

142. Jarrell ST, Vortmeyer AO, Linehan WM, Oldfield EH, Lonser RR (2006) Metastases to hemangioblastomas in von Hippel-Lindau disease. J Neurosurg 105:256–263

143. Nielsen SM et al (2016) Von Hippel-Lindau disease: genetics and role of genetic Counseling in a multiple neoplasia syndrome. J Clin Oncol 34:2172–2181

144. Richard S, Graff J, Lindau J, Resche F (2004) Von Hippel-Lindau disease. Lancet Lond Engl 363:1231–1234

145. Friedrich CA (2001) Genotype-phenotype correlation in von Hippel-Lindau syndrome. Hum Mol Genet 10:763–767

146. Ammerman JM, Lonser RR, Dambrosia J, Butman JA, Oldfield EH (2006) Long-term natural history of hemangioblastomas in patients with von Hippel-Lindau disease: implications for treatment. J Neurosurg 105:248–255

147. Wanebo JE, Lonser RR, Glenn GM, Oldfield EH (2003) The natural history of hemangioblastomas of the central nervous system in patients with von Hippel-Lindau disease. J Neurosurg 98:82–94

148. Vougioukas VI et al (2006) Surgical treatment of hemangioblastomas of the central nervous system in pediatric patients. Childs Nerv Syst 22:1149–1153

149. Boström A et al (2008) Intramedullary hemangioblastomas: timing of surgery, microsurgical technique and follow-up in 23 patients. Eur Spine J 17:882–886

150. Neumann HP et al (1992) Central nervous system lesions in von Hippel-Lindau syndrome. J Neurol Neurosurg Psychiatry 55:898–901

151. Pietilä TA, Stendel R, Schilling A, Krznaric I, Brock M (2000) Surgical treatment of spinal hemangioblastomas. Acta Neurochir 142:879–886

152. Niemelä M et al (1999) Long-term prognosis of haemangioblastoma of the CNS: impact of von Hippel-Lindau disease. Acta Neurochir 141:1147–1156

153. Shirley MD et al (2013) Sturge–weber syndrome and port-wine stains caused by somatic mutation in GNAQ. N Engl J Med 368:1971–1979

154. Comi AM (2007) Update on Sturge-weber syndrome: diagnosis, treatment, quantitative measures, and controversies. Lymphat Res Biol 5:257–264

155. Pascual-Castroviejo I, Pascual-Pascual S-I, Velazquez-Fragua R, Viaño J (2008) Sturge-weber syndrome: study of 55 patients. Can. J Neurol Sci J Can Sci Neurol 35:301–307

156. Sujansky E, Conradi S (1995) Sturge-weber syndrome: age of onset of seizures and glaucoma and the prognosis for affected children. J Child Neurol 10:49–58

157. Kossoff EH, Ferenc L, Comi AM (2009) An infantile-onset, severe, yet sporadic seizure pattern is common in Sturge-weber syndrome. Epilepsia 50:2154–2157

158. Thomas-Sohl KA, Vaslow DF, Maria BL (2004) Sturge-Weber syndrome: a review. Pediatr Neurol 30:303–310

159. Lee JS et al (2001) Sturge-weber syndrome: correlation between clinical course and FDG PET findings. Neurology 57:189–195

160. Hu J et al (2008) MR susceptibility weighted imaging (SWI) complements conventional contrast

enhanced T1 weighted MRI in characterizing brain abnormalities of Sturge-weber syndrome. J Magn Reson Imaging 28:300–307

161. Hoffman HJ, Hendrick EB, Dennis M, Armstrong D (1979) Hemispherectomy for Sturge-weber syndrome. Childs Brain 5:233–248

162. Di Rocco C, Tamburrini G (2006) Sturge-Weber syndrome. Childs Nerv Syst 22:909–921

163. Roach ES et al (1994) Sturge-weber syndrome: recommendations for surgery. J Child Neurol 9:190–192

164. Arzimanoglou A, Aicardi J (1992) The epilepsy of Sturge-weber syndrome: clinical features and treatment in 23 patients. Acta Neurol Scand Suppl 140:18–22

165. Lo Muzio L (2008) Nevoid basal cell carcinoma syndrome (Gorlin syndrome). Orphanet J Rare Dis 3:32

166. Kimonis VE et al (1997) Clinical manifestations in 105 persons with nevoid basal cell carcinoma syndrome. Am J Med Genet 69:299–308

167. Evans DG et al (2010) Birth incidence and prevalence of tumor-prone syndromes: estimates from a UK family genetic register service. Am J Med Genet A 152A:327–332

168. Gorlin RJ, Goltz RW (1960) Multiple nevoid basal-cell epithelioma, jaw cysts and bifid rib. A syndrome. N Engl J Med 262:908–912

169. Takahashi C et al (2009) Germline PTCH1 mutations in Japanese basal cell nevus syndrome patients. J Hum Genet 54:403–408

170. Hahn H et al (1996) Mutations of the human homolog of drosophila patched in the nevoid basal cell carcinoma syndrome. Cell 85:841–851

171. Johnson RL et al (1996) Human homolog of patched, a candidate gene for the basal cell nevus syndrome. Science 272:1668–1671

172. Smith MJ et al (2014) Germline mutations in SUFU cause Gorlin syndrome-associated childhood medulloblastoma and redefine the risk associated with PTCH1 mutations. J Clin Oncol 32:4155–4161

173. Pastorino L et al (2009) Identification of a SUFU germline mutation in a family with Gorlin syndrome. Am J Med Genet A 149A:1539–1543

174. Xie J, Bartels CM, Barton SW, Gu D (2013) Targeting hedgehog signaling in cancer: research and clinical developments. OncoTargets Ther 6:1425–1435

175. Xie J et al (1998) Activating smoothened mutations in sporadic basal-cell carcinoma. Nature 391:90–92

176. Lee Y-W et al (2007) Identification of a novel mutation in the PTCH gene in a Korean family with naevoid basal cell carcinoma syndrome. Clin Exp Dermatol 32:202–203

177. Kieran MW (2014) Targeted treatment for sonic hedgehog-dependent medulloblastoma. NeuroOncol 16:1037–1047

178. Shanley S et al (1994) Nevoid basal cell carcinoma syndrome: review of 118 affected individuals. Am J Med Genet 50:282–290

179. Thalakoti S, Geller T (2015) Basal cell nevus syndrome or Gorlin syndrome. Handb Clin Neurol 132:119–128

180. Bresler SC, Padwa BL, Granter SR (2016) Nevoid basal cell carcinoma syndrome (Gorlin syndrome). Head Neck Pathol 10:119–124

181. Torrelo A et al (2014) Early-onset acral basal cell carcinomas in Gorlin syndrome. Br J Dermatol 171:1227–1229

182. Diociaiuti A et al (2015) Naevoid basal cell carcinoma syndrome in a 22-month-old child presenting with multiple basal cell carcinomas and a fetal rhabdomyoma. Acta Derm Venereol 95:243–244

183. Guha D et al (2018) Management of peripheral nerve sheath tumors: 17 years of experience at Toronto Western Hospital. J Neurosurg 128(4):1226–1234. https://doi.org/10.3171/2017.1.JNS162292

184. Taylor MD et al (2012) Molecular subgroups of medulloblastoma: the current consensus. Acta Neuropathol 123:465–472

185. Ramanathan S, Kumar D, Al Heidous M, Palaniappan Y (2015) Delayed diagnosis of Gorlin syndrome: learning from mistakes! J Pediatr Neurosci 10:359–361

186. Shiohama T et al (2017) Brain morphology in children with nevoid basal cell carcinoma syndrome. Am J Med Genet A 173:946–952

187. Jones EA, Sajid MI, Shenton A, Evans DG (2011) Basal cell carcinomas in Gorlin syndrome: a review of 202 patients. J Skin Cancer 2011:217378

188. Hogan RE, Tress B, Gonzales MF, King JO, Cook MJ (1996) Epilepsy in the nevoid basal-cell carcinoma syndrome (Gorlin syndrome): report of a case due to a focal neuronal heterotopia. Neurology 46:574–576

189. Evans DG et al (1993) Complications of the naevoid basal cell carcinoma syndrome: results of a population based study. J Med Genet 30:460–464

190. Gorlin RJ (2004) Nevoid basal cell carcinoma (Gorlin) syndrome. Genet Med 6:530–539

191. Bree AF, Shah MR, BCNS Colloquium Group (2011) Consensus statement from the first international colloquium on basal cell nevus syndrome (BCNS). Am J Med Genet A 155A:2091–2097

192. Evans DG, Birch JM, Orton CI (1991) Brain tumours and the occurrence of severe invasive basal cell carcinoma in first degree relatives with Gorlin syndrome. Br J Neurosurg 5:643–646

193. Strong LC (1977) Genetic and environmental interactions. Cancer 40:1861–1866

194. Wallin JL, Tanna N, Misra S, Puri PK, Sadeghi N (2007) Sinonasal carcinoma after irradiation for medulloblastoma in nevoid basal cell carcinoma syndrome. Am J Otolaryngol 28:360–362

195. Choudry Q, Patel HC, Gurusinghe NT, Evans DG (2007) Radiation-induced brain tumours in nevoid basal cell carcinoma syndrome: implications for treatment and surveillance. Childs Nerv Syst 23:133–136

196. O'Malley S, Weitman D, Olding M, Sekhar L (1997) Multiple neoplasms following craniospinal irradiation for medulloblastoma in a patient with nevoid basal cell carcinoma syndrome. Case report. J Neurosurg 86:286–288

197. Sartip K, Kaplan A, Obeid G, Kadom N (2013) Neuroimaging of nevoid basal cell carcinoma syndrome (NBCCS) in children. Pediatr Radiol 43:620–627

198. Jain S, Song R, Xie J (2017) Sonidegib: mechanism of action, pharmacology, and clinical utility for advanced basal cell carcinomas. OncoTargets Ther 10:1645–1653

199. Huq AJ et al (2017) Cohort study of Gorlin syndrome with emphasis on standardised phenotyping and quality of life assessment. Intern Med J 47:664–673

Brainstem Tumors in Children

20

Ali S. Haider, James M. Drake, and James T. Rutka

20.1 Introduction

Brainstem tumors are a disparate group of tumors that span the regions of the midbrain to the cervicomedullary junction (Fig. 20.1). They most frequently occur in children and lack a specific gender predilection. Over the past two decades, we have become increasingly more familiar with their characteristic patient symptom complex, their specific neuroimaging features, and a standardized approach to therapy. That said, there are still a number of challenges that are posed by tumors in this critical region of the neuraxis. As each tumor subtype could be the subject of an independent chapter, here, we will review the main patient presentations, the key neuroimaging features, and the goals of surgical and non-operative therapies for children with brainstem tumors.

A. S. Haider · J. M. Drake
Division of Neurosurgery, The Hospital for Sick Children, Toronto, ON, Canada
e-mail: haider@medicine.tamhsc.edu; james.drake@sickkids.ca

J. T. Rutka (✉)
Division of Neurosurgery, The Arthur and Sonia Labatt Brain Tumour Research Centre, The Hospital for Sick Children, Toronto, ON, Canada

Department of Surgery, University of Toronto, Toronto, ON, Canada
e-mail: james.rutka@sickkids.ca

20.2 Midbrain Tumors

20.2.1 Tectal Gliomas

20.2.1.1 Clinical Symptoms and Signs

Tectal gliomas are located in close proximity to the Sylvian aqueduct, and as such, they most often cause hydrocephalus from aqueductal obstruction. Accordingly, children will demonstrate clinical evidence of increased intracranial pressure, including papilledema, nausea, vomiting, headache, visual changes, and/or oculomotor deficits. Rarely, patients may also exhibit signs of ataxia, pyramidal tract dysfunction, and/or other cranial nerve palsies including nystagmus, tremor, diplopia, and Parinaud's syndrome [1].

20.2.1.2 Diagnostics

MRI is considered the gold standard imaging modality for diagnosis of these tumors. Computed tomography (CT) may often miss these lesions as they are isodense to the surrounding brain. Tectal tumors are best appreciated on T2 and FLAIR MR images in which a classic periaqueductal hyperintensity is seen (Fig. 20.2). In the majority of circumstances, tectal tumors are non-enhancing lesions. However, on occasion, they may be dorsally exophytic, cystic, and quite large (Fig. 20.3).

© Springer Nature Switzerland AG 2019
J.-C. Tonn et al. (eds.), *Oncology of CNS Tumors*, https://doi.org/10.1007/978-3-030-04152-6_20

Fig. 20.1 The classification of brainstem tumors in children. Tumors in the brainstem can arise from the midbrain (tectal and tegmental), the pons (focal, diffuse, and dorsally exophytic), and the cervicomedullary region. This classification system has largely been derived from experience with localization of these tumors on imaging studies, particularly MRI

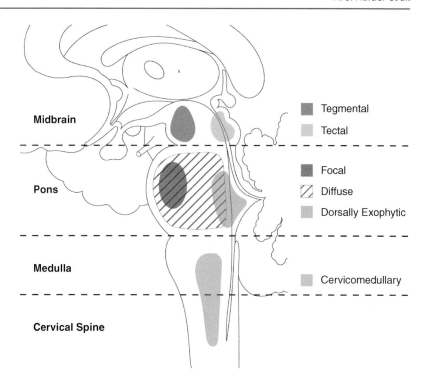

20.2.1.3 Staging and Classification

Tectal tumors can be classified into three groups based on MR appearance and subsequent correlation with neuroendoscopic, histopathologic, and postoperative clinical findings. Group 1 tectal tumors appear on MRI typically as a bulbous tectal mass, isodense on T1-weighted images, and hyperdense on T2-weighted images without gadolinium. Group 2 tectal tumors appear similar to Group 1 along with exophytic growth into the Sylvian aqueduct, further extending into the midbrain tegmentum and diencephalon. Group 3 tectal tumors typically appear as large lesions with mixed intensities on T1-weighted and T2-weighted images along with enhancement on gadolinium. These tumors typically exhibit exophytic growth into the Sylvian aqueduct and third ventricle.

20.2.1.4 Treatment

The preferred management of the majority of children presenting with tectal tumors is endoscopic third ventriculostomy (ETV) to overcome the obstruction of the aqueduct and to permit more physiological cerebrospinal fluid (CSF) drainage [2]. Ventriculoperitoneal (VP) shunting may be required, especially in children less than 1 year of age; however, this can be fraught with complications related to overdrainage in the setting of a child with established macrocephaly. After hydrocephalus is controlled, serial MR imaging is recommended on an annual basis for both ETV-treated and VP-shunted patients. ETVs are known to occlude on occasion requiring repeat fenestrations [3]; and VP shunts may block or disconnect in long-term follow-up. Direct surgical resection of the typical tectal tumor should not be performed. Atypical tectal tumors demonstrating serial growth and enhancement may require a neurosurgical approach, typically an infratentorial supracerebellar, or occipital transtentorial approach. On occasion, intensity-modulated radiation therapy (IMRT) or chemotherapy may be indicated for some of these latter types of tectal tumors.

20.2.1.5 Prognosis/Quality of Life

Children with tectal tumors whose hydrocephalus is well controlled can lead normal lives without significant cognitive or neurodevelopmental issues. The prognosis is typically excellent, although lifelong monitoring of hydrocephalus may be required.

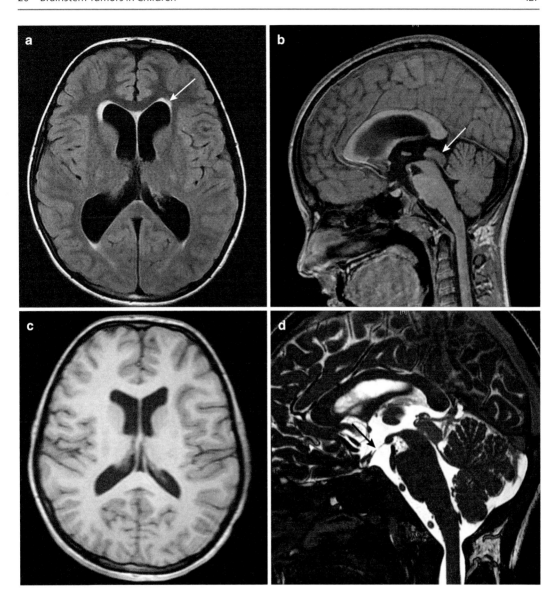

Fig. 20.2 Tectal glioma in an 8-year-old male complaining of headache and vomiting over 6 weeks. (**a**) Axial FLAIR MRI showing enlarged ventricles and periventricular high signal indicative of edema (arrow). (**b**) Sagittal T1 MRI showing mass in tectum creating obstructive hydrocephalus (arrow). (**c**) After endoscopic third ventriculostomy (ETV), the ventricles are smaller, the sulci are seen better, and there was CSF seen over the convexities. (**d**) After ETV, there is now a flow void seen through the third ventricle on the FIESTA MR imaging, indicative of patency of the ventriculostomy (arrow)

20.2.2 Tegmental Tumors

20.2.2.1 Clinical Symptoms and Signs

Tegmental tumors are focal midbrain tumors that typically arise in children less than 14 years of age. They cause symptoms by virtue of their mass effect on the unilateral tegmentum and corticospinal tract causing hemiparesis, oculomotor nerve palsy, and ataxia [4]. In most cases, symptoms can be traced back 6–12 months prior to diagnosis. Occasionally, unilateral tremor is seen, especially in those tumors where extension into the basal ganglia and thalamus are also noted.

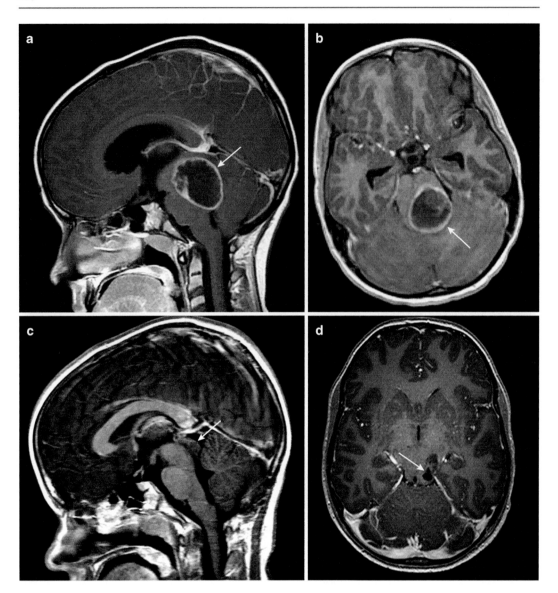

Fig. 20.3 Large, atypical tectal glioma in a 13-year-old male with neurofibromatosis type 1, headache, and vomiting. (**a**) Sagittal contrast-enhanced T1 MRI showing large posterior fossa cystic mass lesion with epicenter in the tectal region (arrow). (**b**) Axial MRI contrast-enhanced MRI depicting extent of involvement of the tectum and the fourth ventricle (arrow). (**c**) Following posterior fossa craniotomy, drainage of the tumor cyst, and removal of the cyst capsule, only small deformation of the tectum is still seen on this T1-weighted contrast-enhanced MRI scan (arrow). (**d**) Postoperative T1-weighted axial MRI with contrast demonstrating origin of the tumor from the tectal region without mass effect (arrow)

20.2.2.2 Diagnostics

The imaging modality of choice is MRI. Tegmental tumors are typically homogeneously enhancing lesions upon the administration of gadolinium (Fig. 20.4). They can be quite large occupying the entire tegmentum and can cause hydrocephalus by virtue of occlusion of the foramina of Monro.

20.2.2.3 Staging and Classification

There is no uniform staging or classification system for midbrain tegmental tumors. Rather, it is

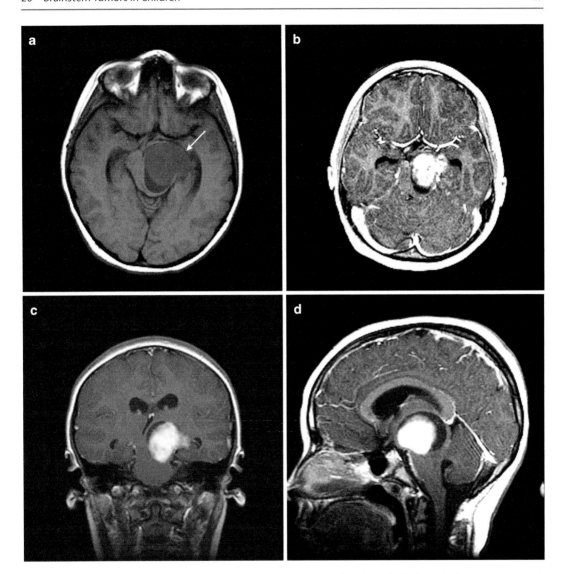

Fig. 20.4 A 12-year-old female with 3-month history of progressive right-sided weakness and ataxia. (**a**) Axial T1 MRI showing mass lesion occupying the left tegmental region of the brainstem (arrow). (**b**) Following contrast administration, the lesion avidly enhances homogeneously. (**c**) Coronal T1 MRI with contrast showing large lesion arising from the left midbrain tegmentum with extension into the thalamus. At times, these lesions are called "thalamopeduncular" lesions. (**d**) Sagittal T1 MRI with contrast demonstrating large, central enhancing mass lesion which typifies focal midbrain gliomas

known that these lesions may extend from the tegmentum to involve the thalamus and are sometimes called "thalamopeduncular" lesions [5].

20.2.2.4 Treatment

Focal tegmental tumors present formidable challenges to the neurosurgeon in terms of approach and long-term management. The majority of lesions are low-grade gliomas. Biopsy can be performed, either framed based or frameless. Options for surgical approaches include trans-Sylvian, transtemporal, or transcallosal depending on the size of the tumor and its presentation to the pial or ventricular surfaces (Fig. 20.5) [5, 6]. Optimal neurosurgical resection is aided through the use of neuronavigation particularly with diffusion tensor

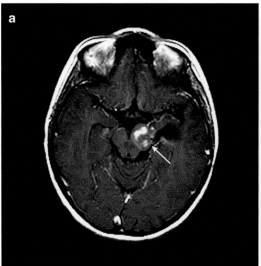

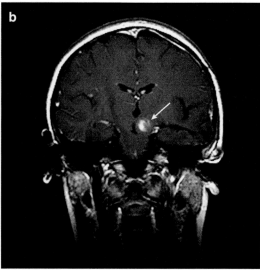

Fig. 20.5 Postoperative MRI in child whose images are shown in Fig. 20.3. A left middle temporal gyrus approach to the lesion was undertaken following temporal craniotomy. Neuronavigation was used to identify the equator of the tumor; and the cavitron was used to debulk the lesion. (**a**) Axial T1 contrast-enhanced MRI showing trajectory to the tumor and small residual that occupies the left tegmen-

tum. (**b**) Coronal MRI with contrast depicting the tract leading from the middle temporal gyrus to the midbrain tumor and small residual. This patient went on to receive chemotherapy in follow-up, and no further surgery was required. There was no new neurological deficit, but transient dysphasia for 2 weeks after surgery

imaging sequences on MR, intraoperative neuronavigation, and intraoperative MRI scanning [7] (Fig. 20.6). The goal of surgery is to achieve a gross total resection of the tumor. Where this is not possible, then a trial of chemotherapy using specific midline low-grade glioma drug therapy becomes possible [6]. At times the BRAF gene may be mutated or fused in low-grade astrocytomas, and this molecular finding offers an opportunity for targeted drug therapy [8]. However, standard low-grade glioma chemotherapy in children is also an option and works well in many instances [8]. If neurosurgical resection and chemotherapy are not sufficient, then intensity-modulated radiation therapy (IMRT) can be delivered.

20.2.2.5 Quality of Life/Prognosis

Children with focal midbrain tumors can do extremely well after aggressive neurosurgical resection of their tumors. If there is residual tumor after surgery and demonstrated regrowth, then several options exist for targeted chemotherapy, conventional chemotherapy, or radiation therapy in older children. With maximum

safe surgery, most children with focal midbrain tumors can lead normal lives. By virtue of the potential for recurrence, serial MR imaging is highly recommended. Overall, the prognosis is good for children with focal midbrain tumors with 90% or higher survival rates at 5 years [5].

20.3 Pontine Tumors

Tumors of the pons in children will typically be gliomas of varying grade malignancy. They can be divided into diffuse intrinsic pontine glioma (DIPG), dorsally exophytic, or focal pontine tumors, based primarily on the neuroradiological findings. Here we will cover DIPG and dorsally exophytic pontine gliomas.

20.3.1 Diffuse Intrinsic Pontine Glioma (DIPG)

DIPGs comprise approximately 70% of all brainstem tumors making them the most common

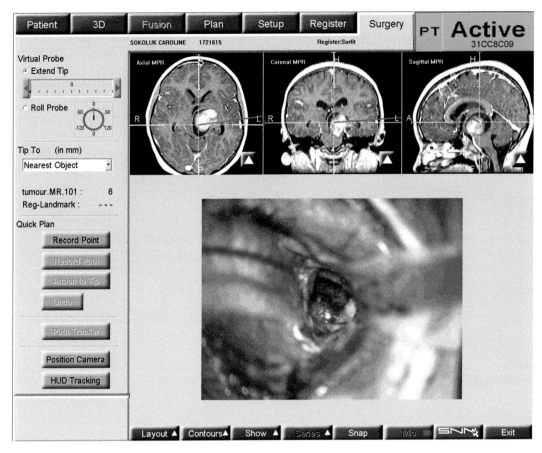

Fig. 20.6 Intraoperative screensaver of case of focal midbrain tumor shown in Figs. 20.3 and 20.4 demonstrating depth of resection with neuronavigation and small corridor of entry through the middle temporal gyrus

form of brainstem tumor. Typically these lesions are high-grade neoplasms, and overall survival is very poor with most children succumbing within 2 years of diagnosis despite all forms of therapy [9]. There is equal sex incidence of DIPGs, and most children are between ages 5 and 10 at time of diagnosis. Interestingly, the molecular genetics of DIPG in childhood are now rather well worked out with novel genetic pathways being identified as drivers of this tumor including ACVR1, H3K27M, PDGB, and several others [10, 11] (Fig. 20.7).

20.3.1.1   Clinical Symptoms and Signs
There is often a rapid appearance of clinical findings including cranial nerve deficits (e.g., facial nerve palsy, VIth nerve palsy causing diplopia), long tract signs, and ataxia. Hydrocephalus may

form causing headaches and a syndrome of raised intracranial pressure, but this is usually a late presenting feature in the course of the disease [9].

20.3.1.2   Diagnostics
The diagnosis of DIPG is most often made by MRI. Frequently, there is diffuse enlargement of the pons occupying 50–75% or more of this region of the brainstem. There may be exophytic components, especially ventrally. Contrast enhancement may exist but is usually patchy and contained within the diffuse swelling of the pons. At times, the basilar artery may be totally engulfed by tumor (Fig. 20.8). Other MR sequences and techniques have been used for DIPG, including MR spectroscopy (MRS) showing lower mean total choline concentration and diffusion tensor imaging (DTI), but these have

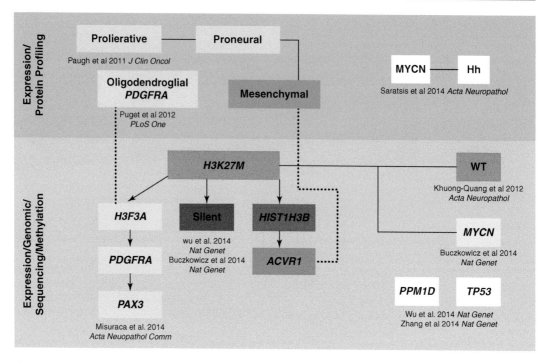

Fig. 20.7 Schematic of molecular genetic characterization of DIPGs. The main genetic drivers of DIPG include MYCN, ACVR1, H3K27M, PDGFRA, and PAX3, among several others (Adapted from Misuraca, Cordero, and Becher, Front Oncol 2015)

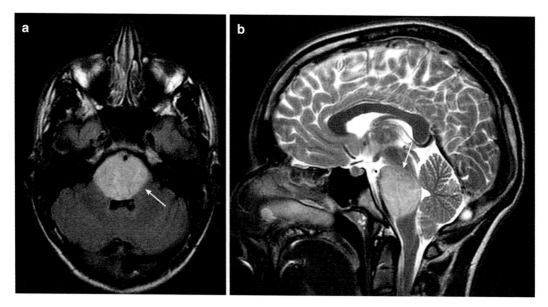

Fig. 20.8 MRI scan of a 14-year-old male with brief history of diplopia, ataxia, and left facial palsy. (**a**) Axial FLAIR MRI showing high signal occupying the entire pons (arrow). (**b**) Sagittal T2 MRI depicting extent of pontine involvement by DIPG (arrow)

not proven reliable in predicting neuropathology of the lesions or outcome.

20.3.1.3 Staging/Classification

There is no generally accepted staging system for children with DIPG. With disease progression, there may be metastases through leptomeningeal seeding to other regions of the brain or to the spinal axis.

20.3.1.4 Treatment

There is no role for direct surgery for the vast majority of children with DIPGs. In addition, for many years, the common practice was not to offer biopsy of DIPGs in children with typically appearing tumors on MRI. Children with a DIPG diagnosis on MRI would move quickly to radiation therapy protocols including the use of IMRT or hyperfractionated radiation therapy [9]. A number of clinical trials have now been performed assessing the role of chemotherapy in DIPG [12, 13]. Chemotherapeutics such as vincristine, CCNU, prednisone, cisplatin, cyclophosphamide, etoposide, and tamoxifen have all been tried but with limited to no effect.

With the recognition that some DIPGs may have atypical features (e.g., child older than 10 years, lateral enhancing tumor with less than 50% brainstem involvement), some centers are now offering stereotactic biopsies for these patients [14, 15]. Stereotactic biopsy can be performed safely, and in groups where molecular genetics can be performed on fresh tumor specimens, there are reasonable expectations of finding new or targetable genetic lesions [16].

Some innovative clinical trials are now being performed on children with DIPG. Souweidane and colleagues have recently published their findings on the use of convection-enhanced delivery (CED) of a radioimmunotherapy agent targeting the glioma-associated B7-H3 antigen, along with a number of other targeted agents, to treat children with DIPG [17–20]. They have shown that the use of CED in children who have already received radiation therapy is both safe and potentially efficacious [17]. In addition, some recent interesting studies have been done with immunotherapy. Benitez-Ribas et al. treated children with DIPG with autologous dendritic cells pulsed with an allogeneic tumoral cell line lysate. They showed that this protocol leads to a definitive immune-generated response and may serve as a promising backbone for future therapy [21]. We have recently shown that the use of magnetic resonance-guided focused ultrasound (MRgFUS) can increase the delivery of chemotherapeutics, specifically doxorubicin, to the brainstem in experimental models [22].

20.3.1.5 Prognosis/Quality of Life

The prognosis of children with DIPG remains poor despite intensive therapies. DIPGs remain highly chemo- and radio-resistant neoplasms. Children normally remain in remission for 6–8 months following the completion of radiation therapy. However, there are some harbingers of a poor prognosis, and these include age less than 2 years at tie of diagnosis, multiple cranial nerve palsies, and rapid onset of symptoms prior to diagnosis.

At times, quality of life is made possible only through the continued use of corticosteroids; however, these should be limited so that children do not suffer some of the feared side effects of these agents. Palliative care approaches should be offered at the time of clear tumor progression after all forms of therapy have been offered and have failed.

20.3.2 Dorsally Exophytic Pontine Gliomas

20.3.2.1 Symptoms and Clinical Signs

Dorsally exophytic pontine gliomas comprise roughly 20% of pediatric brainstem gliomas. They tend to present insidiously, with patients reporting minor symptoms over a 6–12-month time period. Some of the typical symptoms include headaches and vomiting; and ataxia, abducens or facial nerve palsies, and torticollis are some of the typical neurological signs [23].

20.3.2.2 Diagnostics

CT scans may still be used as a quick screening tool. On CT, these lesions are typically hypodense and fill the fourth ventricle. Bright contrast enhancement may be evident as well (Fig. 20.9). MRI has become the standard assessment tool used for children with dorsally exophytic brainstem gliomas. On MRI, a cap of surrounding CSF may be seen dorsolaterally. Ventrally, the tumor will blend into the brainstem, and it is frequently difficult to ascertain where the tumor ends and where the functional components of the brainstem begin. Signal characteristics are of low signal on T1 with high signal on T2 sequences. The tumor edges will generally be consistent between T1 and T2 sequences as compared to diffuse intrinsic lesions where there usually is a larger area of T2 signal abnormality compared to T1. As with CT, there is usually bright enhancement following intravenous contrast administration (Fig. 20.10).

20.3.2.3 Staging and Classification

Dorsally exophytic gliomas are predominantly pilocytic astrocytomas, with rare occurrence of anaplastic, higher-grade lesions, or gangliogliomas. The most consistent area of growth is through the path of least resistance, through the ependyma of the fourth ventricle. These lesions are locally recurrent and rarely show signs of distant dissemination or metastasis.

20.3.2.4 Treatment

Due to modern advances in operative technology and neuroimaging, the majority of dorsally exophytic brainstem gliomas are quite amenable to surgical resection. Whereas these lesions were thought to be inoperable, today dorsally exophytic brainstem gliomas can be approached quite aggressively due to the advent of microneurosurgical techniques, intraoperative neuromoni-

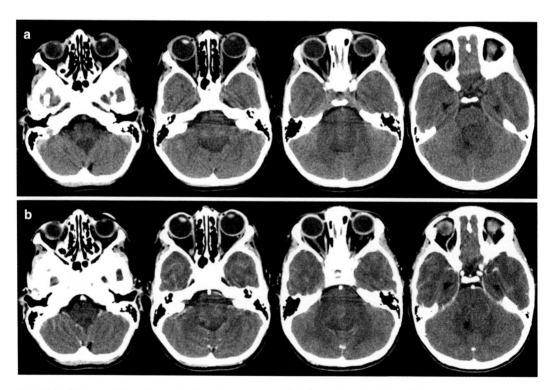

Fig. 20.9 CT scan of dorsally exophytic brainstem glioma in a 12-year-old male with 5-month history of increasing clumsiness, worsening ataxia, and diplopia. (**a**) Axial CT scan without contrast demonstrating subtle slightly low-density lesion filling the fourth ventricle. (**b**) Upon contrast administration, the lesion shows patch, inhomogeneous enhancement. The border of the lesion with the dorsal brainstem is not well appreciated

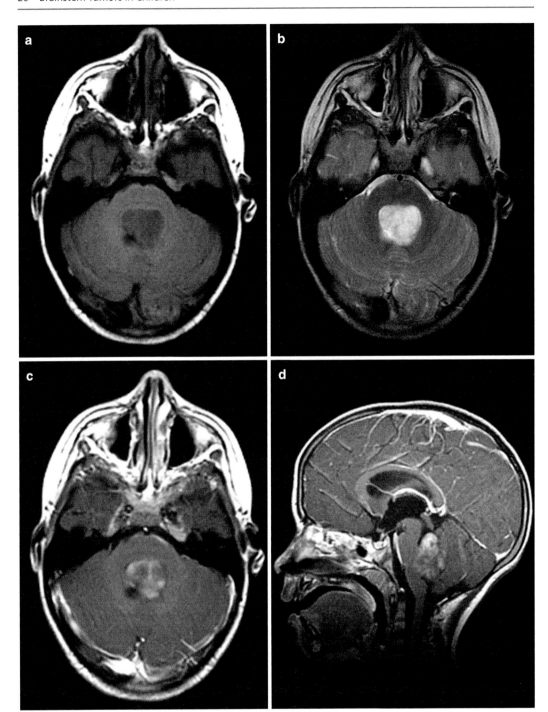

Fig. 20.10 MRI scan of dorsally exophytic brainstem glioma in patient described in Fig. 20.8. (**a**) Axial T1 MRI showing lesion directly opposed with the floor of the fourth ventricle. (**b**) Axial T2 MRI showing high signal intensity lesion in the fourth ventricle. (**c**) Axial T1 MRI with contrast showing somewhat patchy enhancement of the lesion. (**d**) Sagittal T1 MRI with contrast depicting the relationship of the tumor to the floor of the fourth ventricle in better resolution than on CT

toring (IONM), and neuronavigation [7, 24, 25]. Following exposure of the dorsally exophytic mass lesion in the fourth ventricle following standard suboccipital craniotomy and dural opening, tumor is removed stepwise using the ultrasonic aspirator (CUSA), suction, and bipolar cautery (Fig. 20.11). Intraoperative ultrasound is a useful adjunct as well in judging extent of resection,

as is intraoperative MRI. Care must be taken not to resect tumor below the estimated plane of the floor of the fourth ventricle. Decisions on where and when to stop neurosurgical resection are aided by feedback from IONM. Postoperative morbidity is usually noted in the form of exacerbation of existing preoperative ataxia, dysmetria, nystagmus, and cranial nerve dysfunction.

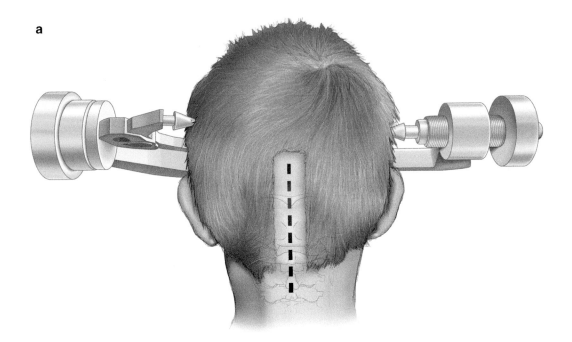

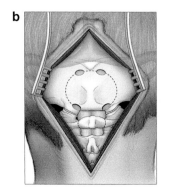
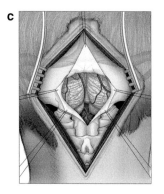
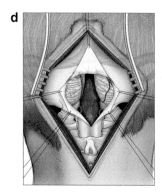

Fig. 20.11 (**a**) Standard midline approach to posterior fossa lesions including dorsally exophytic brainstem glioma. The patient is positioned prone in pin fixation (top image). A small midline hair shave is performed. (**b**) Midline exposure of the occipital region is performed bearing in mind the localization of the transverse sinus on both sides. A craniotomy is performed as shown. Four burr holes are used to prepare the craniotome for bone removal. Care is taken to identify the lip of the foramen magnum so as not to cause a tear in the dura upon using the craniotome. (**c**) The dura is reflected in a Y-shaped manner, and its edges are held back with tack-up sutures. (**d**) The cerebellar hemispheres are gently retracted allowing access to the fourth ventricle. The microscope is used to remove the tumor being careful not to transgress the floor of the fourth ventricle at any time. Alternatively, a telovelar approach can be performed (not shown here)

Radiation therapy may be required for those tumors that have recurred and where further neurosurgical options are limited. Typically, 54 Gy delivered in 30 fractions over 6 weeks is given. Tumor control after radiation therapy has been described as generally favorable in many series [23].

These days, with the known biological targeting of low-grade gliomas in children, dorsally exophytic pontine gliomas may be amenable to chemotherapy. In the past, carboplatin and vincristine have been used. Now, with various BRAF mutations and fusion anomalies discovered, BRAF inhibitor therapy is being explored at this time [26–28].

20.3.2.5 Prognosis/Quality of Life

Overall 5-year survival for the dorsally exophytic pilocytic lesions is good, with rates in most studies of about 95% [23]. Recurrence is recognized even with gross total excision, such that progression-free survival rates at 5 years are between 54 and 72% [23]. Other factors that worsen survival are cranial nerve (particularly abducens) dysfunction at presentation and symptom duration of less than 6 months. Total or subtotal excision of low-grade brainstem lesions has been shown to have an improved outcome compared to partial (<50% of total tumor mass) excision. Long-term neurological function following surgery for dorsally exophytic lesions is generally good, with most patients being either at their presentation baseline or improved.

Although the outcome for the dorsally exophytic pilocytic gliomas is good, the rarer fibrillary gliomas may carry a very poor prognosis. Various novel modalities of treatment are being investigated, including convection-enhanced and slow-flow delivery of chemotherapeutic agents, radiosensitizing agents, gene therapy, and hyperbaric and interstitial radiotherapy. Ultimately, a deeper understanding of the molecular biology of these tumors will lead to improvements in treatment with targeted therapies.

20.3.3 Cervicomedullary Gliomas

20.3.3.1 Symptoms and Clinical Signs

Cervicomedullary gliomas (CMGs) are intramedullary tumors that develop around the craniovertebral junction. They are rare, slow-growing, and histologically benign tumors that typically present with a variety of neurological symptoms including those of lower brainstem dysfunction and those of myelopathy [29]. Patients with tumors located in the medulla typically develop nausea, vomiting, failure to thrive, lower cranial nerve dysfunction, chronic aspiration, sleep apnea, and obstructive hydrocephalus. Tumors located in the upper cervical spine lead to changes in hand preference, gait, and motor regression especially in younger patients. They can also lead to hypo-/hyperreflexia and facial pain. However, independent of anatomical origin, as the tumor expands, patients have a mixture of these signs and symptoms.

20.3.3.2 Diagnostics

Regardless of location, CMGs present with clinical, radiologic, and pathological similarities. MRI is used as an initial diagnostic tool, and tissue diagnosis at the time of surgery leads to the final pathology. On MRI, the majority of CMGs are hypointense to white matter. On T2 and proton density images, they are hyperintense to white matter (Fig. 20.12). On sagittal MRI, CMGs extend from the caudal two thirds of the medulla to the rostral aspect of the cervical cord. They tend to enhance avidly following contrast administration.

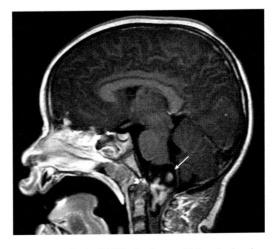

Fig. 20.12 Sagittal MRI of a 6-year-old female showing enhancing lesion of the cervicomedullary junction. This child presented with seizures initially but then went on to display progressive left hemiparesis

CMGs are typically low-grade neoplasms and may be gliomas or gangliogliomas [30]. Occasionally, anaplastic changes may be found in these tumors [29].

20.3.3.3 Classification

There is no standard classification system of CMGs. Since most of these tumors are low-grade, they are inclined to grow circumferentially around pial structures and become redirected at white matter tract interfaces. Thus, the pyramidal decussating fibers and medial lemniscus restrict their spread into the pontomedullary junction and instead direct their growth in the direction of the fourth ventricle. This growth restriction can subsequently lead to well-defined tumor borders and thus easier resection for the surgeon.

20.3.3.4 Treatment

Though conventional treatment for these tumors is by means of surgical resection, there has been a great amount of discussion on the role of radiation and chemotherapy as adjuncts to surgery. The role of surgery is indispensable as it allows the diagnosis to be made via tissue biopsy and decompression of the brainstem and cervical spine, along with treating an associated syrinx or potentially. However, complete resection is often not possible due to poorly defined tumor borders and/or unacceptable risk of neurological deficit. Valuable tools such as ultrasound, intraoperative MRI, stereotaxy, and neurophysiological monitoring are available for achieving maximal resection [7, 24, 25] (Fig. 20.13).

As previously stated, surgery may not be curative in some instances for low-grade lesions and is never curative with high-grade lesions. Radiation therapy (RT) is considered an optional treatment modality for CMGs. It can be used as primary treatment or salvage treatment for low-grade lesions and can be considered in tandem with chemotherapy for primary treatment of

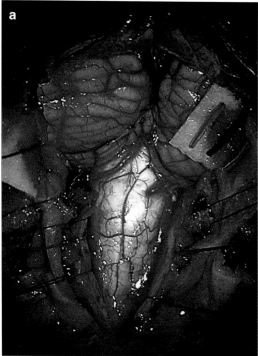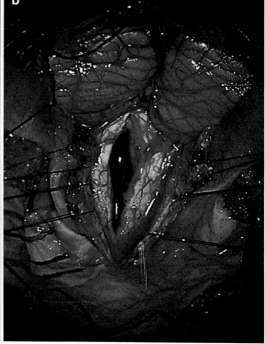

Fig. 20.13 Intraoperative photograph of cervicomedullary glioma in patient described in Fig. 20.11. (a) Following posterior fossa craniotomy and cervical laminotomy, the cervicomedullary glioma is seen. A midline myelotomy was made, and the tumor was debulked cautiously under continuous neuromonitoring, using the CUSA. (b) Immediate post-resection photography showing midline myelotomy and resection of the cervicomedullary glioma

malignant tumors not amenable to surgical resection. A more conservative surgical approach may be indicated for CMGs that demonstrate enhancing tumor tissue among non-enhancing tissue that is continuous with normal cervical spinal cord and/or medulla and/or a poorly delineated tumor/brainstem interface with an abnormal T1 signal extending beyond the apparent tumor into the brainstem on MRI. When these are present on MRI, it is proposed that chemotherapy and/or RT may be superior treatment modalities and provide better survival and neurological outcomes. Chemotherapy alone is typically not considered a standard therapeutic modality but an adjuvant treatment modality in conjunction with surgery and/or salvage treatment for recurrent or progressive tumor [29].

Interestingly, there is a tremendous research focus on the development of novel, targeted therapies based on the specific molecular signature of these tumors. Key tumor molecular markers/pathways have been elucidated, including activation of the ERK/MAPK pathway and identification of KIAA1549-BRAF gene fusions with high frequency [8, 26, 27, 31, 32]. Certain subsets of CMGs are also known to express BRAFV600E mutations. The ERK/MAPK pathway presents a potent area of targeted therapy by MEK inhibitors, which provides a potential alternative treatment modality for patients who are unable to receive maximal resection or do not desire it. Thus, there is tremendous potential for the development of effective targeted therapies as future treatments for CMGs.

20.3.3.5 Prognosis/Quality of Life

CMGs are typically low-grade lesions and thus have favorable overall survival. However, their recurrence rate is high, and they require long-term follow-up to maximize overall survival and neurological preservation. In essence, these tumors take patients down a chronic illness pathway that leads to stepwise deterioration. The goal, of course, is to maximize tumor resection, minimize long-term neurological morbidity, and improve overall quality of life over time.

Interestingly, it has been shown that patients with protracted duration of symptoms prior to diagnosis generally have low-grade tumors with a high probability of long overall survival.

Finally, postoperative cervical sagittal deformity has been reported as a major risk for children undergoing surgery for an intramedullary spinal cord tumor, and this also includes CMGs. At times, instrumented occipito-cervical fusion procedures may be required.

20.4 Conclusions

Brainstem tumors in children are a relatively rare but extremely important subset of brain tumors in children. Their diagnosis is now made fairly accurately on the basis of preoperative MRI scanning which helps apportion these tumors into subgroups affecting the midbrain, pons, and cervicomedullary regions. Despite their critical location, brainstem tumors can now be approached successfully and safely through a number of strategies that have been outlined in this chapter. Tremendous progress has been made in our characterization of the main genetic and epigenetic alterations that affect DIPGs, gangliogliomas, and low-grade gliomas. As a result, there is hope on the horizon that targeted therapy toward activated pathways in these tumors (e.g., BRAF, MAPK, H3KM27, and PDGFB) may provide an additional arm of therapy that will help substantially in improving overall survival and minimizing morbidity in children afflicted with these tumors. In addition, novel drug delivery approaches, such as CED or MRgFUS, should facilitate increased concentrations of targeted therapy into recalcitrant lesions such as DIPG. It is hoped that these approaches will be met with increasing survival advantages among children with these devastating brainstem lesions in particular.

Acknowledgments This chapter was made possible through funds provided from the Canadian Institutes of Health Research, Brainchild, the Wiley Family Foundation, and the Laurie Berman Fund at the Hospital for Sick Children.

References

1. Igboechi C, Vaddiparti A, Sorenson EP, Rozzelle CJ, Tubbs RS, Loukas M (2013) Tectal plate gliomas: a review. Childs Nerv Syst 29:1827–1833

2. Diaz RJ, Girgis FM, Hamiltonn MG (2014) Endoscopic third ventriculostomy for hydrocephalus due to tectal glioma. Can J Neurol Sci 41:476–481

3. Chumas PD, Drake JM, Del Bigio MR (1992) Death from chronic tonsillar herniation in a patient with lumboperitoneal shunt and Crouzon's disease. Br J Neurosurg 6:595–599

4. Vandertop WP, Hoffman HJ, Drake JM, Humphreys RP, Rutka JT, Amstrong DC, Becker LE (1992) Focal midbrain tumors in children. Neurosurgery 31:186–194

5. Broadway SJ, Ogg RJ, Scoggins MA, Sanford R, Patay Z, Boop FA (2011) Surgical management of tumors producing the thalamopeduncular syndrome of childhood. J Neurosurg Pediatr 7:589–595

6. Lee RP, Foster KA, Lillard JC, Klimo P Jr, Ellison DW, Orr B, Boop FA (2017) Surgical and molecular considerations in the treatment of pediatric thalamopeduncular tumors. J Neurosurg Pediatr 20:247–255

7. Ng WH, Mukhida K, Rutka JT (2010) Image guidance and neuromonitoring in neurosurgery. Childs Nerv Syst 26:491–502

8. Packer RJ, Pfister S, Bouffet E, Avery R, Bandopadhayay P, Bornhorst M, Bowers DC, Ellison D, Fangusaro J, Foreman N, Fouladi M, Gajjar A, Haas-Kogan D, Hawkins C, Ho CY, Hwang E, Jabado N, Kilburn LB, Lassaletta A, Ligon KL, Massimino M, Meeteren SV, Mueller S, Nicolaides T, Perilongo G, Tabori U, Vezina G, Warren K, Witt O, Zhu Y, Jones DT, Kieran M (2017) Pediatric low-grade gliomas: implications of the biologic era. Neuro Oncol 19:750–761

9. Mathew RK, Rutka JT (2018) Diffuse intrinsic pontine glioma: clinical features, molecular genetics, and novel targeted therapeutics. J Korean Neurosurg Soc 61:343–351

10. Buczkowicz P, Hoeman C, Rakopoulos P, Pajovic S, Letourneau L, Dzamba M, Morrison A, Lewis P, Bouffet E, Bartels U, Zuccaro J, Agnihotri S, Ryall S, Barszczyk M, Chornenkyy Y, Bourgey M, Bourque G, Montpetit A, Cordero F, Castelo-Branco P, Mangerel J, Tabori U, Ho KC, Huang A, Taylor KR, Mackay A, Bendel AE, Nazarian J, Fangusaro JR, Karajannis MA, Zagzag D, Foreman NK, Donson A, Hegert JV, Smith A, Chan J, Lafay-Cousin L, Dunn S, Hukin J, Dunham C, Scheinemann K, Michaud J, Zelcer S, Ramsay D, Cain J, Brennan C, Souweidane MM, Jones C, Allis CD, Brudno M, Becher O, Hawkins C (2014) Genomic analysis of diffuse intrinsic pontine gliomas identifies three molecular subgroups and recurrent activating ACVR1 mutations. Nat Genet 46:451–456

11. Fontebasso AM, Papillon-Cavanagh S, Schwartzentruber J, Nikbakht H, Gerges N, Fiset PO, Bechet D, Faury D, De Jay N, Ramkissoon LA, Corcoran A, Jones DT, Sturm D, Johann P, Tomita T, Goldman S, Nagib M, Bendel A, Goumnerova L, Bowers DC, Leonard JR, Rubin JB, Alden T, Browd S, Geyer JR, Leary S, Jallo G, Cohen K, Gupta N, Prados MD, Carret AS, Ellezam B, Crevier L, Klekner A, Bognar L, Hauser P, Garami M, Myseros J, Dong Z, Siegel PM, Malkin H, Ligon AH, Albrecht S, Pfister SM, Ligon KL, Majewski J, Jabado N, Kieran MW (2014) Recurrent somatic mutations in ACVR1 in pediatric midline high-grade astrocytoma. Nat Genet 46:462–466

12. Hoffman LM, Veldhuijzen van Zanten SEM, Colditz N, Baugh J, Chaney B, Hoffmann M, Lane A, Fuller C, Miles L, Hawkins C, Bartels U, Bouffet E, Goldman S, Leary S, Foreman NK, Packer R, Warren KE, Broniscer A, Kieran MW, Minturn J, Comito M, Broxson E, Shih CS, Khatua S, Chintagumpala M, Carret AS, Escorza NY, Hassall T, Ziegler DS, Gottardo N, Dholaria H, Doughman R, Benesch M, Drissi R, Nazarian J, Jabado N, Boddaert N, Varlet P, Giraud G, Castel D, Puget S, Jones C, Hulleman E, Modena P, Giagnacovo M, Antonelli M, Pietsch T, Gielen GH, Jones DTW, Sturm D, Pfister SM, Gerber NU, Grotzer MA, Pfaff E, von Bueren AO, Hargrave D, Solanki GA, Jadrijevic Cvrlje F, Kaspers GJL, Vandertop WP, Grill J, Bailey S, Biassoni V, Massimino M, Calmon R, Sanchez E, Bison B, Warmuth-Metz M, Leach J, Jones B, van Vuurden DG, Kramm CM, Fouladi M (2018) Clinical, radiologic, pathologic, and molecular characteristics of long-term survivors of diffuse intrinsic pontine glioma (DIPG): a collaborative report from the International and European Society for Pediatric Oncology DIPG registries. J Clin Oncol 36:1963–1972

13. Truffaux N, Philippe C, Paulsson J, Andreiuolo F, Guerrini-Rousseau L, Cornilleau G, Le Dret L, Richon C, Lacroix L, Puget S, Geoerger B, Vassal G, Ostman A, Grill J (2015) Preclinical evaluation of dasatinib alone and in combination with cabozantinib for the treatment of diffuse intrinsic pontine glioma. Neuro Oncol 17:953–964

14. Puget S, Beccaria K, Blauwblomme T, Roujeau T, James S, Grill J, Zerah M, Varlet P, Sainte-Rose C (2015) Biopsy in a series of 130 pediatric diffuse intrinsic pontine gliomas. Childs Nerv Syst 31:1773–1780

15. Puget, S., Blauwblomme, T., and Grill, J. (2012) Is biopsy safe in children with newly diagnosed diffuse intrinsic pontine glioma? Am Soc Clin Oncol Educ Book 629–633

16. Plessier A, Le Dret L, Varlet P, Beccaria K, Lacombe J, Meriaux S, Geffroy F, Fiette L, Flamant P, Chretien F, Blauwblomme T, Puget S, Grill J, Debily MA, Castel D (2017) New in vivo avatars of diffuse intrinsic pontine gliomas (DIPG) from stereotactic biopsies performed at diagnosis. Oncotarget 8:52543–52559

17. Souweidane MM, Kramer K, Pandit-Taskar N, Zhou Z, Haque S, Zanzonico P, Carrasquillo JA, Lyashchenko SK, Thakur SB, Donzelli M, Turner RS,

Lewis JS, Cheung NV, Larson SM, Dunkel IJ (2018) Convection-enhanced delivery for diffuse intrinsic pontine glioma: a single-centre, dose-escalation, phase 1 trial. Lancet Oncol 19:1040–1050

18. Zhou Z, Singh R, Souweidane MM (2017) Convection-enhanced delivery for diffuse intrinsic pontine glioma treatment. Curr Neuropharmacol 15:116–128

19. Luther N, Zhou Z, Zanzonico P, Cheung NK, Humm J, Edgar MA, Souweidane MM (2014) The potential of theragnostic (1)(2)(4)I-8H9 convection-enhanced delivery in diffuse intrinsic pontine glioma. Neuro Oncol 16:800–806

20. Zhou Z, Luther N, Ibrahim GM, Hawkins C, Vibhakar R, Handler MH, Souweidane MM (2013) B7-H3, a potential therapeutic target, is expressed in diffuse intrinsic pontine glioma. J Neurooncol 111:257–264

21. Benitez-Ribas D, Cabezon R, Florez-Grau G, Molero MC, Puerta P, Guillen A, Paco S, Carcaboso AM, Santa-Maria Lopez V, Cruz O, de Torres C, Salvador N, Juan M, Mora J, La Madrid AM (2018) Immune response generated with the administration of autologous dendritic cells pulsed with an allogenic tumoral cell-lines lysate in patients with newly diagnosed diffuse intrinsic pontine glioma. Front Oncol 8:127

22. Alli S, Figueiredo CA, Golbourn B, Sabha N, Wu MY, Bondoc A, Luck A, Coluccia D, Maslink C, Smith C, Wurdak H, Hynynen K, O'Reilly M, Rutka JT (2018) Brainstem blood brain barrier disruption using focused ultrasound: a demonstration of feasibility and enhanced doxorubicin delivery. J Control Release 281:29–41

23. Pollack IF, Hoffman HJ, Humphreys RP, Becker L (1993) The long-term outcome after surgical treatment of dorsally exophytic brain-stem gliomas. J Neurosurg 78:859–863

24. Stone SS, Rutka JT (2008) Utility of neuronavigation and neuromonitoring in epilepsy surgery. Neurosurg Focus 25:E17

25. Timoney N, Rutka JT (2017) Recent advances in epilepsy surgery and achieving best outcomes using high-frequency oscillations, diffusion tensor imaging, magnetoencephalography, intraoperative neuromonitoring, focal cortical dysplasia, and bottom of sulcus dysplasia. Neurosurgery 64:1–10

26. Green AL, Kieran MW (2015) Pediatric brainstem gliomas: new understanding leads to potential new treatments for two very different tumors. Curr Oncol Rep 17:436

27. Lassaletta A, Zapotocky M, Mistry M, Ramaswamy V, Honnorat M, Krishnatry R, Guerreiro Stucklin A, Zhukova N, Arnoldo A, Ryall S, Ling C, McKeown T, Loukides J, Cruz O, de Torres C, Ho CY, Packer RJ, Tatevossian R, Qaddoumi I, Harreld JH, Dalton JD, Mulcahy-Levy J, Foreman N, Karajannis MA, Wang S, Snuderl M, Nageswara Rao A, Giannini C, Kieran M, Ligon KL, Garre ML, Nozza P, Mascelli S, Raso A, Mueller S, Nicolaides T, Silva K, Perbet R, Vasiljevic A, Faure Conter C, Frappaz D, Leary S, Crane C, Chan A, Ng HK, Shi ZF, Mao Y, Finch E, Eisenstat D, Wilson B, Carret AS, Hauser P, Sumerauer D, Krskova L, Larouche V, Fleming A, Zelcer S, Jabado N, Rutka JT, Dirks P, Taylor MD, Chen S, Bartels U, Huang A, Ellison DW, Bouffet E, Hawkins C, Tabori U (2017) Therapeutic and prognostic implications of BRAF V600E in pediatric low-grade gliomas. J Clin Oncol 35:2934–2941

28. Penman CL, Faulkner C, Lowis SP, Kurian KM (2015) Current understanding of BRAF alterations in diagnosis, prognosis, and therapeutic targeting in pediatric low-grade gliomas. Front Oncol 5:54

29. McAbee JH, Modica J, Thompson CJ, Broniscer A, Orr B, Choudhri AF, Boop FA, Klimo P Jr (2015) Cervicomedullary tumors in children. J Neurosurg Pediatr 16:357–366

30. Janjua MB, Ivasyk I, Pisapia DJ, Souweidane MM (2017) Ganglioglioma of brain stem and cervicomedullary junction: a 50 years review of literature. J Clin Neurosci 44:34–46

31. Garcia MA, Solomon DA, Haas-Kogan DA (2016) Exploiting molecular biology for diagnosis and targeted management of pediatric low-grade gliomas. Future Oncol 12:1493–1506

32. Sturm D, Pfister SM, Jones DTW (2017) Pediatric gliomas: current concepts on diagnosis, biology, and clinical management. J Clin Oncol 35:2370–2377

Supratentorial Lobar Gliomas in Childhood and Adolescence

21

Cassie Kline, Anu Banerjee, and Nalin Gupta

21.1 Epidemiology

Gliomas are the most common type of pediatric brain tumor and include a wide variety of histologies and biologic behaviors. This heterogeneous group of tumors can arise throughout the central nervous system (CNS) but most frequently occur in the supratentorial compartment [1]. Gliomas can be broadly divided into low- and high-grade lesions as defined by WHO classification grades I–IV. Low-grade gliomas (LGG) occur as WHO grades I and II, and high-grade gliomas (HGG) occur as WHO grades III and IV. Glioma describes a variety of histologic groups including astrocytoma, ependymoma, oligodendroglioma, mixed glioma, dysembryoplastic neuroepithelial tumors, and glioblastoma, as well as some more rare histologies.

C. Kline
Division of Hematology/Oncology, Departments of
Pediatrics and Neurology, University of California,
San Francisco, San Francisco, CA, USA
e-mail: Cassie.Kline@ucsf.edu

A. Banerjee
Division of Pediatric Hematology/Oncology,
Departments of Pediatrics and Neurological Surgery,
University of California San Francisco,
San Francisco, CA, USA
e-mail: Anu.Banerjee@ucsf.edu

N. Gupta (✉)
Division of Pediatric Neursurgery, Department of
Neurological Surgery, University of Caliifornia San
Francisco, San Francisco, CA, USA
e-mail: nalin.gupta@ucsf.edu

High-grade gliomas such as anaplastic astrocytomas (AA) and glioblastomas are among the leading causes of cancer-related death in children [2]. Fortunately, LGGs account for 60–80% of supratentorial hemispheric tumors in children; these tumors occur at an incidence of approximately five in one million children per year [3–5]. HGGs account for the remaining 20–40%, with glioblastomas accounting for only about 3% of pediatric brain tumors [1, 6]. Gliomas are more common in white populations, averaging about two times the frequency as compared to black populations [1]. Throughout childhood, the incidence rate of gliomas declines as children age and then increases in incidence once adulthood is reached [1].

Most childhood gliomas are sporadic, although underlying genetic conditions, such as neurofibromatosis type 1 (NF-1), Li-Fraumeni syndrome, tuberous sclerosis complex (TSC), or Turcot syndrome, are known to predispose patients to the development of gliomas. The phenotype of these syndromes is presumed to be dependent upon germline mutations within identified genes, although the origin of the observed phenotypic variability is not well understood in some disorders (e.g., NF-1), and the frequency of glioma occurrence is variable.

A past medical history of brain irradiation is the only established environmental risk factor for the development of gliomas, most often seen in the setting of therapeutic treatment for a prior malignancy. The search for other environmental factors is an active area of research and may reveal other predisposing oncogenic stimuli.

21.2 Symptoms and Clinical Signs

Patients with supratentorial tumors usually present with a combination of symptoms and signs, frequently associated with increased intracranial pressure (ICP) or focal symptoms related to the anatomic location of the tumor. Common symptoms include headache, vomiting, focal motor or sensory deficits, and seizures. Symptoms such as headache and vomiting are often more pronounced in the morning due to increased ICP related to overnight supine positioning with sleep. Focal neurological deficits are present at diagnosis in the majority of cases, with the most common findings being cranial nerve abnormalities and focal weakness. Papilledema may occur secondary to increased intracranial pressure [7].

Patients younger than 3 years of age and those with HGGs typically present with a more rapid progression of symptoms over a period of days to weeks, presumably reflecting rapid tumor growth and associated brain edema [8]. Patients with LGGs are more likely to present with a focal neurologic deficit. However, seizures account for the presenting clinical sign in one third of these patients and are frequently associated with tumors arising from the temporal lobe [9]. Approximately 5–10% of patients present with a rapid neurologic decline, either due to brain herniation or tumor-associated hemorrhage [4]. As with other lesions in the CNS, the physical examination can be helpful in determining the anatomic location of the lesion, but is usually not specific in narrowing the differential diagnosis.

21.3 Diagnostic Studies

The differential diagnosis for any supratentorial tumor includes LGG, HGG, supratentorial primitive neuroectodermal tumor (PNET) or other embryonal tumor, ependymoma, neuronal tumor (gangliocytoma), and, rarely, metastatic tumors, such as lymphoma, neuroblastoma, or sarcoma. Detailed imaging studies are required to define the anatomical relationships between the tumor and surrounding brain, identify the characteristics of the tumor such as infiltrations into the surrounding tissues and associated hemorrhage, and narrow the presumed pathologic diagnosis. Specific imaging studies are also essential for surgical planning and intraoperative neuronavigation.

21.3.1 Computed Tomography

Computed tomography (CT) is usually the first study obtained after a patient presents with symptoms, as this imaging modality is rapid and readily available at most hospitals. Non-contrast images often show the effects of a mass lesion. However, these findings are not limited to tumors and can appear with brain abscesses, acute stroke, or other space-occupying lesions.

Irregular or ring enhancement on cranial CT images following contrast administration reflects the breakdown of the blood-brain barrier and/or tumor neovascularity and is more common with high-grade tumors, such as HGG. However, some low-grade pilocytic astrocytomas can also enhance strongly on post-contrast images. The presence of central necrosis and extension across the midline through the corpus callosum support high-grade tumors. In general, CT images support the diagnosis of a supratentorial glioma but are rarely sufficient by themselves.

CT perfusion studies are helpful in assessing tumor vascularity and, by implication, the pathologic grade. Although magnetic resonance (MR) perfusion studies are more widely used, CT perfusion studies are equally helpful in assessing perfusion without the additional anatomical detail. CT perfusion studies may be particularly useful in delineating grade of tumors that do not illustrate contrast enhancement on MRI. In this setting, perfusion studies such as cerebral blood flow and cerebral blood volume appear to be sensitive and specific to identify WHO grade II versus grade III gliomas [10, 11].

21.3.2 Magnetic Resonance Imaging

High-quality magnetic resonance imaging (MRI), both with and without gadolinium contrast, is essential in the diagnosis of supratentorial gliomas. MRIs of pediatric LGGs frequently reveal a mass with variable enhancement. WHO grade I tumors, pilocytic astrocytomas in particular, are well-circumscribed with enhancement following contrast administration (Fig. 21.1). About 30% of LGGs exhibit cystic changes. Grade II lesions can be locally infiltrative and demonstrate enhancement after contrast administration [12]. The degree of local vasogenic edema is usually minimal with LGG [13]. Imaging of the entire CNS axis is not typically necessary in LGGs given the infrequency of metastasis, but more comprehensive imaging should be considered if concerning clinical symptoms are present.

HGGs are usually isointense or hypointense on T1-weighted images [14]. Contrast enhance-

ment varies from little or none (Fig. 21.2) to a more typical appearance of irregular peripheral enhancement. T2-weighted and FLAIR images usually show increased signal intensity in the surrounding white matter tracts, representing infiltrative tumor and associated vasogenic edema. Areas of necrosis or enhancement support the diagnosis of HGG, although enhancement and cyst formation occurring in LGG can mimic areas of necrosis. Pleomorphic xanthoastrocytomas typically have an enhancing solid component at the cortical surface with a deeper cyst, although more heterogeneous enhancement is occasionally observed. Some HGGs, particularly AA, do not show enhancement and can be quite homogeneous in appearance.

Newer MR techniques have been developed in order to reduce the ambiguity that can occur because of overlapping features observed with conventional sequences. MR perfusion studies are used to assess the tumor blood supply by

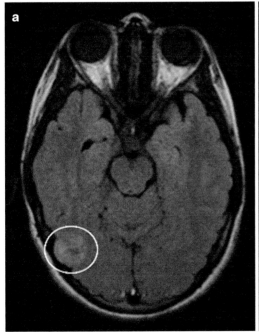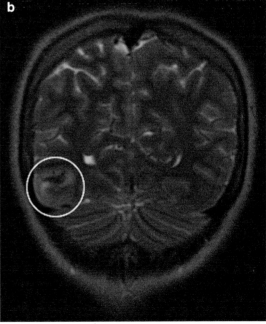

Fig. 21.1 A 13-year-old female who presented with new onset seizures. Imaging revealed right temporal lobe mass with pathology consistent with ganglioglioma, WHO grade I. (**a**) Preoperative axial T2-FLAIR sequence MRI demonstrating well-circumscribed mass within the periphery of the right temporal lobe. (**b**) Preoperative coronal T2-weighted sequence MRI demonstrating some signal intensity. The tumor did not demonstrate enhancement with gadolinium on T1-weighted imaging

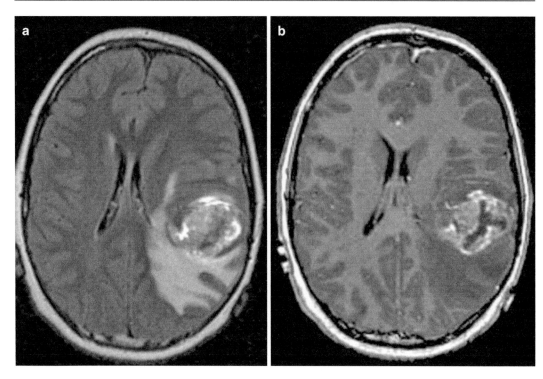

Fig. 21.2 A 14-year-old boy who presented with a progressive history of headaches, dysphasia, and nausea and vomiting. The pathologic diagnosis was glioblastoma. (**a**) Preoperative FLAIR sequence MRI demonstrating a large infiltrative mass in the anterior left parietal lobe with surrounding vasogenic edema with considerable local mass effect. (**b**) A T1-weighted MR image following gadolinium reveals heterogeneous enhancement with a central nonenhancing area consistent with central necrosis

measuring cerebral blood flow and volume and contrast transit time. Increased cerebral blood volume, indicating hypervascularity, may be elevated in areas that do not demonstrate contrast enhancement [14]. LGGs have higher apparent diffusion coefficients and less perfusion on imaging as compared to HGGs and due to their limited local blood flow and lower cellularity [12, 15]. MR spectroscopy (MRS) provides additional metabolic information reflecting different aspects of tumor biology. An increased choline to N-acetylaspartate ratio has been shown to predict a more aggressive malignancy. Presumably, this occurs in high-grade lesions due to increased cell division and turnover with reduced numbers of neurons. On MRS, pilocytic astrocytomas can appear more aggressive than they act, showing increased choline, decreased N-acetylaspartate, and presence of lactate peaks [12]. Increasingly, these modalities are guiding intraoperative biopsies to assure adequate sampling of the most suspicious intratumoral areas [16].

Further, in the posttreatment setting, advanced MR imaging be able to delineate true tumor progression from treatment response and pseudoprogression, particularly when novel therapies such PD-1 inhibition and peptide-based vaccines are used [17]. MR modalities such as diffusion-weighted imaging, MR spectroscopy, MR perfusion, and PET/MR can augment the diagnostic sensitivity and specificity of MR imaging; however, the applicability of these modalities among all patients and in the pediatric setting still requires more experience and research [18].

21.3.3 Genetic Features of Low-Grade Gliomas

While adult and pediatric gliomas have very similar histologic features, the genetic mutations underlying their development are different [19, 20]. For example, pediatric HGGs are more frequently observed to have gains in chromosomes 1q, 2q, and 21q and losses of 6q, 11q, and 16q [21, 22]. Additionally, there may be a correlation in pediatric HGGs between a gain on chromosome 1q and shorter survival, although this was demonstrated in a study where the overall sample size was small (23 patients). Another study found that loss of heterozygosity (LOH) on chromosome 22q, although less common than in adults, occurred in 40% of pediatric AA and 61% of pediatric glioblastoma. LOH at 1p/19q has also been demonstrated to occur much less frequently in pediatric gliomas when compared to adult gliomas [23].

The genetic landscape of pediatric LGG is also quite distinct from that of pediatric HGG. Alterations of *BRAF* resulting in activation of the MAPK signaling pathway are among the most common observed in pediatric LGGs. Mutations or other abnormalities in the *BRAF/MAPK* pathway occur in about 50–80% of all LGG [24, 25]. Activating alterations include *BRAF* V600E and *BRAF:KIAA1549* fusions. *BRAF* V600E mutations can be found in both LGGs and HGGs gliomas, whereas *BRAF:KIAA1549* fusions are almost exclusively seen in LGGs [26]. The specific alterations of *BRAF* correlates strongly with histologic subtype of LGG. For instance, *BRAF* V600E mutations are seen most frequently in pleomorphic xanthoastrocytomas, while *BRAF:KIAA1549* fusions are concentrated in pilocytic astrocytomas [24, 25]. The presence of a *BRAF V600E* mutation in pediatric gliomas suggests that therapy with mutation-specific targeted signaling inhibitors, such as vemurafenib or dabrafenib, will be active.

MYB/MYBL1 mutations are also seen in pediatric LGG. *MYB-QKI* fusions, in particular, carry distinct clinical features including localization to the peripheral cortex, associated with seizures at diagnosis, and an overall good survival prognosis. This molecular and clinical picture is diagnostic of angiocentric gliomas [27, 28].

Germline alterations within the *NF1* and *TSC1/2* tumor suppressor genes are additional molecular abnormalities that predispose children to developing LGGs [29]. In these patients, loss of heterozygosity in a specific cell of origin results in tumor development. Optic pathway glioma is the most common tumor type in patients with NF1, while patients with germline *TSC* mutations are at risk of developing subependymoma giant cell astrocytomas [30]. *NF1* is a negative regulator of *RAS/MAPK* signaling; therefore, loss of all *NF1* expression results in constitutive activation of the pathway and drives tumorigenesis. Similarly, the TSC1/2 complex is a negative regulator of mTOR; loss of *TSC1/2* expression results in unregulated signaling of mTOR [31]. Other mutations seen in pediatric LGG include *FGFR1*, *PIK3CA*, and *TP53* [25]. The frequency of *TP53* is much less than that seen in adults. Methylation of the tumor suppressor gene *PTEN*, resulting in transcriptional silencing of the gene and subsequent activation of the *PI3K* signaling pathway, has also been described in LGGs [32].

21.3.4 Genetic Features of High-Grade Gliomas

Underlying genetic features predisposing patients to the formation of HGGs include mutations in *NF1* (sporadic) and *TP53*. In one analysis of 28 HGG patients, *TP53* mutations were found in 30% of AA and 33% of glioblastomas [23]. Microsatellite instability appears with higher frequency in pediatric primary brain tumors compared to adult brain tumors and correlates with *TP53* mutations. Microsatellite instability and *TP53* mutations predict decreased overall survival [1, 37]. Of the tyrosine kinase receptors, initial data show immunopositivity for *PTEN*, *EGFR*, and *PDGFR* in 20–58% of pediatric HGGs. *PDGFR* and *EGFR* alterations occur with alternate frequency between pediatric and adult gliomas. *PDGFR* alterations occur more frequently in pediatric tumors, while *EGFR* alterations occur more predominantly in adult tumors [22, 33, 34]. Isocitrate dehydrogenase (*IDH1/2*) mutations were previously thought to be isolated to adult gliomas; however, these have now been recently described in a subset of pediatric gliomas and in children as young as 8 years old [35]. *PTEN* mutations appear to have a stronger correlation with decreased survival in pediatric HGGs [36]. Overexpression of O_6 methylguanine DNA methyltransferase (MGMT) expression confers resistance to alkylating chemotherapy and is also predictive of poor survival in pediatric HGG [37].

The histone mutations, *HIST1H3A* (H3.1) and *H3F3A* (H3.3), are common in pediatric gliomas and correlate with diagnosis and prognosis. These genes are involved in chromatin remodeling, and the associated Lys27Met (K27M) or, less frequently, Gly24Arg/Val (G34R/V) mutations in the H3.1 and H3.3 proteins lead to decreased DNA methylation and transcriptional upregulation or downregulation of large number of genes [38, 39]. Although commonly associated with diffuse intrinsic brainstem gliomas (DIPG), sequencing of non-brainstem, midline HGG has identified K27M mutations in up to 70% of patients, with a predominance of tumors bearing K27M mutations localizing to the midline [40, 41]. In contrast, only about 13% of pediatric glioblastomas within the hemispheric cortex carry a G34R/V mutation [40, 42]. The high frequency of H3 K27M mutations in midline gliomas is important diagnostically, as reflected by a newly defined WHO grade IV diagnostic entity, "Diffuse midline glioma, H3 K27M mutant" [43]. The H3.3 K27M variant midline gliomas are associated with the poorest prognoses of all gliomas.

MicroRNA (miRNA) analysis also demonstrates discordance between adult and pediatric gliomas. One study comparing 12 pediatric and 23 adult supratentorial HGG found pediatric HGG clustered separately from adult HGG. Pediatric HGG demonstrated 52% of miRNA were differentially expressed when compared to adult HGG, with a specific upregulation in miR-17-92. In further gene expression analysis, pediatric HGG appears to differentiate themselves from adult HGG in the preferential expression of the Sonic Hedgehog pathway genes: *GLI1*, *CCND1*, *BMP2*, and *SFRP1* [44].

21.4 Staging and Classification

Gliomas include a broad range of tumors of astrocytic, oligodendroglial, and ependymal origin. These specific LGGs are either WHO grades I–II: pilocytic astrocytomas, pleomorphic xanthoastrocytomas, oligodendrogliomas, dsyembryoplastic neuroepithelial tumors, and gangliogliomas. LGG also include rare diagnoses such as diffuse leptomeningeal glioneuronal tumors [45]. HGGs are more limited in classification and consist of anaplastic astrocytoma (WHO grade III) and glioblastoma (WHO grade IV).

Pediatric LGG most commonly occurs as a WHO grade I tumor and thus rarely transforms to more malignant HGG, in contrast to LGGs occurring in adults which more commonly occur as WHO grade II and frequently develop malignant transformation. Most pediatric LGG typically do not disseminate with the exception of pleomorphic xanthoastrocytoma, which tend to be more aggressive and likely to metastasize [46]. An estimated less than 10% of patients with pilocytic astrocytoma develop dissemination, although the prognostic impact of dissemination in this setting is unclear [47]. Unresectable pediatric LGG is typically a lifelong, chronic illnesses, characterized by indolent tumor progression and associated morbidity. Histologic classification of LGG is determined by the subgroup but typically carries low mitotic indices consistent with their low-grade nature.

In contrast to pediatric LGG, HGGs are malignant tumors with an aggressive pattern of growth. Anaplastic astrocytomas are characterized by focal or diffuse hypercellularity with associated nuclear atypia, nuclear pleomorphism, and the presence of mitotic figures. Glioblastomas exhibit many of the same features as AAs but also have a combination of endothelial proliferation and necrosis on histologic examination [4]. Grade III oligodendrogliomas and some pleomorphic xanthoastrocytomas have many of the histologic characteristics similar to HGG and, thus, exhibit a clinical pattern more similar to HGG than LGG.

21.5 Treatment

21.5.1 Surgical

The primary goals of surgery for glioma are to obtain a definitive tissue diagnosis and to achieve gross total resection (GTR) while maintaining neurologic function. The extent of resection affects survival in both LGG and HGG. For instance, complete surgical resection is typically curative for the majority of pediatric patients with LGG [45]. Complete resection also confers improved survival in patients with HGG. Five-year overall survival for AA is 44% following GTR versus 22% after subtotal resection (STR) and for glioblastoma, 26% following GTR versus 4% after STR [48]. Barriers to GTR of HGGs include the infiltrative nature of these tumors and, in some clinical presentations, tumor involvement of eloquent tissue. Modern technologies such as cortical and subcortical mapping improve the likelihood of GTR. Advances in imaging, such as functional MRI (fMRI), positron emission tomography (PET), and diffusion tensor imaging (DTI), are also leading to marked improvements in the resolution and reliability of functional maps [49]. Accurate intraoperative neuronavigation combined with electrophysiological mapping of motor, sensory, and language function has supplanted resections based purely on anatomic landmarks. These advances have contributed to fewer unanticipated neurologic deficits arising from tumor resection.

21.5.2 Chemotherapy

Patients with unresectable, symptomatic LGG are candidates for adjuvant treatment such as chemotherapy. For patients with well controlled or minimal symptoms, a "watchful waiting" approach can also be considered given their typical benign, indolent natural history. Patients with tumor-related symptoms such as visual loss or weakness, however, may benefit from chemotherapy with the goals of stabilization of both tumor growth and symptomatic progression.

Multiple chemotherapy regimens have demonstrated activity in clinical trials, and modern trials have shown activity of biologically targeted agents. Frequently used chemotherapy options include carboplatin, vincristine, and/or vinblastine (VBL) [50–53]. Dosing options for these regimens range from weekly low-dose therapy (i.e., weekly carboplatin/vincristine [CV] combination therapy or vinblastine monotherapy) to monthly high-dose options (i.e., carboplatin monotherapy). Additional chemotherapy treatments include more intensive, multi-agent approaches such as the combination of carboplatin/etoposide, cyclophosphamide/vincristine, and lomustine/procarbazine/vincristine or thioguanine, procarbazine, lomustine, and vincristine (TPCV) [54, 55]. Other agents investigated for the treatment of pediatric LGG include bevacizumab, temozolomide, irinotecan, and cisplatin. Clinical trials in recent years have utilized fewer agents than previous dose-intensive regimens [55–58]. Common side effects include nausea, vomiting, and myelosuppression. Most of these approaches have similar outcomes, with overall survival (OS) ranging from 80 to 100% (Table 21.1). More clinically relevant is the duration of tumor stabilization achieved which typically ranges between 30 and 50% at 3 years [53, 59, 60]. This can be a clinically meaningful outcome in a patient with progressive symptoms, for whom more aggressive therapy with radiation can be associated with high morbidity. For this reason, chemotherapy is often favored as a first-line treatment for symptomatic children at high risk of progressive symptoms. Because multiple chemotherapy regimens demonstrate similar progression-free and overall survival, treatment decisions should be made with consideration of patient factors such as anticipated toxicity, quality of life, and prior treatment.

The benefit of chemotherapy for pediatric HGGs remains unclear (Table 21.2). Although a large, multi-institutional phase III study of adjuvant chemotherapy for pediatric HGGs suggested a benefit with chemotherapy, follow-up studies have been less convincing. Postoperative chemotherapy (CCNU, vincristine, prednisone)

Table 21.1 Completed chemotherapy trials evaluating treatment of supratentorial low grade gliomas

Diagnosis	Chemotherapy	Number of eligible patients	Outcome	Authors
Newly diagnosed and recurrent LGG	CV	37 newly diagnosed 23 recurrent	52% with objective response in recurrent disease 62% with objective response in newly diagnosed disease	[51]
Newly diagnosed, progressive LGG	CV	78	56% objective response 2-year PFS, 75%; 3-year PFS, 68%	[61]
Progressive LGG	Monthly carboplatin	81	28% objective response 85% stable disease 3-year EFS, 64%; 3-year OS, 84%	[60]
Unresectable LGG ± previous treatment	Cisplatin/etopo	34	70% objective response 30% stable disease 3-year PFS, 78%; 3-year OS, 100%	[57]
Progressive LGG	Course 1/4: carboplatin/etopo Course 2/5: cyclophosphamide/vincristine Course 3/6: lomustine/procarbazine/vincristine	10	No patients with progressive disease 100% OS at study follow-up	[54]
Progressive LGG	Cisplatin/etopo (low dose)	37	65% objective response 3-year PFS, 65%; 3-year OS, 97%	[56]
Residual tumor >1.5 cm^2 after resection or progressive LGG	Weekly carbo/vinblastine or day 1 carbo/weekly vinblastine	26 (9 in weekly therapy; 17 in day 1 carbo)	1 PR, 6 MR, 11 SD, 3PD Weekly therapy deemed too toxic due to grade 4 neutropenia	[52]
Progressive/residual LGG in children <10 years	CV or TPCV	274	CV: 5-year EFS, 39%; 5-year OS, 86% TPCV: 5-year EFS, 52%; 5-year OS, 87%	[59]
Recurrent/refractory LGG	Weekly VBL	50	5-year PFS, 42%; 5-year OS, 93%	[53]
Multiply recurrent/progressive LGG (retrospective review)	Bevacizumab Irinotecan	14	86% objective response 100% PFS with active therapy	[58]
Progressive, untreated LGG	Weekly VBL	54	26% objective response 5-year PFS, 53%; 5-year OS, 94%	[62]

in addition to radiation resulted in improved survival in children (5-year OS, 46%) as compared to postoperative radiation alone (5-year OS, 18%) [63, 64]. And, Wolff et al. demonstrated preradiation chemotherapy (cisplatin, etoposide, ifosfamide) also improved survival time [65]. Using the same protocol, Lopez-Aguilar and colleagues found that both pre- and post-radiation chemotherapy improved median survival significantly [66, 67]. Nevertheless, other studies have not shown a survival advantage in using chemotherapy for HGGs [68–71]. In a phase II trial, treatment of patients with recurrent or progressive HGG with temozolomide resulted in minimal radiographic responses, although a small number of patients

Table 21.2 Completed chemotherapy trials evaluating treatment of newly diagnosed supratentorial high-grade gliomas

Diagnosis	Chemotherapy	Number of eligible patients	Outcome	Authors
Newly diagnosed HGG after surgical resection	RT ± CCNU, vincristine, prednisone	58	5-year EFS, 46% in radiation + chemotherapy 5-year EFS, 18% in radiation alone	[63]
Newly diagnosed HGG after surgical resection and radiation	CCNU, vincristine, prednisone (control) or 8-in-1	172 (85 in control; 87 in 8-in-1)	5-year EFS, 33% in control 5-year EFS, 36% in 8-in-1	[64]
Newly diagnosed HGG	Preradiation ifosfamide, carboplatin, etoposide	25	5-year EFS, 56% 5-year OS, 67%	[66]
Newly diagnosed HGG after surgical resection	Preirradiation BCNU, etoposide, cisplatin (number of cycles and order of radiation determined by degree of residual disease)	66	5-year EFS, 16% 5-year OS, 28% 10-year EFS, 13% 10-year OS, 21%	[74]
Newly diagnosed HGG after STR	Pre-RT procarbazine *or* topotecan, concurrent RT + vincristine, adjuvant CCNU + vincristine	40 (13 treated with procarbazine; 14 with topotecan; 13 with RT + adjuvant)	Procarbazine: 3-year EFS, 7.7%; 3-year OS, 7.7% Topotecan: 3-year EFS, 7%; 3-year OS, 14% Overall: 3-year EFS, 10%; 3-year OS, 15%	[75]
Newly diagnosed HGG (age <5 years) after surgical resection	Alternating cycles of carboplatin/procarbazine, cisplatin/etoposide, vincristine/cyclophosphamide	21	5-year EFS, 35% 5-year OS, 59%	[76]
Newly diagnosed HGG after surgical resection	RT + temozolomide, adjuvant temozolomide	90	3-year EFS, 11% 3-year OS, 22%	[77]
Newly diagnosed HGG after surgical resection	RT + temozolomide, adjuvant temozolomide, lomustine	108	1-year EFS, 49% 1-year OS, 72% 3-year EFS, 22%	[73]

RT radiation therapy, *CCNU* chloroethyl-cyclohexyl nitrosourea, *8-in-1* vincristine, carmustine, procarbazine, cytarabine, hydroxyurea, cisplatin, dacarbazine, methylprednisolone delivered in 1 day

did achieve transient disease stabilization with tolerable toxicity [72]. The Children's Oncology Group then followed with a phase II trial of temozolomide for newly diagnosed, nonmetastatic supratentorial HGG. Patients underwent maximal surgical resection followed by radiation with concomitant temozolomide before maintenance therapy with six cycles of lomustine and temozolomide. One-year event-free survival (EFS) was 49% and OS was 72%. This study identified survival benefit with the addition of lomustine as compared to monotherapy with adjuvant temozolomide alone, most pronounced in patients with subtotal resections and positive for MGMT overexpression [73].

21.5.3 Targeted Therapy

In the era of rapid genetic sequencing, the role of biologically targeted therapies has gained significant momentum, with the hope of decreasing side effects and individualizing therapy. The frequent activation of the *MAPK* pathway in LGG has led to considerable interest in utilizing therapies that inhibit activation of this pathway. Specific genetic targets in this pathway include *BRAF* and *MEK*. Sixty to 80% of pediatric LGG demonstrate constitutive activation of the pathway arising from molecular aberrations of *BRAF* or activating fusion proteins (i.e., *BRAF-KIAA1549*). Pathway activating *BRAF* V600E mutations are therapeutic targets that can be inhibited by the pharmacologic agents vemurafenib and dabrafenib. Vemurafenib is currently undergoing evaluation in a phase 0/pilot efficacy study in pediatric patients with *BRAF* V600E mutant gliomas, including LGG (NCT01748149). Tumor regression in *BRAF* V600E mutated pediatric LGG has been shown in response to dabrafenib treatment, with sustained tumor response in 38%. Dabrafenib is currently being evaluated in a phase 1 study (NCT01677741) [78, 79]. Clinical trials are also investigating *MAPK* pathway inhibition driven by *BRAF* fusion abnormalities as well as inhibition of downstream targets such as *MEK*. A phase 1 clinical trial completed by the Pediatric Brain Tumor Consortium evaluated the *MEK1/2* inhibitor, selumetinib, in 38 children with LGG. Eight patients in this cohort exhibited sustained responses [80, 81]. Selumetinib is now being investigated in a phase 2 trial (NCT01089101). Other *MEK1/2* inhibitors with promise in treating pediatric LGG include trametinib and cobimetinib. Cobimetinib is undergoing phase 1 investigation in pediatric patients with *MAPK*-activated CNS tumors (NCT02639546) [82]. Lastly, *mTOR* inhibition with everolimus is undergoing investigation for the treatment of recurrent/refractory pediatric LGG in a phase 2 clinical trial (NCT01734512).

For the treatment of HGG, an effort to inhibit *RAS/MAPK* signaling with the farnesyl transferase inhibitor, tipifarni, did not demonstrate activity as a single agent in pediatric HGG [83]. Erlotinib, an inhibitor of *EGFR* (a compelling biologic target in a wide range of human malignancies including HGG in adults), in combination with temozolomide is well tolerated, but its activity in HGG in children has not been established [84]. Single-agent *EGFR* inhibitor therapy with gefitinb in pediatric HGG has also not demonstrated significant effect promise [85]. Anti-angiogenic agents such as cilengitide have demonstrated activity based on a small population of responding patients in a phase I trial but require further investigation [86]. In the recurrent pediatric HGG setting, a monoclonal antibody directed at *EGFR*, nimotuzumab, has been evaluated and showed clinical promise, resulting in OS of 9 months [87]. However, this agent is not currently readily available in the United States.

21.5.3.1 Novel Investigational Therapy

In addition to new targeted therapies, novel approaches such as convection-enhanced delivery (CED) and immunotherapy are emerging as new treatment strategies for pediatric glioma. Most of these strategies are directed at pediatric HGG, given the continued poor outcomes in this patient population. As efficacy of therapeutic agents directed at the CNS may be affected by the blood-brain barrier, alternate modes of drug delivery are in ongoing clinical investigation including CED. CED is a new mode of drug delivery in which catheters are surgically placed directly into the tumor for infusion of drug. CED has been used to deliver a variety of agents for the treatment of recurrent HGG including TP-38 (a chimeric protein fusing TGF-alpha with pseudomonas exotoxin), cintredekin besudotox, IL-4 pseudomonas exotoxin, paclitaxel, AP 12009 (an antisense oligonucleotide binding TGF-ß2 mRNA), and cotara immunotoxin [87–92]. In children, there is an upcoming clinical trial investigating the use of oncolytic poliovirus given by CED to children with recurrent HGG (NCT03043391).

Immunotherapy agents such as peptide-based vaccines and immunostimulants are also being investigated for the treatment of pediatric HGG. There are currently four ongoing clinical trials looking at the use of peptide-based vaccines or dendritic cell vaccines for the treatment of pediatric HGG. These trials are intended to target proteins unique to the tumor, either intrinsically expressed such as H3.3 K27M mutant protein (NCT 02960230, NCT001130077) or peptides isolated directly from biopsied/resected tumor tissue (NCT02722512, NCT1808820). Immunotherapy via T-cell stimulation with PD-1 (programmed cell death inhibition) is also an ongoing area of research in the treatment of pediatric gliomas (NCT02359565). This approach seems to hold particular promise for patients with gliomas associated with mismatch repair defects [93, 94].

21.5.4 Radiation Therapy

Radiation therapy has demonstrated benefit in phase II prospective studies for pediatric LGG with high rates of long-term progression-free survival. It is important to recognize, however, that radiation therapy is also associated with substantial late complications in pediatric LGG patients, and, thus, its use is often reserved for patients with progressive, disabling symptoms. Similarly, the utility of radiation treatment in prolonging survival for patients with HGGs has been well established [48, 65, 95–99]. Standard radiation therapy consists of 54–60 Gy delivered by opposed external beams. Attempts to limit the damage to normal brain parenchyma have led to the adoption of conformal techniques in more recent years [95]. It should be noted that conformal radiation therapy still relies on a fractionated radiobiological effect. Stereotactic radiosurgery, conversely, utilizes a single treatment with doses in the range of 14–20 Gy. Radiosurgery can be delivered by multiple fixed cobalt sources (Gamma Knife, Elekta AB, Stockholm) or by a mobile linear accelerator (LINAC). In either case, the total dose delivered depends upon the treatment volume. Radiosurgery treatment minimizes the dose beyond the target volume and can be used to boost external beam therapy, usually in the setting of focal and limited recurrent disease [6, 98]. Close proximity to sensitive structures such as the optic nerves or brainstem can reduce the effectiveness of radiosurgery, and in the setting of widespread infiltrative disease or leptomeningeal dissemination, radiosurgery is typically not considered.

21.6 Prognosis and Outcome

Pediatric LGG carries overall good prognoses for long-term survival, particularly if the tumor is able to be completely resected. One comprehensive retrospective review revealed 30-year survival of 4040 children with LGG to be 75%, with only 347 patients dying of their tumor. Increased risk of death related to disease was associated with age <2 years at diagnosis, diagnosis between 1970 and 1989, histology other than pilocytic astrocytoma, tumor location outside the cerebellum, exposure to radiation, and WHO grade II tumor. There did not appear to be statistically significant difference in survival between patients with GTR versus STR [100]. For children unable to achieve complete resection and whom chemotherapy is pursued, LGG can become a chronic, lifelong condition requiring ongoing surveillance to monitor for disease progression. Survivors of LGG typically go on to have high qualities of life; however, those having undergone radiation appear to have the highest of negative quality of life impact [101]. Important questions remain for pediatric LGG patients, including improved understanding of the disease and identification of more effective and less toxic treatment modalities.

In contrast to pediatric LGG and despite therapeutic advances, the overall prognosis for pediatric HGG remains poor. Overall survival for supratentorial HGG is less than 20% at 5 years, with most patients dying within 2 years of diagnosis [102, 103]. Children with glioblastoma, the most aggressive HGG, have a 5-year survival rate of only 5–15% [48, 63, 104]. Anaplastic astrocytoma demonstrates only somewhat improved outcomes with 5-year survival between 20 and 40% [63, 104]. Leptomeningeal dissemination portends an even worse prognosis [105]. Factors predicting a worse prognosis for any HGG include lower performance score at diagnosis, bilateral disease, disease located in the parietal lobes, STR, and radiotherapy dose less than 50 Gy [106]. The importance of central review of pathology in clinical trials measuring survival of pediatric malignant glioma cannot be overemphasized, as significant discordance between institutional diagnosis and central review has been observed in prior trials and is integral to accurate outcome measurements [107]. Pediatric HGG remains a fatal disease, requiring intensive ongoing preclinical and clinical investigation to identify more effective treatments.

References

1. Ostrom QT et al (2014) CBTRUS statistical report: primary brain and central nervous system tumors diagnosed in the United States in 2007-2011. Neuro Oncol 16(Suppl 4):iv1–iv63
2. Ostrom QT et al (2015) CBTRUS statistical report: primary brain and central nervous system tumors diagnosed in the United States in 2008-2012. Neuro Oncol 17(Suppl 4):iv1–iv62
3. Pollack IF (1994) Brain tumors in children. N Engl J Med 331(22):1500–1507
4. Tamber MS, Rutka JT (2003) Pediatric supratentorial high-grade gliomas. Neurosurg Focus 14(2):e1
5. Wessels PH et al (2003) Supratentorial grade II astrocytoma: biological features and clinical course. Lancet Neurol 2(7):395–403
6. Baumann GS et al (1996) Gamma knife radiosurgery in children. Pediatr Neurosurg 24(4):193–201
7. Sievert AJ, Fisher MJ (2009) Pediatric low-grade gliomas. J Child Neurol 24(11):1397–1408
8. Wilne SH et al (2006) The presenting features of brain tumours: a review of 200 cases. Arch Dis Child 91(6):502–506
9. Kemerdere R et al (2014) Low-grade temporal gliomas: surgical strategy and long-term seizure outcome. Clin Neurol Neurosurg 126:196–200
10. Beppu T et al (2011) Prediction of malignancy grading using computed tomography perfusion imaging in nonenhancing supratentorial gliomas. J Neurooncol 103(3):619–627
11. Eastwood JD, Provenzale JM (2003) Cerebral blood flow, blood volume, and vascular permeability of cerebral glioma assessed with dynamic CT perfusion imaging. Neuroradiology 45(6):373–376
12. Zamora C, Huisman TA, Izbudak I (2017) Supratentorial tumors in pediatric patients. Neuroimaging Clin N Am 27(1):39–67
13. Ricci PE, Dungan DH (2001) Imaging of low- and intermediate-grade gliomas. Semin Radiat Oncol 11(2):103–112
14. Chang YW et al (2003) MR imaging of glioblastoma in children: usefulness of diffusion/perfusion-weighted MRI and MR spectroscopy. Pediatr Radiol 33(12):836–842
15. Chalil A, Ramaswamy V (2016) Low grade gliomas in children. J Child Neurol 31(4):517–522
16. Law M et al (2003) Glioma grading: sensitivity, specificity, and predictive values of perfusion MR imaging and proton MR spectroscopic imaging compared with conventional MR imaging. AJNR Am J Neuroradiol 24(10):1989–1998
17. Furtado AD et al (2017) Neuroimaging of peptide-based vaccine therapy in pediatric brain tumors: initial experience. Neuroimaging Clin N Am 27(1):155–166
18. Marner L et al (2017) Clinical PET/MRI in neurooncology: opportunities and challenges from a single-institution perspective. Clin Transl Imaging 5(2):135–149
19. Fernandez C et al (2003) Pilocytic astrocytomas in children: prognostic factors--a retrospective study of 80 cases. Neurosurgery 53(3):544–553; discussion 554–5
20. Ware ML, Berger MS, Binder DK (2003) Molecular biology of glioma tumorigenesis. Histol Histopathol 18(1):207–216
21. Rickert CH et al (2001) Pediatric high-grade astrocytomas show chromosomal imbalances distinct from adult cases. Am J Pathol 158(4):1525–1532
22. Paugh BS et al (2010) Integrated molecular genetic profiling of pediatric high-grade gliomas reveals key differences with the adult disease. J Clin Oncol 28(18):3061–3068
23. Nakamura M et al (2007) Molecular pathogenesis of pediatric astrocytic tumors. Neuro Oncol 9(2):113–123
24. Zhang J et al (2013) Whole-genome sequencing identifies genetic alterations in pediatric low-grade gliomas. Nat Genet 45(6):602–612
25. Johnson A et al (2017) Comprehensive genomic profiling of 282 pediatric low- and high-grade gliomas reveals genomic drivers, tumor mutational burden, and hypermutation signatures. Oncologist 22(12):1478–1490
26. Ryall S, Tabori U, Hawkins C (2017) A comprehensive review of paediatric low-grade diffuse glioma: pathology, molecular genetics and treatment. Brain Tumor Pathol 34(2):51–61
27. Grajkowska W et al (2014) Angiocentric glioma: a rare intractable epilepsy-related tumour in children. Folia Neuropathol 52(3):253–259
28. Bergthold G et al (2016) MYB-QKI rearrangements in angiocentric glioma drive tumorigenicity through a tripartite mechanism. Neuro Oncol 18:iii78
29. Chen YH, Gutmann DH (2014) The molecular and cell biology of pediatric low-grade gliomas. Oncogene 33(16):2019–2026
30. Jozwiak S, Mandera M, Mlynarski W (2015) Natural history and current treatment options for subependymal giant cell astrocytoma in tuberous sclerosis complex. Semin Pediatr Neurol 22(4):274–281
31. Krueger DA et al (2010) Everolimus for subependymal giant-cell astrocytomas in tuberous sclerosis. N Engl J Med 363(19):1801–1811
32. Mueller S et al (2012) PTEN promoter methylation and activation of the PI3K/Akt/mTOR pathway in pediatric gliomas and influence on clinical outcome. Neuro Oncol 14(9):1146–1152

33. Macy ME et al (2012) Clinical and molecular characteristics of congenital glioblastoma. Neuro Oncol 14(7):931–941

34. Sung T et al (2000) Preferential inactivation of the p53 tumor suppressor pathway and lack of EGFR amplification distinguish de novo high grade pediatric astrocytomas from de novo adult astrocytomas. Brain Pathol 10(2):249–259

35. Ferris SP et al (2016) IDH1 mutation can be present in diffuse astrocytomas and giant cell glioblastomas of young children under 10 years of age. Acta Neuropathol 132(1):153–155

36. Raffel C et al (1999) Analysis of oncogene and tumor suppressor gene alterations in pediatric malignant astrocytomas reveals reduced survival for patients with PTEN mutations. Clin Cancer Res 5(12):4085–4090

37. Pollack IF et al (2006) O6-methylguanine-DNA methyltransferase expression strongly correlates with outcome in childhood malignant gliomas: results from the CCG-945 Cohort. J Clin Oncol 24(21):3431–3437

38. Lewis PW et al (2013) Inhibition of PRC2 activity by a gain-of-function H3 mutation found in pediatric glioblastoma. Science 340(6134):857–861

39. Bender S et al (2013) Reduced H3K27me3 and DNA hypomethylation are major drivers of gene expression in K27M mutant pediatric high-grade gliomas. Cancer Cell 24(5):660–672

40. Wu G et al (2012) Somatic histone H3 alterations in pediatric diffuse intrinsic pontine gliomas and non-brainstem glioblastomas. Nat Genet 44(3):251–253

41. Wu G et al (2014) The genomic landscape of diffuse intrinsic pontine glioma and pediatric non-brainstem high-grade glioma. Nat Genet 46(5):444–450

42. Khuong-Quang DA et al (2012) K27M mutation in histone H3.3 defines clinically and biologically distinct subgroups of pediatric diffuse intrinsic pontine gliomas. Acta Neuropathol 124(3):439–447

43. Louis DN, et al (2016) World Health Organization histological classification of tumours of the central nervous system. International Agency for Research on Cancer, Lyon

44. Miele E et al (2014) High-throughput microRNA profiling of pediatric high-grade gliomas. Neuro Oncol 16(2):228–240

45. Sturm D, Pfister SM, Jones DTW (2017) Pediatric gliomas: current concepts on diagnosis, biology, and clinical management. J Clin Oncol 35(21):2370–2377

46. Dodgshun AJ et al (2016) Pediatric pleomorphic xanthoastrocytoma treated with surgical resection alone: clinicopathologic features. J Pediatr Hematol Oncol 38(7):e202–e206

47. Chamdine O et al (2016) Metastatic low-grade gliomas in children: 20 years' experience at St. Jude Children's Research Hospital. Pediatr Blood Cancer 63(1):62–70

48. Wisoff JH et al (1998) Current neurosurgical management and the impact of the extent of resection in the treatment of malignant gliomas of childhood: a report of the Children's Cancer Group trial no. CCG-945. J Neurosurg 89(1):52–59

49. Gupta N, Berger MS (2003) Brain mapping for hemispheric tumors in children. Pediatr Neurosurg 38(6):302–306

50. Shah AC et al (2016) Carboplatin rechallenge after hypersensitivity reactions in pediatric patients with low-grade glioma. Pediatr Blood Cancer 63(1):21–26

51. Packer RJ et al (1993) Carboplatin and vincristine for recurrent and newly diagnosed low-grade gliomas of childhood. J Clin Oncol 11(5):850–856

52. Jakacki RI et al (2011) A phase 1 study of vinblastine in combination with carboplatin for children with low-grade gliomas: a Children's Oncology Group phase 1 consortium study. Neuro Oncol 13(8):910–915

53. Bouffet E et al (2012) Phase II study of weekly vinblastine in recurrent or refractory pediatric low-grade glioma. J Clin Oncol 30(12):1358–1363

54. Bruggers CS, Greene D (2007) A phase 2 feasibility study of sequential, dose intensive chemotherapy to treat progressive low-grade gliomas in children. J Pediatr Hematol Oncol 29(9):602–607

55. Lancaster DL, Hoddes JA, Michalski A (2003) Tolerance of nitrosurea-based multiagent chemotherapy regime for low-grade pediatric gliomas. J Neurooncol 63(3):289–294

56. Massimino M et al (2010) A lower-dose, lower-toxicity cisplatin-etoposide regimen for childhood progressive low-grade glioma. J Neurooncol 100(1):65–71

57. Massimino M et al (2002) High response rate to cisplatin/etoposide regimen in childhood low-grade glioma. J Clin Oncol 20(20):4209–4216

58. Hwang EI et al (2013) Long-term efficacy and toxicity of bevacizumab-based therapy in children with recurrent low-grade gliomas. Pediatr Blood Cancer 60(5):776–782

59. Ater JL et al (2012) Randomized study of two chemotherapy regimens for treatment of low-grade glioma in young children: a report from the Children's Oncology Group. J Clin Oncol 30(21):2641–2647

60. Gururangan S et al (2002) Phase II study of carboplatin in children with progressive low-grade gliomas. J Clin Oncol 20(13):2951–2958

61. Packer RJ et al (1997) Carboplatin and vincristine chemotherapy for children with newly diagnosed progressive low-grade gliomas. J Neurosurg 86(5):747–754

62. Lassaletta A et al (2016) Phase II weekly vinblastine for chemotherapy-naive children with progressive low-grade glioma: a Canadian Pediatric Brain Tumor Consortium Study. J Clin Oncol 34(29):3537–3543

63. Sposto R et al (1989) The effectiveness of chemotherapy for treatment of high grade astrocytoma in children: results of a randomized trial. A report from the Childrens Cancer Study Group. J Neurooncol 7(2):165–177

64. Finlay JL et al (1995) Randomized phase III trial in childhood high-grade astrocytoma comparing vincristine, lomustine, and prednisone with the eight-drugs-in-1-day regimen. Childrens Cancer Group J Clin Oncol 13(1):112–123

65. Wolff JE et al (2002) Preradiation chemotherapy for pediatric patients with high-grade glioma. Cancer 94(1):264–271

66. Lopez-Aguilar E et al (2003) Preirradiation ifosfamide, carboplatin and etoposide (ICE) for the treatment of high-grade astrocytomas in children. Childs Nerv Syst 19(12):818–823

67. Lopez-Aguilar E et al (2000) Preirradiation ifosfamide, carboplatin, and etoposide for the treatment of anaplastic astrocytomas and glioblastoma multiforme: a phase II study. Arch Med Res 31(2):186–190

68. Wolff JE et al (2006) Maintenance treatment with interferon-gamma and low-dose cyclophosphamide for pediatric high-grade glioma. J Neurooncol 79(3):315–321

69. Puchner MJ et al (2000) Surgery, tamoxifen, carboplatin, and radiotherapy in the treatment of newly diagnosed glioblastoma patients. J Neurooncol 49(2):147–155

70. Levin VA et al (2003) Phase III randomized study of postradiotherapy chemotherapy with combination alpha-difluoromethylornithine-PCV versus PCV for anaplastic gliomas. Clin Cancer Res 9(3):981–990

71. Heideman RL et al (1995) Preirradiation chemotherapy with carboplatin and etoposide in newly diagnosed embryonal pediatric CNS tumors. J Clin Oncol 13(9):2247–2254

72. Lashford LS et al (2002) Temozolomide in malignant gliomas of childhood: a United Kingdom Children's Cancer Study Group and French Society for Pediatric Oncology Intergroup Study. J Clin Oncol 20(24):4684–4691

73. Jakacki RI et al (2016) Phase 2 study of concurrent radiotherapy and temozolomide followed by temozolomide and lomustine in the treatment of children with high-grade glioma: a report of the Children's Oncology Group ACNS0423 study. Neuro Oncol 18(10):1442–1450

74. Chastagner P et al (2007) Outcome of children treated with preradiation chemotherapy for a high-grade glioma: results of a French Society of Pediatric Oncology (SFOP) Pilot Study. Pediatr Blood Cancer 49(6):803–807

75. Chintagumpala MM et al (2006) A phase II window trial of procarbazine and topotecan in children with high-grade glioma: a report from the children's oncology group. J Neurooncol 77(2):193–198

76. Dufour C et al (2006) High-grade glioma in children under 5 years of age: a chemotherapy only approach with the BBSFOP protocol. Eur J Cancer 42(17):2939–2945

77. Cohen KJ et al (2011) Temozolomide in the treatment of high-grade gliomas in children: a report from the Children's Oncology Group. Neuro Oncol 13(3):317–323

78. Lassaletta A et al (2016) Profound clinical and radiological response to BRAF inhibition in a 2-month-old diencephalic child with hypothalamic/chiasmatic glioma. Pediatr Blood Cancer 63(11):2038–2041

79. (2017) Dabrafenib effective in pediatric glioma. Cancer Discov 7(1):OF5

80. Banerjee A et al (2014) A phase I study of AZD6244 in children with recurrent or refractory low-grade gliomas: a Pediatric Brain Tumor Consortium report. J Clin Oncol 32(15)

81. Banerjee A et al (2017) A phase I trial of the MEK inhibitor selumetinib (AZD6244) in pediatric patients with recurrent or refractory low-grade glioma: a Pediatric Brain Tumor Consortium (PBTC) study. Neuro Oncol 19(8):1135–1144

82. Grossauer S et al (2016) Concurrent MEK targeted therapy prevents MAPK pathway reactivation during BRAFV600E targeted inhibition in a novel syngeneic murine glioma model. Oncotarget 7(46):75839–75853

83. Fouladi M et al (2007) A phase II study of the farnesyl transferase inhibitor, tipifarnib, in children with recurrent or progressive high-grade glioma, medulloblastoma/primitive neuroectodermal tumor, or brainstem glioma: a Children's Oncology Group study. Cancer 110(11):2535–2541

84. Jakacki RI et al (2008) Pediatric phase I and pharmacokinetic study of erlotinib followed by the combination of erlotinib and temozolomide: a Children's Oncology Group Phase I Consortium Study. J Clin Oncol 26(30):4921–4927

85. Geyer JR et al (2010) A phase I and biology study of gefitinib and radiation in children with newly diagnosed brain stem gliomas or supratentorial malignant gliomas. Eur J Cancer 46(18):3287–3293

86. MacDonald TJ et al (2008) Phase I clinical trial of cilengitide in children with refractory brain tumors: Pediatric Brain Tumor Consortium Study PBTC-012. J Clin Oncol 26(6):919–924

87. Saurez G et al (2009) Clinical experience with nimotuzumab in cuban pediatric patients with brain tumors, 2005 to 2007. MEDICC Rev 11(3):27–33

88. Sampson JH et al (2008) Intracerebral infusion of an EGFR-targeted toxin in recurrent malignant brain tumors. Neuro Oncol 10(3):320–329

89. Vogelbaum MA et al (2007) Convection-enhanced delivery of cintredekin besudotox (interleukin-13-PE38QQR) followed by radiation therapy with and without temozolomide in newly diagnosed malignant gliomas: phase 1 study of final safety results. Neurosurgery 61(5):1031–1037; discussion 1037–8

90. Rand RW et al (2000) Intratumoral administration of recombinant circularly permuted interleukin-4-Pseudomonas exotoxin in patients with high-grade glioma. Clin Cancer Res 6(6):2157–2165

91. Lidar Z et al (2004) Convection-enhanced delivery of paclitaxel for the treatment of recurrent malig-

nant glioma: a phase I/II clinical study. J Neurosurg 100(3):472–479

92. Morrison PF et al (1994) High-flow microinfusion: tissue penetration and pharmacodynamics. Am J Physiol 266(1 Pt 2):R292–R305

93. Bouffet E et al (2016) Immune checkpoint inhibition for hypermutant glioblastoma multiforme resulting from germline biallelic mismatch repair deficiency. J Clin Oncol 34(19):2206–2211

94. Campbell B et al (2016) Hypermutation and neo-antigen formation predict response to immune checkpoint inhibition in childhood biallelic mismatch repair deficient glioblastoma. Neuro Oncol 18:iii59–iii60

95. Merchant TE et al (2002) Preliminary results from a Phase II trail of conformal radiation therapy for pediatric patients with localised low-grade astrocytoma and ependymoma. Int J Radiat Oncol Biol Phys 52(2):325–332

96. Burton EC, Prados MD (2000) Malignant gliomas. Curr Treat Options Oncol 1(5):459–468

97. Gilbert MR et al (2002) A phase II study of temozolomide in patients with newly diagnosed supratentorial malignant glioma before radiation therapy. Neuro Oncol 4(4):261–267

98. Hodgson DC et al (2001) Radiosurgery in the management of pediatric brain tumors. Int J Radiat Oncol Biol Phys 50(4):929–935

99. Wara WM et al (1986) Retreatment of pediatric brain tumors with radiation and misonidazole. Results of a CCSG/RTOG phase I/II study. Cancer 58(8):1636–1640

100. Bandopadhayay P et al (2014) Long-term outcome of 4,040 children diagnosed with pediatric low-grade gliomas: an analysis of the Surveillance Epidemiology and End Results (SEER) database. Pediatr Blood Cancer 61(7):1173–1179

101. Nwachukwu CR et al (2015) Health related quality of life (HRQOL) in long-term survivors of pediatric low grade gliomas (LGGs). J Neurooncol 121(3):599–607

102. Broniscer A, Gajjar A (2004) Supratentorial high-grade astrocytoma and diffuse brainstem glioma: two challenges for the pediatric oncologist. Oncologist 9(2):197–206

103. Gottardo NG, Gajjar A (2008) Chemotherapy for malignant brain tumors of childhood. J Child Neurol 23(10):1149–1159

104. Phuphanich S et al (1984) Supratentorial malignant gliomas of childhood. Results of treatment with radiation therapy and chemotherapy. J Neurosurg 60(3):495–499

105. Vertosick FT Jr, Selker RG (1990) Brain stem and spinal metastases of supratentorial glioblastoma multiforme: a clinical series. Neurosurgery 27(4):516–521; discussion 521–2

106. Hales R et al (2006) Prognostic factors in pediatric high-grade glioma and the importance of accurate pathologic diagnosis. Int J Radiat Oncol Biol Phys 66(3 Suppl 1):S527

107. Pollack IF et al (2003) The influence of central review on outcome associations in childhood malignant gliomas: results from the CCG-945 experience. Neuro Oncol 5(3):197–207

Thalamic Gliomas

22

William B. Lo and James T. Rutka

22.1 Introduction

Pediatric thalamic gliomas present specific challenges in surgical and oncological management. Although the tumor histopathologies are similar to their supratentorial counterparts and are often benign, they are considered as a distinct entity because of its deep-seated anatomical location and therefore relative surgical inaccessibility. Non-glial tumors, though less common, also occur in the thalamic region. Lesions involving the thalamus may arise from the surrounding structures, e.g., the basal ganglia. Thalamic tumors also occur over a wide age spectrum. Non-glial lesions, lesions from surrounding structures and the adult population, are out of the scope of this chapter and will not be discussed.

Historically, thalamic gliomas have been treated somewhat conservatively. In the past few decades, advances in neuroimaging, neuroanesthetics, microsurgical techniques, intraoperative neuronavigation, and neurophysiologic monitoring have enabled the safe surgical resection of some of these lesions, especially the low-grade ones with discrete margins. The multidisciplinary management also includes radiation therapy and chemotherapy, but the standard of care is not well-defined. Treatment should be individualized to patients according to their age, clinical status, and tumor type. Overall, children with thalamic gliomas have good outcome. Recently, further understanding of pediatric low-grade glioma molecular biology has led to the trial of new target therapies such as BRAF and MEK inhibitors. Laser interstitial thermal therapy offers minimally invasive cytoreduction in selected patients.

22.2 Surgical Anatomy of the Thalamus

The thalamus is a nuclear complex that makes up the majority of the diencephalon, which also consists of the hypothalamus, epithalamus, and subthalamus [1]. The thalamus is an important relay center in subserving both the sensory and motor mechanisms. It is also involved in awareness, attention, and other neurocognitive processes such as memory and language. The neural circuitry and the anatomical details are beyond the scope of this chapter. We provide a brief description relevant to the clinicopathologic correlations and surgical approaches to lesions in this area.

W. B. Lo
Division of Neurosurgery, The Hospital for Sick Children, Toronto, ON, Canada

Department of Neurosurgery, Birmingham Children's Hospital, Birmingham, United Kingdom

J. T. Rutka (✉)
Division of Neurosurgery, The Arthur and Sonia Labatt Brain Tumour Research Centre, The Hospital for Sick Children, Toronto, ON, Canada

Department of Surgery, University of Toronto, Toronto, ON, Canada
e-mail: james.rutka@sickkids.ca

© Springer Nature Switzerland AG 2019
J.-C. Tonn et al. (eds.), *Oncology of CNS Tumors*, https://doi.org/10.1007/978-3-030-04152-6_22

The thalamus is divided into symmetrical halves, connected by the mass intermedia. Each half is oval-shaped, measuring $30 \times 20 \times 20$ mm in rostrocaudal, superior-inferior, and lateral dimensions (Fig. 22.1). It is located in the center of the C-shaped lateral ventricle, superior to the brainstem. It is deep to the posterior half of the insula, the inferior part of the pre- and postcentral gyri, and the adjacent part of the superior temporal gyrus [2]. Laterally, the external medullary lamina, a sheet of white matter,

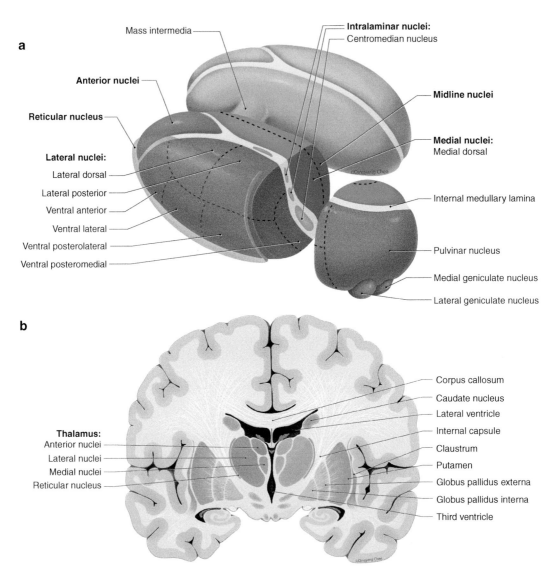

Fig. 22.1 (**a**) Bilateral thalami as seen from the left superoposteriorly. Anatomically, the thalamus is divided by a Y-shaped internal medullary lamina (a white matter band) into three large cell groups: anterior, medial, and lateral. The intralaminar nuclei are found within the lamina, and the reticular nucleus surrounds the thalamus on the dorsolateral side. (**b**) Coronal cross section of the thalamus and the surrounding structures at the level of foramen of Monro. The thalamus is closely related to the internal capsule, the basal ganglia, and the midbrain. In relation to the cerebrospinal fluid (CSF) space, the lateral ventricle wraps around the superior, posterior, and inferior surfaces of the thalamus. The third ventricle is situated between the two halves of the thalamus. The anterior thalamic tubercle forms the posterior edge of the foramen of Monro. The posterolateral part of the pulvinar forms the lateral half of the anterior wall of the atrium, the posteromedial part is in contact with the quadrigeminal cistern, and the inferolateral part forms part of the roof of the ambient cistern

separates the main body of thalamus from the reticular nucleus. Further laterally, the posterior limb of the internal capsule lies between the thalamus and the lentiform complex. The main nuclei, their cortical connection, function, and clinical feature if involved are summarized in Table 22.1.

22.3 Epidemiology

Thalamic tumors constitute approximately 2–5% of all pediatric intracranial tumors, compared with 1% for all ages [3–9]. Glioma is the most common pediatric intracranial tumor [10]. However, the true incidence of pediatric thalamic glioma is unknown, partly due to its relatively uncommon occurrence. Some series included tumors arising from the surrounding structures as well as the thalamus, such as the basal ganglia and other diencephalic structures. This was because of difficulty in distinguishing the two, especially in the pre-MRI era [3, 11–16]. Also, many clinical series include both pediatric and adult populations, which have different tumor biology [3–5, 13, 14, 16–26].

Thalamic tumors have a bimodal age distribution. The first peak is the first and second decades, accounting for >40% of all patients [3, 4, 18, 21]. The second smaller peak is over 40 years [5, 18]. The average age at diagnosis is 8 years [6–8, 11, 12, 15, 19, 27–34]. There does not appear to be a gender predilection [7, 8, 29, 33, 35, 36]. In a 10-year review of the St. Jude experience, 12% of all low-grade gliomas were found in the thalamus, compared with 20% for cerebral hemispheres and 35% for the cerebellum [34]. There is no lateralization bias. The HIT-LGG 1996 study showed that 10% of children with low-grade glioma has a neurofibromatosis type 1 trait and approximately 15% of NF1 patients develop low-grade glioma [37–39].

22.4 Symptoms and Clinical Signs

The average age at presentation for thalamic tumors is 8 years although they can affect children of any age. Over 70% of the patients have a duration of symptoms of <6 months, of which half have a duration of <1 month [7, 11, 28, 29,

31, 33, 35]. The duration of symptoms is shorter in children than adults and in high-grade tumors [3, 4, 36, 40].

The clinical features of thalamic tumors are varied. Common symptoms and signs are raised intracranial pressure (ICP)-related, motor deficits, sensory syndrome, involuntary movements, visual disturbances, and seizures. The pattern is influenced by the exact anatomical location, size, and growth rate of the tumors. The symptoms can be caused by:

1. Raised ICP from tumor mass effect or obstruction of cerebrospinal fluid (CSF) pathway, i.e., hydrocephalus, typically at the posterior third ventricle
2. Focal involvement and dysfunction of thalamic nuclei, mainly the dorsomedial and ventrolateral groups which are separated by the internal medullary lamina
3. Mass effect or infiltration of surrounding structures

22.4.1 Raised Intracranial Pressure

The most common symptoms are caused by raised ICP. Fifty to seventy-five percent of patients present with headache, nausea and vomiting, papilledema, drowsiness, and, in more severe cases, coma [6, 7, 28, 29, 31–33, 35, 41]. In infants, raised ICP can be manifested as macrocephaly, bulging fontanel, and splayed sutures [42]. Hydrocephalus is present in two-thirds of the patients, and 60–75% of patients required CSF diversion surgeries at presentation or soon after initial treatment [6–8, 15, 28, 29, 32, 33, 35, 41]. Tumors arising from the midline structures, i.e., the dorsomedial thalamus, are more likely to cause early CSF pathway obstruction [35, 42]. Raised ICP symptoms from bithalamic tumors are more often caused by tumor volume than hydrocephalus [43].

22.4.2 Motor and Sensory Disturbances

Children typically present with motor and sensory disturbances when the ventrolateral nuclei

Table 22.1 Summary of the thalamic nuclei, their afferent and efferent projections, and their functions and clinical features if they are involved

Anatomical groups	Nuclei	Afferents	Efferents	Functions	Impairment
Anterior	Anterior group of nuclei: Anteroventral (AV) Anteromedial (AM) Anterodorsal (AD)	Mammillothalamic tract, hippocampus, basal forebrain, and brainstem	Cingulate gyrus, also anterior limbic area, parahippocampal gyrus	Learning, acquisition of memory, regulation of alertness, attention	Psychological dysfunction, including aphasia, memory impairment, anomia
Medial	Mediodorsal (MD) [or dorsomedial (DM)]	Prefrontal cortex, olfactory, limbic system, piriform and adjacent cortex, ventral pallidum, amygdala	Prefrontal cortex, also olfactory areas on the orbital surface of the frontal lobe	Executive function, memory, social cognition, emotion	Impaired cognition, memory, recognition, olfaction, wake-sleep cycle, respiratory, vegetative and endocrine circadian activities, decrease in anxiety, tension, aggression, obsessive thinking
Lateral	Ventral anterior (VA)	Ipsilateral globus pallidus, also substantia nigra premotor cortex (area 6) and frontal eye field (area 8)	Prefrontal cortex, also intralaminar thalamic nuclei, frontal lobe, anterior parietal cortex	Modulation of motor function	Hemiparesis
	Ventral lateral (VL)				
	VLo—anterior part (pars oralis) VLc—posterior part (pars caudalis)	Ipsilateral globus pallidus Contralateral deep cerebellar nuclei	Supplementary motor area, also lateral premotor cortex Motor cortex	Modulation, coordination, and learning of movements	Ataxia
	Ventral posterior (VP)				
	Ventral posterolateral (VPl) Ventral posteromedial (VPm) Posterior part of ventral medial nucleus (VMpo)	Medial (sensory) lemniscal and spinothalamic pathways Somatic afferents from the head region, trigeminothalamic pathway, solitary tract	Primary somatic sensory cortex (SI), also second somatic sensory area (SII) Primary somatic sensory cortex, also premotor cortex, frontal eye field, cortical gustatory area, anterior insula	Somatosensation of the body Somatosensation of the head, gustatory sensation	Chronic pain, dystonia

(continued)

Table 22.1 (continued)

Anatomical groups	Nuclei	Afferents	Efferents	Functions	Impairment
	Medial geniculate nucleus (MGN)	Brachium of the inferior colliculi	Primary auditory cortex, also auditory areas of the cortex, adjacent insular and opercular fields	Hearing	Auditory illusion/agnosia
	Lateral geniculate nucleus (LGN)	Optic tract, superior colliculi, also primary visual cortex	Primary visual cortex (area 17)	Vision	Quadranopia, hemianopia
	Lateral dorsal (LD)	Hippocampus	Cingulate cortex	Learning, memory	Impaired learning
	Lateral posterior (LP)	Superior colliculus, primary visual, auditory and somatosensory cortex	Parietal association cortex	Similar to pulvinar	Similar to pulvinar
	Pulvinar	Superior colliculus, subcortical afferents are uncertain	Association areas of parietotemporal cortex, also the prefrontal and orbital frontal cortices and visual association cortex of occipital lobe areas	Coordination of intra- and cross-modal cortical information processing, language	Neglect syndrome
	Intralaminar Anterior (rostral): Central medial Paracentral Central lateral Posterior (caudal): Centromedian Parafasciular	Reticular formation, basal ganglia, also limbic system substantia nigra, spinothalamic tract, superior colliculus	Cerebral cortex, corpus striatum	Mediates cortical activation from the brainstem reticular formation, sensorimotor integration	Thalamic (motor) neglect, bilateral injury to posterior intralaminar nuclei leads to kinetic mutism, apathy and loss of motivation
	Midline nuclei	Hypothalamus, periaqueductal gray matter, spinothalamic tract, reticular formation	Hippocampal formation, amygdala, nucleus accumbens, cingulate, possibly orbitofrontal cortex	Memory, arousal	Regulation of seizure activity
	Reticular	Thalamus, cortex	Thalamus	Attention, samples and gates the information through the thalamus and focuses thalamocortical outputs	

The list is organized according to anatomical location and not by function. There are a total of 50–60 nuclei. Only the main nuclei are listed. The thalamocortical interconnections, corticothalmocortical loops, and intrathalamic networks are complex. Relationships between single thalamic nuclei and single cortical areas are not simple one to one. Single thalamic nuclei can send afferents to multiple cortical areas and vice versa (see Fig. 22.1).

are involved. Motor deficits, usually in the form of hemiparesis, are present in 30–60% of patients. This is usually caused by a tumor from the ventrolateral nuclei that compresses or infiltrates the internal capsule laterally. Interestingly, only 5–25% of patients present with sensory symptoms, although the ventrolateral thalamus contains the major sensory relay nuclei. This can be because young children cannot verbalize these symptoms. A significant proportion of patients, 18–55%, present with mental changes and/or psychological symptoms. These include changes in mood, personality, cognition and behavior, memory impairment, and inattention. The anterior, mediodorsal, intralaminar nuclei, mammillothalamic tract, and fornices are likely to be responsible for these symptoms due to their connections with the frontal cortex and the limbic areas. Bithalamic tumors sometimes present with a more profound clinical constellation of personality changes and/or mental deterioration, although this is less common in children [43, 44]. Only 6–36% of the children present with movement disorder. The most common involuntary movements are tremor, followed by dystonia, chorea, rarely ballismus, and athetoid movements [45]. Considering the proximity to the basal ganglia and the subthalamus, the frequency of extrapyramidal symptoms is low. However, this could be masked by the concurrent hemiparesis. Surprisingly, the classic thalamic syndrome of Dejerine-Roussy, characterized by contralateral hemianesthesia (or hyperesthesia), hemiparesis, hemiataxia, and severe, persistent, paroxysmal, and often intolerable pain, is rare [18, 46].

22.4.3 Visual, Seizure, Endocrine, and Speech Disturbances

Up to half of the children present with visual disturbances. The common ocular findings are ipsilateral poorly reactive miotic pupil, oculomotor nerve palsy, and exotropia, caused by tumor infiltration or compression on the rostral mesencephalic tegmentum [42]. Hemianopsia is the most common visual field defect, caused by the tumor effect on the retrolenticular segment of the internal capsule or the optic radiation. Seizure is a presenting feature in 1–35%. Uncommonly, patients have endocrinopathies due to hypothalamic involvement. The dominant thalamus is shown to be involved in speech generation; thus, patients can present with speech disturbance [47–49].

22.5 Diagnosis

Magnetic resonance imaging is the modality of choice for excluding nonneoplastic lesion and elucidating the exact location and extent of the tumor, its discreteness or infiltrative nature, mass effect on surrounding structures, and presence of hydrocephalus [50]. Nonneoplastic lesions include vascular diseases, infectious/inflammatory diseases, metabolic processes, and other malformations [51, 52]. Advanced imaging modalities, such as MR spectroscopy, positron-emission tomography (PET), and perfusion-weighted imaging (PWI), allow noninvasive evaluation of the malignancy of thalamic gliomas [51, 53, 54]. Imaging is also essential for planning stereotactic biopsy to increase the yield and safe open resection [55].

Thalamic gliomas can be classified as focal, diffuse, or bithalamic [50]. Focal lesions, often pilocytic astrocytomas, are well-circumscribed, tend to expand rather than infiltrate into surrounding white matter, and respect the ependymal surface. Diffuse lesions, often the fibrillary astrocytic type, are less well-demarcated and often infiltrate beyond the thalamus. Bilateral tumors usually are symmetrical, suggestive of de novo bilateral origin, although a unilateral onset with migration across interthalamic commissures is possible. Puget et al. classified thalamic gliomas into three growth patterns, which have different natural histories and specific surgical strategies (Fig. 22.2) [7, 8]:

1. Unilateral thalamic tumors (82%): originating from one thalamus with possible extension to adjacent structures including the brainstem inferiorly (32%) and the contralateral thalamus (4%); it can also be diffuse (28%) [7, 9, 33]

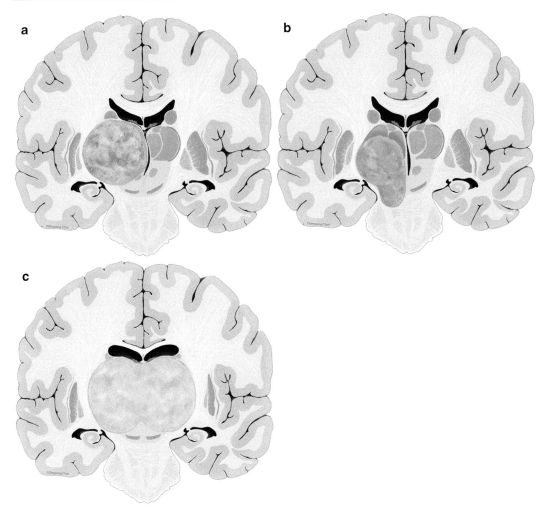

Fig. 22.2 Classification of growth patterns of thalamic glioma. (**a**) Unilateral. This is the commonest growth pattern (80%) and includes both high- and low-grade glioma. It often causes obstruction to the posterior third ventricle causing hydrocephalus. (**b**) Thalamopeduncular. This growth pattern accounts for 10% of thalamic gliomas. (**c**) Bithalamic. This growth pattern accounts for 10% of thalamic gliomas. They are often symmetrical. The growth is typically expansile rather than infiltrative, as shown by the intact internal capsule

2. Thalamopeduncular tumors (9%): arising at the junction of the thalamus and cerebral peduncle, with symmetrical supra- and infratentorial extensions
3. Bilateral thalamic tumors (9%): originating from both thalamus (as opposed to tumors with contralateral extension)

In general, T2-weighted images (T2-WI) have the highest sensitivity for detecting thalamic glioma. T2-WI high intensity indicates microcystic constitution and/or low cellularity, usually found in low-grade astrocytomas [56]. In contrast, T2-WI low intensity indicates high cellularity or hemosiderin deposit, usually seen in highly proliferating areas in high-grade astrocytic and embryonal tumors and germ cell tumors and lymphomas. Heterogeneity suggests possible anaplasia. Pilocytic astrocytomas tend to have discrete margins, while diffuse fibrillary astrocytomas and high-grade tumors (WHO grades II–IV) tend to infiltrate adjacent tissues. Pilocytic astrocytomas typically enhance homogeneously, compared to

anaplastic astrocytomas and glioblastoma mul-
tiformes which enhance heterogeneously.
Tumor cysts are a characteristic feature of pilocytic astrocytoma. On the other hand, perilesional edema is usually seen in high-grade
gliomas, and necrosis is specific of glioblastoma. Colosimo et al. proposed a classification
based on four different CT and MRI patterns
(Table 22.2).

Bithalamic gliomas typically are hyperintense on T2-WI and isointense on T1-WI, possess compact epicenters, and do not enhance
with contrast [33, 43, 52]. They can be homogeneous or heterogeneous. On magnetic resonance
spectroscopy, the increased creatine-phospho-
creatine peak distinguishes bilateral from unilateral tumors and suggests different biology
[53].

Currently, none of the imaging modalities and
tumor radiologic appearances accurately predict
the histology [29]. Furthermore, many tumors do
not have the "typical" appearance, e.g., only
three-quarters of pilocytic astrocytomas contrast
enhanced and two-thirds cystic [7, 33]. Therefore,
a biopsy is required to confirm the diagnosis.

22.6 Histopathology

Glial tumors account for the majority of pediatric
thalamic lesions. On analyzing 486 cases of 14
clinical series, 70% are glial tumors (Table 22.3)
[6–9, 11, 22, 27, 29, 32, 33, 35, 41, 57, 58]. Of
these, 55% are low-grade. The World Health
Organization (WHO) grade I pilocytic astrocytomas account for a quarter of all thalamic gliomas
[7–9, 22, 27, 32, 33, 35, 57]. The remainders are
mainly diffuse (WHO grade II) and rarely pilomyxoid astrocytoma (grade I) and glial-neuronal.
For high-grade glioma, anaplastic astrocytoma
(grade III) is slightly commoner than glioblastoma multiforme (grade IV). The high proportion
of low-grade and pilocytic astrocytoma is consistent with the pattern observed in other anatomical
sites in children [59].

Bilateral thalamic glioma represents a specific
subset where low-grade tumors predominate and
diffuse astrocytoma is more common than pilocytic. In their series of 69 patients at the Hospital
Necker-Enfants Malades in Paris, Puget et al.
reported five of the nine bilateral thalamic gliomas were diffuse astrocytoma and only one was

Table 22.2 Basic neuroimaging patterns of thalamic tumors [27]

Pattern	CT	MRI	Likely diagnosis
1	Hypodense	T1: hypo- to isointense T2: hyperintense Moderate or absent edema, no contrast enhancement	Diffuse fibrillary astrocytoma Infiltration of adjacent structures, despite lack of contrast enhancement suggests anaplastic astrocytoma
2	Solid tumor with or without cystic components, hypodense	T1: hypointense T2: hyperintense Contrast enhancement	Well-defined margin, homogeneous enhancement: pilocytic astrocytoma (or more rarely ganglioglioma) Ill-defined margins, infiltrative, heterogeneous enhancement: anaplastic astrocytoma Above features + extensive edema, necrosis, hemorrhage: glioblastoma, (atypical teratoid rhabdoid tumors in infants)
3	Solid tumor with or without cystic components, calcification	T1: heterogeneous hypointensity T2: hyperintensity Contrast enhancement	Oligodendrogliomas or mixed oligoastrocytoma, but astrocytoma or anaplastic astrocytoma cannot be excluded
4	Solid or predominantly solid, hyperdense	T1: hypo- or isointense T2: hypointense Contrast enhancement Infiltrating the walls of the posterior portion of the third ventricle	Suggestive of germ cell tumor, even if the pineal gland is not involved Lymphoma

Table 22.3 Summary of the histologic types of thalamic tumors

Histologic subtype		Wong et al. [122]	Steinbok et al. [114]	Bilginer et al. [16]	Puget et al. [100]	Reardon et al. [101]	Bernstein et al. [15]
Low-grade		27	29	20	35	23	21
High-grade		34	22	17	25	12	20
Astrocytoma							
	Low-grade						
	Pilocytic	11	13	17	14	9	
	Diffuse	14	7			6	
	Others		2			6	
	High-grade						
	Anaplastic	17	6	2		4	
	Glioblastoma	8	11	11		7	
Oligodendroglioma							
	Low-grade				2		
	High-grade		1	1	4		
Oligoastrocytoma							
	Low-grade				5		
	High-grade						
Xanthoastrocytoma							
DNET		1					
Ganglioglioma			2	1	1	2	
Neurocytoma		1	2		1		
PNET		6		1	2		
Ependymoma							
	Ependymoma		2	2			
	Anaplastic	1	4	1			
Atypical teratoid/rhabdoid tumor		2		1			
Low-grade, increased cellularity (nonspecific)			1				
High-grade, unspecified						1	
No histology		8	21	8	9		19
Total		69	72	45	69	36	60

Pediatric series of more than 30 patients are included.
DNET dysembryoplastic neuroepithelial tumor, *PNET* primitive neuroepithelial tumor

pilocytic [7]. In Wong et al.'s series of 69 children, 4 had bilateral disease, of which 2 were anaplastic and 1 was diffuse astrocytoma [8]. Steinbok reported three bithalamic diffuse astrocytoma and two glioblastoma [33]. Bilginer et al. reported three cases of pilocytic astrocytoma out of the four cases of bithalamic tumor where definitive histology was available [35].

Less commonly, oligodendroglioma and ependymoma account for 4% of all thalamic lesions, respectively. Other rarer tumors include subependymal giant cell astrocytomas, mixed gliomas, dysembryoplastic neuroepithelial tumors, gangliogliomas, neurocytomas, primitive neuroectodermal tumors, atypical teratoid/rhabdoid tumors, germinomas, and lymphomas [51, 60]. Approximately 20% of thalamic tumors do not have a histological diagnosis, because biopsies were inconclusive or not taken. Significant interobserver variability exists [61, 62]. In their Canadian multicenter study, Steinbok et al. reported discrepancies between central and local diagnoses in one-third of the cases [33].

22.7 Genetic Features

Neurofibromatosis type 1 is an autosomal dominant disorder. The NF1 gene, mapped to chromosome 17q11, encodes neurofibromin, a tumor suppressor gene that regulates the RAS signaling pathway. Ten percent of pediatric low-grade glioma is associated with NF1, and 15% of NF1 patients develop low-grade gliomas [37–39].

Within the last decade, advanced molecular techniques have revolutionized our understanding of the tumorigenesis of pediatric glial and glial-neuronal tumors [63–65]. Most mutations and molecular markers are associated with the RAS/RAF/MEK/MAPK (mitogen-activated-protein kinase) intracellular signaling pathway. Pilocytic astrocytomas predominantly contain BRAF-KIAA1549 fusion (70–80%) [63]. On the other hand, diffuse astrocytomas exhibit three mutually exclusive genetic markers: BRAF V600E, *FGFR1*, and *MYB/MYBL1* mutation (each ≈25%), the last one being outside the RAS pathway [26, 66]. The BRAF V600E is also found in high frequency in pleomorphic xanthoastrocytomas and gangliogliomas [67]. The BRAF V600E mutation renders the serine-/threonine-specific protein kinase constitutively active on the downstream MEK without the upstream RAS phosphorylation [68]. It occurs in 17–36% of diencephalic low-grade glioma. Eighty-three percent of thalamopeduncular tumors harbor the BRAF-KIAA1549 fusion [69]. In contrast, in the Canadian study, all of the high-grade gliomas and bithalamic tumors lacked a fusion event [33]. The *H3F3A* K27M mutation in histone H3.3 is found in 30% of pediatric glioblastoma, altering cellular function through an epigenetic mechanism [70, 71]. From a diagnostic point of view, these biological markers stratify tumors which share the same histology and will potentially be included in a more integrated histopathologic-molecular classification [66, 72]. From a prognostic point of view, they predict biological behavior and clinical outcome. Also, they provide target for novel therapeutic agents (see Sects. 22.9.3 and 22.12).

22.8 Treatment

Thalamic gliomas have historically been treated nonsurgically, due to the deep-seated location and the unacceptably high morbidity and mortality associated with surgery. In 1958, Arseni reported a 40% perioperative mortality rate [3]. In the same year, in McKissock and Paine's report of 24 patients, 3 underwent surgery, 2 died in the perioperative period, and the third had a "useless life" [4]. The mainstay of treatment was CSF diversion, in the form of a Torkildsen's ventriculocisternostomy or shunt, followed by radiotherapy. Some groups advised against biopsy, which carried a significant risk [4, 5, 18, 28]. Most of the early series included adults, which harbored different pathologies from children. In the 1980s, as stereotactic techniques improved, biopsy became a minimal requirement. Beks et al. recommended stereotactic biopsy followed by appropriate radiation therapy [36]. Resective surgery was performed when absolutely indicated by raised ICP. Bernstein et al. from The Hospital for Sick Children, Toronto, advocated open biopsy, which allowed diagnosis, potential for partial resection and restoration of normal CSF pathway [29]. Albright also recommended biopsy, decompression of cyst, and occasionally extensive resection [12]. With improving surgical morbidity, the Mayo Clinic, Rochester, Minnesota, stratified the management for low- and high-grade lesions. For low-grade lesions or pilocytic astrocytomas, asymptomatic patients were treated conservatively, and those with neurological deterioration, well-circumscribed tumors, or recurrent cysts would be considered for stereotactic resection [20]. High-grade lesions confirmed by stereotactic biopsy would be treated with radiotherapy [14, 20]. In Drake et al.'s report on their experience in computer- and robot-assisted resection of pediatric thalamic astrocytoma, they felt that radical resection was reasonable [30]. In the 1990s, Hoffman et al. recommended surgery for low-grade lesions and radiotherapy for children older than 5 years with malignant lesions [15, 42]. Cuccia and Monges advocated surgical resection for both benign and anaplastic tumors [6].

In the past two decades, advances in neuroanesthesia, neuroimaging, Cavitron ultrasonic aspirator (CUSA), neuronavigation, intraoperative MRI, ultrasound, and neurophysiologic monitoring have resulted in much safer resective surgery for thalamic glioma. Since the turn of the millennium, the consensus from the contemporary series is that subtotal and sometimes total resection is safe in most cases, with a perioperative mortality of less than 5%. They should be performed for discrete, low-grade unilateral tumors, usually pilocytic, for symptom reversal and improved prognosis [7, 8, 22, 23, 32, 35, 58, 73]. High-grade gliomas should be confirmed by biopsy. Adjuvant chemoradiotherapy should be reserved for high-grade tumors and symptomatic, progressive, or recurrent low-grade tumors. Radiotherapy should be deferred until 3–5 years of age due to its long-term sequelae [74]. Bilateral thalamic tumors represent a special subset. Although they tend to be low-grade, safe effective surgical resection is not possible. Therefore, they are often biopsied and treated accordingly. The management of thalamic glioma is complex and requires a multidisciplinary approach.

22.8.1 Surgery

Neurosurgery is commonly the initial treatment of the tumor and hydrocephalus. Surgical procedures include biopsy, CSF diversion, tumor debulking or resection, and cyst decompression.

22.8.1.1 Biopsy

This is performed using a stereotactic frame or under neuronavigation guidance, either with head fixation or pinless electromagnetic (EM) technology [75]. The EM technology is particularly useful for children younger than 3 years or those who have thin cranium due to long-standing hydrocephalus. Biopsy can also be taken endoscopically as part of the initial CSF diversion surgery [76]. Intraoperative smear or frozen section is useful to confirm lesional samples.

22.8.1.2 CSF Diversion

Hydrocephalus is common, and 60–75% of patients require CSF diversion either as the initial treatment or following resective surgery [6–8, 15, 28, 29, 32, 33, 35, 41]. This can be ventriculoperitoneal shunt or endoscopic third ventriculostomy.

22.8.1.3 Tumor Debulking or Resection

For unilateral low-grade tumors, maximal safe resection is desirable. As mentioned above, several surgical adjuncts have significantly improved the extent of resection and morbidity. White matter tractography, based on diffusion-tensor imaging (using a deterministic algorithm) or other probabilistic algorithm, identifies the posterior limb of the internal capsule (PLIC), which is usually displaced by the glioma anterolaterally but can deviate in other directions or course through in the tumor [24, 77, 78]. This adjunct facilitates the planning of the optimal surgical approach to achieve gross total resection without disrupting the corticospinal tract and causing motor deficit (Fig. 22.3h, i) [69, 77, 79, 80]. Neuronavigation has improved microsurgical precision, but its accuracy decreases with brain shift following loss of CSF and tumor debulking. Intraoperative MRI (IOM) offers nearly real-time images for detection of residual tumors or complications, e.g., hematoma. Zheng et al. reported, with the use of IOM in 38 patients, the gross total resection rate increased from 42.1 to 68.4% and subtotal resection rate from 13.2 to 23.7%, respectively [81]. On the other hand, intraoperative ultrasonography in experienced hands provides real-time imaging of the operative field. Neurophysiologic monitoring, specifically cortical and subcortical stimulation, is another effective adjunct to reduce motor deficit, although it does not prevent speech disturbance or cognitive impairment [82, 83].

The optimal open surgical approach and surgical goal, in terms of extent of resection, are dependent on the laterality, location and size of the tumor, tumor extension, presence of ventriculomegaly, and deviation or infiltration of the internal capsule. Moshel et al. have divided the

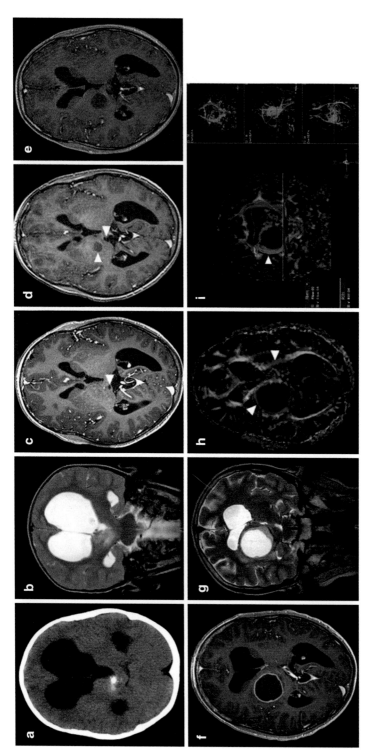

Fig. 22.3 A 3-year-old boy presented with 1-week history of vomiting and a background of macrocephaly. (**a, b**) CT and MRI demonstrated a right thalamic lesion with calcification and obstruction of posterior third ventricle, causing massive hydrocephalus. The hydrocephalus was treated successfully with endoscopic third ventriculostomy (**c, d, e**) Serial imaging at 8, 11, and 13 years of age showing increasing in size of tumor and multiple tumoral cysts (arrowheads), with the development of a left upper limb tremor. A neuronavigation- and ultrasound-guided biopsy was performed at 13 years old, confirming WHO grade I pilocytic astrocytoma. (**f, g**) The tumor cyst continued to expand, and the child developed acute hemiparesis. (**h, i**) Tractography demonstrated the anterolateral displacement of the ipsilateral internal capsule (arrowheads). In the following year, the child underwent ultrasound-guided insertion of Ommaya catheter and reservoir into the tumor cyst. (**j**) Postoperative MRI demonstrating the decompression of the cyst and the catheter tip (arrowhead). Four months later, the hemiparesis did not improve, and the child underwent interhemispheric transcallosal approach and subtotal resection of tumor. (**k, li, j**) Postoperative imaging. The tumor was immunopositive for RAF V600E mutation and negative for H3K27M

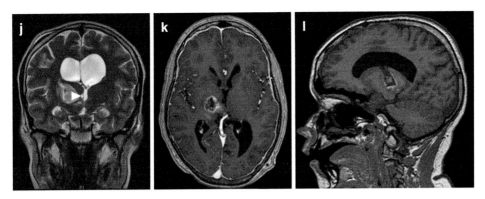

Fig. 22.3 (continued)

thalamic tumors to anterior, posterior superior, and posterior inferior, to aid selection of the ideal surgical approach [23]. Steiger described the thalamus as a tetrahedron. Apart from the ventrolateral surface which abuts the internal capsule and the subthalamic area, the other surfaces are in contact with the ventricles and CSF spaces, providing multiple natural surgical corridors [22]. The common surgical approaches include:

- *Transcortical transventricular* (Figs. 22.3 and 22.4): This approach is the most often used and can be through the frontal, parietal, occipital, and temporal lobe [6, 8, 20, 22–24, 29, 32, 33, 35, 41, 58, 73, 77]. It is most suitable for large tumors with thinning of the cortex and ventricular dilatation. It avoids disruption to the parasagittal veins. The frontal approach is used for superior tumors, and the parieto-occipital is suitable for posterior tumors. However, the corticotomy carries seizure risk and language disturbance on the dominant hemisphere. The transtemporal approach is particularly useful for tumors extending to the mesial temporal region and thalamopeduncular tumors [8, 84]. However, it carries the risk of injuring the corticospinal tract, optic tract, and oculomotor nerve [24, 82].
- *Interhemispheric transcallosal transventricular* (Fig. 22.3): This approach avoids the disruption of the cortex. The callosotomy can be anterior or posterior [6, 8, 24, 29, 33, 35, 41, 58, 73, 85]. This approach is more suitable for tumors protruding into the ventricles causing

hydrocephalus. Careful preoperative study of the parasagittal draining veins and their avoidance is key to prevent venous infarct.
- Yaşargil described the *interhemispheric parasplenial* approach for pulvinar lesions [85]. The *posterior infratentorial supracerebellar* approach is suitable for small tumors in this region, which is accessible from the quadrigeminal cistern [22, 58, 86]. The *occipital transtentorial* and *interhemispheric precuneus* routes are also occasionally used [24, 33, 87].
- *Transsylvian transinsular*: Also popularized by Yaşargil, an opening through the postcentral sulcus allows access to a thalamic tumor that displaces the internal capsule anterolaterally [85].

22.8.1.4 Neuroendoscopy
Neuroendoscopy is also used in surgical management of thalamic glioma, mainly for biopsy, but recently also for resection [76, 88, 89]. Occasionally, an Ommaya reservoir is inserted into a symptomatic tumor cyst, to allow periodic aspiration of cystic fluid (Fig. 22.3).

22.8.1.5 Postoperative Course
Early postoperative complications secondary to dysfunction of the thalamus include reduced conscious level, sensory disturbance, and anomia. Disturbance or damage to the adjacent cortical spinal tract and basal ganglia can cause hemiparesis and ataxia. Depending on the approach, the affected cortical areas, white fiber tracts, and cra-

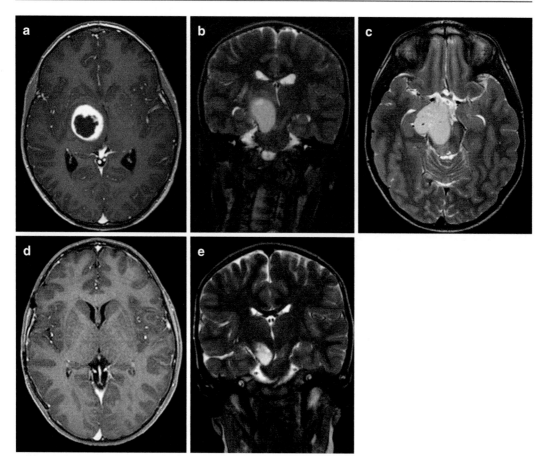

Fig. 22.4 A 9-year-old boy presented with 3-week acute history of left facial, upper, and lower limb weakness, over a 3-month background of slightly slurred speech. He has multiple café au lait macules and axillary frecklings. He was also diagnosed with attention deficiency hyperactivity disorder. In retrospect, the symptoms could be attributed to an organic cause. (**a**, **b**) Axial MRI with contrast and coronal T2-WI demonstrating a ring enhancing right thalamopeduncular tumor. (**c**) The tumor involved the mesial temporal structure. The child underwent a trans-middle-temporal gyrus transventricular approach and subtotal resection of the tumor. (**d**, **e**) Six-month postoperative imaging showing the resection of the thalamic portion and a small residual tumor in the midbrain. The histology was grade I pilocytic astrocytoma, and the BRAF duplication-fusion status was negative. BRAF V600E and H3K27M were also negative by immunohistochemistry. Genetic testing confirmed a variant of the NF1 gene. The boy will be followed up radiologically and will be considered for adjuvant therapy for progressive disease

nial nerves can lead to seizures, dysphasia, visual field deficit, and oculomotor nerve paresis. Hydrocephalus can persist or exacerbate after resection, requiring further surgery (Fig. 22.5).

22.8.1.6 Surgery for Recurrent or Progressive Disease

As surgery provides the most effective local disease control, resection with or without adjuvant chemotherapy should be considered for recurrent low-grade tumors.

22.8.2 Radiation Therapy

For low-grade glioma, surgery remains the mainstay of treatment. So far, no effective radio- or chemotherapy has been clearly demonstrated [33]. The majority of the large oncological studies group thalamic gliomas with other tumors arising from the midline. In a series of 71 children with low-grade glioma, Pollack et al. demonstrated that radiotherapy had no role in patients

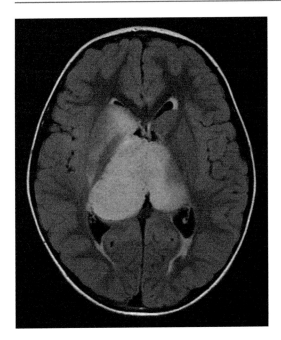

Fig. 22.5 A 6-year-old boy presented with intermittent headache and left arm intentional tremor. The MRI (FLAIR sequence) demonstrated a bilthalamic tumor, right larger than left. The right head of caudate was also involved. The ventricles were slightly enlarged and transependymal edema was present. The internal capsules were preserved. The boy underwent a left frontal endoscopic biopsy and septostomy and then later a left occipital ventriculoperitoneal shunt insertion. The histopathologic diagnosis was WHO grade III anaplastic astrocytoma, immunonegative for H3K27M, p53, and BRAF V600E mutation. The MIB-1 proliferative index was 40%. The boy was commenced on concomitant temozolomide (TMZ) and focal radiation (59.4 Gy) as per the Stupp protocol and to receive maintenance TMZ of an accumulative dose of 12 cycles of 200 mg/m². The boy remained stable clinically and radiologically 15 months after diagnosis

who underwent total resection [90]. Although radiotherapy offered some improvement in progression-free survival for patients with residual tumors, the overall survival did not significantly improve. Furthermore, for "unresectable tumors," upfront radiotherapy increased the risk of overall late deaths by threefold [91]. Considering the significant long-term side effects of endocrinopathy, growth retardation, vasculopathy, neurocognitive impairment, behavioral issues, and secondary neoplasia, most centers only consider radiotherapy for recurrent or progressive inoperable disease [92, 93].

For histologically confirmed high-grade glioma, most centers treat with radiotherapy with or without chemotherapy. The efficacy of radiotherapy in bithalamic low-grade glioma has not been clearly demonstrated [33].

22.8.3 Chemotherapy

For low-grade glioma that requires adjuvant treatment, chemotherapy is preferred over radiation as the first-line option, due to the latter's long-term side effect [74]. It is often indicated in children less than 3–5 years with progressive or in some cases residual disease, to delay the need for radiation. There is currently no standardized chemotherapeutic treatment protocol. The most used combination are carboplatin/vincristine and thioguanine/procarbazine/loustine (CCNU)/vincristine (TPCV) [94–97]. The carboplatin/vincristine combination is particularly effective in children less than 3 years, in which radiotherapy should be delayed. Other non-carboplatin-based regimens include vinblastine monotherapy which has been shown to be effective for refractory, recurrent low-grade gliomas and also unresectable and/or progressive therapy-naïve tumors [98, 99]. The results of temozolomide as mono or part of combination therapy are mixed [100, 101]. Angiogenesis inhibitor bevacizumab-based therapy with or without irinotecan has shown some promising results [102].

For pediatric high-grade gliomas, there is no robust evidence that addition of chemotherapy to radiotherapy improves outcome. The commonly used temozolomide regime is extrapolated from the Stupp protocol validated in the adult population, which is known to exhibit different tumor biology [103]. Although the result from temozolomide monotherapy is disappointing, a recent Phase 2 study from the Children's Oncology Group showed that addition of lomustine to temozolomide improved event-free survival, particularly in children with glioblastoma multiforme, incomplete resection, and overexpression of O^6-DNA methylguanine-methyltransferase (MGMT) [104, 105].

22.9 Prognosis and Outcome

22.9.1 Surgical Morbidity

In the past three decades, the surgical morbidity has much improved and has become acceptable. In the Canadian study, 17 of 39 (43%) of patients who underwent resective surgery for unilateral tumors had no neurological deficits, 38% had motor, and 14% had visual deficits post-resection [33]. Seven (19%) had permanent neurological deficits post-resection (five motor, two visual). Other contemporary series reported similar figures [7, 8].

22.9.2 Overall and Progression-Free Survival

In general, children with thalamic gliomas have longer survivals than adults [5]. Children with thalamic gliomas have a lower survival rate than those with the same tumor at more superficial sites [34, 96]. Armstrong et al. from St. Jude's Children's Research Hospital reported a thalamic low-grade glioma 5-year survival of 47% [106]. A prospective multi-institutional study from the Children's Oncology Group of 518 children reported an 8-year overall survival (OS) of 86% for midline low-grade gliomas, compared to 100% and 96% for cerebellar and cerebral tumors, respectively [107]. The 8-year progression-free survival (PFS) for the three locations were 58, 91, and 75%. In their series of 69 thalamic tumors, Wong et al. reported the 5-, 10-, and 15-year OS for thalamic low-grade astrocytomas to be 87, 87, and 80%. Steinbok et al. reported overall, i.e., including both high- and low-grade, 5-year PFS and OS as 54 and 61%.

In Krishnatry et al.'s report on long-term survival for incompletely resected low-grade gliomas, 20- and 30-year survivals for thalamic tumors are approximately 75 and 60%, significantly lower than those for all locations of 90 and 88% [91]. The report also revealed a bimodal pattern in the thalamic tumor survival curve, with late deaths occurring 10–20 years after diagnosis,

which was not observed in other sites. While 37% of deaths in the first 5 years of diagnosis were attributed to malignant transformation, most of the late deaths are due to effect of therapy.

22.9.3 Prognostic Factors

Prior to the recent discovery of molecular biomarkers, histological grade is the only consistent predictive factor in most studies [7, 9, 33, 35, 40]. In the Canadian multicenter study, Steinbok et al. provided the first multivariate analysis on factors affecting survival [33]. Low-grade unithalamic tumors had a much higher 5-year OS (84%) compared to high-grade tumors (7%). Patients with symptom duration longer than 3 months have better outcome (5-year OS: 86% vs. 42%). Also, 5-year OS was higher for patients who had ≥95% resection than <95% resection or biopsy (80% vs. 52%). The 5-year OS for patients who received some form of adjuvant therapy was 36% and for patients who did not receive adjuvant therapy was 85%. This could be confounded by the observation that patients who received radiation therapy predominantly had high-grade lesions. Despite the above findings, multivariate analysis showed that tumor grade was the only significant factor. Surprisingly, younger age, contrast enhancement, and tumor extension beyond the thalamus do not affect survival [9]. Interesting, Puget et al. found that presence of perilesional edema and unilateral thalamic tumor volume of >30 mL is associated with shorter OS, while presence of a cyst is indicative of a benign tumor and is thus associated with better outcome [7].

High-grade thalamic glioma carries a dismal prognosis. Based on the HIT-GBM trial data for high-grade thalamic glioma, the 1-, 2-, and 5-year OS were 54, 21, and 11% and event-free survival 18, 8, and 7% [40]. No patients had a gross total resection and only 10% had subtotal/partial resection. The extent of resection and early response to chemoradiotherapy were identified as prognostic factors. After taking into account the surgical inaccessibility and thus less extent of resection compared to other nonthalamic supratentorial tumors, the thalamic location is still a poor prognostic factor *per se*. In fact, the survival curve is more similar to that of diffuse pontine glioma, suggesting thalamic gliomas have a different biology from other sites.

Bithalamic glioma carries a significantly poorer prognosis than unithalamic tumors, despite the predominance of low-grade astrocytoma histology [9]. However, it is possible that the large tumors harbor anaplastic areas which were not sampled. Steinbok et al. reported a 5-year overall survival of 37% for bilthalamic tumors compared to 61% for unithalamic tumors [33]. The inferior outcome is likely because safe gross total resection is not possible and response to chemoradiotherapy is poor [7, 33, 35, 43, 108].

Overall, NF1 patients have better outcome than non-NF1 patients, although this difference is likely to be less significant when optic chiasm/hypothalamic tumors are removed from the analysis [109]. The recently identified biomarkers from genomic sequencing have proved to be powerful prognostic factors. BRAF-KIAA1549 is associated with a much better survival and is frequently found in pilocytic astrocytomas and thalamopeduncular tumors but not in high-grade gliomas and bithalamic tumors [26, 33, 63, 110]. BRAF V600E mutation is an independent poor prognostic factor for pediatric low-grade glioma which have undergone gross total or subtotal resection [26, 111, 112]. It is also associated with poor outcome despite administration of radio- or chemotherapy. The 5-year PFS is 22% compared to 52% for BRAF wild type. Furthermore, *CDKN2A* deletion, which results in the escape from the cell cycle regulation, is associated with poor overall and progression-free survival, although its effect is present only in BRAF V600E tumors. Overall, a combination of BRAF V600E and *CDKN2A* deletion and subtotal resection confers a <10% chance of tumor control and poor survival with conventional therapies. The *H3F3A* K27M mutation is found in 30% of pediatric glioblastoma and 80% of diffuse intrinsic pontine gliomas [70, 71]. This mutation is indicative of a malignant course regardless of the histology and treatment.

22.9.4 Malignant Transformation

Unlike their adult counterparts, pediatric low-grade gliomas are less aggressive and do not commonly undergo malignant transformation [113]. In a retrospective population-based cohort study of 886 patients, only 3% of pediatric low-grade gliomas transform to secondary high-grade glioma [114]. None of the high-grade tumors harbored the BRAF-KIAA1549 fusion, but BRAF V600E mutation and CDKN2A deletion are present in 39% and 57%. Strikingly, all BRAF V600E and 80% of CDKN2A alterations can be traced back to the primary low-grade tumors.

22.10 Follow-Up/Specific Problems and Measures

Since most low-grade gliomas are more akin to a chronic disease with a small percentage that transforms, patients should be followed up regularly to assess response to treatment and identify recurrence/progression, so further surgical, adjuvant, and new target therapy can be considered. In our institute, patients with unilateral low-grade glioma who underwent uncomplicated surgery are followed clinically and radiologically at 3, 6, and 12 months and then annually if the disease is stable. Patients with high-grade or bithalamic tumors, or who developed complications, are followed more frequently. The follow-up frequency is also dependent on any concurrent adjuvant therapy timetable. In addition, long-term sequelae from surgery and adjuvant therapy including motor deficit, endocrinopathy, growth retardation, neurocognitive impairment, behavioral issues, and secondary neoplasia should be followed by the various specialties of the multidisciplinary team.

22.11 New Treatment Strategies

Magnetic resonance-guided laser interstitial thermal therapy (MRgLITT) is delivered by a laser applicator which is inserted into the lesion stereotactically [115]. It generates photons which interact with the chromophores in the lesion, causing subsequent excitation of the orbital electrons, and leads to subsequent dissipation of heat. Irreversible thermal damage is time-dependent at a temperature above 45 °C, which is visualized in "real time" using magnetic resonance thermography. MRgLITT is increasingly used for deep-seated lesions, including high-grade gliomas [116–119]. The results in adults are promising, and MRgLITT provides an alternate treatment modality in pediatric thalamic glioma for *de novo* or recurrent tumors when the risk of open surgery is high.

22.12 Future Perspectives

In addition to diagnostic and prognostic function, the BRAF alteration also offers a target for novel therapy [120]. The use of BRAF inhibitor (e.g., dabrafenib) in BRAF V600E tumors which failed to respond to conventional treatments has shown early promising clinical and radiologic results [111, 120–122]. Similar response is also seen with MEK inhibitors (e.g., selumetinib) in BRAF-KIAA1549 fusion tumors [123]. If proven to be effective at longer term, targeted therapy could potentially achieve tumor control or shrinkage without the side effects related to conventional adjuvant therapies [124]. This is important as this group of patients have long survival and thus the side effect burden of chemoradiotherapy is significant. It is even more relevant for NF1 patients, who have less aggressive tumors and thus even longer survival [125]. In the currently planned SIOP-E trial LOGGIC (Low-Grade Glioma in Children), a Phase 3 randomized trial comparing different vinca alkaloids and treatment durations, one arm will include targeted therapy to MAPK activation [66]. Currently, for *H3F3A* K27M mutation, there is no novel therapy on the horizon. Radical surgery should be avoided in these cases.

References

1. Herrero M, Barcia C (2002) Functional anatomy of thalamus and basal ganglia. Childs Nerv Syst 18:386–404
2. Rhoton AL (2002) The cerebrum. Neurosurgery 51(Suppl 1):1–51
3. Arseni C (1958) Tumors of the basal ganglia. Their surgical treatment. Arch Neurol Psychiatry 80:18–24
4. McKissock W, Paine KWE (1958) Primary tumours of the thalamus. Brain 81:41–63
5. Cheek WR, Taveras JM (1966) Thalamic Tumors. J Neurosurg 24:505–513
6. Cuccia V, Monges J (1997) Thalamic tumors in children. Childs Nerv Syst 13:514–521
7. Puget S, Crimmins DW, Garnett MR et al (2007) Thalamic tumors in children: a reappraisal. J Neurosurg 106(5 Suppl):354–362
8. Wong T, Chen H, Liang M et al (2016) Clinical considerations and surgical approaches for low-grade gliomas in deep hemispheric locations: thalamic lesions. Childs Nerv Syst 32:1895–1906
9. Reardon DA, Gajjar A, Sandford RA et al (1998) Bithalamic involvement predicts poor outcome among children with thalamic glial tumors. Pediatr Neurosurg 29:29–35
10. Ostrom QT, Gittleman H, Liao P et al (2015) CBTRUS statistical report: primary brain and central nervous system tumors diagnosed in the United States in 2007-2011. Neuro Oncol 17(Suppl 4):iv1–iv63
11. Martínez-Lage JF, Pérez-espejo MA, Esteban JA (2002) Thalamic tumors: clinical presentation. Childs Nerv Syst 18:405–411
12. Albright AL, Price RA, Guthkelch AN (1985) Diencephalic gliomas of children. A clinicopathologic study. Cancer 55:2789–2793
13. McGirr SJ, Kelly PJ, Scheithauer BW (1987) Stereotactic resection of juvenile pilocytic astrocytomas of the thalamus and basal ganglia. Neurosurgery 20(3):447–452
14. Lyons MK, Kelly PJ (1992) Computer-assisted stereotactic biopsy and volumetric resection of thalamic pilocytic astrocytomas. Report of 23 cases. Stereotact Funct Neurosurg 59:100–104
15. Hoffman HJ, Soloniuk DS, Humphreys R et al (1993) Management and outcome of low-grade astrocytomas of the midline in children: a retrospective review. Neurosurgery 33(6):964–971
16. Franzini A, Leocata F, Cajola L, Servello D, Allegranza A, Broggi G (1994) Low-grade glial tumors in basal ganglia and thalamus: natural history and biological reappraisal. Neurosurgery 35(5):817–821
17. Grigsby PW, Thomas PR, Schwartz HG, Fineberg BB (1989) Multivariate analysis of prognostic factors in pediatric and adult thalamic and brainstem tumor. Int J Radiat Oncol Biol Phys 16:649–655
18. Tovi D, Schisano G, Liljeqvist B (1961) Primary tumors of the region of the thalamus. J Neurosurg 18:730–740
19. Prakash B (1985) Surgical approach to large thalamic gliomas. Acta Neurochir 104:100–104
20. Kelly PJ (1989) Stereotactic biopsy and resection of thalamic astrocytomas.pdf. Neurosurgery 25(2):185–195
21. Krouwer HGJ, Prados MD (1995) Infiltrative astrocytomas of the thalamus. J Neurosurg 82:548–557

22. Steiger H-J, Gotz C, Schmid-Elsaesser R, Stummer W (2000) Thalamic astrocytomas: surgical anatomy and results of a pilot series using maximum microsurgical removal. Acta Neurochir 142:1327–1337

23. Moshel YA, Link MJ, Kelly PJ (2007) Stereotactic volumetric resection of thalamic pilocytic astrocytomas. Neurosurgery 61(1):66–75

24. Sai Kiran NA, Thakar S, Dadlani R et al (2013) Surgical management of thalamic gliomas: case selection, technical considerations, and review of literature. Neurosurg Rev 36:383–393

25. Frank F, Fabrizi AP, Gaist G, Frank-Ricci R, Piazzi M, Spagnolli F (1987) Stereotaxy and thalamic masses. Survey of 44 cases. Appl Neurophysiol 50:243–247

26. Ichimura K, Narita Y, Hawkins CE (2015) Diffusely infiltrating astrocytomas: pathology , molecular mechanisms and markers. Acta Neuropathol 129(6):789–808

27. Albright AL (2004) Feasibility and advisability of resections of thalamic tumors in pediatric patients. J Neurosurg 100(5 Suppl):468–472

28. Hirose G, Lombroso CI, Eisenberg H (1975) Thalamic tumors in childhood. Clinical, laboratory, and therapeutic considerations. Arch Neurol 32:740–744

29. Bernstein M, Hoffman HJ, Halliday WC, Hendrick EB, Humphreys RP (1984) Thalamic tumors in children. Long-term follow-up and treatment guidelines. JNS 61:649–656

30. Drake JM, Joy M, Goldenberg A, Kreindler D (1991) Computer- and robot-assisted resection of thalamic astrocytomas in children.pdf. Neurosurgery 29(1):27–31

31. Fernandez C, Figarella-Branger D, Girard N, Bouvier-labit C, Lena G (2003) Pilocytic astrocytomas in children: prognostic factors-a retrospective study of 80 cases. Neurosurgery 53(3):544–555

32. Baroncini M, Vinchon M, Minéo J-F, Pichon F, Francke J-P, Dhellemmes P (2007) Surgical resection of thalamic tumors in children: approaches and clinical results. Childs Nerv Syst 23:753–760

33. Steinbok P, Gopalakrishnan CV, Hengel AR et al (2016) Pediatric thalamic tumors in the MRI era: a Canadian perspective. Childs Nerv Syst 32:269–280

34. Gajjar A, Sanford RA, Heideman R et al (1997) Low-grade astrocytoma: a decade of experience at St. Jude Children's Research Hospital. J Clin Oncol 15(8):2792–2799

35. Bilginer B, Narin F, Ilkay I, Oguz KK, Söylemezoglu F, Akalan N (2014) Thalamic tumors in children. Childs Nerv Syst 30:1493–1498

36. Beks JWF, Bouma GJ, Journée HL (1987) Tumours of the thalamic region. A retrospective study of 27 cases. Acta Neurochir 85:125–127

37. Gutmann DH, Donahoe J, Brown T, James CD, Perry A (2000) Loss of neurofibromatosis 1 (NF1) gene expression in NF1-associated pilocytic astrocytomas. Neuropathol Appl Neurobiol 26(4):361–367

38. Rodríguez AD, Martos Moreno GÁ, Martín Santo-Domingo Y et al (2015) Phenotypic and genetic features in neurofibromatosis type 1 in children. An Pediatr 83:173–182

39. Hernáiz Driever P, Von Hornstein S, Pietsch T et al (2010) Natural history and management of low-grade glioma in NF-1 children. J Neurooncol 100(2):199–207

40. Kramm CM, Butenhoff S, Rausche U et al (2011) Thalamic high-grade gliomas in children: a distinct clinical subset? Neuro Oncol 13(6):680–689

41. Villarejo F, Amaya C, Díaz CP, Sastre CA, Goyenechea F (1994) Radical surgery of thalamic tumors in children. Childs Nerv Syst 10:111–114

42. Souweidane MM, Hoffman HJ (1996) Current treatment of thalamic gliomas in children. J Neurooncol 28:157–166

43. Di Rocco C, Iannelli A (2002) Bilateral thalamic tumors in children. Childs Nerv Syst 18(8):440–444

44. Partlow GD, Carpio-O'Donovan R, Malanson D, Peters TM (1984) Bilateral thalamic glioma: review of eight cases with personality change and mental deterioration. AJNR 13:1225–1230

45. Krauss JK, Nobbe F, Wakhloo AK, Mohadjer M, Vach W, Mundinger F (1992) Disorders in astrocytomas of the basal ganglia and the thalamus. JNNP 55:1162–1167

46. Dejerine J, Roussy G (1906) Le syndrome thalamique. Rev Neurol 14:521–532

47. Alomar S, King NKK, Tam J, Bari AA, Hamani C, Lozano AM (2017) Speech and language adverse effects after thalamotomy and deep brain stimulation in patients with movement disorders: a meta-analysis. Mov Disord 32(1):53–63

48. Fuertinger S, Horwitz B, Simonyan K (2015) The functional connectome of speech control. PLoS Biol 13(7):1–31

49. Simonyan K, Fuertinger S (2015) Speech networks at rest and in action: interactions between functional brain networks controlling speech production. J Neurophysiol 113:2967–2978

50. Burger PC, Cohen KJ, Rosenblum MK, Tihan T (2000) Pathology of diencephalic astrocytomas. Pediatr Neurosurg 32:214–219

51. Colosimo C, di Lelle GM, Tartaglione T, Riccardi R (2002) Neuroimaging of thalamic tumors in children. Childs Nerv Syst 18:426–439

52. Khanna PC, Iyer RS, Chaturvedi A et al (2011) Imaging bithalamic pathology in the pediatric brain: demystifying a diagnostic conundrum. Am J Roentgenol 197(6):1449–1459

53. Estève F, Grand S, Rubin C et al (1999) MR spectroscopy of bilateral thalamic gliomas. Am J Neuroradiol 20(5):876–881

54. Orphanidou-Vlachou E, Auer D, Brundler MA et al (2013) 1H magnetic resonance spectroscopy in the diagnosis of paediatric low grade brain tumours. Eur J Radiol 82(6):e295–e301

55. Messing-Jünger AM, Floeth FW, Pauleit D et al (2002) Multimodal target point assessment for stereotactic biopsy in children with diffuse bithalamic astrocytomas. Childs Nerv Syst 18:445–449

56. García-Santos JM, Torres S, Martínez-lage JF (2002) Basal ganglia and thalamic tumours: an imaging approximation. Childs Nerv Syst 18:412–425

57. Fernandez C, de Paula AM, Colin C et al (2006) Thalamic gliomas in children: an extensive clinical, neuroradiological and pathological study of 14 cases. Childs Nerv Syst 22:1603–1610

58. Özek MM, Türe U (2002) Surgical approach to thalamic tumors. Childs Nerv Syst 18:450–456

59. Reddy AT, Packer RJ (1999) Chemotherapy for low-grade gliomas. Childs Nerv Syst 15:506–513

60. Kim CH, Paek SH, Park IA, Chi JG, Kim DG (2002) Cerebral germinoma with hemiatrophy of the brain: report of three cases cases. Acta Neurochir (Wien) 144(2):145–150

61. Gilles FH, Tavare CJ, Becker LE et al (2008) Pathologist interobserver variability of histologic features in childhood brain tumors: results from the CCG-945 study. Pediatr Dev Pathol 11:108–117. 07-06-0303 [pii]

62. van den Bent MJ (2010) Interobserver variation of the histopathological diagnosis in clinical trials on glioma: a clinician's perspective. Acta Neuropathol 120(3):297–304

63. Jones DTW, Kocialkowski S, Liu L et al (2008) Tandem duplication producing a novel oncogenic BRAF fusion gene defines the majority of pilocytic astrocytomas. Cancer Res 68(21):8673–8677

64. Pfister S, Janzarik WG, Remke M et al (2008) BRAF gene duplication constitutes a mechanism of MAPK pathway activation in low-grade astrocytomas. J Clin Invest 118:1739–1749

65. Collins VP, Jones DTW, Giannini C (2015) Pilocytic astrocytoma: pathology, molecular mechanisms and markers. Acta Neuropathol 129(6):775–788

66. Packer RJ, Pfster S, Bouffet E et al (2017) Pediatric low-grade gliomas: Implications of the biologic era. Neuro Oncol 19(6):750–761

67. Schindler G, Capper D, Meyer J et al (2011) Analysis of BRAF V600E mutation in 1,320 nervous system tumors reveals high mutation frequencies in pleomorphic xanthoastrocytoma, ganglioglioma and extra-cerebellar pilocytic astrocytoma. Acta Neuropathol 121(3):397–405

68. Davies H, Bignell GR, Cox C et al (2002) Mutations of the BRAF gene in human cancer. Nature 417(6892):949–954

69. Lee RP, Foster KA, Lillard JC et al (2017) Surgical and molecular considerations in the treatment of pediatric thalamopeduncular tumors. J Neurosurg Pediatr 20(3):247–255

70. Venneti S, Santi M, Felicella MM et al (2014) A sensitive and specific histopathologic prognostic marker for H3F3A K27M mutant pediatric glioblastomas. Acta Neuropathol 128(5):743–753

71. Khuong-Quang DA, Buczkowicz P, Rakopoulos P et al (2012) K27M mutation in histone H3.3 defines clinically and biologically distinct subgroups of pediatric diffuse intrinsic pontine gliomas. Acta Neuropathol 124(3):439–447

72. Louis DN, Perry A, Burger P et al (2014) International Society of Neuropathology-Haarlem consensus guidelines for nervous system tumor classification and grading. Brain Pathol 24(5):429–435

73. Albright L (2004) Feasibility and advisability of resections of thalamic tumors in pediatric patients. J Neurosurg 100(5 Suppl Pediatrics):468–472

74. Minturn JE, Fisher MJ (2013) Gliomas in children. Curr Treat Options Neurol 15:316–327

75. Hayhurst C, Byrne P, Eldridge PR, Mallucci CL (2009) Application of electromagnetic technology to neuronavigation: a revolution in image-guided neurosurgery. J Neurosurg 111:1179–1184

76. Selvapandian S (2006) Endoscopic management of thalamic gliomas. Minim Invasive Neurosurg 49:194–196

77. Broadway SJ, Ogg RJ, Scoggins MA, Sanford R, Patay Z, Boop FA (2011) Surgical management of tumors producing the thalamopeduncular syndrome of childhood. J Neurosurg Pediatr 7:589–595

78. Farquharson S, Tournier J-D, Calamante F et al (2013) White matter fiber tractography: why we need to move beyond DTI. J Neurosurg 118(6):1367–1377

79. Moshel YA, Elliott RE, Monoky DJ, Wisoff JH (2009) Role of diffusion tensor imaging in resection of thalamic juvenile pilocytic astrocytoma. J Neurosurg Pediatr 4:495–505

80. Celtikci E, Celtikci P, Fernandes-cabral DT, Ucar M, Fernandez-miranda JC, Borcek AO (2017) High-definition fiber tractography in evaluation and surgical planning of thalamopeduncular pilocytic astrocytomas in pediatric population: case series and review of literature. World Neurosurg 98: 463–469

81. Zheng X, Xu X, Zhang H et al (2016) A preliminary experience with use of intraoperative magnetic resonance imaging in thalamic glioma surgery: a case series of 38 patients. World Neurosurg 89:434–441

82. Carrabba G, Bertani G, Cogiamanian F et al (2016) Role of intraoperative neurophysiologic monitoring in the resection of thalamic astrocytomas. World Neurosurg 94:50–56

83. Coppola A, Tramontano V, Basaldella F, Arcaro C, Squintani G, Sala F (2016) Intra-operative neurophysiological mapping and monitoring during brain tumour surgery in children: an update. Childs Nerv Syst 32(10):1849–1859

84. Foley R, Boop F (2017) Tractography guides the approach for resection of thalamopeduncular tumors. Acta Neurochir (Wien) 159(6):1597–1601

85. Yaşargil MG (1996) Midline tumors (corpus callosum, septum pellucidum, basal ganglia, diencephalon, and brainstem). In: Microneurosurgery, vol 4B. Thieme, Stuttgart

86. Yaşargil MG, Türe U, Yaşargil DCH (2005) Surgical anatomy of supratentorial midline lesions. Neurosurg Focus 18(6B):1–9

87. Akiyama O, Matsushima K, Gungor A et al (2016) Microsurgical and endoscopic approaches to the pulvinar. J Neurosurg 127:1–16

88. Akiyama Y, Wanibuchi M, Mikami T et al (2015) Rigid endoscopic resection of deep-seated or intraventricular brain tumors. Neurol Res 37(3):278–282

89. Brokinkel B, Yavuz M, Warneke N et al (2017) Endoscopic management of a low-grade thalamic glioma: a safe alternative to open microsurgery? Acta Neurochir 159(7):1237–1240

90. Pollack IF, Claassen D, Al-Shboul Q, Janosky JE, Deutsch M (1995) Low-grade gliomas of the cerebral hemispheres in children: an analysis of 71 cases. J Neurosurg 82:536–547

91. Krishnatry R, Zhukova N, Stucklin ASG, Pole JD (2016) Clinical and treatment factors determining long-term outcomes for adult survivors of childhood low-grade glioma: a population-based study. Cancer 122:1261–1269

92. Siffert J, Allen JC (2000) Late effects of therapy of thalamic and hypothalamic tumors in childhood: vascular. Neurobehavioral and Neoplastic 10128:105–111

93. Müller K, Gnekow A, Falkenstein F et al (2013) Radiotherapy in pediatric pilocytic astrocytomas: a subgroup analysis within the prospective multicenter study HIT-LGG 1996 by the German Society of Pediatric Oncology and Hematology (GPOH). Strahlenther Onkol 189:647–655

94. Packer RJ, Ater J, Allen J et al (1997) Carboplatin and vincristine chemotherapy for children with newly diagnosed progressive low-grade gliomas. J Neurosurg 86:747–754

95. Prados MD, Edwards MSB, Rabbitt J, Lamborn K, Davis RL, Levin VA (1997) Treatment of pediatric low-grade gliomas with a nitrosourea-based multiagent chemotherapy regimen. J Neurooncol 32:235–241

96. Ater JL, Zhou T, Holmes E et al (2012) Randomized study of two chemotherapy regimens for treatment of low-grade glioma in young children: a report from the Children's Oncology Group. J Clin Oncol 30:2641–2647

97. Gnekow AK, Walker DA, Kandels D et al (2017) A European randomised controlled trial of the addition of etoposide to standard vincristine and carboplatin induction as part of an 18-month treatment programme for childhood (≤16 years) low grade glioma—a final report. Eur J Cancer 81:206–225

98. Bouffet E, Jakacki R, Goldman S et al (2012) Phase II study of weekly vinblastine in recurrent or refractory pediatric low-grade glioma. J Clin Oncol 30:1358–1363

99. Lassaletta A, Scheinemann K, Zelcer SM et al (2016) Phase II weekly vinblastine for chemotherapy-naïve children with progressive low-grade glioma: a Canadian pediatric brain tumor consortium study. J Clin Oncol 34:3537–3543

100. Gururangan S, Fisher MJ, Allen JC et al (2007) Temozolomide in children with progressive low-grade glioma. Neuro Oncol 9:161–168

101. Chintagumpala M, Eckel SP, Krailo M et al (2015) A pilot study using carboplatin, vincristine, and temozolomide in children with progressive/symptomatic low-grade glioma: a Children's Oncology Group study. Neuro Oncol 17(8):1132–1138

102. Hwang EI, Jakacki R, Fisher MJ et al (2013) Long-term efficacy and toxicity of bevacizumab-based therapy in children with recurrent low-grade gliomas. Pediatr Blood Cancer 60:776–782

103. Stupp R, Mason WP, van den Bent MJ et al (2005) Radiotherapy plus concomitant and adjuvant temozolomide for glioblastoma. N Engl J Med 352(10):987–996

104. Jakacki RI, Cohen KJ, Buxton A et al (2016) Phase 2 study of concurrent radiotherapy and temozolomide followed by temozolomide and lomustine in the treatment of children with high-grade glioma: a report of the Children's Oncology Group ACNS0423 study. Neuro Oncol 18(10):1442–1450

105. Cohen KJ, Pollack IF, Zhou T et al (2011) Temozolomide in the treatment of high-grade gliomas in children: a report from the Children's Oncology Group. Neuro Oncol 13(3):317–323

106. Armstrong GT, Conklin HM, Huang S et al (2011) Survival and long-term health and cognitive outcomes after low-grade glioma. Neuro Oncol 13(2):223–234

107. Wisoff JH, Sanford RA, Heier LA et al (2011) Primary neurosurgery for pediatric low-grade gliomas: a prospective multi-institutional study from the Children's Oncology Group. Neurosurgery 68(6):1548–1554

108. Menon G, Nair S, Sudhir J, Rao BR, Krishnakumar K (2010) Bilateral thalamic lesions. Br J Neurosurg 24:566–571

109. Ater JL, Xia C, Mazewski CM et al (2016) Nonrandomized comparison of neurofibromatosis type 1 and non-neurofibromatosis type 1 children who received carboplatin and vincristine for progressive low-grade glioma: a report from the Children's Oncology Group. Cancer 122(12):1928–1936

110. Hawkins C, Walker E, Mohamed N et al (2011) BRAF-kiaa1549 fusion predicts better clinical outcome in pediatric low-grade astrocytoma. Clin Cancer Res 17(14):4790–4799

111. Lassaletta A, Zapotocky M, Mistry M et al (2017) Therapeutic and prognostic implications of BRAF V600E in pediatric low-grade gliomas. J Clin Oncol 35(25):2934–2941

112. Ho CY, Mobley BC, Gordish-Dressman H et al (2015) A clinicopathologic study of diencephalic pediatric low-grade gliomas with BRAF V600 mutation. Acta Neuropathol 130(4):575–585

113. Jones DTW, Mulholland SA, Pearson DM et al (2011) Adult grade II diffuse astrocytomas are genetically distinct from and more aggressive than their paediatric counterparts. Acta Neuropathol 121(6):753–761

114. Mistry M, Zhukova N, Merico D et al (2015) BRAF mutation and CDKN2A deletion define a clinically distinct subgroup of childhood secondary high-grade glioma. J Clin Oncol 33(9):1015–1022

115. Tovar-spinoza Z, Choi H (2016) MRI-guided laser interstitial thermal therapy for the treatment of low-grade gliomas in children: a case-series review, description of the current technologies and perspectives. Childs Nerv Syst 32(10):1947–1956

116. Missios S, Bekelis K, Barnett GH (2015) Renaissance of laser interstitial thermal ablation. Neurosurg Focus 38:E13

117. Banerjee C, Snelling B, Berger MH, Shah A, Ivan ME, Komotar RJ (2015) The role of magnetic resonance-guided laser ablation in neurooncology. Br J Neurosurg 29(2):192–196

118. Mohammadi AM, Hawasli AH, Rodriguez A et al (2014) The role of laser interstitial thermal therapy in enhancing progression-free survival of difficult-to-access high-grade gliomas: a multicenter study. Cancer Med 3:971–979

119. Hawasli AH, Bagade S, Shimony JS, Miller-Thomas M, Leuthardt EC (2013) Magnetic resonance imaging-guided focused laser interstitial thermal therapy for intracranial lesions: single-institution series. Neurosurgery 73:1007–1017

120. Lassaletta A, Guerreiro Stucklin A, Ramaswamy V et al (2016) Profound clinical and radiological response to BRAF inhibition in a 2-month-old diencephalic child with hypothalamic/chiasmatic glioma. Pediatr Blood Cancer 63(11):2038–2041

121. Kieran MW, Hargrave DR, Cohen KJ et al (2015) Phase 1 study of dabrafenib in pediatric patients (pts) with relapsed or refractory BRAF V600E high- and low-grade gliomas (HGG, LGG), Langerhans cell histiocytosis (LCH), and other solid tumors (OST). J Clin Oncol 33:10004

122. Robinson GW, Orr BA, Gajjar A (2014) Complete clinical regression of a BRAF V600E-mutant pediatric glioblastoma multiforme after BRAF inhibitor therapy. BMC Cancer 14(1):258

123. Banerjee A, Jakacki RI, Onar-Thomas A et al (2017) A phase I trial of the MEK inhibitor selumetinib (AZD6244) in pediatric patients with recurrent or refractory low-grade glioma: a Pediatric Brain Tumor Consortium (PBTC) study. Neuro Oncol 19(8):1135–1144

124. Kieran M, Bouffet E, Tabori U et al (2016) The first study of dabrafenib in pediatric patients with BRAF V600–mutant relapsed or refractory low-grade gliomas [abstract, ESMO 2016 Congress]. Ann Oncol 27:1–36

125. Perilongo G, Moras P, Carollo C et al (1999) Spontaneous partial regression of low-grade glioma in children with neurofibromatosis-1: a real possibility. J Child Neurol 14(6):352–356.

Optic Pathway Gliomas

23

Ian F. Pollack

23.1 Epidemiology

Optic pathway tumors account for about 5% of brain tumors in children [1]. The majority of tumors are diagnosed during the first decade of life, and a sizeable subgroup occurs in children with NF1, where they are often detected asymptomatically during regular screening examinations [2]. NF1 results from mutations in a gene on chromosome 17q11.2 that encodes neurofibromin, a GTPase activator [3] that favors the conversion of the active GTP-bound form of Ras to the inactive GDP-bound form. By interfering with this conversion, the mutated gene promotes persistent activation of the Ras/RAF/MEK (MAPK/ERK kinase)/MAPK (mitogen-activated protein kinase) signalling pathway, a common feature of pilocytic astrocytomas. At least 15% of children with NF1 have optic pathway tumors on MRI [4].

Although the vast majority of childhood optic pathway gliomas are low grade histologically (i.e., World Health Organization Grades I and II) [5], their growth characteristics can vary widely [6]. In children with NF1, these tumors are often detected incidentally and show gradual or, occasionally, no enlargement over time and in rare cases exhibit shrinkage, suggesting that these lesions can have indolent or, in some cases, decelerating growth kinetics [7]. In contrast, the majority of the non-NF1-associated optic pathway tumors enlarge without treatment, in some cases slowly and in others, particularly in infants, quite rapidly, producing progressive visual compromise and, in larger lesions, neurological impairment and symptoms of increased intracranial pressure (ICP) [2]. In addition to the association between age and prognosis, lesions that involve the hypothalamus carry a worse prognosis than those restricted to one or both optic nerves, and large lesion size, which characterizes many optic-hypothalamic tumors, has also been associated with an adverse prognosis [6, 8].

23.2 Symptoms and Signs

The initial manifestations of an optic pathway glioma are influenced by the age of the child and tumor location. Tumors involving a single optic nerve often exhibit proptosis and unilateral visual loss. Tumors arising from the optic chiasm, a common mode of involvement in children with NF1, also typically present with visual deterioration, which is often bilateral. In milder cases, this symptom can be challenging to detect in young children without serial examinations, since many young patients do not report a visual problem until their acuity is poor. Such patients may

I. F. Pollack (✉)
Department of Neurosurgery, Children's Hospital of Pittsburgh, University of Pittsburgh School of Medicine, Pittsburgh, PA, USA
e-mail: ian.pollack@chp.edu

© Springer Nature Switzerland AG 2019
J.-C. Tonn et al. (eds.), *Oncology of CNS Tumors*, https://doi.org/10.1007/978-3-030-04152-6_23

exhibit an esotropia, nystagmus, or poor visual fixation when one eye is covered or demonstrate optic atrophy on fundoscopy, despite a paucity of clinical complaints. In contrast, children with large tumors involving the chiasm and hypothalamus often present with overt signs of increased ICP from local mass effect and obstructive hydrocephalus, reflecting occlusion of the foramen of Monro. In older children, optic pathway tumors with hypothalamic involvement can also manifest with endocrine abnormalities, such as growth delay or precocious puberty, weight gain from hyperphagia, and personality changes. In contrast, infants with large hypothalamic tumors may exhibit macrocephaly, increased ICP, and failure to thrive in conjunction with the so-called diencephalic syndrome with emaciation in association with virtual absence of subcutaneous fat. Larger tumors may also lead to focal neurological deficits from compression of the sensorimotor pathways and upper cranial nerves.

23.3   Diagnostics

Magnetic resonance imaging (MRI) is the diagnostic test of choice to detect an optic pathway tumor, although if unavailable, computerized tomography (CT) may be used to provide useful preliminary information. MRI also delineates the vessels of the circle of Willis, which often avoids the need for an angiogram if surgery is contemplated. A number of characteristic lesion types may be seen. The mildest abnormalities, typically seen in patients with NF1, consist only of thickening of one or both optic nerves [4]; although most such lesions are low-grade gliomas, others may simply represent hyperplasia of the optic nerve sheath. Other patients exhibit a globular thickening of the optic nerves and chiasm (Fig. 23.1a) that may occur in conjunction with T2 signal abnormalities that extend along the optic pathways, often as far as the occipital lobes, and may reach superiorly into the hypothalamus. Although biopsy of such lesions is usually not required to establish the diagnosis in the setting of NF1, those lesions that have been biopsied have typically been found to be low-grade

gliomas histologically [9, 10]. Finally, a third group of patients present with a large mass lesion involving the optic chiasm and hypothalamus that may extend upward into the third ventricle, laterally into the temporal fossa, anteriorly beneath the frontal lobes, and posteriorly into the perimesencephalic region [11] (Fig. 23.1b). In such cases, a diagnosis of a low-grade glioma is inferred, but a biopsy may be warranted to exclude other less likely etiologies, such as germ cell tumors or, in cystic cases, craniopharyngiomas.

Because the majority of optic pathway tumors are low-grade astrocytomas, they are typically hypodense on CT and hypointense on T1-weighted MRI in comparison to the surrounding brain. After administration of contrast medium, some tumors show uniform enhancement, whereas others have mixed signal characteristics reflecting associated cystic components. Although the majority of cases are unifocal, approximately 5% of tumors exhibit dissemination throughout the neuraxis [12], and if this is suspected, spinal MRI may be warranted to assess the pattern of spread, and a cytological examination may be considered, provided there are no ICP-related contraindications.

If the child is clinically stable, a comprehensive neuro-ophthalmologic evaluation is warranted; hypothalamic tumors also merit an endocrinologic evaluation. The ophthalmologic evaluation should include fundoscopy and evaluation of visual fixation in infants; in older children, a formal assessment of visual acuity and visual fields is also recommended. Visual evoked responses are considered helpful in some institutions. Endocrinologic evaluation should include assessments of cortisol and thyroid hormone production, with institution of appropriate cortisol and thyroid hormone replacement, if warranted, including provision of stress doses of corticosteroids during the perioperative period, if surgery is considered. Prolactin levels are often elevated secondary to compression of the pituitary stalk. Diabetes insipidus is uncommon with optic pathway gliomas at initial presentation and if present should raise the possibility that the mass is some other histology. Evaluation of the growth

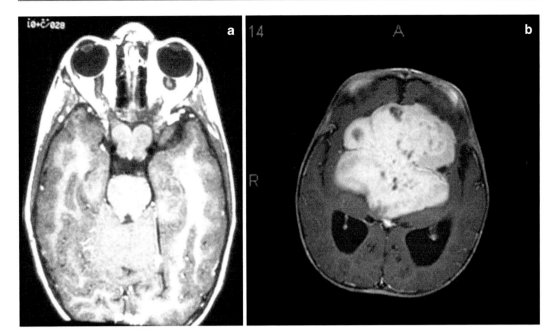

Fig. 23.1 This series of MR images illustrates the diverse manifestations of optic-hypothalamic gliomas. (**a**) Globular enlargement of the optic chiasm is depicted in a child with NF1. In this patient, T2 signal abnormality was seen along the optic tracts bilaterally. (**b**) A massive chiasmatic-hypothalamic glioma shows bright enhancement with intravenous contrast

hormone and gonadotrophic hormone hypothalamopituitary axes are beneficial but are more likely to show actionable abnormalities after the completion of therapy, such as surgery or radiation therapy. In older children, detailed neuropsychological assessments may also be helpful, since these tumors and their associated treatment may cause cognitive impairment as well as neurobehavioral issues that warrant ongoing management.

23.4 Staging and Classification

The vast majority of optic pathway tumors in children are low-grade gliomas, and most of these are pilocytic astrocytomas, with the remainder consisting of gangliogliomas and low-grade nonpilocytic astrocytomas, such as fibrillary and pilomyxoid astrocytomas [5, 13], the latter of which are considered Grade II in current classifications. In older teenagers and adults, anaplastic optic gliomas have been described, although such tumors are rare in younger children, unless the

patient previously received radiotherapy [14] and are beyond the scope of this chapter.

In general, staging of the neuraxis is not required in patients with optic gliomas. As noted earlier, a small percentage of non-NF1-related visual pathway tumors exhibit leptomeningeal dissemination [12], and some investigators have recommended at least a spinal MRI for patients with large chiasmatic-hypothalamic lesions. Similarly, because patients with NF1 can manifest with other lesions throughout the neuraxis, some investigators favor obtaining a total neuraxis MRI as a component of the initial diagnostic work-up.

In recent years, the molecular characteristics of the tumor have come to assume an increasingly important role in treatment planning. Studies over the last decade have demonstrated that pilocytic astrocytomas commonly have low-level copy number gains involving the BRAF locus, often reflecting one of several translocation events between the BRAF gene and the KIAA1549 gene [15, 16]. Another subset of tumors has activating mutations in the BRAF gene, most commonly the BRAF[v600E] mutant [15–17], and a separate group has translocations involving the RAF gene or alterations of other upstream regulators of MAPK signalling [18], the most common being the neurofibromin mutation seen in NF1-related tumors. Taken together, more than 80% of pilocytic astrocytomas have alterations in at least one component of the MAPK signalling pathway, which provides a series of novel molecular targets for therapeutic intervention, highlighting the clinical importance of molecular characterization in the overall classification of these tumors.

23.5 Treatment

23.5.1 General Considerations

The optimal management for optic gliomas has evolved substantially over the years. Before the era of high-resolution CT and MRI, optic pathway tumors were generally detected after the onset of overt symptoms, such as visual impairment, hypothalamic dysfunction, or increased ICP, which clearly mandated therapeutic intervention. However, in the current era, many lesions, particularly in children with NF1, are now detected in asymptomatic or minimally symptomatic children in whom the natural history after incidental detection on screening examinations is unpredictable in any given child. In such patients with characteristic involvement of the anterior visual pathway, the diagnosis can be established without the need for biopsy [2, 9], and serial surveillance imaging may be the most prudent course.

Several studies have reported the results of expectant management in patients with NF1 who had optic pathway tumors that were either asymptomatic or minimally symptomatic with mild visual loss or precocious puberty [9, 10, 19]. Hoffman et al. noted that, in a series of 15 such patients who either had no therapy or only a diagnostic biopsy, 13 had stable disease at long-term follow-up [9]. Similarly, Listernick et al. noted that only 3 of 33 asymptomatic or minimally symptomatic patients with optic pathway tumors

exhibited progressive tumor growth or deteriorating vision after diagnosis with a median follow-up of 2.4 years [19]. These and other studies suggest that optic gliomas in children with NF1 have a distinctly more indolent course than in those without this disorder [8, 20]. In view of the unpredictable growth in any given case, periodic imaging surveillance is warranted until the natural history can be established conclusively.

In that context, it is important to recognize that a subset of children with NF1 will manifest progressive visual impairment, and in such children chemotherapeutic interventions may be beneficial [20], since the likelihood of disease control was actually superior to that in children without NF1 in the recent large Children's Oncology Group trial [20].

Another important caveat is that in non-NF1 patients with an isolated chiasmatic-hypothalamic lesion without extension along the optic tracts or radiations, the diagnosis cannot be confidently made based on MRI alone, and histological confirmation is warranted to rule out other histologies that may require vastly different treatments. In selected cases with substantial exophytic growth, surgical debulking may also achieve prompt relief of intracranial mass effect and improvement of neurological symptoms [11].

23.5.2 Surgery

Because most optic pathway gliomas cannot be completely resected without significant morbidity, and many can be diagnosed based on MRI alone and remain indolent or respond well to adjuvant therapy, the operative indications for extensive resection have become increasingly limited in recent years. Historically, surgical resection was often advocated for tumors that were thought to be restricted to a single optic nerve if there was evidence of severe visual compromise and proptosis, to prevent "spread" to the chiasm and contralateral side [6, 21]. However, because many of these lesions arise in patients with NF1, who almost always have bilateral abnormalities on MRI, the rationale for prophylactic resection of a unilaterally more apparent

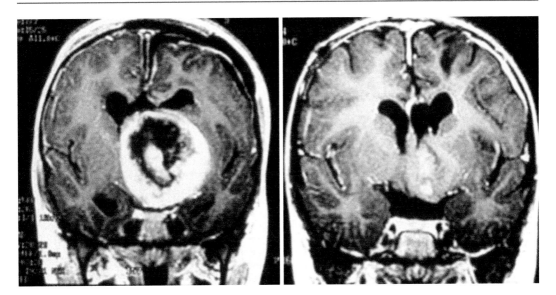

Fig. 23.2 Left: Large hypothalamic glioma that was treated with biopsy and limited debulking, followed by carboplatin and vincristine. Right: Follow-up MRI scan upon completion of induction chemotherapy. The patient's tumor continued to regress during treatment, but ultimately progressed off therapy 5 years later, and again responded to treatment with the above agents

tumor no longer applies in many cases, and such patients are often treated initially with adjuvant therapy. In their historical literature review, Alvord and Lofton commented that patients with NF1 appeared to have a high incidence of intracranial tumor "recurrence" after removal of an affected optic nerve [6], which is not surprising in view of the current MRI data. However, in the rare patient with an optic nerve glioma that is truly unilateral, in whom proptosis and severe visual loss are apparent, surgical resection of the involved nerve from the globe to the chiasm may be a reasonable treatment approach.

Optic gliomas in patients without a diagnosis of NF1 generally involve the optic chiasm and hypothalamus, and, in such cases, the goals of surgery are to establish a histological diagnosis and, if feasible, to relieve local mass effect. A third goal that has become more relevant over time is the need to define the molecular characteristics of the tumor, which may influence adjuvant treatment options. Diagnosis can often be achieved by minimally invasive strategies, such as endoscopic or stereotactic biopsy, but in some situations, an open approach may be preferred. Because most tumors will respond to adjuvant therapy (Fig. 23.2), many centers now prefer to obtain a biopsy, reserving resection for lesions that grow despite medical therapy and exhibit increasing mass effect. In some instances, a well-timed tumor debulking will stabilize the patient sufficiently that additional chemotherapy or irradiation can be administered, leading to long-term disease control.

However, for certain tumors with significant neurological compromise or bilateral ventricular obstruction from tumor growing exophytically from the optic chiasm and hypothalamus, extensive resection may be preferred as an initial intervention [6, 9, 11]. In such cases, the operative approach is determined by the growth pattern of the tumor. For lesions mushrooming anteriorly or above the chiasm and displacing the third ventricle posteriorly, a subfrontal and interhemispheric approach may be combined with opening the lamina terminalis. For lesions extending more posterosuperiorly into the third and possibly lateral ventricles, a transcallosal approach allows access to the dome of the tumor and re-establishment of intraventricular CSF flow pathways. Finally, for more laterally projecting tumors, a pterional and/or subtemporal approach can provide access to the bulk of the tumor. Although complete resection is not feasible because these lesions infiltrate the optic chiasm and hypothalamus, substantial cytoreduction can sometimes be achieved [9, 11]. Because these tumors often engulf arteries of the circle of Willis, care must be taken during the resection to avoid injury to these vessels. Although several groups have advocated a general management approach of surgery for children with large tumors growing exophytically from the optic chiasm [9, 11], it remains uncertain whether the long-term results in terms of disease stability and functional outcome are superior to those achieved with more conservative management approaches [22].

23.5.3 Radiotherapy

Radiation therapy has long been used for the treatment of optic pathway tumors [6, 10, 23, 24]. This approach provides excellent results in terms of disease stabilization and tumor regression and can result in improvement in visual function if the visual loss is not long-standing. For example, Pierce et al. [10] reported 6-year progression-free and overall survival rates of 88 and 100% in 24 children with symptomatic chiasmal gliomas who received >4500 cGy of radiotherapy. Vision improved in 7 patients and remained stable in 14 [10]. However, radiation can produce significant cognitive and endocrine deficits [25–27] and places the patient at risk for radiation-induced malignancies [14] and vasculopathy, such as moyamoya syndrome [28, 29]. Patients with NF1 are at particular risk of developing these complications. One review found that 9 of 18 (50%) patients with NF1 who received radiotherapy as treatment for an optic pathway tumor developed second tumors as compared to 8 of 40 patients (20%) who were not treated with radiotherapy [30].

As a way to reduce these risks, there has been increasing interest in using conformal techniques to more precisely deliver radiation to the tumor and a narrow margin while limiting doses to the surrounding brain. Stereotactic radiosurgery [31], which administers a high dose of radiation

in a single fraction, has demonstrated efficacy against progressive low-grade gliomas, but because this approach is generally not applicable for lesions greater than 3 cm in diameter, and dose reduction is required for irradiating the optic apparatus, this technique has been applied very selectively for chiasmatic-hypothalamic gliomas. However, new methods of delivering fractionated radiotherapy to a conformal treatment volume using three-dimensional image-based treatment planning and narrow peritumoral margins (i.e., stereotactic radiotherapy) do appear to have broad applicability for these tumors as a strategy to theoretically reduce treatment-induced morbidity without sacrificing long-term disease control [32, 33]. This approach has been applied in a pilot study involving 50 children with progressive low-grade gliomas, in whom the target included the preoperative tumor volume with a 2-mm margin, with doses ranging from 5000 to 5800 cGy in standard fractions. After a median follow-up of 6.9 years, the progression-free survival rate was 82.5% at 5 years and 65% at 8 years. The overall survival rate was 97.8% at 5 years and 82% at 8 years. Six patients had local progression, two of which evolved to higher-grade lesions, and five had dissemination; there were no marginal failures [33]. However, extended follow-up will be needed to determine whether these approaches are truly beneficial in terms of maintaining progression-free survival and functional status. This strategy was evaluated in detail in a larger cohort in the Children's Oncology Group (COG) ACNS0221 study, although final results are pending at this point.

23.5.4 Chemotherapy

In view of the known sequelae of irradiation, chemotherapy has come to assume an increasing role in the management of optic pathway tumors, particularly for patients younger than 10 years of age [8, 34–40], in whom the long-term risks of radiotherapy-induced cognitive and endocrine impairment are particularly high and the potential benefits of avoiding, or at least deferring, radiotherapy are substantial. A variety of regimens have been employed, with response rates of 20–80% and response or stabilization rates of 75–100% [8, 34–40]. In one of the earliest pilot studies, Packer et al. [36] administered 6 8-week cycles of actinomycin D and vincristine to 24 patients with a median time to disease progression of 3 years in the 9 patients who initially presented with tumor growth; 15 other children remained progression-free with a median follow-up of 3.1 years. Based on these encouraging initial results, a variety of other regimens have subsequently been examined. One regimen that has been extensively evaluated combines carboplatin and vincristine (Fig. 23.2). In a multi-institutional study in 78 children with unresectable, progressive disease (median age, 3.1 years), 44 patients showed an objective response to treatment, and 29 had stable disease, allowing a significant delay in radiotherapy in more than 85% of children. Progression-free survival at 3 years was $68 \pm 7\%$ [35]. A second regimen that has been widely employed combines thioguanine, procarbazine, CCNU, and vincristine (TPCV) [37, 40]. In the initial pilot study, this combination was utilized in 19 infants and young children, 12 at the time of diagnosis and 7 after tumor progression. Fifteen patients either responded to therapy or stabilized. The median time to tumor progression was 30.3 months with a 5-year survival rate of 82.7% [37]. The efficacy and tolerability of these two regimens were compared in the COG A9952 study [8]. The results with the TPCV regimen were nominally superior, but did not reach statistical significance based on a stratified log-rank test. For both regimens, younger age, larger tumor size, and involvement of the diencephalon were adverse prognostic factors.

The efficacy of the carboplatin/vincristine regimen in children with NF1-associated low-grade gliomas was also assessed in the COG A9952 study [20]. Such children were nonrandomly assigned to the carboplatin/vincristine arm because of concerns about the increased risk of secondary leukemias from alkylating agents, which has provided a rationale for avoiding such agents in frontline regimens. The notable observation from this study was the much lower rate of disease progression among the NF1 cohort compared to non-NF1 group that received either regimen in the randomized component of the trial, highlighting the impact of NF1 status on the pace of disease growth.

Other agents that have shown activity against low-grade gliomas include vinblastine [41–43], temozolomide [38], and the combination of temozolomide and carboplatin [39]. Antiangiogenic agents, such as lenalidomide [44] and bevacizumab [45], have also been observed to have activity in pilot studies to treat these tumors.

More recently, agents designed to interfere with the constitutively activated BRAF signalling pathway of these tumors [46] have been evaluated. In a phase 1 dose-finding study with selumetinib, 20% of children had objective tumor responses, and 2-year progression-free survival was $69 \pm 9.8\%$ among patients treated at the recommended phase 2 dose [47]. These encouraging results have formed a foundation for a phase 2 study of this agent that stratifies enrollment based on tumor molecular features (e.g., BRAF translocation, BRAF activating mutations, NF1 mutations), which is incorporating detailed molecular and imaging analyses to define the response and disease control rates in different tumor subsets.

23.6 Prognosis/Quality of Life

Although most optic pathway gliomas of childhood are histologically benign, the inherent unresectability of these lesions leads to a substantially worse prognosis than for other low-grade gliomas that are more amenable to resection. Gliomas restricted to the optic nerves rarely prove fatal [6] but can lead to progressive visual compromise. In contrast, chiasmatic-hypothalamic gliomas can eventually lead to extensive morbidity and, in some cases, mortality. In a large postoperative natural history study conducted by the Children's Cancer Group and Pediatric Oncology Group (9891/8930), 4-year progression-free survival was approximately 50% for patients with chiasmatic-hypothalamic gliomas, with a 4-year overall survival of 90% [48]. These percentages were comparable to those of other low-grade gliomas that were not amenable to total resection. In a single institution review of children with hypothalamic and/or chiasmatic gliomas, the 6-year overall survival rate was $86 \pm 5\%$ and was not affected by initial treatment [49]. Symptomatic chiasmatic-hypothalamic tumors in NF1 patients seem to carry a more favorable prognosis for long-term disease control than comparable tumors in patients without NF1 [9, 20, 49, 50]. For example, Hoffman et al. noted that whereas only 1 of 23 patients with NF1 and optic-hypothalamic glioma died of disease progression, 7 of 39 patients without NF1 died ($p = 0.045$) [9]. Deliganis et al. [50] also noted that time to progression among children with newly diagnosed symptomatic optic pathway gliomas arising in association with NF1 was substantially longer than for patients with sporadic tumors (8.4 years versus 2.4 years, respectively). With an average follow-up of 10.2 years, only 5 of 16 patients with NF1 exhibited disease progression [50]. A similar progression-free survival advantage was also noted in the A9952 study following treatment with carboplatin-vincristine chemotherapy [20]. In addition, a small subset of tumors exhibit spontaneous regression in the absence of surgical or adjuvant therapy [7].

A disappointing feature of these tumors is that given the fact that there is almost always residual disease after surgery, chemotherapy, and radiation, there is a substantial incidence of late tumor progression, particularly in the non-NF1 subgroup, a factor that is not well captured on studies having less than 10 years of follow-up. Although actuarial survival rates of 70–90% have been reported at 10 years [23, 24], in the literature review by Alvord and Lofton, the cumulative frequency of progression and death was noted to progressively increase with follow-up times up to 20 years, by which time approximately 40% of children had died [6]. This fits with anecdotal observations that a subset of children diagnosed within the first few years of life die of recurrent, increasingly aggressive, disease in young adulthood. In some cases, this reflects malignant progression of the original tumor, potentially from prior irradiation [14, 33], or a secondary malignancy from prior therapy, but in other cases the tumor remains histologically benign, although increasingly invasive.

Although detailed quality-of-life studies in surviving patients have been lacking in the literature, it is clear that long-term survivors have a high incidence of visual, cognitive, behavioral, and endocrinological morbidity, as a result of both the tumor itself and its treatment with surgery and irradiation. In one report of 33 patients treated with relatively conservative surgery and a combination of irradiation and chemotherapy, 5 patients had died, 5 were functionally blind, 14 had useful vision in only one eye, and all but 12 required endocrine replacement; only half had completed or were in school [22]. Another follow-up report on 38 children with low-grade gliomas treated between 1994 and 2000 found that 61% of children had neurologic or endocrine impairments, 45% required special education or remedial help in school, and 10% had severe disabilities [51]. The frequency and severity of the disabilities depended on tumor location, age, and disease recurrence. Patients who have received radiotherapy are also at risk for second malignancies within the treatment volume and radiation-induced vasculopathy. It remains to be determined whether these outcomes are improved with a policy of more limited surgery and initial treatment with chemotherapy or biological therapy or with the use of more conformally directed irradiation. The results of COG ACNS0221 study and the ongoing studies of BRAF pathway inhibitors may help to address these issues.

23.7 Follow-Up/Specific Problems and Measures

There are no objective standards for follow-up in children with optic pathway tumors. In general, for children with NF1 who have newly diagnosed, asymptomatic tumors, where intervention is deferred until there is either clinical or radiographic progression, follow-up MRI and ophthalmological evaluations may be performed 3–4 months after diagnosis. If these are stable, follow-up evaluations may gradually extend to yearly intervals, depending on the age of the child and the size and enhancement characteristics of the tumor. Once the child is past the middle school years, the likelihood of tumor progression appears to decrease, particularly for those tumors that are non-enhancing or have lost their enhancement, and surveillance imaging can often be performed less frequently. For non-NF1 patients, who generally present with symptomatic tumors and are enrolled on a course of therapy, follow-up evaluations are performed at approximately 3-month intervals for the first year (with the specific timing defined by the protocol being followed, typically occurring at the completion of chemotherapy induction, completion of every two or three courses of therapy, or completion of irradiation). After completion of a therapeutic regimen, evaluations may be performed at 4- to 6-month intervals for the next few years if the patient is stable and subsequently on an annual basis. A transient increase in the size and enhancement of the lesion within a year of completing radiation therapy is common and, unless progressive, should not be assumed to represent treatment failure or malignant degeneration. The full effect of irradiation is often not seen for up to 2 years.

If clinically indicated, follow-up endocrinological evaluations are also warranted to detect delayed dysfunction of the hypothalamopituitary axis, which is a particular concern in patients who have received radiotherapy and those with progressive disease. In view of the high risk of cognitive and behavioral abnormalities in children with these tumors, neuropsychological evaluation is helpful if not essential to identify educational resources as well as accommodations for visual and cognitive impairments that may be required to optimize long-term functional outcome.

23.8 Future Perspectives

A major advance during the last 20 years has been the widespread incorporation of chemotherapy into the initial management of symptomatic, progressive, or high-risk chiasmatic-hypothalamic gliomas. A9952 compared the activity and tolerability of two active treatment regimens, carboplatin and vincristine versus 6-thioguanine, procarbazine, CCNU, and vincristine, and subsequent studies have examined other chemotherapeutic agents, which also have activity. A large pilot study, which should be nearing publication, has tested the safety of conformally administered irradiation for tumors in children older than 10 years and those younger than 10 years who have disease progression after initial chemotherapy. As an essential element in evaluating the success of these approaches for improving not only the duration but also the quality of survival, these studies incorporate analyses of endocrine and functional status, using validated quality-of-life indicators.

More recent advances have come in the form of biological therapy for these tumors. A series of studies evaluated antiangiogenic agents, such as lenalidomide [44] and bevacizumab [45], in the management of these tumors. More recently, the widespread detection of mutations and gene fusions affecting mediators within the MAP kinase signalling pathway has opened the possibility for precision medicine-based molecularly targeted therapies for these tumors. The preliminary results have been extremely exciting [47] and have provided an impetus for larger-scale studies designed to determine whether particular patterns of genomic alterations correlate with treatment response. Lastly, recent studies have demonstrated a potential role for immunotherapy in children with treatment-refractory low-grade gliomas, targeting antigens overexpressed in the tumor relative to the normal brain. In one pilot study, objective imaging responses were noted in 5 of 13 evaluable children and immunological responses in 12 of 12 [52], and a phase II study is in progress to further evaluate these intriguing observations.

Acknowledgments This work was supported in part by NIH grant 1R01CA187219, the Pediatric Low-Grade Glioma Initiative via the National Brain Tumor Society, and the Connor's Cure Fund, the Ian Yagoda's Friends Foundation, and the Translational Brain Tumor Fund of the Children's Hospital of Pittsburgh Foundation.

References

1. Pollack IF (1994) Brain tumors in children. N Engl J Med 331(22):1500–1507
2. Pollack IF (2014) Neurofibromatosis 1 and 2. In: Albright AL, Pollack IF, Adelson PD (eds) Principles and practice of pediatric neurosurgery, 3rd edn. Thieme, New York, pp 626–641
3. Xu GF, O'Connell P, Viskochil D, Cawthon R, Robertson M, Culver M et al (1990) The neurofibromatosis type 1 gene encodes a protein related to GAP. Cell 62(3):599–608
4. FJ DM Jr, Ramsby G, Greenstein R, Langshur S, Dunham B (1993) Neurofibromatosis type 1: magnetic resonance imaging findings. J Child Neurol 8(1):32–39
5. Louis DN, Perry A, Reifenberger G, von Deimling A, Figarella-Branger D, Cavenee WK et al (2016) The 2016 World Health Organization classification of tumors of the central nervous system: a summary. Acta Neuropathol 131(6):803–820
6. Alvord EC Jr, Lofton S (1988) Gliomas of the optic nerve or chiasm. Outcome by patients' age, tumor site, and treatment. J Neurosurg 68(1):85–98
7. Perilongo G, Moras P, Carollo C, Battistella A, Clementi M, Laverda A et al (1999) Spontaneous partial regression of low-grade glioma in children with neurofibromatosis-1: a real possibility. J Child Neurol 14(6):352–356
8. Ater JL, Zhou T, Holmes E, Mazewski CM, Booth TN, Freyer DR et al (2012) Randomized study of two chemotherapy regimens for treatment of low-grade glioma in young children: a report from the Children's Oncology Group. J Clin Oncol 30(21):2641–2647
9. Hoffman HJ, Humphreys RP, Drake JM, Rutka JT, Becker LE, Jenkin D et al (1993) Optic pathway/hypothalamic gliomas: a dilemma in management. Pediatr Neurosurg 19(4):186–195
10. Pierce SM, Barnes PD, Loeffler JS, McGinn C, Tarbell NJ (1990) Definitive radiation therapy in the management of symptomatic patients with optic glioma. Survival and long-term effects. Cancer 65(1):45–52
11. Wisoff JH, Abbott R, Epstein F (1990) Surgical management of exophytic chiasmatic-hypothalamic tumors of childhood. J Neurosurg 73(5):661–667
12. Hukin J, Siffert J, Velasquez L, Zagzag D, Allen J (2002) Leptomeningeal dissemination in children with progressive low-grade neuroepithelial tumors. Neuro Oncol 4(4):253–260
13. Tihan T, Fisher PG, Kepner JL, Godfraind C, McComb RD, Goldthwaite PT et al (1999) Pediatric astrocytomas with monomorphous pilomyxoid features and a less favorable outcome. J Neuropathol Exp Neurol 58(10):1061–1068
14. Dirks PB, Jay V, Becker LE, Drake JM, Humphreys RP, Hoffman HJ et al (1994) Development of anaplastic changes in low-grade astrocytomas of childhood. Neurosurgery 34(1):68–78
15. Jones DT, Kocialkowski S, Liu L, Pearson DM, Backlund LM, Ichimura K et al (2008) Tandem duplication producing a novel oncogenic BRAF fusion gene defines the majority of pilocytic astrocytomas. Cancer Res 68(21):8673–8677
16. Pfister S, Janzarik WG, Remke M, Ernst A, Werft W, Becker N et al (2008) BRAF gene duplication constitutes a mechanism of MAPK pathway activation in low-grade astrocytomas. J Clin Invest 118(5):1739–1749
17. Horbinski C, Nikiforova MN, Hagenkord JM, Hamilton RL, Pollack IF (2012) Interplay among BRAF, p16, p53, and MIB1 in pediatric low-grade gliomas. Neuro Oncol 14(6):777–789
18. Jones DT, Kocialkowski S, Liu L, Pearson DM, Ichimura K, Collins VP (2009) Oncogenic RAF1 rearrangement and a novel BRAF mutation as alternatives to KIAA1549:BRAF fusion in activating the MAPK pathway in pilocytic astrocytoma. Oncogene 28(20):2119–2123
19. Listernick R, Charrow J, Greenwald M, Mets M (1994) Natural history of optic pathway tumors in children with neurofibromatosis type 1: a longitudinal study. J Pediatr 125(1):63–66
20. Ater JL, Xia C, Mazewski CM, Booth TN, Freyer DR, Packer RJ et al (2016) Nonrandomized comparison of neurofibromatosis type 1 and non-neurofibromatosis type 1 children who received carboplatin and vincristine for progressive low-grade glioma: a report from the Children's Oncology Group. Cancer 122(12):1928–1936
21. Housepian EM, Chi TL (1993) Neurofibromatosis and optic pathways gliomas. J Neurooncol 15(1):51–55
22. Sutton LN, Molloy PT, Sernyak H, Goldwein J, Phillips PL, Rorke LB et al (1995) Long-term outcome of hypothalamic/chiasmatic astrocytomas in children treated with conservative surgery. J Neurosurg 83(4):583–589
23. Kovalic JJ, Grigsby PW, Shepard MJ, Fineberg BB, Thomas PR (1990) Radiation therapy for gliomas of the optic nerve and chiasm. Int J Radiat Oncol Biol Phys 18(4):927–932
24. Rodriguez LA, Edwards MS, Levin VA (1990) Management of hypothalamic gliomas in children: an analysis of 33 cases. Neurosurgery 26(2):242–246; discussion 6–7
25. Donahue B (1992) Short- and long-term complications of radiation therapy for pediatric brain tumors. Pediatr Neurosurg 18(4):207–217
26. Livesey EA, Hindmarsh PC, Brook CG, Whitton AC, Bloom HJ, Tobias JS et al (1990) Endocrine disorders following treatment of childhood brain tumours. Br J Cancer 61(4):622–625
27. Lustig RH, Post SR, Srivannaboon K, Rose SR, Danish RK, Burghen GA et al (2003) Risk factors for the development of obesity in children surviving brain tumors. J Clin Endocrinol Metab 88(2):611–616
28. Grill J, Couanet D, Cappelli C, Habrand JL, Rodriguez D, Sainte-Rose C et al (1999) Radiation-induced cerebral vasculopathy in children with neu-

rofibromatosis and optic pathway glioma. Ann Neurol 45(3):393–396

29. Kestle JR, Hoffman HJ, Mock AR (1993) Moyamoya phenomenon after radiation for optic glioma. J Neurosurg 79(1):32–35

30. Sharif S, Ferner R, Birch JM, Gillespie JE, Gattamaneni HR, Baser ME et al (2006) Second primary tumors in neurofibromatosis 1 patients treated for optic glioma: substantial risks after radiotherapy. J Clin Oncol 24(16):2570–2575

31. Grabb PA, Lunsford LD, Albright AL, Kondziolka D, Flickinger JC (1996) Stereotactic radiosurgery for glial neoplasms of childhood. Neurosurgery 38(4):696–701; discussion 2

32. Nishihori T, Shirato H, Aoyama H, Onimaru R, Komae T, Ishii N et al (2002) Three-dimensional conformal radiotherapy for astrocytic tumors involving the eloquent area in children and young adults. J Neurooncol 60(2):177–183

33. Marcus KJ, Goumnerova L, Billett AL, Lavally B, Scott RM, Bishop K et al (2005) Stereotactic radiotherapy for localized low-grade gliomas in children: final results of a prospective trial. Int J Radiat Oncol Biol Phys 61(2):374–379

34. Gururangan S, Cavazos CM, Ashley D, Herndon JE 2nd, Bruggers CS, Moghrabi A et al (2002) Phase II study of carboplatin in children with progressive low-grade gliomas. J Clin Oncol 20(13):2951–2958

35. Packer RJ, Ater J, Allen J, Phillips P, Geyer R, Nicholson HS et al (1997) Carboplatin and vincristine chemotherapy for children with newly diagnosed progressive low-grade gliomas. J Neurosurg 86(5):747–754

36. Packer RJ, Sutton LN, Bilaniuk LT, Radcliffe J, Rosenstock JG, Siegel KR et al (1988) Treatment of chiasmatic/hypothalamic gliomas of childhood with chemotherapy: an update. Ann Neurol 23(1):79–85

37. Petronio J, Edwards MS, Prados M, Freyberger S, Rabbitt J, Silver P et al (1991) Management of chiasmal and hypothalamic gliomas of infancy and childhood with chemotherapy. J Neurosurg 74(5):701–708

38. Nicholson HS, Kretschmar CS, Krailo M, Bernstein M, Kadota R, Fort D et al (2007) Phase 2 study of temozolomide in children and adolescents with recurrent central nervous system tumors: a report from the Children's Oncology Group. Cancer 110(7):1542–1550

39. Chintagumpala M, Eckel SP, Krailo M, Morris M, Adesina A, Packer R et al (2015) A pilot study using carboplatin, vincristine, and temozolomide in children with progressive/symptomatic low-grade glioma: a Children's Oncology Group study. Neuro Oncol 17(8):1132–1138

40. Mishra KK, Squire S, Lamborn K, Banerjee A, Gupta N, Wara WM et al (2010) Phase II TPDCV protocol for pediatric low-grade hypothalamic/chiasmatic gliomas: 15-year update. J Neurooncol 100(1):121–127

41. Lafay-Cousin L, Holm S, Qaddoumi I, Nicolin G, Bartels U, Tabori U et al (2005) Weekly vinblastine in pediatric low-grade glioma patients with carboplatin allergic reaction. Cancer 103(12):2636–2642

42. Lassaletta A, Scheinemann K, Zelcer SM, Hukin J, Wilson BA, Jabado N et al (2016) Phase II weekly vinblastine for chemotherapy-naive children with progressive low-grade glioma: a Canadian Pediatric Brain Tumor Consortium Study. J Clin Oncol 34(29):3537–3543

43. Singh G, Wei XC, Hader W, Chan JA, Bouffet E, Lafay-Cousin L (2013) Sustained response to weekly vinblastine in 2 children with pilomyxoid astrocytoma associated with diencephalic syndrome. J Pediatr Hematol Oncol 35(2):e53–e56

44. Warren KE, Goldman S, Pollack IF, Fangusaro J, Schaiquevich P, Stewart CF et al (2011) Phase I trial of lenalidomide in pediatric patients with recurrent, refractory, or progressive primary CNS tumors: Pediatric Brain Tumor Consortium study PBTC-018. J Clin Oncol 29(3):324–329

45. Gururangan S, Fangusaro J, Poussaint TY, McLendon RE, Onar-Thomas A, Wu S et al (2014) Efficacy of bevacizumab plus irinotecan in children with recurrent low-grade gliomas—a Pediatric Brain Tumor Consortium study. Neuro Oncol 16(2):310–317

46. Kolb EA, Gorlick R, Houghton PJ, Morton CL, Neale G, Keir ST et al (2010) Initial testing (stage 1) of AZD6244 (ARRY-142886) by the Pediatric Preclinical Testing Program. Pediatr Blood Cancer 55(4):668–677

47. Banerjee A, Jakacki RI, Onar-Thomas A, Wu S, Nicolaides T, Young Poussaint T et al (2017) A phase I trial of the MEK inhibitor selumetinib (AZD6244) in pediatric patients with recurrent or refractory low-grade glioma: a Pediatric Brain Tumor Consortium (PBTC) study. Neuro Oncol 19(8):1135–1144

48. Wisoff JH, Sanford RA, Heier LA, Sposto R, Burger PC, Yates AJ et al (2011) Primary neurosurgery for pediatric low-grade gliomas: a prospective multi-institutional study from the Children's Oncology Group. Neurosurgery 68(6):1548–1554; discussion 54–5

49. Foulad M, Wallace D, Langston JW, Mulhern R, Rose SR, Gajjar A et al (2003) Survival and functional outcome of children with hypothalamic/chiasmatic tumors. Cancer 97(4):1084–1092

50. Deliganis AV, Geyer JR, Berger MS (1996) Prognostic significance of type 1 neurofibromatosis (von Recklinghausen Disease) in childhood optic glioma. Neurosurgery 38(6):1114–1118; discussion 8–9

51. Aarsen FK, Paquier PF, Reddingius RE, Streng IC, Arts WF, Evera-Preesman M et al (2006) Functional outcome after low-grade astrocytoma treatment in childhood. Cancer 106(2):396–402

52. Pollack IF, Jakacki RI, Butterfield LH, Hamilton RL, Panigrahy A, Normolle DP et al (2016) Immune responses and outcome after vaccination with glioma-associated antigen peptides and poly-ICLC in a pilot study for pediatric recurrent low-grade gliomas. Neuro Oncol 18(8):1157–1168

Ganglioglioma

24

Christian Dorfer

24.1 Introduction

According to the World Health Organization gangliogliomas are classified as well-differentiated and slowly growing neuroepithelial tumors. They were first identified by Perkins in 1926 as a distinct type of intracranial neoplasms with a biphasic morphologic pattern composed of dysplastic neuronal cell elements (i.e., ganglion cells) and neoplastic glial cell elements (i.e., glioma cells) [41]. They account for only 0.5% of all central nervous system tumors and 1–5% of all pediatric CNS tumors [1, 5, 8, 55]. They typically occur in young patients with median ages ranging from 8 to 26 years [5, 17], and there is a prevalence of male compared to female patients (1.25:1.0) [17].

They can occur throughout the CNS with the following predilection sites in descending frequency: temporal lobe (68%), frontal lobe (10%), parietal lobe (9%), cerebellum (6%), brainstem (4%), and spinal cord (3%) [17, 35, 60].

When considering gangliogliomas as a group, they represent a benign clinical entity with 5 and 10 year overall survival rates of >90% and 80%, respectively. However, from a clinical perspective, ganglioglioma may be separately discussed depending on their location as supratentorial, posterior fossa, and spinal tumors.

C. Dorfer (✉)
Department of Neurosurgery, Medical University of Vienna, Vienna, Austria
e-mail: christian.dorfer@meduniwien.ac.at

24.2 Supratentorial Tumors

24.2.1 Symptoms and Clinical Signs

In the supratentorial compartment, about 70% of all tumors are located in the temporal lobe involving its mesial structures, and seizures are the most common presenting symptom [17]. The prevalent temporal location, direct cortico/subcortical involvement, and slow tumor growth all contribute to the high rate of seizures associated with GG. Even more, gangliogliomas can be identified as a structural lesion underlying chronic temporal lobe epilepsy in 20–40% of patients in cohorts that undergo neurosurgery [35]. The pathogenic mechanism underlying the epileptogenesis in ganglioglioma is poorly understood. It is either the neuronal component of the tumor itself that may contribute to the epileptic activity or the tumor-associated epileptic changes of the adjacent brain [7, 58].

A clinical presentation other than seizures is far less frequent and includes focal neurological deficits mainly in parietal and deeply located tumors as well as symptoms of increased intracranial pressure (5%) [31, 61].

24.2.2 Imaging

24.2.2.1 MRI

Supratentorial ganglioglioma typically present as solid or solid-cystic tumors (50–50%) [26].

© Springer Nature Switzerland AG 2019
J.-C. Tonn et al. (eds.), *Oncology of CNS Tumors*, https://doi.org/10.1007/978-3-030-04152-6_24

The cystic wall of the lesions is hypointense on T1-weighted images, hyperintense on T2-weighted images, and isointense on T2FLAIR and DWI, and the wall shows no contrast medium uptake after Gd-DTPA administration. The signal of the cyst content is commonly higher than CSF on T2-weighted images indicating higher protein levels and viscosity.

The solid parts typically show a high signal on proton-density-weighted images and hyperintensity on T2-weighted images. Zentner et al. also reported T2 tumor iso-hypointensity in 32% of their patients [61]. On T1-weighted images they are usually isointense. Gadolinium enhancement has been reported in 12–44% of the cases and is usually moderate and homogeneous; perifocal edema is usually absent. Anaplastic GG is often more infiltrative on MRI and demonstrates a higher degree of enhancement and peritumoral edema. Calcifications on CCT are commonly seen (50%) [26, 31]. Scalloping of the calvarium may be seen adjacent to superficially located tumors.

24.2.3 Histology and Molecular Biology

24.2.3.1 Histopathology

The histopathological hallmark of gangliogliomas is a combination of neuronal and glial cell elements with a wide variety in the morphological spectrum from a predominately neuronal phenotype toward variants with a prominent glial population [61]. The pathogenesis of gangliogliomas is thought to have originated from a dysplastic precursor lesion, which is supported by the fact that gangliogliomas harbor a typical expression of the stem cell epitope CD34.

From radiological and surgical experiences, gangliogliomas are attributed to be well demarcated from the adjacent brain parenchyma; however, histopathological examinations revealed a more complex picture [43]. At first, gangliogliomas tend to permeate the preexisting cytoarchitecture, such as neocortex, hippocampus, and amygdala. Second, the stem cell epitope CD34, which has evolved as a helpful diagnostic marker

in gangliogliomas, could be observed in isolated tumor satellite clusters in the adjacent normal brain without obvious connection to the main tumor [6].

The neuronal component is typically characterized by dysplastic neurons with a loss of the cytoarchitectural organization, abnormal subcortical localization, clustered appearance, cytomegaly, and perimembranous-aggregated Nissl substance.

The glial component is the proliferative cell population and defines its biological behavior [46]. Histopathological features are calcifications, extensive lymphoid infiltrates along perivascular spaces or within the tumor parenchyma, and a prominent capillary network. There is a wide range of the morphological phenotype resembling fibrillary astrocytomas, oligodendrogliomas, or pilocytic astrocytomas, and correct diagnosis is sometimes challenging.

This histological variability is also reflected by a variance in the immunoreactivity for CD34. Whereas most tumors in the temporal lobe exhibit CD34 positivity, about 50% of the tumors in other brain regions are CD34-negative tumors [8]. This may point toward a different pathogenic mechanism between temporal gangliogliomas and others. The fact, that CD34 is abundantly expressed in the developing brain, but not in the neuroepithelial cell elements in adults, may support the speculation that the precursor cells of the temporal gangliogliomas may be different from gangliogliomas in the rest of the brain [6, 57, 59].

Other markers that have been established for immunostaining in gangliogliomas were neuronal marker proteins such as MAP2, NeuN, neurofilaments, and synaptophysin as well as GFAP and S-100 for the glial component. Semiquantitative estimation of the Ki67-labeling index can be used to characterize the biological behavior of the tumor [43, 57, 59]. Typically, gangliogliomas show a very low proliferation index (>1%).

24.2.3.2 Genetics

So far, comprehensive genetic data of gangliogliomas that could enhance our understanding of the molecular biology both from an epileptogenic and oncologic view is limited. Several gene expression profiles have been analyzed in recent years, the results of which are, however, hampered by the limited comparability due to different study designs [2, 18, 48].

Gains of chromosome 5 and 7 are the most frequently detected genetic alterations [42]. IGH1/2 and TP53 mutations are generally absent. Xu et al., for instance, used GTG-banding, SKY, and molecular karyotyping using genome-wide SNP arrays and detected losses within chromosomes 10, 13, and 22 as well as gains within chromosome 5, 7, 8, and 12. Notably, they documented a low frequent unbalanced nonreciprocal translocation t(1;18)(q21;q21). This translocation resulted in loss of chromosomal sequence 18q21, which encodes ion channels possibly indicating involvement in cortical excitability [60]. Accordingly, Fassunke et al. reported a series of deregulated genes in ganglioglioma related to aberrant development of neuronal precursors, which were grouped in five different categories: chromatin state regulation and transcription factors (CDY1 and Bcl11A downregulation), intracellular signal transduction (HSJ2, ARF3, ST6GalNAc4, and PRKCB1 downregulation), extracellular signal transduction and cell adhesion (NELL2 downregulation, MMP2, and PLAT upregulation), cell cycle and proliferation control (TP53-inducible protein 3, and TRIB1 upregulation), and development and differentiation (NGFR, p75 and BDNF upregulation, LMO4, and LDB2 downregulation) [18].

Recently, the BRAF V600E mutation was identified in approximately 20–60% of gangliogliomas [13, 49]. BRAF is a member of the RAS/RAF/MEK/ERK signal transduction cascade involved in transmitting extracellular signals to the nucleus. Mutations in BRAF have been detected in up to 7% of human neoplasms. In primary human brain tumors, the most frequent BRAF mutation is a tandem duplication and fusion with the KIAA1549 gene found in the majority of childhood pilocytic astrocytomas [19, 23]. The BRAF V600E mutation has also been reported [15, 16]. Koelsche et al. demonstrated predominant expression of mutated BRAF protein by the neuronal tumor compartment indicat-

ing that the neuronal compartment is crucially involved in the pathogenesis of gangliogliomas [29]. Contrary, in a series by Dahiya et al., 72% revealed BRAF staining of both glial and neuronal cellular populations, which would support the notion that both cellular components may be derived from a common progenitor cell [13]. Furthermore, Koelsch et al. showed small nests of BRAF-staining positive cells distant from the main tumor without any connection to the primary tumor similar to the aforementioned findings seen with CD34 staining [29].

In addition, the BRAF V600E status seems to have implications for the expected rate of tumor recurrence and prognosis. In a series by Dahiyra et al., positive BRAF V600E staining was associated with shorter recurrence-free survival [13].

From an epileptogenic point of view, deregulation of the mTOR pathway, which is critical to cell growth and proliferation during development of the cerebral cortex, was hypothesized to play a role in the development of chronic seizures associated with GG [12]. The abnormal activation of mTOR pathway may contribute to apoptosis signaling pathway and premature activation of mechanisms of neurodegeneration. In this regard, a high level of apoptosis has been reported in both the neuronal and glial component indicating its role in epileptogenesis [42].

24.2.4 WHO Grading and Recurrences

Most GG correspond to WHO grade I. Some GG with anaplastic features in their glial component are classified as WHO grade III but represent only 1–5% of all GGs [34]. An intermediate WHO grade II (formerly labeled as atypical GG) has not been established in the current 2016 classification. Some authors, however, do advocate that grading of GG should be three-tiered instead of two-tiered. Majores et al., for example, applied the diagnosis of atypical GG to tumors that had increased cellularity, nuclear pleomorphism, and increased proliferative activity but lacked definitive criteria for anaplasia, such as palisading necrosis or a brisk mitotic count [36]

(Majores). On the basis of their data, a distinction of WHO grade II GG from grades I and III did provide a valuable prognostic information as the 5-year overall survival rate was 92% for WHO grade I, 70% for grade II, and 30% for grade III tumors [36].

Ganglioglioma recurrences are relatively common (up to 30%), but the information regarding histological and molecular factors predicting recurrence are scarce. In case of relapse, tumors can undergo malignant transformation, with a rate ranging from 2 to 5% [36] (Majores). There are three larger studies addressing predictors of recurrence, specifically [13, 35, 36] (Luyken, Dahiya, Majores). In a series by Dahiya et al., 15 out of 53 patients with WHO grade I ganglioglioma exhibit tumor recurrence, with a 5-year event-free survival rate of 70% and a mean follow-up period over 4 years. They demonstrated that hypercellularity, the lack of an oligodendroglial component, the presence of a moderate to marked chronic inflammatory cell infiltrate, microvascular proliferation, and BRAF V600E mutation correlate with shorter recurrence-free survival. They argued that these findings could be designated as atypical features implicating a WHO grade II classification [13]. In the largest series pertaining gangliogliomas so far, Luyken et al. saw increased cellularity, conspicuous nuclear pleomorphism in glial cell elements, and microvascular proliferation as parameters for tumor recurrence [35]. In the third series by Majores et al., a gemistocytic component, the absence of protein droplets, and intralesional CD34 staining were associated with shorter progression free survival [36].

24.2.5 Treatment

24.2.5.1 Surgery

From an oncological point of view, maximal safe resection is the best strategy for patients harboring gangliogliomas [11, 30, 53, 61]. Because tumors are usually noninfiltrative and well demarcated from the normal tissue, gross total resection is often feasible in the hemispheric location. In the largest series of 402 patients so far, the 10-year local control rates were 89% after gross total resection compared to 52% after subtotal resection [45]. In the series of Luyken et al., including 184 patients with both grade I and II tumors, patients who received a complete resection had a significantly longer 7.5-year recurrence-free survival rate than those who received a partial resection (99% versus 92%) [35]. In children a recent series by Haydon et al. confirmed the improved recurrence-free survival from greater extent of resection with volumetric analysis [24].

With regard to the epilepsy outcome for patients with chronic seizures, the debate whether lesionectomy, i.e., resection of the tumor, or resection of various amounts of adjacent brain tissue is ongoing.

Many groups have provided data regarding seizure outcomes after surgical treatment of patients with ganglioglioma-associated seizures, which represent the vast majority of patients with supratentorial tumors (80–90%) [54]. The most consistent finding across these studies is that increased extent of resection increases seizure freedom. Specifically, gross total resection was found to be better than subtotal resection [3, 40, 51, 53]. Overall, the seizure control rate is reported to be between 59 and 84% [30, 31, 35].

While intraoperative electrocorticography (ECoG) is commonly used in lesional epilepsy surgery to identify potential extratumoral epileptogenic zones, the benefit of applying ECoG in GG and tailoring the resection according to the ECoG findings has not been consistently confirmed [25, 40, 53]. Particularly, in temporal tumors, where several surgical options including anteromesial resection, mesial resection, and lateral neocortical resections can be discussed, the best option in the individual patient is difficult to assess [56]. For temporomesial tumors some researchers have found simple lesionectomy to be sufficient, while others advocate additional resection in cases of MRI-identifiable hippocampal lesions or intraoperative findings of epileptiform activity on ECOG [9, 21, 28].

24.2.5.2 Adjuvant Treatment

The role of adjuvant treatment is poorly defined and very controversial. For example, upfront radiotherapy in patients with subtotally resected tumors has been reported to increase the local tumor control rate from 52% after subtotal resection up to 65% after subtotal resection followed by radiotherapy [45]. However, most physicians would be very reluctant to administer radiotherapy, because of the potential radiation-related morbidity in long-term survivors. This is of particular concern in children and young adults. In the rare event of malignant progression, radiotherapy as well as chemotherapy represent accepted treatment options. In a large series of 184 supratentorial GGs reported by Lyken et al., adjuvant radiotherapy and chemotherapy were administered to only 4 patients (2 after initial surgery and after malignant progression in 2 patients). One child in this series was treated with chemotherapy after undergoing incomplete resection of a WHO grade I tumor. The median follow-up duration for the 184 patients was 8 years (ranging from 1 to 14 years). The calculated 7.5-year survival rate was 98%, and the 7.5-year recurrence-free survival rate was 97% [35].

24.3 Posterior Fossa Tumors

24.3.1 Symptoms and Clinical Signs

The clinical presentation of posterior fossa gangliogliomas depends on the structures involved. Pure cerebellar lesions are rare, and they are more often hemispheric than vermian and can also be incidental findings. If symptoms occur, they typically present with slowly progressive cerebellar signs eventually associated with ataxia and gait disturbances.

Brainstem lesions are more common in posterior fossa gangliogliomas than pure cerebellar lesions. In most cases they are located within the brainstem with extension into the cerebellar peduncles and frequent exophytic portions in the fourth ventricle or the cerebellopontine angle, which have also been called transitional forms [4]. Depending on the location, they commonly present with cranial nerve deficits and ataxia but also focal motor and sensory long tract impairments. Signs of raised intracranial pressure and hydrocephalus are less common [44].

24.3.2 Imaging

Posterior fossa gangliogliomas can be subdivided into cerebellar and brainstem location. In cerebellar gangliogliomas the hemispheres are more commonly involved than the vermis. Brainstem tumor most frequently arise from the medulla oblongata, but can be found from the tectal plate down to the cervicomedullary junction [62]. Cerebellar GG tends to be well-circumscribed, while brainstem GG frequently shows ill-defined tumor margins. Peritumoral edema is more typical for brainstem GGs.

The MRI features of infratentorial gangliogliomas compared to their supratentorial counterparts were a larger size at presentation, less cystic components (20%), and more pronounced contrast enhancement [33]. The solid portions demonstrate isointensity or slightly hypointensity on T1WI and heterogeneous hyperintensity on T2WI. The majority of brainstem GGs do enhance after gadolinium administration and frequently show a diffuse pattern, which was referred to as "paintbrush" pattern [62].

24.3.3 Histology and Molecular Biology

In general, the histological diagnosis of GG in posterior fossa location shares the same criteria as for the supratentorial tumors. Recently, Gupta et al. suggested to divide the GG of the posterior fossa into two distinct morphological groups, namely, classic ganglioglioma, Group 1, and pilocytic astrocytoma with focal gangliocytic differentiation, Group 2 [22]. While Group 1 is characterized by dysmorphic ganglion cells with atypical glial cells, aggregates of perivascular lymphocytes, eosinophilic granular bodies, and a fibrillary phenotype with diffuse infiltration of the adjacent brain parenchyma, Group 2 showed features of a classic pilocytic astrocytoma with foci of gangliocytic differentiation. They typically display a glial element with a biphasic architecture alternating between solid areas of piloid cells and more cystic regions with variable myxoid degeneration.

In addition to these morphological differences, Groups 1 and 2 quite clearly separated from each other on a molecular basis. While Group 2 tumors revealed a BRAF duplication and KIAA 1549-BRAF fusion gene in 82% of their cases, none of the Group 1 tumors did. At the same time, 43% of the Group 1 tumors had a BRAF V600E mutation but none in Group 2.

24.3.4 Treatment

24.3.4.1 Surgery

The best treatment of this rare disease is based on an individual case-by-case decision, and any definitive conclusion that could be drawn from the literature or consensus in their optimal management is lacking. In general, posterior fossa GGs have a less favorable outcome as compared to ST ones and are considered to have a fivefold increased risk of recurrence compared to equivalent tumors in the cerebral hemisphere [10, 24, 32]. From the study of the SEER database, Dudley et al. found that BS location was associated with worse 5-year survival compared to spinal cord and all other locations independent from the extent of resection [17]. In a mixed series with 58 adults and children reported by Lang et al., 9 were located in the BS. For these BS GGs that were all low-grade, the overall survival (OS) was 78% at 5 years, and the progression free survival was 53% at 3 years. A GTR was achieved in three of the nine BS tumors [31]. Given the fact that adjuvant therapy has shown limited benefit so far, maximal safe resection has gained widespread acceptance.

In this regard, it seems quite obvious that a GG of the cerebellar hemisphere is more easily amenable to gross total resection than with brainstem involvement and that not all patients with brainstem GG benefit equally from an attempted resection [31, 62]. In a series of 33 posterior fossa

GGs by Puget et al., 12% of the tumors were located within the cerebellar hemisphere/vermis. According to their experience, pure cerebellar GG should be treated similarly to pilocytic astrocytomas in this region with the aim of gross total resection [44]. This is a statement many authors would agree with.

In brainstem GG, however, with the various location and growth pattern of the tumors in the reported series, agreement is less intuitive. Pan et al. tried to acknowledge the notion that the growth pattern itself may predict the clinical course and classified the brainstem GG in their series into three types: exophytic, intrinsic, and endo-exophytic. They found that endo-exophytic tumors exhibit significantly lower event-free survival rates than the other two types, even after adjusting the effect of extent of resection [39].

Some authors advocated that removal of the enhancing portion of the tumor could result in long event-free survival even in the absence of any further treatment [4, 44].

24.3.4.2 Adjuvant Treatment

For patient with progressive tumors and malignant progression, adjuvant treatment with chemotherapy and radiotherapy has been reported, but the benefit has not been systematically investigated. In general, recurrent tumors are re-operated on to optimize the extent of resection as well as to obtain a second pathologic diagnosis [26]. When radiation is required, treatment doses and volumes are typically selected by analogy to low-grade glial neoplasms with conformal radiation delivery doses ranging from 45 to 54 Gy in 1.7–2.0 Gy/day fractions. For anaplastic tumors treatment doses up to 60 Gy are applied, but the dose response of these lesions remains poorly defined. Alternatively, radiosurgery poses an option [52].

Chemotherapy should be considered for patients with persistent recurrent low- and high-grade tumors not amenable to re-resection or reirradiation [38]. Responses have been reported both in children and adults after nitrosoureas, temozolomide, etoposide, carboplatin, and cyclophosphamide. Targeted therapy with BRAF inhibitors has been reported to be useful in patients with GGs and BRAF V600E mutation, for instance, in brainstem GG vemurafenib in combination with chemotherapy as reported by Rush et al. or alone as shown by del Bufalo et al. [14, 47]. Based on these and other experiences, a pilot clinical trial of vemurafenib against BRAF V600E-mutant recurrent or refractory low-grade glioma in children has started [14] (clinicaltrials. gov NCT 0174 8149). Furthermore, another BRAF inhibitor, dabrafenib, has shown a good response [50].

24.4 Spinal Tumors

24.4.1 Imaging

Spinal cord GGs are exceedingly rare, accounting for less than 10% of all intramedullary neoplasms [37]. Within the spinal cord, GG most frequently occurs in the cervical cord including the craniospinal junction and the medulla oblongata, although they can occur throughout the entire length of the spinal cord [20]. Evaluation of GG with MR mostly demonstrates a circumscribed solid or mixed solid-cystic mass often extending over multiple levels of the spinal cord with hypointensity on T1 and hyperintensity on T2. Based on imaging alone, it is very challenging to differentiate a ganglioglioma from the far more commonly seen tumor types, namely, astrocytoma and ependymoma. Astrocytoma and ependymoma share many similar features to ganglioglioma, including T2 hyperintensity, enhancement, tumoral cysts, and cord edema. Poorly defined margins may be more suggestive of astrocytoma, while a central location in the spinal cord, hemorrhage, and hemosiderin staining are often seen with ependymoma.

24.4.2 Symptoms and Clinical Signs

GG typically presents with slowly progressing myelopathy. Patients with acute neurological deficits due to intra-/peritumoral bleeding have been reported but were the exception. Scoliosis or neck deviation is a commonly seen phenomenon.

24.4.3 Histology and Molecular Biology

The vast majority of spinal cord GGs represent WHO grade I tumors characterized by low to moderate cellularity [20]. The astrocytic component shows variable cytology, mainly piloid or microcystic, typically GFAP and MAP2C positive. In about two thirds eosinophilic granular bodies and in about one third of the cases, Rosenthal fibers can be identified [20]. In a series by Gessi et al., tumors further showed abundant hyalinized vessels (14%), calcifications (14%), and lymphocytic inflammatory infiltrates (28%). Forty-two percent in their series displayed an abundant neuronal component with dysmorphic ganglion cells, which showed a wide variety in their morphology. Most cells displayed irregular-shaped nuclei and variably large plump cytoplasms with aggregated Nissl substance. They commonly appear in small clusters scattered within the tumor. Perisomatic positivity for synaptophysin and cytoplasmatic expression of chromogranin A helps to distinguish between the dysplastic neurons from preexisting normal neurons [20].

As in their cerebral counterparts, mitotic figures are rarely seen in spinal GG, and the proliferation index varies between 1 and 4%. Anaplastic gangliogliomas (WHO III) were encountered more frequently than in cerebral GG reaching 16% in a series by Gessi et al. [20].

Although spinal GGs share similar morphological features with their cerebral counterparts, they apparently display different molecular features. In spinal GG BRAF V600E mutation and KIAA 1549-BRAF fusion are rarely seen (11%). In the study by Gupta et al., four spinal GGs were classified as "pilocytic astrocytoma with gangliocytic component." All four showed KIAA-BRAF fusion, but no BRAF V600E mutations [22]. Notably, two anaplastic GGs in the series by Gessi et al. showed positivity for antibody against mutated H3.3K27M protein, which according to the new WHO 2016 classification represents a distinct tumor entity, namely, diffuse glioma of the midline H3K27M [41].

24.4.4 Surgical Treatment

Extensive resection seems to be the most important factor for progression free and overall survival. However, this should not be attempted at the expense of severe permanent morbidity [27]. In the to date largest series of spinal cord GG, Jallo et al. reported a 5-year survival rate of 67% in a series of 56 patients that had gross total (46 cases) or subtotal (10 cases) tumor resection. Operative morbidity in this series was low reaching 28% [27].

In contrast, Lang et al. suggested that the tumor location per se and not the degree of resection influenced the recurrence rate. Gross total tumor removal in 29 out of 30 patients did not prevent tumor recurrence in 47% of the cases. The 10-year survival rate was 87% suggesting a rather indolent clinical course despite the recurrence [31].

References

1. Adachi Y, Yagishita A (2008) Gangliogliomas: characteristic imaging findings and role in the temporal lobe epilepsy. Neuroradiology 50(10):829–834. https://doi.org/10.1007/s00234-008-0410-x
2. Aronica E, Boer K, Becker A, Redeker S, Spliet WG, van Rijen PC, Wittink F, Breit T, Wadman WJ, Lopes da Silva FH, Troost D, Gorter JA (2008) Gene expression profile analysis of epilepsy-associated gangliogliomas. Neuroscience 151(1):272–292. https://doi.org/10.1016/j.neuroscience.2007.10.036
3. Aronica E, Leenstra S, van Veelen CW, van Rijen PC, Hulsebos TJ, Tersmette AC, Yankaya B, Troost D (2001) Glioneuronal tumors and medically intractable epilepsy: a clinical study with long-term follow-up of seizure outcome after surgery. Epilepsy Res 43(3):179–191
4. Baussard B, Di Rocco F, Garnett MR, Boddaert N, Lellouch-Tubiana A, Grill J, Puget S, Roujeau T, Zerah M, Sainte-Rose C (2007) Pediatric infratentorial gangliogliomas: a retrospective series. J Neurosurg 107(4 Suppl):286–291. https://doi.org/10.3171/PED-07/10/286
5. Becker AJ, Wiestler OD, Figarella-Branger D, Blumcke I (2007) Ganglioglioma and gangliocytoma. In: Louis DN, Ohgaki H, Wiestler OD, Cavenee WK (eds) WHO classification of tumours of the central nervous system, 4th edn. International Agency for Research on Cancer, Lyon, pp 103–105
6. Blumcke I, Giencke K, Wardelmann E, Beyenburg S, Kral T, Sarioglu N, Pietsch T, Wolf HK, Schramm J, Elger CE, Wiestler OD (1999) The CD34 epitope is expressed in neoplastic and malformative lesions associated with chronic, focal epilepsies. Acta Neuropathol 97(5):481–490
7. Blumcke I, Lobach M, Wolf HK, Wiestler OD (1999) Evidence for developmental precursor lesions in epilepsy-associated glioneuronal tumors. Microsc Res Tech 46(1):53–58. https://doi.org/10.1002/(SICI)1097-0029(19990701)46:1<53::AID-JEMT5>3.0.CO;2-0
8. Blumcke I, Wiestler OD (2002) Gangliogliomas: an intriguing tumor entity associated with focal epilepsies. J Neuropathol Exp Neurol 61(7):575–584
9. Cataltepe O, Turanli G, Yalnizoglu D, Topcu M, Akalan N (2005) Surgical management of temporal lobe tumor-related epilepsy in children. J Neurosurg 102(3 Suppl):280–287. https://doi.org/10.3171/ped.2005.102.3.0280
10. Chan MH, Kleinschmidt-Demasters BK, Donson AM, Birks DK, Foreman NK, Rush SZ (2012) Pediatric brainstem gangliogliomas show overexpression of neuropeptide prepronociceptin (PNOC) by microarray and immunohistochemistry. Pediatr Blood Cancer 59(7):1173–1179. https://doi.org/10.1002/pbc.24232
11. Compton JJ, Laack NN, Eckel LJ, Schomas DA, Giannini C, Meyer FB (2012) Long-term outcomes for low-grade intracranial ganglioglioma: 30-year experience from the Mayo Clinic. J Neurosurg 117(5):825–830. https://doi.org/10.3171/2012.7.JNS111260
12. Crino PB (2011) mTOR: a pathogenic signaling pathway in developmental brain malformations. Trends Mol Med 17(12):734–742. https://doi.org/10.1016/j.molmed.2011.07.008
13. Dahiya S, Haydon DH, Alvarado D, Gurnett CA, Gutmann DH, Leonard JR (2013) BRAF(V600E) mutation is a negative prognosticator in pediatric ganglioglioma. Acta Neuropathol 125(6):901–910. https://doi.org/10.1007/s00401-013-1120-y
14. del Bufalo F, Carai A, Figa-Talamanca L, Pettorini B, Mallucci C, Giangaspero F, Antonelli M, Badiali M, Moi L, Bianco G, Cacchione A, Locatelli F, Ferretti E, Mastronuzzi A (2014) Response of recurrent BRAFV600E mutated ganglioglioma to vemurafenib as single agent. J Transl Med 12:356. https://doi.org/10.1186/s12967-014-0356-1
15. Dias-Santagata D, Lam Q, Vernovsky K, Vena N, Lennerz JK, Borger DR, Batchelor TT, Ligon KL, Iafrate AJ, Ligon AH, Louis DN, Santagata S (2011) BRAF V600E mutations are common in pleomorphic xanthoastrocytoma: diagnostic and therapeutic

implications. PLoS One 6(3):e17948. https://doi.org/10.1371/journal.pone.0017948

16. Dougherty MJ, Santi M, Brose MS, Ma C, Resnick AC, Sievert AJ, Storm PB, Biegel JA (2010) Activating mutations in BRAF characterize a spectrum of pediatric low-grade gliomas. Neuro Oncol 12(7):621–630. https://doi.org/10.1093/neuonc/noq007

17. Dudley RW, Torok MR, Gallegos DR, Mulcahy-Levy JM, Hoffman LM, Liu AK, Handler MH, Hankinson TC (2015) Pediatric low-grade ganglioglioma: epidemiology, treatments, and outcome analysis on 348 children from the surveillance, epidemiology, and end results database. Neurosurgery 76(3):313–319. ; discussion 319; quiz 319–320. https://doi.org/10.1227/NEU.0000000000000619

18. Fassunke J, Majores M, Tresch A, Niehusmann P, Grote A, Schoch S, Becker AJ (2008) Array analysis of epilepsy-associated gangliogliomas reveals expression patterns related to aberrant development of neuronal precursors. Brain 131(Pt 11):3034–3050. https://doi.org/10.1093/brain/awn233

19. Forshew T, Tatevossian RG, Lawson AR, Ma J, Neale G, Ogunkolade BW, Jones TA, Aarum J, Dalton J, Bailey S, Chaplin T, Carter RL, Gajjar A, Broniscer A, Young BD, Ellison DW, Sheer D (2009) Activation of the ERK/MAPK pathway: a signature genetic defect in posterior fossa pilocytic astrocytomas. J Pathol 218(2):172–181. https://doi.org/10.1002/path.2558

20. Gessi M, Dorner E, Dreschmann V, Antonelli M, Waha A, Giangaspero F, Gnekow A, Pietsch T (2016) Intramedullary gangliogliomas: histopathologic and molecular features of 25 cases. Hum Pathol 49:107–113. https://doi.org/10.1016/j.humpath.2015.09.041

21. Giulioni M, Galassi E, Zucchelli M, Volpi L (2005) Seizure outcome of lesionectomy in glioneuronal tumors associated with epilepsy in children. J Neurosurg 102(3 Suppl):288–293. https://doi.org/10.3171/ped.2005.102.3.0288

22. Gupta K, Orisme W, Harreld JH, Qaddoumi I, Dalton JD, Punchihewa C, Collins-Underwood R, Robertson T, Tatevossian RG, Ellison DW (2014) Posterior fossa and spinal gangliogliomas form two distinct clinicopathologic and molecular subgroups. Acta Neuropathol Commun 2:18. https://doi.org/10.1186/2051-5960-2-18

23. Hasselblatt M, Riesmeier B, Lechtape B, Brentrup A, Stummer W, Albert FK, Sepehrnia A, Ebel H, Gerss J, Paulus W (2011) BRAF-KIAA1549 fusion transcripts are less frequent in pilocytic astrocytomas diagnosed in adults. Neuropathol Appl Neurobiol 37(7):803–806. https://doi.org/10.1111/j.1365-2990.2011.01193.x

24. Haydon DH, Dahiya S, Smyth MD, Limbrick DD, Leonard JR (2014) Greater extent of resection improves ganglioglioma recurrence-free survival in children: a volumetric analysis. Neurosurgery 75(1):37–42. https://doi.org/10.1227/NEU.0000000000000349

25. Hu WH, Ge M, Zhang K, Meng FG, Zhang JG (2012) Seizure outcome with surgical management of epileptogenic ganglioglioma: a study of 55 patients. Acta

Neurochir 154(5):855–861. https://doi.org/10.1007/s00701-011-1259-z

26. Im SH, Chung CK, Cho BK, Wang KC, Yu IK, Song IC, Cheon GJ, Lee DS, Kim NR, Chi JG (2002) Intracranial ganglioglioma: preoperative characteristics and oncologic outcome after surgery. J Neurooncol 59(2):173–183

27. Jallo GI, Freed D, Epstein FJ (2004) Spinal cord gangliogliomas: a review of 56 patients. J Neurooncol 68(1):71–77

28. Jooma R, Yeh HS, Privitera MD, Gartner M (1995) Lesionectomy versus electrophysiologically guided resection for temporal lobe tumors manifesting with complex partial seizures. J Neurosurg 83(2):231–236. https://doi.org/10.3171/jns.1995.83.2.0231

29. Koelsche C, Wohrer A, Jeibmann A, Schittenhelm J, Schindler G, Preusser M, Lasitschka F, von Deimling A, Capper D (2013) Mutant BRAF V600E protein in ganglioglioma is predominantly expressed by neuronal tumor cells. Acta Neuropathol 125(6):891–900. https://doi.org/10.1007/s00401-013-1100-2

30. Krouwer HG, Davis RL, McDermott MW, Hoshino T, Prados MD (1993) Gangliogliomas: a clinicopathological study of 25 cases and review of the literature. J Neurooncol 17(2):139–154

31. Lang FF, Epstein FJ, Ransohoff J, Allen JC, Wisoff J, Abbott IR, Miller DC (1993) Central nervous system gangliogliomas. Part 2: clinical outcome. J Neurosurg 79(6):867–873. https://doi.org/10.3171/jns.1993.79.6.0867

32. Lindsay AJ, Rush SZ, Fenton LZ (2014) Pediatric posterior fossa ganglioglioma: unique MRI features and correlation with BRAF V600E mutation status. J Neurooncol 118(2):395–404. https://doi.org/10.1007/s11060-014-1450-1

33. Lou X, Gui QP, Sun L, Wu NZ, Lyu JH, Ma L (2016) Comparisons of MR findings between supratentorial and infratentorial gangliogliomas. Clin Neuroradiol 26(1):65–71. https://doi.org/10.1007/s00062-014-0333-3

34. Lucas JT Jr, Huang AJ, Mott RT, Lesser GJ, Tatter SB, Chan MD (2015) Anaplastic ganglioglioma: a report of three cases and review of the literature. J Neurooncol 123(1):171–177. https://doi.org/10.1007/s11060-015-1781-6

35. Luyken C, Blumcke I, Fimmers R, Urbach H, Wiestler OD, Schramm J (2004) Supratentorial gangliogliomas: histopathologic grading and tumor recurrence in 184 patients with a median follow-up of 8 years. Cancer 101(1):146–155. https://doi.org/10.1002/cncr.20332

36. Majores M, von Lehe M, Fassunke J, Schramm J, Becker AJ, Simon M (2008) Tumor recurrence and malignant progression of gangliogliomas. Cancer 113(12):3355–3363. https://doi.org/10.1002/cncr.23965

37. Miller DC (2000) Surgical pathology of intramedullary spinal cord neoplasms. J Neurooncol 47(3):189–194

38. Mohile N, Raizer JJ (2006) Chemotherapy for glioneural tumors. In: Newton HB (ed) Handbook of

brain tumor chemotherapy. Elsevier, Amsterdam, pp 432–438

39. Pan CC, Chen X, Xu C, Wu WH, Zhang P, Wang Y, Wu T, Tang J, Xiao XR, Wu Z, Zhang JT, Zhang LW (2016) Brainstem gangliogliomas: prognostic factors, surgical indications and functional outcomes. J Neurooncol 128(3):445–453. https://doi.org/10.1007/s11060-016-2131-z

40. Park YS, Kim DS, Shim KW, Kim JH, Choi JU (2008) Factors contributing to resectability and seizure outcomes in 44 patients with ganglioglioma. Clin Neurol Neurosurg 110(7):667–673. https://doi.org/10.1016/j.clineuro.2008.03.017

41. Perkins OC (1926) Gangliogliomas. Arch Pathol Lab Med 2:11–17

42. Prabowo AS, van Thuijl HF, Scheinin I, Sie D, van Essen HF, Iyer AM, Spliet WG, Ferrier CH, van Rijen PC, Veersema TJ, Thom M, Schouten-van Meeteren AY, Reijneveld JC, Ylstra B, Wesseling P, Aronica E (2015) Landscape of chromosomal copy number aberrations in gangliogliomas and dysembryoplastic neuroepithelial tumours. Neuropathol Appl Neurobiol 41(6):743–755. https://doi.org/10.1111/nan.12235

43. Prayson RA, Khajavi K, Comair YG (1995) Cortical architectural abnormalities and MIB1 immunoreactivity in gangliogliomas: a study of 60 patients with intracranial tumors. J Neuropathol Exp Neurol 54(4):513–520

44. Puget S, Alshehri A, Beccaria K, Blauwblomme T, Paternoster G, James S, Dirocco F, Dufour C, Zerah M, Varlet P, Sainte-Rose C (2015) Pediatric infratentorial ganglioglioma. Childs Nerv Syst 31(10):1707–1716. https://doi.org/10.1007/s00381-015-2860-x

45. Rades D, Zwick L, Leppert J, Bonsanto MM, Tronnier V, Dunst J, Schild SE (2010) The role of postoperative radiotherapy for the treatment of gangliogliomas. Cancer 116(2):432–442. https://doi.org/10.1002/cncr.24716

46. Rumana CS, Valadka AB, Contant CF (1999) Prognostic factors in supratentorial ganglioglioma. Acta Neurochir 141(1):63–68; discussion 68–69

47. Rush S, Foreman N, Liu A (2013) Brainstem ganglioglioma successfully treated with vemurafenib. J Clin Oncol 31(10):e159–e160. https://doi.org/10.1200/JCO.2012.44.1568

48. Samadani U, Judkins AR, Akpalu A, Aronica E, Crino PB (2007) Differential cellular gene expression in ganglioglioma. Epilepsia 48(4):646–653. https://doi.org/10.1111/j.1528-1167.2007.00925.x

49. Schindler G, Capper D, Meyer J, Janzarik W, Omran H, Herold-Mende C, Schmieder K, Wesseling P, Mawrin C, Hasselblatt M, Louis DN, Korshunov A, Pfister S, Hartmann C, Paulus W, Reifenberger G, von Deimling A (2011) Analysis of BRAF V600E mutation in 1,320 nervous system tumors reveals high mutation frequencies in pleomorphic xanthoastrocytoma, ganglioglioma and extra-cerebellar pilocytic astrocytoma. Acta Neuropathol 121(3):397–405. https://doi.org/10.1007/s00401-011-0802-6

50. Shih KC, Shastry M, Williams JT, Jelsma PF, Abram SR, Ayyanar K, Burris HA 3rd, Infante JR (2014) Successful treatment with dabrafenib (GSK2118436) in a patient with ganglioglioma. J Clin Oncol 32(29):e98–e100. https://doi.org/10.1200/JCO.2013.48.6852

51. Sommer B, Wimmer C, Coras R, Blumcke I, Lorber B, Hamer HM, Stefan H, Buchfelder M, Roessler K (2015) Resection of cerebral gangliogliomas causing drug-resistant epilepsy: short- and long-term outcomes using intraoperative MRI and neuronavigation. Neurosurg Focus 38(1):E5. https://doi.org/10.3171/2014.10.FOCUS14616

52. Song JY, Kim JH, Cho YH, Kim CJ, Lee EJ (2014) Treatment and outcomes for gangliogliomas: a single-center review of 16 patients. Brain Tumor Res Treat 2(2):49–55. https://doi.org/10.14791/btrt.2014.2.2.49

53. Southwell DG, Garcia PA, Berger MS, Barbaro NM, Chang EF (2012) Long-term seizure control outcomes after resection of gangliogliomas. Neurosurgery 70(6):1406–1413.; ; discussion 1404–1413. https://doi.org/10.1227/NEU.0b013e3182500a4c

54. van Breemen MS, Wilms EB, Vecht CJ (2007) Epilepsy in patients with brain tumours: epidemiology, mechanisms, and management. Lancet Neurol 6(5):421–430. https://doi.org/10.1016/S1474-4422(07)70103-5

55. Ventureyra E, Herder S, Mallya BK, Keene D (1986) Temporal lobe gangliogliomas in children. Childs Nerv Syst 2(2):63–66

56. Wallace D, Ruban D, Kanner A, Smith M, Pitelka L, Stein J, Vannemreddy PS, Whisler WW, Byrne RW (2013) Temporal lobe gangliogliomas associated with chronic epilepsy: long-term surgical outcomes. Clin Neurol Neurosurg 115(4):472–476. https://doi.org/10.1016/j.clineuro.2012.05.034

57. Wolf HK, Muller MB, Spanle M, Zentner J, Schramm J, Wiestler OD (1994) Ganglioglioma: a detailed histopathological and immunohistochemical analysis of 61 cases. Acta Neuropathol 88(2):166–173

58. Wolf HK, Roos D, Blumcke I, Pietsch T, Wiestler OD (1996) Perilesional neurochemical changes in focal epilepsies. Acta Neuropathol 91(4):376–384

59. Wolf HK, Wiestler OD (1993) Surgical pathology of chronic epileptic seizure disorders. Brain Pathol 3(4):371–380

60. Xu LX, Holland H, Kirsten H, Ahnert P, Krupp W, Bauer M, Schober R, Mueller W, Fritzsch D, Meixensberger J, Koschny R (2015) Three gangliogliomas: results of GTG-banding, SKY, genome-wide high resolution SNP-array, gene expression and review of the literature. Neuropathology 35(2):148–157. https://doi.org/10.1111/neup.12176

61. Zentner J, Wolf HK, Ostertun B, Hufnagel A, Campos MG, Solymosi L, Schramm J (1994) Gangliogliomas: clinical, radiological, and histopathological findings in 51 patients. J Neurol Neurosurg Psychiatry 57(12):1497–1502

62. Zhang S, Ai L, Chen XZ, Wang K (2016) Radiological evaluation of infratentorial gangliogliomas in various anatomic locations of the cerebellum and brainstem. Clin Neuroradiol 27(3):319–327. https://doi.org/10.1007/s00062-015-0495-7

Cerebellar Astrocytomas

25

Michael C. Dewan and John C. Wellons III

25.1 Epidemiology

The term cerebellar astrocytoma typically refers to the WHO grade I lesion within the cerebellum known also as a cerebellar pilocytic astrocytoma or cerebellar juvenile pilocytic astrocytoma (JPA). However, cerebellar astrocytomas may be fibrillary instead of pilocytic or may show more malignant histological characteristics. Although pilocytic astrocytomas may occur throughout the brain or spinal cord, they mainly occur in the posterior fossa, particularly in the cerebellum, and those occurring in the cerebellum tend to be cystic with a mural nodule. Currently, brain tumors are the most common solid organ cancer of the pediatric population. Approximately 10–15% of all pediatric brain tumors and over 25% of posterior fossa tumors in children will be identified as a cerebellar JPA [1, 2]. Aggressive, safe surgical resection is the mainstay of therapy, both at initial diagnosis and in the event of recurrence. Adjuvant chemotherapy or radiation is rarely used for patients with progressive unresectable tumors but does play a role in therapy for malignant tumors.

25.2 Symptoms and Clinical Signs

Most commonly, pediatric cerebellar astrocytomas present with symptomatic hydrocephalus. The typical history is that of a gradually worsening headache with vomiting over weeks to months. A more rapid presentation suggests a faster-growing and therefore more malignant lesion, but this observation is certainly no rule. The mean age at presentation for children with cerebellar low-grade gliomas is 6–8 years old, and no significant gender predilection exists [1]. Other symptoms can be broadly categorized into those secondary to hydrocephalus, cerebellar dysfunction, or surrounding brain dysfunction. In addition to headache and vomiting, hydrocephalus may manifest as lethargy, papilledema, a unilateral or bilateral sixth nerve palsy, or an enlarging head circumference in young children whose sutures are open. Those symptoms related to cerebellar dysfunction include dysmetria, ataxia, titubation, and nystagmus, and those due to compression of surrounding neural structures include cranial nerve palsies, hemiparesis, gait disturbances, and pyramidal signs. Neck pain, head tilt, vertigo, and even seizures have been reported as presenting symptoms [3–5].

M. C. Dewan · J. C. Wellons III (✉)
Department of Neurosurgery, Vanderbilt University
Medical Center, Nashville, TN, USA
e-mail: michael.dewan@vumc.org;
jay.wellons@vumc.org

© Springer Nature Switzerland AG 2019
J.-C. Tonn et al. (eds.), *Oncology of CNS Tumors*, https://doi.org/10.1007/978-3-030-04152-6_25

25.3 Diagnostics

25.3.1 Synopsis

Oftentimes, the first imaging study obtained on children with persistent headaches and/or vomiting through their pediatrician's clinic or the emergency department is a CT scan. If abnormalities are seen, the child should then undergo an MRI of the brain with and without gadolinium administration. Findings suggestive of a cerebellar astrocytoma do not warrant spine imaging initially. Histological confirmation obviates the need for MRI imaging of the spine in the absence of symptoms referable to the spinal cord, cauda equina, or nerve roots. If, however, preoperative history or imaging is suggestive of ependymoma or medulloblastoma, then the child should undergo a complete spinal MRI with and without contrast either preoperatively or no less than 2 weeks postoperatively to allow the blood to clear from the operative procedure. An MRI of the brain with and without gadolinium is performed within the first 24–48 h postoperatively to evaluate resection status and to rule out immediate surgical complications.

The "classic" juvenile pilocytic astrocytoma occurs in the cerebellar hemisphere but also can be seen in the cerebellar median or paramedian structures. They are intrinsic to the brain and may cause mass effect on surrounding structures, including the fourth ventricle, the cerebellar peduncles, the brain stem, or the cranial nerves of the cerebellopontine angle. The demarcation from the surrounding brain parenchyma is usually distinct. These lesions can also present as noncystic solid vermian or hemispheric lesions with mass effect, that like their cystic counterparts are intrinsic, usually with an identifiable border from the surrounding brain.

25.3.2 Computerized Tomography (CT)

On a noncontrasted CT scan, a cerebellar JPA will typically appear as a cyst within the cerebellar hemisphere containing a nodule of varying size. Hydrocephalus due to obstruction of the fourth ventricle or aqueduct may be present. The nodule will enhance with contrast, but the cyst wall is variable. Calcification is present in only 10% [6]. Cerebellar JPAs may also be solid, mostly homogenously enhancing lesions as well and may also occur in the vermis or other midline cerebellar structures.

25.3.3 Magnetic Resonance Imaging (MRI)

The pre- and postoperative radiographic study of choice for assessment of tumor volume is an MRI with and without gadolinium administration. If the use of neuronavigation is anticipated (e.g., brainstem involvement), obtaining thin slice MR images is necessary. As in CT, the most common imaging characteristics of cerebellar JPAs are of a cystic lesion with an enhancing "mural nodule" on T1-weighted, gadolinium-enhanced imaging with variable enhancement of the cyst wall (Fig. 25.1). Without administration

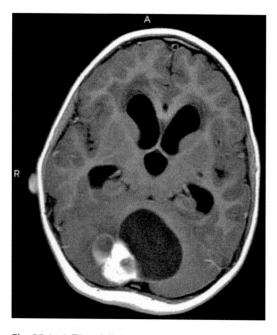

Fig. 25.1 A T1 gadolinium-enhanced axial MRI depicting a large, enhancing mural nodule with a cyst causing mass effect on the surrounding brain. Note the absence of enhancement of the cyst wall as well as the obvious hydrocephalus

of gadolinium, the nodule and/or cyst contents are hypo- or isointense on T1-weighted imaging and on T2-weighted imaging tend to be hyperintense [6]. Effacement of the fourth ventricle (Fig. 25.2) with triventricular hydrocephalus is commonly observed. Solid noncystic cerebellar JPAs tend to follow the same enhancement characteristics. Differentiation among cerebellar JPA, ependymomas, and medulloblastomas can be made with apparent diffusion coefficient maps, wherein the less cellular JPA has a higher ADC value (increased diffusion of water) than the more cellular ependymoma or medulloblastoma, which has a lower ADC value (restricted diffusion of water) [7].

25.4   Staging and Classification

25.4.1   Synopsis

The classic cerebellar JPA is considered WHO grade I and treated by surgical excision only. Fibrillary astrocytomas are WHO grade II tumors and are treated by surgical excision as well but historically have been noted to have a poorer outcome [1] Malignant cerebellar tumors are considered grade III or IV, require adjuvant therapy, and have a much worse outcome. These tumors, however, are far less common, comprising approximately 5% of all cerebellar astrocytomas [5].

25.4.2   Histopathology

Cerebellar JPAs may have a "biphasic pattern" in which loose cystic glial tissue is present in addition to areas of compact tissue often containing Rosenthal fibers. While pathognomonic, the combination of these two patterns is rare, and the presence of both is not mandatory for the diagnosis. Oftentimes, the hair-like processes of the bipolar cells can be seen on smear preparation. The loose glial tissue may contain microcysts or granular bodies, and the compact tissue may consist of bipolar cells in addition to Rosenthal fibers. Of note, Rosenthal fibers are intracytoplasmic eosinophilic hyaline masses and are not specific to JPA as they may be present in gliosis as well as in Alexander's disease (a primary disease of the white matter).

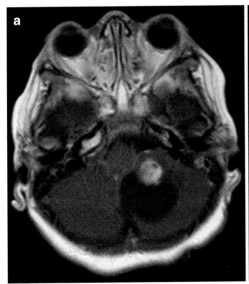
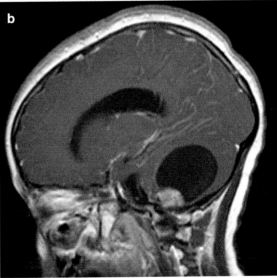

Fig. 25.2   (**a** and **b**). Axial (**a**) and sagittal (**b**) T1 gadolinium-enhanced MR images demonstrate a left cerebellar hemispheric cystic mass with a contrast-enhancing nodule causing mass effect on the brainstem anteriorly and effacing the fourth ventricle and cerebral aqueduct

Importantly, mitosis and vascular hyperproliferation may occur, but do not correlate with malignancy [8].

Fibrillary astrocytomas consist of fibrillary astrocytes on a loosely structured tumor matrix with microcysts, low to moderate cellular density, rare mitoses, and possible nuclear atypia [1]. Margins may be less distinct [2]. Malignant cerebellar astrocytomas exhibit greater nuclear atypia, mitotic figures, proliferation of endothelium, and necrosis [2, 9].

Pilocytic astrocytomas are heavily GFAP (glial fibrillary acid protein) positive and also positive for S-100 protein and OLIG2 [10]. The Ki-67 proliferative index is universally low in JPA though more aggressive astrocytomas are associated with a higher index [10]. The predictive value of MIB-1 staining is controversial. While MIB-1 staining may be helpful in establishing the proliferation rate in a particular tumor, it does not appear to correlate with the outcome of JPAs [8]. Evidence exists that it may help predict biological activity in higher-grade tumors [5].

25.4.3 Molecular Biology

With advances in gene amplification and molecular marking over the last decade, the diagnosis and classification of pilocytic astrocytomas (PA) have evolved significantly. Most PAs demonstrate modifications in the Ras/RAF/mitogen-activated protein kinase (MAPK)/extracellular signal-regulated kinase (ERK) pathway. In mammalian cells, this pathway assists in the regulation of cell growth, proliferation, and apoptosis [11]. Between 60 and 90% of cerebellar pilocytic astrocytomas demonstrate a duplication at 7q34 which results in fusion of two genes, KIAA1549 and BRAF [12]. The KIAA1549-BRAF fusion causes a constitutive activation of the kinase functionality of the Ras/ERK pathway, thereby catalyzing cell proliferation [13]. Numerous other genetic alterations have been described in a minority of PAs including those involving KRAS [14], FGFR1 [15], and MYB [11], as well as point mutations of BRAF itself [16] and a similar genetic fusion involving FAM131B and BRAF [17].

While the molecular biology surrounding PAs is better understood, how that knowledge influences treatment—and ultimately prognosis—is less clear. To date, a correlation between the presence of the KIAA1549-BRAF fusion and overall survival has not been established [18]. Even less clinical data has matured regarding the rarer point mutations and fusions found in a subpopulation of cerebellar astrocytomas. With time, targeted treatment regimens will likely be founded on our genetic understanding of these tumors, but in the meantime the clinical value of genetic alterations is largely limited to diagnostic and classification purposes.

25.5 Treatment

25.5.1 Synopsis

Timing of surgical excision is based upon the clinical status of the patient, the availability of capable and competent resources, and surgeon preference. Patient presenting with decompensated and progressive hydrocephalus warrant urgent CSF diversion via external ventricular drainage, followed by surgical resection within 12–24 h. Lethargic children with signs of brain stem compression or acute herniation unresponsive to ventriculostomy placement should be taken to the OR urgently. Patients presenting with less urgent symptoms and who respond to steroid therapy or who present without symptoms are admitted and treated electively within a period of days. The paradigm varies according to institution and surgeon, but is ultimately driven by the child's clinical status and response to stabilizing measures.

25.5.2 Surgery

The placement of a preoperative external ventricular drain (EVD) depends upon clinical presentation and surgeon preference. For lesions not causing hydrocephalus, foregoing prophylactic external CSF drainage is reasonable as most patients do not require chronic CSF diversion. At the authors' institution, for patients with moderate or severe hydrocephalus, an EVD is inserted through a separate sterile preparation in the operating room just prior to the formal tumor resection. Kocher's point [19] on the nondominant hemisphere is preferred, and the catheter is tunneled subcutaneously and connected to an adjustable closed drainage system. The anesthesia team is carefully counseled on EVD etiquette before and during the case. Generally, we allow 10–15 cm^3 of CSF egress preoperatively, clamp the drain, and then evaluate the need for further drainage as the case proceeds. Alternatively, the ventriculostomy may be placed from a posterior trajectory—such as Frazier's point [20]—in the same surgical preparation as the posterior fossa craniotomy. If the EVD is placed intraoperatively, the posterior approach may save time relative to an anteriorly placed drain. However, since the postoperative drain weaning period often consists of several days in a supine or sitting position, the authors feel the anterior approach is better tolerated in the pediatric population.

After induction and intubation, steroids, mannitol, and antibiotics are administered. Anesthesia preparation includes two large bore intravenous lines, an arterial catheter, a bladder catheter, an esophageal temperature probe, and a well-taped endotracheal tube to avoid loosening from surgical preparation or dependent positioning. After EVD placement if necessary and following application of the Mayfield clamp on the superior temporal line of both sides, the child is flipped to the prone position on chest and iliac crest rolls. Due to the risk of venous air embolus and to surgeon arm fatigue, the sitting position is not used at our institution. The head is slightly elevated, and the neck gently flexed ensuring adequate space between the chin and chest. Excessive neck flexion can compromise venous drainage at the jugular outlet and should be avoided. After final positioning and head immobilization, breath sounds, line orientation, and EVD status are all confirmed by the anesthesia team.

A small strip of hair beginning just above the inion is clipped. Betadine solution is applied in layers and allowed to dry. Sterile towels and an iodine-impregnated clear drape are then applied to the surgical site. The incision spans from the inion to the spinous process of C2. Electrocautery is used to dissect in the midline fascial plane between the paraspinous muscles. The muscle attachments to C2 are left intact to minimize discomfort postoperatively unless the entrance into the fourth ventricle has descended to this level. A muscle cuff may be left at the superior nuchal line for reattachment of the suboccipital muscles during closure, depending on the degree of cerebellum that must be exposed. The muscle is carefully dissected off of the suboccipital bone while meticulously coagulating or waxing any venous channels through the bone. The dissection is taken just wider than the width of the foramen magnum for midline approaches and adjusted to one side for paramedian approaches. Careful subperiosteal dissection along the posterior arch of C1 is performed, avoiding the nearby vertebral artery and encircling venous plexus. In infants and young children, this posterior arch may be incompetent in the midline or cartilaginous. The loose tissue spanning the distance between the suboccipital bone and the ring of C1 is also carefully dissected until the posterior atlanto-occipital ligament is exposed. Utilizing two initial paramedian burr holes, a single-piece craniotomy is fashioned using a high-speed drill. The posterior arch of C1 is removed with rongeurs. The dura is opened in a Y-shaped fashion, the operating microscope is brought into the field, and a self-retraction system is placed. If the tumor is within the fourth ventricle and accessible via the foramen of Magendie, an attempt is made to avoid significantly disrupting the vermis. However, tumor resection should not be compromised by inadequate exposure. Otherwise, the cortical incision is made in the hemisphere, and the lesion is entered. Intraoperative ultrasound may be used to identify the lesion or its cystic component and help guide the approach.

For tumors that occur in the most lateral portion of the hemisphere, a retromastoid approach may be chosen. The child is induced as above and then placed into the lateral decubitus position with the operative side up. A curvilinear incision is made posterior to the auricle, and the myocutaneous flap is reflected anteriorly, exposing the asterion and superior margin of the mastoid tip. After placement of a single burr hole just inferior and posterior to the junction of the transverse and sigmoid sinuses, a high-speed drill with foot plate is used to create a craniotomy overlying the approximate area of the tumor. Neuronavigation can assist in the delineation of the craniotomy borders; however, after dural opening and CSF egress, its reliability may be compromised by brain shift. The decision to replace bone is surgeon dependent. Lastly, for tumors centered in the superior aspect of the cerebellum, consideration should be given to an infratentorial, supracerebellar approach, the details of which are not addressed in this chapter.

The shortest route through viable cortex should be taken to approach the lesion. It should be mentioned here that occasionally despite adequately controlled end tidal CO_2 and normal ICP as measured by direct ventricular monitoring, the cerebellum may appear to be under pressure and even herniate through the initial dural opening. If a cystic component to the tumor exists, a ventricular needle with a stylet may be used with or without ultrasound guidance to puncture the cyst and reduce the pressure within the posterior fossa if deemed necessary. This maneuver then affords a safe and controlled approach to the tumor.

Frequently, the tumor tissue maintains a clear demarcation from surrounding white and gray matter. The suction/bipolar technique or the ultrasonic surgical aspirator is used for tumor resection. Conventional wisdom does not mandate removal of the cyst wall if it is not enhancing and has a smooth appearance. In fact, it is rare that enhancing cyst walls will be removed unless they appear on gross inspection to have obvious tumor burden. In tumors that are near the fourth ventricle, a cotton surgical patty is placed along the floor to assist with intraoperative localization and protection of critical brain stem structures. This simple maneuver affords the surgeon a constant reminder of the location of the floor of the fourth ventricle and hence the brain stem, but does not replace constant reorientation, particularly after surgical table adjustment. Once seen, the cerebral aqueduct may be carefully plugged with a small cotton ball to prevent blood entering the third ventricle. Careful inspection of the postoperative tumor bed, including the "lip" of the cerebellum underneath the retractor blades, is necessary to avoid small portions of tumor being left behind.

Pericranium from the occipital region above the muscle cuff is harvested and sewn into the dural opening, and the bone flap is replaced with heavy silk sutures. The muscle and fascia are closed along the midline and reattached to the previously left cuff along the superior nuchal line. The soft tissue and skin are closed, and a sterile dressing is placed. After emergence from general anesthesia, the patient convalesces in the intensive care unit with frequent neurological evaluations. The EVD is initially allowed to drain at 10 cm H_2O and is gradually weaned over the next 2–5 days, depending on the individual child's CSF absorptive capability. Steroids are tapered as well.

Beyond brainstem dysfunction resulting from a deep tumor adherent to traversing cranial nerves or their nuclei, notable surgical morbidity consists primarily of hydrocephalus, CSF leak, and cerebellar mutism. Postoperative hydrocephalus and its management are discussed in the section on "Follow-Up Care." CSF leak can be avoided by ensuring a watertight closure with autologous graft sewn along the dural edges. Persistent leakage despite meticulous closure is usually a harbinger of hydrocephalus and warrants radiologic evaluation of ventricular volume. Cerebellar mutism (CM) is a curious form of delayed, transient akinetic mutism with dysarthria that occurs in up to a third of posterior fossa resections [21]. The incidence of CM is lower for JPA, occurring in 2–9% of patients and associated with deeper lesions adjacent to the fourth ventricle floor, the superior cerebellar peduncle, and/or involving the dentate nucleus [22–24]. The treatment is supportive, and most patients will regain functional speech with mild, persistent motor phonation deficits [21].

25.5.3 Radiation

No role exists for standard radiation therapy as a primary treatment for cerebellar JPAs, as a standard adjunct to gross total resection (GTR), or as a means of treating residual resectable disease. This is particularly true for young children, where neurocognitive deficits following radiosurgery are more pronounced. Following GTR, radiation to the tumor bed offers no clinical benefit in low-grade astrocytoma, while risking undue morbidity [23]. The use of radiation therapy in the setting of residual unresectable tumor is an active area of research that has demonstrated favorable results in small, uncontrolled series [4, 25, 26]. In the earliest series of children undergoing salvage treatment with stereotactic radiosurgery (SRS), short-term control was excellent and morbidity mild [26]. Recent evidence with long-term follow-up suggests that salvage SRS offers favorable disease control in surgically unresectable residual disease with infrequent and mild toxicity [25].

Malignant transformation of posterior fossa astrocytomas in children has been associated with previous radiotherapy to the area [2]. The literature regarding malignant cerebellar astrocytomas is sparse, but the consensus has been that these patients receive postoperative radiation therapy in a manner similar to supratentorial high-grade gliomas [1]. Evidence of CSF dissemination of malignant disease warrants irradiation to the craniospinal axis [2]. The damaging long-term effects of whole-brain radiation on the developing brain are well known and have no role in today's treatment of cerebellar astrocytoma.

25.5.4 Chemotherapy

There is no role for chemotherapy as a primary treatment for cerebellar JPA. As the underlying biological mechanisms underpinning JPA are better elucidated, targeted molecular therapy may be a viable strategy for post-surgical residual disease. In patients with progressive nonresectable low-grade gliomas of the optic apparatus, diencephalon, brain stem, and other less surgically accessible regions, chemotherapy demonstrates variable efficacy [1]. Single-agent treatment, including high-dose cyclophosphamide, carboplatin, and etoposide, have provided periods of stable disease, and combination chemother-

apy has provided some degree of radiological response [1]. A protocol combining carboplatin and vincristine is used at many institutions for patients with unresectable or progressive noncerebellar pilocytic astrocytomas. The protocol is well tolerated, and survival rates are encouraging but rarely indicated for patients with cerebellar JPA unless they have progressive unresectable lesions. Malignant cerebellar glial tumors are treated with chemotherapy regiments similar to those for supratentorial high-grade gliomas of childhood [1].

25.6 Prognosis/Quality of Life

A safe gross total resection is the goal of surgery, and over 95% of these children remain alive at 25 years. Approximately 10% demonstrate spontaneous recurrence after GTR, though following repeat total resection, the long-term survival for low-grade cerebellar astrocytoma remains excellent [23]. The majority of recurrences will occur in the first 3 years [1], though late recurrence beyond 10 years has been described [23]. In up to one quarter of cerebellar astrocytomas, a gross total resection is not possible without risking significant neurological morbidity [27]. Residual tumor has a reported 30–100% chance of enlarging on follow-up imaging [2]. Experience dictates that small amounts of residual tumor will often remain stable or involute over time, and there are case series reporting 14–45% incidence of tumor regression after subtotal resection of a JPA [28–30]. However, subtotal resections do reduce the progression-free survival [3, 31]. Desai et al. found that the extent of tumor resection, a vermian location of the tumor, and the histological grade are negatively correlated with survival [3]. Histopathology appears to be the strongest predictor of outcome [5, 31]. Bristot et al. report four cases of malignant cerebellar astrocytomas treated with varying degrees of surgical excision, radiation therapy, and chemotherapy. One mortality occurred in the immediate postoperative phase; two who underwent subtotal excision followed by radiation died at 5 and 10 months. The one who underwent total excision, chemotherapy, and craniospinal radiation with a boost to the tumor bed was alive at 13 months but did have signs of pathological progression [9]. In a large series of cerebellar glial tumors, the Mayo Clinic reported an average overall survival of children with grade III and grade IV tumors of 2.3 and 0.8 years, respectively, despite adjuvant radiation or chemotherapy [31].

The quality of life in these patients has traditionally thought to be good, particularly when compared to children who have undergone resection and adjuvant treatment of a medulloblastoma, ependymoma, or supratentorial tumor [32]. Adults who underwent JPA resection in childhood, generally match their peers in terms of energy level, academic achievement, autonomy, and sense of well-being [22, 32]. Mild cognitive difficulties were more common, however, in the JPA cohort, as were mild problems with balance and fine motor skills [22]. In the vast majority of patients who enjoy long-term survival following cerebellar astrocytoma resection, Kulkarni et al. found the most important predictors of a decreased quality of life were the presence of a CSF shunt and lower socioeconomic status [33].

25.7 Follow-Up Care

Tumor recurrence following GTR of low-grade cerebellar astrocytoma occurs in a minority of patients (3–9%) and may occur with diminishing frequency from time of initial resection [23]. In addition to the immediate postoperative enhanced MRI, we obtain studies at 3 months then at 6-month intervals twice, then yearly for 4 years, and then every 2 years. This is institution-dependent and may be modified based on residual tumor or presence of a CSF shunt [34]. As a more conservative surveillance regimen, the demonstration of tumor absence on two postoperative MRIs separated by at least 3 months has shown a strong negative likelihood ratio of recurrence [35]. As with all surveillance studies, disease monitoring must be weighed against cost, convenience, and patient risk.

Prior studies have reported a 10–50% rate of CSF shunting despite adequate tumor resection

[1, 2]. Over the past two decades, endoscopic third ventriculostomy (ETV) has been used with greater frequency to treat post-resection hydrocephalus with favorable results [36–38]. The nature of the hydrocephalus influences the treatment modality. For hydrocephalus due to persistent obstruction at the level of the cerebral aqueduct or fourth ventricular outlet despite adequate and safe tumor resection, ETV should be strongly considered. For hydrocephalus believed to be due to poor absorption at the level of the arachnoid granulations, a VPS is a more viable long-term option. For hydrocephalus secondary to posterior fossa tumor, a recent meta-analysis suggested greater treatment durability and less complications in patients treated via ETV than those with a shunt [39]. Inherent bias and non-equivalent comparison groups, however, prevent drawing strong conclusions. Further study on this topic is necessary, particularly as the presence of a shunt has been showed to be among the most important predictors of quality of life in a disease that carries a long-term overall survival. If residual tumor is present and hydrocephalus is persistent and due to CSF pathway obstruction, consideration should be given to a safe secondary resection in lieu of ETV or shunt placement. While several groups have published on the topic [40, 41], there is little role for preoperative ETV in patients with obstructive hydrocephalus from a cerebellar astrocytomas, since as many as 83–88% of patients do not need permanent CSF diversion after tumor resection [42, 43].

25.8 Future Perspectives

Cerebellar astrocytomas are one of the most common brain tumors of childhood. The vast majority are low-grade, termed juvenile pilocytic astrocytoma. Surgical resection remains the treatment of choice, and a gross total resection carries an excellent long-term prognosis without additional therapy needed. For residual disease or unresectable recurrence, targeted radiosurgery and chemotherapy may improve progression-free survival. The less common high-grade astrocytoma likewise mandates maximal safe surgical resection; adjuvant chemotherapy and radiation improve overall survival. Beyond histologic grade, extent of resection and the presence of persistent hydrocephalus are the most important prognostic factors—both for survival and quality of life. Laboratory investigations to identify effective adjuvant therapies for disease unamenable to surgical cure are underway. Similarly, novel methods to prevent and treat comorbidities like post-resection hydrocephalus and cerebellar mutism remain a focus for surgeon-scientists.

References

1. Reddy AT, Mapstone TB (2001) Cerebellar astrocytomas. In: McLone DG (ed) Pediatric neurosurgery, pp 835–843
2. Steinbok P, Mutat A (1999) Cerebellar astrocytomas. In: Albright L, Pollack I, Adelson D (eds) Principles and practice of pediatric neurosurgery. Thieme Medical Publisher, Inc., New York, pp 641–662
3. Desai KI, Nadkarni TD, Muzumdar DP, Goel A (2001) Prognostic factors for cerebellar astrocytomas in children: a study of 102 cases. Pediatr Neurosurg 35(6):311–317
4. Hadjipanayis CG, Kondziolka D, Gardner P, Niranjan A, Dagam S, Flickinger JC et al (2002) Stereotactic radiosurgery for pilocytic astrocytomas when multimodal therapy is necessary. J Neurosurg 97(1):56–64
5. Medlock MD (2001) Infratentorial astrocytoma. In: Keating RF, Goodrich JT, Packer RJ (eds) Tumors of the pediatric central nervous system. Thieme Medical Publishers, Inc., New York, pp 199–205
6. Osborn AG (1994) Diagnostic neuroradiology. Mosby, St. Louis
7. Rumboldt Z, Camacho DLA, Lake D, Welsh CT, Castillo M (2006) Apparent diffusion coefficients for differentiation of cerebellar tumors in children. AJNR Am J Neuroradiol 27(6):1362–1369
8. Burger PC, Scheithauer BW, Vogel FS (2002) Surgical pathology of the nervous system and its coverings. Churchill Livingstone, Philadelphia
9. Bristot R, Raco A, Vangelista T, Delfini R (1998) Malignant cerebellar astrocytomas in childhood experience with four cases. Childs Nerv Syst 14(10):532–536
10. Matyja E, Grajkowska W, Stępień K, Naganska E (2016) Heterogeneity of histopathological presentation of pilocytic astrocytoma—diagnostic pitfalls. A review. Folia Neuropathol 3:197–211
11. Tatevossian RG, Lawson ARJ, Forshew T, Hindley GFL, Ellison DW, Sheer D (2010) MAPK pathway activation and the origins of pediatric low-grade astrocytomas. J Cell Physiol 222(3):509–514
12. Bergthold G, Bandopadhayay P, Bi WL, Ramkissoon L, Stiles C, Segal RA et al (2014) Pediatric low-grade gliomas: how modern biology reshapes the clinical field. Biochim Biophys Acta 1845(2):294–307
13. Bar EE, Lin A, Tihan T, Burger PC, Eberhart CG (2008) Frequent gains at chromosome 7q34 involving BRAF in pilocytic astrocytoma. J Neuropathol Exp Neurol 67(9):878–887
14. Gajjar A, Pfister SM, Taylor MD, Gilbertson RJ (2014) Molecular insights into pediatric brain tumors have the potential to transform therapy. Clin Cancer Res 20(22):5630–5640
15. Jones DTW, Hutter B, Jäger N, Korshunov A, Kool M, Warnatz H-J et al (2013) Recurrent somatic alterations of FGFR1 and NTRK2 in pilocytic astrocytoma. Nat Genet 45(8):927–932
16. Schindler G, Capper D, Meyer J, Janzarik W, Omran H, Herold-Mende C et al (2011) Analysis of BRAF V600E mutation in 1,320 nervous system tumors reveals high mutation frequencies in pleomorphic xanthoastrocytoma, ganglioglioma and extracerebellar pilocytic astrocytoma. Acta Neuropathol 121(3):397–405
17. Cin H, Meyer C, Herr R, Janzarik WG, Lambert S, Jones DTW et al (2011) Oncogenic FAM131B-BRAF fusion resulting from 7q34 deletion comprises an alternative mechanism of MAPK pathway activation in pilocytic astrocytoma. Acta Neuropathol 121(6):763–774
18. Sadighi Z, Slopis J (2013) Pilocytic astrocytoma: a disease with evolving molecular heterogeneity. J Child Neurol 28(5):625–632
19. Tillmanns H (1908) Something about puncture of the brain. Br Med J (Clin Res Ed) 2:983–984
20. Lee CK, Tay LL, Ng WH, Ng I, Ang BT (2008) Optimization of ventricular catheter placement via posterior approaches: a virtual reality simulation study. Surg Neurol 70(3):274–277; discussion 277–8
21. Tamburrini G, Frassanito P, Chieffo D, Massimi L, Caldarelli M, Di Rocco C (2015) Cerebellar mutism. Childs Nerv Syst 31(10):1841–1851
22. Ait Khelifa-Gallois N, Laroussinie F, Puget S, Sainte-Rose C, Dellatolas G (2014) Long-term functional outcome of patients with cerebellar pilocytic astrocytoma surgically treated in childhood. Brain Inj 29(3):366–373
23. Due-Tønnessen BJ, Lundar T, Egge A, Scheie D (2013) Neurosurgical treatment of low-grade cerebellar astrocytoma in children and adolescents: a single consecutive institutional series of 100 patients. J Neurosurg Pediatr 11(3):245–249
24. Sergeant A, Kameda-Smith MM, Manoranjan B, Karmur B, Duckworth J, Petrelli T et al (2017) Analysis of surgical and MRI factors associated with cerebellar mutism. J Neurooncol 30(10):375–314
25. Trifiletti DM (2017) Evaluation of outcomes after stereotactic radiosurgery for pilocytic astrocytoma. J Neurooncol 134(2):297–302
26. Grabb PA, Lunsford LD, Albright AL, Kondziolka D, Flickinger JC (1996) Stereotactic radiosurgery

for glial neoplasms of childhood. Neurosurgery 38(4):696–701; discussion 701–702

27. Steinbok P, Mangat JS, Kerr JM, Sargent M, Suryaningtyas W, Singhal A et al (2013) Neurological morbidity of surgical resection of pediatric cerebellar astrocytomas. Childs Nerv Syst 29(8):1269–1275

28. Due-Tønnessen BJ, Helseth E, Scheie D, Skullerud K, Aamodt G, Lundar T (2002) Long-term outcome after resection of benign cerebellar astrocytomas in children and young adults (0–19 years): report of 110 consecutive cases. Pediatr Neurosurg 37(2):71–80

29. Gunny RS, Hayward RD, Phipps KP, Harding BN, Saunders DE (2005) Spontaneous regression of residual low-grade cerebellar pilocytic astrocytomas in children. Pediatr Radiol 35(11):1086–1091

30. Palma L, Celli P, Mariottini A (2004) Long-term follow-up of childhood cerebellar astrocytomas after incomplete resection with particular reference to arrested growth or spontaneous tumour regression. Acta Neurochir (Wien) 146(6):581–588; discussion 588

31. Morreale VM, Ebersold MJ, Quast LM, Parisi JE (1997) Cerebellar astrocytoma: experience with 54 cases surgically treated at the Mayo Clinic, Rochester, Minnesota, from 1978 to 1990. J Neurosurg 87(2):257–261

32. Pompili A, Caperle M, Pace A, Ramazzotti V, Raus L, Jandolo B et al (2002) Quality-of-life assessment in patients who had been surgically treated for cerebellar pilocytic astrocytoma in childhood. J Neurosurg 96(2):229–234

33. Kulkarni AV, Piscione J, Shams I, Bouffet E (2013) Long-term quality of life in children treated for posterior fossa brain tumors. J Neurosurg Pediatr 12(3):235–240

34. Saunders DE, Phipps KP, Wade AM, Hayward RD (2005) Surveillance imaging strategies following surgery and/or radiotherapy for childhood cerebellar low-grade astrocytoma. J Neurosurg 102(2 Suppl):172–178

35. Alford R (2016) Postoperative surveillance of pediatric cerebellar pilocytic astrocytoma. J Neurooncol 130(1):53–62

36. Sainte-Rose C, Cinalli G, Roux FE, Maixner R, Chumas PD, Mansour M et al (2001) Management of hydrocephalus in pediatric patients with posterior fossa tumors: the role of endoscopic third ventriculostomy. J Neurosurg 95(5):791–797

37. Ray P, Jallo GI, Kim RYH, Kim B-S, Wilson S, Kothbauer K et al (2005) Endoscopic third ventriculostomy for tumor-related hydrocephalus in a pediatric population. Neurosurg Focus 19(6):E8

38. El-Ghandour NMF (2011) Endoscopic third ventriculostomy versus ventriculoperitoneal shunt in the treatment of obstructive hydrocephalus due to posterior fossa tumors in children. Childs Nerv Syst 27(1):117–126

39. Dewan MC, Lim J, Shannon CN, Wellons JC III (2017) The durability of endoscopic third ventriculostomy and ventriculoperitoneal shunts in children with hydrocephalus following posterior fossa tumor resection: a systematic review and time-to-failure analysis. J Neurosurg Pediatr 19(5):578–584

40. El Beltagy MA, Kamal HM, Taha H, Awad M, El Khateeb N (2010) Endoscopic third ventriculostomy before tumor surgery in children with posterior fossa tumors, CCHE experience. Childs Nerv Syst 26(12):1699–1704

41. Azab W, Al-Sheikh T, Yahia A (2013) Preoperative endoscopic third ventriculostomy in children with posterior fossa tumors: an institution experience. Turk Neurosurg 23(3):359–365

42. Due-Tønnessen BJ, Helseth E (2007) Management of hydrocephalus in children with posterior fossa tumors: role of tumor surgery. Pediatr Neurosurg 43(2):92–96

43. Fritsch MJ, Doerner L, Kienke S, Mehdorn HM (2005) Hydrocephalus in children with posterior fossa tumors: role of endoscopic third ventriculostomy. J Neurosurg 103(1 Suppl):40–42

Rare Childhood Tumors: Desmoplastic Infantile Ganglioglioma and Pleomorphic Xanthoastrocytoma

Gregory W. Albert

26.1 Desmoplastic Infantile Ganglioglioma

Desmoplastic infantile ganglioglioma (DIG) and a related entity, desmoplastic infantile astrocytoma (DIA), are very rare tumors found almost exclusively in infants. Taratuto et al. were the first to describe this entity. Their initial report in 1984 documented six patients, ages 1.5–9 months old, who all presented with solid/cystic tumors which involved the cerebral cortex and the meninges and had unique histological features. They gave this new tumor the name "superficial cerebral astrocytoma" [1]. Three years later, VandenBerg et al. reported an additional 11 patients with similar radiographic and pathologic findings. They gave this entity the name "desmoplastic infantile ganglioglioma" [2].

26.1.1 Epidemiology

DIG and DIA are very rare brain tumors of infancy. A recent review of the literature identified 107 reported cases of these entities. The

G. W. Albert (✉)
Division of Neurosurgery, Arkansas Children's Hospital, Little Rock, AR, USA

Department of Neurosurgery, University of Arkansas for Medical Sciences, Little Rock, AR, USA
e-mail: galbert2@uams.edu

patients ranged in age from 5 days to 4 years old although most patients were below 18 months of age at diagnosis. DIG showed a slight male predominance although there did not seem to be a gender predilection for DIA [3].

26.1.2 Molecular Biology and Pathology

The WHO classification lists DIA and DIG as grade I neoplasms [4]. The original report of DIG described two components of the tumors, an extracerebral, dural-based component that demonstrated cells in fascicles with strong reticulin positivity and a cortical component with features typical of proliferating astrocytes [1]. Grossly, these tumors are firm due to the desmoplasia [3]. They tend to be associated with large cysts with the solid portion being superficial, involving superficial cortex and leptomeninges with attachment to the dura. In DIA, the neoplastic cells are all astrocytic, while DIG will have neoplastic neurons, typically ganglion cells, in addition to neoplastic astrocytes. The desmoplastic leptomeninges display a mixture of fibroblastic spindle cells and neoplastic neuroepithelial cells within a reticulin network. Anaplasia may be present but does not seem to affect the overall outcome [4] (Fig. 26.1).

Given the rarity of DIG and DIA, limited genomic and molecular data is available. However,

J.-C. Tonn et al. (eds.), *Oncology of CNS Tumors*, https://doi.org/10.1007/978-3-030-04152-6_26

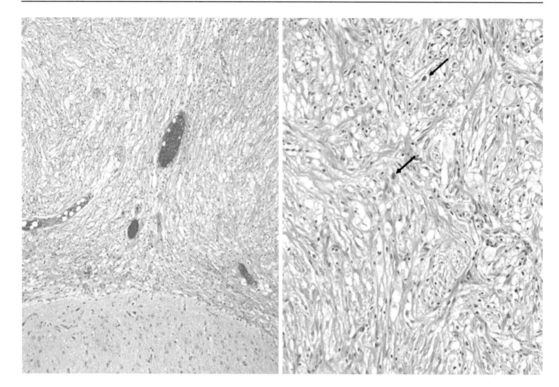

Fig. 26.1 Desmoplastic infantile ganglioglioma (H&E; original magnification, left panel ×100, right panel ×200). Left: A spindle-cell neoplasm (center and top) with low cellularity is seen on the brain (bottom) surface. Right: Prominent desmoplasia is represented by bright eosinophilic collagen bundles. Scattered plump ganglion cells (arrows) with large nuclei are present. (Images and caption courtesy Dr. Murat Gokden)

there have been no consistent mutations identified. These same studies do suggest, however, that DIG and DIA are histologic variants of the same entity, rather than two distinct tumor types [5].

26.1.3 Presentation

Infants will often present with a short duration of symptoms, perhaps only 3–6 months. Older children may present with a clinical history that is somewhat longer at about 6–9 months. Symptoms primarily occur as a result of mass effect. Infants with open fontanelles and sutures will develop rapid head growth and bulging of the anterior fontanelle. Later in the clinical course, the infant may develop upgaze paresis. Calvarial remodeling may occur over the tumor. In addition to signs and symptoms of increased intracranial pressure, older children may present with focal neurological deficits [3]. Overall, the most common pre-

senting signs and symptoms are rapid increase in the head circumference (56.3%), seizures (30%), and vomiting (11%). Children over 2 years of age are more likely than infants to present with seizures (71% versus 17%) [6].

26.1.4 Imaging

On computed tomography (CT) scanning of the head, these lesions are mixed solid and cystic. The solid component may be iso- or hyperdense but will enhance avidly with contrast [7]. Transfontanelle ultrasound is rarely performed in these patients. However, if this study is done, it may demonstrate a cystic component along with a solid portion that is hypoechoic compared to the brain. The adjacent vasogenic edema can appear hyperechoic [8].

As with all patients suspected of harboring a brain tumor, magnetic resonance imaging (MRI) is the imaging study of choice for the identification of DIG or DIA. The tumors are typically supratentorial, although other intracranial locations have been reported. They are mixed solid and cystic with thickened meninges overlying the lesion. The solid component is typically superficial and isointense on T1 sequences but can be hyper-, iso-, or hypointense on T2 imaging. The solid component of the tumor and the thickened meninges enhance strongly with contrast. Hemorrhage is rarely present. DIG and DIA can also exhibit diffusion restriction, likely due to the hypercellular nature of the solid portion of the tumor [9] (Fig. 26.2).

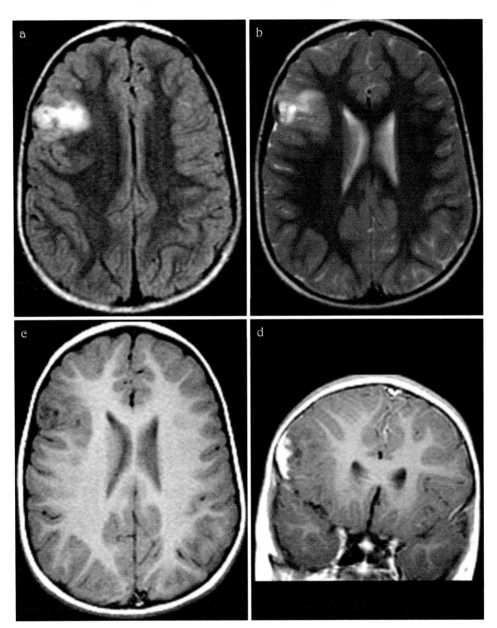

Fig. 26.2 Axial FLAIR (**a**), T2 (**b**), T1 (**c**), and post-contrast coronal T1-weighted images show cortically based mixed cystic and solid right frontal lesion with intense parenchymal and dural enhancement. Thinning of the inner table is seen adjacent to the tumor. (Images and caption courtesy Dr. Charles Glasier)

26.1.5 Treatment and Prognosis

The principle treatment for DIG is surgical resection. The goal of surgery should be gross total resection. This goal, however, is not always achieved. These tumors can be quite extensive, potentially involving eloquent cortex. In addition, the dura of the skull base or venous sinuses may be involved, thus limiting the extent of dural resection. Finally, the young of age of these patients may preclude extensive surgery due to blood loss [3].

With gross total resection, long-term progression-free survival is expected. With subtotal resection, close follow-up is recommended as regrowth can occur. However, in these cases, the residual may remain quiescent for an extended period of time [3]. Regression of residual tumor after subtotal resection has also been shown to occur [10]. Chemotherapy can be considered in the case of tumor recurrence that is not amenable to surgical resection but this approach has not been shown to be of benefit. Of the 107 patients reported in the literature, there was a 6% mortality rate. Three of these patients died of respiratory compromise and hypothalamic dysfunction related to hypothalamic tumors. Another patient presented with disseminated disease. The other two patients died of causes thought unrelated to the primary tumor [3].

Although these tumors are typically benign, more malignant presentations and courses have been reported. Cases with intracranial and spinal leptomeningeal spread are fortunately rare [11–13]. There are also case reports of late malignant transformation to glioblastoma in patients who had previously undergone gross total resection of DIG/DIA [14, 15].

26.2 Pleomorphic Xanthoastrocytoma

Pleomorphic xanthoastrocytoma (PXA) first appeared in the second edition of the WHO classification of central nervous system tumors in 1993. The name is derived from the histo-logic appearance with varying cell morphology (pleomorphism) and astrocytic cells with intracellular lipid deposits (xanthoastrocytes). Early reports of this entity classified the tumors as fibrous xanthomas, presuming that the tissue was of mesenchymal origin. It was not until the discovery of glial fibrillary acidic protein (GFAP) in 1977–1978 that these tumors were reclassified as astrocytic [16]. The name "pleomorphic astrocytoma" was proposed by Kepes et al. in their 1979 report of 12 patients, primarily children, who predominantly had good clinical outcomes [17]. However, in retrospect, the first recorded resection of a PXA was by Mr. Hugh Cairns in 1930. The patient was 24 years old at the time of presentation and survived for 40 years after surgery before succumbing to tuberculosis [18].

26.2.1 Epidemiology

Fewer than 1% of patients with primary brain tumors have a PXA. A recent analysis of data from the Surveillance, Epidemiology, and End Results (SEER) database identified 214 patients. The patients were predominantly children at the time of diagnosis with 50% being 20 years of age or younger with a median age at diagnosis of 20.5 years. However, the range of ages was considerable, from infancy up to 86 years of age. There was a slight female predominance with 54% of the tumors occurring in women. Ninety-nine percent of the tumors were supratentorial with the temporal lobe being the most common location harboring 39% of the lesions. The remaining tumors in the SEER database were cerebellar [19]. A two center review identified 74 cases of PXA. In this study, there was a slight male predominance (54%) with a median age at diagnosis of 21.5 years and a range of 5–73 years. Again, the most common location was the temporal lobe (35%) [20]. Although exceedingly rare, spinal cord [21, 22], cerebellopontine angle [23], sellar [24], suprasellar [25], tectal [26], pineal region [27, 28], and retinal PXA [29] have been reported.

26.2.2 Molecular Biology and Pathology

The WHO classifies PXA as a grade II neoplasm. Macroscopically, these tumors are typically solid and cystic, located superficially in the brain with leptomeningeal extension. Microscopically, the neoplastic cells are pleomorphic with intermixed spindled cells, mononucleated giant astrocytes, and multinucleated giant astrocytes. The nuclei will frequently demonstrate inclusions and prom-inent nucleoli. As implied in the name, the tumor also contains xanthomatous cells containing lipid droplets. Granular cells and lymphocytes are also frequently present. Silver staining will demon-strate a network of reticulin fibers. Anaplastic PXA is a WHO grade III neoplasm that has the histologic features of PXA but also demonstrates five or more mitoses per ten high-powered fields. Necrosis is more likely to be present in anaplastic PXA than grade II PXA but is not a criterion for anaplasia by itself [30, 31] (Fig. 26.3).

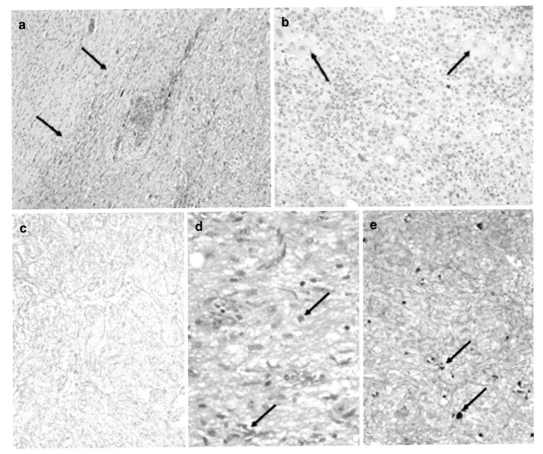

Fig. 26.3 Pleomorphic xanthoastrocytoma (**a**, **b**, **d**, **e**, **h** and **e**, original magnifications, ×100, ×200, ×400, and ×40, respectively; (**c**), reticulin, original magnification, ×200): (**a**) Hypercellular neoplasm (bottom right) has a well-defined border (arrows) with the surrounding neu-roglial tissue (top left) and, in this field, shows a fas-cicular growth pattern. (**b**) Large, atypical cells with xanthomatous cytoplasm (arrows) create a pleomorphic appearance. (**c**) Reticulin fibers are seen to encircle individual cells. (**d**) Rosenthal fibers (arrows) and (**e**) microcalcifications (arrows) suggest a low-grade neo-plasm in spite of the prominent atypical and pleomor-phism. (Images and caption courtesy Dr. Murat Gokden)

BRAF (serine threonine kinase v-RAF murine sarcoma viral oncogene homologue B1) mutations have been identified in a number of human cancers including brain tumors. In some of these neoplasms, most notably melanoma, BRAF inhibitors have been used as part of the treatment regimen with good success. Among brain tumors, PXA and craniopharyngioma demonstrate the highest rates of BRAF mutations [32]. The BRAF V600E mutation was first identified in PXA independently by two research groups in 2011. They showed rates of this mutation of 60–66% of PXA and 17–65% of anaplastic PXA [33, 34]. Mutation of BRAF appears to be associated with temporal lobe location, increased reticulin fiber deposition, and increased CD34 expression in PXA [35].

26.2.3 Presentation

The majority of patients with PXA have seizures which are seen in 57–79% of patients at presentation. Other presenting symptoms are due to increased intracranial pressure and/or focal neurological deficits [20, 36–38]. PXA accounts for 1.6–3.6% of brain tumors causing epilepsy in children [39, 40].

26.2.4 Imaging

As with all brain tumors, the imaging study of choice is MRI. These tumors are typically located in a superficial location near the cortex. They characteristically are mixed solid and cystic, although cystic tumors with enhancing walls and entirely solid tumors have been described. The solid component is usually adjacent to the leptomeningeal surface of the brain and demonstrates enhancement with intravenous contrast. Often, peritumoral edema is seen as well [41, 42] (Fig. 26.4).

26.2.5 Treatment and Prognosis

Surgical resection is the mainstay of therapy for PXA. The goal of surgery should be gross total resection (GTR) as this improves progression-free survival (PFS). Those patients undergoing subtotal resection (STR) or biopsy alone had a 5-year PFS of 41.7%, whereas GTR was associated with a 5-year PFS of 84.9%. Looking exclusively at pediatric PXA patients, the 5-year PFS are 41.7% and 92.3% for STR/biopsy and GTR, respectively. The 5-year overall survival (OS) does not seem to be impacted by the extent of resection but is impacted by the grade of the tumor. Grade II PXA patients have a 5-year OS of 90.4% compared to 57.1% for grade III anaplastic PXA patients. The effect of BRAF mutation status on OS could not be determined due to the small number of patients [20]. Transformation of PXA into glioblastoma has been reported [43, 44].

Adjuvant therapy is not recommended for patients who undergo GTR of a grade II PXA. Chemotherapy and/or radiation therapy may be recommended for patients with grade III PXA or incompletely resected grade II PXA. Temozolomide, an oral alkylating agent, is the chemotherapy traditionally used [37]. More recently, BRAF inhibitors (murafenib, dabrafenib, vemurafenib) have been proposed as potential therapeutic agents for patients whose tumors contain the BRAF V600E mutation. The experience with these medications in PXA and anaplastic PXA is limited to case reports and case series of patients with recurrent disease, mostly of the anaplastic variety [45–49].

Acknowledgments I would like to thank Dr. Murat Gokden, UAMS Department of Pathology and Chief of Neuropathology, for the pathology images and captions. I would like to thank Dr. Charles Glasier, UAMS Department of Radiology and ACH Chief of Neuroradiology, for the radiographs.

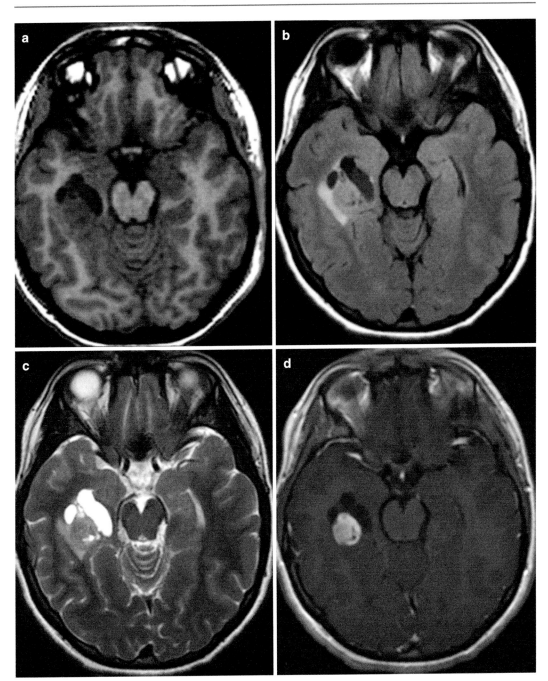

Fig. 26.4 Axial T1 (**a**), FLAIR (**b**), T2 (**c**), and post-contrast T1 (**d**) show a mixed cystic and solid left temporal lobe mass without significant perilesional edema. The lesion did not exhibit restricted diffusion. The solid component demonstrated intense contrast enhancement. (Images and caption courtesy Dr. Charles Glasier)

References

1. Taratuto AL, Monges J, Lylyk P, Leiguarda R (1984) Superficial cerebral astrocytoma attached to dura. Report of six cases in infants. Cancer 54(11):2505–2512

2. VandenBerg SR, May EE, Rubinstein LJ, Herman MM, Perentes E, Vinores SA, Collins VP, Park TS (1987) Desmoplastic supratentorial neuroepithelial tumors of infancy with divergent differentiation potential ("desmoplastic infantile gangliogliomas"). Report on 11 cases of a distinctive embryonal tumor with favorable prognosis. J Neurosurg 66(1):58–71. https://doi.org/10.3171/jns.1987.66.1.0058

3. Bianchi F, Tamburrini G, Massimi L, Caldarelli M (2016) Supratentorial tumors typical of the infantile age: desmoplastic infantile ganglioglioma (DIG) and astrocytoma (DIA). A review. Childs Nerv Syst 32(10):1833–1838. https://doi.org/10.1007/s00381-016-3149-4

4. Brat DJ, VandenBerg SR, Figarella-Branger D, Reuss DE (2016) Desmoplastic infantile astrocytoma and ganglioglioma. In: Louis DN, Ohgaki H, Wiestler OD, Cavenee WK (eds) WHO classification of tumours of the central nervous system. International Agency for Research on Cancer, Lyon, pp 144–146

5. Gessi M, Zur Mühlen A, Hammes J, Waha A, Denkhaus D, Pietsch T (2013) Genome-wide DNA copy number analysis of desmoplastic infantile astrocytomas and desmoplastic infantile gangliogliomas. J Neuropathol Exp Neurol 72(9):807–815. https://doi.org/10.1097/NEN.0b013e3182a033a0

6. Hummel TR, Miles L, Mangano FT, Jones BV, Geller JI (2012) Clinical heterogeneity of desmoplastic infantile ganglioglioma: a case series and literature review. J Pediatr Hematol Oncol 34(6):e232–e236. https://doi.org/10.1097/MPH.0b013e3182580330

7. Tenreiro-Picon OR, Kamath SV, Knorr JR, Ragland RL, Smith TW, Lau KY (1995) Desmoplastic infantile ganglioglioma: CT and MRI features. Pediatr Radiol 25(7):540–543

8. Lababede O, Bardo D, Goske MJ, Prayson RA (2001) Desmoplastic infantile ganglioglioma (DIG): cranial ultrasound findings. Pediatr Radiol 31(6):403–405. https://doi.org/10.1007/s002470100459

9. Jurkiewicz E, Grajkowska W, Nowak K, Kowalczyk P, Walecka A, Dembowska-Bagińska B (2014) MR imaging, apparent diffusion coefficient and histopathological features of desmoplastic infantile tumors—own experience and review of the literature. Childs Nerv Syst 31(2):251–259. https://doi.org/10.1007/s00381-014-2593-2

10. Takeshima H, Kawahara Y, Hirano H, Obara S-I, Niiro M, Kuratsu J-I (2003) Postoperative regression of desmoplastic infantile gangliogliomas: report of two cases. Neurosurgery 53(4):979–984. https://doi.org/10.1227/01.NEU.0000084165.60662.6D

11. Uro-Coste E, Ssi-Yan-Kai G, Guilbeau-Frugier C, Boetto S, Bertozzi AI, Sevely A, Lolmede K, Delisle MB (2009) Desmoplastic infantile astrocytoma with benign histological phenotype and multiple intracranial localizations at presentation. J Neuro-Oncol 98(1):143–149. https://doi.org/10.1007/s11060-009-0075-2

12. Darwish B, Arbuckle S, Kellie S, Besser M, Chaseling R (2007) Desmoplastic infantile ganglioglioma/astrocytoma with cerebrospinal metastasis. J Clin Neurosci 14(5):498–501. https://doi.org/10.1016/j.jocn.2006.01.024

13. Taranath A, Lam A, Wong CKF (2005) Desmoplastic infantile ganglioglioma: a questionably benign tumour. Australas Radiol 49(5):433–437. https://doi.org/10.1111/j.1440-1673.2005.01479.x

14. Loh J-K, Lieu A-S, Chai C-Y, Howng S-L (2011) Malignant transformation of a desmoplastic infantile ganglioglioma. Pediatr Neurol 45(2):135–137. https://doi.org/10.1016/j.pediatrneurol.2011.04.001

15. Phi JH, Koh EJ, Kim S-K, Park S-H, Cho B-K, Wang K-C (2011) Desmoplastic infantile astrocytoma: recurrence with malignant transformation into glioblastoma: a case report. Childs Nerv Syst 27(12):2177–2181. https://doi.org/10.1007/s00381-011-1587-6

16. Kepes JJ (1993) Pleomorphic xanthoastrocytoma: the birth of a diagnosis and a concept. Brain Pathol (Zurich, Switzerland) 3(3):269–274

17. Kepes JJ, Rubinstein LJ, Eng LF (1979) Pleomorphic xanthoastrocytoma: a distinctive meningocerebral glioma of young subjects with relatively favorable prognosis. A study of 12 cases. Cancer 44(5):1839–1852

18. Geddes JF, Swash M (1999) Hugh Cairns, Dorothy Russell and the first pleomorphic xanthoastrocytoma? Br J Neurosurg 13(2):174–177

19. Perkins SM, Mitra N, Fei W, Shinohara ET (2012) Patterns of care and outcomes of patients with pleomorphic xanthoastrocytoma: a SEER analysis. J Neuro-Oncol 110(1):99–104. https://doi.org/10.1007/s11060-012-0939-8

20. Ida CM, Rodriguez FJ, Burger PC, Caron AA, Jenkins SM, Spears GM, Aranguren DL, Lachance DH, Giannini C (2014) Pleomorphic xanthoastrocytoma: natural history and long-term follow-up. Brain Pathol 25(5):575–586. https://doi.org/10.1111/bpa.12217

21. Das S, Yip S, Hukin J, Cochrane D, Dunham C (2014) Pleomorphic xanthoastrocytoma of the spinal cord: case report and literature review. Clin Neuropathol 33(3):190–196. https://doi.org/10.5414/NP300689

22. Nakamura M, Chiba K, Matsumoto M, Ikeda E, Toyama Y (2006) Pleomorphic xanthoastrocytoma of the spinal cord. Case report. J Neurosurg Spine 5(1):72–75. https://doi.org/10.3171/spi.2006.5.1.72

23. Kurschel S, Lellouch-Tubiana A, Kulkarni AV, Sainte-Rose C (2006) Pleomorphic xanthoastrocytoma of the cerebellopontine angle in a child. Childs Nerv Syst 22(11):1479–1482. https://doi.org/10.1007/s00381-006-0164-x

24. Arita K, Kurisu K, Tominaga A, Sugiyama K, Sumida M, Hirose T (2002) Intrasellar pleomorphic xanthoastrocytoma: case report. Neurosurgery

51(4):1079–1082, discussion 1082. https://doi.org/10.1227/01.NEU.0000029023.74222.56

25. Jiang G-Y, Yu J-H, Zhang X-Y, Qi X-L, Sun Y-S (2016) Pleomorphic xanthoastrocytoma arising from the suprasellar region: a report of two cases. J Clin Neurosci 33(C):228–231. https://doi.org/10.1016/j.jocn.2016.04.018

26. Suzuki Y, Akiyama Y, Kimura Y, Sugita S, Hasegawa T, Mikuni N (2016) Pleomorphic Xanthoastrocytoma with anaplastic features in the Tectal region in a young adult patient: a case report. World Neurosurg 94(C):580.e511–580.e515. https://doi.org/10.1016/j.wneu.2016.07.110

27. Srinivas BH, Uppin MS, Panigrahi MK, Saradhi MV, Rani YJ, Challa S (2010) Pleomorphic xanthoastrocytoma of the pineal region. J Clin Neurosci 17(11):1439–1441. https://doi.org/10.1016/j.jocn.2010.02.022

28. Thakar S, Sai Kiran NA, Ghosal N, Hegde AS (2011) Pleomorphic xanthoastrocytoma: a new differential diagnosis for a pediatric pineal neoplasm. Brain Tumor Pathol 29(3):168–171. https://doi.org/10.1007/s10014-011-0076-7

29. Zarate JO, Sampaolesi R (1999) Pleomorphic xanthoastrocytoma of the retina. Am J Surg Pathol 23(1):79–81

30. Giannini C, Paulus W, Louis DN, Liberski PP, Figarella-Branger D, Capper D (2016) Pleomorphic xanthoastrocytoma. In: Louis DN, Ohgaki H, Wiestler OD, Cavenee WK (eds) WHO classification of tumours of the central nervous system. International Agency for Research on Cancer, Lyon, pp 94–97

31. Giannini C, Paulus W, Louis DN, Liberski PP, Figarella-Branger D, Capper D (2016) Anaplastic pleomorphic xanthoastrocytoma. In: Louis DN, Ohgaki H, Wiestler OD, Cavenee WK (eds) WHO classification of tumours of the central nervous system. International Agency for Research on Cancer, Lyon, pp 98–99

32. Berghoff AS, Preusser M (2014) BRAF alterations in brain tumours. Curr Opin Neurol 27(6):689–696. https://doi.org/10.1097/WCO.0000000000000146

33. Dias-Santagata D, Lam Q, Vernovsky K, Vena N, Lennerz JK, Borger DR, Batchelor TT, Ligon KL, Iafrate AJ, Ligon AH, Louis DN, Santagata S (2011) BRAF V600E mutations are common in pleomorphic xanthoastrocytoma: diagnostic and therapeutic implications. PLoS One 6(3):e17948. https://doi.org/10.1371/journal.pone.0017948.t003

34. Schindler G, Capper D, Meyer J, Janzarik W, Omran H, Herold-Mende C, Schmieder K, Wesseling P, Mawrin C, Hasselblatt M, Louis DN, Korshunov A, Pfister S, Hartmann C, Paulus W, Reifenberger G, von Deimling A (2011) Analysis of BRAF V600E mutation in 1320 nervous system tumors reveals high mutation frequencies in pleomorphic xanthoastrocytoma, ganglioglioma and extra-cerebellar pilocytic astrocytoma. Acta Neuropathol 121(3):397–405. https://doi.org/10.1007/s00401-011-0802-6

35. Koelsche C, Sahm F, Wöhrer A, Jeibmann A, Schittenhelm J, Kohlhof P, Preusser M, Romeike B, Dohmen-Scheufler H, Hartmann C, Mittelbronn M, Becker A, von Deimling A, Capper D (2014) BRAF-mutated pleomorphic xanthoastrocytoma is associated with temporal location, reticulin fiber deposition and CD34 expression. Brain Pathol 24(3):221–229. https://doi.org/10.1111/bpa.12111

36. Oh T, Kaur G, Madden M, Bloch O, Parsa AT (2014) Pleomorphic xanthoastrocytomas: institutional experience of 18 patients. J Clin Neurosci 21(10):1767–1772. https://doi.org/10.1016/j.jocn.2014.04.002

37. Gallo P, Cecchi PC, Locatelli F, Rizzo P, Ghimenton C, Gerosa M, Pinna G (2013) Pleomorphic xanthoastrocytoma: long-term results of surgical treatment and analysis of prognostic factors. Br J Neurosurg 27(6):759–764. https://doi.org/10.3109/02688697.2013.776666

38. Rao AAN, Laack NN, Giannini C, Wetmore C (2010) Pleomorphic xanthoastrocytoma in children and adolescents. Pediatr Blood Cancer 55(2):290–294. https://doi.org/10.1002/pbc.22490

39. Prayson RA (2010) Tumours arising in the setting of paediatric chronic epilepsy. Pathology 42(5):426–431. https://doi.org/10.3109/00313025.2010.493870

40. Fallah A, Weil AG, Sur S, Miller I, Jayakar P, Morrison G, Bhatia S, Ragheb J (2015) Epilepsy surgery related to pediatric brain tumors: Miami children's hospital experience. J Neurosurg Pediatr 16(6):675–680. https://doi.org/10.3171/2015.4.PEDS14476

41. Yu S, He L, Zhuang X, Luo B (2011) Pleomorphic xanthoastrocytoma: MR imaging findings in 19 patients. Acta Radiol (Stockholm, Sweden: 1987) 52(2):223–228. https://doi.org/10.1258/ar.2010.100221

42. Moore W, Mathis D, Gargan L, Bowers DC, Klesse LJ, Margraf L, Koral K (2014) Pleomorphic xanthoastrocytoma of childhood: MR imaging and diffusion MR imaging features. AJNR Am J Neuroradiol 35(11):2192–2196. https://doi.org/10.3174/ajnr.A4011

43. Vu TM, Liubinas SV, Gonzales M, Drummond KJ (2012) Malignant potential of pleomorphic xanthoastrocytoma. J Clin Neurosci 19(1):12–20. https://doi.org/10.1016/j.jocn.2011.07.015

44. Nakajima T, Kumabe T, Shamoto H, Watanabe M, Suzuki H, Tominaga T (2005) Malignant transformation of pleomorphic xanthoastrocytoma. Acta Neurochir 148(1):67–71. https://doi.org/10.1007/s00701-005-0549-8

45. Chamberlain MC (2013) Salvage therapy with BRAF inhibitors for recurrent pleomorphic xanthoastrocytoma: a retrospective case series. J Neuro-Oncol 114(2):237–240. https://doi.org/10.1007/s11060-013-1176-5

46. Hofer S, Berthod G, Riklin C, Rushing E, Feilchenfeldt J (2015) BRAF V600E mutation: a treatable driver mutation in pleomorphic xanthoastrocytoma (PXA). Acta Oncol 55(1):122–123. https://doi.org/10.3109/0284186X.2015.1021428

47. Lee EQ, Ruland S, LeBoeuf NR, Wen PY, Santagata S (2016) Successful treatment of a progressive BRAF V600E-mutated anaplastic pleomorphic xanthoastrocytoma with vemurafenib monotherapy. J Clin Oncol Off J Am Soc Clin Oncol 34(10):e87–e89. https://doi.org/10.1200/JCO.2013.51.1766

48. Migliorini D, Aguiar D, Vargas M-I, Lobrinus A, Dietrich P-Y (2017) BRAF/MEK double blockade in refractory anaplastic pleomorphic xanthoastrocytoma. Neurology 88(13):1291–1293. https://doi.org/10.1212/WNL.0000000000003767

49. Brown NF, Carter T, Mulholland P (2017) Dabrafenib in BRAFV600-mutated anaplastic pleomorphic xanthoastrocytoma. CNS Oncol 6(1):5–9. https://doi.org/10.2217/cns-2016-0031

Ependymoma in the Children

27

Shobhan Vachhrajani and Corey Raffel

27.1 Introduction

Ependymomas are rare tumors of neuroectodermal origin and are the third most common pediatric brain tumors following astrocytoma and medulloblastoma. They arise from radial glial-like stem cells in the subventricular zone (SVZ), lining the fourth ventricle and within the spinal cord [1]. Typical tumor location differs between adults and children: most childhood ependymomas are intracranial, while in adults they more commonly occur in the spinal cord. They are located infratentorially in up to two-thirds of pediatric cases, most often arising from the floor of the fourth ventricle. The remaining one-third occur equally divided between the spinal cord and cerebral hemispheres [2]. This chapter focuses on pediatric intracranial ependymoma.

Surgical resection remains the foundation of therapy. Gross total resection greatly enhances the chances for long-term survival. Complete removal is often difficult however, due to tumor origination from, or infiltration into, the floor of the fourth ventricle and/or adherence to critical adjacent neural structures, such as the cranial nerves. Surgical decision-making is therefore complicated by the conflicting goals of gross total resection and improved survival vs. the risk of significant neurological deficit due to tumor location.

These tumors are typically resistant to chemotherapy and irradiation and may recur even 10–20 years after initial resection. Radiation is used to treat residual tumor and historically was withheld from children under 3 years of age, but this paradigm is shifting. Defining optimal treatment strategies has been challenging due to the relatively low incidence of these tumors and difficulties in associating tumor grade with outcome. Recently devised molecular classification schemes may define specific therapeutic targets, potentially resulting in improved outcomes for these patients. Multi-institutional cooperative studies using this data are ongoing.

27.2 Epidemiology

Intracranial ependymomas account for 7% of all glial neoplasms. In adults, approximately 2% of all intracranial tumors are ependymomas, but in children ependymomas are more common and comprise 6–12% of all primary brain tumors.

S. Vachhrajani
Department of Neurosurgery, Dayton Children's
Hospital, Dayton, OH, USA

Boonshoft School of Medicine, Wright State
University, Dayton, OH, USA
e-mail: vachhrajanis@childrensdayton.org

C. Raffel (✉)
Department of Neurological Surgery, University of
California, San Francisco, San Francisco, CA, USA
e-mail: corey.raffel@ucsf.edu

© Springer Nature Switzerland AG 2019
J.-C. Tonn et al. (eds.), *Oncology of CNS Tumors*, https://doi.org/10.1007/978-3-030-04152-6_27

They are located intracranially in >90% of children. Approximately 20–30% of all posterior fossa tumors in children are ependymomas. Intracranial ependymoma is the third most common histological type of brain tumor in children after astrocytoma and medulloblastoma [3].

The majority of pediatric ependymomas, approximately 60–75%, occur in the infratentorial compartment in or near the fourth ventricle. In 50% of these cases, the tumor extends into the subarachnoid space of the cisterna magna or cerebellopontine angle or infiltrates into the upper cervical spinal cord or medulla. Supratentorial ependymomas are equally divided between the parenchyma of the cerebral hemispheres and the ventricles and more commonly arise in the lateral ventricle (75%) than the third ventricle (25%).

Data from the Surveillance, Epidemiology, and End Results database suggests that the overall incidence of ependymoma is approximately 0.3/100,000 patient-years [4]. The incidence of pediatric ependymoma in North America is 2–4/1,000,000. The reported incidence of intracranial ependymoma has increased 35% since 1973, perhaps resulting from improvements in diagnosis. Typically, ependymoma presents between 3 and 6 years of age with a peak incidence at approximately 4 years. They occur in males slightly more often than females (1.4:1) [3–6].

The cause of these tumors remains unknown. No environmental factor has been implicated. Similarities between DNA sequences of ependymoma and simian virus 40 (SV40) raised the possibility of contaminated polio vaccines leading to the development of ependymoma. Polyoma viruses, including JC and BK viruses, have been implicated in tumorigenesis in laboratory studies. This has not been replicated in human investigation [7].

Approximately 2–5% of patients with neurofibromatosis type 2 harbor ependymomas where they occur almost exclusively within the spinal cord. As such, alterations in the NF2 gene may be present in the spinal but not intracranial ependymomas [2, 8]. In a recent molecular genetic analysis of 18 sporadic pediatric intracranial ependymomas, normal NF2 genes were found. In one family without NF2 who had a predisposition to ependymomas and meningiomas, there was loss of a gene locus distinct from the region on chromosome 22 responsible for NF2. Loss or mutations of the p53 locus on chromosome 17p do not appear to play a significant role in the development of ependymomas, in contrast to other gliomas. Amplification of the MDM2 gene and overexpression of its gene product mdm2 were found in 35% and 96% of ependymoma specimens, respectively. The MDM2 protein may be an important regulator of p53-mediated tumor growth. More malignant grades of ependymoma have increased proliferation indices, greater capacity to migrate, more matrix metalloprotease activity, as well as greater expression of VEGF [9–12].

27.3 Signs and Symptoms

The clinical presentation of pediatric ependymoma is nonspecific and depends on the size, location, malignancy of the tumor, and patient age. As these lesions typically present in younger children, behavioral symptoms including lethargy, irritability, and decreased social interaction may manifest. Hydrocephalus is commonly associated with posterior fossa lesions due to obstruction of CSF flow through the fourth ventricle. Occasionally Robin's rule, comprising vomiting often in the absence of nausea followed by headache, is the presenting syndrome. Some patients may present with a midline posterior fossa syndrome: frequent headaches that are worse in the morning, vomiting, lethargy, irritability, and decline in school or work performance combined with truncal or gait ataxia. These syndromes are not pathognomonic of ependymoma and may result from the presence of other posterior fossa tumors. Truncal ataxia is more commonly observed than appendicular ataxia due the usual midline location. Mass effect upon, or invasion into, the floor of the inferior fourth ventricle near the area postrema may lead to intractable vomiting. An extensive gastrointestinal evaluation is often performed prior to neuroimaging because of the prominence of these complaints. Symptoms often become more persistent as the tumor gets larger. Symptoms may be present for as long as 3 years before diagnosis; a longer symptomatic interval has been associated with a more favorable prognosis owing to lower-grade tumors.

Presenting signs are generally dependent on tumor location. In infratentorial lesions, common signs include papilledema, nystagmus, diplopia from sixth nerve palsy, and change in visual acuity. In as many as 35% of patients, lower cranial nerve paresis is seen, often as a result of tumor extension through the foramen of Luschka into the cerebellopontine angle and lateral medullary cistern. Rarely, a head tilt and neck pain resulting from impaction of the cerebellar tonsils into the cervical spinal canal may occur.

Supratentorial tumors usually present as large masses with signs and symptoms of increased intracranial pressure. Focal signs and seizures are less common and have been reported to occur in about one-third of patients [13]. Younger patients with supratentorial tumors may present only with an abnormally rapid increase in head circumference. If these symptoms persist without treatment, opisthotonos, bradycardia, and even apnea may result.

In adults, intracranial ependymomas most often arise in the cerebral hemispheres or in relation to the lateral and third ventricle. As such, the most common symptoms are headache, diplopia, hemiparesis, and seizures. Tumors of the lateral ventricle may expand slowly and cause nonspecific and indolent symptoms, most commonly cognitive impairment or memory difficulties. Rarely, the patient may present with an acute spontaneous hemorrhage into the tumor or subarachnoid space resulting in severe headache and alteration of consciousness.

Ependymomas may metastasize throughout the cerebrospinal fluid (CSF) pathways, although this is generally a feature of recurrence rather than presentation. Seeding of the CSF occurs in 9.6–12% of intracranial ependymomas, although some small series have quoted this figure as high as 33% [14–16]. Risk factors for dissemination are infratentorial tumors, high-grade tumors, younger age, and inability to achieve a gross total resection [17]. Presenting symptoms referable to the spinal cord or nerve root from spinal drop metastases are extremely rare in ependymoma [14].

27.4 Diagnostics

27.4.1 Magnetic Resonance Imaging

MRI is the imaging modality of choice for lesions in the posterior fossa. MRI best defines the tumor and its relation to normal anatomy, including the brainstem, spinal cord, and cerebellopontine angle, with high-resolution images in multiple planes; these can be used with neuronavigation systems to aid in surgical planning. Intracranial ependymoma characteristically appears as an inhomogeneous mass arising from the inferior floor of the fourth ventricle, filling this space. They have a propensity to project through the foramen of Luschka into the cerebellopontine angle and through the foramen of Magendie into the cervical spinal canal; this can help to differentiate ependymoma from other posterior fossa pathology. The vertebral and/or posterior inferior cerebellar arteries may be displaced or encased by the tumor. Similarly, cranial nerves may also be encased. This pattern of subarachnoid spread may be responsible for the protracted symptoms seen in many patients prior to presentation.

Ependymoma most commonly appears as an inhomogeneous mass, isointense or hypointense on T1-weighted imaging (85%) and isointense or hyperintense on T2-weighted imaging or proton density-weighted imaging. Gadolinium contrast enhancement is also inhomogeneous (Fig. 27.1). Calcification may be seen in up to 50% of intracranial lesions [18]. Diffusion-weighted imaging (DWI) in conjunction with apparent diffusion coefficient (ADC) maps may help to differentiate between posterior fossa pathologies and may help to predict tumor grade. Increased cellularity within the solid component of tumor leads to restricted diffusion, and the degree of diffusion restriction tends to fall somewhere between that seen with medulloblastoma and pilocytic astrocytoma [5]. A recent French study suggested that relative ADC and relative cerebral blood volume, as obtained from perfusion-weighted MRI, could

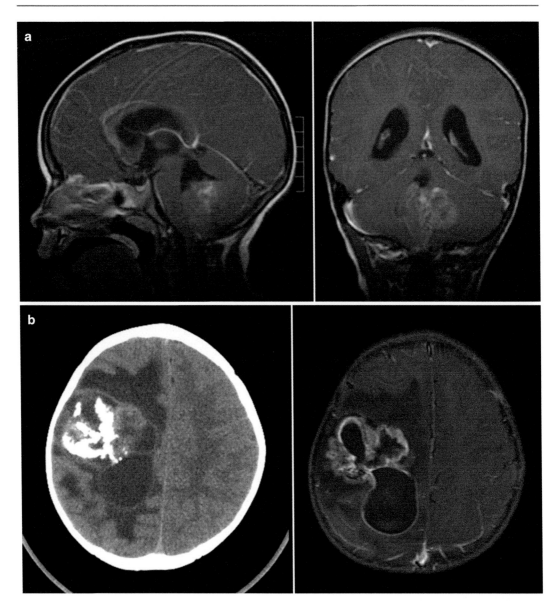

Fig. 27.1 (**a**) MR image of an infratentorial ependymoma with heterogeneous, irregular contrast enhancement arising to posterior brainstem closely associated to floor of fourth ventricle. The fourth ventricle is expanded by the presence of the tumor and causes hydrocephalus secondary to obstruction of the Sylvian aqueduct. (**b**) CT and MR image of large calcified right posterior frontal ependymoma in infant presenting with lethargy and macrocephaly

predict histologic grade and disease-free survival [19]. The fast imaging employing steady-state acquisition (FIESTA) imaging sequence uses extremely short time to relaxation intervals between radio-frequency pulses and allows for high-contrast resolution of low-intensity cranial nerves and blood vessels against a high-intensity background of CSF.

Magnetic resonance spectroscopy (MRS) has also been used in an attempt to improve diagnostic accuracy and could be used to differentiate among pediatric posterior fossa tumors. Astrocytoma has a decreased ratio of N-acetylaspartate (NAA) to choline ratio compared to normal brain. Ependymoma has an even lower ratio than astrocytoma, and medulloblastoma has the lowest ratio. This is in keeping with NAA serving as a marker of neuronal viability [5]. MRS was previously shown to have a sensitivity of 0.75 and positive predictive value of 0.6 when comparing ratios of metabolites and using creatinine as the internal reference standard. Neural network-based algorithms utilizing MRS in combination with standard MR imaging, patient age, and tumor size may predict histology with 95% accuracy [20]. A more recent study using linear discriminant analysis and combined DWI and MRS using water rather than creatinine as an internal reference standard improved the predictive accuracy to 100% [21]. Medulloblastomas exhibit elevated tau and choline peaks with restricted diffusion (high DWI signal). An elevated glutamate plus glutamine and myoinositol peaks distinguish ependymoma from infiltrating and pilocytic astrocytomas. The increased height of the myoinositol peak in lower-grade gliomas distinguishes infiltrating astrocytoma and pilocytic astrocytoma.

As mentioned above, ependymomas rarely show dissemination at time of diagnosis. Nonetheless, obtaining this information preoperatively can aid in surgical planning, as it can guide the aggressiveness of surgical resection. A less aggressive surgical approach may be justified in the presence of disseminated disease. MRI scan of the entire spine should be obtained preoperatively whenever possible. Artifacts from blood products deposited during posterior fossa surgery may make interpretation difficult if imaging is obtained postoperatively. Infants and small children may be, however, very ill at presentation, and sedation to obtain a spinal study may be unwise. In this circumstance, staging spinal MRI may be deferred to after surgery. It is best to wait 2 weeks after surgery to minimize postsurgical artifact.

27.4.2 Computed Tomography

CT remains a quick and effective means of diagnosing posterior fossa tumors in children. It is often more readily available than MRI, and the speed of image acquisition can obviate the need for sedation, although the establishment of rapid single-sequence MRI protocols has alleviated this concern in many centers. Ependymomas have the same or increased X-ray attenuation compared to cerebellar cortex (75–80%) and are homogeneous in X-ray attenuation. Hemorrhage of varying ages may be present in 10–13% of tumors. Calcification is present in ependymomas with a reported frequency of 25–50% and is better defined with CT than MRI. Cysts and necrotic regions within (47%) or related to the tumor appear with low density. Fourth ventricular tumors are often (24%) surrounded by a halo of edema or CSF. This imaging finding is not specific to ependymoma and may be seen with other tumor types. Administration of contrast leads to at least partial heterogeneous and irregular contrast enhancement in virtually all ependymomas.

Supratentorial tumors are frequently very large (>4 cm in 80%) at diagnosis. They are intraventricular in 24%, periventricular in 29%, parenchymal in 41%, and extra-axial in 6%. Enhancement characteristics are similar to infratentorial tumors. Supratentorial ependymomas may have a low-density necrotic center (47%) mimicking a malignant glioma.

Imaging findings on MRI and CT are nonspecific. The sensitivity for correctly identifying an ependymoma on conventional MR imaging is 0.5 and the specificity 0.81 [20]. The differential diagnosis of a posterior fossa mass in a child includes medulloblastoma, choroid plexus papilloma, dorsally exophytic brainstem glioma, and pilocytic astrocytoma. There are, however, some imaging features that may suggest ependymoma. The presence of desmoplastic development and a tumor-vermis cleavage plane in an isodense appearing posterior fossa tumor is highly suggestive of ependymoma, as medulloblastoma more commonly originates at the roof of the fourth ventricle and is usually hyperdense on CT. Pilocytic astrocytoma is more commonly cystic with a brightly enhancing mural nodule that usually occurs laterally in the cerebellar hemispheres. Dorsally exophytic fibrillary astrocytomas may not enhance and commonly distort the anatomy of the brainstem itself. Subependymomas are smaller, less calcified, and noncystic compared to ependymoma and typically present in older patients.

27.4.3 Pathology

Grossly, ependymomas are soft, fleshy, reddish-gray, discrete tumors most often without a well-defined capsule. When calcified, they have whitish flecks of mineralization; rarely is there a large solid calcified mass. As on imaging, they are found commonly in the fourth ventricle extending into the lateral recesses and into the subarachnoid space of the lateral medullary cistern through the foramen of Luschka and/or into the cisterna magna and upper cervical spinal canal through the foramen of Magendie. Occasionally, ependymomas may invade brain tissue and exhibit cystic elements, necrotic regions, or hemorrhage.

On histologic examination, ependymomas are typically well-circumscribed, moderately cellular tumors with uniform cells. They exhibit little nuclear pleomorphism and rare mitoses. The tumors can exhibit a typical or classical morphology, or they can show heterogeneous features. The diagnostic feature is the ependymal rosette, a ring of polygonal cells surrounding a central canal. Characteristic features include dichromatous patterns of small, epithelium-like cells merging with bipolar, fibrillated cells with perivascular pseudorosette formation. Combinations of perivascular pseudorosette, papillary clusters, calcification, and intranuclear inclusions may be identified in varying amounts in different regions of the tumor (Fig. 27.2). Signs of malignancy can obscure the classical appearance of perivascular rosettes. Significant mitotic activity, nuclear polymorphism, and variations in the shape of the cell membranes generally characterize high-grade tumors. The number of mitoses, labeling indices of proliferation markers, and cell density has been considered good parameters for prognostic purposes [22].

Typical ependymoma cells demonstrate cilia in a 9 + 2 arrangement, microlumina, microvilli, and long, interdigitating intercellular adhesive plaque-type junctions (zonula adherens) on the lateral surface. Apical and lateral portions of these cells surrounding the microlumina are clearly different from the tight junctions (zona occludens) of epithelial tumors. Zonula adherens structures contain numerous 10 nm intermediate filaments occasionally forming thick bundles and resemble an ultrastructural correlate for glial fibrillary acidic protein (GFAP) in astrocytic tumors. These intermediate filaments positive for GFAP can be shown with colloidal gold immuno-electron microscopy. Rosette cell gatherings occur around small electron lucent lumina that are filled with numerous microvilli. Electron microscopy is not always required to make a diagnosis but can be used to confirm or establish a diagnosis when light microscopic appearance is atypical. On immunohistochemistry, ependymoma cells stain positive for GFAP and occasionally stain positive for vimentin and epithelial membrane antigen (EMA). Stains for neuron-associated proteins such as synaptophysin are rarely positive [23]. A study by the Childhood Brain Tumor Consortium yielded 26 histological features and 5 factors that may provide a method for quantifying the histological heterogeneity of these tumors [24]. Predicting behavior based on histology has been controversial because the microscopic pattern appears to be of limited value in establishing a prognosis [25].

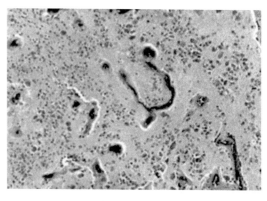

Fig. 27.2 Histologic example of a perivascular pseudorosette characteristic of ependymoma. These originate from tumor cells arranged radially around blood vessels

27.5 Grading and Molecular Classification

Cancer stem cells, a rare subgroup of transformed stem cells, are likely responsible for the development and growth of many brain tumors. Although phenotypically similar, they differ in their patterns of self-renewal and differentiation. This phenomenon has been reliably demonstrated in hematologic malignancies and for embryonal and astrocytic brain tumors [1].

Ependymomas arise from ependymal or subependymal cell layers surrounding the ventricles and central canal of the spinal cord. The cell of origin is likely a radial glial-like cancer stem cell, and restricted populations of these radial glial cells are the cell of origin of different anatomic subgroups of ependymomas. In vitro study has shown that histologically identical but genetically distinct tumors arise from different subpopulations of progenitor cells in their tissue of origin. Tumors from the supratentorial region, fourth ventricle, and spinal cord exhibit distinct patterns of gene expression and chromosome gain and loss that correlates with the anatomical location of the tumor but not with clinical parameters or histologic grade [1].

Histologic classification of ependymoma has classically comprised four broad categories. The classic or benign ependymoma (WHO grade II) has four subtypes distinguished as cellular, papillary, clear cell, and tanycytic. Cellular ependymomas are hypercellular with narrow perivascular pseudorosettes, uniform cellular appearance, and low proliferative activity. Notably this subgroup has been removed from the 2016 WHO classification given its overlap with standard WHO grade I ependymoma [26]. Papillary ependymomas are rare and contain tubovillous architecture as their distinguishing feature. Clear cell ependymomas have clear cytoplasm with a perinuclear halo and closely mimic oligodendroglioma, central neurocytoma, clear cell carcinoma, and hemangioblastoma. Immunoreactivity to GFAP and features on electron microscopy will usually distinguish it from these other tumor types. Tanycytic ependymomas consist of elongated cells arranged in fascicles with variable cell density. They resemble tanycytes, cells with elongated cytoplasmic process extending to ependymal surfaces. Rosettes and pseudorosettes are poorly delineated, and these tumors must be distinguished from astrocytomas.

Anaplastic ependymomas are malignant tumors (WHO grade III) and contain large numbers of mitotic figures, necrosis, and vascular proliferation. Anaplastic tumors show histological evidence of anaplasia, including high cellularity, nuclear atypia, hyperchromatism, and high mitotic activity. Vascular proliferation, necrosis, and CSF seeding are more common in these tumor types. These tumors will occasionally lose their structural features and exhibit necrosis and pseudopalisading, with immunostaining and electron microscopy required to distinguish from other malignant gliomas. There is a tremendous variation in the relative incidence of grade II vs grade III lesions, with series quoting ratios between 17:1 and 1:7 [25]. The difficulties encountered even by experienced neuropathologists in grading these lesions is well reported in the literature, and the wide variability in the outcome seemingly unrelated to tumor grade is likely due to this phenomenon.

Other categories of ependymoma, including myxopapillary and subependymoma, are discussed in other chapters. Historically, ependymoblastoma was combined in series with ependymoma. This is a rare, malignant, embryonal brain tumor arising from periventricular neuroepithelial cells called ependymoblasts. In the 2016 WHO classification, these tumors are named based on their C19MC amplification status: those with amplification present are classified as embryonal tumor with multilayered rosettes (ETMR), C19MC-altered; those without such amplification are referred to as ETMR, not otherwise specified (NOS) [26].

27.5.1 Molecular Classification

A number of issues have plagued the histologic grading of intracranial ependymoma. Inconsistency in determining grade, even among experienced neuropathologists, has led to poor reproducibility of grading data which in turn renders the association of grade with outcome more difficult [25]. Intratumoral heterogeneity, whereby distinct areas of differing histologic grade exist within the same tumor, makes it challenging to discern which component will drive overall tumor biology in that particular patient [8]. The application of criteria for anaplasia has been uneven in many studies, and many studies report small cohorts with poor generalizability [25, 27]. Finally the anatomic compartment may also confound grading [6, 8, 28]. Consequently the association of histologic tumor grade to outcome remains largely unknown. A Children's Oncology Group review found that only 9/32 studies was tumor grade associated with overall survival and in their own study was found not to be a predictive factor [27]. This leaves clinicians unclear on how to optimally treat patients based on histologic tumor grade.

This uncertainty has led to the development of a molecular classification of ependymoma that aims to better stratify patients and determine optimal management paradigms. Although histologically similar, lesions from different compartments are easily delineated due to distinct genetic, transcriptional, and epigenetic programs [28–33]. Cross-species analysis has proven that these differences may be the result of differing developmental and cellular origins [1, 32, 34]. The methods by which the nine ependymoma molecular subgroups were derived are beyond the scope of this chapter and however are available in the landmark article by Pajtler et al. [8].

The nine subgroups are equally divided between the three anatomic compartments in which these tumors are found: spine (SP), supratentorial (ST), and posterior fossa (PF). Within each compartment exists a molecular signature of WHO grade I subependymoma; these were found in adults only. In the spine were also lesions matching histologically classified myxopapillary ependymoma (SP-MPE) and WHO grade II/III ependymoma (SP-EPN).

In the posterior fossa, clinically distinct groups A and B (PF-EPN-A and PF-EPN-B) were identified through retrospective study.

Group A lesions were located more laterally and were therefore harder to completely resect, and recurrence rates were consequentially higher. These lesions were more commonly found in infants and younger children. Group A tumors display a balanced genomic profile, with increased occurrence of chromosome 1q gain compared to group B tumors. Group B tumors tended to be located in the midline and were found in adolescents and young adults. These carried a more favorable prognosis. This subgroup displays a number of cytogenetic abnormalities often involving whole chromosomes or chromosomal arms. These include loss of chromosomes 1, 2, 3, 6, 8, 10, 14q, 17q, and 22q; they may also exhibit gains of chromosomes 4, 5q, 7, 9, 11, 12, 15q, 18, 20, and 21q [28]. The strongest predictor of poor outcome in patients of all ages was being in the PF-EPN-A subgroup; a substantial portion of patients in the PF-EPN-B subgroup were cured with complete surgical resection [35].

The majority of supratentorial tumors show fusion between the C11ORF95 and RELA genes; these tumors are placed in the ST-EPN-RELA group. The most recent WHO classification scheme has also recognized these as a distinct group [26]. RELA fusion-positive lesions are found in children and adults. The last subgroup, ST-EPN-YAP1, contains recurrent fusions to the oncogene YAP1 and is predominantly found in children. Early retrospective analysis has suggested that these patients may have an excellent prognosis [8]. Of note, there remains a heterogeneous group of supratentorial tumors that do not possess either RELA or YAP1 fusions. Further study will be required to better characterize these lesions.

A recently convened consensus conference aimed to operationalize this molecular classification for clinical use. Figure 27.3 summarizes the consensus statements from the group and suggests evidence-based management options for each of the intracranial ependymoma subgroups [6]. Most notably, histologic grading is no longer recommended for treatment decision-making outside of clinical trials. This represents

General Consensus Statements

1. Outside of clinical trials, treatment decisions should not be based on grading (II vs III)
2. ST and PF ependymomas are different diseases although the impact on therapy is still evolving
3. Central radiological and histological review should be a principal component of future clinical trials
4. Molecular subgrouping should be part of all clinical trials henceforth
5. Submission of fresh-frozen tumor samples as well as of blood samples will be mandatory in future clinical trials

Subgroup Consensus Statements

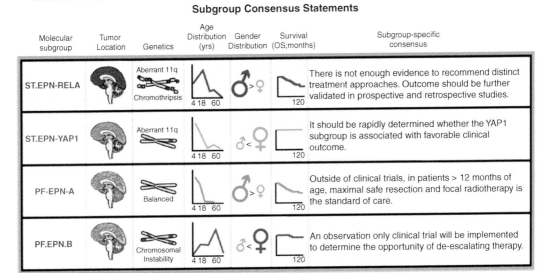

Molecular subgroup	Tumor Location	Genetics	Age Distribution (yrs)	Gender Distribution	Survival (OS;months)	Subgroup-specific consensus
ST.EPN-RELA		Aberrant 11q / Chromothripsis	4 18 60	♂ > ♀	120	There is not enough evidence to recommend distinct treatment approaches. Outcome should be further validated in prospective and retrospective studies.
ST.EPN-YAP1		Aberrant 11q	4 18 60	♂ < ♀	120	It should be rapidly determined whether the YAP1 subgroup is associated with favorable clinical outcome.
PF-EPN-A		Balanced	4 18 60	♂ > ♀	120	Outside of clinical trials, in patients > 12 months of age, maximal safe resection and focal radiotherapy is the standard of care.
PF.EPN.B		Chromosomal Instability	4 18 60	♂ < ♀	120	An observation only clinical trial will be implemented to determine the opportunity of de-escalating therapy.

Fig. 27.3 Consensus statements for the management of intracranial ependymoma based on molecular subgrouping. Used with permission from Pajtler et al. [6]

a paradigm shift in the way that intracranial ependymoma is managed.

studies are underway to better align subgrouping, treatment, and outcomes [6].

27.6 Treatment

Despite aforementioned changes in the classification and its impact on management and outcome, surgery remains the mainstay of treatment for intracranial ependymoma. Radical resection has been shown to be the most important prognostic factor affecting survival in multiple studies. Encasement of vessels and cranial nerves has led to complete resection being achieved only in 50% of patients in recent series [5]. As such adjuvant therapy may be required. Implementation of the previously described molecular classification is likely to change currently administered treatment regimens; a number of multicenter

27.6.1 Surgery

Surgery, with the goal of maximal safe resection, is the preferred initial treatment modality for pediatric ependymoma. Surgery provides tissue for diagnosis, reduces local mass effect, reduces tumor burden, and can open obstructed CSF pathways. Improvements in neurosurgical technique and anesthesia have reduced operative mortality to less than 3% of cases. Complete removal of tumor remains the only universally accepted prognostic factor. Historical figures suggest 5-year overall survival with complete removal of up to 80% compared to 50% for STR [36, 37]. Complete removal of the tumor decreases the rate of spinal seeding from 9.5 to

3.3% compared to subtotal removal, another reason for aggressive removal of the primary tumor at the first operation [38]. Factors preventing complete removal include adherence to, and invasion into, the floor of the fourth ventricle, adherence to cranial nerves, and invasion of the surrounding brain. The rate of complete removal is highest when the tumor is located in the roof of the fourth ventricle (~100%) compared to mid-floor (85%) and lateral recess tumors (50%). Even if complete resection is achieved at the initial operation, recurrence of tumor most commonly occurs in the region of prior surgery.

Surgical approach is dependent on the location of the tumor. In young children, where tumors most commonly originate in the fourth ventricle, they can be resected through a midline suboccipital craniotomy or craniectomy in the prone or sitting position. Complete removal is more difficult for tumors located in the lateral recess and cerebellopontine and cerebellomedullary cisterns, as tumors here commonly involve the cranial nerves. Complete removal may be more easily achieved in supratentorial cases. Supratentorial tumors are approached through a standard craniotomy with the exact approach determined by tumor location. Lateral ventricular tumors and those in noneloquent regions have the highest likelihood of complete resection. Complication rates between patients receiving total and subtotal resection are reported to be no different, implying that experience and intraoperative judgment are important in achieving good postoperative outcome.

CSF diversion prior to tumor resection is generally unnecessary, even with documented hydrocephalus at presentation. These patients can be managed with steroids until the definitive surgical procedure. If the patient presents with acute neurological deterioration, an external ventricular drain (EVD) should be placed to control hydrocephalus. Upward herniation following EVD or shunt placement has been reported in this context; the minimal amount of CSF necessary to improve clinical status should be removed. Resection of tumor is the preferred means of reestablishing obstructed CSF pathways. At the time of surgical resection, an EVD may be placed

to assist with brain relaxation prior to durotomy. The external ventricular drain is weaned over the next several days following surgery. Despite aggressive tumor removal, up to 40% of patients will have persistent hydrocephalus requiring permanent CSF diversion [39].

A postoperative MRI should be obtained within 72 h to assess the extent of resection. Surgical impression agrees with radiographic assessment of tumor removal in only 68% of cases. Second-look surgery is justified for removal of residual tumor if it can be performed with low morbidity [40]. In the setting of recurrence, repeat surgical resection is still the treatment of choice for accessible lesions and has been shown to result in improved long-term outcomes.

Postoperative complications are related to tumor location and include cranial nerve palsies, increased ataxia, mutism, and rarely death. Morbidity, primarily related to the involvement of the brainstem and cranial nerves, has decreased but has been reported as high as 50% [41]. Current mortality rates are less than 3%. Cerebellar mutism and pseudobulbar palsy may develop within the first postoperative week but usually resolve over 1–3 months. For reasons that are not clear, this complication is far more common with resection of medulloblastoma as compared to ependymoma [42].

27.6.2 Radiation Therapy

Intracranial ependymal tumors are relatively radioresistant. Data on survival after surgery alone versus surgery followed by radiation has not been analyzed in a randomized clinical trial. Nonetheless, radiation therapy has been considered the standard of care for patients with nondisseminated ependymoma, with the aim of decreasing local recurrence. This is particularly true for patients with posterior fossa lesions, those in whom tumors have been subtotally resected, WHO grade III tumors, and for all patients with disseminated disease. Whether all patients with gross total resection of supratentorial grade II ependymomas, as defined by postoperative

MR imaging, should receive irradiation is not clear. Regardless, there is a consensus in North America that the most effective treatment for localized ependymoma is surgery followed by adjuvant radiation therapy [43]. This approach in children greater than 3 years of age leads to the progression-free survival of 50–60% at 5 years.

The current standard of care comprises a conformal, local fractionated radiation dose of 54–59.4 Gy with a 1 cm margin delivered over 25–30 fractions. The treatment fields should cover the tumor bed to minimize long-term radiation damage. Craniospinal irradiation, in which 36–39.6 Gy is administered to the whole neuraxis with an additional boost of 54–59.4 Gy to primary and metastatic sites, offers survival advantage and is used when spinal seeding is radiologically or pathologically evident. Cure rates for ependymoma disseminated at diagnosis is unknown but is estimated to be 20–30% at 5 years and more likely in patients with limited disease burdens [44]. Re-irradiation of recurrent ependymoma has demonstrated significant survival benefit but at the cost of intellectual function [45].

As expected, radiotherapy has deleterious effects on growth, hearing, endocrinologic function, and CNS development when administered to children. It is inversely proportional to the patient's age at the time of irradiation. The effect on cognitive function has a statistically significant relationship to three-dimensional dosimetry to the supratentorial brain. Until recently, radiation therapy in children under the age of 3 years was avoided. Results from St. Jude's Children's Research Hospital, however, showed improved progression-free survival, 69.5% at 3 years, and excellent functional outcomes by neurologic, endocrine, and cognitive measures in 48 children less than 3 years of age [44]. This led to a Children's Oncology Group trial (ACNS0121), and preliminary results released in 2015 show favorable results, even in young children, associated with histologic grade and extent of resection [46]. Final results of this study are pending. For anatomically challenging lesions, particularly laterally located infant tumors, proton beam therapy has also been tried with local control rates at 3–5 years of approximately 80%, with overall survival reaching 95% in one series [47–49].

Several recent series with a small number of patients have reported good outcome in children with low-grade intracranial ependymoma who did not receive irradiation after a gross total resection. The option of close observation and delaying radiation until signs of tumor progression are evident may be useful to avoid the long-term complications of cognitive and endocrine dysfunction. As such, reserving radiotherapy for relapses or subtotally resected lesions may be a reasonable therapeutic option. Use of molecular subtyping is likely to aid decision-making in this regard.

27.6.3 Chemotherapy

Chemotherapy has remained unsuccessful in the treatment of ependymoma. Studies of postoperative chemotherapy in children under 3 years of age, in an attempt to delay radiation, have demonstrated 5-year progression-free survival figures of at most 42%, with most regimens cisplatin and etoposide based [50]. With 5-year progression-free survival reaching almost 80% after radiotherapy even in young children, most centers have abandoned chemotherapy for children over 12 months of age. The currently ongoing ACNS0831 trial aims to evaluate the role of neo-adjuvant chemotherapy with second-look surgery using vincristine, etoposide, cisplatin, and cyclophosphamide. As such, no chemotherapeutic regimen is considered to be the standard of care and should be used only within the context of a clinical trial. For those with recurrent disease, salvage therapy must be individually considered and may consist of second surgery, radiosurgery, or re-irradiation in addition to chemotherapy [51].

27.6.4 Radiosurgery

There is scant evidence for treating pediatric intracranial ependymoma with stereotactic radiosurgery (SRS). The literature does contain several retrospective reports of its use for residual or recurrent disease. Due to their uncontrolled nature, there is considerable variation among the studies with respect to progression-free survival, with ranges from 22 to 42% being reported [52]. Most experience suggests that local control of focally recurrent ependymoma is possible with SRS although patients often fail with the subsequent development of disseminated disease or distant tumor progression. It is unknown whether stereotactic radiosurgery leads to improved survival with less morbidity compared to reoperation at time of local recurrence. The improved normal tissue dosimetry and perceived theoretical advantage of proton and other heavy particle beam modalities in reducing side effects have not been investigated in the treatment of childhood intracranial ependymoma.

27.6.5 Treatment by Molecular Classification

None of the aforementioned literature on treatment and its efficacy has taken into account the now validated molecular classification of ependymoma. The results of previous studies may be confounded by clinical differences in response to treatment between the subgroups that were previously undefined; prior studies accounted only for historical demographics, extent of resection, and WHO grade [6]. Work on associating treatment-related outcomes to molecular subgrouping has already begun. A recent retrospective study of four multicenter cohorts of posterior fossa ependymoma showed that patients uniformly derived benefit from maximal safe resection but that those with PF-EPN-A tumors showed poor outcomes even with adjuvant radiotherapy [35]. Given that PF-EPN-A tumors generally occur in younger children and in more challenging locations, it has been recommended that these patients be treated in specialized centers by experienced surgeons. For those older than 12 months being treated outside of clinical trials, maximal safe resection and

adjuvant focal radiotherapy should be the standard of care [6]. By contrast, a large proportion of those with PF-EPN-B tumors did not recur after complete resection even without radiotherapy; there is a consensus recommendation for a randomized trial examining observation vs. upfront focal radiation to the resection cavity after complete resection. This may permit therapy to be stepped down in this subgroup of patients [6, 35]. Differences in biological pathways may also provide opportunities for targeted therapies. PF-EPN-A tumors have shown activation of several cancer-related networks including angiogenesis (HIF-1α signalling, VEGF signalling, cell migration), PDGF signalling, MAPK signalling, EGFR signalling, TGF-β signalling, integrin signalling, extracellular matrix assembly, tyrosine receptor kinase signalling, and RAS/small GTPase signalling. In contrast, group B tumors were defined by genes involving ciliogenesis and microtubule formation and mitochondria and oxidative metabolism [28].

The data regarding supratentorial tumors is less clear and is contaminated by a number of studies that vary in patient age groups, treatments administered, and availability of molecular data. Progression-free survival in historical studies of completely resected supratentorial ependymoma, including WHO grade III tumors, has been as high as 85% at 5 years without the need for radiotherapy; however these groups have often included adults and children [53, 54]. In a retrospective analysis of molecularly defined supratentorial tumors, with samples collected over 20 years, those in the ST-EPN-RELA group demonstrated poor prognosis independent of degree of resection, with 5-year PFS of 29% and OS of 75%. This group also included adults however. Those in the ST-EPN-YAP1 group had much better prognosis, with 5-year PFS of 66% and OS of 100% [8]. Further molecular study of well-documented trial cohorts and retrospective cohorts is ongoing to better define optimal treatment and outcome data for supratentorial ependymoma.

27.7 Conclusion

Pediatric ependymoma continues to be a challenging disease for neurosurgeons, neuro-oncologists, and neuropathologists. Surgery remains the primary modality of treatment, with focal adjuvant radiotherapy as the standard of care for posterior fossa lesions. Historical data is now ripe for revision with the introduction of a robust molecular classification system that continues to be clinically validated. The identification of specific drug targets based on the genetic profiles of the various subgroups has the potential to open a vast new array of therapeutic options for an increasingly heterogeneous disease that previously had limited management options.

References

1. Taylor MD, Poppleton H, Fuller C, Su X, Liu Y, Jensen P et al (2005) Radial glia cells are candidate stem cells of ependymoma. Cancer Cell 8(4):323–335
2. Kilday JP, Rahman R, Dyer S, Ridley L, Lowe J, Coyle B et al (2009) Pediatric ependymoma: biological perspectives. Mol Cancer Res 7(6):765–786
3. Ostrom QT, Gittleman H, Liao P, Rouse C, Chen Y, Dowling J et al (2014) CBTRUS statistical report: primary brain and central nervous system tumors diagnosed in the United States in 2007-2011. Neuro-Oncology 16(Suppl 4):iv1–i63
4. McGuire CS, Sainani KL, Fisher PG (2009) Incidence patterns for ependymoma: a surveillance, epidemiology, and end results study. J Neurosurg 110(4):725–729
5. Dorfer C, Tonn J, Rutka JT (2016) Ependymoma. a heterogeneous tumor of uncertain origin and limited therapeutic options Handb Clin Neurol 134:417–431
6. Pajtler KW, Mack SC, Ramaswamy V, Smith CA, Witt H, Smith A et al (2017) The current consensus on the clinical management of intracranial ependymoma and its distinct molecular variants. Acta Neuropathol 133(1):5–12
7. Bergsagel DJ, Finegold MJ, Butel JS, Kupsky WJ, Garcea RL (1992) DNA sequences similar to those of simian virus 40 in ependymomas and choroid plexus tumors of childhood. N Engl J Med 326(15):988–993
8. Pajtler KW, Witt H, Sill M, Jones DT, Hovestadt V, Kratochwil F et al (2015) Molecular classification of ependymal tumors across all CNS compartments, histopathological grades, and age groups. Cancer Cell 27(5):728–743
9. McLendon RE, Lipp E, Satterfield D, Ehinger M, Austin A, Fleming D et al (2015) Prognostic marker analysis in pediatric intracranial ependymomas. J Neurooncol 122(2):255–261
10. Preusser M, Wolfsberger S, Haberler C, Breitschopf H, Czech T, Slavc I et al (2005) Vascularization and expression of hypoxia-related tissue factors in intracranial ependymoma and their impact on patient survival. Acta Neuropathol 109(2):211–216
11. Snuderl M, Chi SN, De Santis SM, Stemmer-Rachamimov AO, Betensky RA, De Girolami U et al (2008) Prognostic value of tumor microinvasion and metalloproteinases expression in intracranial pediatric ependymomas. J Neuropathol Exp Neurol 67(9):911–920
12. Wagemakers M, Sie M, Hoving EW, Molema G, de Bont ES, den Dunnen WF (2010) Tumor vessel biology in pediatric intracranial ependymoma. J Neurosurg Pediatr 5(4):335–341
13. Allen JC, Siffert J, Hukin J (1998) Clinical manifestations of childhood ependymoma: a multitude of syndromes. Pediatr Neurosurg 28(1):49–55
14. Yuh EL, Barkovich AJ, Gupta N (2009) Imaging of ependymomas: MRI and CT. Childs Nerv Syst 25(10):1203–1213
15. Salazar OM (1983) A better understanding of CNS seeding and a brighter outlook for postoperatively irradiated patients with ependymomas. Int J Radiat Oncol Biol Phys 9(8):1231–1234
16. Qian X, Goumnerova LC, De Girolami U, Cibas ES (2008) Cerebrospinal fluid cytology in patients with ependymoma: a bi-institutional retrospective study. Cancer 114(5):307–314
17. Figarella-Branger D, Civatte M, Bouvier-Labit C, Gouvernet J, Gambarelli D, Gentet JC et al (2000) Prognostic factors in intracranial ependymomas in children. J Neurosurg 93(4):605–613
18. Choudhri AF, Siddiqui A, Klimo P Jr (2016) Pediatric cerebellar tumors: emerging imaging techniques and advances in understanding of genetic features. Magn Reson Imaging Clin N Am 24(4):811–821
19. Tensaouti F, Ducassou A, Chaltiel L, Sevely A, Bolle S, Muracciole X et al (2016) Prognostic and predictive values of diffusion and perfusion MRI in paediatric intracranial ependymomas in a large national study. Br J Radiol 89(1066):20160537
20. Arle JE, Morriss C, Wang ZJ, Zimmerman RA, Phillips PG, Sutton LN (1997) Prediction of posterior fossa tumor type in children by means of magnetic resonance image properties, spectroscopy, and neural networks. J Neurosurg 86(5):755–761
21. Schneider JF, Confort-Gouny S, Viola A, Le Fur Y, Viout P, Bennathan M et al (2007) Multiparametric differentiation of posterior fossa tumors in children using diffusion-weighted imaging and short echo-time 1H-MR spectroscopy. J Magn Reson Imaging 26(6):1390–1398
22. Raghunathan A, Wani K, Armstrong TS, Vera-Bolanos E, Fouladi M, Gilbertson R et al (2013) Histological predictors of outcome in ependymoma are dependent on anatomic site within the central nervous system. Brain Pathol 23(5):584–594

23. Pfister S, Hartmann C, Korshunov A (2009) Histology and molecular pathology of pediatric brain tumors. J Child Neurol 24(11):1375–1386

24. Sobel EL, Gilles FH, Leviton A, Tavare CJ, Hedley-Whyte ET, Rorke LB et al (1996) Survival of children with infratentorial neuroglial tumors. The childhood brain tumor consortium. Neurosurgery 39(1):45–54. discussion -6

25. Ellison DW, Kocak M, Figarella-Branger D, Felice G, Catherine G, Pietsch T et al (2011) Histopathological grading of pediatric ependymoma: reproducibility and clinical relevance in European trial cohorts. J Negat Results Biomed 10:7

26. Louis DN, Perry A, Reifenberger G, von Deimling A, Figarella-Branger D, Cavenee WK et al (2016) The 2016 World Health Organization classification of tumors of the central nervous system: a summary. Acta Neuropathol 131(6):803–820

27. Tihan T, Zhou T, Holmes E, Burger PC, Ozuysal S, Rushing EJ (2008) The prognostic value of histological grading of posterior fossa ependymomas in children: a Children's Oncology Group study and a review of prognostic factors. Mod Pathol 21(2):165–177

28. Witt H, Mack SC, Ryzhova M, Bender S, Sill M, Isserlin R et al (2011) Delineation of two clinically and molecularly distinct subgroups of posterior fossa ependymoma. Cancer Cell 20(2):143–157

29. Carter M, Nicholson J, Ross F, Crolla J, Allibone R, Balaji V et al (2002) Genetic abnormalities detected in ependymomas by comparative genomic hybridisation. Br J Cancer 86(6):929–939

30. Dyer S, Prebble E, Davison V, Davies P, Ramani P, Ellison D et al (2002) Genomic imbalances in pediatric intracranial ependymomas define clinically relevant groups. Am J Pathol 161(6):2133–2141

31. Korshunov A, Witt H, Hielscher T, Benner A, Remke M, Ryzhova M et al (2010) Molecular staging of intracranial ependymoma in children and adults. J Clin Oncol 28(19):3182–3190

32. Parker M, Mohankumar KM, Punchihewa C, Weinlich R, Dalton JD, Li Y et al (2014) C11orf95-RELA fusions drive oncogenic NF-kappaB signalling in ependymoma. Nature 506(7489):451–455

33. Wani K, Armstrong TS, Vera-Bolanos E, Raghunathan A, Ellison D, Gilbertson R et al (2012) A prognostic gene expression signature in infratentorial ependymoma. Acta Neuropathol 123(5):727–738

34. Johnson RA, Wright KD, Poppleton H, Mohankumar KM, Finkelstein D, Pounds SB et al (2010) Cross-species genomics matches driver mutations and cell compartments to model ependymoma. Nature 466(7306):632–636

35. Ramaswamy V, Hielscher T, Mack SC, Lassaletta A, Lin T, Pajtler KW et al (2016) Therapeutic impact of cytoreductive surgery and irradiation of posterior fossa Ependymoma in the molecular era: a retrospective multicohort analysis. J Clin Oncol 34(21):2468–2477

36. Pollack IF, Gerszten PC, Martinez AJ, Lo KH, Shultz B, Albright AL et al (1995) Intracranial ependymomas of childhood: long-term outcome and prognostic factors. Neurosurgery 37(4):655–666; discussion 66-7

37. Rousseau P, Habrand JL, Sarrazin D, Kalifa C, Terrier-Lacombe MJ, Rekacewicz C et al (1994) Treatment of intracranial ependymomas of children: review of a 15-year experience. Int J Radiat Oncol Biol Phys 28(2):381–386

38. Shu HK, Sall WF, Maity A, Tochner ZA, Janss AJ, Belasco JB et al (2007) Childhood intracranial ependymoma: twenty-year experience from a single institution. Cancer 110(2):432–441

39. Riva-Cambrin J, Detsky AS, Lamberti-Pasculli M, Sargent MA, Armstrong D, Moineddin R et al (2009) Predicting postresection hydrocephalus in pediatric patients with posterior fossa tumors. J Neurosurg Pediatr 3(5):378–385

40. Massimino M, Solero CL, Garre ML, Biassoni V, Cama A, Genitori L et al (2011) Second-look surgery for ependymoma: the Italian experience. J Neurosurg Pediatr 8(3):246–250

41. Cochrane DD, Gustavsson B, Poskitt KP, Steinbok P, Kestle JR (1994) The surgical and natural morbidity of aggressive resection for posterior fossa tumors in childhood. Pediatr Neurosurg 20(1):19–29

42. Doxey D, Bruce D, Sklar F, Swift D, Shapiro K (1999) Posterior fossa syndrome: identifiable risk factors and irreversible complications. Pediatr Neurosurg 31(3):131–136

43. Merchant TE, Li C, Xiong X, Kun LE, Boop FA, Sanford RA (2009) Conformal radiotherapy after surgery for paediatric ependymoma: a prospective study. Lancet Oncol 10(3):258–266

44. Merchant TE, Mulhern RK, Krasin MJ, Kun LE, Williams T, Li C et al (2004) Preliminary results from a phase II trial of conformal radiation therapy and evaluation of radiation-related CNS effects for pediatric patients with localized ependymoma. J Clin Oncol 22(15):3156–3162

45. Bouffet E, Hawkins CE, Ballourah W, Taylor MD, Bartels UK, Schoenhoff N et al (2012) Survival benefit for pediatric patients with recurrent ependymoma treated with reirradiation. Int J Radiat Oncol Biol Phys 83(5):1541–1548

46. Merchant TE, Bendel AE, Sabin N, Burger PC, Wu S, Boyett JM (2015) A phase II trial of conformal radiation therapy for pediatric patients with localized ependymoma, chemotherapy prior to second surgery for incompletely resected ependymoma and observation for completely resected, differentiated, supratentorial ependymoma. Int J Radiat Oncol Biol Phys 93(3):S1

47. Macdonald SM, Sethi R, Lavally B, Yeap BY, Marcus KJ, Caruso P et al (2013) Proton radiotherapy for pediatric central nervous system ependymoma: clinical outcomes for 70 patients. Neuro-Oncology 15(11):1552–1559

48. Sato M, Gunther JR, Mahajan A, Jo E, Paulino AC, Adesina AM et al (2017) Progression-free survival

of children with localized ependymoma treated with intensity-modulated radiation therapy or proton-beam radiation therapy. Cancer 123(13):2570–2578

49. Ares C, Albertini F, Frei-Welte M, Bolsi A, Grotzer MA, Goitein G et al (2016) Pencil beam scanning proton therapy for pediatric intracranial ependymoma. J Neurooncol 128(1):137–145

50. Grundy RG, Wilne SA, Weston CL, Robinson K, Lashford LS, Ironside J et al (2007) Primary postoperative chemotherapy without radiotherapy for intracranial ependymoma in children: the UKCCSG/SIOP prospective study. Lancet Oncol 8(8):696–705

51. Merchant TE, Boop FA, Kun LE, Sanford RA (2008) A retrospective study of surgery and reirradiation for recurrent ependymoma. Int J Radiat Oncol Biol Phys 71(1):87–97

52. Kano H, Yang HC, Kondziolka D, Niranjan A, Arai Y, Flickinger JC et al (2010) Stereotactic radiosurgery for pediatric recurrent intracranial ependymomas. J Neurosurg Pediatr 6(5):417–423

53. Ghia AJ, Mahajan A, Allen PK, Armstrong TS, Lang FF Jr, Gilbert MR et al (2013) Supratentorial grosstotally resected non-anaplastic ependymoma: population based patterns of care and outcomes analysis. J Neurooncol 115(3):513–520

54. Venkatramani R, Dhall G, Patel M, Grimm J, Hawkins C, McComb G et al (2012) Supratentorial ependymoma in children: to observe or to treat following gross total resection? Pediatr Blood Cancer 58(3):380–383

Medulloblastoma

28

Claudia M. Kuzan-Fischer, Isabelle Ferry,
Ana S. Guerreiro Stucklin, and Michael D. Taylor

28.1 Introduction and Epidemiology

Medulloblastoma and other embryonal brain tumors such as atypical teratoid/rhabdoid tumors (AT/RT) represent the most frequent malignant central nervous system (CNS) tumors in children below 4 years and the second in children and adolescents up to 19 years [1]. These malignant neoplasias share common characteristics, such as undifferentiated cell morphology and an ability to disseminate throughout the CNS making those malignancies highly aggressive and particularly challenging to cure. The large majority of embryonal brain tumors are medulloblastomas; they account for around 10% of all pediatric brain tumors and are the most common malignant childhood posterior fossa tumor [2]. Predominantly occurring in children with a median age of 6 years and showing a male gender bias, medulloblastomas are prevalent across the entire age spectrum but rare in adults [2, 3]. In the United States, the incidence rate reported in children up to 9 years is 6 per million children compared to 0.6 per million adults [4]. Medulloblastoma etiology is largely unknown, and although potential risk factors such as epidemiological, environmental, and infectious factors have been studied, there is not yet any clear evidence [5]. Genetic predisposition is reported in up to 13% of medulloblastoma patients [6]. Several cancer predisposition syndromes, including Gorlin

Claudia M. Kuzan-Fischer and Isabelle Ferry contributed equally to this work.

C. M. Kuzan-Fischer · I. Ferry
Developmental and Stem Cell Biology Program, The Hospital for Sick Children, Toronto, ON, Canada

The Arthur and Sonia Labatt Brain Tumour Research Centre, The Hospital for Sick Children,
Toronto, ON, Canada
e-mail: cmk9015@med.cornell.edu; i-ferry@o-lambret.fr

A. S. Guerreiro Stucklin
Developmental and Stem Cell Biology Program, The Hospital for Sick Children, Toronto, ON, Canada

The Arthur and Sonia Labatt Brain Tumour Research Centre, The Hospital for Sick Children,
Toronto, ON, Canada

Division of Haematology/Oncology, The Hospital for Sick Children, Toronto, ON, Canada
e-mail: ana.stuecklin@kispi.uzh.ch

M. D. Taylor (✉)
Developmental and Stem Cell Biology Program, The Hospital for Sick Children, Toronto, ON, Canada

The Arthur and Sonia Labatt Brain Tumour Research Centre, The Hospital for Sick Children,
Toronto, ON, Canada

Department of Surgery, University of Toronto,
Toronto, ON, Canada

Department of Laboratory Medicine and Pathobiology, University of Toronto,
Toronto, ON, Canada

Division of Neurosurgery, The Hospital for Sick Children, Toronto, ON, Canada
e-mail: mdtaylor@sickkids.ca

© Springer Nature Switzerland AG 2019
J.-C. Tonn et al. (eds.), *Oncology of CNS Tumors*, https://doi.org/10.1007/978-3-030-04152-6_28

syndrome, Turcot syndrome, and the Li-Fraumeni syndrome, are associated with an increased risk of medulloblastoma [7, 8], and it was the study of these diseases that first suggested the molecular basis of medulloblastoma (MB) pathogenesis [9].

28.2 Pathology and Molecular Subgroups

The updated 2016 WHO classification of CNS tumors recently moved to an integrated diagnosis, including histology and genetics. All medulloblastomas are classified as WHO grade IV, which is the highest malignant tumor grade [10]. Long-established histological variants, which are the classic, the desmoplastic nodular (D/N), and the anaplastic/large cell (LCA) medulloblastomas as well as the medulloblastomas with extensive nodularity (MBEN), are still part of the present classification [10]. The main histological variant is classic medulloblastoma characterized by sheets of small cells with a high nuclear-to-cytoplasmic ratio, followed by D/N and LCA with variable frequencies across age groups [3].

Genome- and epigenome-wide tumor profiling studies have changed our understanding of medulloblastoma biology. Molecular insights and phenotype-genotype correlations have offered new perspectives in medulloblastoma characterization by redefining this tumor entity. It has been widely accepted and consensually defined that medulloblastoma consists of at least four entities: Wnt/Wingless (WNT), Sonic Hedgehog (SHH), Group 3, and Group 4 [11]. Each subgroup is characterized by specific genetic alterations, histological variants, patient demographics, and clinical outcomes [11, 12] (Table 28.1). Indeed, molecular subgroup affiliation has a direct correlation with survival and should be considered for patient risk assessment, adjustment of treatment, and development of specific subgroup therapies [13].

28.2.1 WNT Medulloblastoma

WNT represent the rarest subgroup and account for only 11% of all medulloblastoma tumors [3].

WNT medulloblastomas typically occur in older children and teenagers with a peak incidence around 10 years of age and a balanced sex ratio (1:1) [3]. WNT tumors are thought to arise from cells of the dorsal brain stem and are rarely metastatic at diagnosis [3, 11, 14]. The majority of WNT tumors have a deletion of one copy of chromosome 6 (monosomy 6), while further copy number alterations are rare [3, 12]. Hyperactivation of the WNT signaling pathway is often due to the presence of somatic mutations in the *CTNNB1* gene which leads to nuclear accumulation of a mutant beta-catenin 1 protein that is resistant to degradation [11]. In addition to the *CTNNB1* mutations, *TP53*, *SMARCA4*, and *DDX3X* mutations are also reported in WNT patients [15–18].

28.2.2 SHH Medulloblastoma

SHH medulloblastomas constitute ~33% of all medulloblastomas [3]. SHH medulloblastomas have a bimodal incidence, mostly occurring in infants under 3 years and teenagers and young adults older than 16 years of age; they do not show gender bias [3, 11]. SHH medulloblastomas frequently arise laterally, within the cerebellar hemispheres, and metastases are present at diagnosis in about 25% of cases [3, 14]. Histologically, D/N and MBEN variants are almost exclusively described in this subgroup. However, SHH tumors can also present with classic or LCA histological variants [15]. Mutations in the components of the Sonic Hedgehog signaling pathway, such as *PTCH1, SMO, and SUFU*, lead to "SHH pathogenesis" [19]. *PTCH1* mutations are described across all age groups, whereas mutations in *SUFU* are more often present in infants and adult tumors more frequently harbor mutations in *SMO. GLI2* and *MYCN* amplifications as well as *TP53* mutations are also often reported in SHH tumors [19].

28.2.3 Group 3 Medulloblastoma

Group 3 medulloblastomas account for 25% of all medulloblastomas and are typically diagnosed in

Table 28.1 Clinical and molecular features of the four medulloblastoma subgroups [3, 11, 15, 20]

Molecular subgroup:	WNT	SHH	Group 3	Group 4
Percentage	10%	30%	25%	35%
Age group				
Gender ratio (♂:♀)	♂:♀	♂:♀	♂♂:♀	♂♂:♀
Histology	Classic, rarely LCA	Classic, desmoplastic nodular, LCA, MBEN	Classic, LCA	Classic, LCA
WHO grade	IV	IV	IV	IV
Cells of origin	Lower rhombic lip progenitor cells	Cerebellar granule neuron precursor cells of the external granule-cell layer	Unknown	Unknown
Typical anatomic location	Brainstem, fourth ventricle	Cerebellar hemispheres	Midline, fourth ventricle	Midline, fourth ventricle
Metastasis at diagnosis	Rarely (5–10%)	Uncommonly (15–20%)	Very frequently (40–45%)	Frequently (35–40%)
Pattern of recurrence	Rarely local or metastatic	Local	Metastatic	Metastatic
Prognosis	Very good	Infants good, others intermediate	Poor	Intermediate
Key genetic alterations	*CTNNB1*, *DDX3X*, *SMARCA4*, *TP53* mutation	*PTCH1*, *SMO*, *SUFU*, *TP53* mutation *GLI2*, *MYCN* amplification	*GFI1*, *GFI1B* activation, *MYC*, *PVT1*, *OTX-2* amplification, *SMARCA4* mutation	*KDM6A* mutation, *SNCAIP* duplication *CDK6*, *MYCN* amplification *GFI1*, *GFI1B* activation
Cytogenetics	Monosomy 6	3q gain 9q, 10q, 17p loss	i17q 1q, 7, 18 gain 10q, 11, 16q, 17p loss	i17q 7q, 18q gain 8p, 11p, X loss
Gene expression	WNT signaling	SHH signaling	Photoreceptor/GABAergic signature	Neuronal/Glutamatergic signature

infants and children (peak incidence is between 3 and 5 years) with a male preponderance (2:1) [3]. Classic and LCA histological variants are only reported in this subgroup, which also presents with the highest prevalence of metastasis at diagnosis (up to 45%) [3, 20]. The tumor usually arises in the midline of the cerebellum. A GABAergic and photoreceptor pathway transcriptional signature characterizes this subgroup [11]. These tumors present multiple copy number and chromosomal structural alterations, for example, gain of iso-chromosome 17q (i17q), which correlates with worse outcome [20, 21]. Mutation in *SMARCA4*, enhancer activation of *GFI1* and *GFI1B* [22], and amplifications of *MYC*, *PVT1*, or *OTX-2* are other alterations in oncogenic drivers reported in Group 3 tumors [16, 20].

28.2.4 Group 4 Medulloblastoma

The most common subgroup of medulloblastoma is Group 4, accounting for 35% of all medulloblastoma tumors [3]. Group 4 medulloblastomas develop across all age groups with a peak incidence around 9 years of age and are three times more frequent in males [3, 20]. The most common histological variant is classic medulloblastoma. Group 4 medulloblastomas usually arise in the cerebellar midline, and metastatic disease at diagnosis is seen in 35–40% of patients [3]. Although Group 4 tumors make up to one third of all medulloblastomas, the biology of this subgroup is not well understood; gene expression studies suggest a role for neuronal and glutaminergic pathways. The most common mutation involves *KDM6A*, a gene located on the X chromosome and which encodes a histone demethylase (H3K27) [16]. Additionally, *CDK6* (cyclin-dependent kinase 6) and *MYCN* amplifications, as well as *SNCAIP* duplications, are commonly described [20]. Frequently identified cytogenetic alterations are isochromosome 17q, as well as loss of 11q and the X chromosome [20, 21].

28.3   Clinical Presentation

Children and teenagers with medulloblastoma often present with symptoms of obstructive noncommunicating hydrocephalus due to the cerebellar tumor location in close proximity to the fourth brain ventricle and obstruction of the CSF flow causing an increase in intracranial pressure (ICP) [23]. In infants, open cranial sutures are protective against the increasing intracranial pressure and, to a certain degree, provide a compliant intracranial space. Thus, infants typically present with hydrocephalus causing progressive asymptomatic macrocephaly and bulging of fontanelles [24] and nonspecific symptoms such as lethargy, irritability, feeding difficulties, and developmental delay. The gradual closure of the cranial sutures in children and adolescents leads to a reduced tolerance to increased ICP and can typically cause headaches (especially in the early morning upon awakening) accompanied by vomiting and lethargy [25]. In severe cases, Cushing's triad consisting of increased blood pressure, bradycardia, and irregular breathing can occur and require emergent diagnostic and therapeutic action [26]. Papilledema can occur in medulloblastoma patients with hydrocephalus but is often a late sign.

Due to the localization of medulloblastomas in the posterior fossa, cerebellar symptoms, such as dysmetria, dysarthria, and ataxia, are common findings at presentation. Midline cerebellar masses are often associated with truncal ataxia, whereas patients with lateral tumors located in the cerebellar hemispheres more frequently present with limb ataxia showing abnormal findings in the finger-nose-finger, alternating movements and heel-to-shin testing. Diplopia can be observed due to sixth cranial nerve palsy, which can present as a result of a direct involvement of the cranial nerve or as a consequence of nerve damage due to increased ICP [27].

In the rare event of tumor bleeding, patients usually show an acute onset of symptoms. Cerebellar hemorrhages in the pediatric population are scarce and should always raise suspicion for an underlying neoplasm. The differential diagnosis for medulloblastoma in children includes other pediatric posterior fossa tumors such as pilocytic astrocytoma, ependymoma, and atypical teratoid/rhabdoid tumors. Evaluation with imaging and tissue collection during tumor resection for histopathology and molecular analyses are crucial for a definitive diagnosis.

The time from onset of symptoms to the diagnosis is, on average, 4 weeks [28]. Generally, rapid disease progression in patients correlates with a shorter time to diagnosis and a worse outcome [29]. Interestingly, the pre-diagnostic interval of patients with Group 4 and WNT tumors is distinctly longer compared to other medulloblastoma subgroups [28].

28.4   Imaging Characteristics

Medulloblastomas show specific neuroradiological features in CT and MR imaging. CT usually represents the initial imaging modality to diagnose patients with medulloblastoma. On noncontrast CT scans, medulloblastomas present as hyperdense posterior fossa tumors surrounded by peritumoral edema, which homogenously enhance following contrast administration. The majority of medulloblastomas arise from the vermis with close contact to the fourth brain ventricle, often causing an obstructive, high-pressure hydrocephalus with enlargement of the brain ventricles (in up to 95% of cases) [30].

MRI is the imaging modality of choice for staging (whole neuroaxis required), surgical planning, and follow-up examination as it provides good soft-tissue contrast and is superior to other modalities regarding the detection of meningeal dissemination. The standard MRI protocol for children with an undiagnosed posterior fossa tumor consists of T1- and T2-weighted, T1-weighted post-contrast, FLAIR (fluid-attenuated inversion recovery), and diffusion sequences. Medulloblastomas appear on T1-weighted images as iso- to hypointense masses with sharply defined margins. On T2-weighted and FLAIR sequences, medulloblastomas typically present hyperintense to the gray matter. Heterogeneous enhancement is usually detectable after contrast administration on T1-weighted images. Diffusion-weighted images show restricted diffusion caused by disturbed mobility of water molecules in the hypercellular medulloblastomas [31] (Fig. 28.1).

While large cysts and necrosis are typical characteristics of pilocytic astrocytomas, medulloblastomas can also present with smaller, often multiple, cysts [30]. Detection of calcification and extension of the tumor into the foraminae Luschkae and Magendii are more common in patients with ependymoma; however, when present, medulloblastoma should still be considered as a differential diagnosis [32].

28.4.1 Subgroup-Specific Features

Tumor location in the cerebellar peduncles and cerebellopontine angle, often extending into the fourth ventricle, is predictive for WNT medulloblastoma [33]. On MRI, WNT tumors present as well-defined masses with highly restricted diffusion; leptomeningeal metastases are commonly not detectable at diagnosis [34]. Medulloblastomas of the SHH subgroup are frequently located in the cerebellar hemispheres [33]. They often appear as well-circumscribed tumors, show extensive enhancement after contrast administration, and present with restriction on diffusion-weighted MRI images [34]. In contrast to the laterally located SHH medulloblastomas, Group 3 and Group 4 tumors typically arise in the midline often causing an obstructive hydrocephalus. Patients with tumors of these subgroups more often present with metastatic disease at the time of diagnosis. The typical appearance of Group 3 medulloblastomas on MRI is a high-contrast mass with ill-defined

tumor margins. On the contrary, Group 4 tumors typically show minimal to no enhancement on MR imaging. Imaging features such as mineralization, edema, necrosis, cysts, and hemorrhage are not significantly overrepresented in any of the four molecular subgroups [33].

28.5 Staging and Risk Stratification

Most studies completed over the last two decades have performed a risk assessment based on clinical criteria: age at diagnosis, metastatic status at diagnosis, extent of surgical resection, and (in some studies) histology. Brain and spine MRIs with and without gadolinium as well as CSF analysis are required to assess the metastatic disease at diagnosis. Extent of surgical resection is evaluated by postoperative MRI, and presence of more than $1.5 \ cm^2$ of tumor is defined as local residual disease. Nowadays, based on their age and the presence or absence of residual disease (metastatic and/or local), patients are divided into two categories: high and average risk. High-risk patients are infants (under 3 years of age) or non-infants with a local residual disease $>1.5 \ cm^2$ and/or dissemination; all other patients are considered average risk.

Future tumor staging will integrate the four main subgroups of medulloblastoma as well as new biomarkers (specific key genetic aberrations and cytogenetic alterations) in order to refine risk stratification for children and teenagers up to 17 years of age [13]. Integration of these biological findings correlates with outcome and allows a more robust and detailed tumor risk stratification. New risk groups of patients have recently been proposed based on the prognosis: >90% survival for low risk, 75–90% survival for standard risk, 50–75% survival for high risk, and < 50% survival for very high risk [13]. Low-risk patients are WNT patients (below 16 years old) and Group 4 patients with localized disease and whole chromosome 11 loss. Standard-risk patients are all patients with localized disease and one of the following molecular tumor profiles: non-MYCN-amplified SHH tumors, non-MYC-amplified

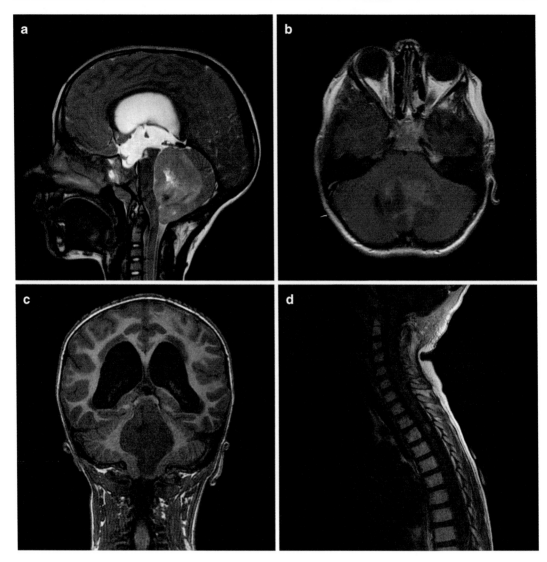

Fig. 28.1 MRI of a pediatric patient with medulloblastoma in close proximity to the fourth ventricle. (**a**) Sagittal T2-weighted image, the tumor is mildly hyperintense compared to the normal cerebellum tissue. (**b**) Post-contrast axial T1-weighted image, the tumor is partially enhancing. (**c**) Coronal T1-weighted image shows a hydrocephalic enlargement of the brain ventricles. (**d**) Sagittal T1-weighted post-gadolinium image shows leptomeningeal dissemination on the surface of the spinal cord

Group 3 tumors, and Group 4 medulloblastomas without chromosome 11 loss. High-risk patients are Group 4 and SHH patients with metastatic disease, as well as MYCN-amplified SHH patients with localized disease. Very high-risk patients are patients with *TP53* mutated-SHH tumors and children with disseminated Group 3 tumors [13] (Fig. 28.2).

28.6 Treatment

The current standard of care for pediatric medulloblastoma patients is a multimodal treatment consisting of maximal safe tumor resection, adjuvant chemotherapy, and for children over 3 years of age, radiotherapy to the whole craniospinal axis [15, 35].

CURRENT RISK STRATIFICATION OF MEDULLOBLASTOMA PATIENTS BASED ON CLINICAL CRITERIA*

Risk assessment	Clinical criteria
Standard risk	IF: ☑ non-metastatic **AND** ☑ < 1.5cm² of residual tumor
High risk	IF: ☑ metastatic **OR** ☑ > 1.5cm² of residual tumor

*For children > 3 years

Metastatic status defined by the Chang classification	
M0	No gross nodular or laminar subarachnoid or haematogenous metastasis
M1	Microscopic tumor cells found in CSF
M2	Gross nodular or laminar seeding in the cerebellum, cerebral subarachnoid space, or in the third or fourth ventricles
M3	Gross nodular or laminar seeding in the spinal subarachnoid space
M4	Extra-neuraxial metastasis

POTENTIAL FUTURE RISK STRATIFICATION OF MEDULLOBLASTOMA PATIENTS BASED ON MOLECULAR AND CLINICAL CRITERIA*

Risk assessment	WNT	SHH	Group 3	Group 4
Low risk (>90% survival)	IF: ☑ non-metastatic			IF: ☑ non-metastatic **AND** ☑ chromosome 11 loss
Standard risk (75-90% survival)		IF: ☑ non-metastatic **AND** ☑ TP53 WT **AND** ☑ No MYCN amplification	IF: ☑ non-metastatic **AND** ☑ No MYC amplification	IF: ☑ non-metastatic **AND** ☑ no chromosome 11 loss
High risk (50-75% survival)		IF: ☑ metastatic **AND** ☑ TP53 WT – **OR** – ☑ non-metastatic **AND** ☑ MYCN amplification		IF: ☑ metastatic
Very high risk (<50% survival)		IF: ☑ TP53 mutation	IF: ☑ metastatic **AND** ☑ MYC amplification	

Fig. 28.2 Current and potential future risk stratification for children with medulloblastoma: from the clinic to the molecular era [5, 13]

28.6.1 Surgery

Surgery is a key aspect of effective treatment for patients with medulloblastoma. The main objectives of surgical therapy are maximum safe tumor resection, hydrocephalus treatment, decompression of the brain stem, and other critical neighboring structures such as the cranial nerves and tissue collection for diagnosis and molecular tumor profiling.

The treatment of obstructive hydrocephalus often has priority, as most patients with medulloblastoma present with symptoms of increased ICP at the time of diagnosis. There are different therapeutic options for surgical treatment of hydrocephalus: The temporary implantation of an external ventricular drain (EVD), the placement of a permanent ventriculoperitoneal shunt (VP-shunt), an endoscopic third ventriculostomy (ETV), and early tumor resection with perioperative treatment with steroids. As only 30% of all medulloblastoma patients show hydrocephalus after tumor resection, a prediction tool—the Canadian Preoperative Prediction Rule for Hydrocephalus (CPPRH)—has been developed to identify the patients at high risk for persistent hydrocephalus. The CPPRH described by Cambrin et al. consists of the following criteria: Age < 2 years, presence of papilledema, degree of hydrocephalus, presence of cerebral metastases, and preoperative estimation of tumor pathology. The prediction tool supports the neurosurgeon with patient counseling, planning of the pre-resectional CSF diversion and evaluation of the required intensity of postoperative hydrocephalus surveillance [36]. Children classified as low risk for postresection hydrocephalus may be treated conservatively, with or without an intraoperative EVD. The implantation of an EVD during tumor resection as well as intensive postoperative monitoring is recommended for all high-risk patients; a preoperative ETV can also be evaluated [37]. Patients with SHH, Group 3, and Group 4 tumors require CSF diversion surgery more often than patients with a WNT medulloblastoma. The lack of metastases at the time of diagnosis and the older age of patients with WNT medulloblastoma are likely important factors in the decreased risk

of hydrocephalus development in this MB subgroup [38].

The typical approach in order to resect a posterior fossa tumor has the child in prone position; the head is flexed allowing an easier approach to the craniocervical junction. A median suboccipital craniotomy is performed following a midline incision and the dissection of the soft tissue. A C1 laminectomy is required in order to create space for a Y-shaped dura opening. The transvermian and the telovelar approaches are the most common routes to access a tumor located in the fourth ventricle. Early visualization of the floor of the fourth ventricle is crucial to avoid damage to the underlying brain stem. The resection of tumor tissue infiltrating the floor of the fourth ventricle involving the brain stem should be avoided as brain stem damage can lead to severe neurological complications, including cranial nerve dysfunction and fatal cardiorespiratory failure. The tumor tissue is commonly removed using a cavitron ultrasonic surgical aspirator (CUSA). Before closure, the neurosurgeon ensures sufficient hemostasis of the resection cavity [24].

Neuro-navigation systems and intraoperative imaging are helpful and support the neurosurgeon in terms of orientation within the operative site and detection of residual tumor. This increases the likelihood of a safe total or near-total resection and reduces the risk of postoperative neurological morbidity and the necessity of early second-look surgery; however, these advantages come at a price of longer anesthesia and operating times [39].

When subgroup affiliation is taken into account, gross total resection, defined as no visible remaining tumor tissue on postoperative MR images, has no or minimal survival advantage in medulloblastoma patients compared to near-total resection with <1.5 cm^2 remaining tumor tissue on the postoperative scan. Patients with Group 4 medulloblastoma possibly benefit from gross total resection compared to subtotal resection (≥1.5 cm^2 tumor remaining) in terms of an increased progression-free survival; nonetheless, no difference was observed in overall survival. For this reason, neurosurgeons are advised to perform maximum safe tumor resection, considering that aggressive surgery should be avoided at the risk of increased postoperative neurological deficiencies [40].

28.6.2 Postoperative Care

After posterior fossa surgery, patients require close surveillance, including repetitive neurological examinations at a specialized intensive care unit. Due to the limited space in the posterior fossa compared to the supratentorial region, complications such as a postoperative hemorrhage can quickly lead to a life-threatening situation. Therefore, unexpected neurological deficits or sudden deterioration of the patient's condition should always be evaluated for acute hydrocephalus, postoperative hemorrhage, and cerebellar edema using CT imaging. Delayed extubation can be considered in cases of extended operating time or manipulation of the cranial nerves during surgery; however, close monitoring of the patient must be ensured. An EVD provides the opportunity to closely observe the ICP curve and to drain CSF in case of increased ICP.

Complications after posterior fossa surgery are common but not yet fully understood. Posterior fossa syndrome (PFS)—also known as cerebellar mutism—presents in up to one third of children undergoing posterior fossa surgery. Patients typically develop symptoms within the first few days after surgery, presenting with irritability, mutism, behavioral changes, language deficits, and ataxia. The underlying pathophysiology remains unclear; however, there are some studies that describe an increased incidence of PFS following damage to the dentatothalamocortical pathways and/or the dentate nuclei. The duration of symptoms is variable; some pediatric medulloblastoma patients show only transient deficiencies, whereas others have to cope with persistent deficits [41].

More general symptoms such as headaches, vomiting, and neck pain are frequently present in children who have undergone posterior fossa surgery. The causes of postoperative headaches are multifactorial and can be due to pneumocephalus and intraventricular blood, among others. Vomiting can be explained by side effects of anesthesia, adjuvant chemo- and radiotherapy, as well as acute postoperative hydrocephalus. Neck pain is commonly provoked by intraoperative muscle damage and should be distinguished from neck pain due to meningeal irritation. Other possible complications following posterior fossa surgery are meningitis, CSF leakage, and wound infection [42]. Close monitoring and regular medical examinations allow for early diagnosis and treatment of postoperative complications.

28.6.3 Adjuvant Radiotherapy

The long-term survival of patients with medulloblastoma increased significantly after the introduction of craniospinal irradiation described by Paterson and Farr in 1953 [43]. Based on current knowledge, early adjuvant radiotherapy is recommended, as delayed radiation is associated with worse outcome [44]. Treatment of residual tumor cells at the primary site and the prevention of leptomeningeal dissemination are the main goals of adjuvant craniospinal irradiation. Radiation protocols have been adjusted over time in order to improve overall survival and reduce long-term side effects.

With the implementation of the most recent, risk-adapted regimens, the total radiation dose has been decreased for average-risk patients over 3 years of age, with no survival disadvantage given that adjuvant chemotherapy is administered [45]. Children older than 3 years of age with average-risk disease commonly receive 23.4 Gy of craniospinal irradiation (CSI) and a boost to the tumor bed with up to 54 Gy, whereas a dose of 36 Gy CSI and a boost of 54 Gy to the primary site are considered standard protocols for high-risk patients with extensive disease (> 3 years old). New protocols, such as the ACNS1422 study from the Children's Oncology Group (COG) and the PNET 5 study from the International Society of Pediatric Oncology (SIOP), will treat low-risk patients with WNT medulloblastoma with even more reduced CSI doses (NCT02066220, NCT02066220).

Irradiation treatment is avoided in children under 3 years of age as it is associated with severe sequelae. Common side effects of radiotherapy to the developing brain include neurocognitive deficits, sensorineural hearing loss, and endocrinopathies due to dysfunction of the pituitary and thyroid glands [46, 47]. Studies investigating a further reduction of the overall radiation dose and boost volumes in order to reduce radiation toxicity and improve long-term survival are ongoing [48].

28.6.4 Adjuvant Chemotherapy

Adjuvant chemotherapy has proven to be a survival benefit in average risk as well as high-risk patients and is therefore part of the current standard treatment protocols of all medulloblastoma patients.

Several trials have shown that children with average-risk disease benefit from an adjuvant multimodal therapy consisting of craniospinal radiation as described above and postradiation chemotherapy, including combinations of cisplatin, vincristine, cyclophosphamide, and/ or lomustine. The efficacy of combination chemotherapy allowed a reduction of total radiation dose from 36 to 23.4 Gy, maintaining an overall survival of children with average-risk disease above 85% [49, 50]. The St. Jude's clinical trial SJMB96 showed similar results based on craniospinal radiation and cyclophosphamide-based high-dose chemotherapy cycles with tandem autologous stem cell rescue [51].

A more intense radiotherapy with 36 Gy to the neuroaxis and a boost to the primary site with up to 54 Gy is still the cornerstone of treatment of patients with high-risk disease. The drugs shown to be of benefit to patients with high-risk disease are the same used to treat average-risk disease. The POG 9031 study compared in a randomized fashion the efficacy of chemotherapy pre- and postirradiation and found no significant difference between the two regimens, with 5-year overall survival around 75% [52]. Other studies have shown that neoadjuvant chemotherapy and delayed irradiation may in fact be associated with a survival disadvantage [53] and thus the standard practice remains of using chemotherapy after craniospinal irradiation. The clinical

trial SJMB96 showed similar survival results in high-risk patients given a combination treatment consisting of radiotherapy followed by an early high-dose four-cycle cyclophosphamide-based chemotherapy [51]. There is evidence that carboplatin can have a radiosensitizing effect with a survival advantage in high-risk patients [54].

The postsurgical treatment of infants under 3 years of age is especially challenging and consists of chemotherapy-based approaches, as radiation treatment should be avoided due to its devastating effects on the developing brain. It has been shown that a prolonged remission in medulloblastoma patients <3 years of age can be achieved by postoperative chemotherapy, especially in children with desmoplastic histology (which belongs exclusively to the SHH subgroup) and without initial metastases [55]. The Head Start clinical trials use a brief high-dose myeloablative chemotherapy followed by autologous stem cell rescue [56]. The CCG99703 study of the Children's Cancer Group is comparable and includes a high-dose myeloablative chemotherapy consisting of three induction cycles of cisplatin, cyclophosphamide, etoposide, and vincristine followed by three consolidation cycles of carboplatin and thiotepa with consecutive autologous stem cell rescue [57].

28.6.5 Molecular Therapeutic Targets

Based on epidemiological, genetic, and transcriptional differences and the identification of key signaling pathways, four molecular medulloblastoma subgroups were described in 2010 [11]. The WNT and SHH pathways have been studied extensively using molecular analyses of primary tumor samples and specific animal models in order to identify new molecular targets and agents for selective therapies. The smoothened (SMO) inhibitor vismodegib showed promising results in the treatment of patients with SHH medulloblastoma [58], and its effect is currently being further investigated in the St. Jude's clinical trial SJMB012 (NCT01878617). Key molecules of other overexpressed signaling pathways such as the AKT and TGF-β represent promising molecular targets and new therapeutic opportunities for patients with SHH medulloblastoma [59].

Efforts are underway to de-escalate the treatment of patients with WNT medulloblastoma as this subgroup has a good prognosis with low risk for recurrence and metastasis. Therefore, even though molecular targets of the WNT signaling pathway have been identified, there is currently no strong indication to further investigate these therapeutic options [60]. Furthermore, the clinical trial NCT02212574 is currently ongoing and is evaluating the feasibility of a treatment consisting of only surgery and chemotherapy.

Compared to the well-studied drivers of the WNT and SHH medulloblastomas, there are a lack of key targetable molecules for Group 3 and Group 4 medulloblastomas due to a shortage of spontaneous mouse models hindering their identification. BET bromodomain inhibitors [61] and inhibitors of the PI3K/AKT signaling pathway [62], as well as the combination treatment consisting of gemcitabine and pemetrexed, showed promising preclinical results in the treatment of MYC-driven mouse models [63] and possibly represent a therapeutic potential for patients with Group 3 medulloblastoma. Due to the development of drug resistance with monotherapy, combined targeted therapies may be administered with conventional chemotherapy to favor improved outcomes and decreased resistance.

Patient stratification based on the biology and the molecular characteristics of the tumor will open the door for subgroup-specific treatment in the future. The goal of specific treatment is an improvement of overall survival and quality of life in long-term survivors.

28.7 Recurrence and Metastatic Disease

Medulloblastoma recurrences tend to occur with a specific location, incidence, and timeline across the different subgroups. At the time of relapse, tumors can arise locally in the posterior fossa or as metastases, most commonly through leptomeningeal dissemination. A significant proportion of SHH tumors recur locally at the primary site of the disease, whereas the majority of Group 3 and Group 4 medulloblastomas relapse with metastatic disease. WNT tumors rarely recur [64]. SHH and Group 3 tumors tend to recur early, with a shorter survival when compared to Group 4 tumors [64]. Metastatic disease at presentation is a prognostic factor that correlates with poor outcome. Previously irradiated Group 3 and Group 4 tumors are typically metastatic at time of relapse and often incurable [64]. Interestingly, metastasis and primary tumors share the same subgroup affiliation, and medulloblastoma subgroup affiliation stays stable at the time of recurrence [64, 65]. However, even if subgroup affiliation is conserved (over time and between locations), recent genetic comparison between treatment-naïve primary tumors and recurrent tumors found significant clonal divergence and selection of genetic events through treatment [66]. At the time of relapse, MYCN amplifications and TP53 mutations may emerge and become therapeutic targets [67]. This significant biological and temporal heterogeneity across subgroups and between primary and relapse tumors has important potential therapeutic and diagnostic implications. At the time of relapse for all tumors, a biopsy should be performed, especially if targeted therapies are an option [13].

28.8 Prognosis and Quality of Life

Overall 5-year survival for medulloblastoma patients has reached 60–80% using a combination of maximal safe resection, craniospinal radiation (in children older than 3 years), and chemotherapy [13]. Outcome greatly correlates with tumor subgroup affiliation and is significantly different across the medulloblastoma subgroups [3]. Patients younger than 16 years of age presenting with WNT tumors have an excellent prognosis, over 90% event-free survival at 5 years with current standard of treatment [15]. SHH patient outcomes can be highly correlated with patient age and/or TP53 status. Infants generally have a good prognosis, and children with TP53 mutated tumors a dismal prognosis compared to TP53 wild-type tumors [68]. Group 3 patients present with a globally poor outcome using current treatment modalities [35]. Dissemination, *MYC* amplification, and i17q are factors that must be taken into consideration because they confer a less favorable prognosis for Group 3 patients [21]. Group 4 tumor patients have an intermediate prognosis [35], and loss of chromosome 11 is a favorable biomarker [21].

Although current standard therapies cure a large number of medulloblastoma patients, the majority of survivors suffer with long-term side effects including neurological, otological, endocrine, and psychosocial impairments, as well as higher risk of developing secondary malignancies [69]. Important neurological morbidity related to the treatment modalities impacts these patients in their daily life [70, 71]. Radiation therapy, especially in the youngest children, impacts the quality of life of these patients, and radiation avoidance in infants as well as proton therapy advances may improve the global neurological outcome of medulloblastoma patients [72–74]. Long-term quality of life studies and potential interventions to decrease treatment burden are under investigation [75, 76]. By implementing recent biological findings, future studies will evaluate the possibility of adjusting conventional and specific therapies, in order to treat newly diagnosed medulloblastomas and prevent relapse with the goal of maintaining the best outcome while decreasing toxicities and long-term side effects.

28.9 Future Perspective and Challenges

There has been much improvement in the treatment of patients with medulloblastoma since the first description by Bailey and Cushing in 1926; however, recurrent and metastatic medulloblastomas remain a challenge. Extensive molecular analyses resulted in the identification of the four medulloblastoma subgroups and opened the door for biology-based risk stratification of patients. Recently, a further breakdown into 12 medulloblastoma subtypes has been suggested [77]. The detection of subgroup- and subtype-specific ther-

apeutic targets opens the door for specific treatments resulting in improved survival and reduced treatment-related toxicity. Scientists as well as clinicians are focused on the development of more efficient treatment protocols, which can be implemented in new clinical trials. Assessment of treatment toxicity and resulting long-term sequelae as well as functional outcomes will be essential in future trials and improve the quality of life for long-term survivors [78].

Development of new treatment regimens for the often still fatal recurrent disease, based on preclinical research on therapy-naïve primary tumors, has proven unsuccessful as therapeutic targets discovered at disease presentation may no longer play a major role at the time of relapse. Therefore, the indication for re-biopsy at the time of recurrence should be evaluated if a targeted treatment is considered as a therapeutic option [13].

Acknowledgments The authors would like to thank Stacey Krumholtz, Medical Illustrator at The Hospital for Sick Children, Toronto, for the design of the figure and tables and Dr. Craig Daniels Ph.D for editing the manuscript.

References

1. Ostrom QT, Gittleman H, Xu J, Kromer C, Wolinsky Y, Kruchko C et al (2016) CBTRUS statistical report: primary brain and other central nervous system tumors diagnosed in the United States in 2009-2013. Neuro-Oncology 18(suppl_5):v1–v75
2. Ostrom QT, Gittleman H, Fulop J, Liu M, Blanda R, Kromer C et al (2015) CBTRUS statistical report: primary brain and central nervous system tumors diagnosed in the United States in 2008-2012. Neuro-Oncology 17(Suppl 4):iv1–iv62
3. Kool M, Korshunov A, Remke M, Jones DT, Schlanstein M, Northcott PA et al (2012) Molecular subgroups of medulloblastoma: an international meta-analysis of transcriptome, genetic aberrations, and clinical data of WNT, SHH, Group 3, and Group 4 medulloblastomas. Acta Neuropathol 123(4):473–484
4. Smoll NR, Drummond KJ (2012) The incidence of medulloblastomas and primitive neurectodermal tumours in adults and children. J Clin Neurosci 19(11):1541–1544
5. Massimino M, Biassoni V, Gandola L, Garre ML, Gatta G, Giangaspero F et al (2016) Childhood medulloblastoma. Crit Rev Oncol Hematol 105:35–51

6. Zhang J, Walsh MF, Wu G, Edmonson MN, Gruber TA, Easton J et al (2015) Germline mutations in predisposition genes in pediatric cancer. N Engl J Med 373(24):2336–2346

7. Evans G, Burnell L, Campbell R, Gattamaneni HR, Birch J (1993) Congenital anomalies and genetic syndromes in 173 cases of medulloblastoma. Med Pediatr Oncol 21(6):433–434

8. Villani A, Malkin D, Tabori U (2012) Syndromes predisposing to pediatric central nervous system tumors: lessons learned and new promises. Curr Neurol Neurosci Rep 12(2):153–164

9. Taylor MD, Mainprize TG, Rutka JT (2000) Molecular insight into medulloblastoma and central nervous system primitive neuroectodermal tumor biology from hereditary syndromes: a review. Neurosurgery 47(4):888–901

10. Louis DN, Perry A, Reifenberger G, von Deimling A, Figarella-Branger D, Cavenee WK et al (2016) The 2016 World Health Organization Classification of tumors of the central nervous system: a summary. Acta Neuropathol 131(6):803–820

11. Taylor MD, Northcott PA, Korshunov A, Remke M, Cho YJ, Clifford SC et al (2012) Molecular subgroups of medulloblastoma: the current consensus. Acta Neuropathol 123(4):465–472

12. Northcott PA, Korshunov A, Witt H, Hielscher T, Eberhart CG, Mack S et al (2011) Medulloblastoma comprises four distinct molecular variants. J Clin Oncol 29(11):1408–1414

13. Ramaswamy V, Remke M, Bouffet E, Bailey S, Clifford SC, Doz F et al (2016) Risk stratification of childhood medulloblastoma in the molecular era: the current consensus. Acta Neuropathol 131(6):821–831

14. Gibson P, Tong Y, Robinson G, Thompson MC, Currle DS, Eden C et al (2010) Subtypes of medulloblastoma have distinct developmental origins. Nature 468(7327):1095–1099

15. Gajjar AJ, Robinson GW (2014) Medulloblastoma-translating discoveries from the bench to the bedside. Nat Rev Clin Oncol 11(12):714–722

16. Jones DT, Jager N, Kool M, Zichner T, Hutter B, Sultan M et al (2012) Dissecting the genomic complexity underlying medulloblastoma. Nature 488(7409):100–105

17. Lindsey JC, Hill RM, Megahed H, Lusher ME, Schwalbe EC, Cole M et al (2011) TP53 mutations in favorable-risk Wnt/Wingless-subtype medulloblastomas. J Clin Oncol 29(12):e344–e346. author reply e7-8

18. Robinson G, Parker M, Kranenburg TA, Lu C, Chen X, Ding L et al (2012) Novel mutations target distinct subgroups of medulloblastoma. Nature 488(7409):43–48

19. Kool M, Jones DT, Jager N, Northcott PA, Pugh TJ, Hovestadt V et al (2014) Genome sequencing of SHH medulloblastoma predicts genotype-related response to smoothened inhibition. Cancer Cell 25(3):393–405

20. Northcott PA, Jones DT, Kool M, Robinson GW, Gilbertson RJ, Cho YJ et al (2012) Medulloblastomics:

the end of the beginning. Nat Rev Cancer 12(12):818–834

21. Shih DJ, Northcott PA, Remke M, Korshunov A, Ramaswamy V, Kool M et al (2014) Cytogenetic prognostication within medulloblastoma subgroups. J Clin Oncol 32(9):886–896

22. Northcott PA, Lee C, Zichner T, Stutz AM, Erkek S, Kawauchi D et al (2014) Enhancer hijacking activates GFI1 family oncogenes in medulloblastoma. Nature 511(7510):428–434

23. Kumar V, Phipps K, Harkness W, Hayward RD (1996) Ventriculo-peritoneal shunt requirement in children with posterior fossa tumours: an 11-year audit. Br J Neurosurg 10(5):467–470

24. Sutton LN, Phillips PC, Molloy PT (1996) Surgical management of medulloblastoma. J Neurooncol 29(1):9–21

25. Lee M, Wisoff JH, Abbott R, Freed D, Epstein FJ (1994) Management of hydrocephalus in children with medulloblastoma: prognostic factors for shunting. Pediatr Neurosurg 20(4):240–247

26. Stevens RD, Shoykhet M, Cadena R (2015) Emergency neurological life support: intracranial hypertension and herniation. Neurocrit Care 23(Suppl 2):S76–S82

27. Millard NE, De Braganca KC (2016) Medulloblastoma. J Child Neurol 31(12):1341–1353

28. Ramaswamy V, Remke M, Shih D, Wang X, Northcott PA, Faria CC et al (2014) Duration of the pre-diagnostic interval in medulloblastoma is subgroup dependent. Pediatr Blood Cancer 61(7):1190–1194

29. Gerber NU, von Hoff K, von Bueren AO, Treulieb W, Deinlein F, Benesch M et al (2012) A long duration of the prediagnostic symptomatic interval is not associated with an unfavourable prognosis in childhood medulloblastoma. Eur J Cancer 48(13):2028–2036

30. Eran A, Ozturk A, Aygun N, Izbudak I (2010) Medulloblastoma: atypical CT and MRI findings in children. Pediatr Radiol 40(7):1254–1262

31. Fruehwald-Pallamar J, Puchner SB, Rossi A, Garre ML, Cama A, Koelblinger C et al (2011) Magnetic resonance imaging spectrum of medulloblastoma. Neuroradiology 53(6):387–396

32. Tortori-Donati P, Fondelli MP, Rossi A, Cama A, Caputo L, Andreussi L et al (1996) Medulloblastoma in children: CT and MRI findings. Neuroradiology 38(4):352–359

33. Perreault S, Ramaswamy V, Achrol AS, Chao K, Liu TT, Shih D et al (2014) MRI surrogates for molecular subgroups of medulloblastoma. Am J Neuroradiol 35(7):1263–1269

34. Raybaud C, Ramaswamy V, Taylor MD, Laughlin S (2015) Posterior fossa tumors in children: developmental anatomy and diagnostic imaging. Childs Nerv Syst 31(10):1661–1676

35. Ramaswamy V, Remke M, Adamski J, Bartels U, Tabori U, Wang X et al (2016) Medulloblastoma subgroup-specific outcomes in irradiated children: who are the true high-risk patients? Neuro-Oncology 18(2):291–297

36. Riva-Cambrin J, Detsky AS, Lamberti-Pasculli M, Sargent MA, Armstrong D, Moineddin R et al (2009) Predicting postresection hydrocephalus in pediatric patients with posterior fossa tumors. J Neurosurg Pediatr 3(5):378–385

37. Lin CT, Riva-Cambrin JK (2015) Management of posterior fossa tumors and hydrocephalus in children: a review. Childs Nerv Syst 31(10):1781–1789

38. Schneider C, Ramaswamy V, Kulkarni AV, Rutka JT, Remke M, Tabori U et al (2015) Clinical implications of medulloblastoma subgroups: incidence of CSF diversion surgery. J Neurosurg Pediatr 15(3):236–242

39. Choudhri AF, Klimo P Jr, Auschwitz TS, Whitehead MT, Boop FA (2014) 3T intraoperative MRI for management of pediatric CNS neoplasms. Am J Neuroradiol 35(12):2382–2387

40. Thompson EM, Hielscher T, Bouffet E, Remke M, Luu B, Gururangan S et al (2016) Prognostic value of medulloblastoma extent of resection after accounting for molecular subgroup: a retrospective integrated clinical and molecular analysis. Lancet Oncol 17(4):484–495

41. Tamburrini G, Frassanito P, Chieffo D, Massimi L, Caldarelli M, Di Rocco C (2015) Cerebellar mutism. Childs Nerv Syst 31(10):1841–1851

42. Dubey A, Sung WS, Shaya M, Patwardhan R, Willis B, Smith D et al (2009) Complications of posterior cranial fossa surgery—an institutional experience of 500 patients. Surg Neurol 72(4):369–375

43. Paterson E, Farr RF (1953) Cerebellar medulloblastoma: treatment by irradiation of the whole central nervous system. Acta Radiol 39(4):323–336

44. Rieken S, Mohr A, Habermehl D, Welzel T, Lindel K, Witt O et al (2011) Outcome and prognostic factors of radiation therapy for medulloblastoma. Int J Radiat Oncol Biol Phys 81(3):e7–e13

45. von Hoff K, Rutkowski S (2012) Medulloblastoma. Curr Treat Options Neurol 14(4):416–426

46. Uday S, Murray RD, Picton S, Chumas P, Raju M, Chandwani M et al (2015) Endocrine sequelae beyond 10 years in survivors of medulloblastoma. Clin Endocrinol 83(5):663–670

47. Frange P, Alapetite C, Gaboriaud G, Bours D, Zucker JM, Zerah M et al (2009) From childhood to adulthood: long-term outcome of medulloblastoma patients. The Institut Curie experience (1980-2000). J Neurooncol 95(2):271–279

48. Moxon-Emre I, Bouffet E, Taylor MD, Laperriere N, Scantlebury N, Law N et al (2014) Impact of craniospinal dose, boost volume, and neurologic complications on intellectual outcome in patients with medulloblastoma. J Clin Oncol 32(17):1760–1768

49. Packer RJ, Gajjar A, Vezina G, Rorke-Adams L, Burger PC, Robertson PL et al (2006) Phase III study of craniospinal radiation therapy followed by adjuvant chemotherapy for newly diagnosed average-risk medulloblastoma. J Clin Oncol 24(25):4202–4208

50. Lannering B, Rutkowski S, Doz F, Pizer B, Gustafsson G, Navajas A et al (2012) Hyperfractionated versus conventional radiotherapy followed by chemotherapy in standard-risk medulloblastoma: results from the randomized multicenter HIT-SIOP PNET 4 trial. J Clin Oncol 30(26):3187–3193

51. Gajjar A, Chintagumpala M, Ashley D, Kellie S, Kun LE, Merchant TE et al (2006) Risk-adapted craniospinal radiotherapy followed by high-dose chemotherapy and stem-cell rescue in children with newly diagnosed medulloblastoma (St Jude Medulloblastoma-96): long-term results from a prospective, multicentre trial. Lancet Oncol 7(10):813–820

52. Tarbell NJ, Friedman H, Polkinghorn WR, Yock T, Zhou T, Chen Z et al (2013) High-risk medulloblastoma: a pediatric oncology group randomized trial of chemotherapy before or after radiation therapy (POG 9031). J Clin Oncol 31(23):2936–2941

53. Kortmann RD, Kuhl J, Timmermann B, Mittler U, Urban C, Budach V et al (2000) Postoperative neoadjuvant chemotherapy before radiotherapy as compared to immediate radiotherapy followed by maintenance chemotherapy in the treatment of medulloblastoma in childhood: results of the German prospective randomized trial HIT '91. Int J Radiat Oncol Biol Phys 46(2):269–279

54. Jakacki RI, Burger PC, Zhou T, Holmes EJ, Kocak M, Onar A et al (2012) Outcome of children with metastatic medulloblastoma treated with carboplatin during craniospinal radiotherapy: a Children's Oncology Group Phase I/II study. J Clin Oncol 30(21):2648–2653

55. Rutkowski S, Bode U, Deinlein F, Ottensmeier H, Warmuth-Metz M, Soerensen N et al (2005) Treatment of early childhood medulloblastoma by postoperative chemotherapy alone. N Engl J Med 352(10):978–986

56. Dhall G, Grodman H, Ji L, Sands S, Gardner S, Dunkel IJ et al (2008) Outcome of children less than three years old at diagnosis with non-metastatic medulloblastoma treated with chemotherapy on the "Head Start" I and II protocols. Pediatr Blood Cancer 50(6):1169–1175

57. Cohen BH, Geyer JR, Miller DC, Curran JG, Zhou T, Holmes E et al (2015) Pilot study of intensive chemotherapy with peripheral hematopoietic cell support for children less than 3 years of age with malignant brain tumors, the CCG-99703 phase I/II study. A report from the Children's Oncology Group. Pediatr Neurol 53(1):31–46

58. Rudin CM, Hann CL, Laterra J, Yauch RL, Callahan CA, Fu L et al (2009) Treatment of medulloblastoma with hedgehog pathway inhibitor GDC-0449. N Engl J Med 361(12):1173–1178

59. de Bont JM, Packer RJ, Michiels EM, den Boer ML, Pieters R (2008) Biological background of pediatric medulloblastoma and ependymoma: a review from a translational research perspective. Neuro-Oncology 10(6):1040–1060

60. Northcott PA, Dubuc AM, Pfister S, Taylor MD (2012) Molecular subgroups of medulloblastoma. Expert Rev Neurother 12(7):871–884

61. Bandopadhayay P, Bergthold G, Nguyen B, Schubert S, Gholamin S, Tang Y et al (2014) BET bromodo-

main inhibition of MYC-amplified medulloblastoma. Clin Cancer Res 20(4):912–925

62. Pei Y, Moore CE, Wang J, Tewari AK, Eroshkin A, Cho YJ et al (2012) An animal model of MYC-driven medulloblastoma. Cancer Cell 21(2):155–167

63. Morfouace M, Shelat A, Jacus M, Freeman BB 3rd, Turner D, Robinson S et al (2014) Pemetrexed and gemcitabine as combination therapy for the treatment of Group3 medulloblastoma. Cancer Cell 25(4):516–529

64. Ramaswamy V, Remke M, Bouffet E, Faria CC, Perreault S, Cho YJ et al (2013) Recurrence patterns across medulloblastoma subgroups: an integrated clinical and molecular analysis. Lancet Oncol 14(12):1200–1207

65. Wang X, Dubuc AM, Ramaswamy V, Mack S, Gendoo DM, Remke M et al (2015) Medulloblastoma subgroups remain stable across primary and metastatic compartments. Acta Neuropathol 129(3):449–457

66. Morrissy AS, Garzia L, Shih DJ, Zuyderduyn S, Huang X, Skowron P et al (2016) Divergent clonal selection dominates medulloblastoma at recurrence. Nature 529(7586):351–357

67. Hill RM, Kuijper S, Lindsey JC, Petrie K, Schwalbe EC, Barker K et al (2015) Combined MYC and P53 defects emerge at medulloblastoma relapse and define rapidly progressive, therapeutically targetable disease. Cancer Cell 27(1):72–84

68. Zhukova N, Ramaswamy V, Remke M, Pfaff E, Shih DJ, Martin DC et al (2013) Subgroup-specific prognostic implications of TP53 mutation in medulloblastoma. J Clin Oncol 31(23):2927–2935

69. Packer RJ, Zhou T, Holmes E, Vezina G, Gajjar A (2013) Survival and secondary tumors in children with medulloblastoma receiving radiotherapy and adjuvant chemotherapy: results of Children's Oncology Group trial A9961. Neuro-Oncology 15(1):97–103

70. Fay-McClymont TB, Ploetz DM, Mabbott D, Walsh K, Smith A, Chi SN et al (2017) Long-term neuropsychological follow-up of young children with

medulloblastoma treated with sequential high-dose chemotherapy and irradiation sparing approach. J Neurooncol 133(1):119–128

71. King AA, Seidel K, Di C, Leisenring WM, Perkins SM, Krull KR et al (2017) Long-term neurologic health and psychosocial function of adult survivors of childhood medulloblastoma/PNET: a report from the Childhood Cancer Survivor Study. Neuro-Oncology 19(5):689–698

72. Lafay-Cousin L, Bouffet E, Hawkins C, Amid A, Huang A, Mabbott DJ (2009) Impact of radiation avoidance on survival and neurocognitive outcome in infant medulloblastoma. Curr Oncol 16(6):21–28

73. Lafay-Cousin L, Smith A, Chi SN, Wells E, Madden J, Margol A et al (2016) Clinical, pathological, and molecular characterization of infant medulloblastomas treated with sequential high-dose chemotherapy. Pediatr Blood Cancer 63(9):1527–1534

74. Yock TI, Yeap BY, Ebb DH, Weyman E, Eaton BR, Sherry NA et al (2016) Long-term toxic effects of proton radiotherapy for paediatric medulloblastoma: a phase 2 single-arm study. Lancet Oncol 17(3):287–298

75. Kulkarni AV, Piscione J, Shams I, Bouffet E (2013) Long-term quality of life in children treated for posterior fossa brain tumors. J Neurosurg Pediatr 12(3):235–240

76. Piscione PJ, Bouffet E, Mabbott DJ, Shams I, Kulkarni AV (2014) Physical functioning in pediatric survivors of childhood posterior fossa brain tumors. Neuro-Oncology 16(1):147–155

77. Cavalli FMG, Remke M, Rampasek L, Peacock J, Shih DJH, Luu B et al (2017) Intertumoral heterogeneity within medulloblastoma subgroups. Cancer Cell 31(6):737–754. e6

78. Kuzan-Fischer CM, Guerreiro Stucklin AS, Taylor MD (2017) Advances in genomics explain medulloblastoma behavior at the bedside. Neurosurgery 64(CN_suppl_1):21–26

Dysembryoplastic Neuroectodermal Tumors

Aurelia Peraud, Jörg-Christian Tonn, and James T. Rutka

29.1 Epidemiology

Dysembryoplastic neuroectodermal or neuroepithelial tumor (DNET) was initially described by Daumas-Duport et al. [1] in 1988 as a mixed tumor with glial and neuronal elements and has been included in the World Health Organization classification of brain tumors as a separate entity [2].

It is considered as hamartomatous, low-grade lesion (WHO grade I) due to the dysplastic appearance of the lesion and the surrounding cortex. It constitutes about 1.2% of all pediatric intracranial tumors [3]. They mainly occur in the temporal lobe followed by the frontal and occipital lobe or the cerebellum and brain stem [4]. Macroscopically, DNETs are most of the time confined to the cerebral cortex but may extend into the adjacent white matter. DNETs typically manifest during childhood or early adulthood with medically refractory epileptic seizures. The seizure focus is frequently in the temporal location, and the lesion most often found in the temporal lobe, followed by the frontal lobes, and is only rarely located in other lobes. Associated cranial bone deformities with thinning of the overlying calvarium may be present. Histologically, DNETs are characterized by the presence of a specific element and by a nodular component. The specific elements consist of oligodendroglia-like cells that are distributed within a mucinous matrix, in which normal and dysplastic ganglion-like neurons appear to be floating ("floating neurons"). Although increased cellularity and some pleomorphism may be present, these lesions are devoid of anaplastic features. Based on the results of immunohistochemical studies, DNETs are considered to originate from progenitor cells with potential for glial and neuronal differentiation. The surgical outcome is excellent. Even after subtotal resection recurrences are rare.

A. Peraud (✉)
Neurochirurgische Klinik, Klinikum Großhadern, Munich, Germany
e-mail: aurelia.peraud@med.uni-muenchen.de

J.-C. Tonn
Department of Surgery, University Hospital Ludwig Maximilian University Munich, Munich, Germany
e-mail: Joerg.Christian.Tonn@med.uni-muenchen.de

J. T. Rutka
Division of Neurosurgery, The Arthur and Sonia Labatt Brain Tumour Research Centre, The Hospital for Sick Children, Toronto, ON, Canada

Department of Surgery, University of Toronto, Toronto, ON, Canada
e-mail: James.rutka@sickkids.ca

29.2 Symptoms and Clinical Signs

By far the most common presenting symptom in patients with DNETs is seizures, followed by headache [5, 6]. The seizures usually begin before the age of 20 years, occasionally as infan-

© Springer Nature Switzerland AG 2019
J.-C. Tonn et al. (eds.), *Oncology of CNS Tumors*, https://doi.org/10.1007/978-3-030-04152-6_29

tile spasm. The type of seizure depends on the location and age of the patient but is most often a partial seizure with or without secondary generalization. Patients with frontal lobe DNET may have psychosis as well as seizures. Focal neurological deficits are lacking. There are some reports describing an association with phakomatosis like neurofibromatosis type 1 [7]. Although DNET is commonly associated with cortical dysplasia, and some delay of early developmental milestones may be apparent, the involvement of the cortex is not severe enough to cause significant mental retardation [8].

29.3 Diagnostics

All imaging modalities show the cortical topography of the lesion, with MR images being superior for diagnosis. DNETs are typically well-circumscribed lesions with gyral or nodular configuration and hypointense on T1- and hyperintense on T2-weighted images relative to gray matter. They lead to an enlargement of the involved gyrus but cause no mass effect. Cystic components can be seen in about 30% with focal enhancement in 16–66% [4, 9–11]. An extension into the white matter is noted in about 40%, and blurring of the gray-white matter interface has been contributed to invasion, cortical dysgenesis, and dysmyelination (Fig. 29.1). These tumors may be hypo- to isodense to gray matter on CT images and have cysts in up to 7.5% and calcifications in up to 36% [12]. Focal contrast enhancement is possible in around 20%. Erosion of the temporal fossa and calvarial scalloping are reported in 44–60% of cortically based tumors [12]. DNETs are angiographically occult, occasionally avascular masses. They demonstrate a hypoperfused area on SPECT imaging with no thallium uptake and a low methionine uptake on PET, unlike other low-grade gliomas [13].

Extraoperative electrocorticographic recordings from subdural electrodes demonstrated that the ictal onset zone in patients with temporal DNETs was more frequent in the adjacent tissues of the tumor (88.9%) than within the tumor or in the mesial temporal area (66.7%) [14].

29.4 Staging and Classification

DNETs correspond histologically to WHO grade I and are composed of a glial and a neuronal component. They show some similarities with other mixed glioneuronal tumors like ganglioglioma, glioneuronal hamartoma, or tuberous lesion but have typical histological criteria with a nodular architecture and the presence of a specific element. The specific glioneuronal element has a columnar appearance oriented perpendicular to the cortical surface. The columns are formed of axon bundles that are lined with oligo dendrocyte-like cells. Neurons with normal cytology appear to float in an eosinophilic matrix between these columns ("floating neurons") [15, 16]. Despite the benign clinical course, nuclear atypias, monstrous cells, and foci of necrosis and mitosis can be found [17]. Three different variants of DNET have been distinguished: the simple, the complex, and the so-called nonspecific form. These variants raise different problems in terms of their histological diagnosis; however, this histological subclassification has no clinical or therapeutic implication. Although DNETs share histological features with diffuse astrocytic and oligodendroglial tumors, they never demonstrate IDH mutation nor 1p/19q co-deletion. V600E mutations of the BRAF gene have been reported in up to 20% [18]. Alterations in the MAP kinase pathway (FGFR1) were recently reported [18]. A coexistence with pilocytic astrocytoma has been described [19].

The simple form consists of the unique glioneuronal element, which may be surrounded by isolated neoplastic oligodendrocytes. In the complex form, glial nodules are seen in association with the specific glioneuronal element and/ or foci of cortical dysplasia. The glial component seen in the complex form has a highly variable appearance with a nodular or diffuse pattern, making a differentiation among conventional gliomas difficult. The nonspecific form lacks the diagnostic glioneuronal component and the multinodular architecture but demonstrates similar clinical presentation and neuroradiological profile and does not grow on long-term follow-up.

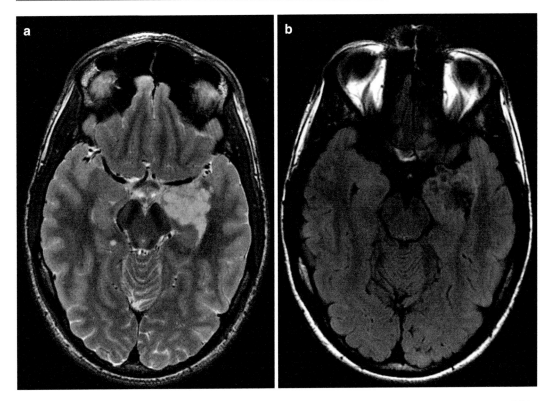

Fig. 29.1 Left temporal DNET of a 15-year-old girl. The tumor led to an enlargement of the involved gyrus, exhibits nodular growth pattern, and is hyperintense on T2-weighted (**a**) and FLAIR (**b**) MR images

29.5   Treatment

29.5.1 Surgery

Surgical resection of the lesion is the sole reasonable therapeutic option in DNETs. Controversies exist about whether the extent of resection has any impact on seizure outcome. Some authors believe that even with partial resection, an improvement of seizure activity and of developmental delay can be achieved [20], while others strongly recommend complete resection of the lesion, including the epileptogenic area, to obtain excellent seizure control [4, 21]. Surgical planning and resection of lesions close to eloquent cortical areas can be facilitated with the use of neuronavigation (Fig. 29.2). Ictal SPECT investigations revealed hyperperfused areas of focal cortical dysplasia associated with DNET, indicating intrinsic epi-

leptogenicity. Kameyama et al. therefore advocate excision of the DNET and the epileptogenic area of the focal cortical dysplasia [14, 22]. But even with incomplete resection, tumors remain stable over many years.

29.5.2 Radiotherapy

Before its description as a separate entity, DNET was usually diagnosed as low-grade astrocytoma, oligodendroglioma, mixed oligoastrocytoma, or ganglioglioma. As a result, patients were treated with radiotherapy and chemotherapy. The lesion is most likely curable by surgical excision alone; adjuvant therapy is not needed. But close clinical and radiological follow-up is recommended because of the rare chance of tumor recurrence or even malignant transformation reported by some authors [23–25]. The publication of Rushing

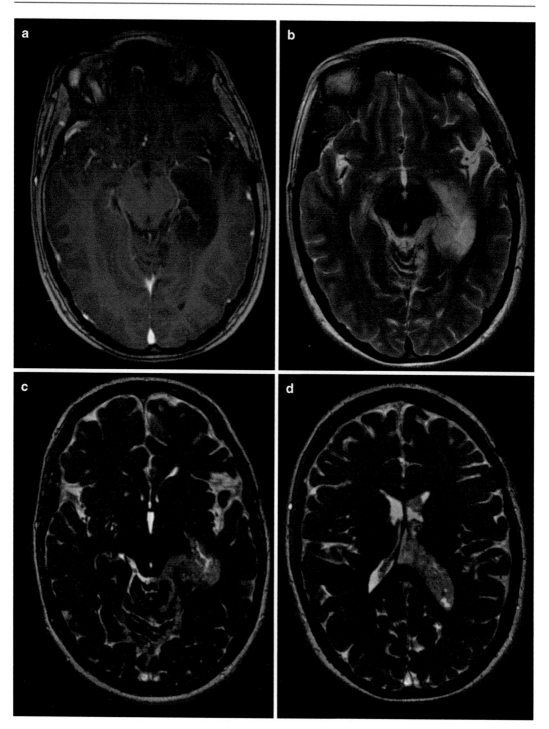

Fig. 29.2 Multifocal DNET in a 12-year-old girl with supra- and infratentorial manifestation. The temporomesial lesion exhibits some faint contrast enhancement on axial T1-weighted images (**a**). The tumor led to an enlargement of the temporomesial gyrus and blurring of the gray-white matter interface on T2-weighted images (**b**). The multifocal tumor appearance is best visualized on CISS 3D images with nodular growth pattern and extension within the lateral ventricle and on the cerebellar surface (**c, d**)

et al. reports about a 14-year-old boy initially diagnosed with a mixed oligoastrocytoma who received combined radio- and chemotherapy and developed an anaplastic astrocytoma 3 years later. Review of the initial biopsy showed typical histological features of the complex form of a DNET [25].

29.6 Prognosis/Quality of Life

The overall prognosis for patients with DNETs is excellent, and the lesion remains stable without progression over many years even after subtotal resection [1, 26]. Tumor recurrences or malignant transformation of the lesion is very unlikely, although single case reports exist [24, 25]. Multifocal (supra- and infratentorial) tumor appearance is described [6]. Seizure outcome is best after early and complete resection of the lesion and, if present, the epileptogenic area of focal cortical dysplasia [21]. Patients with a dual pathology of DNET and hippocampal sclerosis or focal cortical dysplasia seem to do worse with regard to seizure control [27].

29.7 Follow-Up/Specific Problems and Measures

Irrespective of the extent of surgical resection, multiple reports confirm neither clinical nor radiological evidence of recurrence in any patient. Nevertheless, the outcome with regard to seizures is discussed controversially in the literature. Most authors recommend resecting not only the tumor but also the adjacent dysplastic cortex in order to obtain a seizure-free life for the patient, while some could not prove any benefit with extensive resection.

References

1. Daumas-Duport C, Scheithauer BW, Chodkiewicz JP, Laws ER Jr, Vedrenne C (1988) Dysembryoplastic neuroepithelial tumor: a surgically curable tumor of young patients with intractable partial seizures. Report of thirty-nine cases. Neurosurgery 23:545–556
2. Louis DN, Perry A, Reifenberger G, von Deimling A, Figarella-Branger D, Cavenee WK, Ohgaki H, Wiestler OD, Kleihues P, Ellison DW (2016) The 2016 World Health Organization classification of tumors of the central nervous system: a summary. Acta Neuropathol 131:803–820
3. Sukheeja D, Mehta J (2016) Dysembryoplastic neuroepithelial tumor: a rare brain tumor not to be misdiagnosed. Asian J Neurosurg 11:174
4. O'Brien DF, Farrell M, Delanty N, Traunecker H, Perrin R, Smyth MD, Park TS, The Children's Cancer and Leukaemia Group (2007) The Children's Cancer and Leukaemia Group guidelines for the diagnosis and management of dysembryoplastic neuroepithelial tumours. Br J Neurosurg 21:539–549
5. Holthausen H, Blumcke I (2016) Epilepsy-associated tumours: what epileptologists should know about neuropathology, terminology, and classification systems. Epileptic Disord 18:240–251
6. Yang AI, Khawaja AM, Ballester-Fuentes L, Pack SD, Abdullaev Z, Patronas NJ, Inati SK, Theodore WH, Quezado MM, Zaghloul KA (2014) Multifocal dysembryoplastic neuroepithelial tumours associated with refractory epilepsy. Epileptic Disord 16:328–332
7. Lellouch-Tubiana A, Bourgeois M, Vekemans M, Robain O (1995) Dysembryoplastic neuroepithelial tumors in two children with neurofibromatosis type 1. Acta Neuropathol 90:319–322
8. Raymond AA, Halpin SF, Alsanjari N, Cook MJ, Kitchen ND, Fish DR, Stevens JM, Harding BN, Scaravilli F, Kendall B et al (1994) Dysembryoplastic neuroepithelial tumor. Features in 16 patients. Brain 117(Pt 3):461–475
9. Bulakbasi N, Kocaoglu M, Sanal TH, Tayfun C (2007) Dysembryoplastic neuroepithelial tumors: proton MR spectroscopy, diffusion and perfusion characteristics. Neuroradiology 49:805–812
10. Fernandez C, Girard N, Paz Paredes A, Bouvier-Labit C, Lena G, Figarella-Branger D (2003) The usefulness of MR imaging in the diagnosis of dysembryoplastic neuroepithelial tumor in children: a study of 14 cases. AJNR Am J Neuroradiol 24:829–834
11. Paudel K, Borofsky S, Jones RV, Levy LM (2013) Dysembryoplastic neuroepithelial tumor with atypical presentation: MRI and diffusion tensor characteristics. J Radiol Case Rep 7:7–14
12. Stanescu Cosson R, Varlet P, Beuvon F, Daumas Duport C, Devaux B, Chassoux F, Fredy D, Meder JF (2001) Dysembryoplastic neuroepithelial tumors: CT, MR findings and imaging follow-up: a study of 53 cases. J Neuroradiol 28:230–240
13. Rheims S, Rubi S, Bouvard S, Bernard E, Streichenberger N, Guenot M, Le Bars D, Hammers A, Ryvlin P (2014) Accuracy of distinguishing between dysembryoplastic neuroepithelial tumors and other epileptogenic brain neoplasms with [(1)(1)C]methionine PET. Neuro-Oncology 16:1417–1426
14. Seo DW, Hong SB (2003) Epileptogenic foci on subdural recording in intractable epilepsy patients with

temporal dysembryoplastic neuroepithelial tumor. J Korean Med Sci 18:559–565

15. Daumas-Duport C (1993) Dysembryoplastic neuro-epithelial tumours. Brain Pathol 3:283–295

16. Kleihues P, Louis DN, Scheithauer BW, Rorke LB, Reifenberger G, Burger PC, Cavenee WK (2002) The WHO classification of tumors of the nervous system. J Neuropathol Exp Neurol 61:215–225; discussion 226–219

17. Cabiol J, Acebes JJ, Isamat F (1999) Dysembryoplastic neuroepithelial tumor. Crit Rev Neurosurg 9:116–125

18. Fina F, Barets D, Colin C, Bouvier C, Padovani L, Nanni-Metellus I, Ouafik L, Scavarda D, Korshunov A, Jones DT, Figarella-Branger D (2017) Droplet digital PCR is a powerful technique to demonstrate frequent FGFR1 duplication in dysembryoplastic neuroepithelial tumors. Oncotarget 8:2104–2113

19. Nasit JG, Shah P, Zalawadia H (2016) Coexistent dysembryoplastic neuroepithelial tumour and pilocytic astrocytoma. Asian J Neurosurg 11:451

20. Kim SK, Wang KC, Hwang YS, Kim KJ, Cho BK (2001) Intractable epilepsy associated with brain tumors in children: surgical modality and outcome. Childs Nerv Syst 17:445–452

21. Kameyama S, Fukuda M, Tomikawa M, Morota N, Oishi M, Wachi M, Kanazawa O, Sasagawa M, Kakita A, Takahashi H (2001) Surgical strategy and outcomes for epileptic patients with focal cortical dysplasia or dysembryoplastic neuroepithelial tumor. Epilepsia 42(Suppl 6):37–41

22. Zentner J, Hufnagel A, Wolf HK, Ostertun B, Behrens E, Campos MG, Elger CE, Wiestler OD, Schramm J (1997) Surgical treatment of neoplasms associated with medically intractable epilepsy. Neurosurgery 41:378–386; discussion 386–377

23. Hammond RR, Duggal N, Woulfe JM, Girvin JP (2000) Malignant transformation of a dysembryoplastic neuroepithelial tumor. Case report. J Neurosurg 92:722–725

24. Heiland DH, Staszewski O, Hirsch M, Masalha W, Franco P, Grauvogel J, Capper D, Schrimpf D, Urbach H, Weyerbrock A (2016) Malignant transformation of a dysembryoplastic neuroepithelial tumor (DNET) characterized by genome-wide methylation analysis. J Neuropathol Exp Neurol 75:358–365

25. Rushing EJ, Thompson LD, Mena H (2003) Malignant transformation of a dysembryoplastic neuroepithelial tumor after radiation and chemotherapy. Ann Diagn Pathol 7:240–244

26. Markowska-Woyciechowska A, Zub L, Jarus-Dziedzic K, Rabczynski J, Paradowski B, Budrewicz S, Jablonski P (2000) [Dysembryoplastic neuro-epithelial tumor (DNT)—case report and literature review]. Neurol Neurochir Pol 34:1031–1038

27. Luyken C, Blumcke I, Fimmers R, Urbach H, Elger CE, Wiestler OD, Schramm J (2003) The spectrum of long-term epilepsy-associated tumors: long-term seizure and tumor outcome and neurosurgical aspects. Epilepsia 44:822–830

Craniopharyngioma: Current Classification, Management, and Future Directions

30

Zohreh Habibi, Deya Abu Reesh, and James T. Rutka

30.1 Introduction

Craniopharyngioma is one of the most challenging brain tumors, located in sellar/suprasellar region in close proximity to the optic apparatus and hypothalamus. Although histologically low grade, the tumor can be locally aggressive and serve as a source of considerable morbidity due to compression and/or adherence to nearby structures. Morbidity can also arise after treatment by any modality. Accordingly, the optimum management of craniopharyngioma has been the subject of controversy between neurosurgeons for more than one decade.

Z. Habibi
Division of Neurosurgery, Hospital for Sick Children, Toronto, ON, Canada

Department of Surgery, University of Toronto, Toronto, ON, Canada

Department of Neurosurgery, Children's Medical Center, Tehran University of Medical Sciences, Tehran, Iran
e-mail: z-habibi@sina.tums.ac.ir

D. A. Reesh
Division of Neurosurgery, Hospital for Sick Children, Toronto, ON, Canada

Department of Surgery, University of Toronto, Toronto, ON, Canada

J. T. Rutka (✉)
Department of Surgery, University of Toronto, Toronto, ON, Canada

Division of Neurosurgery, The Arthur and Sonia Labatt Brain Tumour Research Centre, The Hospital for Sick Children, Toronto, ON, Canada
e-mail: james.rutka@sickkids.ca

30.2 History and Nomenclature

The first report compatible with a craniopharyngioma dates back to 1857, when Friedrich Albert von Zenker, a German pathologist, defined a cystic suprasellar lesion containing cholesterol crystals and squamous epithelium [6]. About five decades later, Jakob Erdheim described the histopathological features of a kind of squamous tumor in suprasellar area, later named after him as "Erdheim tumors" [29]. Before and after these epochs, different terms have been coined to the cystic-solid calcified mass of suprasellar region, including Rathke's pouch tumor, Rathke's cleft tumor, epithelioma, adamantinoma, ameloblastoma, craniopharyngeal pouch tumors, and Erdheim tumors [6]. The term "craniopharyngioma" was first used by Charles Frazier and later became popular by Harvey Cushing in 1932 [6].

30.3 Epidemiology

The overall world incidence of craniopharyngioma in children and adult is estimated to be 0.5–2 cases per million per year [62, 66]. The tumor has a bimodal age distribution, peaking between 5 and

© Springer Nature Switzerland AG 2019
J.-C. Tonn et al. (eds.), *Oncology of CNS Tumors*, https://doi.org/10.1007/978-3-030-04152-6_30

14 years in children and between 50 and 74 years in adults. Approximately half of the cases will present during childhood and adolescence [62]. Although craniopharyngioma is a rather rare entity, comprising only 1.2–4.6% of all intracranial tumors, it is considered as the most common non-glial intracranial tumor in children with a rate of 10% of all pediatric brain tumors [14].

The sex distribution of craniopharyngioma may be slightly male-dominant, and data regarding geographic distribution is not consistent [37].

30.4 Origin and Embryogenesis

Craniopharyngioma is an embryonal tumor arising from epithelial remnants of stomodeum and primitive oropharyngeal mucosa [79]. The normal development of the oropharynx starts at the beginning of the second month of gestation, when the invagination of the primitive squamous mucosa forms the median *adeno*hypophysis and the lateral dental lamina strands [78]. The hypophyseal-pharyngeal duct starts to be formed at the same time, via fusion of the *neuro*hypophysis and buccopharyngeal membrane [3]. The neurohypophysis arises from an outpouching at the junction of the diencephalon and mesencephalon. The buccopharyngeal membrane forms an ectodermal outpouching, Rathke's pouch, which

projects to the neurohypophysis. These two structures fuse at gestational age of 8 weeks, forming the tubular structure that further collapses into the solid anterior infundibulum [3]. The remnants of embryonal derivatives of these structures are generally considered as the origin of craniopharyngioma (Fig. 30.1) [69, 79].

30.5 Histopathology and Molecular Pathology

Craniopharyngiomas are low-grade epithelial neoplasms that histologically imitate tissues derived from the embryonic oral mucosa [79]. There are two histopathological patterns of tumor, namely, adamantinomatous and papillary types. The adamantinomatous subtype resembles ameloblastoma in the jaw bone in terms of many histological and molecular features, as well as local destruction, slow-growing pattern, and rare malignant transformation [7, 79].

Adamantinomatous craniopharyngiomas (ACPs) occur in children more often than adults and comprise the main subtype of tumor in the pediatric age group [5]. The histological pattern of ACPs usually includes whorls, cords, and lobules, with stellate reticulum and palisading peripheral columnar epithelium [58]. The basal palisading cells are columnar or

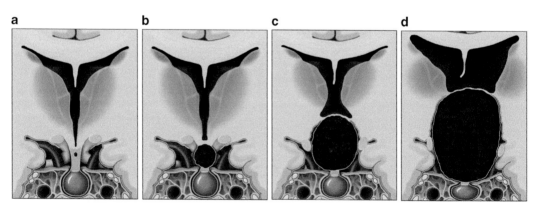

Fig. 30.1 Progressive growth of craniopharyngioma, in the coronal section of the brain in the region of the lateral ventricles, third ventricle, and foramen of Monro. Craniopharyngioma arises from epithelial remnants of the stomodeum and primitive oropharyngeal mucosa. Remnants of these mucosal elements lead to embryonal derivatives along the hypophyseal-pharyngeal duct leading to craniopharyngioma formation (**a**). These elements can then grow over time at first occupying the sellar region (**b**). But with further expansion, suprasellar growth is found (**c**), followed by invagination of the floor of the third ventricle (**d**)

Fig. 30.2
Histopathology of
adamantinomatous
craniopharyngioma, as
seen primarily in
children. There are
whorls, cords, and
lobules with palisading
peripheral columnar
epithelium. Squamous
cell epithelial elements
are also seen. Calcium
deposition is found not
infrequently, as shown
here. Magnification,
×150

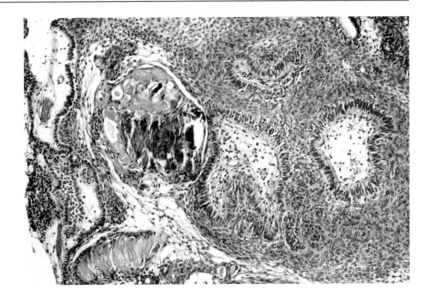

polygonal at the periphery, but the squamous cell pattern becomes more loosely textured and reticular toward the internal layers (Fig. 30.2) [92]. The presence of "wet" keratin is the diagnostic feature of this subtype. ACPs occasionally invade into the normal brain parenchyma and show finger-like interdigitation of the tumor in the surrounding gliotic layer adjacent the tumor [92].

Papillary craniopharyngiomas (PCPs) mainly occur in adults and have a distinct histological appearance, displaying monomorphic squamous epithelium, fibrovascular cores, thin capillary blood vessels, and scattered immune cells [22].

The cystic component of tumor contains brownish-yellow fluid with an appearance resembling machinery oil. Histopathologically, glittering cholesterol crystals can be found in this fluid accompanied with desquamated epithelial cells, keratin, protein, and blood by-products [59].

Recently, molecular markers of craniopharyngioma have been investigated and are similar to those of ameloblastoma and some other derivatives of the Rathke's pouch [7]. The two histopathological subtypes of craniopharyngioma have been shown to carry different molecular markers [1]. About 75% of patients with ACPs harbor recurrent activating mutations in exon 3 of CTNNB1, the gene encoding beta-

catenin [2]. Increased expression of sonic hedgehog (SHH) gene and PTCH1 receptor has been detected in ACPs as well [2]. On the other hand, nearly all PCP tumors have had recurrent mutations in the oncogene BRAF (V600E) which affects the MAP kinase/ERK signaling pathway [11, 12]. Most recently, the expression of PD-L1 and PD-1 was quantified in craniopharyngiomas, and it was shown that all ACP and PCP samples expressed PD-L1. PD-L1 was predominantly expressed by the cyst-lining cells in the ACP subtype, while in PCP it was highly expressed by tumor cells surrounding the stromal fibrovascular cores [21]. ACP also exhibited intrinsic PD-1 expression in the whorled epithelial cells with nuclear-localized beta-catenin which are considered as stem-like population [21]. Prognostic utility of these molecular markers and potential targeted therapies for both subtypes of craniopharyngioma are under investigations [21, 58].

30.6 Sellar and Suprasellar Anatomy

Understanding the anatomy of sellar and suprasellar area is the main key to choose the best surgical approach for craniopharyngiomas (Fig. 30.3).

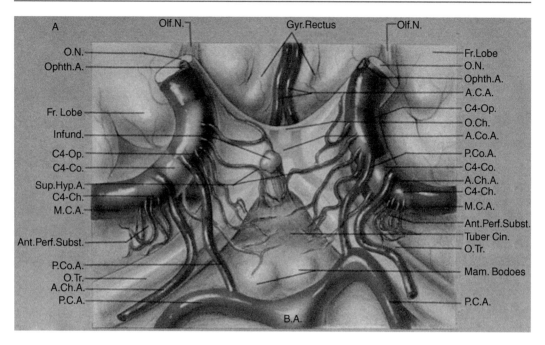

Fig. 30.3 The sellar and suprasellar regions are critical to the understanding of the growth and surgical management of craniopharyngioma. Key neurovascular elements include the optic nerves, optic chiasm, and optic tracts. The intracranial carotid artery lies just lateral to the optic nerves. The pituitary stalk is shown beneath the optic chiasm. The middle cerebral arteries and the anterior cerebral and communicating arteries are found above the optic chiasm. (Reproduced with permission: Gibo et al., Microsurgical anatomy of the supraclinoid portion of the internal carotid artery. J Neurosurg 55: 560–74, 1981)

30.6.1 Sphenoid Sinus and Sella Turcica

The sella turcica is located in the center of the cranial base and occupies the central part of the sphenoid bone. It is bounded anteriorly by the tuberculum sellae and posteriorly by the dorsum sellae. The diaphragma sellae covers the roof of the sella turcica, except for a small central opening in its center which transmits the pituitary stalk. Intercavernous venous connections may be found in the margins of the diaphragma, named on the basis of their relationship to the pituitary gland. The anterior intercavernous sinuses pass anterior, and the posterior intercavernous sinuses pass behind the gland [72].

The body of the sphenoid bone is more or less cubical and contains the sphenoid sinus which separates the sellae turcica above from the nasal cavity [72]. The sphenoid sinus has considerable variations in size, shape, and degree of pneumatization. It presents as minute cavities at birth and undergoes pneumatization and further enlargement as age advances. Thin septa divide the sphenoid sinus into unequal parts that may vary greatly in size, shape, thickness, location, completeness, and relation to the sellar floor [72]. The carotid artery frequently produces a prominence into the lateral wall of sphenoid sinus, the optic canals protrude into the superolateral portion of the sinus, and the second division of the trigeminal nerve protrudes into the inferolateral part [73]. In both sides of sphenoid sinus, the lateral wall of cavernous sinuses extends from the superior orbital fissure in front to the apex of the petrous bone behind. It contains the horizontal portion of the carotid artery and a segment of the abducens nerve, while the oculomotor and trochlear nerves and the ophthalmic division of the trigeminal nerve are located in the roof and lateral wall [72].

30.6.2 Suprasellar Area

The suprasellar region corresponds to the anterior incisural space that opens bilaterally into the Sylvian fissures. The anterior incisural space composes of the interpeduncular cistern, which is located between the cerebral peduncles and the dorsum sellae, and more anteriorly the chiasmatic cistern which is located below the optic chiasm. The two cisterns are separated by membrane of Liliequist which is an arachnoidal sheet extending from the dorsum sellae to the mammillary bodies. The components of the floor of the third ventricle in the suprasellar area, from anterior to posterior, include the optic chiasm, infundibulum of the hypothalamus, tuber cinereum, mammillary bodies, posterior perforated substance, and a part of the tegmentum. In the anterior wall of the third ventricle, the lamina terminalis stretches upward from the upper surface of the chiasm toward the corpus callosum [72].

The optic and oculomotor nerves, carotid arteries, and branches of circle of Willis pass through the suprasellar region. The optic nerves emerge from the optic canals under the falciform ligaments and medial to the anterior clinoid processes and are directed posterior, superior, and medial toward the optic chiasm. After the chiasm, the optic tracts continue in a posterolateral direction. From the surgical point of view, the normal chiasm overlies the diaphragma sellae and the pituitary gland, while the prefixed and postfixed chiasm overlies the tuberculum sellae and dorsum sellae, respectively [73]. The carotid artery exits the cavernous sinus beneath and slightly lateral to the optic nerve and then courses posterolaterally toward its bifurcation into the anterior and middle cerebral arteries below the anterior perforated substance. The anterior cerebral artery is then directed anteromedially above the optic nerve and chiasm to reach the interhemispheric fissure, joining to the opposite anterior cerebral artery via the anterior communicating artery. The ophthalmic artery, posterior communicating artery, and anterior choroidal artery are also in suprasellar region, arising consecutively from the supraclinoid carotid artery. The posterior part of the circle of Willis and the bifurcation of the basilar artery into the posterior cerebral arteries are located in the posterior part of the suprasellar area below the floor of the third ventricle [72, 73].

30.7 Classification

Different classification systems have been described for craniopharyngioma considering its many anatomical, radiological, or surgical characteristics.

30.7.1 Anatomical Classification

Anatomical subclassification is perhaps the most commonly used classification system of craniopharyngioma. This system is often used to choose the most appropriate surgical approach for surgical resection. In this classification scheme, four groups are defined based on their location, origin, and growth pattern [61]:

(a) The intrasellar subtype originates from the intrasellar part of the stalk and frequently enlarges the sellar floor.
(b) The prechiasmatic subtype originates from the anterior part of the stalk and grows in an upward direction, elevating the optic chiasm and anterior communicating artery.
(c) The retrochiasmatic subtype originates from the posterior part of the stalk and grows up toward the posterior fossa, while optic chiasm and anterior communicating artery remain in their normal positions.
(d) The intra-third ventricle subtype originates from the floor of the third ventricle.

30.7.2 Preoperative Classification Based on Hypothalamic Involvement

This classification, described by Puget in 2007, aims to develop a risk-based treatment algorithm in patients with craniopharyngiomas by assessing the grade of hypothalamic involvement. In this grading system, three groups were defined according to preoperative MR images [71]:

(a) Grade 0, no hypothalamic involvement is detected.
(b) Grade 1, the hypothalamus is abutted or displaced by tumor.
(c) Grade 2, the hypothalamic is involved so that the hypothalamus is no longer identifiable on images.

30.7.3 Endoscopic Classification Based on the Infundibulum Topography

This classification scheme is based on the relationships of the tumor to the infundibulum as observed in the endoscopic endonasal surgical field. In this scheme, tumors are categorized into four types according to their suprasellar extension [47]:

(a) Type I is preinfundibular, bounding posteriorly by the infundibulum.
(b) Type II is transinfundibular, extending into the infundibulum.
(c) Type III is retroinfundibular, extending behind the gland and stalk. This type has two subdivisions:
   • IIIa, extending into the third ventricle
   • IIIb, extending into the interpeduncular cistern
(d) Type IV is isolated to the third ventricle and/ or optic recess and is not accessible via an endonasal approach.

30.8   Clinical Presentations

Due to the proximity of craniopharyngiomas to critical neurovascular structures in the suprasellar cistern and the affinity of tumors for attachment to these tissues, a vast spectrum of clinical presentations may occur via being either compressed or invaded by tumor. The symptoms of

pediatric craniopharyngioma are often delayed, enabling the tumors to reach a considerable size to produce symptoms [62]. Furthermore, the distribution of symptoms may be different among children and adults. Children usually present with endocrine dysfunction, insidious visual loss, symptoms from raised intracranial pressure, and papilledema, while adults consistently have visual symptoms [4, 5, 15].

30.8.1 Visual Disturbance

Impairment of vision is the most common finding in children with craniopharyngioma on admission. Between 66% and 86% of the patients present with visual problems at initial disease presentation [38, 86]. Patients with prechiasmatic tumors are more probable to have reduced visual acuity, field defects, and optic atrophy [77]. At ophthalmological examination, the rates of unilaterally/bilaterally decreased visual acuity and visual field defects are 80% and 79%, respectively [86]. Visual loss or field cuts can be attributed to the compression-related disruption of axoplasmic flow and demyelination in the anterior visual pathways [83]. Extraocular muscle deficit due to paresis of cranial nerves three and six is uncommon, occurring in only 5% of patients [86]. Papilledema and pale optic disc may be noted in 16% and 40% of fundoscopic examinations, respectively [38].

30.8.2 Endocrinopathies

Because of the disturbance in function of the hypothalamic-pituitary axis due to compression, distortion, or invasion of the infundibulum, a significant number of patients with craniopharyngioma present with at least one hormonal deficit [43, 74]. Patients with intrasellar craniopharyngioma have more endocrine deficiencies at presentation than those who have tumors restricted to the third ventricle [52]. In children with craniopharyngioma, disturbances in growth hormone (75%), gonadotropins (40%), thyroid-stimulating hormone (TSH) (25%), and adrenocorticotropic hormone (ACTH) (25%) can be found in descending order of frequency [63]. Symptoms and signs of endocrinological dysfunction include short stature, asthenia, delay in puberty, and sexual dysfunction [74]. Preoperative central diabetes insipidus, presenting as polydipsia and polyuria, is found in 17–27% of all patients [63].

30.8.3 Hydrocephalus and Craniopharyngioma

Obstructive hydrocephalus, caused by the extension of the tumor into the third ventricle, is a common finding at diagnosis and can be detected on initial imaging in up to 54% of pediatric tumors [37]. Hydrocephalus has been considered as a poor prognostic factor and usually presents as symptoms of raised ICP, including headache, nausea and vomiting, and papilledema [3, 76]. The higher incidence of hydrocephalus in children rather than adults can be attributed to larger size of tumor and cystic components [46]. Even so, hydrocephalus is the most common life-threatening treatable condition in craniopharyngioma, which can be managed via CSF diversion or tumor debulking [37].

30.8.4 Hypothalamic Damage

Hypothalamus is a collection of multiple specialized nuclei, integrating signals from the viscera, bloodstream, brainstem, and retina, and subsequently exerts control over the hemostasis of the body via hormonal and autonomic output [23]. Insults to these signals may cause sleep disorders and somnolence associated with either melatonin deficiency or disruption of normal circadian rhythm. Abnormalities of thirst (both excess and reduced thirst) because of injury to osmoreceptors located in anterior hypothalamus, thermal dysregulation, hyperphagia, and inappropriate energy storage can also occur [23]. The extent of morbidities and the rate of mortality in patients with craniopharyngioma are more than what is normally estimated in patients with panhypopituitarism, suggesting that the hypothalamic interactions and autonomic signals may play some roles [85].

30.8.5 Obesity and Craniopharyngioma

Hypothalamic obesity occurs in 60–80% of patients with craniopharyngiomas and is associated with increased mortality [68]. The hypothalamic obesity syndrome is considered as intractable weight gain which is unresponsive to diet or exercise and may be associated with somnolence, rage, and hyperphagia [75]. The syndrome is caused by damage to the ventromedial nuclei (VMH) as the site of exerting control over energy balance or the injury of the paraventricular nucleus which results in hyperphagia [75]. Receptors in the VMH and arcuate nucleus of median eminence receive hormonal signals from periphery, including leptin from adipose tissue, insulin from the pancreas, ghrelin from the stomach, and peptide YY from the intestine. Consequently, these receptors exert a negative feedback via forming melanocortin products as the key regulators of energy balance. Damage to this feedback system can interfere with satiety and energy storage, leading to hyperinsulinism and obesity [56].

30.8.6 Neurocognitive and Behavioral Deficits

Neurocognitive and behavioral deficits at initial presentation of pediatric-onset craniopharyngioma range from 10 to 33% [75] and consist of developmental delays, confusion, impaired memory, slow mentation, academic disorders, depression, and excessive fatigue [16, 38]. The symptoms are induced by mass effect on the frontotemporal lobes secondary to a large tumor or hydrocephalus and predict a poor prognosis [4, 15].

30.9 Clinical Evaluations

Considering the spectrum of different clinical manifestations in patients with craniopharyngioma, a thorough and comprehensive clinical evaluation is mandated before any therapeutic attempt. The evaluations should be repeated on a regular basis following treatment or according to the individualized patients' clinical features.

30.9.1 Neurological Examination

Although uncommon in patients with cranio-pharyngioma, monoplegia and hemiplegia have been reported in 6% of patients at their initial presentation [5]. Visual and olfactory hallucinations, seizures, and dementia have been rarely reported, as well [40]. Consequently, a detailed neurological examination including the level of consciousness, motor and sensory testing, and cranial nerves examinations is recommended.

30.9.2 Visual Evaluations

Although ophthalmological impairments are common in children with craniopharyngioma, they are usually not the main complaints, because children may not notice a mild alteration in their vision [3, 24]. Formal neuro-ophthalmologic tests, including best corrected visual acuity (BCVA) and visual field (VF) examination, should be obtained as preoperative baseline. In children, BCVA is tested using either LogMAR or preferential looking charts based on patient's age, and VF is tested with Goldmann perimetry when the child is cooperative enough to perform the test [27]. Extraocular muscles should be tested as well, and funduscopy should be performed to detect papilledema and optic disc paleness resulting from increased intracranial pressure.

30.9.3 Endocrine Evaluations

Baseline measurements of all the hypothalamic-pituitary axis hormones should be obtained, and response of the hypothalamic-pituitary axis to intravenous administration of stimulators should be evaluated preoperatively and followed post-operatively [3, 43]. Accordingly, plasma prolactin, TSH, T4, GH, LH, FSH, testosterone, estradiol, ACTH, and 8 AM plasma cortisol level should be tested [40]. Serum and urine electrolytes and osmolarity should be examined, as well [40].

30.9.4 Neuroimaging

Craniopharyngioma is characteristically a complex lesion, and the images often show polycystic architecture with a variety of signal intensities and enhancement patterns.

Although nowadays magnetic resonance imaging (MRI) is the mainstay of neuroimaging studies, computerized tomography (CT) is an important adjunct to detect the presence and extent of calcification (Fig. 30.4) [37]. This modality also demonstrates hydrocephalus in case of acute deterioration. Coronal and sagittal reconstructions of the skull base and sella frequently demonstrate the secondary skull bony changes [3, 20].

MRI is the imaging modality of choice. A combination of sequences in multiple planes provides a detailed anatomy of the tumor and its relationship to the surrounding neurovascular structures and aids in surgical planning (Fig. 30.5) [19]. The tumor size, shape, and consistency; the relation with the hypothalamus, chiasmatic cistern, or third ventricle; and the location within the sella turcica can be evaluated on the midsagittal

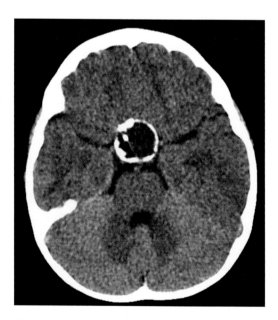

Fig. 30.4 Calcification is a common finding on CT scans of patients with craniopharyngioma. Here, a cystic cranio-pharyngioma is shown with peripheral cyst wall calcification in the suprasellar region on plain CT

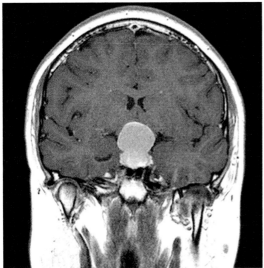
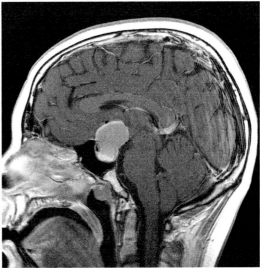
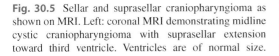

Fig. 30.5 Sellar and suprasellar craniopharyngioma as shown on MRI. Left: coronal MRI demonstrating midline cystic craniopharyngioma with suprasellar extension toward third ventricle. Ventricles are of normal size. Right: sagittal MRI of same patient showing relationship of the craniopharyngioma to the mammillary bodies, the anterior communicating artery, and the optic nerves which are displaced superiorly

and coronal T1-/T2-weighted MRI scans [70]. Gadolinium administration reveals enhancement of the solid components of the tumor and cystic walls [19].

The relationship of the lesion to the vasculature anatomy of suprasellar area is assessed with CT angiography and MR angiography [3].

Recently, diffusion tensor imaging (DTI) tractography has been successfully used to track the hypothalamohypophyseal tract (HHT) through the pituitary stalk in patients with craniopharyngioma [90]. Comparing the location of the tract with the intraoperative view, DTI could consistently localize the pituitary stalk in 87.5% of preoperative images [90].

30.9.5 Neuropsychological Evaluations

Neuropsychological assessments, with a focus on memory recall, should be a component of the clinical management for children with craniopharyngioma [16]. Cognitive functioning can be assessed using the Wechsler Intelligence Scale for Children III [91], while language and verbal memory are evaluated by either the Wide Range Assessment of Memory and Learning or the Boston Naming Test [16, 44, 45]. Visuospatial processing can be tested using the Rey-Osterrieth Complex Figure (ROCF) test and the Developmental Test of Visual Motor Integration [9, 16].

30.10 Therapeutic Decision-Making: Conservative Versus More Aggressive Approaches

Craniopharyngioma is a challenging entity, and due to its unpredictable natural history and long-term sequelae of various treatments, the ideal management has been constantly debated over several generations of neurosurgeons [37]. Recent advances in the management of craniopharyngioma, including stereotactic radiotherapy, chemotherapy, and intracystic drug instillation, have added to the armamentarium to treat this complex tumor. Even with these adjunctive treatment measures, surgical resection still plays an important role as the mainstay of treatment in many cases. Many clinical series have advocated for gross total resection (GTR) to reduce the risk of tumor recurrence, because when the tumor recurs, the choices of treatment strategies becomes somewhat complicated [93]. On the other hand, in other reports, craniopharyngiomas are considered unresectable lesions, and cannot be totally excised with acceptable morbidity, and a recommendation for a more conservative neurosurgical approach followed by radiation therapy or intracystic treatment is given [8, 17, 25]. High rates of recurrence despite GTR have been reported, as well [84]. Complete tumor removal may be hindered by the interdigitation of tumor cells into adjacent gliotic tissue or the existence of inevitable blind spots in the field of surgery [76]. Taken together, in the absence of Class I evidence, the answer to the question of which is the best mode of therapy for craniopharyngioma is not yet known [76]. However, as neurosurgeons, we must focus on preserving quality of life as well as long-term tumor control and survival [1].

The ongoing debate regarding the use of "aggressive" or "less invasive" surgical approaches, at least, has the benefit of suggesting that treatment plans should be customized to the individual patient and tumor characteristics. Indeed, neurosurgical expertise and tumor relationships with the normal neuroanatomy are often the ultimate determinants of the degree of resection [1]. External and endocavitary radiation therapy, proton beam therapy, intracystic sclerotherapy, chemotherapy, or even targeted therapy can further take part in the treatment paradigm. Novel risk-adapted treatment strategies have focused on the following main goals: (a) relief of raised intracranial pressure, (b) reversal of visual compression symptoms, (c) restoration or substitution of pituitary hormone deficits plus all other supplement-supportive measures, and (d) prevention of tumor regrowth/progression while minimizing acute and long-term morbidity and mortality [62].

30.11 Surgery

To choose the most appropriate surgical approach, the key considerations include the anatomical class of tumor (sellar, prechiasmatic, retrochiasmatic, or intraventricular), relationship to the chiasm, hypothalamic attachment, and the position of the infundibulum. For complex tumors combined approaches may be employed [1].

30.11.1 Microscopic Transcranial Approaches

There are several transcranial routes that can be used to remove craniopharyngioma, categorized as frontolateral (pterional-frontotemporal and modified orbitozygomatic) or midline anterior (transcallosal, interhemispheric, and unilateral/bifrontal/subfrontal transbasal) (Fig. 30.6) [1].

The frontotemporal-pterional approach is familiar for most neurosurgeons, providing the shortest working distance to the suprasellar area by removing the lateral sphenoid wing and opening the Sylvian fissure [1, 33]. The tumor is first decompressed through the prechiasmatic space by opening the tumor capsule and draining the cysts and then is carefully dissected from the vital neurovascular structures of the suprasellar region. For parts of tumor extending into the third ventricle, the lamina terminalis can be opened [1]. The orbitozygomatic (OZ) extension can be applied by further removal of the superior orbital rim and zygomatic arch to provide a greater exposure of basilar apex and posterior part of the suprasellar region with less brain traction [34].

Subfrontal transbasal approach, either unilateral or bifrontal, provides a direct *midline* trajectory toward the lamina terminalis and is appropriate for tumors of sellar and prechiasmatic origin with extension into the anterior third ventricle (Fig. 30.7) [55]. Optic nerves and optic chiasm can be exposed by opening the chiasmatic and opticocarotid corridors. After debulking the tumor and cystic components, the capsule is gently dissected from the hypothalamus, and the

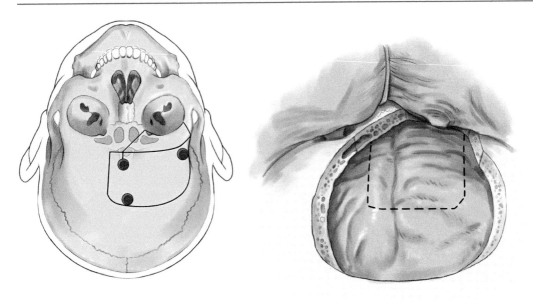

Fig. 30.6 Artist's sketch of right frontal craniotomy including removal of the frontal orbital bar. The craniotomy is taken just over the midline to the left. The dura is opened as shown to enable access to the basal frontal and interhemispheric regions

calcified components which are attached to optic apparatus are removed with meticulous microdissection. Once the lamina terminalis is opened to gain access to the intraventricular portion of the tumor, the plane should be sustained between the tumor capsule and the walls of the ventricle to accomplish dissection and removal of the tumor (Fig. 30.8) [1].

Interhemispheric transcallosal and transcortical approaches are typically used for craniopharyngiomas within the third ventricle or with a significant third ventricular component. The latter may be preferred in the presence of ventriculomegaly [1]. A right-side parasagittal craniotomy is performed anterior to the motor strip (no more than 2 cm behind the coronal suture) with the left edge extending beyond the sagittal sinus. The dura is opened with special attention to large cortical veins entering the superior sagittal sinus, and the dural flap is reflected medially along the sinus. A small callosotomy is performed 1–2 cm behind the tip of the genu in transcallosal approach, and in transcortical approach a small

corticotomy is made in the right frontal cortex directing down toward the right lateral ventricle [26]. Entry into the third ventricle may take the interforniceal, transforaminal, or subchoroidal routes. Following tumor debulking, dissection outside the capsule, resection, and hemostasis are performed in sequence. The placement of an external ventricular drain is recommended [1].

Several important points should be made here which apply to all approaches:

1. For complex craniopharyngiomas, neuronavigation is a useful adjunct to ensure the neurosurgeon remains on target during critical phases of the operation.
2. The plane between the tumor capsule and either the walls of the ventricle or arachnoid membrane of the brain should be maintained throughout the procedure.
3. Static brain retraction should be minimized as much as possible.
4. Bipolar cautery near the optics nerves and chiasm should be performed with caution.

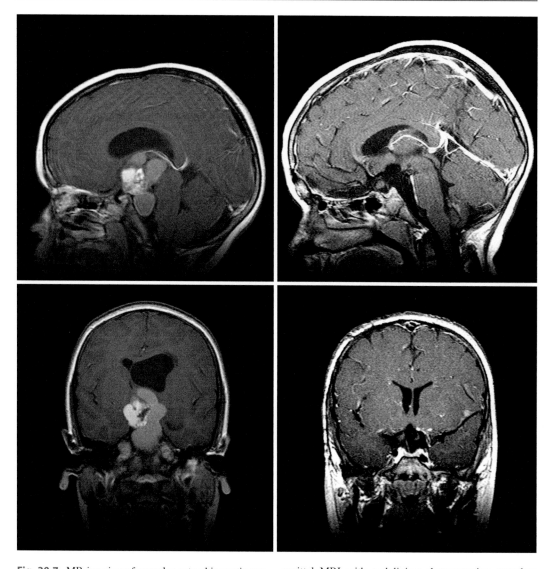

Fig. 30.7 MR imaging of complex retrochiasmatic cra-niopharyngioma. Top left: sagittal MRI showing cystic and solid elements with extension behind the clivus compressing the pons and invagination of the third ventricle. Bottom left: coronal MRI demonstrating unilateral ventricular dilatation and right leaning solid tumor. Top right: sagittal MRI with gadolinium demonstrating complete resection of the craniopharyngioma and preservation of the pituitary stalk. The optic chiasm is also seen on this image. Bottom right: coronal MRI with gadolinium demonstrating complete resection of the tumor and normal-sized ventricles

5. The membrane of Liliequist forms a safe barrier between the posteroinferior margin of the tumor and the basilar artery, posterior cerebral arteries, P1 perforating vessels, and brainstem, as it is intact at initial removal in nearly all cases.

6. If the stalk is to be sectioned, it should be done as distally as possible from the hypothalamus to enable the remnant of the stalk to recover and produce antidiuretic hormone (ADH)

7. After removal of the tumor, hemostasis and closure should be meticulous to prevent postoperative hematoma formation and CSF leak.

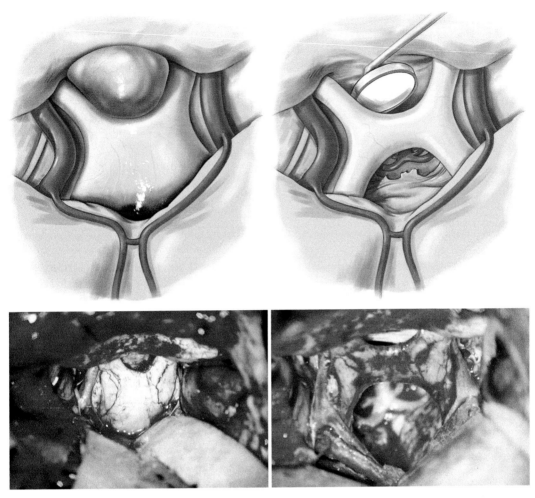

Fig. 30.8 Neurosurgical steps to removing a retrochiasmatic craniopharyngioma. Top left: Artist's sketch from a unilateral subfrontal approach, the right frontal brain is gently retracted, and the lamina terminalis comes into view. The A1 segments of the anterior cerebral arteries and the anterior communicating artery are shown. Prechiasmatic craniopharyngioma is also seen. Bottom left: intraoperative photograph showing right and left optic nerves, the left intracranial carotid artery, and the left anterior cerebral artery. The region of the lamina ter-minalis is visualized. Top right: Artist's sketch following the complete removal of craniopharyngioma showing the bilateral optic nerves and tracts. The lamina terminalis is open, and the basilar artery complex of arteries is seen. Beneath these, the brainstem is found. A micro-mirror is used to ensure that the craniopharyngioma has been removed completely. Bottom right: intraoperative photograph showing removal of the craniopharyngioma with visualization of the bilateral posterior cerebral arteries and the superior cerebellar arteries from the basilar artery

30.11.2 Endoscopic Transsphenoidal Approach in Children

The intimate contact of the sphenoid sinus with the nasal cavity below and the sellar cavity above has made the transsphenoidal route to be accepted as an alternative operative approach to the tumors of this region [72]. Although endoscopic endonasal approach (EEA) seems to be more challenging in the pediatric population due to the small size of the conchal sphenoid sinuses, a careful review of the preoperative images will determine whether the approach is feasible for each patient [1]. A bilateral approach is commonly conducted, often with the aid of an otolaryngologist, raising the nasoseptal flap and subsequently providing visualization with endoscope through one naris, while microsurgical instruments introduced through the other [47]. Bony decompression is then done, including removal of the medial clinoid processes (demarcated by the medial opticocarotid recesses) to access the opticocarotid cistern [47]. After opening the dura, tumor debulking is performed followed by mobilization of the capsule and extracapsular dissection. At closing, the nasoseptal flap with vascular supply from the nasoseptal artery is used for reconstruction of the cranial defect [39].

30.11.3 Less Invasive Surgical Options for Cystic Craniopharyngioma

Intracapsular radioisotope instillation is one of the oldest adjuvant therapies for parasellar tumors, first described in 1912 as radium seeds implantation in the resection cavity of a pituitary tumor [6, 41]. Nowadays, cystic craniopharyngiomas can be managed with repeated aspirations, followed by intracystic instillations of therapeutic substances via an Ommaya reservoir (Fig. 30.9) [17, 88]. The reservoir is connected to an intracystic catheter which can be placed by

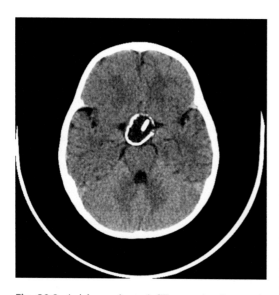

Fig. 30.9 Axial, unenhanced CT scan showing cystic craniopharyngioma into which an Ommaya reservoir catheter has been placed for instillation of interferon-alpha for cystic therapy

craniotomy under direct vision, endoscopic assistance, or stereotactic technique [8]. Different substances have been used for intracystic treatment, including radioisotopes such as ^{32}phosphorus, bleomycin, and interferon-α (INFα) [8, 25, 89]. At this time, INFα has been found to have the best risk-benefit ratio [8]. Intracystic therapies should remain within the cyst and should not cause any injury to the surrounding brain tissues in the event of extravasation [49]. A permeability study is usually performed a few days after catheter implantation prior to starting intracystic instillations in this regard [8].

30.11.4 Postsurgical Management of Electrolytes and Endocrine Disturbance

At diagnosis of craniopharyngioma, antidiuretic hormone (ADH) deficiency is seen in 9–38% of the patients [40]. After surgery, most of the patients develop a kind of water-electrolyte equilibrium disorder, which should be managed meticulously. Central diabetes insipidus (DI) is the most common type of electrolyte imbalance after surgery which can be temporary or permanent, whereas the syndrome of inappropriate secretion of antidiuretic hormone (SIADH) and cerebral salt-wasting syndrome (CSWS) are acute phase disorders, usually resolve within the first month of surgery and rarely become permanent [36, 53].

Central DI is diagnosed if plasma osmolality is above 300 mOsm/kg associated with urine osmolality less than 700 mOsm/kg [40]. In central DI, serum uric acid is also elevated to a value greater than 5 µg/dL, because of impaired urate clearance due to the loss of action of vasopressin on the kidney [74]. Desmopressin acetate (DDAVP) is the mainstay of treatment, being available as both intranasal forms and oral preparations. Due to the proximity of some craniopharyngiomas to the osmoreceptors for thirst in the hypothalamus, some DI patients may develop postoperative abnormal thirst as either polydipsia or adipsia [23]. Both conditions make the management of DI to be more challenging. Adipsic DI can be potentially fatal due to severe hypernatremia. These patients should be given enough fluids and of the appropriate tonicity, as determined by weighing twice daily. On the other hand, the management of polydipsic patients is also difficult. Administration of DDAVP can be dangerous in this situation, since continuous drinking may lead to water intoxication and significant hyponatremia [40].

In contrary to DI, SIADH is characterized by low plasma osmolality and low serum sodium (<135 mEq/L), in association with inappropriate urine concentration (urinary osmolality >100 mOsm/kg) [23]. Normal or low urine volume, clinical signs of euvolemia or hypervolemia, and normal or slightly elevated natriuresis (>20 mEq/L) should be noticed to distinguish SIADH from cerebral salt wasting [23]. Frequently, SIADH is quickly followed by DI, making the management roughly complicated [53]. The appropriate treatment for SIADH is water restriction based on daily weights, urinary specific gravity, serum electrolytes, and osmolality [23].

The diagnostic criteria for CSWS are hyponatremia, polyuria with signs of dehydration and hypovolemia, and elevated natriuresis (>40 mEq/L). The treatment of CSWS is to provide the patient with enough water and sodium based on daily weighs and accurate monitoring of the serum electrolytes and osmolality [23].

In the preoperative planning for the craniopharyngioma surgery, it is recommended that all children with ACTH deficiency should receive stress doses of corticosteroid [40]. The level of thyroid hormones should be corrected before operation, as well. Following surgery, corticosteroids and prophylactic anticonvulsants should be prescribed, and pituitary deficiencies need to be investigated and meticulously replaced. It should be also noted that either ACTH deficiency or TSH deficiency may mask the presentation of DI, and the clinical and laboratory features of DI may appear once these deficiencies are replaced [40].

30.11.5 Surgical Outcome

The first cases of successful resection of the so-called Erdheim tumor were via transsphenoidal approaches [6]. Though Cushing was among the pioneers of transsphenoidal surgeries for pituitary tumors, he employed and extended the transcranial approach for resection of craniopharyngioma because of the better outcomes and fewer complications of this approach during his career [6]. As a result, the outcome and complications of craniopharyngioma treatment have always been informed by the surgical approaches chosen by the neurosurgeons to remove this tumor.

The rate of gross total resection (GTR) of craniopharyngioma is reported to be 59–83.5% [80, 86]. Endoscopic surgeries have achieved acceptable rates of GTR which can be comparable to transcranial approaches, though concerns still remain regarding CSF leak complications [47]. The extent of surgical resection may be influenced by the histological subtypes. The adamantinomatous type is more probable to be cystic and calcified, larger at presentation, and adherent to the adjacent neural tissue, making the surgical resection more challenging. In contrary, the papillary subtype is better circumscribed, less infiltrative, and more amenable to gross total resection [1]

Among patients who undergo GTR for craniopharyngiomas, 50–100% of cases may develop pituitary dysfunction, and up to 50% may experience visual deterioration [46]. The surgical mortality rate within 30 days of surgery, ranges between 1.1 and 4.2% [80, 88].

The major question, not answered by the current evidence, is whether patients with large, invasive craniopharyngiomas would be best managed by subtotal resection followed by radiation therapy rather than by attempted complete resection with the likelihood of further morbidities because of injury to the adjacent structures [76].

30.12 Radiation Therapy

Even if surgical intervention is considered as the initial step in the management of many craniopharyngiomas, the fine balance between further neurological deficit and complete tumor resection has led to the use of various noninvasive forms of therapy. Radiation therapy is often applied in cases of STR or tumor recurrence [48, 88].

Although contemporary strategies favor maximal safe resection followed by adjuvant RT, there are still concerns regarding radiation-induced toxicities, including vascular changes, cognitive deficits, and secondary malignancies [10]. Additional issues with RT in craniopharyngioma are that craniopharyngioma consists of both solid and cystic parts and responses to radiation may be different between the two components [38]. The potential risk also exists for cyst enlargement during or after RT. Though often followed by regression without the need for additional treatment, an enlarging cyst may cause compressive symptoms and signs by exerting effects on nearby cranial nerves or vascular structures [50].

30.12.1 External Radiation Therapy

The current standard of care at many treatment centers is photon-based intensity-modulated radiation therapy (IMRT), which is a modern technique in an effort to spare surrounding normal tissues from high doses of radiation [38, 50]. Using image-guided techniques, important adjacent normal structures particularly the cochlea, brainstem, temporal lobes, pituitary gland, optic chiasm, and optic nerves are contoured and optimally spared while maintaining sufficient coverage of treatment volume. The patient is immobilized with a customized thermoplastic mask, and an image-guided method is taken to choose the clinical target volume (CTV), consisting of the gross tumor volume and postoperative tumor bed, plus a 1 cm margin. The planning target volume (PTV) encompasses the CTV plus a 3–5 mm margin and generally receives a median radiation dose of 50.4 Gy in 28 fractions [38]. Tumor control with appropriate dose planning has been more than 90% [60].

30.12.2 Endocavitary Radiation Therapy

Endocavitary/intracavitary irradiation with a beta-emitter (^{186}Re, ^{32}P, ^{198}Au, or ^{90}Y) is used to treat cystic components of craniopharyngiomas [25].

Intracystic instillation of radioactive agents is performed using stereotactic techniques. The response of lesions to endocavitary irradiation, including either complete cyst resolution or reduction in size, has been reported to be 71–88% [88, 89].

30.12.3 Stereotactic Radiosurgery

Stereotactic radiosurgery [SRS] is a rather recent therapeutic option for craniopharyngioma, aiming to improve the effectiveness and reduce the morbidity associated with radiation therapy. The irradiation is delivered using either the linear accelerator (LINAC) or Gamma Knife (GK) [88]. To achieve a sharper dose gradient between tumor and normal adjacent tissues, a kind of stereotactic system is employed for target localization and treatment planning. For craniopharyngioma, 1–5 radiation courses are used with a mean marginal dose of 12 Gy [88]. Due to the proximity of the tumors to the optic apparatus, only exposure of 8–10 Gy to the optic pathway is tolerable to avoid visual damage [51]. The rate of tumor control with SRS has been 90% for solid tumors, 88% for cystic tumors, and 60% for mixed craniopharyngiomas [1].

30.12.4 CyberKnife Radiosurgery

The CyberKnife consists of a miniature lightweight linear accelerator mounted on a robotic arm with six degrees of freedom of movement, so that photon beams can be targeted with submillimeter accuracy [65]. Using an image-guided control loop with target tracking capabilities, the system can adjust for patient movement and obviates the use of invasive frames to stabilize the patient [88]. In this method, it is possible to keep the dose experienced by the optic apparatus in each session to less than 5 Gy. The rate of tumor control with CyberKnife has been reported as high as 91% [88].

30.12.5 Proton Beam Therapy

Though IMRT still accounts for the current standard of care at many centers, the superior dose profiles provided by proton beam therapy (PBT) have increased the popularity of this modality in a number of brain tumor types [10, 57]. Proton beam radiotherapy is a specific form of conformal external beam therapy by the positively charged particle which significantly reduces damage to the surrounding healthy tissues. High-energy proton passes through tissue with minimal loss of energy until reaching the calculated maximal depth in tumor, where it delivers the majority of its energy, while radiation does not go beyond the tumor [10]. The dose to the optic pathway is kept below 55 Cobalt Gray Equivalent (CGE) with minimal impact on the optic apparatus [57]. With proton therapy in craniopharyngioma, survival and disease control have been equivalent to IMRT [10].

30.13 Chemotherapy

Because of the histologically benign nature of craniopharyngioma, systemic chemotherapy is seldom considered in craniopharyngioma [54]. However, systemic chemotherapeutic courses using vincristine, BiCNU (carmustine), procarbazine, and Adriamycin (doxorubicin) have been successfully applied in cases with recurrent craniopharyngiomas, especially for those in whom there is a contraindication to receive irradiation [13, 54]. Nowadays, intracystic instillation of chemical agents like bleomycin and INF-α seems to be more popular than systemic chemotherapy [8, 49]. Clinical studies have shown that intracystic treatment with the INF-α is a simple method with a very low cost that achieves tumor control in 76% of cases [17].

30.14 Diagnosis and Management in the Era of Genomics and Targeted Therapy

While craniopharyngiomas are traditionally treated with surgery and radiation, targeted therapy is a novel option with probable lower morbidities compared with the traditional treatments [58]. The two histological subtypes of craniopha-

ryngioma are identified by different molecular profiles, requiring distinct forms of targeted therapy. BRAF V600E mutations in papillary craniopharyngioma have made this subtype targetable using BRAF/MEK inhibitors [11, 12]. Similarly, the increased expression of sonic hedgehog (SHH) and its receptor PTCH1 in adamantinomatous subtypes may provide a promising way for targeted therapy with SHH pathway inhibitors such as vismodegib [2]. Both subtypes of craniopharyngioma might be targeted successfully with PD-1/PD-L1 inhibition, because high expression of PD-L1 has been detected in tumor cells of the cyst wall in ACP and tumor cells surrounding the stromal fibrovascular cores in PCP [21]. Tumor cells of cystic craniopharyngiomas have been recently found to express vascular endothelial growth factor (VEGF) to a higher degree than solid tumors, rendering them a target for VEGF inhibitions [87]. Likewise, epidermal growth factor (EGF) gene activation has been demonstrated in the adamantinomatous craniopharyngioma, which may be another opportunity for future treatment with EGFR inhibitors [2]. Molecular profiles of BRAF wild-type craniopharyngiomas and ameloblastomas have been shown to share mutations of fibroblast growth factor receptor (FGFR) genes and additional mutations with potentials for further targeted therapies [7].

However, more experimental and clinical studies will be needed to evaluate targeted therapies in patients with craniopharyngioma.

30.15 Long-Term Disease Control Following Different Therapeutic Approaches

Craniopharyngiomas characteristically tend to recur after treatment owing to tumor attachments to the nearby structures and interdigitation of tumor cells within the adjacent brain tissues [48]. Tumor recurrence after GTR occurs in 13–14.1% of cases, while 33–64.9% of cases with STR or partial resection may experience tumor recurrence [80, 86]. The 10-year recurrence-free survival has been reported as 74–81% after GTR, 41–42% after partial removal, and 83–90% after a combination of surgery and radiotherapy [88]. Hence, despite the lower survival rate in partial resection, further addition of radiation therapy has improved the rate to the values roughly equal to survival rate after GTR. With IMRT, as adjuvant treatment or salvage for relapse after surgery, the 10-year overall survival (OS) and progression-free survival (PFS) were 83.8% ± 8.9% and 60.7% ± 13%, respectively [38]. The 10-year survival rate following PBT has been reported as 72%, with the 10-year local control rate of 85% [30]. In a multi-institutional analysis of patients treated with PBT or IMRT, no difference was found in survival, disease control, and toxicity between two groups [10]. Accordingly, with partial resection and applying a kind of radiation therapy, the rate of 10-year local control ranges between 70 and 100% which is comparable to that of GTR [48].

The standardized overall mortality rate in craniopharyngioma patients varies between 2.88 and 9.28 [62]. Young children have been shown to have a worse prognosis compared to adults, with the standardized mortality ratio being 17 and 3.5, respectively [1].

30.16 Outcome and Quality of Life

Although long-term survival for patients with pediatric craniopharyngiomas has been as high as 80–90%, the tumor itself or the treatment modalities may lead to significant morbidities in this population [75]. The Craniopharyngioma Clinical Status Scale (CCSS) was developed in 2010 to assess preoperative function and posttreatment outcome of childhood craniopharyngioma across the five axes of neurological examination, visual status, pituitary function, hypothalamic dysfunction, and educational/occupational status [28].

Neurological deficit may occur as the result of compression exerted by tumor on the adjacent tissues or intraoperative injury to the nearby neurovascular structures. Intraoperative impairments can be created by venous/arterial infarction, retraction edema, and prolonged pericallosal artery retraction [1]. Seizure occasionally occurs after surgery and can be considered as a source of

neurological symptoms affecting the quality of life even though recurring long-term seizures seldom ensue [77]. Cerebrovascular complications can be seen in long-term follow-up of patients with craniopharyngioma. Adult-onset craniopharyngioma patients experience up to a 19-fold higher cerebrovascular mortality compared to the general population [85]. Also in children with craniopharyngiomas, vasculopathies of the brain, including moyamoya syndrome, have been reported [38].

Visual impairment can profoundly affect the quality of life. Reversing the visual compression symptoms is one of the main goals in the management of craniopharyngioma. Among patients who have had visual disturbance at presentation, 44% were shown to improve in long-term follow-up after surgical decompression and IMRT, 44% remained stable, and 12% experienced worsening [38]. It is worth considering that a significant correlation was found between the visual impairments with increasing volume of irradiation (specifically PTV) and numbers of surgical interventions [38].

Preserving endocrine function to the highest extent possible and correcting any established hormonal deficiency are among essential long-term strategies to improve outcome in patients with craniopharyngioma. Endocrine dysfunction may be exacerbated after surgical interventions or radiation therapy. In long-term follow-up, the rate of endocrine deficiency has increased from 42% at presentation to more than 70% after surgical procedures and before IMRT and sequentially to 88% panhypopituitarism after receiving irradiation [38]. Hormonal deficiency should be meticulously monitored and corrected. Hypocortisolism and hypothyroidism have serious physical and occasionally cognitive consequences [40]. Moreover, both short stature (GH deficiency) and delayed puberty (LH/FSH deficiency) might have inverse effects on the child's self-esteem and quality of life. Among all hormonal therapies, there are some concerns regarding GH replacement in patients with residual tumor. Most pediatric endocrinologists recommend to start GH only 1 year after cure of the tumor is documented [40].

Hypothalamic impairments, pathological or treatment induced, have major impact on prognosis and quality of life in craniopharyngioma patients. Increased mortality and morbidity because of cardiovascular diseases can be attributed to hypothalamic lesion rather than the tumor itself [40, 64]. Changes in circadian rhythm, lack of physical activities, disorders in energy balance and metabolism, decreased satiety leading to severe obesity, and insulin resistance are consequences of hypothalamic damage and can contribute to overall increased morbidities and cerebrovascular deaths [40]. Nonalcoholic fatty liver disease (NAFLD) is a severe, previously underestimated sequela in childhood-onset craniopharyngioma with hypothalamic obesity, occurring in about half of this population and considered as another source of morbidity [42]. The rate of postsurgical hypothalamic obesity has been reported as high as 61% 1 year after surgery [82]. Treatment of hypothalamic obesity remains limited, controversial, and difficult. Surgical bariatric methods of gastrointestinal bypass are efficient but debated in the pediatric population because of medical, ethical, and legal considerations [64]. A variety of pharmaceutical agents like octreotide and dextroamphetamine have been used with roughly promising results [40]. Beloranib, a selective methionine aminopeptidase-2 inhibitor that significantly reduces food intake, has resulted in progressive weight loss in patients with hypothalamic obesity [81]. Even so, initial assessment of risk factors and applying hypothalamus-sparing strategies are recommended for prevention of further hypothalamic damage [64].

Functional status, academic skills, and professional abilities may be affected in patients previously treated for craniopharyngioma. Long-term survivors of childhood craniopharyngioma were shown to have a lower level of education [32]. A variety of cognitive deficits which inversely affect the functional outcome have been documented after treatment of craniopharyngiomas, including lower performance IQ scores, difficulties in problem-solving tasks, and memory impairment [16]. Patients with hypothalamic involvement are generally more affected [32]. In

neurocognitive assessments, problems in the retrieval of learned information can be detected in patients who have undergone surgery but who have not yet received irradiation [16]. Since many such patients are subsequently planned for radiotherapy, additional deficits in cognitive and memory functioning might be anticipated. Long-term assessments after IMRT showed that increase in irradiation volume (specifically PTV) was significantly associated with neurocognitive deficits [38]. In a long-term follow-up study, a relationship was found between cognitive deficits and alterations of microstructural white matter detected with DTI in several neural pathways [31]. Changes in the right uncinate fasciculus were shown to have adverse effect on performance in general knowledge, while cingulum fiber alterations were associated with loss of episodic visual memory, visuospatial ability, executive function, and processing speed [31]. Volumetric evaluations also demonstrated that smaller hippocampal volume and microstructural white matter alterations in hippocampus were associated with decline in general knowledge and episodic visual memory in patients with craniopharyngioma [31]. Despite all mentioned mechanisms, 62.5% of patients were reported to do well in school or have active careers [38]. Overall, periodic neuropsychological assessments, with a specific focus on memory, should be a component of the medical management plan for each patient [16].

30.17 Future Landscapes

It is quite likely that the future of craniopharyngioma therapy may rest in the realm of molecular and microenvironmental investigations and interventions. Targeted therapies for craniopharyngiomas are on their way, in the light of molecular profiling for the subtypes of craniopharyngioma [12, 21, 35].

The role of the local inflammatory microenvironment in craniopharyngioma development is still under investigations. Preoperative inflammatory markers including WBC, lymphocyte, and prognostic nutritional index (PNI) have higher levels in peripheral blood samples of patients with craniopharyngioma [18]. The pattern of preoperative inflammatory markers presents differently in the two histological subtypes of craniopharyngioma, as the papillary and adamantinomatous types have higher neutrophil count and platelet count, respectively [18]. Elevated levels of interleukin 6 (IL-6), IL1α, tumor necrosis factor, and α-defensin 1–3 in the cyst fluid have been detected [67, 94]. Each of these inflammatory markers may serve as a potential avenue for future developments in targeted therapy [37, 94].

30.18 Conclusions

Craniopharyngioma remains as one of the most difficult brain tumors to treat in both children and adults. In this chapter, we have stressed the importance of a multidisciplinary work-up and investigation prior to neurosurgical intervention. The pendulum still swings back and forth between aggressive neurosurgical resection versus more conservative surgical management and tumor control using local cyst instillation therapies and radiation therapy. An individualized patient care plan is essential at the moment for all patients with craniopharyngioma. In this way, the maximum, safe neurosurgical procedure can be performed while minimizing untoward patient morbidity.

References

1. Alli S, Isik S, Rutka JT (2016) Microsurgical removal of craniopharyngioma: endoscopic and transcranial techniques for complication avoidance. J Neurooncol 130(2):299–307
2. Apps JR, Martinez-Barbera JP (2016) Molecular pathology of adamantinomatous craniopharyngioma: review and opportunities for practice. Neurosurg Focus 41(6):E4
3. Balogun JA, Rutka JT (2015) Surgery of craniopharyngiomas in children. In: Kenning TJ, Evans JJ (eds) Craniopharyngiomas. Comprehensive diagnosis, treatment and outcome. Elsevier, New York, pp 459–477
4. Banna M (1973) Craniopharyngioma in adults. SurgNeurol 1:202–204
5. Banna M, Hoare RD, Stanley P, Till K (1973) Craniopharyngioma in children. J Pediatr 83(5):781–785
6. Barkhoudarian G, Laws ER (2013) Craniopharyngioma: history. Pituitary 16:1–8
7. Bartels S, Adisa A, Aladelusi T, Lemound J, Stucki-Koch A, Hussein S, Kreipe H, Hartmann C, Lehmann U, Hussein K (2018) Molecular defects in BRAF wild-type ameloblastomas and craniopharyngiomas differences in mutation profiles in epithelial-derived oropharyngeal neoplasms. Virchows Arch 472(6):1055–1059. https://doi.org/10.1007/s00428-018-2323-3
8. Bartels U, Laperriere N, Bouffet E, Drake J (2012) Intracystic therapies for cystic craniopharyngioma in childhood. Front Endocrinol (Lausanne) 3:39
9. Bernstein JH, Waber DP (1996) Developmental Scoring System for the Rey-Osterrieth Complex Figure. Professional manual. Psychological Assessment Resources, Lutz
10. Bishop AJ, Greenfield B, Mahajan A, Paulino AC, Okcu MF, Allen PK, Chintagumpala M, Kahalley LS, McAleer MF, McGovern SL, Whitehead WE, Grosshans DR (2014) Proton beam therapy versus conformal photon radiation therapy for childhood craniopharyngioma: multi-institutional analysis of outcomes, cyst dynamics, and toxicity. Int J Radiat Oncol Biol Phys 90(2):354–361
11. Brastianos PK, Santagata S (2016) Endocrine tumors: BRAF V600E mutations in papillary craniopharyngioma. Eur J Endocrinol 174(4):R139–R144
12. Brastianos PK, Taylor-Weiner A, Manley PE, Jones RT, Dias-Santagata D, Thorner AR, Lawrence MS, Rodriguez FJ, Bernardo LA, Schubert L, Sunkavalli A, Shillingford N, Calicchio ML, Lidov HG, Taha H, Martinez-Lage M, Santi M, Storm PB, Lee JY, Palmer JN, Adappa ND, Scott RM, Dunn IF, Laws ER Jr, Stewart C, Ligon KL, Hoang MP, Van Hummelen P, Hahn WC, Louis DN, Resnick AC, Kieran MW, Getz G, Santagata S (2014) Exome sequencing identifies BRAF mutations in papillary craniopharyngiomas. Nat Genet 46:161–165
13. Bremer AM, Nguyen TQ, Balsys R (1984) Therapeutic benefits of combination chemotherapy with vincristine, BCNU, and procarbazine on recurrent cystic craniopharyngioma. I Ncuroomol 2:47–51
14. Bunin GR, Surawicz TS, Witman PA, Preston-Martin S, Davis F, Bruner JM (1998) The descriptive epidemiology of craniopharyngioma. J Neurosurg 89(4):547–551
15. Carmel PW, Antunes JL, Chang CH (1982) Craniopharyngiomas in children. Neurosurgery 11:382–389
16. Carpentieri SC, Waber DP, Scott RM, Goumnerova LC, Kieran MW, Cohen LE, Kim F, Billett AL, Tarbell NJ, Pomeroy SL (2001) Memory deficits among children with craniopharyngiomas. Neurosurgery 49(5):1053–1057
17. Cavalheiro S, Di Rocco C, Valenzuela S, Dastoli PA, Tamburrini G, Massimi L, Nicacio JM, Faquini IV,

Ierardi DF, Silva NS, Pettorini BL, Toledo SR (2010) Craniopharyngiomas: intratumoral chemotherapy with interferon-α: a multicenter preliminary study with 60 cases. Neurosurg Focus 28(4):E1

18. Chen M, Zheng SH, Yang M, Chen ZH, Li ST (2018) The diagnostic value of preoperative inflammatory markers in craniopharyngioma: a multicenter cohort study. J Neurooncol 138(1):113–122. https://doi.org/10.1007/s11060-018-2776-x.

19. Cohen M, Bartels U, Branson H, Kulkarni AV, Hamilton J (2013) Trends in treatment and outcomes of pediatric craniopharyngioma, 1975-2011. Neuro Oncol 15(6):767–774

20. Cook DJ, Rutka JT (2009) Craniopharyngiomas: neurosurgical management. In: Hanna YE, DeMonte F (eds) Comprehensive management of skull base tumors. Informa Healthcare, New York, pp 573–581

21. Coy S, Rashid R, Lin JR, Du Z, Donson AM, Hankinson TC, Foreman NK, Manley PE, Kieran MW, Reardon DA, Sorger PK, Santagata S (2018) Multiplexed immunofluorescence reveals potential PD-1/PD-L1 pathway vulnerabilities in craniopharyngioma. Neuro Oncol 20(8):1101–1112. https://doi.org/10.1093/neuonc/noy035

22. Crotty TB, Scheithauer BW, Young WF Jr, Davis DH, Shaw EG, Miller GM, Burger PC (1995) Papillary craniopharyngioma: a clinicopathological study of 48 cases. J Neurosurg 83:206–214

23. Crowley RK (2011) Hypothalamic disease in craniopharyngioma patients [MD Thesis]. Royal College of Surgeons in Ireland, Dublin

24. Defoort-Dhellemmes S, Moritz F, Bouacha I, Vinchon M (2006) Craniopharyngioma: ophthalmological aspects at diagnosis. J Pediatr Endocrinol Metab JPEM 19(Suppl 1):321–324

25. Derrey S, Blond S, Reyns N, Touzet G, Carpentier P, Gauthier H, Dhellemmes P (2008) Management of cystic craniopharyngiomas with stereotactic endocavitary irradiation using colloidal 186Re: a retrospective study of 48 consecutive patients. Neurosurgery 63:1045–1053

26. Desai KI, Nadkarni TD, Muzumdar DP, Goel AH (2002) Surgical management of colloid cyst of the third ventricle—a study of 105 cases. Surg Neurol 57:295–302

27. Drimtzias E, Falzon K, Picton S, Jeeva I, Guy D, Nelson O, Simmons I (2014) The ophthalmic natural history of paediatric craniopharyngioma: a long-term review. J Neurooncol 120(3):651–656

28. Elliott RE, Sands SA, Strom RG, Wisoff JH (2010) Craniopharyngioma Clinical Status Scale: a standardized metric of preoperative function and posttreatment outcome. Neurosurg Focus 28:E2

29. Erdheim J (1904) Uber hypophysenganggeschwwuste und hirncholesteatome. Gerold, Wien

30. Fitzek MM, Linggood RM, Adams J, Munzenrider JE (2006) Combined proton and photon irradiation for craniopharyngioma: long-term results of the early cohort of patients treated at Harvard Cyclotron Laboratory and Massachusetts General Hospital. Int J Radiat Oncol Biol Phys 64:1348–1354

31. Fjalldal S, Follin C, Svärd D, Rylander L, Gabery S, Petersen Å, Van Westen D, Sundgren P, Bjorkman-Burtscher I, Lätt J, Ekman B, Johanson A, Erfurth EM (2018) Microstructural white matter alterations and hippocampal volumes are associated with cognitive deficits in craniopharyngioma. Eur J Endocrinol 178(6):577–587. https://doi.org/10.1530/EJE-18-0081

32. Fjalldal S, Holmer H, Rylander L, Elfving M, Ekman B, Osterberg K, Erfurth EM (2013) Hypothalamic involvement predicts cognitive performance and psychosocial health in long-term survivors of childhood craniopharyngioma. J Clin Endocrinol Metabol 98(8):3253–3262

33. Gerganov V, Metwali H, Samii A, Fahlbusch R, Samii M (2014) Microsurgical resection of extensive craniopharyngiomas using a frontolateral approach: operative technique and outcome. J Neurosurg 120:559–570

34. Golshani KJ, Lalwani K, Delashaw JB, Selden NR (2009) Modified orbitozygomatic craniotomy for craniopharyngioma resection in children. J Neurosurg Pediatr 4:345–352

35. Gong J, Zhang H, Xing S, Li C, Ma Z, Jia G, Hu W (2014) High expression levels of CXCL12 and CXCR4 predict recurrence of adamanti-nomatous craniopharyngiomas in children. Cancer Biomark 14(4):241–251

36. González Briceño L, Grill J, Bourdeaut F, Doz F, Beltrand J, Benabbad I, Brugières L, Dufour C, Valteau-Couanet D, Guerrini-Rousseau L, Aerts I, Orbach D, Alapetite C, Samara-Boustani D, Pinto G, Simon A, Touraine P, Sainte-Rose C, Zerah M, Puget S, Elie C, Polak M (2014) Water and electrolyte disorders at long-term post-treatment follow-up in paediatric patients with suprasellar tumours include unexpected persistent cerebral salt-wasting syndrome. Horm Res Paediatr 82(6):364–371

37. Graffeo CS, Perry A, Link MJ, Daniels DJ (2018) Pediatric craniopharyngiomas: a primer for the skull base surgeon. J Neurol Surg B 79(1):65–80

38. Greenfield BJ, Okcu MF, Baxter PA, Chintagumpala M, Teh BS, Dauser RC, Su J, Desai SS, Paulino AC (2015) Long-term disease control and toxicity outcomes following surgery and intensity modulated radiation therapy (IMRT) in pediatric craniopharyngioma. Radiother Oncol 114(2):224–229

39. Hadad G, Bassagasteguy L, Carrau RL, Mataza JC, Kassam A, Snyderman CH, Mintz A (2006) A novel reconstructive technique after endoscopic expanded endonasal approaches: vascular pedicle nasoseptal flap. Laryngoscope 116:1882–1886

40. Halac I, Zimmerman D (2005) Endocrine manifestations of craniopharyngioma. Childs Nerv Syst 21(8–9):640–648

41. Hirsch O (1912) Die operative behandlung von hypophysistumoren: Nach endonasalen methoden. Arch Laryngol Rhinol 26:529–686

42. Hoffmann A, Bootsveld K, Gebhardt U, Daubenbuchel AM, Sterkenburg AS, Muller HL (2015) Nonalcoholic fatty liver disease and fatigue in long-term survivors of childhood-onset craniopharyngioma. Eur J Endocrinol 173(3):389–397

43. Hopper N, Albanese A, Ghirardello S, Maghnie M (2006) The pre-operative endocrine assessment of craniopharyngiomas. JPEM 19(Suppl 1):325–327

44. Jastak S (1990) Wide range assessment of memory and learning. Adams and Sheslow, New York

45. Kaplan E, Goodglass H, Weintraub S (1983) Boston naming test. Lea & Febiger, Philadelphia

46. Karavitaki N, Brufani C, Warner JT, Adams CB, Richards P, Ansorge O, Shine B, Turner HE, Wass JA (2005) Craniopharyngiomas in children and adults: systematic analysis of 121 cases with long-term follow-up. Clin Endocrinol (Oxf) 62(4):397–409

47. Kassam AB, Gardner PA, Snyderman CH, Carrau RL, Mintz AH, Prevedello DM (2008) Expanded endonasal approach, a fully endoscopic transnasal approach for the resection of midline suprasellar craniopharyngiomas: a new classification based on the infundibulum. J Neurosurg 108:715–728

48. Klimo P Jr, Venable GT, Boop FA, Merchant T (2015) Recurrent craniopharyngioma after conformal radiation in children and the burden of treatment. J Neurosurg Pediatr 15:499–505

49. Lafay-Cousin L, Bartels U, Raybaud C, Kulkarni AV, Guger S, Huang A, Bouffet E (2007) Neuroradiological findings of bleomycin leakage in cystic craniopharyngioma. J Neurosurg 107(4 Suppl):318–323

50. Lamiman K, Wong KK, Tamrazi B, Nosrati JD, Olch A, Chang EL, Kiehna EN (2016) A quantitative analysis of craniopharyngioma cyst expansion during and after radiation therapy and surgical implications. Neurosurg Focus 41(6):E15

51. Leber KA, Berglöff J, Pendl G (1998) Dose-response tolerance of the visual pathways and cranial nerves of the cavernous sinus to stereotactic radiosurgery. J Neurosurg 88:43–50

52. Lee YY, Wong TT, Fang YT, Chang KP, Chen YW, Niu DM (2008) Comparison of hypothalamopituitary axis dysfunction of intrasellar and third ventricular craniopharyngiomas in children. Brain Dev 30(3):189–194

53. Lehrnbecher T, Muller-Scholden J, Danhauser-Leistner I, Sorensen N, von Stockhausen HB (1998) Perioperative fluid and electrolyte management in children undergoing surgery for craniopharyngioma. A 10-year experience in a single institution. Childs Nerv Syst 14(6):276–279

54. Lippens RJ, Rotteveel JJ, Otten BJ, Merx H (1998) Chemotherapy with Adriamycin@ (doxorubicin) and CCNU@ (lomustine) in four children with recurrent craniopharyngiomaEur. J Paediatr Neurol 2(5):263–268

55. Liu JK, Christiano LD, Gupta G, Carmel PW (2010) Surgical nuances for removal of retrochiasmatic craniopharyngiomas via the transbasal subfrontal translamina terminalis approach. Neurosurg Focus 28:E6

56. Iughetti L, Bruzzi P (2011) Obesity and craniopharyngioma. Ital J Pediatr 16(37):38

57. Luu QT, Loredo LN, Archambeau JO, Yonemoto LT, Slater JM, Slater JD (2006) Fractionated proton radiation treatment for pediatric craniopharyngioma: preliminary report. Cancer J 12:155–159

58. Martinez-Gutierrez JC, D'Andrea MR, Cahill DP, Santagata S, Barker FG 2nd, Brastianos PK (2016) Diagnosis and management of craniopharyngiomas in the era of genomics and targeted therapy. Neurosurg Focus 41(6):E2

59. Miller DC (1994) Pathology of craniopharyngiomas: clinical import of pathological findings. Pediatr Neurosurg 21(Suppl 1):11–17

60. Minniti G, Saran F, Traish D, Soomal R, Sardell S, Gonsalves A, Ashley S, Warrington J, Burke K, Mosleh-Shirazi A, Brada M (2007) Fractionated stereotactic conformal radiotherapy following conservative surgery in the control of craniopharyngiomas. Radiother Oncol 82:90–95

61. Morisako H, Goto T, Goto H, Bohoun CA, Tamrakar S, Ohata K (2016) Aggressive surgery based on an anatomical subclassification of craniopharyngiomas. Neurosurg Focus 41(6):E10

62. Müller HL (2016) Risk-adapted treatment and followup management in childhood-onset craniopharyngioma. Expert Rev Neurother 16(5):535–548

63. Muller HL (2008) Childhood craniopharyngioma. Recent advances in diagnosis, treatment and follow-up. Horm Res 69:193–202

64. Muller HL (2016) Craniopharyngioma and hypothalamic injury: latest insights into consequent eating disorders and obesity. Curr Opin Endocrinol Diabetes Obes 23(1):81–89

65. Murphy MJ, Chang SD, Gibbs IC, Le QT, Hai J, Kim D, Martin DP, Adler JR Jr (2003) Patterns of patient movement during frameless image-guided radiosurgery. Int J Radiat Oncol Biol Phys 55:1400–1408

66. Nielsen EH, Feldt-Rasmussen U, Poulsgaard L, Kristensen LO, Astrup J, Jorgensen JO, Bjerre P, Andersen M, Andersen C, Jorgensen J, Lindholm J, Laurberg P (2011) Incidence of craniopharyngioma in Denmark (n = 189) and estimated world incidence of craniopharyngioma in children and adults. J Neurooncol 104:755–763

67. Pettorini BL, Inzitari R, Massimi L, Tamburrini G, Caldarelli M, Fanali C, Cabras T, Messana I, Castagnola M, Di Rocco C (2010) The role of inflammation in the genesis of the cystic component of craniopharyngiomas. Childs Nerv Syst 26(12):1779–1784

68. Poretti A, Grotzer MA, Ribi K, Schonle E, Boltshauser E (2004) Outcome of craniopharyngioma in children: long-term complications and quality of life. Dev Med Child Neurol 46:220–229

69. Prabhu VC, Brown HG (2005) The pathogenesis of craniopharyngiomas. Childs Nerv Syst 21(8–9):622–627

70. Prieto R, Pascual JM, Rosdolsky M, Barrios L (2018) Preoperative assessment of craniopharyngioma

adherence: magnetic resonance imaging findings correlated with the severity of tumor attachment to the hypothalamus. World Neurosurg 110:e404–e426

71. Puget S, Garnett M, Wray A, Grill J, Habrand JL, Bodaert N, Zerah M, Bezerra M, Renier D, Pierre-Kahn A, Sainte-Rose C (2007) Pediatric craniopharyngiomas: classification and treatment according to the degree of hypothalamic involvement. J Neurosurg 106(1 Suppl):3–12

72. Rhoton AL Jr (2002) The sellar region. Neurosurgery 51(4 Suppl):S335–S374

73. Rhoton AL Jr (2001) Anatomy of the pituitary gland and sellar region. In: Thapar K, Kovacs K, Scheithauer BW, Lloyd RV (eds) Diagnosis and management of pituitary tumors. Humana Press, Totowa

74. Robinson AG, Verbalis JG (2003) Posterior pituitary gland. In: Larsen PR, Kronenberg HM, Melmed S, Polonsky KS (eds) Williams textbook of endocrinology. Elsevier, Philadelphia, pp 281–329

75. Rosenfeld A, Arrington D, Miller J, Olson M, Gieseking A, Etzl M, Harel B, Schembri A, Kaplan A (2014) A review of childhood and adolescent craniopharyngiomas with particular attention to hypothalamic obesity. Pediatr Neurol 50(1):4–10

76. Rutka JT (2002) Craniopharyngioma. J Neurosurg 97:1–2

77. Rutka JT, Hoffman HJ, Drake JM, Humphreys RP (1992) Suprasellar and sellar tumors in childhood and adolescence. Neurosurg Clin N Am 3:803–820

78. Schiebler TH, Schmidt W, Zilles K (1995) Anatomie. Springer, Berlin

79. Sekine S, Takata T, Shibata T, Mori M, Morishita Y, Noguchi M, Uchida T, Kanai Y, Hirohashi S (2004) Expression of enamel proteins and LEF1 in adamantinomatous craniopharyngioma: evidence for its odontogenic epithelial differentiation. Histopathology 45:573–579

80. Shi XE, Wu B, Fan T, Zhou ZQ, Zhang YL (2008) Craniopharyngioma: surgical experience of 309 cases in China. Clin Neurol Neurosurg 110: 151–159

81. Shoemaker A, Proietto J, Abuzzahab MJ, Markovic T, Malloy J, Kim DD (2017) A randomized, placebo-controlled trial of beloranib for the treatment of hypothalamic injury-associated obesity. Diabetes Obes Metab 19(8):1165–1170

82. Sorva R (1988) Children with craniopharyngioma. Early growth failure and rapid postoperative weight gain. Acta Paediatr Scand 77(4):587–592

83. Stark KL, Kaufman B, Lee BC, Primack J, Tychsen L (1999) Visual recovery after a year of craniopharyngioma-related amaurosis: report of a nine-year-old child and a review of pathophysiologic mechanisms. JAAPOS 3:366–371

84. Tomita T, McLone DG (1993) Radical resections of childhood craniopharyngiomas. Pediatr Neurosurg 19(1):6–14

85. Tomlinson JW, Holden N, Hills RK, Wheatley K, Clayton RN, Bates AS, Sheppard MC, Stewart PM (2001) Association between premature mortality and hypopituitarism. West Midlands Prospective Hypopituitary Study Group. Lancet 357(9254):425–431

86. Van Effenterre R, Boch AL (2002) Craniopharyngioma in adults and children: a study of 122 surgical cases. J Neurosurg 97:3–11

87. Vaquero J, Zurita M, de Oya S, Coca S, Morales C, Salas C (1999) Expression of vascular permeability factor in craniopharyngioma. J Neurosurg 91:831–834

88. Veeravagu A, Lee M, Jiang B, Chang SD (2010) The role of radiosurgery in the treatment of craniopharyngiom. Neurosurg Focus 28(4):E11

89. Voges J, Sturm V, Lehrke R, Treuer H, Gauss C, Berthold F (1997) Cystic craniopharyngioma: long-term results after intracavitary irradiation with stereotactically applied colloidal betaemitting radioactive sources. Neurosurgery 40:263–270

90. Wang F, Jiang J, Zhang J, Wang Q (2017) Predicting pituitary stalk position by in vivo visualization of the hypothalamo-hypophyseal tract in craniopharyngioma using diffusion tensor imaging tractography. Neurosurg Rev 41(3):841–849. https://doi.org/10.1007/s10143-017-0933-x.

91. Wechsler D (1991) WISC-III: Wechsler Intelligence Scale for children, 3rd edn. Psychological Corp, San Antonio

92. Weiner HL, Wisoff JH, Rosenberg ME, Kupersmith MJ, Cohen H, Zagzag D, Shiminski-Maher T, Flamm ES, Epstein FJ, Miller DC (1994) Craniopharyngiomas: a clinicopathological analysis of factors predictive of recurrence and functional outcome. Neurosurgery 35:1001–1010

93. Yasargil MG, Curcic M, Kis M, Siegenthaler G, Teddy PJ, Roth P (1990) Total removal of craniopharyngiomas. Approaches and long-term results in 144 patients. J Neurosurg 73(1):3–11

94. Zitvogel L, Galluzzi L, Kepp O, Smyth MJ, Kroemer G (2015) Type I interferons in anticancer immunity. Nat Rev Immunol 15(7):405–414

Intracranial Germ Cell Tumors

31

Seung-Ki Kim, Ji Hoon Phi, Sung-Hye Park,
and Kyu-Chang Wang

31.1 Epidemiology

The incidence data of IGCT shows intriguing geographic differences. The incidence of IGCT is higher in East Asian countries than in western countries. Data from the Korean Central Cancer Registry (KCCR) show that the incidence of IGCT is 3.4/million/year [1]. International and North American data show an overall incidence of 2.7/million/year in Japan, 1.0/million/year in the United Kingdom and Germany, and 0.6/million/year in the United States [2]. In a study comparing the IGCT incidence in different racial populations living in the United States, a signifi-cantly higher incidence was observed in Asian/Pacific islanders than in Caucasians. The relative risks were 2.25 for males and 3.04 for females [3]. Because IGCT develops predominantly in children and adolescents, the high incidence of IGCT in East Asia is more prominent in these age groups. In KCCR data, IGCT constitutes 12.5% of all brain tumors in patients under 19 years, second only to astrocytic tumors [1]. In a population-based study from Japan, the incidence of IGCT in children under 15 years of age is 5.0/million/year, and IGCT accounts for 14.3% of all brain tumors [4].

The most frequent age range for IGCT diagnosis is puberty. The majority of patients are within 10–25 years of age. However, a second incidence peak is evident in young infants; IGCTs, which comprise mostly mature and immature teratomas, are the most common congenital brain tumors found in utero and during early infancy. There is a consistent male predominance in the IGCT incidence. In KCCR data, overall male-to-female incidence rate ratio (IRR) of IGCT is 4.53:1 [1]. In the Surveillance, Epidemiology, and End Results (SEER) data, the male-to-female IRR of malignant IGCT is 3.9:1 [5]. Male predominance is more exaggerated in pineal tumors (16.0:1) than in suprasellar tumors (2.1:1). However, for nonmalignant IGCTs, which comprise only mature teratomas, the male-to-female IRR is 1.4:1, reflecting a high incidence of teratomas in young females [5]. In infants, IGCTs are more

S.-K. Kim (✉)
Division of Pediatric Neurosurgery, Seoul National University Children's Hospital,
Seoul, Republic of Korea

Department of Neurosurgery, Seoul National University College of Medicine,
Seoul, Republic of Korea
e-mail: nsthomas@snu.ac.kr

J. H. Phi · K.-C. Wang
Division of Pediatric Neurosurgery, Seoul National University Children's Hospital,
Seoul, Republic of Korea
e-mail: kcwang@snu.ac.kr

S.-H. Park
Department of Pathology, Seoul National University Hospital, Seoul, Republic of Korea
e-mail: shparknp@snu.ac.kr

© Springer Nature Switzerland AG 2019
J.-C. Tonn et al. (eds.), *Oncology of CNS Tumors*, https://doi.org/10.1007/978-3-030-04152-6_31

common in females, and teratomas are the predominant subtype.

Extragonadal GCT tends to develop in sites along the midline of the body, such as the head, neck, mediastinum, and sacrococcyx. IGCT follows this rule. The majority of IGCTs develop in midline structures around the third ventricle, i.e., the pineal or suprasellar regions. Approximately 33–66% of IGCTs arise in the pineal region, and 23–35% arise from the suprasellar area [2]. Approximately 10–14% of IGCTs develop in the basal ganglia and these IGCTs are often bilateral [6, 7]. Rarely, IGCTs develop in the cerebrum, cerebellum, and brainstem [8]. Klinefelter syndrome and Down syndrome are associated with a higher risk of extragonadal GCT, and there are some reports of IGCT developing in the background of each syndrome [9, 10].

31.2 Pathology and Molecular Genetics

IGCT is currently classified into seven histologic subtypes: germinoma, embryonal carcinoma, yolk sac tumor (endodermal sinus tumor), choriocarcinoma, teratoma, teratoma with malignant transformation, and mixed GCT (Table 31.1). The classification is based on the histologic similarity of GCTs to embryonic and extraembryonic tissues. In 1965, Teilum proposed the germ cell theory of GCT based on studies of testicular GCT [11]. In Teilum's concept, seminoma and the other subtypes (non-seminomas) develop hierar-

Table 31.1 The current (2016 revised) WHO classification of CNS GCT, based on histological element of the tumor

Germ cell tumors	ICD-10 codes
Germinoma	9064/3
Embryonal carcinoma	9070/3
Yolk sac tumor	9071/3
Choriocarcinoma	9100/3
Teratoma	9080/1
Mature	9080/0
Immature	9080/3
Teratoma with malignant transformation	9084/3
Mixed germ cell tumor	9085/3

chically from germ cells (seminoma), totipotent cells (embryonal carcinoma), extraembryonic structures (yolk sac tumor/choriocarcinoma), and embryonic tissues (teratoma). Later, extragonadal GCTs were found to have almost the same histologic features as their testicular counterparts [12]. Thus, they can be classified with the same scheme: germinoma and various nongerminomatous GCTs (NGGCTs) in hierarchical orders. According to the germ cell theory, extragonadal GCTs including IGCT arise from ectopic primordial germ cells (PGCs) entrapped in the midline of the body during embryonic migration of the PGCs from the hindgut to the gonadal ridges [12]. However, a mouse and rat teratoma model, in which a graft of embryonic tissues produces teratoma and teratocarcinoma, supports pluripotent stem cells rather than PGCs as cell of origin [13, 14]. Sano questioned the validity of the germ cell theory in view of prognosis because the most undifferentiated tumor, germinoma, has better prognosis and more differentiated choriocarcinomas and yolk sac tumors have worse prognoses [15]. Oosterhuis et al. proposed the dual ancestry theory in which infantile teratomas/yolk sac tumors are derived from remnant stem cells and other GCTs, most arising after puberty, are of germ cell origin [12]. Recently, genomic DNA methylation profiling in IGCTs has provided new evidence for this origin. Germinoma shows global hypomethylation in the genome that is distinct from the hypermethylation of NGGCT [16]. This hypomethylation pattern of germinoma is similar to that of migrating PGCs, supporting the germ cell origin of the tumor. In contrast, NGGCTs with DNA hypermethylation are derived from more primitive blast cells (epiblasts, hypoblasts, and trophoblasts) [16].

Germinoma comprises monotonous primitive germ cells with varying amounts of lymphocytes and histiocytes. Granulomas are prominent in a quarter of cases (Fig. 31.1). Occasionally, beta-human chorionic gonadotropin (β-hCG) secreting syncytiotrophoblasts is present without intervening cytotrophoblasts. Germinoma cells are immunoreactive for placental alkaline phosphatase (PLAP), c-Kit (CD117), OCT4, and NANOG (Table 31.2). However, c-Kit is also

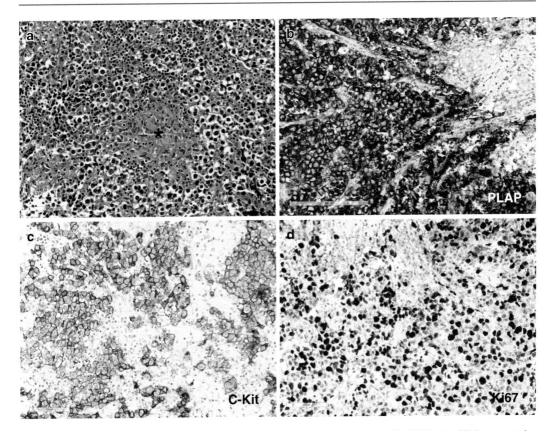

Fig. 31.1 (**a**) The high-power view of germinoma shows large neoplastic cells with small lymphoplasma cell infiltration and granuloma (asterisk). The nuclei of tumor cells are vesicular and contain prominent nucleoli. (**b**) Placental alkaline phosphatase (PLAP) is positive in the cytoplasm of the neoplastic germ cell (×200). (**c**) c-Kit immunostaining is positive in the membrane of the neoplastic germ cells (×200). (**d**) Ki-67 is positive in most neoplastic nuclei, suggesting a high proliferation index (×200)

Table 31.2 Immunohistochemical findings of the germ cell tumors

	PLAP	c-Kit	OCT4	NANOG	SOX2	Pan-CK	EMA	αFP	β-hCG	CD30	CEA
Germinoma	+++	+++	+++	+++	−	−/+	−	−	−	−	−
Embryonal carcinoma	+++	+++	+++	+++	+++	++++	−	+	+	+++	−
Yolk sac tumor	++	++	−	−	−	++++	−	+++	−	−	−/+
Choriocarcinoma	++	++	−	−	−	++++	++	−	++++	−	+

PLAP placental alkaline phosphatase, *c-Kit* CD117, *pan-CK* pan-cytokeratin, *EMA* epithelial membrane antigen, *αFP* alpha-fetoprotein, *β-hCG* β-human chorionic gonadotropin, *CEA* carcinoembryonic antigen

positive in other malignant GCTs, and OCT4 and NANOG are also positive in embryonal carcinomas. Therefore, when a panel of embryonic stem cell transcription factors is used, it is useful to distinguish germinoma from NGGCT: the signature of germinoma is OCT4+, NANOG+, and SOX2− and that of embryonal carcinoma is OCT4+, NANOG+, and SOX2+ [17]. Although isochromosome 12p is the most common chromosomal abnormality in testicular GCTs found in 80% of cases, it is observed in only 20–25% of IGCTs [18, 19]. Targeted sequencing has been used to show that 60% of germinomas harbor mutually exclusive KIT/RAS mutations. The mutation is rare in NGGCTs (8.6%) [20]. Next-generation sequencing has also been used to identify mutations in the KIT/RAS signaling pathway, including KIT, KRAS, NRAS, and CBL, in more than 50% of IGCTs [21]. Somatic mutations in the AKT/mTOR pathway, including a copy number gain of the AKT locus, were found in 19% of IGCTs. Interestingly, a germline variant of JMJD1C, a histone demethylase and coactivator of the androgen receptor, was found in 16% of IGCTs, indicating the presence of a genomic risk of IGCT development [21].

Embryonal carcinoma comprises epithelial cells that resemble those of the embryonic disc and that grow in one or more of several patterns, namely, glandular, tubular, papillary, and solid patterns. The neoplastic cells are large and primitive, and they show alpha-fetoprotein (AFP) and CD30 reactivity (Fig. 31.2). The yolk sac tumor is a histopathologically heterogeneous neoplasm. Reticular patterns are formed by a loose, basophilic, myxoid stroma harboring a meshwork of microcystic, labyrinthine spaces lined by clear or flattened epithelial cells with cytoplasmic PAS-positive, diastase-resistant hyaline globules. Papillary fibrovascular projections that are lined by an epithelial layer, called Schiller-Duval bodies, are found (Fig. 31.3). Choriocarcinoma shows an admixture of cytotrophoblasts, syncytiotrophoblasts, and extravillous trophoblasts (Fig. 31.3). Primary central nervous system (CNS) choriocarcinoma is rare in the pure form and is usually found associated with other germ cell components.

Teratomas are subdivided into mature and immature teratomas. Mature teratomas are cystic tumor and rarely solid tumors that are composed exclusively of mature, adult-type tissues derived from two or three embryonic germ layers. The most common ectodermal components are the skin, brain, and choroid plexus. Mesenchymal derivatives include the cartilage, bone, adipose tissue, and both skeletal and smooth muscles. Cysts lined by enteric and respiratory epithelia are the usual endodermal components. Mitotic activity is low or absent. Immature teratomas contain variable amount of immature, embryonal-type neuroectodermal (primitive neuroepithelial) tissue. Based on the quantity of the immature neuroepithelial component, immature teratomas are graded from 1 to 3 [22]. To enhance reproducibility, a two-tiered grading system that divides immature teratomas into low grade (grade 1) and high grade (grades 2 and 3) has been proposed. Adequate sampling of the primary tumor and of all resected implants is crucial for histological grading. SOX2, a neural stem cell marker, is robustly expressed in the primitive neuroectodermal tissue of immature teratomas and may be helpful toward quantitative grading (Fig. 31.4) [23]. CNS immature teratomas have been reported to undergo spontaneous differentiation into fully mature somatic-type tissues over time.

Teratomas with malignant transformation are teratomas (usually mature) with various non-

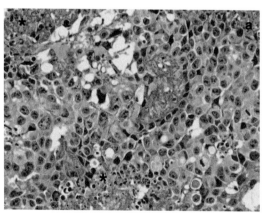
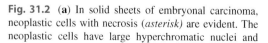
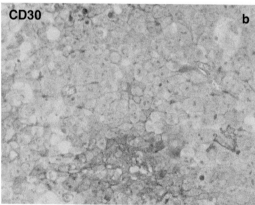

Fig. 31.2 (**a**) In solid sheets of embryonal carcinoma, neoplastic cells with necrosis (*asterisk*) are evident. The neoplastic cells have large hyperchromatic nuclei and prominent nucleoli. The cytoplasm is amphiphilic or eosinophilic (×200). (**b**) CD30 is strongly positive in the neoplastic cell membrane (×200)

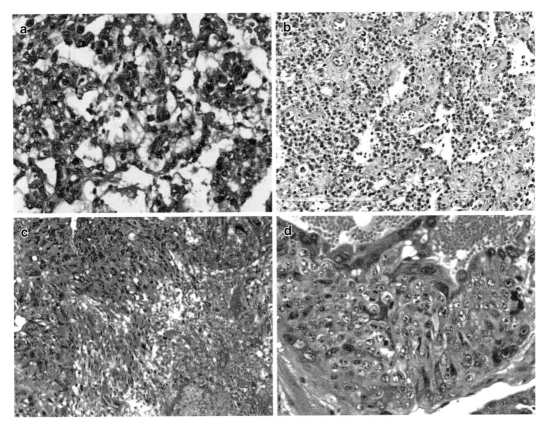

Fig. 31.3 (**a**) The yolk sac tumor shows a reticular pattern with numerous eosinophilic globules (×100). (**b**) The Schiller-Duval body is composed of a central fibrovascular core with a covering single layer of cuboidal tumor cells (×400). (**c**) The choriocarcinoma shows sheets or nests of atypical tumor cells with extensive hemorrhagic necrosis (×100). (**d**) The neoplastic cells of choriocarcinoma are composed of an admixture of cytotrophoblasts, syncytiotrophoblastic giant cells, and extravillous trophoblasts (×400)

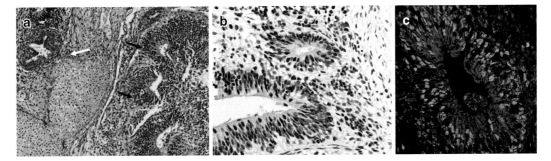

Fig. 31.4 (**a**) The immature teratoma shows immature neuroepithelial tubules (*black arrows*), and mature teratoma components, such as cartilage islands, fibrous stroma, and a benign gland (*white arrow*) (×100). (**b**) SOX2, a transcription factor regulating neural stem cell fate, is highly expressed in the primitive neuroepithelial tubules of immature teratomas (SOX2 immunostaining, ×400). (**c**) The cells in the primitive neuroepithelial tubules co-expressed neural stem cell markers, SOX2 and nestin (immunofluorescence; SOX2 green, nestin red, DAPI blue; ×400)

germ cell malignant tumors of epithelial and mesenchymal origin. The most common sarcoma is rhabdomyosarcoma, and rarely undifferentiated sarcoma is present. For epithelial malignancies, squamous cell carcinomas are frequently included, and rarely, adenosarcomas are present.

Mixed GCTs comprise at least two different germ cell elements of which at least one is primitive (Fig. 31.5). The most common association, between a germinoma and a teratoma, has been estimated to occur in one-fifth of all reported cases. Other mixtures of germinomas and yolk sac tumors, immature or mature teratomas with embryonal carcinomas, and/or choriocarcinomas may also be present. The relative percentage of each tumor type should be delineated.

Interestingly, in two patients, the germinoma and NGGCT components in their mixed GCTs shared the same genetic mutations while maintaining a distinct methylation profiling [21]. It is likely that mixed GCTs develop from early stem cells acquiring a critical genetic mutation or that mixed GCTs arise from PGCs that develop into germinoma and then dedifferentiate into NGGCTs by epigenetic reprogramming [21].

Based on disease prognosis, IGCTs have been classified into three prognosis groups [24]. The good prognosis group includes pure germinomas and mature teratomas, and patients in this group have an excellent long-term survival. The intermediate prognosis group includes germinomas with elevated β-hCG, immature teratomas, teratoma with malignant transformations, and mixed

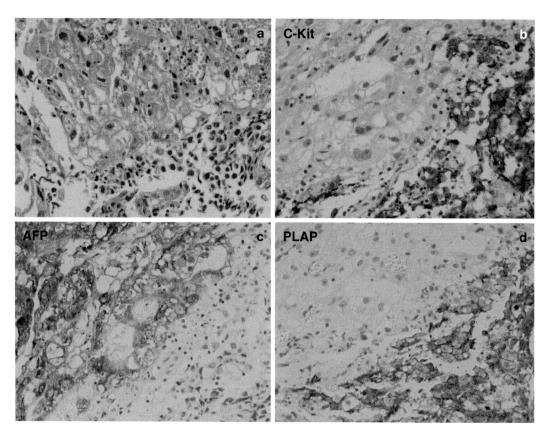

Fig. 31.5 (a) This mixed germ cell tumor is composed of the yolk sac tumor (*upper*) and germinoma (*lower*) (×200). (**b–d**) The germinoma cells are immunoreactive for c-Kit and placental alkaline phosphatase (PLAP), while the cells of the yolk sac tumor are completely nega-

tive for both antibodies. α-fetoprotein (αFP) is immunoreactive in the neoplastic cells of the yolk sac tumor but negative in the germinoma cells (**b**, c-Kit; **c**, αFP; **d**, PLAP immunostaining; **b–d**, ×200)

GCTs mainly composed of germinoma and teratoma. Malignant NGGCTs such as embryonal carcinomas, yolk sac tumors, choriocarcinomas, and mixed GCTs mainly composed of these tumors belong to the poor prognosis group. The position of germinomas with elevated β-hCG in the intermediate prognosis group has been questioned because compared with pure germinomas, no difference in survival has been consistently reported [25, 26].

31.3 Presentation

The symptoms and signs of an IGCT are dependent on the tumor size, location, and accompanying hydrocephalus. For pineal GCTs, upward gaze palsy and Parinaud's syndrome are commonly observed. Obstruction of the cerebral aqueduct by the mass causes hydrocephalus which elicits headache, nausea, vomiting, and visual disturbance with elevated intracranial pressure. Older children can exhibit progressive cognitive deterioration and poor school performance. Rapid progression of hydrocephalus and a decreased level of consciousness are sometimes observed when the diagnosis is delayed. Suprasellar GCTs usually present with endocrinopathy. The most common endocrinopathy is diabetes insipidus (DI) [27]. Central DI can precede the appearance of a mass on brain MRI by months to years. This so-called occult germinoma is difficult to diagnose because there is no visible lesion to biopsy [28]. Frequently, disappearance of the normal bright signal of posterior hypophysis is the only sign found on MRI. Other endocrinopathies include growth retardation, precocious puberty, and delayed puberty [27]. However, panhypopituitarism is uncommon for suprasellar GCT. A typical symptom of basal ganglia GCT is progressing hemiparesis with an insidious onset [7]. Spasticity can develop following Wallerian degeneration of the pyramidal tract.

31.4 Diagnosis

The diagnosis of IGCT is based on typical symptomatology, age, sex, tumor markers, imaging, and surgical biopsy. Elevated levels of tumor markers, β-hCG and AFP, in the serum and/or CSF offer a great opportunity for a noninvasive diagnosis of IGCT. An elevated β-hCG level indicates choriocarcinoma, and an increased level of AFP indicates a yolk sac tumor. In embryonal carcinoma, both tumor markers are elevated. Germinoma is double-marker negative, but a mild elevation of β-hCG (50–100 mU/mL) is often observed in germinoma patients because of the presence of syncytiotrophoblasts in germinoma. The prognostic significance of mildly elevated serum/CSF β-hCG in germinoma is controversial. Teratomas are also double-marker negative, but immature teratomas can secrete varying degrees of both tumor markers, possibly due to the presence of tiny amounts of choriocarcinoma and/or yolk sac tumor tissue within them [29]. In the same patient, the CSF β-hCG level tends to be higher than the serum β-hCG level, and the serum AFP level is usually higher than the CSF AFP level. It is preferable to check the serum and CSF tumor markers on the same day [30]. It is controversial whether CSF collection via the lumbar or ventricular route is more advantageous, but in one study, the β-hCG level was much higher in the lumbar than ventricular CSF [31]. Tumor markers can also be utilized for disease surveillance after treatments are finished.

CT is useful for visualization of calcification, fat tissue, and acute hemorrhage. The presence of dense calcification and fat tissues in tumors suggest that teratoma and the presence of hemorrhage favors choriocarcinoma. Brain MRI is the imaging method of choice for the diagnosis of IGCT. Germinomas are frequently solid with an slightly high density on CT and an iso- or low signal intensity on T1-weighted MR images (Fig. 31.6). Surrounding edema is absent or minimal, and there is usually a strong homogeneous enhancement. Calcification is absent or minimal in the extrapineal regions. Generally, the neuroimaging features are close to those of the lymphomas. However, patients with lymphoma are typically much older. Some of them may have a small cystic portion. If the surrounding brain shows evidence of atrophy or Wallerian degeneration, germinoma is favored. NGGCTs

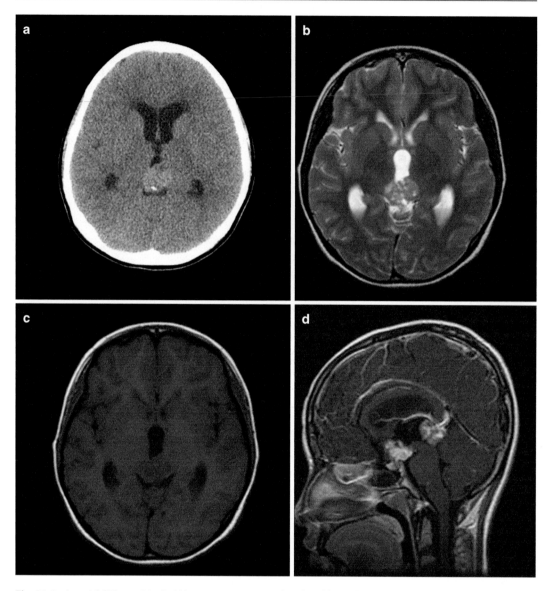

Fig. 31.6 An axial CT scan (**a**) of a bifocal germinoma in a 14-year-old boy shows a slightly high-density mass with focal calcification in the pineal region. The mass exhibits iso-signal intensities in the (**b**) T2- and (**c**) T1-weighted images. Masses in the pineal and suprasellar region are enhanced by gadolinium (**d**)

tend to be more heterogeneous than germinomas (Fig. 31.7). NGGCTs are frequently huge, and surrounding edema is more prominent. Teratomas are heterogeneous, and the degree of enhancement is variable (Fig. 31.8).

For pineal GCTs, differential diagnoses include pineal parenchymal tumor, benign pineal cyst, glioma, and cavernous malformation. If a female teenager has a pineal mass, it is less likely to be an IGCT because the male-to-female ratio in pineal GCTs is very high. For suprasellar GCTs, optic pathway glioma, craniopharyngioma, Langerhans cell histiocytosis (LCH), and lymphocytic hypophysitis should be differentiated. Suprasellar GCTs are frequently occult, or only mild thickening of the pituitary stalk is observed despite persisting symptoms of DI [32]. Loss of the bright white signal in

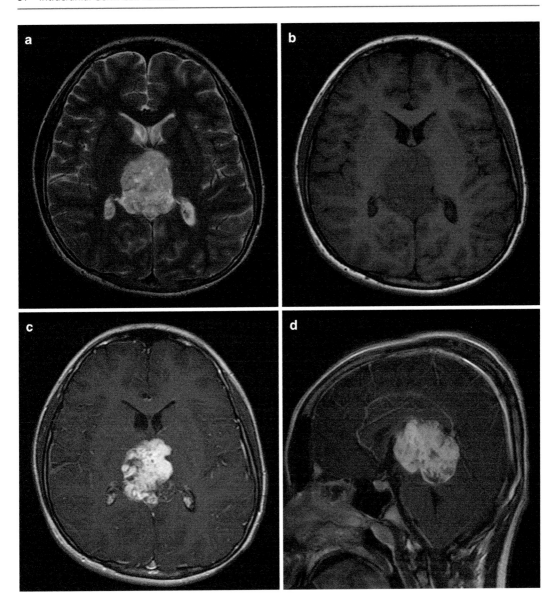

Fig. 31.7 MR images of a pineal non-germinomatous germ cell tumor in a 12-year-old boy. The serum alphafetoprotein (AFP) level was elevated to 329 ng/mL. The mass is huge and shows heterogeneously high signal intensities in (**a**) a T2-weighted image and shows iso- to low signal intensities in (**b**) a nonenhanced T1-weighted image. The mass is well enhanced with gadolinium (**c, d**)

posterior hypophysis is characteristic, but it is also observed in idiopathic central DI. If surgical biopsy is not feasible, the recommendation is to wait and repeat the brain MRI and serum/CSF tumor marker exam every 3–6 months [28]. Approximately 6–41% of IGCTs present with double lesions in both suprasellar and pineal areas (Fig. 31.6) [33]. These so-called bifocal

GCTs have been regarded as almost a pathognomonic sign of germinoma, negating the need for surgical biopsy [34]. However, some patients with bifocal GCTs are found to have mixed GCT [33]. Therefore, even for bifocal lesions, surgical biopsy is also recommended if tumor markers are not elevated. It is highly controversial whether bifocal GCTs involve a synchronous

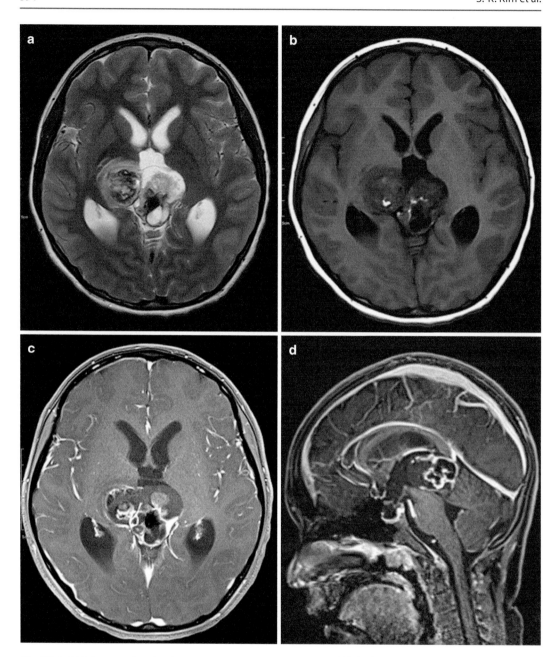

Fig. 31.8 MR images of a pineal mature teratoma in a 10-year-old boy. (**a**) The T2-weighted image shows a large, partially cystic heterogeneous mass in the pineal region. (**b**) In the nonenhanced T1-weighted image, there are areas of high signal intensity indicating the presence of fatty tissues. (**c**, **d**) The enhancement pattern is focal and heterogeneous reflecting diverse tissue components in the teratoma

development or metastatic spread of the disease [33, 35]. Basal ganglia GCT is also frequently occult in onset with an insidious, protracted clinical course [36]. In such a patient, MRI shows only a patchy, nonspecific T2 high signal abnormality in the basal ganglia with atrophy of caudate nucleus, cerebral peduncle, and cerebral hemisphere [7]. ^{11}C-methionine PET is helpful for diagnosis and guiding a biopsy target [37] (Fig. 31.9).

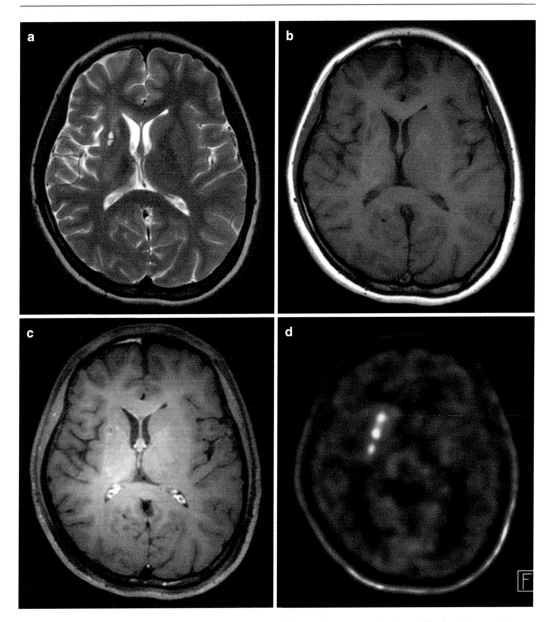

Fig. 31.9 MR images of a basal ganglia germinoma in a 15-year-old girl show small cystic lesions in the right basal ganglia (**a**, **b**). Atrophic changes of the right caudate nucleus and right hemisphere are noted. (**c**) Faint gado-linium enhancement is observed in the lesions and epen-dymal linings. (**d**) The lesion shows high uptake on ^{11}C-methionine PET

Approximately 5–35% of IGCT cases have metastatic dissemination at diagnosis [2]. Therefore, M staging is important for assessing disease severity and treatment guidance. Evaluation of spinal MRI (with enhancement) is mandatory for all IGCT patients. However, unlike medulloblastoma, IGCT that usually spreads into the ventricles, with a far less proportion, has spinal dissemination. CSF cytology is usually examined with tumor markers via lumbar punctures if not medically contraindicated.

It is widely accepted that IGCTs can be diagnosed based on tumor marker studies and imaging findings. Elevated serum/CSF tumor markers combined with typical MRI findings provides a relatively accurate diagnosis of IGCT and its subtype (usually NGGCTs). However, surgical biopsy is required for marker-negative lesions such as germinomas and teratomas. Sometimes, another brain tumor mimics the typical radiological findings of IGCTs [38]. Molecular genomic information can be obtained by surgical biopsy of the tumor tissue, which will be crucial in future clinical trials.

31.5 Treatment

Treatment of IGCT is multidisciplinary and combines surgery, chemotherapy, and radiation therapy with all other supportive domains. The role of surgery for IGCTs consists of management of hydrocephalus, surgical biopsy, direct surgical excision, and second-look operation for residual lesions. Management of hydrocephalus should be the first consideration because many patients with IGCT have hydrocephalus and related symptoms. If overt obstructive hydrocephalus is present, CSF diversion before the start of therapy is required. For pineal GCTs, endoscopic third ventriculostomy (ETV) is most widely applied. For suprasellar GCT, ETV is rarely feasible,

and extraventricular drainage (EVD) or shunt is recommended. Permanent ventriculoperitoneal shunt is losing favors because CSF pathway can be reopened after a short course of chemotherapy by tumor shrinkage [30]. If one or both foramina of Monro are occluded by a mass, endoscopic septostomy can be combined with CSF diversion.

For marker-negative lesions, a surgical biopsy is indicated. Suprasellar and pineal lesions can be approached using an endoscopic procedure. Accompanying hydrocephalus and ventricular enlargement facilitates endoscopic access to the mass. The transsphenoidal route or open craniotomy is utilized for smaller lesions with collapsed ventricles. Transsphenoidal approach can be applied for suprasellar lesions (Fig. 31.10), and the occipital transtentorial, supracerebellar infratentorial, or interhemispheric transcallosal transventricular approaches can be used for pineal lesions. The basal ganglia lesion is usually biopsied using the stereotactic method.

Mature and immature teratomas should be surgically removed, completely if possible. The prognosis for mature teratoma is excellent. Immature teratoma, especially of higher histologic grade, requires adjuvant therapy after surgical removal. For other malignant NGGCTs, the indication for radical surgery is not clear but

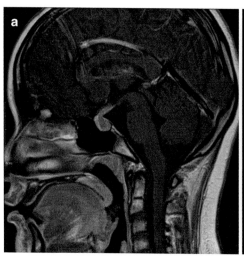
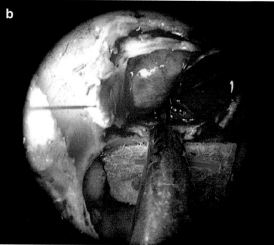

Fig. 31.10 Endoscopic transsphenoidal biopsy of a germinoma (**a**). The pituitary stalk is markedly thickened, and the normal pituitary gland is anteriorly displaced by the tumor beneath the diaphragm sellae. (**b**) Intraoperative view. After elevating the normal pituitary gland, gray-colored germinoma tissue is observed

must be limited to cytoreduction or to removal of teratomatous component (in mixed GCTs) that is not chemo- and radiosensitive. Growing teratoma syndrome refers to the phenomenon whereby the mature or immature teratoma component grows substantially during or after adjuvant chemo/radiation therapies for malignant GCTs [39]. It is supposed that the malignant components are eradicated by chemo/radiation therapies but that the teratoma components that are insensitive to the therapies remain and grow. Clinically, in this situation, teratomas grow rapidly to form a huge mass with a characteristic honeycomb appearance comprising multiple small cysts and micro-hemorrhages (Fig. 31.11).

Germinoma is highly sensitive to chemotherapy and radiotherapy. Previously, craniospinal irradiation up to 36 Gy with a tumor boost of approximately 15 Gy was the standard therapy for localized germinoma [40]. Because craniospinal radiotherapy yielded an excellent outcome (long-term survival rate > 90%), a radiation volume and/or dose reduction has been continuously attempted. As the majority of patients with IGCT are children and adolescents, radiotherapy sequelae such as endocrinopathy, vasculopathy, and cognitive decline are of particular concern. An extensive review of the published data has shown that whole brain or whole ventricular radiotherapy yields slightly more relapse (7.6%) than craniospinal irradiation with tumor boost (3.8%). The difference in spinal relapse rates is not significant. Focal radiotherapy should be avoided because focal radiotherapy has a far higher relapse rate (23.3%) [40]. Currently, whole brain or whole ventricular radiotherapy with reduced dose is widely accepted for localized germinoma. Radiation to the tumor with a dose range of 36–39 Gy and to the whole brain/ventricles with a range of 19.5–24 Gy, with or without chemotherapy, provides excellent tumor control [41–43]. For disseminated germinoma, craniospinal irradiation is required.

Pre-radiation chemotherapy has been adopted in many protocols. Recently, the published SIOP CNS GCT 96 trial showed that chemotherapy followed by reduced volume and dose radiotherapy produced comparable outcome to that of cranio-spinal irradiation alone [44]. The main purpose of chemotherapy for intracranial germinoma is to reduce the radiotherapy dose and enhance the quality of life of the patient [30]. The most commonly used chemotherapeutic agents for IGCT regimens are carboplatin, cisplatin, etoposide, ifosfamide, bleomycin, and cyclophosphamide. Chemotherapy alone for intracranial germinoma has been tested but resulted in a high failure rate [45, 46]. Currently, the ongoing North American Children's Oncology Group trial, ACNS1123, states that for localized germinomas, four cycles of chemotherapy with carboplatin and etoposide should be given and followed by 18-Gy radiation to the whole ventricle and a 12-Gy boost to the tumor-involved field. In the European SIOP CNS GCT II trial, localized germinoma is treated with four cycles of chemotherapy with an alternating schedule of carboplatin/etoposide and ifosfamide/etoposide and, after reevaluation, delivery of risk-adapted radiotherapy (24-Gy whole ventricular irradiation for complete remission plus a 16- to 30-Gy boost to the tumor bed for non-complete remission).

The prognosis of NGGCTs is worse than for germinomas. In two large retrospective studies published in the 1990s, the 5-year survival rates of malignant NGGCT were 27 and 38% [24, 47]. A multimodal, intensified treatment with surgical resection, chemotherapy, and craniospinal radiotherapy has improved the treatment outcome of NGGCT greatly. In retrospective studies on NGGCT, a Korean group reported a 10-year overall survival of 74.6%, and a Taiwanese center reported a 6-year overall survival rate of 79.5% [48, 49]. The importance of resective surgery for intracranial NGGCT has been questioned. In the German MAKEI89 trial, surgery was not important, but craniospinal radiotherapy and a higher cisplatin dose were critical for the outcome [50]. Therefore, for NGGCTs, the current standard is chemotherapy to shrink the tumor volume followed by craniospinal irradiation. The goal of chemotherapy for NGGCT is not to reduce the radiation dose but to maximize the chance of cure [30]. Recently, the published Children's Oncology Group's phase II trial adopted six cycles of chemotherapy followed by 36 Gy of craniospinal

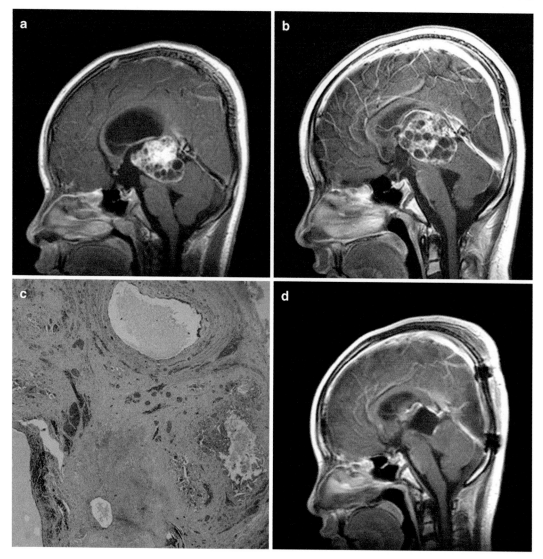

Fig. 31.11 Growing teratoma syndrome from a non-germinomatous germ cell tumor. An 8-year-old boy presented with precocious puberty. A tumor marker exam showed that serum AFP was 103 ng/mL, serum β-hCG was 655 mU/mL, and CSF αFP and β-hCG were 118 ng/mL and 1350 mU/mL, respectively. (**a**) The gadolinium-enhanced MRI revealed a solid and cystic enhancing pineal mass that was 3 cm in size and severe ventriculomegaly. Endoscopic third ventriculostomy and biopsy were performed. The histological diagnosis was a yolk sac tumor. He underwent chemotherapy and craniospinal irradiation. (**b**) The follow-up MRI after chemotherapy and radiotherapy showed the paradoxically increased size of the enhancing multi-lobulated cystic mass despite normalized tumor markers. Second-look surgery achieved gross total removal of the tumor. (**c**) The pathological specimen obtained at second-look surgery. Mature elements of the endoderm-derived cuboidal to columnar epithelium lined cystic lesions and mature mesenchymal components were found. There were scattered foreign body granulomas, suggesting a post-necrotic or degenerating process of malignant elements with chemotherapy (×40). (**d**) He had no evidence of recurrence at the 28-month follow-up visit after the second operation

irradiation with an 18-Gy boost to the tumor bed [51]. Second-look surgery and high-dose chemotherapy with stem cell rescue were also applied to patients with residual lesions before radio-

therapy. However, a reduction in the radiation volume/dose is being sought in current clinical trials. In ACNS1123, after six cycles of chemotherapy, patients with NGGCT undergo an evaluation, and if complete remission is evident, the patients receive radiotherapy comprising 30.6 Gy to the whole ventricle and a 23.4-Gy boost to the involved field. In the SIOP CNS GCT II trial, whole ventricular irradiation is also applied to nonmetastatic, standard risk NGCCT patients.

Second-look surgery is frequently performed for NGGCT patients if a residual lesion is found after chemotherapy. The purpose of second-look surgery is to evaluate the response to chemotherapy, to relocate the patient to stratified protocols, and to remove the residual teratoma component to prevent or avert the growing teratoma syndrome. The utility of second-look surgery has been debated. In a report of ten second-look surgeries, five were performed for teratomas and five were for scar tissues [52]. Another study reported that teratoma was found in five of seven second-look surgeries [53]. However, second-look surgery can be avoided for an asymptomatic, stable, or diminishing residual lesion with normalized tumor markers because the lesion most likely represents scar tissue [54]. The timing of second-look surgery is not uniform. In North American and European countries, second-look surgery is generally performed between chemotherapy and radiotherapy, whereas in Japan, second-look surgery tends to be performed after completion of chemotherapy and radiation therapy [30].

31.6 Long-Term Follow-Up

The prognosis of IGCT, especially of germinoma, is excellent. The long-term survival rate of germinoma reaches 95–100%. Therefore, treatment of IGCT has evolved to decrease the toxicity of therapies and to enhance the quality of life. Diabetes insipidus, which is common to suprasellar germinoma, tends to persist after complete remission of the tumor. After radiotherapy, growth hormone deficiency and other hormone deficits are commonly observed [41]. Therefore, endocrinological consultation and examination before and after treatment are required for IGCT patients. Prolonged surveillance for tumor recurrence may be required because delayed recurrence of germinoma after 5–10 years of

remission is reported [55–57]. The possibility of radiation-induced secondary malignancy should be considered. Psychological and neurocognitive development can be negatively affected in treated children and adolescents. Decline of working memory, processing speed, and visual memory over time has been reported in patients during longitudinal follow-up [58].

31.7 Perspectives

The diagnosis and treatment of IGCT have been developed heavily due to multidisciplinary and collaborative efforts. For germinomas, various measures to enhance patients' quality of life while maintaining current cure rates will be attempted. For NGGCT, we still have a long way to go to raise the survival rate. Genetic aberrations and epigenetic profiling need to be incorporated into the current pathological classification. To facilitate molecular genomic research and better disease stratification, surgical biopsy will be more important for IGCT. Above all, IGCT is a relatively rare brain tumor type, and more collaborative research and clinical trials are required.

References

1. Dho YS, Jung KW, Ha J, Seo Y, Park CK, Won YJ et al (2017) An updated nationwide epidemiology of primary brain tumors in Republic of Korea, 2013. Brain Tumor Res Treat 5(1):16–23
2. Murray MJ, Horan G, Lowis S, Nicholson JC (2013) Highlights from the Third International Central Nervous System Germ Cell Tumour symposium: laying the foundations for future consensus. Ecancermedicalscience 7:333
3. Poynter JN, Fonstad R, Tolar J, Spector LG, Ross JA (2014) Incidence of intracranial germ cell tumors by race in the United States, 1992-2010. J Neuro-Oncol 120(2):381–388
4. Makino K, Nakamura H, Yano S, Kuratsu J (2010) Population-based epidemiological study of primary intracranial tumors in childhood. Childs Nerv Syst 26(8):1029–1034
5. McCarthy BJ, Shibui S, Kayama T, Miyaoka E, Narita Y, Murakami M et al (2012) Primary CNS germ cell tumors in Japan and the United States: an analysis of 4 tumor registries. Neuro-Oncology 14(9):1194–1200

6. Sonoda Y, Kumabe T, Sugiyama S, Kanamori M, Yamashita Y, Saito R et al (2008) Germ cell tumors in the basal ganglia: problems of early diagnosis and treatment. J Neurosurg Pediatr 2(2):118–124

7. Phi JH, Cho BK, Kim SK, Paeng JC, Kim IO, Kim IH et al (2010) Germinomas in the basal ganglia: magnetic resonance imaging classification and the prognosis. J Neuro-Oncol 99(2):227–236

8. Koh EJ, Phi JH, Park SH, Kim IO, Cheon JE, Wang KC et al (2009) Mixed germ cell tumor of the midbrain. Case report. J Neurosurg Pediatr 4(2):137–142

9. Matsumura N, Kurimoto M, Endo S, Fukuda O, Takaku A (1998) Intracranial germinoma associated with Down's syndrome. Report of 2 cases. Pediatr Neurosurg 29(4):199–202

10. Prall JA, McGavran L, Greffe BS, Partington MD (1995) Intracranial malignant germ cell tumor and the Klinefelter syndrome. Case report and review of the literature. Pediatr Neurosurg 23(4):219–224

11. Teilum G (1965) Classification of endodermal sinus tumour (mesoblatoma vitellinum) and so-called "embryonal carcinoma" of the ovary. Acta Pathol Microbiol Scand 64(4):407–429

12. Oosterhuis JW, Stoop H, Honecker F, Looijenga LH (2007) Why human extragonadal germ cell tumours occur in the midline of the body: old concepts, new perspectives. Int J Androl 30(4):256–263; discussion 63–4.

13. Sobis H, Vandeputte M (1976) Yolk sac-derived rat teratomas are not of germ cell origin. Dev Biol 51(2):320–323

14. Solter D, Dominis M, Damjanov I (1980) Embryo-derived teratocarcinoma. II. Teratocarcinogenesis depends on the type of embryonic graft. Int J Cancer 25(3):341–343

15. Sano K (1999) Pathogenesis of intracranial germ cell tumors reconsidered. J Neurosurg 90(2):258–264

16. Fukushima S, Yamashita S, Kobayashi H, Takami H, Fukuoka K, Nakamura T et al (2017) Genome-wide methylation profiles in primary intracranial germ cell tumors indicate a primordial germ cell origin for germinomas. Acta Neuropathol 133(3):445–462

17. Santagata S, Ligon KL, Hornick JL (2007) Embryonic stem cell transcription factor signatures in the diagnosis of primary and metastatic germ cell tumors. Am J Surg Pathol 31(6):836–845

18. Sukov WR, Cheville JC, Giannini C, Carlson AW, Shearer BM, Sinnwell JP et al (2010) Isochromosome 12p and polysomy 12 in primary central nervous system germ cell tumors: frequency and association with clinicopathologic features. Hum Pathol 41(2):232–238

19. Okada Y, Nishikawa R, Matsutani M, Louis DN (2002) Hypomethylated X chromosome gain and rare isochromosome 12p in diverse intracranial germ cell tumors. J Neuropathol Exp Neurol 61(6):531–538

20. Fukushima S, Otsuka A, Suzuki T, Yanagisawa T, Mishima K, Mukasa A et al (2014) Mutually exclusive mutations of KIT and RAS are associated with KIT mRNA expression and chromosomal instability in primary intracranial pure germinomas. Acta Neuropathol 127(6):911–925

21. Wang L, Yamaguchi S, Burstein MD, Terashima K, Chang K, Ng HK et al (2014) Novel somatic and germline mutations in intracranial germ cell tumours. Nature 511(7508):241–245

22. O'Connor DM, Norris HJ (1994) The influence of grade on the outcome of stage I ovarian immature (malignant) teratomas and the reproducibility of grading. Int J Gynecol Pathol 13(4):283–289

23. Phi JH, Park SH, Paek SH, Kim SK, Lee YJ, Park CK et al (2007) Expression of Sox2 in mature and immature teratomas of central nervous system. Mod Pathol 20(7):742–748

24. Matsutani M, Sano K, Takakura K, Fujimaki T, Nakamura O, Funata N et al (1997) Primary intracranial germ cell tumors: a clinical analysis of 153 histologically verified cases. J Neurosurg 86(3):446–455

25. Ogino H, Shibamoto Y, Takanaka T, Suzuki K, Ishihara S, Yamada T et al (2005) CNS germinoma with elevated serum human chorionic gonadotropin level: clinical characteristics and treatment outcome. Int J Radiat Oncol Biol Phys 62(3):803–808

26. Shibamoto Y, Takahashi M, Sasai K (1997) Prognosis of intracranial germinoma with syncytiotrophoblastic giant cells treated by radiation therapy. Int J Radiat Oncol Biol Phys 37(3):505–510

27. Jorsal T, Rorth M (2012) Intracranial germ cell tumours. A review with special reference to endocrine manifestations. Acta Oncol (Stockholm, Sweden) 51(1):3–9

28. Mootha SL, Barkovich AJ, Grumbach MM, Edwards MS, Gitelman SE, Kaplan SL et al (1997) Idiopathic hypothalamic diabetes insipidus, pituitary stalk thickening, and the occult intracranial germinoma in children and adolescents. J Clin Endocrinol Metab 82(5):1362–1367

29. Phi JH, Kim SK, Park SH, Hong SH, Wang KC, Cho BK (2005) Immature teratomas of the central nervous system: is adjuvant therapy mandatory? J Neurosurg 103(6 Suppl):524–530

30. Murray MJ, Bartels U, Nishikawa R, Fangusaro J, Matsutani M, Nicholson JC (2015) Consensus on the management of intracranial germ-cell tumours. Lancet Oncol 16(9):e470–e477

31. Legault G, Allen JC (2013) Potential role of ventricular tumor markers in CNS germ cell tumors. Pediatr Blood Cancer 60(10):1647–1650

32. Kato T, Sawamura Y, Tada M, Murata J, Abe H, Shirato H et al (1998) Occult neurohypophyseal germinomas in patients presenting with central diabetes insipidus. Neurosurg Focus 5(1):e6

33. Phi JH, Kim SK, Lee J, Park CK, Kim IH, Ahn HS et al (2013) The enigma of bifocal germ cell tumors in the suprasellar and pineal regions: synchronous lesions or metastasis? J Neurosurg Pediatr 11(2):107–114

34. Lafay-Cousin L, Millar BA, Mabbott D, Spiegler B, Drake J, Bartels U et al (2006) Limited-field radiation for bifocal germinoma. Int J Radiat Oncol Biol Phys 65(2):486–492

35. Reddy AT, Wellons JC 3rd, Allen JC, Fiveash JB, Abdullatif H, Braune KW et al (2004) Refining the staging evaluation of pineal region germinoma using neuroendoscopy and the presence of preoperative diabetes insipidus. Neuro-Oncology 6(2):127–133

36. Takeda N, Fujita K, Katayama S, Uchihashi Y, Okamura Y, Nigami H et al (2004) Germinoma of the basal ganglia. An 8-year asymptomatic history after detection of abnormality on CT. Pediatr Neurosurg 40(6):306–311

37. Sudo A, Shiga T, Okajima M, Takano K, Terae S, Sawamura Y et al (2003) High uptake on 11C-methionine positron emission tomographic scan of basal ganglia germinoma with cerebral hemiatrophy. AJNR Am J Neuroradiol 24(9):1909–1911

38. Phuakpet K, Larouche V, Hawkins C, Huang A, Tabori U, Bartels UK et al (2016) Rare presentation of supratentorial primitive neuroectodermal tumors mimicking bifocal germ cell tumors: 2 case reports. J Pediatr Hematol Oncol 38(2):e67–e70

39. Kim CY, Choi JW, Lee JY, Kim SK, Wang KC, Park SH et al (2011) Intracranial growing teratoma syndrome: clinical characteristics and treatment strategy. J Neuro-Oncol 101(1):109–115

40. Rogers SJ, Mosleh-Shirazi MA, Saran FH (2005) Radiotherapy of localised intracranial germinoma: time to sever historical ties? Lancet Oncol 6(7):509–519

41. Odagiri K, Omura M, Hata M, Aida N, Niwa T, Ogino I et al (2012) Treatment outcomes, growth height, and neuroendocrine functions in patients with intracranial germ cell tumors treated with chemoradiation therapy. Int J Radiat Oncol Biol Phys 84(3):632–638

42. Cheng S, Kilday JP, Laperriere N, Janzen L, Drake J, Bouffet E et al (2016) Outcomes of children with central nervous system germinoma treated with multi-agent chemotherapy followed by reduced radiation. J Neuro-Oncol 127(1):173–180

43. Cho J, Choi JU, Kim DS, Suh CO (2009) Low-dose craniospinal irradiation as a definitive treatment for intracranial germinoma. Radiother Oncol 91(1):75–79

44. Calaminus G, Kortmann R, Worch J, Nicholson JC, Alapetite C, Garre ML et al (2013) SIOP CNS GCT 96: final report of outcome of a prospective, multinational nonrandomized trial for children and adults with intracranial germinoma, comparing craniospinal irradiation alone or with chemotherapy followed by focal primary site irradiation for patients with localized disease. Neuro-Oncology 15(6):788–796

45. da Silva NS, Cappellano AM, Diez B, Cavalheiro S, Gardner S, Wisoff J et al (2010) Primary chemotherapy for intracranial germ cell tumors: results of the third international CNS germ cell tumor study. Pediatr Blood Cancer 54(3):377–383

46. Kellie SJ, Boyce H, Dunkel IJ, Diez B, Rosenblum M, Brualdi L et al (2004) Intensive cisplatin and cyclophosphamide-based chemotherapy without radiotherapy for intracranial germinomas: failure of a primary chemotherapy approach. Pediatr Blood Cancer 43(2):126–133

47. Sawamura Y, Ikeda J, Shirato H, Tada M, Abe H (1998) Germ cell tumours of the central nervous system: treatment consideration based on 111 cases and their long-term clinical outcomes. Eur J Cancer (Oxford, England: 1990) 34(1):104–110

48. Kim JW, Kim WC, Cho JH, Kim DS, Shim KW, Lyu CJ et al (2012) A multimodal approach including craniospinal irradiation improves the treatment outcome of high-risk intracranial nongerminomatous germ cell tumors. Int J Radiat Oncol Biol Phys 84(3):625–631

49. Lai IC, Wong TT, Shiau CY, Hu YW, Ho DM, Chang KP et al (2015) Treatment results and prognostic factors for intracranial nongerminomatous germ cell tumors: single institute experience. Childs Nerv Syst 31(5):683–691

50. Calaminus G, Bamberg M, Jurgens H, Kortmann RD, Sorensen N, Wiestler OD et al (2004) Impact of surgery, chemotherapy and irradiation on long term outcome of intracranial malignant non-germinomatous germ cell tumors: results of the German Cooperative Trial MAKEI 89. Klin Padiatr 216(3):141–149

51. Goldman S, Bouffet E, Fisher PG, Allen JC, Robertson PL, Chuba PJ et al (2015) Phase II trial assessing the ability of neoadjuvant chemotherapy with or without second-look surgery to eliminate measurable disease for nongerminomatous germ cell tumors: a Children's Oncology Group Study. J Clin Oncol 33(22):2464–2471

52. Weiner HL, Lichtenbaum RA, Wisoff JH, Snow RB, Souweidane MM, Bruce JN et al (2002) Delayed surgical resection of central nervous system germ cell tumors. Neurosurgery 50(4):727–733; discussion 33–4.

53. Ogiwara H, Kiyotani C, Terashima K, Morota N (2015) Second-look surgery for intracranial germ cell tumors. Neurosurgery 76(6):658–661; discussion 61–2.

54. Souweidane MM, Krieger MD, Weiner HL, Finlay JL (2010) Surgical management of primary central nervous system germ cell tumors: proceedings from the Second International Symposium on Central Nervous System Germ Cell Tumors. J Neurosurg Pediatr 6(2):125–130

55. Hanakita S, Takenobu A, Kambe A, Watanabe T, Shin M, Teraoka A (2012) Intramedullary recurrence of germinoma in the spinal cord 15 years after complete remission of a pineal lesion. J Neurosurg Spine 16(5):513–515

56. Ohno M, Narita Y, Miyakita Y, Shibui S (2016) The necessity of long-term follow-up including spinal examination after successful initial treatment of intracranial germinoma: case reports. Childs Nerv Syst 32(3):547–551

57. Sivasubramaniam V, Zebian B, Thakur B, Saran F, Chandler C (2016) Germinoma recurrence in the conus medullaris 12 years after remission of primary intracranial lesion in the pituitary. J Clin Neurosci 25:150–152

58. Mabbott DJ, Monsalves E, Spiegler BJ, Bartels U, Janzen L, Guger S et al (2011) Longitudinal evaluation of neurocognitive function after treatment for central nervous system germ cell tumors in childhood. Cancer 117(23):5402–5411

Choroid Plexus Tumors

32

Mark M. Souweidane

32.1 Introduction

Derived from choroid plexus epithelium and vascularized by choroidal arteries, choroid plexus tumors (CPTs) are primary intraventricular brain tumors of neuroectodermal origin with a papillary pattern resembling nonneoplastic choroid plexus. CPTs include both benign choroid plexus papilloma (CPP) and malignant choroid plexus carcinoma (CPC), as well as an intermediate-grade CPT called atypical choroid plexus papilloma (APP).

Although its principle location is at the parenchymal-ventricular junction within all four ventricles, the choroid plexus, embryonically, is derived from the ventricular epithelium along certain segments of the neural tube. It is first to form in the fourth ventricle, followed by the lateral ventricles, and finally in the third ventricle. With its main function to produce cerebrospinal fluid (CSF), the choroid plexus contains a superficial layer of cuboidal epithelium linked by tight junctions overlying a basal membrane that covers a papillary-shaped mesenchymal stromal core, which is formed by leptomeningeal cells, fenestrated blood vessels, and con-

nective tissue distributed in a loose pattern over an extracellular matrix. Immunohistochemical studies have shown ubiquitous aquaporin-1 (AQP-1) expression in line with its main function of CSF production. Other roles of the choroid plexus are autoimmune inflammation, epithelial cells express major histocompatibility complex classes I and II; and a primary constituent of the blood-brain barrier due to intercellular zonula occludens connections [1].

32.2 Epidemiology

CPTs are rare childhood tumors with an approximate incidence of 0.3 cases per one million persons per year with approximately 1500 cases diagnosed annually; however, the annual incidence in the pediatric age group is 3–5% and up to 12% in children less than 2 years old [2–7]. Overall, CPTs make up 0.3–0.6% of all brain tumors. With up to 70% occurring in children and half in those less than 2 years of age, CPTs make up 2–4% of all pediatric intracranial tumors and 10–23% of all pediatric tumors in children less than 1 year old with some case reports even suggesting congenital findings of CPT by ultrasound [2, 8]. There are no known race or sex preponderance and no known difference between CPP and CPC in regard to sex, age, symptoms, or lesion location [9]. Reports have found one region in Southern Brazil with a higher incidence of CPC

M. M. Souweidane (✉)
Department of Neurological Surgery, Weill Cornell
Medical College and Memorial Sloan-Kettering
Cancer Center, New York, NY, USA
e-mail: mmsouwei@med.cornell.edu

© Springer Nature Switzerland AG 2019
J.-C. Tonn et al. (eds.), *Oncology of CNS Tumors*, https://doi.org/10.1007/978-3-030-04152-6_32

where the median age is 3.5 years at diagnosis and a male preponderance (1.2:1). This geographic aberrancy in presentation is mainly due to higher incidence of an allele (R337H) associated with the TP53 gene [10, 11].

In children, the most common location for these tumors is within the lateral ventricle, whereas, in adults, CPTs are more commonly infratentorial (fourth ventricle and cerebellopontine angle) [11–13]. Although the primary location is intraventricular, ectopic extraventricular locations of CPTs have been reported, including the suprasellar or pineal regions [13–16]. Overall, CPPs make up the majority of CPTs with about 80%. For the more aggressive CPTs, 15% are APPs, and <5% are CPCs, which mainly occur in infants in about 80% of cases [17].

The recurrence of CPP after surgical resection and the progression from CPP to CPC are rare; however, cases of both have been reported. Following resection of CPP, one study found a 6% recurrence rate, possibly overestimated due to non-specific initial classification of tumor. In the literature, there are eight cases reported of CPP to CPC progression. This malignant transformation is correlated with mitotic activity and ki-67 proliferation index. Those tumors exhibiting these qualities should be monitored closely [18–20].

32.3 Clinical Features

For most patients with CPT, the most common presenting symptom is hydrocephalus. Because of the intraventricular location of CPTs, patient may remain asymptomatic until the lesion results in overproduction of CSF and/or interfere with CSF pathways resulting in hydrocephalic symptoms, which thereby results in insidious intracranial hypertensive symptoms such as headaches, nausea, vomiting, irritability, and/or visual disturbances [21, 22]. In one series, 33 of 38 children presented with hydrocephalus [23–25]. Further signs and symptoms indicative of hydrocephalus include increased intracranial pressure (ICP), seizures, hemorrhage, focal neurologic deficits, and constitutional symptoms. On physical examination, the most common finding is papilledema. Infants and younger children typically present with irritability, lethargy, bulging fontanelle, macrocephaly, protruding scalp veins, and/or suture diastasis. For those CPTs arising in the third ventricle, patients may present with endocrinologic dysfunction, including obesity, precocious puberty, diabetes insipidus, menstrual irregularity in older children, psychosis, or bobblehead doll syndrome [23–27]. Most severely, intratumoral hemorrhage or acute hydrocephalus may result in a sudden deterioration of consciousness.

32.4 Pathology

The World Health Organization (WHO) classifies CPTs based on histologic criteria as choroid plexus papilloma, WHO grade I (CPP); atypical choroid plexus papilloma, WHO grade II (APP); and choroid plexus carcinoma, WHO grade III (CPC) [28].

CPPs are benign and usually curable with surgical gross total resection. Histologically and radiographically, CPPs demonstrate the papillary architecture of nonneoplastic choroid plexus, with "cauliflower-like" morphology, but the papillary fronds are hypercellular and stratified, with flattening of the usual cobblestone surface pattern of normal choroidal tissue (Fig. 32.1). CPPs are well-circumscribed intraventricular masses that do not typically intrude into adjacent brain parenchyma. They can have cystic or hemorrhagic components but demonstrate very low or absent mitotic activity [28–35].

APPs show increased proliferative activity relative to CPP, typically defined as two or more mitoses per ten randomly selected high-power fields (HPFs), and by definition do not meet histological criteria for CPC. Overall, APP has an increased risk of recurrence compared to CPP. Of note, the risk of recurrence relative to the degree of proliferation may not be identical for all age groups, with children less than 3 years of age showing more tolerance for an increased mitotic activity [36].

By definition, CPCs exhibit at least four out of five histologically aggressive features: frequent mitoses (typically defined as five or more

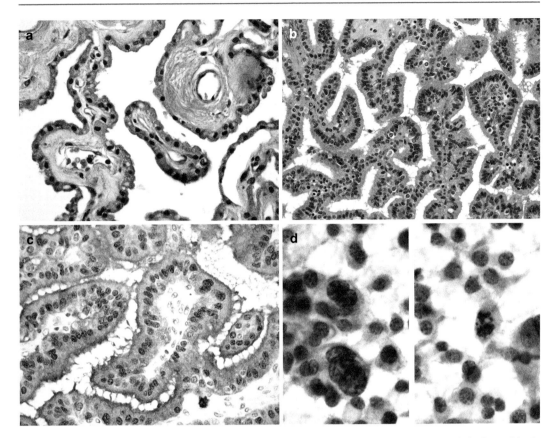

Fig. 32.1 (a) Nonneoplastic choroid plexus showing simple epithelial layer with cobblestone-like surface; (b) CPP showing more complex papillary architecture, increased cellularity, and flat epithelial luminal surface; (c) staining for S100 which is characteristically positive in addition to cytokeratin staining and transthyretin; (d) CPC on intraoperative squash preparation showing increased nuclear pleomorphism (left) and mitotic activity (right)

mitoses per ten randomly selected HPFs), nuclear pleomorphism, hypercellularity, sheetlike architectural growth, and necrosis. CPCs may demonstrate diffuse invasion of the adjacent brain parenchyma [28]. These features are associated with the increased risk of recurrence and dissemination that is seen in CPC. At the time of diagnosis, disseminated disease, which can be traced along the CSF pathways, ranges from 20 to 70% and is associated with a poor prognosis in CPC [24, 37–40].

Although CPTs can usually be diagnosed using only standard hematoxylin and eosin staining, immunohistochemistry may facilitate the diagnosis when the histological differential diagnosis includes metastatic carcinoma or tumors arising intracranially with papillary features, such as the papillary variant of ependymoma, papillary meningioma, and papillary endolymphatic sac tumor of the cerebellopontine angle [17, 41]. For example, CPTs are frequently positive for CK7, S100, and/or transthyretin. These immunohistochemical stains must be interpreted in the appropriate context as none are specific for CPT and they also do not demonstrate complete sensitivity. Kir7.1, a potassium channel found in normal choroid plexus, and stanniocalcin 1, a protein involved in calcium homeostasis, are both typically expressed and have been shown to be relatively sensitive and specific for CPT [42–44]. In contrast to ependymomas, strong GFAP expression is not typical in CPT, and EMA staining does not demonstrate the dot-like microluminal staining characteristic of ependymal differentiation. Decreased labeling for S100 and transthyretin may be seen with higher-grade tumors. For CPC, the differential diagnosis may include atypical teratoid/rhabdoid tumors (AT/RT) and supratentorial embryonal tumors of the CNS. Staining for the nuclear antigen integrase interactor 1 (INI1) may be used to exclude AT/RT, which is characterized in the vast majority of cases by loss of INI1 expression with associated alterations of the *SMARCB1* locus [28, 45–47]. In difficult cases, methylation profiling may prove to be of increasing clinical utility [48].

32.5 Etiology and Pathogenesis

CPTs usually occur sporadically; however, they are also seen in the setting of recognized syndromic associations [41]. Chromosomal abnormalities have been identified, and aberration patterns differ according to the degree of anaplasia. Chromosomal imbalances, including gains, losses, or duplications, have been identified in tumor tissue chromosomes 1, 4, 5, 7, 9, 10, 12, 14, 18, and 20. One large study including 149 CPC patients identified an association between a gain of chromosome 9 and loss of chromosome 10 with prolonged survival, whereas, another study noted a 12q loss of function associated with poor survival [49, 50].

The most recognized syndrome associated with increased risk of CPC is Li-Fraumeni syndrome, characterized by an autosomal dominant TP53 germline mutation [42, 43, 51]. The incidence of this cancer-predisposing syndrome is about 1 in 20,000, and reports have documented coincidental CPC with other carcinomas in patients with Li-Fraumeni syndrome. One study of 42 patients with CPC found TP53 mutations in 50% of patients. Furthermore the quantitative and qualitative status of TP53 was predictive of survival [42, 51–53]. Another syndrome associated with the development of CPT is Aicardi syndrome, a triad of callosal agenesis, infantile spasms, and chorioretinal lacunae [54–58].

More recently, platelet-derived growth factor receptor (PDGFR), a receptor normally expressed in choroid plexus tissue, has been identified in the pathogenesis of CPTs. In CPCs, the PDGFR beta isoform is highly phosphorylated compared to CPPs and thereby promotes cell proliferation when bound [52, 53, 59–63]. Two genes, TWIST1, a p53 suppressor, and Notch 3, an oncogene, are also associated with CPT development [64].

32.6 Diagnostic Imaging

Diagnostic imaging for CPTs included contrast computed tomography (CT), magnetic resonance imaging (MRI), magnetic resonance spectroscopy (MRS), magnetic resonance angiography (MRA), and catheter-based cerebral angiography. Usually, CPTs are initially evaluated by computed tomography (CT) and show a lobulated intraventricular tumor with "cauliflower-like" edges sharply demarcated from the surround parenchyma. Brain CT with contrast exhibits an intense homogeneously enhancing mass. The tumors in infancy that occur in the lateral ventricles are frequently voluminous with mass effect and ependymal expansion [65]. Possible findings on CT include cyst formations, calcification, hemorrhage, and/or perilesional edema [66]. Given the association with hydrocephalus, ventriculomegaly is nearly always present.

For perioperative evaluation, MRI is used preoperatively to assess tumor vascularization and for metastatic evaluation. Postoperatively, MRI is employed to determine the extent of resection and for recurrence monitoring. On MRI, T1-weighted sequences display the tumor as isointense or slightly hypointense with uniform enhancement on postcontrast sequences (Fig. 32.2). T2-weighted sequences display the tumor as a heterogeneous iso- to hyperintense intraventricular mass (Fig. 32.3). Complete neuraxis imaging is recommended preoperatively to rule out dissemination, which is identified by linear or nodular leptomeningeal enhancement [67].

MRS is used to highlight the difference between normal choroid plexus, high-grade, and low-grade tumors. CPPs demonstrate a single elevated myoinositol, while CPCs have a choline and lactate peak with decreased *N*-acetyl aspartate level [68, 69].

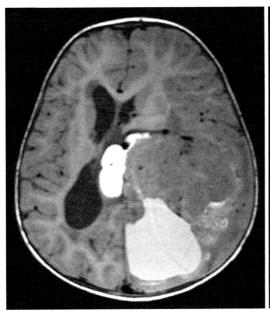
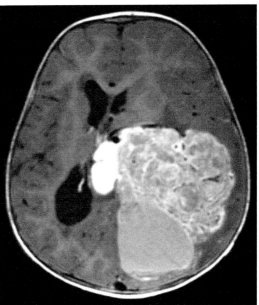

Fig. 32.2 T1-weighted MRI without contrast (left) and with contrast (right) of choroid plexus carcinoma in a 1-year-old male. Large, enhancing, lobulated mass centered within the left parietal lobe with surrounding tumoral proteinaceous cysts, resulting in significant mass effect upon the ventricular system with rightward midline shift and entrapment and dilatation of the right lateral ventricle and left temporal horn

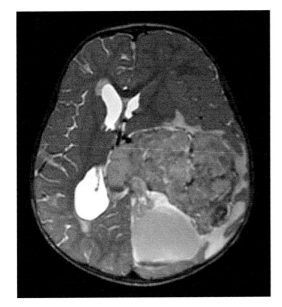

Fig. 32.3 T2-weighted MRI of choroid plexus carcinoma in 1-year-old male

32.7 Treatment

In most cases, CPPs that undergo gross total resection (GTR) are considered cured [9]. Following total removal of CPPs, several patient series have reported a 5-year survival of 100% without adjuvant chemotherapy and a 10-year survival rate up to 85%. Fortunately, GTR is possible in the majority of patients. In several series including patients with CPP, complete resection was achieved in 100% of patients [23, 70–75]. Nevertheless, long-term follow-up and radiographic monitoring are required given reports of relapse following GTR [9, 11, 70, 73, 76–79].

CPCs, on the other hand, are malignant tumors, more likely to locally recur and metastasize, and therefore come with a poor prognosis [17]. Because of their vascularity and invasion, GTR is more challenging in patients with CPC; however various studies have shown the extent of resection directly correlated with survival. Compared to CPPs, CPC surgeries achieve GTR less than 50% of the time [71]. For CPCs, those patients with a GTR had a survival rate of 84%, while those with a subtotal resection had a survival rate of 18% [80]. Moreover, the 5-year survival rates range from 11 to 86% following GTR and adjuvant therapy, while a subtotal resection drops the 5-year survival to less than 20% (68%). In a meta-analysis of resection percentage among the subtypes of CPTs, researchers observed GTR in 80% of CPPs, 61% of APPs, and 49% of CPCs [81]. Overall, for these malignant CPTs, an aggressive surgical resection is recommended, and oftentimes a "second-look" operation is considered [38, 82].

Metastatic CPTs, mainly from disseminated CPCs, have an incidence of 12–50%, with a pattern of drop metastasis through physiologic CSF pathways [11, 38, 83, 84]. For all patients diagnosed with CPTs, complete neuraxis imaging with MRI to evaluate for dissemination and genetic testing for TP53 mutations is recommended [67, 85, 86].

32.7.1 Surgery

Gross total surgical resection is the single most important prognostic variable irrespective of histologic type in the treatment of CPTs (Fig. 32.4) [21, 87–89]. That said, due to the deep location and proximity to vascular structures of these lesions, CPTs, and especially CPCs, are technically demanding operations that, despite technical advances, from diagnostic imaging to neuroanesthesia, come with significant risk of intraoperative hemorrhage and a mortality rate up to 25% [23]. Prior to surgery, arterial access for continuous blood pressure monitoring and adequate venous access for possible rapid intraoperative fluid and blood transfusion must be secured. Blood loss is of particular concern both due to the intense vascularization of these tumors and the very low circulating blood volumes (80 mL/kg) in young children affected by CPTs. For this reason, blood, fresh frozen plasma, platelets, and fibrinogen are all mandatory prior to incision. Due to this hemorrhagic risk, microneurosurgical techniques must be employed to apply gen-

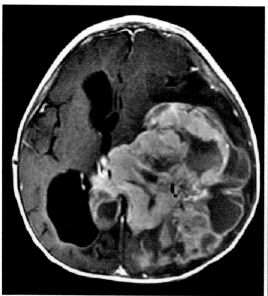
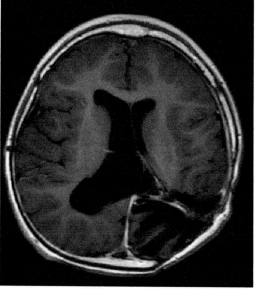

Fig. 32.4 Choroid plexus carcinoma in an 8-month-old male. Preoperative T1-weighted MRI with contrast (left) and postoperative (right) T1-weighted MRI with contrast in patient who underwent tumor embolization and second-look surgery for tumor resection following systemic induction chemotherapy (cyclophosphamide, etoposide, vincristine) with gross total resection. After undergoing consolidation chemotherapy and involved field radiation (4005 cGy), the child remains alive at 102 months post-diagnosis

erous coagulation to the tumor surface prior to dissection or debulking and to isolate vascular pedicles early. For CPC resection, some reports recommend a two-stage approach beginning with a biopsy, followed by neoadjuvant chemotherapy and then "second-look surgery." This approach has been documented to reduce the tumor vascularity and overall dimension, making total tumor removal safer and more feasible [38, 82].

Postoperatively, despite complete tumor removal, patients may require a ventriculoperitoneal shunt (VPS) for treatment of symptomatic hydrocephalus or subdural fluid collections [90–92]. In 1 study, 9 of 38 patients required permanent CSF diversion following CPT removal [23], while other studies state 30–50% of patients may require a VPS postoperatively [9]. Although rare, CSF diversion resulting in abdominal metastasis has been reported [85]. Another adverse surgical effect of CPT removal is the development of subdural fluid collections, which occasionally require a VPS for CSF diversion. Surgeons have recommended filling the ventricles with saline prior to closing, closing corticectomy with pial

sutures or fibrin glue, or placing temporary external ventricular drain in order to minimize the risk of post-resection subdural collections [23, 93].

Although not the mainstay of treatment, neuroendoscopic surgery has a clear role in the management of CPTs. Given that these tumors are mainly intraventricular, endoscopic approaches come with the well-recognized advantages—minimal parenchymal disruptions, improved visualization, and favorable cosmetics—as well as the benefit of also treating hydrocephalus and possibly decreasing the need for VPS placement [94, 95]. A purely endoscopic approach logically is best suited for isolated tumors of the third ventricle owing to their comparatively small size and early onset of occlusive hydrocephalus (Fig. 32.5) [95, 96].

32.7.2 Interventional Neuroradiology

As for most neurosurgical conditions, interventional neuroradiology (INR) is making continu-

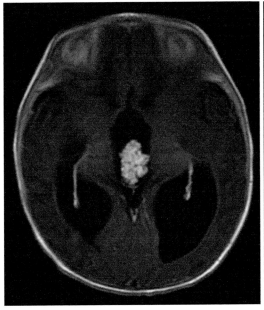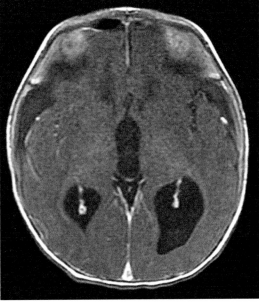

Fig. 32.5 Third ventricular choroid plexus papilloma (WHO Grade I) in a 16-month-old male. Preoperative T1-weighted MRI with contrast (left) and postoperative (right) T1-weighted MRI with contrast in patient who underwent right frontal endoscopic approach for tumor resection with gross total resection and improved ventriculomegaly

ous technological advancements toward treating neurosurgical conditions, and the same applies to CPTs. There are currently both diagnostic and therapeutic roles for INR in the management of CPTs. Given the variety of locations of CPTs, hypertrophied choroidal vessels, single or multiple, can arise from anterior or posterior circulation [97–106]. The tumor dependency on a dominant vascular pattern is illustrated in a case report of a 3-month-old who underwent embolization for her third ventricular CPT. The embolization resulted in complete regression of the tumor in 7 months [98]. Although CPTs have characteristic high vascularization and seemingly well-suited for embolization, reported success rates for meaningful embolization are low due to a variety of factors [107–109]. Notably, choroidal vessels feeding CPTs are elongated, tortuous, and narrow, not to mention usually provide solitary blood supply to the optic pathways and internal capsule [23, 98, 106]. Furthermore, the patient population do not make ideal INR candidates due to the low body mass and required contrast load and radiation burden necessary for INR.

32.7.3 Radiation Therapy

The role of radiotherapy for CPTs is most accepted in patients with CPC and especially in those who have undergone a subtotal resection and leptomeningeal metastatic disease. Postoperative radiotherapy, in the form of craniospinal irradiation, has been shown to increase survival time in both complete and subtotal resections of CPC [110, 111]. Moreover, a literature review of 524 patients who underwent GTR for CPC identified a 5-year survival period of 68% with postoperative radiation and 16% without radiation [110]. That said, regardless of radiation, the prognosis following an incomplete CPC resection is dismal [11]. Due to the adverse cognitive and endocrinologic effects as well as the risk of radiation-induced secondary malignancies, radiation is commonly withheld in younger patients (under 3 years of age) or unless there is metastatic/progression of disease [110, 112]. Due to both the

rarity of CPTs and the potential for adjacent radiation complications, intensity-modulated radiation therapy, often used to maximize therapeutic ratio for other primary brain tumors, has been used in CPT radiotherapy to limit exposure to nearby organs and structures [113, 114].

32.7.4 Chemotherapy

Similar to radiation therapy, the role of chemotherapy in the treatment of CPTs remains unclear, and its application has been mostly focused on the treatment of CPCs. In a meta-analysis of 857 CPTs with 247 CPCs, chemotherapy improved survival from 24.4 to 54.8% in CPC patients who had subtotal resections [75, 81]. Following GTR, chemotherapy, usually a combination of etoposide, cyclophosphamide, vincristine, and/or platinum agents, may increase survival rate [37, 38, 74, 82]. In one series treating CPC, two to six cycles of ifosfamide, carboplatinum, and etoposide were used and resulted in an overall decrease in expression of cell cycle proteins [71]. Furthermore, preoperative chemotherapy has been suggested in order to reduce tumor size and vascularity, thereby reducing intraoperative bleeding during resection and associated consequences [4, 115–117]. "Second-look" surgery is playing an increasing role after neoadjuvant chemotherapy in malignancies in infants. Postoperatively, in patients with subtotal resection, adjuvant chemotherapy has been shown to delay the need for radiation therapy [75, 118].

32.8 Outcome/Conclusions

Due to the rarity of these tumors and the variety of treatment options, CPTs continue to be challenging tumors in a mainly pediatric population. Through a multidisciplinary approach among international collaborators of neuroscientists, neuro-oncologists, neurointerventionalists, radiation oncologists, and neurosurgeons, advancements toward new and innovative therapies are underway for improving the care and management of this poorly prognostic disease.

References

1. Wolburg H, Paulus W (2010) Choroid plexus: biology and pathology. Acta Neuropathol 119(1):75–88
2. Custodio G, Taques GR, Figueiredo BC, Gugelmin ES, Figueiredo MM, Watanabe F, Pontarolo R, Lalli E, Torres LF (2011) Increased incidence of choroid plexus carcinoma due to the germline TP53 R337H mutation in southern Brazil. PLoS One 6(3):e18015
3. Clair SK, Humphreys RP, Pillay PK, Hoffman HJ, Blaser SI, Becker LE (1991) Current management of choroid plexus carcinoma in children. Pediatr Neurosurg 17(5):225–233
4. Jooma R, Grant N (1983) Third ventricle choroid plexus papillomas. Pediatr Neurosurg 10(4):242–250
5. Body G, Darnis E, Soutoul JH, Pourcelot D, Santini JJ, Gold F (1990) Choroid plexus tumors: antenatal diagnosis and follow-up. J Clin Ultrasound 18(7):575–578
6. Koh EJ, Wang KC, Phi JH, Lee JY, Choi JW, Park SH, Park KD, Kim IH, Cho BK, Kim SK (2014) Clinical outcome of pediatric choroid plexus tumors: retrospective analysis from a single institute. Childs Nerv Syst 30(2):217–225
7. Jänisch W, Staneczek W (1989) Primary tumors of the choroid plexus. Frequency, localization and age. Zentralbl Allg Pathol 135(3):235–240
8. Cassinari V, Bernasconi V (1963) Tumori della parte anteriore del terzo ventricolo. Acta Neurochir 11(2):236–271
9. Keating RF, Goodrich JT, Packer RJ (eds) (2001) Tumors of the pediatric central nervous system. Thieme, New York
10. Wolff JE, Sajedi M, Brant R, Coppes MJ, Egeler RM (2002) Choroid plexus tumours. Br J Cancer 87(10):1086
11. Carter AB, Price DL Jr, Tucci KA, Lewis GK, Mewborne J, Singh HK (2001) Choroid plexus carcinoma presenting as an intraparenchymal mass: case report. J Neurosurg 95(6):1040–1044
12. Koeller KK, Sandberg GD (2002) From the archives of the AFIP: cerebral intraventricular neoplasms: radiologic-pathologic correlation. Radiographics 22(6):1473–1505
13. Dhillon RS, Wang YY, McKelvie PA, O'Brien B (2013) Progression of choroid plexus papilloma. J Clin Neurosci 20(12):1775–1778
14. Kimura M, Takayasu M, Suzuki Y, Negoro M, Nagasaka T, Nakashima N, Sugita K (1992) Primary choroid plexus papilloma located in the suprasellar region: case report. Neurosurgery 31(3):563–566
15. Rickert CH, Paulus W (2001) Tumors of the choroid plexus. Microsc Res Tech 52(1):104–111
16. McGirr SJ, Ebersold MJ, Scheithauer BW, Quast LM, Shaw EG (1988) Choroid plexus papillomas: long-term follow-up results in a surgically treated series. J Neurosurg 69(6):843–849
17. Ang LC, Taylor AR, Bergin D, Kaufmann JC (1990) An immunohistochemical study of papillary tumors in the central nervous system. Cancer 65(12):2712–2719
18. Niikawa S, Ito T, Murakawa T, Hirayama H, Ando T, Sakai N, Yamada H (1993) Recurrence of choroid plexus papilloma with malignant transformation. Neurol Med Chir 33(1):32–35
19. Jeibmann A, Wrede B, Peters O, Wolff JE, Paulus W, Hasselblatt M (2007) Malignant progression in choroid plexus papillomas. J Neurosurg 107(3 Suppl):199–202
20. Rickert CH, Wiestler OD, Paulus W (2002) Chromosomal imbalances in choroid plexus tumors. Am J Pathol 160(3):1105–1113
21. Ellenbogen RG, Winston KR, Kupsky WJ (1989) Tumors of the choroid plexus in children. Neurosurgery 25(3):327–335
22. Eisenberg HM, McComb JG, Lorenzo AV (1974) Cerebrospinal fluid overproduction and hydrocephalus associated with choroid plexus papilloma. J Neurosurg 40(3):381–385
23. Hawkins JC III (1980) Treatment of choroid plexus papillomas in children: a brief analysis of twenty years' experience. Neurosurgery 6(4):380–384
24. Matson DD, Crofton FD (1960) Papilloma of the choroid plexus in childhood. J Neurosurg 17(6):1002–1027
25. Raimondi AJ, Gutierrez FA (1975) Diagnosis and surgical treatment of choroid plexus papillomas. Pediatr Neurosurg 1(2–3):81–115
26. Hopper KD, Foley LC, Nieves NL, Smirniotopoulos JG (1987) The interventricular extension of choroid plexus papillomas. Am J Neuroradiol 8(3):469–472
27. Carlotti CG, Salhia B, Weitzman S, Greenberg M, Dirks PB, Mason W, Becker LE, Rutka JT (2002) Evaluation of proliferative index and cell cycle protein expression in choroid plexus tumors in children. Acta Neuropathol 103(1):1–10
28. Louis DN, Perry A, Reifenberger G, Von Deimling A, Figarella-Branger D, Cavenee WK, Ohgaki H, Wiestler OD, Kleihues P, Ellison DW (2016) The 2016 World Health Organization classification of tumors of the central nervous system: a summary. Acta Neuropathol 131(6):803–820. Aquilina K, Nanra JS, Allcutt DA, Farrell M (2005) Choroid plexus adenoma: case report and review of the literature. Childs Nerv Syst 21(5):410–415
29. Buccoliero AM, Bacci S, Mennonna P, Taddei GL (2004) Pathologic quiz case: infratentorial tumor in a middle-aged woman. Arch Pathol Lab Med 128(12):1448–1450
30. Corcoran GM, Frazier SR, Prayson RA (2001) Choroid plexus papilloma with osseous and adipose metaplasia. Ann Diagn Pathol 5(1):43–47
31. Gaudio RM, Tacconi L, Rossi ML (1998) Pathology of choroid plexus papillomas: a review. Clin Neurol Neurosurg 100(3):165–186
32. Ikota H, Tanaka Y, Yokoo H, Nakazato Y (2011) Clinicopathological and immunohistochemical study of 20 choroid plexus tumors: their histological diversity and the expression of markers useful for differentiation from metastatic cancer. Brain Tumor Pathol 28(3):215–221

33. Tena-Suck ML, López-Gómez M, Salinas-Lara C, Arce-Arellano RI, Renbao-Bojorquez D (2006) Psammomatous choroid plexus papilloma: three cases with atypical characteristics. Surg Neurol 65(6):604–610

34. Watanabe K, Ando Y, Iwanaga H, Ochiai C, Nagai M, Okada K, Watanabe N (1995) Choroid plexus papilloma containing melanin pigment. Clin Neuropathol 14(3):159–161

35. Gupta N (2003) Choroid plexus tumors in children. Neurosurg Clin 14(4):621–631

36. Thomas C, Ruland V, Kordes U, Hartung S, Capper D, Pietsch T, Gerß J, Wolff JE, Paulus W, Hasselblatt M (2015) Pediatric atypical choroid plexus papilloma reconsidered: increased mitotic activity is prognostic only in older children. Acta Neuropathol 129(6):925–927

37. Britz GW, Kim DK, Loeser JD (1996) Hydrocephalus secondary to diffuse villous hyperplasia of the choroid plexus: case report and review of the literature. J Neurosurg 85(4):689–691

38. McCall T, Binning M, Blumenthal DT, Jensen RL (2006) Variations of disseminated choroid plexus papilloma: 2 case reports and a review of the literature. Surg Neurol 66(1):62–67

39. Geerts Y, Gabreels F, Lippens R, Merx H, Wesseling P (1996) Choroid plexus carcinoma: a report of two cases and review of the literature. Neuropediatrics 27(3):143–148

40. Santos MM, Souweidane MM (2015) Purely endoscopic resection of a choroid plexus papilloma of the third ventricle: case report. J Neurosurg Pediatr 16(1):54–57

41. Gopal P, Parker JR, Debski R, Parker JC Jr (2008) Choroid plexus carcinoma. Arch Pathol Lab Med 132(8):1350–1354

42. Qualman SJ, Shannon BT, Boesel CP, Jacobs D, Jinkens C, Hayes J (1992) Ploidy analysis and cerebrospinal fluid nephelometry as measures of clinical outcome in childhood choroid plexus neoplasia. Pathol Annu 27:305

43. Barreto AS, Vassallo J, Queiroz LD (2004) Papillomas and carcinomas of the choroid plexus: histological and immunohistochemical studies and comparison with normal fetal choroid plexus. Arq Neuropsiquiatr 62(3A):600–607

44. Smith ZA, Moftakhar P, Malkasian D, Xiong Z, Vinters HV, Lazareff JA (2007) Choroid plexus hyperplasia: surgical treatment and immunohistochemical results. Case report. J Neurosurg 107(3 Suppl):255–262

45. Kepes JJ, Collins J (1999) Choroid plexus epithelium (normal and neoplastic) expresses synaptophysin. A potentially useful aid in differentiating carcinoma of the choroid plexus from metastatic papillary carcinomas. J Neuropathol Exp Neurol 58(4):398–401

46. Paulus W, Jänisch W (1990) Clinicopathologic correlations in epithelial choroid plexus neoplasms: a study of 52 cases. Acta Neuropathol 80(6):635–641

47. Tabori U, Shlien A, Baskin B, Levitt S, Ray P, Alon N, Hawkins C, Bouffet E, Pienkowska M, Lafay-Cousin L, Gozali A (2010) TP53 alterations determine clinical subgroups and survival of patients with choroid plexus tumors. J Clin Oncol 28(12):1995–2001

48. Capper D, Jones DT, Sill M, Hovestadt V, Schrimpf D, Sturm D, Koelsche C, Sahm F, Chavez L, Reuss DE, Kratz A (2018) DNA methylation-based classification of central nervous system tumours. Nature 555(7697):469

49. Krutilkova V, Trkova M, Fleitz J, Gregor V, Novotna K, Krepelova A, Sumerauer D, Kodet R, Siruckova S, Plevova P, Bendova S (2005) Identification of five new families strengthens the link between childhood choroid plexus carcinoma and germline TP53 mutations. Eur J Cancer 41(11):1597–1603

50. Ruland V, Hartung S, Kordes U, Wolff JE, Paulus W, Hasselblatt M (2014) Choroid plexus carcinomas are characterized by complex chromosomal alterations related to patient age and prognosis. Genes Chromosom Cancer 53(5):373–380

51. Aicardi J (2005) Aicardi syndrome. Brain Dev 27(3):164–171

52. Engels EA, Katki HA, Nielsen NM, Winther JF, Hjalgrim H, Gjerris F, Rosenberg PS, Frisch M (2003) Cancer incidence in Denmark following exposure to poliovirus vaccine contaminated with simian virus 40. J Natl Cancer Inst 95(7):532–539

53. Hosoya KI, Hori S, Ohtsuki S, Terasaki T (2004) A new in vitro model for blood–cerebrospinal fluid barrier transport studies: an immortalized choroid plexus epithelial cell line derived from the tsA58 SV40 large T-antigen gene transgenic rat. Adv Drug Deliv Rev 56(12):1875–1885

54. Muchardt C, Sardet C, Bourachot B, Onufryk C, Yaniv M (1995) A human protein with homology to Saccharomyces cerevisiae SNF5 interacts with the potential helicase hbrm. Nucleic Acids Res 23(7):1127–1132

55. Sévenet N, Sheridan E, Amram D, Schneider P, Handgretinger R, Delattre O (1999) Constitutional mutations of the hSNF5/INI1 gene predispose to a variety of cancers. Am J Hum Genet 65(5):1342–1348

56. Versteege I, Sévenet N, Lange J, Rousseau-Merck MF, Ambros P, Handgretinger R, Aurias A, Delattre O (1998) Truncating mutations of hSNF5/INI1 in aggressive paediatric cancer. Nature 394(6689):203

57. Wade PA, Wolffe AP (1999) Transcriptional regulation: SWItching circuitry. Curr Biol 9(6):R221–R224

58. Andrae J, Gallini R, Betsholtz C (2008) Role of platelet-derived growth factors in physiology and medicine. Genes Dev 22(10):1276–1312

59. Enge M, Wilhelmsson U, Abramsson A, Stakeberg J, Kühn R, Betsholtz C, Pekny M (2003) Neuron-specific ablation of PDGF-B is compatible with normal central nervous system development and astroglial response to injury. Neurochem Res 28(2):271–279

60. Hellstrom M, Lindahl P, Abramsson A, Betsholtz C (1999) Role of PDGF-B and PDGFR-beta in recruitment of vascular smooth muscle cells and pericytes

during embryonic blood vessel formation in the mouse. Development 126(14):3047–3055

61. Kaminski WE, Lindahl P, Lin NL, Broudy VC, Crosby JR, Hellström M, Swolin B, Bowen-Pope DF, Martin PJ, Ross R, Betsholtz C (2001) Basis of hematopoietic defects in platelet-derived growth factor (PDGF)-B and PDGF β-receptor null mice. Blood 97(7):1990–1998

62. Koos B, Paulsson J, Jarvius M, Sanchez BC, Wrede B, Mertsch S, Jeibmann A, Kruse A, Peters O, Wolff JE, Galla HJ (2009) Platelet-derived growth factor receptor expression and activation in choroid plexus tumors. Am J Pathol 175(4):1631–1637

63. Safaee M, Oh MC, Bloch O, Sun MZ, Kaur G, Auguste KI, Tihan T, Parsa AT (2012) Choroid plexus papillomas: advances in molecular biology and understanding of tumorigenesis. Neuro-Oncology 15(3):255–267

64. Bergsagel DJ, Finegold MJ, Butel JS, Kupsky WJ, Garcea RL (1992) DNA sequences similar to those of simian virus 40 in ependymomas and choroid plexus tumors of childhood. N Engl J Med 326(15):988–993

65. Asai A, Hoffman HJ, Matsutani M, Takakura K (1991) Choroid plexus tumors in infancy. No shinkei geka. Neurol Surg 19(1):21–26

66. Horská A, Ulug AM, Melhem ER et al (2001) Proton magnetic resonance spectroscopy of choroid plexus tumors in children. J Magn Reson Imaging 14(1):78–82

67. Donovan DJ, Prauner RD (2005) Shunt-related abdominal metastases in a child with choroid plexus carcinoma: case report. Neurosurgery 56(2):E412

68. Krieger MD, Panigrahy A, McComb JG, Nelson MD, Liu X, Gonzalez-Gomez I, Gilles F, Bluml S (2005) Differentiation of choroid plexus tumors by advanced magnetic resonance spectroscopy. Neurosurg Focus 18(6):1–4

69. Bettegowda C, Adogwa O, Mehta V, Chaichana KL, Weingart J, Carson BS, Jallo GI, Ahn ES (2012) Treatment of choroid plexus tumors: a 20-year single institutional experience. J Neurosurg Pediatr 10(5):398–405

70. Packer RJ, Perilongo G, Johnson D, Sutton LN, Vezina G, Zimmerman RA, Ryan J, Reaman G, Schut L (1992) Choroid plexus carcinoma of childhood. Cancer 69(2):580–585

71. Zuccaro G, Sosa F, Cuccia V, Lubieniecky F, Monges J (1999) Lateral ventricle tumors in children: a series of 54 cases. Childs Nerv Syst 15(11–12):774–785

72. Zuccaro G, Taratuto AL, Monges J (1986) Intracranial neoplasms during the first year of life. Surg Neurol 26(1):29–36

73. Pierga JY, Kalifa C, Terrir-Lacombe MJ et al (1993) Carcinoma of the choroid plexus: a pediatric experience. Med Pediatr Oncol 21:480–487

74. Souweidane MM, Johnson JH, Lis E (1999) Volumetric reduction of a choroid plexus carcinoma using preoperative chemotherapy. J Neuro-Oncol 43(2):167–171

75. Wrede B, Liu P, Wolff JE (2007) Chemotherapy improves the survival of patients with choroid plexus carcinoma: a meta-analysis of individual cases with choroid plexus tumors. J Neuro-Oncol 85(3):345–351

76. Due-Tønnessen B, Helseth E, Skullerud K, Lundar T (2001) Choroid plexus tumors in children and young adults: report of 16 consecutive cases. Childs Nerv Syst 17(4–5):252–256

77. Krishnan S, Brown PD, Scheithauer BW, Ebersold MJ, Hammack JE, Buckner JC (2004) Choroid plexus papillomas: a single institutional experience. J Neuro-Oncol 68(1):49–55

78. Lafay-Cousin L, Keene D, Carret AS, Fryer C, Brossard J, Crooks B, Eisenstat D, Johnston D, Larouche V, Silva M, Wilson B (2011) Choroid plexus tumors in children less than 36 months: the Canadian Pediatric Brain Tumor Consortium (CPBTC) experience. Childs Nerv Syst 27(2):259–264

79. McEvoy AW, Harding BN, Phipps KP, Ellison DW, Elsmore AJ, Thompson D, Harkness W, Hayward RD (2000) Management of choroid plexus tumours in children: 20 years experience at a single neurosurgical centre. Pediatr Neurosurg 32(4):192–199

80. Nagib MG, O'Fallon MT (2000) Lateral ventricle choroid plexus papilloma in childhood: management and complications. Surg Neurol 54(5):366–372

81. Fitzpatrick LK, Aronson LJ, Cohen KJ (2002) Is there a requirement for adjuvant therapy for choroid plexus carcinoma that has been completely resected? J Neuro-Oncol 57(2):123–126

82. Kumar R, Singh S (2005) Childhood choroid plexus papillomas: operative complications. Childs Nerv Syst 21(2):138–143

83. Yoshida K, Sato K, Kitai R, Hashimoto N, Kubota T, Kikuta KI (2013) Coincident choroid plexus carcinoma and adrenocortical tumor in an infant. Brain Tumor Pathol 30(2):104–108

84. Ahn SS, Cho YD (2007) Spinal drop metastasis from a posterior fossa choroid plexus papilloma. J Korean Neurosurg Soc 42(6):475

85. Daly MB, Axilbund JE, Buys S, Crawford B, Farrell CD, Friedman S, Garber JE, Goorha S, Gruber SB, Hampel H, Kaklamani V (2010) Genetic/familial high-risk assessment: breast and ovarian. J Natl Compr Cancer Netw 8(5):562–594

86. Dohrmann GJ, Collias JC (1975) Choroid plexus carcinoma: case report. J Neurosurg 43(2):225–232

87. Claire B, Philippe T, Arielle LT, Chantal K, Alain PK, Eric B (1998) Choroid plexus carcinomas in childhood: clinical features and prognostic factors. Neurosurgery 42(3):470–475

88. Sharma R, Rout D, Gupta AK, Radhakrishnan VV (1994) Choroid plexus papillomas. Br J Neurosurg 8(2):169–177

89. Pencalet P, Sainte-Rose C, Lellouch-Tubiana A, Kalifa C, Brunelle F, Sgouros S, Meyer P, Cinalli G, Zerah M, Pierre-Kahn A, Renier D (1998) Papillomas and carcinomas of the choroid plexus in children. J Neurosurg 88(3):521–528

90. Ghatak NR, McWhorter JM (1976) Ultrastructural evidence for CSF production by a choroid plexus papilloma. J Neurosurg 45(4):409–415

91. Husag L, Costabile G, Probst C (1984) Persistent hydrocephalus following removal of choroid plexus papilloma of the lateral ventricle. Neurochirurgia 27(03):82–85

92. McDonald JV (1969) Persistent hydrocephalus following the removal of papillomas of the choroid plexus of the lateral ventricles: report of two cases. J Neurosurg 30(6):736–740

93. Greenberg ML (1999) Chemotherapy of choroid plexus carcinoma. Childs Nerv Syst 15(10):571–577

94. Haliasos N, Brew S, Robertson F, Hayward R, Thompson D, Chakraborty A (2013) Pre-operative embolisation of choroid plexus tumours in children. Part II. Observations on the effects on CSF production. Childs Nerv Syst 29(1):71–76

95. Reddy D, Gunnarsson T, Scheinemann K, Provias JP, Singh SK (2011) Combined staged endoscopic and microsurgical approach of a third ventricular choroid plexus papilloma in an infant. Minim Invasive Neurosurg 54(05/06):264–267

96. Snider C, Suh JH, Murphy ES (2018) Choroid plexus tumors. In: Adult CNS radiation oncology. Springer, Cham, pp 299–306

97. Lafay-Cousin L, Mabbot DJ, Halliday W et al (2010) Use of ifosfamide, carboplatin, and etoposide chemotherapy in choroid plexus carcinoma. J Neurosurg Pediatr 5(6):615–621

98. Wolff JE, Sajedi M, Coppes MJ, Anderson RA, Egeler RM (1999) Radiation therapy and survival in choroid plexus carcinoma. Lancet 353(9170):2126

99. Davis LE (1924) A physio-pathologic study of the choroid plexus with the report of a case of villous hypertrophy. J Med Res 44(5):521

100. Ceddia A, Di CR, Carlucci A (1993) Hypersecretive congenital hydrocephalus due to choroid plexus villous hypertrophy associated with controlateral papilloma. Minerva Pediatr 45(9):363–367

101. Casey KF, Vries JK (1989) Cerebral fluid overproduction in the absence of tumor or villous hypertrophy of the choroid plexus. Childs Nerv Syst 5(5):332–334

102. Iplikcioglu AC, Bek S, Gökduman CA, Bıkmaz K, Cosar M (2006) Diffuse villous hyperplasia of choroid plexus. Acta Neurochir 148(6):691–694

103. Bucholz RD, Pittman T (1991) Endoscopic coagulation of the choroid plexus using the Nd: YAG laser: initial experience and proposal for management. Neurosurgery 28(3):421–427

104. Philips MF, Shanno G, Duhaime AC (1998) Treatment of villous hypertrophy of the choroid plexus by endoscopic contact coagulation. Pediatr Neurosurg 28(5):252–256

105. Welch K, Strand R, Bresnan M, Cavazzuti V (1983) Congenital hydrocephalus due to villous hypertrophy of the telencephalic choroid plexuses: case report. J Neurosurg 59(1):172–175

106. Wind JJ, Bell RS, Bank WO, Myseros JS (2010) Treatment of third ventricular choroid plexus papilloma in an infant with embolization alone: case report. J Neurosurg Pediatr 6(6):579–582

107. Otten ML, Riina HA, Gobin YP, Souweidane MM (2006) Preoperative embolization in the treatment of choroid plexus papilloma in an infant: case report. J Neurosurg Pediatr 104(6):419–421

108. Trivelato FP, Manzato LB, Rezende MT, Barroso PM, Faleiro RM, Ulhôa AC (2012) Preoperative embolization of choroid plexus papilloma with Onyx via the anterior choroidal artery. Childs Nerv Syst 28(11):1955–1958

109. Hoffman C, Riina HA, Stieg P, Allen B, Gobin YP, Santillan A, Souweidane M (2011) Associated aneurysms in pediatric arteriovenous malformations and the implications for treatment. Neurosurgery 69(2):315–322

110. Mazloom A, Wolff JE, Paulino AC (2010) The impact of radiotherapy fields in the treatment of patients with choroid plexus carcinoma. Int J Radiat Oncol Biol Phys 78(1):79–84

111. Chow E, Reardon DA, Shah AB, Jenkins JJ, Langston J, Heideman RL, Sanford RA, Kun LE, Merchant TE (1999) Pediatric choroid plexus neoplasms. Int J Radiat Oncol Biol Phys 44(2):249–254

112. Taylor MB, Jackson RW, Hughes DG, Wright NB (2001) Magnetic resonance imaging in the diagnosis and management of choroid plexus carcinoma in children. Pediatr Radiol 31(9):624–630

113. Safaee M, Clark AJ, Bloch O, Oh MC, Singh A, Auguste KI, Gupta N, McDermott MW, Aghi MK, Berger MS, Parsa AT (2013) Surgical outcomes in choroid plexus papillomas: an institutional experience. J Neuro-Oncol 113(1):117–125

114. Johnson DL (1989) Management of choroid plexus tumors in children. Pediatr Neurosurg 15(4):195–206

115. Wrede B, Hasselblatt M, Peters O, Thall PF, Kutluk T, Moghrabi A, Mahajan A, Rutkowski S, Diez B, Wang X, Pietsch T (2009) Atypical choroid plexus papilloma: clinical experience in the CPT-SIOP-2000 study. J Neuro-Oncol 95(3):383–392

116. Razzaq AA, Cohen AR (1997) Neoadjuvant chemotherapy for hypervascular malignant brain tumors of childhood. Pediatr Neurosurg 27(6):296–303

117. Duffner PK, Kun LE, Burger PC, Horowitz ME, Cohen ME, Sanford RA, Krischer JP, Mulhern RK, James HE, Rekate HL, Friedman HS (1995) Postoperative chemotherapy and delayed radiation in infants and very young children with choroid plexus carcinomas. Pediatr Neurosurg 22(4):189–196

118. Postovsky S, Vlodavsky E, Eran A, Guilburd J, Arush MW (2007) Secondary glioblastoma multiforme after treatment for primary choroid plexus carcinoma in childhood. J Pediatr Hematol Oncol 29(4):248–252

Atypical Teratoid Rhabdoid Tumors

33

Holly Lindsay and Annie Huang

33.1 Epidemiology

Central nervous system (**CNS**) atypical teratoid rhabdoid tumors (**ATRTs**) are World Health Organization (**WHO**) grade IV malignant embryonal tumors that almost exclusively affect children with a median age at diagnosis of 12–18 months. These tumors constitute up to 20% of CNS tumors

H. Lindsay, MD, MS
Department of Pediatrics, Division of Hematology/
Oncology, Baylor College of Medicine,
Houston, TX, USA

Texas Children's Cancer Center, Texas Children's
Hospital, Houston, TX, USA
e-mail: hblindsa@texaschildrens.org

A. Huang, MD, PhD (✉)
Arthur and Sonia Labatt Brain Tumour Research
Centre, Hospital for Sick Children,
Toronto, ON, Canada

Department of Cell Biology, Hospital for Sick
Children, Toronto, ON, Canada

Department of Laboratory Medicine and
Pathobiology, Faculty of Medicine, University of
Toronto, Toronto, ON, Canada

Department of Medical Biophysics, Faculty of
Medicine, University of Toronto,
Toronto, ON, Canada

Department of Paediatrics, University of Toronto,
Toronto, ON, Canada

Division of Hematology/Oncology, Hospital for Sick
Children, Toronto, ON, Canada
e-mail: Annie.huang@sickkids.ca

diagnosed prior to 3 years of age and are the most common malignant CNS tumor diagnosed in children younger than 12 months of age [1–6]. ATRTs historically have a dismal median survival of only 6–18 months, with the lowest survival rates seen in infants [3–10]. The mean 5-year overall survival (**OS**) rate between 2001 and 2010 for patients with ATRT was only 28% [3]. Cerebral spinal fluid metastases or other disseminated disease occur in up to 30% of patients at the time of diagnosis, worsening prognosis [5–9, 11–13].

33.2 Clinical Presentation

Similar to other CNS tumors, ATRTs present with clinical signs and symptoms reflecting the anatomic location of the primary mass. ATRTs may occur anywhere in the neuroaxis including the fourth ventricle, cerebrum, basal ganglia, pineal gland, and spine, though approximately 50% of ATRT arises from the posterior fossa. Patients with posterior fossa ATRT often present with symptoms of obstructive hydrocephalus including early morning headaches, emesis, and lethargy. Supratentorial tumors may also present with signs and symptoms of increased intracranial pressure in addition to seizures, visual changes, or hemiparesis. The clinical presentation of ATRT may also include ataxia, cranial nerve palsies, irritability, motor deficits, failure to thrive, and regression of milestones. In infants and young children with open cranial sutures, ATRT may present simply with a rapidly enlarging head circumference. Given the malignant behavior of ATRTs, symptoms typically last only days to weeks before a patient presents to clinical attention [11, 12].

33.3 Diagnostic Imaging

Imaging characteristics are relatively nonspecific in differentiating ATRT from other high-grade CNS neoplasms. CT scans classically demonstrate hyperdense masses, occasionally accompanied by fine calcifications. On MRI, ATRT is often invasive and may have areas of necrosis, hemorrhage, calcification, or cysts, leading to strong but heterogeneous uptake of gadolinium contrast (Fig. 33.1). Around half of the ATRTs demonstrate peritumoral edema. ATRT typically demonstrates hypodensity on T1 sequences and variable iso-/hypodensity on T2 images and is diffusion restricted. On MR spectroscopy, these tumors are characterized by marked elevation of choline on long echo times and lactate + lipid and choline peaks on short echo times [11, 14–16].

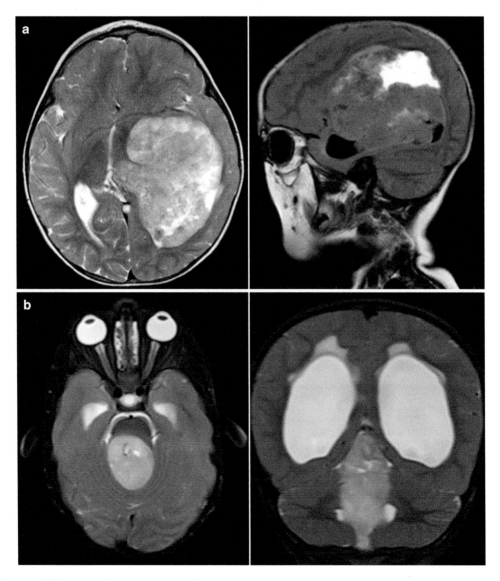

Fig. 33.1 MRI images after contrast administration showing a supratentorial (**a**) and intratentorial (**b**) location of ATRT. (**c**) MRI demonstrating large cystic area in an infratentorial ATRT. Images courtesy of Texas Children's Hospital

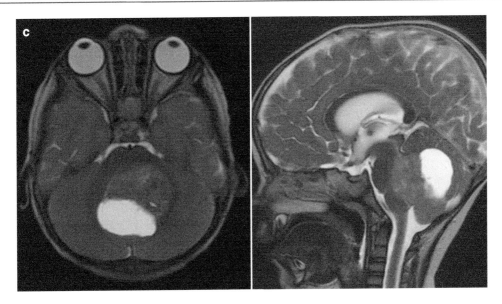

Fig. 33.1 (continued)

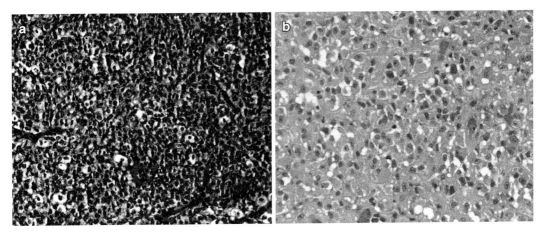

Fig. 33.2 H&E images of ATRT showing sheets of small round blue cells (**a**) and classic rhabdoid cells (**b**). Images courtesy of Dr. Cynthia Hawkins, Hospital for Sick Children

33.4 Histopathology

ATRT was pathologically defined as an independent tumor entity distinct from primitive neuroectodermal tumor and medulloblastoma in the 1980s. Macroscopically, ATRTs are classically large, fleshy tumors, often reddish gray in color. Microscopically, ATRTs may appear similar to malignant rhabdoid tumors of the kidney or soft tissues with predominantly bland small round blue cells. ATRTs characteristically have nests of sheets of rhabdoid cells, with an eccentric round

nucleus, prominent nucleolus, vesicular chromatin, eosinophilic cytoplasmic inclusion, plump cell body with abundant cytoplasm, and distinct cell borders (Fig. 33.2). These cells may be sparse in a background of more classic epithelial, neuroectodermal, or mesenchymal tumor cells. Necrosis and hemorrhage are frequently seen in ATRT but are not required for pathologic diagnosis. Rhabdoid tumor cells classically express epithelial membrane antigen, vimentin, and smooth-muscle actin as assessed by immunohistochemical (**IHC**) staining and are negative for desmin expression. Ki-67 ranges from 50 to

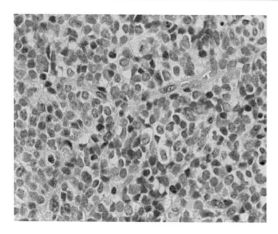

Fig. 33.3 IHC image of ATRT with negative staining for SMARCB1/INI1/BAF47. Note internal positive control of tumor vasculature. Image courtesy of Hospital for Sick Children

100% [2, 9–11, 13, 17–21]. The WHO CNS tumor classification requires loss of nuclear SMARCB1/INI1/BAF47 or SMARCA4/BRG1 expression as detected by IHC for a diagnosis of ATRT (Fig. 33.3) [9, 19, 20, 22].

33.5 SWI/SNF Biology and Genomic Features of ATRTs

SWI/SNF chromatin remodeling complexes function to dynamically regulate chromatin structure in an ATP-dependent manner and consequently play an essential role in controlling gene expression. SWI/SNF complexes are encoded by 26 genes and composed of 10–15 subunits. Each complex includes a catalytic ATP subunit (either SMARCA4 or SMARCA2) and three core subunits (SMARCB1, BAF155, and BAF170) in addition to variant subunits that depends on the cell context. These complexes utilize ATP to remodel nucleosome structure both by ejecting and inserting histone octamers and by nucleosome sliding enabling different transcription factors and other regulatory proteins to access promoter and enhancer regions to regulate gene expression. The SWI/SNF complex has been implicated in many cellular processes including control of cell identity, cell cycle,

mitotic spindle maintenance, and cell differentiation and proliferation [2, 4, 6, 8, 23–28]. It is estimated up to 20% of human cancers, including ATRTs, have a mutation in one of the SWI/SNF genes, a rate approaching that of *TP53,* the most common mutated tumor suppressor gene in human cancers [6, 24, 26–28].

SMARCB1 (SWI/SNF, a matrix-associated, actin-dependent regulator of chromatin, subfamily b, member 1) is located at chromosome 22q11.23 and is also known as *hSNF5, INI1,* and *BAF47* [1, 2, 5, 6, 8, 9, 11, 13, 19, 20, 23, 25, 28–34]. Wild-type *SMARCB1* functions as a potent tumor suppressor and controls expression of cyclin D1 to regulate cell cycle progression [23, 24, 28]. Loss of SMARCB1 via gene mutations or deletions leads to SWI/SNF complex dysfunction and unregulated cell cycle entry and consequent uncontrolled cell proliferation, to promote ATRT tumorigenesis [2, 23, 26, 27]. Mouse model studies show loss of *SMARCB1* alone can drive formation of brain tumors and soft tissue sarcomas that resemble human rhabdoid tumors, underscoring a central role for this gene in the biology of these malignancies.

The vast majority of ATRTs studied to date exhibit biallelic SMARCB1 loss-of-function alterations, while a minority (2–5%) are altered in *SMARCA4* [6, 9, 13, 20, 28, 33]. Exome sequencing studies of ATRTs have generally showed no recurrent coding mutations other than in the *SMARCB1* or *SMARCA4* genes, highlighting these as important etiologic driver genes [8, 13, 28, 30, 31]. In contrast to the coding genome, a much higher mutation rate has been reported in nonprotein-coding regions of the ATRT genome, the nature of which remains to be fully studied. Genetic mechanisms targeting *SMARCB1,* which are quite varied and predominantly structural, may include large or focal homozygous deletions, whole-arm chromosome 22 gains and losses, and complex inter- and intrachromosomal gene rearrangements [6, 8, 13, 30, 35]. About 40% of *SMARCB1* alterations in ATRTs are point mutations targeting any of the nine exons, with no evident mutational "hot spots". With the routine use of SMARCB1/INI1/BAF47 IHC in pathology diagnosis, *SMARCB1* genetic analyses have generally been only undertaken for workup of heritable disease. Due to the spectrum of genetic alterations targeting *SMARCB1*, a diagnostic workup will include SNP arrays for large deletion events or multiple ligation-mediated PCR (MLPA) analyses to pick up small deletions or exon duplication events. In the absence of structural alterations, complete sequencing of exons 1–9 is needed to rule out genetic alterations in *SMARCB1*.

33.6 Molecular Subgroups

The clinical heterogeneity seen in ATRT had until recently been difficult to explain with only recurrent *SMARCB1* alterations detected in these tumors. Early gene expression studies performed on a small cohort of 18 tumors were the first to suggest ATRTs may comprise molecular sub-types. Birks et al. reported that ATRTs segregated into four clusters based on gene expression signatures and observed that down-regulation of neuronal differentiation genes and enrichment of bone morphogenetic protein (**BMP**) signaling in two clusters correlated with significantly shorter survival [34]. Torchia et al. extended these initial observations with an integrated transcriptional and clinicopathologic analyses of a larger cohort and also identified two broad ATRT subgroups. Group 1 tumors showed enrichment of genes regulating brain and neural development and increased activation of the NOTCH developmental signaling pathway. Group 2 ATRT showed low expression of neural lineage markers but enrichment of genes involved in mesenchymal differentiation and BMP signaling. The group 1 neurogenic tumors had superior OS and a higher proportion of patients with supratentorial tumors than the group 2 mesenchymal tumors, in which the predominant tumor location was infratentorial and the tumors demonstrated a more aggressive, treatment-resistant phenotype [32]. Their follow-up study with unsupervised cluster analyses of methylation microarray data demonstrated that the heterogeneous group 2 could be subdivided into two groups: 2a and 2b

[35]. Similarly, Pascal et al. reported three molecular subgroups of ATRT in an independent DNA methylation and gene expression-based study, which they named TYR, SHH, and MYC. ATRT-TYR correlates with molecular subgroup 2a and is defined by overexpression of tyrosinase as well as other melanosomal markers and ciliogenesis genes. ATRT-SHH correlates with subgroup 1 and is characterized by overexpression of sonic hedgehog signaling pathway genes including *MYCN* and *GLI2*. ATRT-MYC, which correlates with subgroup 2b, demonstrates overexpression of *MYC* and *HOX* cluster genes [8].

Currently, there is an international consensus that ATRT is comprised of three epigenetic subgroups. These molecular subgroups exhibit subtype-specific patterns of copy number alterations and mechanisms of *SMARCB1* loss, suggesting unique mechanisms of tumor initiation and pathogenesis. Group 1 ATRT/ATRT-SHH, which arise as supratentorial tumors in toddlers at a median age of 24 months, are genomically characterized by focal/subgenic genomic alterations *SMARCB1*. Group 1 ATRT/ATRT-SHH additionally have recurrent chromosome 14 gains and chromosome 19 losses. Group 2a ATRT/ATRT-TYR most commonly occur infratentorially and are found most frequently in younger children with a median age of 12 months. This subgroup has significantly lower level of CpG island methylation than the other groups, which are characterized by hypermethylated genomes. Additionally, compared to the other two molecular subgroups, *SMARCB1* loss in group 2a ATRT/ATRT-TYR tumors is more frequently associated with large chromosome 22q deletions and chromosome 22 monosomy. Group 2b ATRT/ATRT-MYC occurs supratentorially, infratentorially, or in the spine and comprise the majority of ATRTs diagnosed in children >3 years old. This subgroup is characterized by large chromosome 22 deletions encompassing *SMARCB1* and has more focal genomic alterations and copy number losses across multiple chromosomes than the other groups. At this time no subgroup association with gender or metastatic status at presentation has been identified [8, 35].

33.7 Rhabdoid Tumor Predisposition Syndrome

Rhabdoid tumor predisposition syndrome (**RTPS**) type 1 is defined by germline mutations in *SMARCB1* and is noted in up to 10–35% of patients with ATRT. Patients with RTPS type 2 have *SMARCA4* germline mutations; the exact percentage of patients with SMARCA4-deficient ATRT with RTPS type 2 has not been well defined. Both types of RTPS are inherited in an autosomal dominant manner; the second hit in the tumor cells can be caused either by a mutation or through loss of heterozygosity in the wild-type allele [6, 19, 20, 23, 25, 32, 33].

Patients with RTPS type 1 classically present at a younger age (4–5 months vs. 13–18 months) and with more extensive disease compared to patients with rhabdoid tumors resulting from de novo *SMARCB1* genomic alterations [6, 19, 20, 25, 33]. Incomplete penetrance and gonadal mosaicism have been noted in RTPS type 1 families [25]. Patients with RPTS type 2 have a much shorter survival (3 months compared to 24 months) than patients with sporadic ATRT [33]. Patients with SMARCA4-deficient ATRT are more likely to have an underlying germline *SMARCA4* abnormality compared to the rates of germline *SMARCB1* alterations detected in patients with SMARCB1-deficient ATRT [33].

In addition to rhabdoid tumors, RTPS type 1 patients are also at increased risk of schwannomas, malignant peripheral nerve sheath tumors, and meningiomas. Patients with RTPS type 1 are recommended to have an MRI every 3 months from birth to 5 years. Whole-body MRIs should be considered up to age 5 years, though at an undetermined frequency, while abdominal ultrasounds should be repeated every 3 months up to age 5 years. These guidelines remain in evolution as adults presenting with these rare diseases are increasingly reported.

RTPS type 2 patients are at increased risk of small cell carcinoma of the ovary, hypercalcemic type, in addition to rhabdoid tumors. Patients with RTPS type 2 are not currently recommended to have brain or abdominal tumor screening due to the lower penetrance of the *SMARCA4* muta-tion for the development of rhabdoid tumors, though an every 6-month abdominal ultrasound to assess for ovarian tumors in females should be considered. Additionally, prophylactic oophorectomy should be considered postpuberty in these women [20].

33.8 Treatment Approaches and Outcomes

ATRT was historically considered a fatal disease with only recent increasing reports of survival using more intensive regimens. ATRT therapy generally involves maximal surgery followed by radiation therapy (**XRT**) and systemic conventional or high-dose chemotherapy with or without addition of intrathecal chemotherapy. The young age of most patients at diagnosis often limits the use of XRT [1, 7, 8, 32]. With exception of the recently completed Children's Oncology Group ACNS0333 study, no large prospective data for ATRT exist; consequently, therapy-related disease outcomes are based solely on registry data or small clinical trials with limited follow-up data (Table 33.1). Thus a standard, best treatment regimen for ATRT remains to be established.

To date ATRT chemotherapy has been based either on a doxorubicin- and dactinomycin-based sarcoma backbone or a cisplatin- and cyclophosphamide-containing CNS embryonal tumor regimen, with both types of regimens reporting similar, general long-term survival [4]. In a small prospective institutional trial run by the Dana-Farber Cancer Institute, 20 ATRT patients were treated postoperatively with a systemic sarcoma-based chemotherapy regimen combined with intrathecal chemotherapy and XRT. They reported a 2-year event-free survival (**EFS**) of 53 ± 13% and OS of 70 ± 10% for the 12/20 patients who successfully completed therapy. Patients who had undergone a gross total resection demonstrated a significantly higher 2-year OS of 91 ± 9%. Patient status beyond 2 years has not yet been reported [7]. The European rhabdoid tumor registry (**EU-RHAB**) registry-based Rhabdoid 2007 study, which also employed a

Table 33.1 Overview of selected ATRT clinical trials

Treatment protocol	ACNS0333 (Children's Oncology Group)	CCG-9921 (Children's Cancer Group) [37]	Dana-Farber Cancer Institute regimen [7]	Head start III [42]	Korean experience [46]	Medical University of Vienna regimen [43]
Accrual years	2008–2013	1993–1997	2004–2006	2003–2009	2005–2010	1992–2012
Patient numbers	Pending	28	25 (20 evaluable)	19	9	9
Standard-dose chemotherapy	2 cycles of induction: Cisplatin, cyclophosphamide, etoposide, 8 g/m² methotrexate, vincristine	5 cycles of induction: Regimen A: cisplatin, cyclophosphamide, etoposide, vincristine Regimen B: carboplatin, etoposide, ifosfamide, vincristine 8 cycles of maintenance: carboplatin, cyclophosphamide, etoposide, vincristine	5 phases of treatment: Cisplatin, cyclophosphamide, dactinomycin, doxorubicin, temozolomide, vincristine	5 cycles of induction: Cisplatin, cyclophosphamide, etoposide, 270–400 mg/kg methotrexate, temozolomide, vincristine	6 cycles of induction: Carboplatin, cisplatin, cyclophosphamide, etoposide, ifosfamide	3 cycles: Cisplatin, cyclophosphamide, doxorubicin, etoposide, 5 g/m² methotrexate, ifosfamide, vincristine
High-dose chemotherapy with autologous stem cell rescue	3 cycles of consolidation: carboplatin, thiotepa	No	No	1 cycle: carboplatin, etoposide, thiotepa	2 cycles: (1) carboplatin, etoposide, thiotepa; (2) cyclophosphamide, melphalan	1 cycle: carboplatin, etoposide, thiotepa
Radiation therapy	Focal for M0 disease, age-adjusted craniospinal recommended for M+ disease	Only if metastatic at diagnosis or residual tumor after induction	Focal if M0, craniospinal if M+ once ≥3 years old	Only if 6–10 years old or residual tumor after induction	Yes	Focal
Intrathecal chemotherapy	No	No	Yes: Ara-C/ hydrocortisone/ methotrexate	No	No	Yes: varying combinations of cytarabine, etoposide, mafosfamide, methotrexate
Survival data	Pending	5-year EFS: 14 ± 7% 5-year OS: 29 ± 9%	2-year EFS: 53 ± 13% 2-year OS: 70 ± 10%	3-year EFS: 21 ± 9% 3-year OS: 26 ± 10%	3-year EFS: 0% 3-year OS: 53.3 ± 17.3%	5-year EFS: 88.9 ± 10.5% 5-year OS: 100%

sarcoma chemotherapy backbone combined with XRT and intraventricular chemotherapy, reported a 6-year EFS of 45 ± 9% and OS of 46 ± 10% for 31 patients [36].

In early studies, ATRT patients were treated with conventional-dose embryonal-type therapy. The prospective Children's Cancer Group 9921 study, which aimed to defer XRT for children younger than 3 years of age with all malignant brain tumor diagnoses, treated children with completely resected, nonmetastatic disease with conventional-dose chemotherapy. In contrast, patients with residual or metastatic tumor had XRT delayed until they turned 3 years old or completed eight cycles of maintenance chemotherapy. The 5-year EFS for 28 ATRT patients enrolled on this study was only 14 ± 7%, while the OS rate was 29 ± 9% [4, 37]. Similar outcomes were noted in the Pediatric Oncology group study 9933/34, which also evaluated the role of chemotherapy to delay XRT in children younger than 3 years old at diagnosis [38]. St. Jude Children's Research Hospital reported 2-year EFS and OS rates for children diagnosed at 3 years and older of 78 ± 14% and 89 ± 11% after treatment with postsurgical craniospinal XRT and alkylator-based chemotherapy. However survival of children <3 years old treated heterogeneously, though mostly without XRT, was much poorer, with 2-year EFS and OS rates of 11 ± 6% and 17 ± 8% [2].

The dismal outcome of embryonal brain tumors, including ATRT, with conventional chemotherapy led to the development of the Children's Cancer Group study 99703. This treatment regimen demonstrated the safety of utilizing three cycles of high-dose chemotherapy following conventional chemotherapy [39]. Reports of outcome on 42 patients from an early ATRT patient registry suggested extent of surgery and high-dose chemotherapy were positive prognosticators [40]. The Head Start studies utilized high-dose chemotherapy and demonstrated that long-term survival was possible for patients with ATRT without the need for XRT [41, 42]. A Canadian national registry study compared outcomes for 40/50 ATRT patients treated variably over a 12-year period with conventional chemotherapy, high-dose chemotherapy,

and intrathecal chemotherapy, with or without XRT, and also observed short median progression time of 5.5 months and 2-year OS of 36.4 ± 7.7% for all patients. However, they also observed better patient outcomes with complete surgery (2-year OS 60% ± 12.6 vs. 21.7% ± 8.5, $p = 0.03$) or high-dose chemotherapy (2-year OS 47.9% ± 12.1 vs. 27.3% ± 9.5, $p = 0.036$) and noted that 50% of long-term survivors received only high-dose chemotherapy without XRT [12]. The Medical University of Vienna reported on nine patients treated on the MUV-ATRT protocol with a highly intensive regimen comprised of conventional sarcoma-type regimen with intrathecal chemotherapy followed by high-dose chemotherapy and focal XRT in all patients. This group reported a 5-year EFS of 88.9 ± 10.5% and an OS rate of 100% [43].

Preliminary reports of the largest prospective single-arm upfront ATRT trial from the Children's Oncology group which enrolled 65 patients suggest promising results with a 99703-based high-dose chemotherapy regimen combined with focal XRT. In this study, it preliminarily appears that the sequence of XRT does not impact patient outcomes [4].

33.9   Clinical Prognostic Factors

Identification of reliable treatment and patient-related prognostic factors in ATRTs is challenged by the rare nature of this disease, as much of the clinical data collected has spanned decades of improvement in surgical and imaging methods as well as the adoption of high-dose and intrathecal chemotherapy for brain tumors. Evaluation of prognostic factors is also challenged by heterogeneous therapeutic combination used across studies and bias toward less aggressive or palliative approaches in younger patients or those with more extensive disease. Patient age, tumor location, and the tumor bed volume have also significantly influenced the timing and use of focal or craniospinal XRT. Consequently, the prognostic impact of patient age, metastatic status, extent of surgery, high-dose chemotherapy, intrathecal chemotherapy, and XRT reported to date must be interpreted with these limitations in mind.

33.9.1 Age at Diagnosis and Presence of Metastases

A National Cancer Database analysis of retrospective data on over 350 ATRT patients treated diversely indicated better 5-year OS of 37.5% for children ≥3 years old as compared to 27.5% ($p < 0.001$) for <3 years old at diagnosis. Children with localized disease had a 5-year OS of 33.5%, compared to 19.5% for those with metastatic disease ($p = 0.03$). Univariate analysis of gender, race, tumor location, or tumor size at presentation was not significant; however multivariate analysis suggested patients ≥3 years old had improved survival irrespective of metastatic disease or use of XRT as compared to patients ≤2 years old at presentation [10]. Similarly, a study from the National Cancer Institute's Surveillance, Epidemiology, and End Results (**NCI SEERS**) database, which analyzed data from >140 ATRT patients, reported median OS of 3 and 13 months, respectively, in patients with localized and metastatic disease ($p = 0.0001$) [5].

33.9.2 Extent of Surgery and XRT

Although gross total tumor resection is the standard surgical recommendation for ATRT, the prognostic impact of surgical extent has not been consistently demonstrated. Several studies reported extent of surgery was not prognostic of EFS and/or OS [2, 5, 44]. In contrast, however, a meta-analysis found that complete surgical tumor removal correlated with a longer mean OS of 21.3 months compared to 12.3 months in patients who had undergone only partial tumor resection [21].

The use of XRT in ATRT is highly contentious due to the very young patient population. The clinical benefits of XRT have been reported in various individual and combined retrospective analyses including the NCI SEERS database study [5]. In addition, a meta-analysis indicated that addition of XRT to conventional chemotherapy prolonged OS for ATRT ($p = 0.097$) [21]. A pooled data review of 332 ATRT patients also showed an improved EFS and OS for patients who had XRT compared to those treated with chemotherapy alone [44]. In the St. Jude Children's Research Hospital experience of ATRT treatment in children ≥3 years, the 2-year OS rate was 12 ± 7% in patients treated postoperatively only with chemotherapy compared to 90 ± 10% in those who received both XRT and chemotherapy [2]. Further data from this group suggest delay of XRT was associated with higher rates of both local and metastatic disease recurrence [45]. However, a population of long-term survivors of ATRT treated without XRT has also been increasingly reported [12, 40–44, 46–48]. Consequently, the impact of high-dose chemotherapy and tumor biology on need for XRT remains to be clarified. As focal XRT has generally been applied to children <3 years old as compared to children ≥3 years old, who typically receive craniospinal XRT, these data must be interpreted with respect to the average age of patients treated. Due to differences in the use and specifics of XRT in published studies and clinical trials, the ideal timing, field, and dose of XRT for infants and children with ATRT remain unclear.

In addition to the well-documented neurocognitive morbidities associated with administering XRT to infants and young children, the radiation oncology group at MD Anderson Cancer Center highlighted another XRT-related side effect [1, 8, 32, 49]. Of 31 patients with ATRT who received proton beam XRT, 5 patients (16%) developed clinical findings and brainstem imaging changes within 4 months post XRT consistent with brainstem necrosis. 4 of these patients received only local XRT without any planned XRT to the brainstem, while the fifth patient received craniospinal XRT [49]. Whether these proton XRT-related effects are influenced by type of chemotherapy given remains unknown.

33.9.3 High-Dose and Intrathecal Chemotherapy

High-dose chemotherapy followed by autologous stem cell rescue has been increasingly used to avoid or delay XRT in ATRT patients [41–44, 46–48]. A Canadian ATRT registry report indicated superior survival for patients treated with high-dose chemotherapy vs. conventional chemotherapy, with a 2-year OS rate of 47.9 ± 12.1% vs. 27.3 ± 9.5 ($p = 0.036$), respectively [12]. This finding has also been reported in a pooled analysis of 332 ATRT patients [44]. However, preliminary results from the prospective ACN0333 study which indicate improved survival for ATRT patients compared to historical conventional-dose regimens also suggest high-dose chemotherapy alone may not benefit all ATRT patients and highlight the impact of specific tumor biology on therapeutic response.

Various single- and multi-agent intrathecal chemotherapies have been utilized in attempts to delay or spare XRT in ATRT patients. An ATRT patient pooled data review demonstrated a statistically significant benefit in OS for patients treated with intrathecal chemotherapy [44]. Additionally, a meta-analysis of ATRT treatment studies showed patients who received intrathecal chemotherapy as a component of treatment had significantly higher OS rates compared to those who did not receive this treatment modality (64% vs. 17.3%, $p < 0.0001$) [21]. However, given the great diversity of overall treatment regimens as well as specific intrathecal chemotherapies utilized, the benefit of intrathecal therapy can also not be clearly determined.

33.10 Preclinical Models

Several ATRT cell lines have been generated and utilized in the published literature for *in vitro* drug testing, molecular pathway analyses, and implantation into animals to generate xenograft models [50–52]. Homozygous deletion of *SMARCB1* in mice results in early embryonal lethality, while heterozygous gene loss predisposes mice to develop sarcomas and rhabdoid tumors, including in intracranial locations [53–56]. A genetically engineered mouse model of ATRT has been generated by ablating *SMARCB1* from GFAP-positive progenitor cells in the developing CNS of mice with background p53 loss. Tumors histopathologically resembling ATRT formed in the murine cerebellum and demon-

strated leptomeningeal dissemination [54]. Another genetically engineered ATRT mouse model was created in Rosa-Cre mice by inactivating both copies of *SMARCB1* between E6 and E10; resultant tumors were histopathologically and biologically similar to human ATRT [57]. An ATRT mouse model has also been generated through conditional inactivation of *SMARCB1* in neural crest cells on E9.5 [58]. Numerous groups continue to generate ATRT cell lines, animal models, and three-dimensional organoids in order to further biological understanding of this tumor and perform preclinical evaluations of new compounds and novel therapeutic combinations.

33.11 Targeted Therapies for ATRTs

Despite highly intensive therapy, survival remains poor for the majority of ATRT patients, underscoring the need for more specific agents targeted to tumor biology. High-throughput *in vitro* drug screens and biological studies have identified a number of kinases as well as developmental and epigenetic signaling pathways as attractive therapeutic targets for ATRTs.

33.11.1 Kinases

Aurora Kinase A is a serine/threonine protein kinase involved in the regulation of mitosis. Overexpression of Aurora Kinase A can induce oncogenesis in experimental models and has been noted in various tumor pathologies including ATRT [4, 6, 59–61]. Preclinical *in vitro* studies showed that inhibition of Aurora Kinase A induced ATRT cell death via induction of apoptosis and also sensitized the cells to XRT [60]. Based on observations of significant disease regression in two recurrent ATRT patients, St. Jude Children's Research Hospital has commenced an active treatment protocol for patients with either newly diagnosed or recurrent ATRT utilizing the Aurora Kinase A inhibitor Alisertib [61, 62].

Both single-agent preclinical studies and recent high-throughput drug screens by Chauvin et al.

demonstrate that rhabdoid tumor cells are broadly sensitive to inhibition of tyrosine kinases. Chauvin and colleagues showed that the broad tyrosine kinase inhibitor pazopanib reduces growth of rhabdoid tumor cells and xenografts [63]. Sorafenib and sunitinib, two tyrosine kinase inhibitors in clinical use, have been shown to inhibit ATRT cell growth in a dose-dependent manner [64]. The Pediatric Oncology Experimental Therapeutics Investigators' Consortium group performed drug screening on three ATRT cell lines. Lapatinib, a HER2 and EGFR dual tyrosine kinase inhibitor, demonstrated *in vitro* cytotoxicity against the ATRT cell lines at low IC_{50}s. *In vivo* testing in ATRT xenografts demonstrated inhibition of tumor growth in the lapatinib-treated animals [65]. Treatment of rhabdoid tumor cell lines with imatinib, a tyrosine kinase inhibitor against c-ABL, c-Kit, and platelet-derived growth factor, reduced cell proliferation [66]. Vatalanib, a broad-spectrum tyrosine kinase inhibitor, reduced the growth of ATRT cell lines grow both in traditional monolayer cell culture and as spheroids [67]. Interestingly Torchia et al. showed that the specific sensitivity of group 2 ATRT cells to multi-tyrosine kinase inhibitors dasatinib and nilotinib was associated with differential epigenetic regulation and expression of PDGFRB in group 2 but not group 1 ATRT cells, thus underscoring the need and potential to tailor targeted agents to ATRT sub-type-specific biology in future trials [35].

33.11.2 Epigenetic Inhibitors

EZH2 is the catalytic subunit of Polycomb Repressive Complex 2 (**PRC2**), a protein complex which catalyzes trimethylation of histone 3 at lysine 27 (**H3K27me3**) and antagonizes normal SWI/SNF function in chromatin remodeling. Loss of SMARCB1 in ATRT leads to increased intra-tumoral expression of EZH2 and consequent tumorigenesis due to epigenetic dysregulation and uncontrolled cell cycle entry [23, 24, 26–28, 68–72]. EZH2 is important for neovascularization, oncogenesis, and cancer stem cell self-renewal. Silencing of EZH2 is known to inhibit cancer cell invasion and migration [6, 28, 70,

72–75]. Various chemical EZH2 inhibitors have shown preclinical efficacy in animal models of extracranial malignant rhabdoid tumors and in *in vitro* ATRT model systems [6, 68, 75, 76]. Tazemetostat, a pharmacologically active EZH2 inhibitor, is currently being evaluated as a single agent for the treatment of recurrent ATRT through both an industry-sponsored study and as a component of the National Cancer Institute-/Children's Oncology Group-sponsored Pediatric MATCH trial [62]. In addition to EZH2, preclinical studies suggest inhibitors of histone methyl transferases and bromodomain proteins are also attractive targets in ATRTs [35].

33.11.3 Cell Cycle Regulators

Loss of SMARCB1 leads to upregulation of Cyclin D1 and other related cell cycle pathway genes. Cyclin D1 inhibitors have demonstrated *in vitro* and *in vivo* preclinical activity against ATRT, suggesting cell cycle regulators as potential clinically relevant target for ATRTs [4, 6, 23, 77]. Preclinical data with the CDK4/6 inhibitor palbociclib demonstrated prolongation of ATRT xenograft survival when administered in combination or after the administration of XRT [78]. Palbociclib and other CDK4/6 inhibitors are currently under consideration for testing in a prospective Children's Oncology Group ATRT trial.

33.11.4 Lineage/Developmental Signaling Pathways

Cell line and human tumor studies suggest that oncogenic lineage-associated pathways may represent attractive ATRT targets. Specifically, Torchia et al. showed lineage-specific differences and responses of cell lines derived from different ATRT molecular sub-types to inhibition of NOTCH and BMP signaling [35]. SMARCB1 loss also leads to activation of the Hedgehog signaling pathway and increased GLI1 expression, which has also been demonstrated to be enriched in group 1/SHH ATRTs [6, 79, 80]. Indeed, suppression of GLI1 with arsenic trioxide has been shown to inhibit ATRT cell line and xenograft growth [80]. SMARCB1 and SMARCA4 are also known to regulate WNT/β-Catenin pathway targets suggesting these as additional potential therapeutic targets [6, 81, 82].

Additional proposed molecular targets for ATRT include insulin-like growth factor, FGF signaling, potassium channels, histone deacetylases, and polo-like kinase 1 [4, 6, 52, 64, 65, 83, 84]. Given the molecular heterogeneity ATRT and the demonstrated sub-type specific therapeutic vulnerabilities of this tumor, consideration of ATRT molecular sub-types will be important for all future therapeutic evaluations.

33.12 Summary/Future Prospects

ATRT remains a disease with poor survival outcomes despite aggressive treatment strategies of surgery, chemotherapy, and XRT. However, recent advances in the understanding of ATRT molecular pathophysiology as well as awareness of inter-tumoral epigenetic differences may allow risk-stratified and targeted, subgroup-specific treatment in the near future. Upcoming clinical trials will need to further establish phenotypic differences between molecular subgroups and refine our understanding of targetable biologic alterations in ATRT. Furthermore, the development of new preclinical subgroup-specific models will be important to validate the tumorigenic roles of these molecular targets and guide future clinical investigations.

References

1. De Amorim Bernstein K et al (2013) Early clinical outcomes using proton radiation for children with central nervous system atypical teratoid rhabdoid tumors. Int J Radiat Oncol Biol Phys 86:114–120. https://doi.org/10.1016/j.ijrobp.2012.12.004
2. Tekautz TM et al (2005) Atypical teratoid/rhabdoid tumors (ATRT): improved survival in children 3 years of age and older with radiation therapy and high-dose alkylator-based chemotherapy. J Clin Oncol 23:1491–1499. https://doi.org/10.1200/JCO.2005.05.187
3. Ostrom QT et al (2014) The descriptive epidemiology of atypical teratoid/rhabdoid tumors in the United States, 2001-2010. Neuro Oncol 16:1392–1399. https://doi.org/10.1093/neuonc/nou090
4. Ginn KF, Gajjar A (2012) Atypical teratoid rhabdoid tumor: current therapy and future directions. Front Oncol 2:114. https://doi.org/10.3389/fonc.2012.00114
5. Buscariollo DL, Park HS, Roberts KB, Yu JB (2012) Survival outcomes in atypical teratoid rhabdoid tumor for patients undergoing radiotherapy in a surveillance, epidemiology, and end results analysis. Cancer 118:4212–4219. https://doi.org/10.1002/cncr.27373
6. Fruhwald MC, Biegel JA, Bourdeaut F, Roberts CW, Chi SN (2016) Atypical teratoid/rhabdoid tumors-current concepts, advances in biology, and potential future therapies. Neuro Oncol 18:764–778. https://doi.org/10.1093/neuonc/nov264
7. Chi SN et al (2009) Intensive multimodality treatment for children with newly diagnosed CNS atypical teratoid rhabdoid tumor. J Clin Oncol 27:385–389. https://doi.org/10.1200/JCO.2008.18.7724
8. Johann PD et al (2016) Atypical teratoid/rhabdoid tumors are comprised of three epigenetic subgroups with distinct enhancer landscapes. Cancer Cell 29:379–393. https://doi.org/10.1016/j.ccell.2016.02.001
9. Dufour C et al (2012) Clinicopathologic prognostic factors in childhood atypical teratoid and rhabdoid tumor of the central nervous system: a multicenter study. Cancer 118:3812–3821. https://doi.org/10.1002/cncr.26684
10. Fischer-Valuck BW et al (2017) Assessment of the treatment approach and survival outcomes in a modern cohort of patients with atypical teratoid rhabdoid tumors using the National Cancer Database. Cancer 123:682–687. https://doi.org/10.1002/cncr.30405
11. Reddy AT (2005) Atypical teratoid/rhabdoid tumors of the central nervous system. J Neurooncol 75:309–313. https://doi.org/10.1007/s11060-005-6762-8
12. Lafay-Cousin L et al (2012) Central nervous system atypical teratoid rhabdoid tumours: the Canadian Paediatric Brain Tumour Consortium experience. Eur J Cancer 48:353–359. https://doi.org/10.1016/j.ejca.2011.09.005
13. Fuller CE (2016) All things rhabdoid and SMARC: an enigmatic exploration with Dr Louis P. Dehner. Semin Diagn Pathol 33:427–440. https://doi.org/10.1053/j.semdp.2016.08.003
14. Bruggers CS, Moore K (2014) Magnetic resonance imaging spectroscopy in pediatric atypical teratoid rhabdoid tumors of the brain. J Pediatr Hematol Oncol 36:e341–e345. https://doi.org/10.1097/MPH.0000000000000041
15. Nowak J et al (2018) Magnetic resonance imaging surrogates of molecular subgroups in atypical teratoid/rhabdoid tumor (ATRT). Neuro Oncol 20:1672–1679. https://doi.org/10.1093/neuonc/noy111
16. Warmuth-Metz M et al (2008) CT and MR imaging in atypical teratoid/rhabdoid tumors of the central nervous system. Neuroradiology 50:447–452. https://doi.org/10.1007/s00234-008-0369-7

17. Rorke LB, Packer RJ, Biegel JA (1996) Central nervous system atypical teratoid/rhabdoid tumors of infancy and childhood: definition of an entity. J Neurosurg 85:56–65. https://doi.org/10.3171/jns.1996.85.1.0056

18. Rorke LB, Packer R, Biegel J (1995) Central nervous system atypical teratoid/rhabdoid tumors of infancy and childhood. J Neurooncol 24:21–28

19. Bruggers CS et al (2011) Clinicopathologic comparison of familial versus sporadic atypical teratoid/rhabdoid tumors (AT/RT) of the central nervous system. Pediatr Blood Cancer 56:1026–1031. https://doi.org/10.1002/pbc.22757

20. Foulkes WD et al (2017) Cancer surveillance in Gorlin syndrome and rhabdoid tumor predisposition syndrome. Clin Cancer Res 23:e62–e67. https://doi.org/10.1158/1078-0432.CCR-17-0595

21. Athale UH, Duckworth J, Odame I, Barr R (2009) Childhood atypical teratoid rhabdoid tumor of the central nervous system: a meta-analysis of observational studies. J Pediatr Hematol Oncol 31:651–663. https://doi.org/10.1097/MPH.0b013e3181b258a9

22. Louis DN et al (2016) The 2016 World Health Organization classification of tumors of the central nervous system: a summary. Acta Neuropathol 131:803–820. https://doi.org/10.1007/s00401-016-1545-1

23. Wilson BG, Roberts CW (2011) SWI/SNF nucleosome remodellers and cancer. Nat Rev Cancer 11:481–492. https://doi.org/10.1038/nrc3068

24. Wang X, Haswell JR, Roberts CW (2014) Molecular pathways: SWI/SNF (BAF) complexes are frequently mutated in cancer—mechanisms and potential therapeutic insights. Clin Cancer Res 20:21–27. https://doi.org/10.1158/1078-0432.CCR-13-0280

25. Eaton KW, Tooke LS, Wainwright LM, Judkins AR, Biegel JA (2011) Spectrum of SMARCB1/INI1 mutations in familial and sporadic rhabdoid tumors. Pediatr Blood Cancer 56:7–15. https://doi.org/10.1002/pbc.22831

26. Shain AH, Pollack JR (2013) The spectrum of SWI/SNF mutations, ubiquitous in human cancers. PLoS One 8:e55119. https://doi.org/10.1371/journal.pone.0055119

27. Kadoch C et al (2013) Proteomic and bioinformatic analysis of mammalian SWI/SNF complexes identifies extensive roles in human malignancy. Nat Genet 45:592–601. https://doi.org/10.1038/ng.2628

28. Kim KH, Roberts CW (2014) Mechanisms by which SMARCB1 loss drives rhabdoid tumor growth. Cancer Genet 207:365–372. https://doi.org/10.1016/j.cancergen.2014.04.004

29. Woehrer A et al (2010) Incidence of atypical teratoid/rhabdoid tumors in children: a population-based study by the Austrian Brain Tumor Registry, 1996–2006. Cancer 116:5725–5732. https://doi.org/10.1002/cncr.25540

30. Hasselblatt M et al (2013) High-resolution genomic analysis suggests the absence of recurrent genomic alterations other than SMARCB1 aberrations in atypical teratoid/rhabdoid tumors. Genes Chromosomes Cancer 52:185–190. https://doi.org/10.1002/gcc.22018

31. Lee RS et al (2012) A remarkably simple genome underlies highly malignant pediatric rhabdoid cancers. J Clin Invest 122:2983–2988. https://doi.org/10.1172/JCI64400

32. Torchia J et al (2015) Molecular subgroups of atypical teratoid rhabdoid tumours in children: an integrated genomic and clinicopathological analysis. Lancet Oncol 16:569–582. https://doi.org/10.1016/S1470-2045(15)70114-2

33. Hasselblatt M et al (2014) SMARCA4-mutated atypical teratoid/rhabdoid tumors are associated with inherited germline alterations and poor prognosis. Acta Neuropathol 128:453–456. https://doi.org/10.1007/s00401-014-1323-x

34. Birks DK et al (2011) High expression of BMP pathway genes distinguishes a subset of atypical teratoid/rhabdoid tumors associated with shorter survival. Neuro Oncol 13:1296–1307. https://doi.org/10.1093/neuonc/nor140

35. Torchia J et al (2016) Integrated (epi)-genomic analyses identify subgroup-specific therapeutic targets in CNS Rhabdoid Tumors. Cancer Cell 30:891–908. https://doi.org/10.1016/j.ccell.2016.11.003

36. Bartelheim K et al (2016) Improved 6-year overall survival in AT/RT—results of the registry study Rhabdoid 2007. Cancer Med 5:1765–1775. https://doi.org/10.1002/cam4.741

37. Geyer JR et al (2005) Multiagent chemotherapy and deferred radiotherapy in infants with malignant brain tumors: a report from the Children's Cancer Group. J Clin Oncol 23:7621–7631. https://doi.org/10.1200/JCO.2005.09.095

38. Strother DR et al (2014) Benefit from prolonged dose-intensive chemotherapy for infants with malignant brain tumors is restricted to patients with ependymoma: a report of the Pediatric Oncology Group randomized controlled trial 9233/34. Neuro Oncol 16:457–465. https://doi.org/10.1093/neuonc/not163

39. Cohen BH et al (2015) Pilot study of intensive chemotherapy with peripheral hematopoietic cell support for children less than 3 years of age with malignant brain Tumors, the CCG-99703 phase I/II study. A report from the Children's Oncology Group. Pediatr Neurol 53:31–46. https://doi.org/10.1016/j.pediatrneurol.2015.03.019

40. Hilden JM et al (2004) Central nervous system atypical teratoid/rhabdoid tumor: results of therapy in children enrolled in a registry. J Clin Oncol 22:2877–2884. https://doi.org/10.1200/JCO.2004.07.073

41. Gardner SL et al (2008) Intensive induction chemotherapy followed by high dose chemotherapy with autologous hematopoietic progenitor cell rescue in young children newly diagnosed with central nervous system atypical teratoid rhabdoid tumors. Pediatr Blood Cancer 51:235–240. https://doi.org/10.1002/pbc.21578

42. Zaky W et al (2014) Intensive induction chemotherapy followed by myeloablative chemotherapy with

autologous hematopoietic progenitor cell rescue for young children newly-diagnosed with central nervous system atypical teratoid/rhabdoid tumors: the head start III experience. Pediatr Blood Cancer 61:95–101. https://doi.org/10.1002/pbc.24648

43. Slavc I et al (2014) Atypical teratoid rhabdoid tumor: improved long-term survival with an intensive multi-modal therapy and delayed radiotherapy. The Medical University of Vienna experience 1992–2012. Cancer Med 3:91–100. https://doi.org/10.1002/cam4.161

44. Schrey D et al (2016) Multimodal therapy in children and adolescents with newly diagnosed atypical teratoid rhabdoid tumor: individual pooled data analysis and review of the literature. J Neurooncol 126:81–90. https://doi.org/10.1007/s11060-015-1904-0

45. Pai Panandiker AS et al (2012) Sequencing of local therapy affects the pattern of treatment failure and survival in children with atypical teratoid rhabdoid tumors of the central nervous system. Int J Radiat Oncol Biol Phys 82:1756–1763. https://doi.org/10.1016/j.ijrobp.2011.02.059

46. Park ES et al (2012) Tandem high-dose chemotherapy and autologous stem cell transplantation in young children with atypical teratoid/rhabdoid tumor of the central nervous system. J Korean Med Sci 27:135–140. https://doi.org/10.3346/jkms.2012.27.2.135

47. Nicolaides T et al (2010) High-dose chemotherapy and autologous stem cell rescue for atypical teratoid/rhabdoid tumor of the central nervous system. J Neurooncol 98:117–123. https://doi.org/10.1007/s11060-009-0071-6

48. Finkelstein-Shechter T et al (2010) Atypical teratoid or rhabdoid tumors: improved outcome with high-dose chemotherapy. J Pediatr Hematol Oncol 32:e182–e186. https://doi.org/10.1097/MPH.0b013e3181dce1a2

49. McGovern SL et al (2014) Outcomes and acute toxicities of proton therapy for pediatric atypical teratoid/rhabdoid tumor of the central nervous system. Int J Radiat Oncol Biol Phys 90:1143–1152. https://doi.org/10.1016/j.ijrobp.2014.08.354

50. Xu J, Margol A, Asgharzadeh S, Erdreich-Epstein A (2015) Pediatric brain tumor cell lines. J Cell Biochem 116:218–224. https://doi.org/10.1002/jcb.24976

51. Hashizume R et al (2010) Morphologic and molecular characterization of ATRT xenografts adapted for orthotopic therapeutic testing. Neuro Oncol 12:366–376. https://doi.org/10.1093/neuonc/nop033

52. Narendran A et al (2008) Establishment of atypical-teratoid/rhabdoid tumor (AT/RT) cell cultures from disseminated CSF cells: a model to elucidate biology and potential targeted therapeutics. J Neurooncol 90:171–180. https://doi.org/10.1007/s11060-008-9653-y

53. Guidi CJ et al (2001) Disruption of Ini1 leads to peri-implantation lethality and tumorigenesis in mice. Mol Cell Biol 21:3598–3603. https://doi.org/10.1128/MCB.21.10.3598-3603.2001

54. Ng JM et al (2015) Generation of a mouse model of atypical teratoid/rhabdoid tumor of the central

nervous system through combined deletion of Snf5 and p53. Cancer Res 75:4629–4639. https://doi.org/10.1158/0008-5472.CAN-15-0874

55. Roberts CW, Galusha SA, McMenamin ME, Fletcher CD, Orkin SH (2000) Haploinsufficiency of Snf5 (integrase interactor 1) predisposes to malignant rhabdoid tumors in mice. Proc Natl Acad Sci U S A 97:13796–13800. https://doi.org/10.1073/pnas.250492697

56. Klochendler-Yeivin A et al (2000) The murine SNF5/INI1 chromatin remodeling factor is essential for embryonic development and tumor suppression. EMBO Rep 1:500–506. https://doi.org/10.1093/embo-reports/kvd129

57. Han ZY et al (2016) The occurrence of intracranial rhabdoid tumours in mice depends on temporal control of Smarcb1 inactivation. Nat Commun 7:10421. https://doi.org/10.1038/ncomms10421

58. Vitte J, Gao F, Coppola G, Judkins AR, Giovannini M (2017) Timing of Smarcb1 and Nf2 inactivation determines schwannoma versus rhabdoid tumor development. Nat Commun 8:300. https://doi.org/10.1038/s41467-017-00346-5

59. Katayama H, Brinkley WR, Sen S (2003) The Aurora kinases: role in cell transformation and tumorigenesis. Cancer Metastasis Rev 22:451–464

60. Venkataraman S et al (2012) Targeting Aurora kinase A enhances radiation sensitivity of atypical teratoid rhabdoid tumor cells. J Neurooncol 107:517–526. https://doi.org/10.1007/s11060-011-0795-y

61. Wetmore C et al (2015) Alisertib is active as single agent in recurrent atypical teratoid rhabdoid tumors in 4 children. Neuro Oncol 17:882–888. https://doi.org/10.1093/neuonc/nov017

62. www.clinicaltrials.gov.

63. Chauvin C et al (2017) High-throughput drug screening identifies pazopanib and clofilium tosylate as promising treatments for malignant rhabdoid tumors. Cell Rep 21:1737–1745. https://doi.org/10.1016/j.celrep.2017.10.076

64. Jayanthan A, Bernoux D, Bose P, Riabowol K, Narendran A (2011) Multi-tyrosine kinase inhibitors in preclinical studies for pediatric CNS AT/RT: evidence for synergy with topoisomerase-I inhibition. Cancer Cell Int 11:44. https://doi.org/10.1186/1475-2867-11-44

65. Singh A et al (2013) Profiling pathway-specific novel therapeutics in preclinical assessment for central nervous system atypical teratoid rhabdoid tumors (CNS ATRT): favorable activity of targeting EGFR-ErbB2 signaling with lapatinib. Mol Oncol 7:497–512. https://doi.org/10.1016/j.molonc.2013.01.001

66. Koos B et al (2010) The tyrosine kinase c-Abl promotes proliferation and is expressed in atypical teratoid and malignant rhabdoid tumors. Cancer 116:5075–5081. https://doi.org/10.1002/cncr.25420

67. Messerli SM, Hoffman MM, Gnimpieba EZ, Bhardwaj RD (2017) Therapeutic targeting of PTK7 is cytotoxic in atypical teratoid rhabdoid tumors. Mol Cancer Res 15:973–983. https://doi.org/10.1158/1541-7786.MCR-16-0432

68. Alimova I et al (2013) Inhibition of EZH2 suppresses self-renewal and induces radiation sensitivity in atypical rhabdoid teratoid tumor cells. Neuro Oncol 15:149–160. https://doi.org/10.1093/neuonc/nos285

69. Venneti S et al (2011) Malignant rhabdoid tumors express stem cell factors, which relate to the expression of EZH2 and Id proteins. Am J Surg Pathol 35:1463–1472. https://doi.org/10.1097/PAS.0b013e318224d2cd

70. Wilson BG et al (2010) Epigenetic antagonism between polycomb and SWI/SNF complexes during oncogenic transformation. Cancer Cell 18:316–328. https://doi.org/10.1016/j.ccr.2010.09.006

71. Ezponda T, Licht JD (2014) Molecular pathways: deregulation of histone H3 lysine 27 methylation in cancer-different paths, same destination. Clin Cancer Res 20:5001–5008. https://doi.org/10.1158/1078-0432.CCR-13-2499

72. Kim KH, Roberts CW (2016) Targeting EZH2 in cancer. Nat Med 22:128–134. https://doi.org/10.1038/nm.4036

73. Smits M et al (2011) Down-regulation of miR-101 in endothelial cells promotes blood vessel formation through reduced repression of EZH2. PLoS One 6:e16282. https://doi.org/10.1371/journal.pone.0016282

74. Crea F et al (2012) EZH2 inhibition: targeting the crossroad of tumor invasion and angiogenesis. Cancer Metastasis Rev 31:753–761. https://doi.org/10.1007/s10555-012-9387-3

75. Knutson SK et al (2013) Durable tumor regression in genetically altered malignant rhabdoid tumors by inhibition of methyltransferase EZH2. Proc Natl Acad Sci U S A 110:7922–7927. https://doi.org/10.1073/pnas.1303800110

76. Kurmasheva RT et al (2017) Initial testing (stage 1) of tazemetostat (EPZ-6438), a novel EZH2 inhibitor, by the Pediatric Preclinical Testing Program. Pediatr Blood Cancer 64. https://doi.org/10.1002/pbc.26218

77. Smith ME et al (2011) Therapeutically targeting cyclin D1 in primary tumors arising from loss of Ini1. Proc Natl Acad Sci U S A 108:319–324. https://doi.org/10.1073/pnas.0913297108

78. Hashizume R et al (2016) Inhibition of DNA damage repair by the CDK4/6 inhibitor palbociclib delays irradiated intracranial atypical teratoid rhabdoid tumor and glioblastoma xenograft regrowth. Neuro Oncol 18:1519–1528. https://doi.org/10.1093/neuonc/now106

79. Jagani Z et al (2010) Loss of the tumor suppressor Snf5 leads to aberrant activation of the Hedgehog-Gli pathway. Nat Med 16:1429–1433. https://doi.org/10.1038/nm.2251

80. Kerl K et al (2014) Arsenic trioxide inhibits tumor cell growth in malignant rhabdoid tumors in vitro and in vivo by targeting overexpressed Gli1. Int J Cancer 135:989–995. https://doi.org/10.1002/ijc.28719

81. Mora-Blanco EL et al (2014) Activation of beta-catenin/TCF targets following loss of the tumor suppressor SNF5. Oncogene 33:933–938. https://doi.org/10.1038/onc.2013.37

82. Chakravadhanula M et al (2015) Wnt pathway in atypical teratoid rhabdoid tumors. Neuro Oncol 17:526–535. https://doi.org/10.1093/neuonc/nou229

83. Alimova I et al (2017) Targeting polo-like kinase 1 in SMARCB1 deleted atypical teratoid rhabdoid tumor. Oncotarget 8:97290–97303. https://doi.org/10.18632/oncotarget.21932

84. Tang Y et al (2014) Epigenetic targeting of Hedgehog pathway transcriptional output through BET bromodomain inhibition. Nat Med 20:732–740. https://doi.org/10.1038/nm.3613

Part IV

Spinal Neurooncology and Peripheral Nerve Tumors

Jörg-Christian Tonn, Manfred Westphal

Intramedullary Tumors

34

Manfred Westphal

34.1 Definition

Intramedullary tumors may arise in the spinal cord from the intrinsic cell types therein (intra-axial lesions) or get into the spinal cord as metastases from systemic cancer (extra-axial lesion). Intra-axial intramedullary tumors are gliomas and are classified like the intrinsic brain tumors according to the WHO grading system in their respective chapters but have no chapter of their own [35]. Corresponding to the intracranial compartment, ependymomas, astrocytomas, oligodendrogliomas, and glioneuronal tumors are found also in the intramedullary segment of the central nervous system. Hemangioblastomas are frequently also found in the spinal cord and are truly intramedullary but as they arise from the surface are almost an invagination into the cord, displacing and compressing the fiber tracts rather than dissecting them. Tumors are called purely intramedullary from the level of C1 downward to the end of the cord at the level of the conus. Tumors of the filum terminale without extension into the conus will in this context not be considered intramedullary.

Depending on their location, tumors are cervical, cervicothoracic, thoracic, thoracolumbar, and conal.

M. Westphal (✉)
Department of Neurosurgery, University of Hamburg, University Hospital Eppendorf, Hamburg, Hamburg, Germany
e-mail: westphal@uke.de

Upward extensions into the medulla oblongata will be called cervicomedullary, and further extension into the pons will lead to a tumor being classified as pontomedullary.

34.1.1 Epidemiology and Etiology

Intramedullary tumors affect all ages and races. They are mostly spontaneous and not associated with specific syndromes. There is a higher incidence of intramedullary ependymomas in patients with neurofibromatosis type II [46] and with multiple hemangioblastomas in patients with von Hippel-Lindau disease, both hereditary syndromes. In general, the majority of the adult patients are between 20 and 50 years of age. Ependymomas are more frequent in children, becoming less frequent with age, whereas astrocytic tumors increase with age.

Intramedullary tumors recapitulate the whole histological spectrum of intracranial neuropathology. Likewise, there is no associated etiology for any of the tumors as there are no fundamental epidemiological clues for the cerebral tumors.

34.1.2 Histology and Molecular Genetics

The relative proportions of the different histologies within the spectrum of tumors occurring in

© Springer Nature Switzerland AG 2019
J.-C. Tonn et al. (eds.), *Oncology of CNS Tumors*, https://doi.org/10.1007/978-3-030-04152-6_34

Table 34.1 Spectrum of intramedullary lesions (1984–2017) (*n* = 438)

Intra-axial	*N* = 273 (60%)	Extra-axial	*N* = 165 (40%)
Ependymoma	170 (62.3%)	Cavernoma	48 (29.1%)
Hemangioblastoma	68 (41.2%)	Lipoma	11 (6.7%)
Astrocytoma I–II	57 (20.9%)	Metastasis	23 (13.9%)
Astrocytoma III/IV	27 (9.98%)	Teratoma	2 (1.2%)
Oligodendroglioma	4 (1.5%)	Tumefactive inflammation	4 (2.4%)
Ganglioglioma/cytoma	12 (4.4%)	Intramedullary cyst	9 (5.5%)
Melanocytoma	3 (1.3%)		

the spinal cord tissue are slightly different from the brain tissue. In contrast to the brain, ependymomas are the major group, followed by astrocytomas, gangliocytomas, and hemangioblastomas. Lipomas are not really considered neoplastic but are still slowly expanding lesions and need to be discussed in the context of management of spinal cord lesions. This spectrum is reflected by our own departmental series which is very similar to other large series (Table 34.1).

There is no report on fundamental, specific molecular genetic differences between spinal cord tumors and cerebral tumors except for ependymomas which in a proposed new classification would be called SP-EPN and show more often than any other loss of parts of chromosome 22q which is the locus of the NF2 gene for which there is a known association [45]. These differences, however, do not indicate a different etiology or cell lineage [32]. Hemangioblastomas in the spinal cord are known to carry mutations of the VHL gene as do hemangioblastomas elsewhere in the central nervous system [52].

34.1.3 Diagnostics

The onset of neurological symptoms is usually very slow, and the symptoms may erroneously be seen in the context of fatigue or exhaustion so that they are not taken seriously. The feeling of "heaviness" in the legs, some tingling in one extremity, the sensation as if a cuff were inflated around an arm or a leg, and occasional numbness are not considered severe enough to be aggressively pursued because there are many other transient indispositions which may cause the same. Only with progressive loss of neurological

function and the gradual development of a transverse syndrome, patients will be subjected to more aggressive diagnostics including spinal imaging. The field of intramedullary pathologies has been revolutionized since the routine availability of the MRI in the late 1980s. Since then, diagnosis and differential diagnosis have become much more rapid and definitive and can safely guide the appropriate therapy. Because diagnosis of an intramedullary lesion will in many cases lead to surgery, the imaging should include the craniocervical junction or the sacrum so that the exact level of the lesion can be determined even in cases of vertebral variations. Imaging can be supported by electrophysiology which can provide an estimate of how severely some fiber tracts might already be damaged. In many cases one side is more affected than the other. The analysis of cerebrospinal fluid may also be of help when as a differential diagnosis an inflammatory process needs to be considered although myelitis may go on for a long time without any reflection in the CSF. An acute inflammation shows a marked discrepancy of lesion size, and the dynamics of symptoms and a rapid onset and progression of symptoms in the absence of hemorrhage and a lesion with little mass effect are almost certainly inflammatory. Tumefactive inflammatory lesions are rare [38, 67].

As a rule of thumb, all tumorous lesions show a considerable mass effect and distend the medulla to an extent easily seen on sagittal MRI because of narrowing of the perimedullary CSF space, best depicted in a T2-weighted series.

Ependymomas show a very diverse appearance [6, 36, 59]. Because of their origin from the central canal, they are usually centrally located and displace the medulla in a concentric pattern which is best seen on axial images. Rarely can they break their coat of fiber tracts and protrude dorsally or ventrally through the dorsal midline sulcus (Fig. 34.1) in which case they are called exophytic [18]. That, however, is a rather unusual presentation, and other differential diagnoses (i.e., amelanotic melanocytoma) have to be con-

sidered and evaluated by exhaustive immunohistochemistry after resection (Fig. 34.2). Ependymomas are normally contained within the cord and are either solid or homogeneously enhancing with gadolinium (Fig. 34.3), or as in most cases, there will be polar cysts which can extend three to four levels beyond the tumor

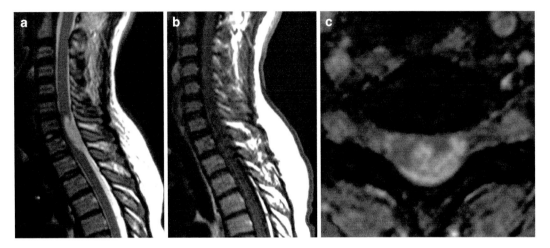

Fig. 34.1 Sagittal MR scans (**a**, **b**) of an atypical cervicothoracic ependymoma which shows homogeneous contrast enhancement and can be seen to be exophytic in the axial scans (**c**). The tumor part which covers the surface of the cord could be completely lifted up and showed no sign of infiltration

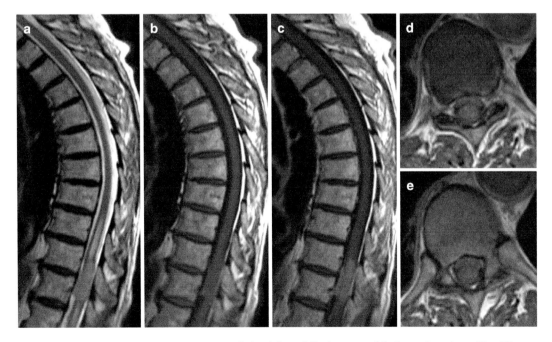

Fig. 34.2 Very similar MRI appearance (**a–c** saggital and **d**, **e** axial) of a tumor of the lower thoracic cord in a 74-year-old male which upon scrutinous immunohistochemistry turned out to be an amelanotic melanocytoma

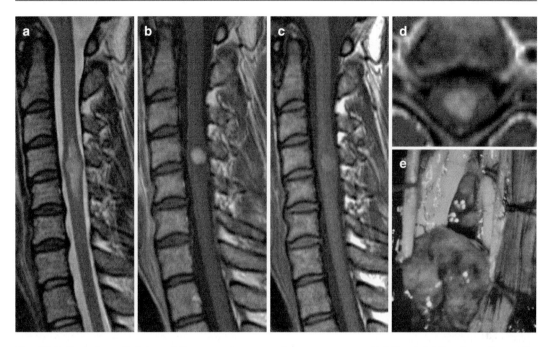

Fig. 34.3 Typical small intramedullary ependymoma showing again the uniform enhancement, central location, focal distension of the cord, and polar edema (**a–c**). These tumors are very well delineated (**d**) and can be usually removed in toto (**e**)

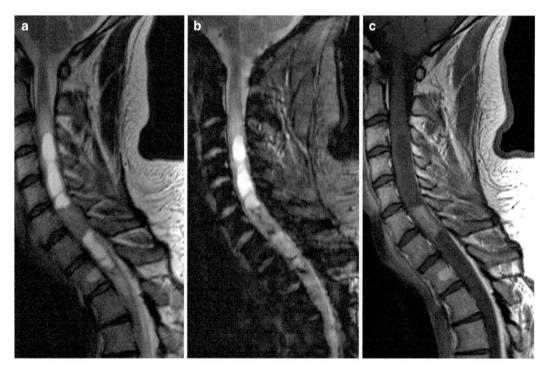

Fig. 34.4 Typical intramedullary ependymoma with inhomogeneous polar cysts which impresses like septated syringomyelia (**a**, **b**). The tumor itself is a contrast-enhancing mass which appears to be taking up the whole transverse diameter of the cord with no proper cord tissue (**c–f**)

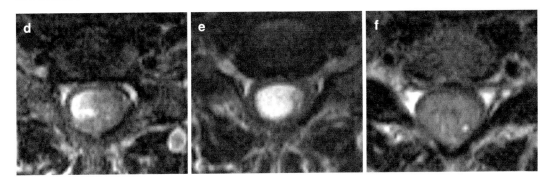

Fig. 34.4 (continued)

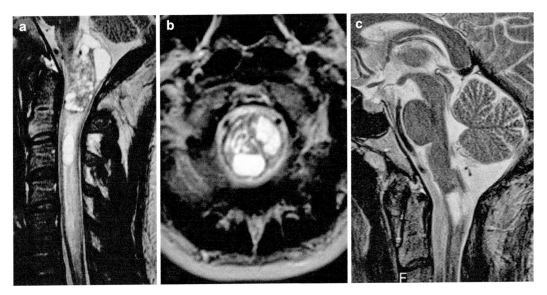

Fig. 34.5 Ependymoma of the craniocervical junction (**a**) which is associated with polar as well as intratumoral cysts (**b**). Despite the impressive size, even such lesions can be removed without neurological deficits (**c**). The inhomogeneous appearance in such cases is indicative of regressive changes which allow for optimal distinction between tumor and the proper cord tissue during microsurgical dissection

poles (Fig. 34.4) and are the most discriminating feature from other etiologies [29]. The syringomyelia which may appear septated is usually communicating. In addition, some tumors may show regressive changes within themselves like degenerative cysts or signs of older hemorrhages (Fig. 34.5). When infiltration of surrounding structures from exophytic growth is present, an anaplastic lesion is to be suspected. Whatever the appearance of an ependymoma is, it will most likely be relatively easy to remove it completely (see below). Therefore that diagnosis should not be missed to adequately counsel the patients.

Under no circumstance should patients be told by therapists who are not dealing with these lesions on a regular basis that, based on a dramatic neuroradiological presentation, they have an untreatable lesion. It should be standard that MR images from intramedullary lesions are sent for consultation to experienced neuroradiologists especially because of the very heterogeneous spectrum of appearances. Incidental findings may be counselled to wait and see and be treated only at the time of progression in imaging or developing symptoms, but patients with progressive symptoms should be advised for treatment.

In anaplastic lesions, dissemination may occur early or be present at the time of diagnosis. In such cases at the latest in the follow-up situation, the MRI should cover all of the spinal canal.

Astrocytomas are also heterogeneous in their appearance [6, 16, 22], but in contrast to ependymomas, they are asymmetrical and located off-center which is in agreement with symptoms of more laterality than in the mostly central ependymomas. Pilocytic astrocytomas (WHO I) can enhance homogeneously with contrast media, which have some patchy enhancement or no enhancement at all (Figs. 34.6, 34.7, and 34.8). The nature of their growth is hard to predict from the MRI where the axial images as far as definitive margins are concerned can be just the opposite intraoperatively as what is seen in the images. In cases which are endophytic, a clean resection plane may be present allowing for radi-

cal removal, but in other cases, despite suggestive axial images, no dissection plane can be found, and only a debulking is possible. In cases in which very diffuse growth with Gd enhancement is seen, only a biopsy may be possible. A biopsy is, however, definitely indicated to exclude other lesions which might have other treatment options and to determine the grade because there is rare progression to anaplasia in pilocytic tumors and adjuvant options may need to be considered.

Diffuse astrocytomas (WHO II) regularly do not enhance, show diffuse growth in all MRI sequences, and show some kind of edema (T2 abnormality) extending far beyond the main tumor mass. Like in the intrinsic lesions of the brain, this could be indicative of continuous tumor spread, and these tumors are known to extend eventually far upward into the medulla oblongata or the pons where they cause terminal problems [54].

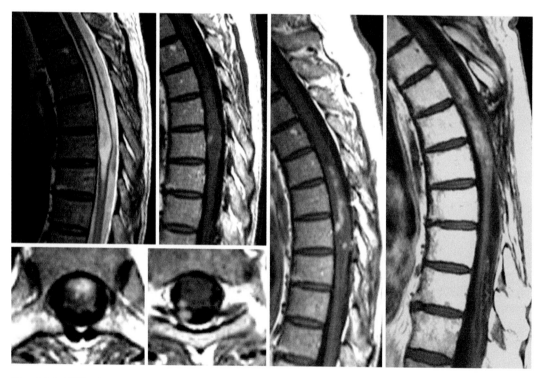

Fig. 34.6 Diffusely growing pilocytic astrocytoma which has profusely infiltrated through the whole cord with only minimal affection of the fiber tracts. At several points the tumor has broken out of the cord forming little solid nodules on the surface which were removed to secure the diagnosis (left panels). Upon progression after 2 years (middle panel), the patient sought an attempt at removal against advice and was left paraplegic. This was followed by radiation which somewhat stabilized the upward extension for 12 years (right panel)

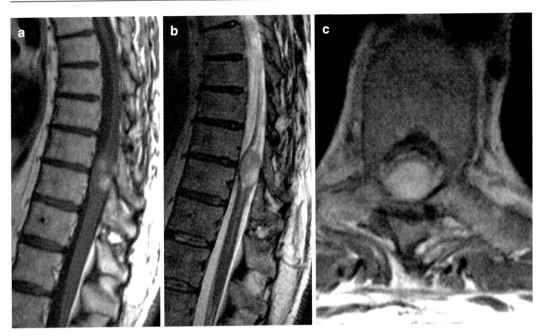

Fig. 34.7 Recurrent pilocytic astrocytoma which had be gross totally resected 8 years prior to the shown scans. The lesion appears also homogeneously contrast enhancing but lacks polar cysts (**a**, **b**). Upon reoperation by the same sur-geon, the whole interface between tumor and residual cord (**c**) was found to be an area of broad invasion, not allowing radical resection

Anaplastic astrocytomas are rare (Fig. 34.9). They are suspected in the presence of a relatively short and rapidly progressive history of neurological defects, affecting one side more than the other, and an MRI with diffuse distension, no polar cysts, patchy but strong contrast enhancement, T2 changes much beyond the distended part of the medulla, and signs of necrosis as in intracerebral glioblastoma. Because of the rarity of these lesions and their heterogeneous imaging nature, the differential diagnosis has to relate to the case history, but definitive certainty can only be obtained from histological evaluation. A very short history and a lesion with hypointense center and rim enhancement may be a primary glioblastoma, looking very similar to an intracranial lesion (Fig. 34.10).

Glioneuronal tumors are nodular, inhomogeneously enhancing lesions which may have a cyst [47] (Fig. 34.11). They can cause very pronounced distension of the medulla and even enlargement of the spinal canal which already indicates their dysontogenetic nature and long presence. They can go along with hemiatrophy of the whole body when located in the upper cervical region or of the legs when located in the thoracic region (Fig. 34.12).

Intramedullary hemangioblastomas are nearly always associated with a cystic component which can extend over many levels, while the angioblastoma is only the size of a small pea or a grain of rice [15, 40] (Fig. 34.13). When located at the surface, they can grow within a cyst which indents the medulla (Fig. 34.14) but can also be without a cystic component. Upon gadolinium application they stain intensely. In the T2-weighted sequences, it may be possible to see distended vessels on the surface of the medulla which are usually the draining veins. Angiography can confirm the diagnosis but should only be performed mainly if there is an attempt to do a preoperative embolization (see below). To make the diagnosis is easy for sporadic cases and unequivocal when a known von Hippel-Lindau disease is present.

Intramedullary metastases are becoming more frequent [48]. They are typically associated with a

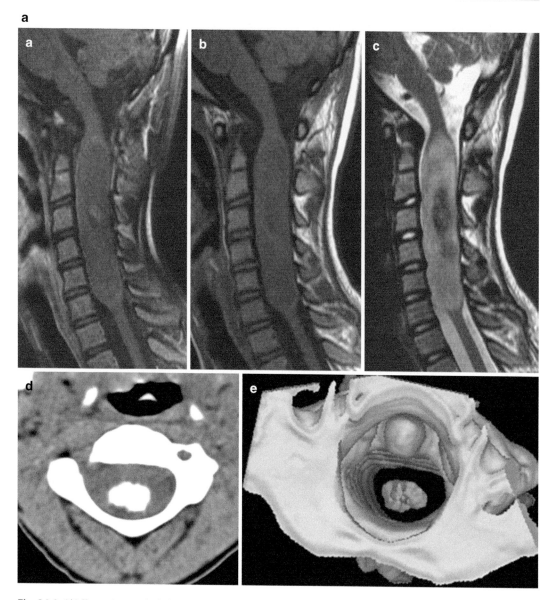

Fig. 34.8 (**A**) Extensive cervical pilocytic astrocytoma of a 14-year-old boy which showed a long calcified nucleus as seen as a hypointense area in the MRI (**a–c**) and on axial (**d**) as well as spiral (**e**) CT. This case could only be extensively debulked in the absence of a clear dissection plane. The long surgical exposure led to the development of a swan neck already within 1 year postoperatively despite laminotomy, requiring eventual stabilization (see further below, Fig. 34.23a). (**B**) Extensive diffusely growing cervical astrocytoma with only minor sensory deficits in the right hand in a 37-year-old male. A homogeneous nodule are at the right side was removed (arrow) and the histology confirmed and upon inspection it could be seen that strings of spinal cord tissue were interspersed with diffuse tumor, as was already suggested by the MRI, best seen on the axial images

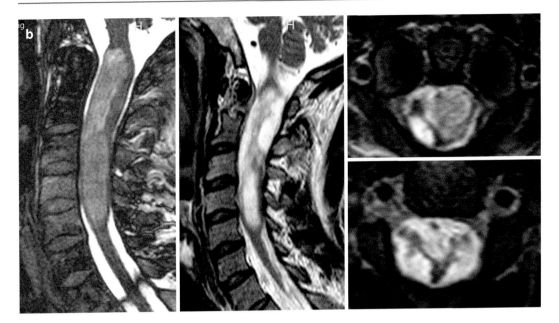

Fig. 34.8 (continued)

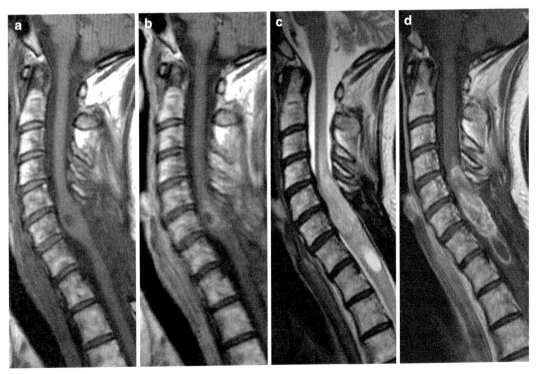

Fig. 34.9 Recurrent anaplastic astrocytoma in a 56-year-old woman. A diffuse enlargement of the cervical cord is seen as well as inhomogeneous contrast enhancement (**a**, **b**). Without further option for resection or radiation, the patient underwent chemotherapy but still progressed to a picture which is consistent with glioblastoma (**c**, **d**)

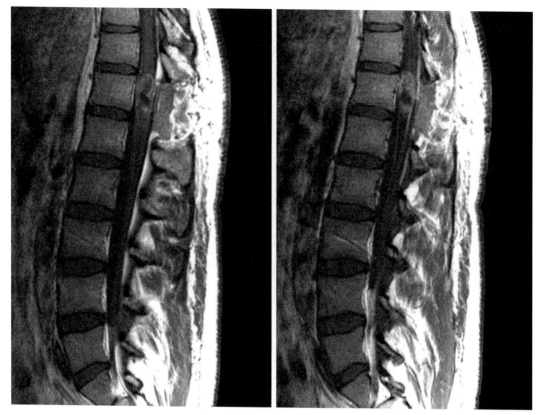

Fig. 34.10 Recurrent glioblastoma 3 months after combined radiochemotherapy with exactly the same appearance as the original tumor (not shown). The tumor is inside the conus, presented with a rapidly developing weakness in the legs, urinary problems, and pain which is the most instructive clinical sign

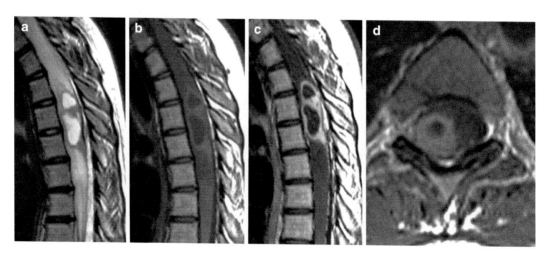

Fig. 34.11 Excentric, cystic intramedullary lesion with contrast enhancement in a massively distended cord (**a–c**). In the presence of very slowly progressing symptoms which retrospectively had a history of years, only a well-differentiated process is to be suspected, and in this case the histology turned out to be gangliocytoma. Intraoperatively the lesion turned out to be gangliocytoma and could only be debulked as the lesion is isomorphic with the tissue of the cord and offers no dissection plane despite the sharp demarkation in the axial MRI (**d**)

Fig. 34.12 Incidental finding of an intramedullary lesion (**a, b**) in a 40-year-old woman. Retrospectively she reported that all her life her left side was somewhat weaker, and upon physical examination she revealed a marked hemihypotrophy which can be seen in direct comparison of the hands (**c**). The lesion was never biopsied, but a glioneuronal dysontogenic lesion is the most likely histology

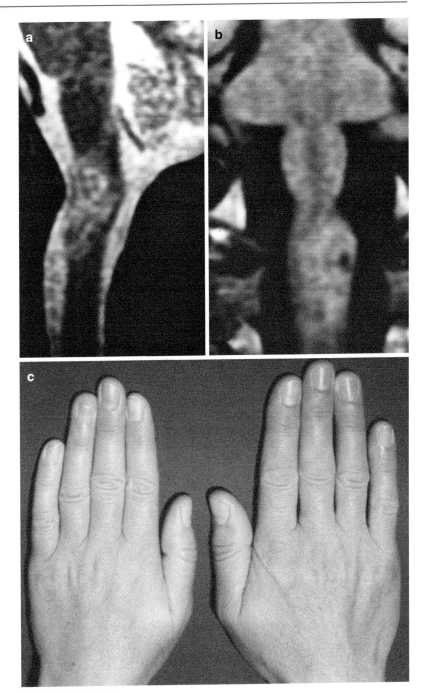

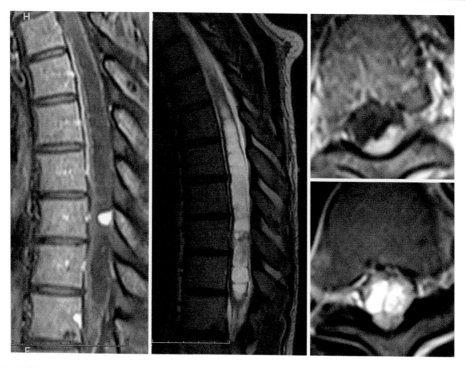

Fig. 34.13 MRI showing a massive syringomyelia in a 54-year-old woman associated with a strongly contrast-enhancing small non-von Hippel-Lindau hemangioblastoma. After removal, the syrinx collapsed

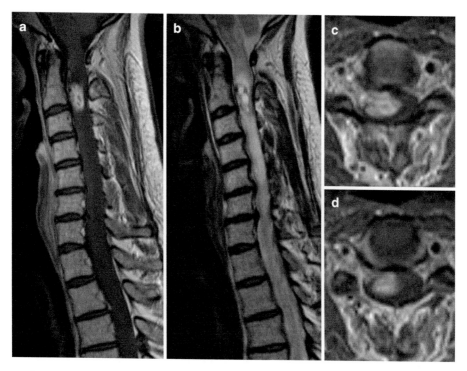

Fig. 34.14 Contrast enhancing, presumably intramedullary tumor with a polar cyst which was thought to be an ependymoma (**a, b**). Intraoperatively it was found to be a hemangioblastoma which needed to be approached from a far lateral exposure with transection of the dentate ligament. No prominent blood vessels were seen, and the only clue to the possible differential diagnosis was the broad attachment to the surface of the cord (**c, d**)

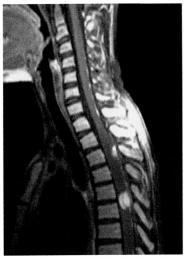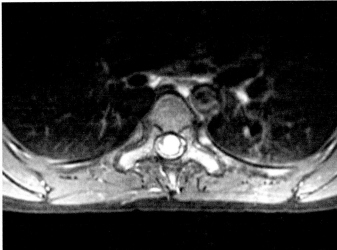

Fig. 34.15 Multiple dorsal intramedullary lesions with strong Gd enhancement of which the lesion in the middle thoracic region had caused rapid neurological deteriora-tion so that it needed to be removed showing a MPNST-like lesion. Just 6 months prior to this, a left temporal anaplastic astrocytoma was removed

known systemic cancer and can be truly intramed-ullary from hematogenic metastases as well as invading the medulla from the surface after break-ing the pial membrane in the context of meningeal carcinomatosis. They have no typical neuroimag-ing characteristics, and the diagnosis is based on the context of the systemic disease. Primary intra-medullary melanoma has been reported, but it is unresolved whether this is truly a primary lesion or cancer with unknown primary which is not infrequently found in melanoma due to the postu-lated immunogenicity outside the CNS.

Intramedullary neurinomas are reported but very rare. Likewise related tumors, like the malignant peripheral nerve sheath tumor, are very rare but when present may occur at multiple sites, originating from the dorsal root entry zone and from there extending intramedullarly (Fig. 34.15).

Intramedullary lipomas show a characteristic pattern of signal intensities in T1 and T2 which allow the diagnosis without histology [28, 34]. In most cases, the lipoma is exophytic as a very intense mass in T1, but it may also be intramedul-lary, mimicking syrigomyelia on some sequences (Fig. 34.16).

Benign teratoma may also occur in the spinal cord, preferentially at the level of the conus, show a very inhomogeneous pattern (Fig. 34.17), and in some cases contain all types of tissues like car-tilage, glandular tissue, and enteral mucosa or muscle but all inside a cystic compartment. The wall being assimilated to the cord, as in cranial tumors is left behind during surgical removal and over long periods of decades may lead to an "expected" recurrence.

34.2 Differential Diagnosis

The most important differential diagnoses are inflammation and arteriovenous fistula [10, 33, 65].

Inflammatory lesions are mostly excentric and have diffuse margins, weak contrast enhance-ment, and most often a spindle-shaped extension

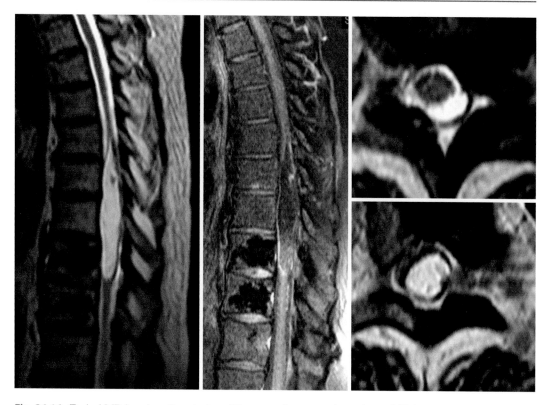

Fig. 34.16 Typical MR imaging of a spinal cord lipoma which is partially exophytic and else distended the cord so that only a thin shell remained allowing for a wedge decompression using a CO2 laser, to "melt" the lipoma until the interface with the cord which can bear important nutritive vessels appeared

rather than a nodular appearance (Fig. 34.18). They may be most easily mistaken for an anaplastic astrocytoma. Very frequently there is only a relatively short history of clinical symptoms (subacute onset) which is disproportional to the usually limited extent of the lesion when compared to the ratio of size to symptoms in tumorous lesions. Apart from the case history, the next clue is the complete absence or only negligible extent of mass effect. CSF examination may be normal, but obtaining CSF is warranted to try and find inflammatory cells or clues from inflammatory markers. PET has been used to differentiate between differentiated and anaplastic lesions as well as vascular and inflammatory, but the results despite providing some hints are not superior to less involved imaging techniques [42].

The other very important differential diagnosis is that of a congestive myelopathy due to an arteriovenous malformation. Spinal dural AV fistula may cause such congestion and if left undiagnosed and untreated will result in gliotic changes in the medulla which may lead to necrotic changes. Therefore the disease, before the elucidation of is cause, was known as necrotizing myelitis (Fig. 34.19). The neuroradiological signs are clear because there are distended blood vessels on the surface of the medulla and a homogeneous central edema on T2 which may affect almost the whole spinal cord (Fig. 34.20). When this is not recognized and erroneously biopsied, the wrong diagnosis may even become consolidated histologically because of the gliotic changes associated with persistent congestive myelopathy which can resemble low-grade glioma.

Finally it has to be mentioned that the spinal cord is considered to be less tolerant to radiation than other tissues and that therefore there is a considerable risk for radiation-induced myelopathy [27, 37] which is mostly due to irradiation to the immediate surroundings like in vertebral metastases [49]. Also, when radiation for thyroid cancer or lesions in the mediastinum requires

Fig. 34.17 Benign
teratoma which is well
demarcated and very
inhomogeneous in its
signal intensity

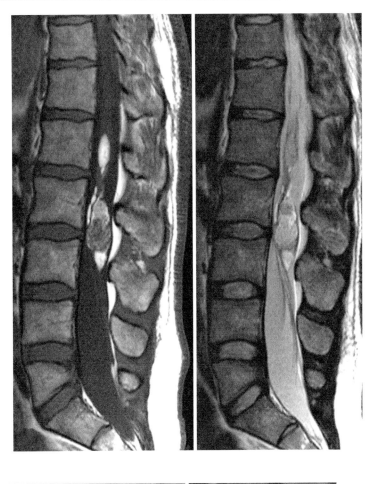

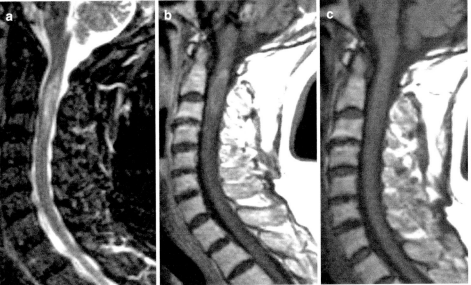

Fig. 34.18 Male patient with a diffusely enhancing, ill-defined lesion in the cervical spinal cord and a rapid onset of symptoms. The absence of a cord distension together with the rapid onset of the neurological problems is a characteristic for an inflammatory lesion (**a, b**). This proved to be the case and the lesion resolved over the course of a year (**c**)

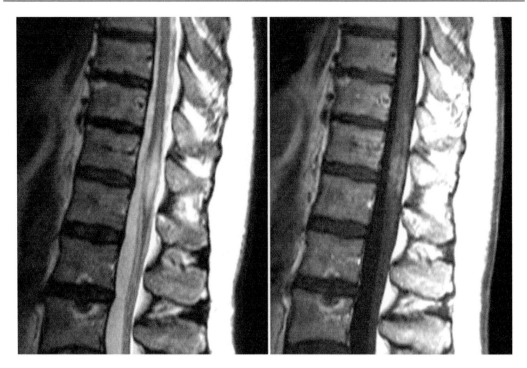

Fig. 34.19 Spinal MRI of a male patient with a long history of leg weakness, sensory deficit, and genitourinary impairment. In the absence of neuroradiological signs for an arteriovenous lesion, a biopsy was performed which showed arterialized veins, and the histology showed a necrotizing myelitis consistent with long-standing SDAVF in which the nidus may have spontaneously obliterated, leaving the severely impaired cord with luxury perfusion

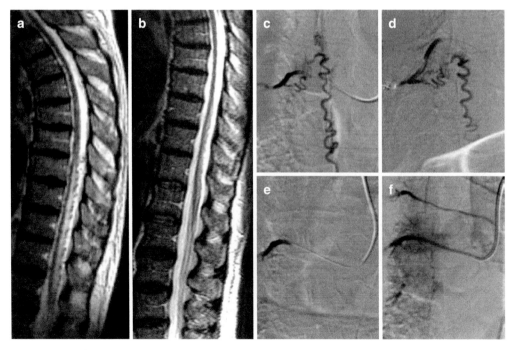

Fig. 34.20 A patient with the typical features of a spinal dural arteriovenous fistula. There is an edema in most of the thoracic cord but only very little mass effect (**a**). In this case, there is a very pronounced venous congestion which should lead to the correct diagnosis already on MRI. Angiography identifies the fistulous point (**c**, **d**), whereupon the fistula can be eliminated by transection (**e**, **f**), whereupon the edema resolves (**b**)

high-dose radiation and a considerable amount of dose is going through the spinal canal, radiation necrosis may be produced. In imaging it imposes malignant glioma, and there is also a relatively short history of progressive neurological deficit. However, the case history and the analysis of the radiation plans should clear the situation [2]. Often the fatty degeneration of the vertebral bodies is seen right in the area of medullary pathology. Induction of a secondary malignancy should be ruled out because of the time course which is much more rapid for radiation necrosis than for a radiation-induced malignancy. This diagnosis should become much less frequent due to the improved conformal radiation techniques [51].

34.2.1 Treatment and Prevention

Treatment of spinal cord tumors is mostly surgical but may for some subgroups involve also radiation and/or chemotherapy, especially in lymphomas (see there).

Ependymomas can be completely removed by established and refined microsurgical approaches [8, 13, 14, 56]. There is a well-demarcated dissection plane, and the ends are frequently delineated by cysts. There is a tapering sleeve of gliosis around the cysts at the ends which extends into the central canal which during surgery is severed, thereby preventing any upward or downward spread. The approach is through a midline incision and then dissection along the surface from pole to pole which in most cases of ependymoma allows for an en bloc resection (Fig. 34.21). The vascular supply always comes from the anterior spinal artery through the ventral sulcus, and injury to that vessel is the major pitfall for surgery. The tolerance to disturbances of the vascular supply also varies at different levels of the cord. The cervical region is rich in supply from above and below because of feeders to the anterior spinal artery from different levels. The mid-thoracic region in contrast is less rich in vascular supply and therefore much more vulnerable (Westphal et al., unpublished observation). Dissection as with all other medullary

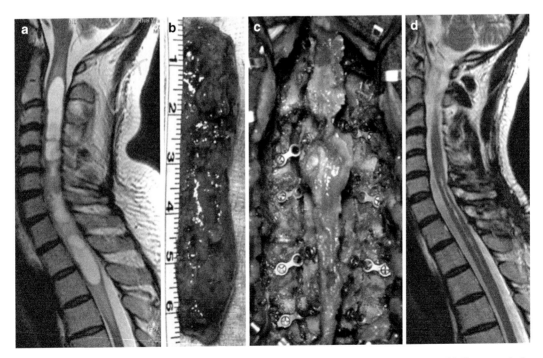

Fig. 34.21 Extensive, typical cervical ependymoma (**a**). Developing the lesion from the polar cysts along a dissection plane to the fiber tracts, the lesion can be developed in one piece (**b**). Postoperative stability is optimized by reinsertion of the en bloc laminotomy (**c**). Postoperatively the cysts are usually completely collapsed (**d**), and also the alignment is highly satisfactory

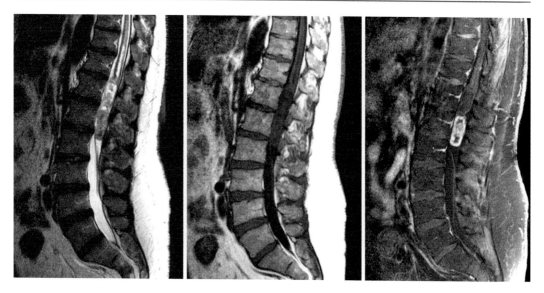

Fig. 34.22 The lowest possible form of an intramedullary ependymoma grade II in a young man which is at the junction between cord and filum terminale but has an upper pole in the conus and an accompanying syringomyelia with a distinct border between tumor and adjacent gliosis

pathologies can be monitored by intraoperative electrophysiology of the motor and somatosensory evoked potentials, making the complete resection safer [31, 41]. In some cases, the signal quality may be severely impaired already at the outset of surgery, and in such cases, monitoring is not helpful and deterioration of signal unpredictive of outcome (Westphal et al., unpublished observation). For grade II lesions, there is a high cure rate after complete removal. The polar cysts are coated with a gliosis but not tumor and should not be removed. They may extend several levels beyond the tumor proper and need to be left untouched and will resolve after resection of the solid tumor even when they seem to be distant from the tumor mass as in conal ependymomas at the origin of the filum terminale (Fig. 34.22). Especially with a conus ependymoma, a holocord syringomyelia has been reported [55].

For anaplastic ependymoma (WHO grade III) lesions, the rate of recurrence is considerable [21, 50]. The anaplastic lesions should also receive other therapies such as radiation [23] and/or chemotherapy [5, 9] although no standardized regimen has been established.

Follow-up with MRI is done for grade II in yearly intervals up to 6 years and then biannually thereafter. Recurrence after 10 years is extremely unlikely. For grade III lesions, follow-up is in 6 months intervals for the first 2 years and then annually until year 6 and then as in the grade II lesions. Should there be a recurrence, a reoperation should be considered.

The removal of pilocytic astrocytomas (PA) may be attempted, and feasibility depends on the growth pattern, whether a tumor grows endophytically or diffusely. In an endophytic tumor, complete removal may be possible (Fig. 34.23 b), but when growing diffusely, only a biopsy or debulking is possible (Figs. 34.6 and 34.8) or a dural expansion after biopsy. Additional therapies can be extrapolated from the supratentorial lesions where radiation and chemotherapy have been introduced [4]. Radiation therapy should, however, be withheld and only used as a last resort because of the vulnerability of the cord to high doses of radiation in conventional and stereotactic techniques [66]. The patients are regularly followed as for low-grade ependymomas, and whenever there is progression, repeated decompressions may be reconsidered. Upward extension is possible, but usually the distension at the original level causing eventually a complete transverse syndrome is more typical. Although there may be a complete removal, recurrence/progression is more likely because of the more infiltrative nature

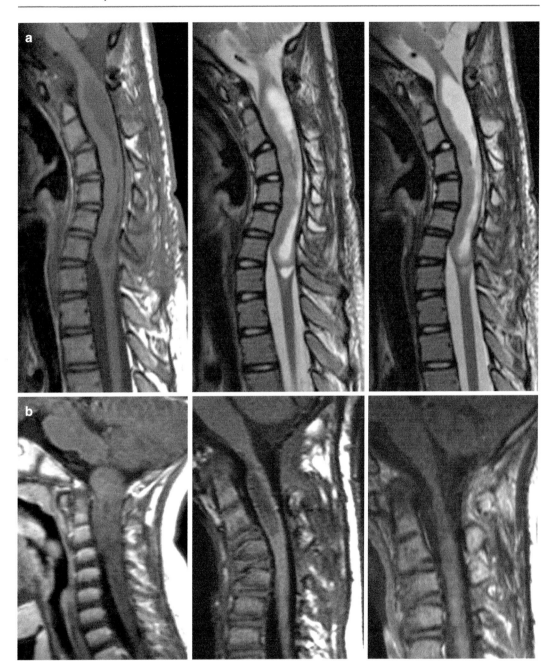

Fig. 34.23 (**a**) Follow-up of a large pilocytic astrocytoma (Fig. 34.8) which was only debulked and developed a beginning swan neck deformity so that eventually a spinal stabilization and postural correction with dorsal and ventral instrumentation had to be performed (**b**). Large pilocytic astrocytoma in the cervicomedullary junction a 4-year-old child (left panel) which could be completely removed (middle panel) because of a favorable dissection plane. As seen more frequently in young children, there was, however, malalignment of the cervical spine and the indication of a developing swan neck (middle panel). Before surgical intervention, specific and intensive physiotherapy was administered leading to lasting stabilization and realignment (right panel)

of the tumors compared to ependymomas (Fig. 34.6). Histological progression in intramedullary PA to "anaplastic" intramedullary PA is extremely rare but seen rather as an increase in anaplastic features rather than a change in WHO grade [11] with that issue still being a matter of debate for spinal as well as intracranial lesions. Leptomeningeal spread has also been reported [1].

Astrocytomas of WHO grades II to IV are also removed as far as possible to gain time and secure the diagnosis [16, 22]. There are no series for adjuvant therapies for low-grade tumors (WHO II) which allow conclusions [17]. Patients are followed and re-decompressed when necessary and permissible. Upward extension with progressive involvement of additional levels is common. As with the intracerebral astrocytomas, there is progression to higher grades (II to III or IV and III to IV), and then chemotherapy and radiation may be given as a palliative therapy according to the Stupp regimen [58]. The postoperative course of grade II patients may be stable for several years, whereas the course of the anaplastic tumors is rapidly progressive [30] leading eventually to lower brain stem dysfunction due to upward extension. As ultimate measure, cutting the cord above the level of the tumor in cases with already complete paraplegia ("cordectomy") has been attempted and very controversially discussed, but in anecdotal cases, long-term control could be achieved [63]. This is in contrast to larger series reporting generally poor outcome for spinal cord glioblastoma even with radiation "cordotomy" [57].

Oligodendrogliomas are very rare so that there is no series which reports on the efficacy of procarbazine/CCNU/vincristine chemotherapy which has proven to be highly successful in the treatment of cranial oligodendrogliomas [61]. According to recent studies for cranial tumors, temozolamide may also be used for chemotherapy in these cases.

Glioneuronal tumors when found accidentally and suspected because of the absence of any symptoms or dynamics of neurological deficits may be observed. When symptoms and clinical course justify intervention, surgery is the only option, and when gross total resection is achieved, this may lead to a long-term remission [13, 25, 47]. The surgeon has to be prepared for an isomorphic lesion which has no gliotic boundaries, is only slightly off-color from the fiber tracts, and without distinct change in consistency as it is really glioneuronal and very similar to the original tissue matrix of the cord. Therefore decompression may be the only possibility in some cases. In this respect, these lesions are very different from the supratentorial compartment where they can be resected within a safety boundary of normal white matter in most cases, guided by intraoperative imaging like ultrasound or MRI. Such tolerance does not exist in the spinal cord because the fiber tracts are certain to be contained somewhere in the periphery of the tumor tissue which in MRI or in the intraoperative ultrasound appears abnormal in its signal characteristics.

Hemangioblastomas are surgically removed, mostly without prior embolization [60, 62, 64]. The symptoms which are more frequently from the syringomyelia-like cyst [44] than from the tumor usually reverse after removal. The tumors arise at the pial level, and when that plane is circumcised, first obliterating the feeding vessels, the tumors can usually be moved out of their gliotic boundary which protects the fiber tracts so that surgery is safe and should be preferred to any other theoretically possible measures like radiosurgery or sole embolization. Surgical removal achieves 96% stable long-term control, whereas the value of radiosurgery beyond plain feasibility remains to be evaluated, especially for long-term myelopathy [7]. Restraint is advisable especially for the multiple hemangiomas found in the patients with von Hippel-Lindau, to only treat clearly symptomatic lesions and not all that are present on the scans but may remain asymptomatic [52, 62]. The dynamics are very asynchronous, and some lesions may be silent for many years, whereas others suddenly appear and become symptomatic. The cause of this is unknown.

Lipomas may become symptomatic but are difficult to treat. Their interface with the cord is assimilated to the pia and cannot be dissected in most cases without causing damage to the surface vasculature. Because of progressive symptoms, sometimes a partial resection of up to 70% of the mass or dural expansion is performed [28] to ease the pressure in the compartment.

Teratomas are a very rare pathology and are mature in the vast majority of the cases. When symptomatic due to a growing cystic compartment, they will be partially resected, but when very adherent to the cord or the conus/filum interface where they tend to occur more often than elsewhere, remnants may be left behind without any future necessity for other kinds of therapy, especially no radiation except for immature lesions.

Surgical treatment of spinal cord lesion has to follow some general rules. The first concerns the indication for treatment which should be made early because a favorable prognostic parameter is the neurological status of the patient with better prognosis in better performance patients [43]. Whenever possible, an en bloc laminotomy with reinsertion of the segment (laminoplasty) is to be preferred to laminectomy, and in multilevel exposures it is mandatory. Although the need for subsequent stabilization appears to be independent from the choice between laminectomy and laminoplasty [20], laminoplasty offers an easier dissection plane, should repeat surgery be necessary for a recurrent lesion. In cervical exposures, the farther the exposure is extended laterally, the more muscles are detached, and the more danger is there for a swan neck deformity [3, 24]. This needs some-

times to be corrected with later stabilization but can sometimes be prevented with immediate and consequent physiotherapy which has to be closely watched by the physicians who take care of the patients between follow-up visits (Fig. 34.23). Development of a swan neck deformity is more frequent in children [68] and more frequent when the lesion itself causes muscular weakness like an infiltrative glioma and when the exposure is long, involving three or more levels (Fig. 34.23). When no exposure of the whole cord is needed, minimal exposures for lesions presenting at the surface like hemangioblastoma will be sufficient and thus avoid any biomechanical concerns [39].

Radiation therapy as such is reserved for the respective anaplastic tumors [26]. After initial reports [53] spinal radiosurgery is becoming increasingly refined but mostly with radiation to the vertebral elements [27, 51] not yet including extensive consideration for intrinsic lesions like residual pilocytic or ependymoma grade II. The evaluation of larger series generally acknowledges that spinal stereotactic radiosurgery is feasible and safe but that surgery is still the primary option [19].

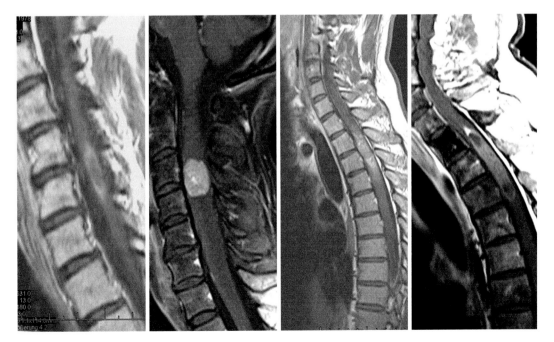

Fig. 34.24 Imaging of four different spinal metastases from left to right: cervical intramedullary metastasis of a mammary carcinoma surrounding edema, upper cervical nodular metastasis of a mammary carcinoma, cervicotho-racic metastasis of a non-small cell lung cancer, and at the far right intramedullary metastasis of a prostate carcinoma over several levels

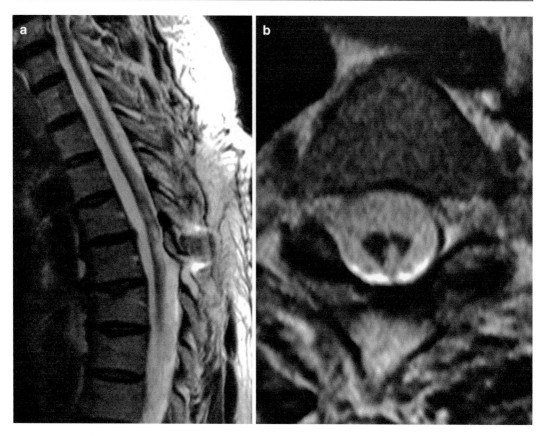

Fig. 34.25 Postoperative MRI of a patient with a mid-thoracic ependymoma. Although an attempt was made to close the arachnoid, it has to be postulated that "sticky surfaces" remained which adhered to the dural opening and suture so that eventually the surface of the exposure became adherent. Because of segmental, movement-associated pain, a revision was performed 8 years after the initial surgery where the cord was dissected from tight scarry adhesions to the dura

As spinal metastases become more frequent (Fig. 34.24), there is a need to define the therapeutic options. Intramedullary metastases occur in late disease stages, and therefore no risks should be taken. As symptoms develop rapidly, urgent surgery, sometimes even acute intervention, is to be considered, but any indication for treatment has to be seen in the context of the whole oncological situation. Metastases tend to irritate their edematous vulnerable cord surroundings, and fiber tracts will be immediately on the surface of the lesion so that debulking is the first step, and then it has to be evaluated on an individual basis whether the remaining shell can be completely peeled off the cord or is left when a good decompression is achieved. This measure will be followed by radiation and/or chemotherapy, and without having to worry about late effects of radiation, this affects the palliation and stabilization aimed for in these patients.

After removal of an intramedullary lesion, care should be taken to close the pia or at least the arachnoid. We have observed a case in which adhesions formed to the dura which led to a "suspended" or tethered appearance of the myelon in the area of exposure. Within years this led to posture-dependent pain and required a revision (Fig. 34.25).

34.3 Prognosis

The prognosis of intramedullary tumors depends very much on the histology but also on the time of diagnosis. Sporadic, single hemangioblastomas when completely resected have an excellent prognosis. Also ependymomas grade II also have an excellent prognosis, especially when they are detected early. Patients can expect to be cured with minor sensory deficits or dysesthesias which can originate from the manipulation of the dorsal columns. Glioblastoma has the worst prognosis, no matter what is done therapeutically.

The prognosis is mixed for anaplastic ependymomas, non-resectable pilocytic astrocytomas, and slowly progressive glioneuronal tumors. Regular follow-up is warranted to determine possible time points for repeated intervention.

The functional prognosis of the patients depends also on the tolerance of the spinal cord for therapeutic interventions at the time of diagnosis, and that is greatly reduced when the patients are in poor grade according to Cooper and Epstein. Once a patient through a long history of misconceptions about his condition has become wheelchair bound before the diagnosis is established, the chances for the patient to get out of it are almost nil. For other patients, who even in the most optimal clinical setting suffer from a deterioration from a surgical procedure, advise has to be given that regeneration takes place over a period of about 2 years and that for that time at least there should be intense physiotherapy to get to the best possible postoperative result which may be much better than the preoperative status.

References

1. Abel TJ, Chowdhary A, Thapa M, Rutledge JC, Geyer JR, Ojemann J, Avellino AM (2006) Spinal cord pilocytic astrocytoma with leptomeningeal dissemination to the brain. Case report and review of the literature. J Neurosurg 105:508–514
2. Allison R, Vaughan J, Thurber A, Rajecki M, Vongtama V, Barry T (1999) Spinal cord dose is higher than expected in head and neck radiation. Med Dosim 24:135–139
3. Alvisi C, Borromei A, Cerisoli M, Giulioni M (1988) Long-term evaluation of cervical spine disorders following laminectomy. J Neurosurg Sci 32:109–112
4. Aryan HE, Meltzer HS, Lu DC, Ozgur BM, Levy ML, Bruce DA (2005) Management of pilocytic astrocytoma with diffuse leptomeningeal spread: two cases and review of the literature. Childs Nerv Syst 21:477–481
5. Balmaceda C (2000) Chemotherapy for intramedullary spinal cord tumors. J Neurooncol 47:293–307
6. Bourgouin PM, Lesage J, Fontaine S, Konan A, Roy D, Bard C, Del Carpio O'Donovan R (1998) A pattern approach to the differential diagnosis of intramedullary spinal cord lesions on MR imaging. AJR Am J Roentgenol 170:1645–1649
7. Bridges KJ, Jaboin JJ, Kubicky CD, Than KD (2017) Stereotactic radiosurgery versus surgical resection for spinal hemangioblastoma: a systematic review. Clin Neurol Neurosurg 154:59–66
8. Brotchi J (2002) Intrinsic spinal cord tumor resection. Neurosurgery 50:1059–1063
9. Chamberlain MC (2002) Salvage chemotherapy for recurrent spinal cord ependymoma. Cancer 95:997–1002
10. Choi KH, Lee KS, Chung SO, Park JM, Kim YJ, Kim HS, Shinn KS (1996) Idiopathic transverse myelitis: MR characteristics. AJNR Am J Neuroradiol 17:1151–1160
11. Collins VP, Tihan T, VandenBerg SR, Burger PC, Hawkins C, Jones D, Giannini G, Rodriguez F, Figarella-Branger D (2016) Pilocytic astrocytoma. In: Louis DN (ed) WHO classification of tumours of the central nervous system. IARC Press, Lyon, pp 80–89
13. Constantini S, Miller DC, Allen JC, Rorke LB, Freed D, Epstein FJ (2000) Radical excision of intramedullary spinal cord tumors: surgical morbidity and long-term follow-up evaluation in 164 children and young adults. J Neurosurg Spine 93:183–193
14. Cristante L, Herrmann HD (1994) Surgical management of intramedullary spinal cord tumors: functional outcome and sources of morbidity. Neurosurgery 35:69–74.; ; discussion 74–76
15. Cristante L, Herrmann HD (1999) Surgical management of intramedullary hemangioblastoma of the spinal cord. Acta Neurochir (Wien) 141:333–339.; ; discussion 339–340
16. Epstein FJ, Farmer JP, Freed D (1992) Adult intramedullary astrocytomas of the spinal cord. J Neurosurg 77:355–359
17. Hassall TE, Mitchell AE, Ashley DM (2001) Carboplatin chemotherapy for progressive intramedullary spinal cord low-grade gliomas in children: three case studies and a review of the literature. Neuro Oncol 3:251–257
18. Hentschel SJ, McCutcheon IE, Ginsberg L, Weinberg JS (2004) Exophytic ependymomas of the spinal cord. Acta Neurochir (Wien) 146:1047–1050
19. Hernandez-Duran S, Hanft S, Komotar RJ, Manzano GR (2016) The role of stereotactic radiosurgery in the treatment of intramedullary spinal cord neoplasms: a systematic literature review. Neurosurg Rev 39:175–183.; ; discussion 183
20. Hersh DS, Iyer RR, Garzon-Muvdi T, Liu A, Jallo GI, Groves ML (2017) Instrumented fusion for spinal deformity after laminectomy or laminoplasty for resection of intramedullary spinal cord tumors in pediatric patients. Neurosurg Focus 43:E12
21. Hoshimaru M, Koyama T, Hashimoto N, Kikuchi H (1999) Results of microsurgical treatment for intramedullary spinal cord ependymomas: analysis of 36 cases. Neurosurgery 44:264–269

22. Houten JK, Cooper PR (2000) Spinal cord astrocytomas: presentation, management and outcome. J Neurooncol 47:219–224

23. Isaacson SR (2000) Radiation therapy and the management of intramedullary spinal cord tumors. J Neurooncol 47:231–238

24. Ishida Y, Suzuki K, Ohmori K, Kikata Y, Hattori Y (1989) Critical analysis of extensive cervical laminectomy. Neurosurgery 24:215–222

25. Jallo GI, Freed D, Epstein FJ (2004) Spinal cord gangliogliomas: a review of 56 patients. J Neurooncol 68:71–77

26. Juthani RG, Bilsky MH, Vogelbaum MA (2015) Current management and treatment modalities for intramedullary spinal cord tumors. Curr Treat Options in Oncol 16:39

27. Katsoulakis E, Jackson A, Cox B, Lovelock M, Yamada Y (2017) A detailed dosimetric analysis of spinal cord tolerance in high-dose spine radiosurgery. Int J Radiat Oncol Biol Phys 99:598–607

28. Kim CH, Wang KC, Kim SK, Chung YN, Choi YL, Chi JG, Cho BK (2003) Spinal intramedullary lipoma: report of three cases. Spinal Cord 41:310–315

29. Kim DH, Kim JH, Choi SH, Sohn CH, Yun TJ, Kim CH, Chang KH (2014) Differentiation between intramedullary spinal ependymoma and astrocytoma: comparative MRI analysis. Clin Radiol 69:29–35

30. Kim MS, Chung CK, Choe G, Kim IH, Kim HJ (2001) Intramedullary spinal cord astrocytoma in adults: postoperative outcome. J Neurooncol 52:85–94

31. Kothbauer K, Deletis V, Epstein FJ (1997) Intraoperative spinal cord monitoring for intramedullary surgery: an essential adjunct. Pediatr Neurosurg 26:247–254

32. Lamszus K, Lachenmayer L, Heinemann U, Kluwe L, Finckh U, Hoppner W, Stavrou D, Fillbrandt R, Westphal M (2001) Molecular genetic alterations on chromosomes 11 and 22 in ependymomas. Int J Cancer 91:803–808

33. Lee M, Epstein FJ, Rezai AR, Zagzag D (1998) Nonneoplastic intramedullary spinal cord lesions mimicking tumors. Neurosurgery 43:788–794.; ; discussion 785–794

34. Lee M, Rezai AR, Abbott R, Coelho DH, Epstein FJ (1995) Intramedullary spinal cord lipomas. J Neurosurg 82:394–400

35. Loius DN, Ohgaki H, Wiestler OD, Cavenee WK, Ellison DW, Figarella-Branger D, Perry A, Reifenberger G, von Deimling A. WHO classification of tumors of the central nervous system. Revised 4th ed. Lyon: IARC Press; 2016.

36. Lowe GM (2000) Magnetic resonance imaging of intramedullary spinal cord tumors. J Neurooncol 47:195–210

37. Macbeth FR, Wheldon TE, Girling DJ, Stephens RJ, Machin D, Bleehen NM, Lamont A, Radstone DJ, Reed NS (1996) Radiation myelopathy: estimates of risk in 1048 patients in three randomized trials of palliative radiotherapy for non-small cell lung cancer. The Medical Research Council Lung Cancer Working Party. Clin Oncol (R Coll Radiol) 8:176–181

38. Makary MS, Kirsch CF (2014) Tumefactive demyelinating disease with isolated spinal cord involvement. Acta Radiol Short Rep 3:2047981614539324

39. Mende KC, Kratzig T, Mohme M, Westphal M, Eicker SO (2017) Keyhole approaches to intradural pathologies. Neurosurg Focus 43:E5

40. Miller DC (2000) Surgical pathology of intramedullary spinal cord neoplasms. J Neurooncol 47:189–194

41. Morota N, Deletis V, Constantini S, Kofler M, Cohen H, Epstein FJ (1997) The role of motor evoked potentials during surgery for intramedullary spinal cord tumors. Neurosurgery 41:1327–1336

42. Naito K, Yamagata T, Arima H, Abe J, Tsuyuguchi N, Ohata K, Takami T (2015) Qualitative analysis of spinal intramedullary lesions using PET/CT. J Neurosurg Spine 23:613–619

43. Nakamura M, Ishii K, Watanabe K, Tsuji T, Takaishi H, Matsumoto M, Toyama Y, Chiba K (2008) Surgical treatment of intramedullary spinal cord tumors: prognosis and complications. Spinal Cord 46:282–286

44. Pai SB, Krishna KN (2003) Secondary holocord syringomyelia with spinal hemangioblastoma: a report of two cases. Neurol India 51:67–68

45. Pajtler KW, Witt H, Sill M, Jones DT, Hovestadt V, Kratochwil F, Wani K, Tatevossian R, Punchihewa C, Johann P, Reimand J, Warnatz HJ, Ryzhova M, Mack S, Ramaswamy V, Capper D, Schweizer L, Sieber L, Wittmann A, Huang Z, van Sluis P, Volckmann R, Koster J, Versteeg R, Fults D, Toledano H, Avigad S, Hoffman LM, Donson AM, Foreman N, Hewer E, Zitterbart K, Gilbert M, Armstrong TS, Gupta N, Allen JC, Karajannis MA, Zagzag D, Hasselblatt M, Kulozik AE, Witt O, Collins VP, von Hoff K, Rutkowski S, Pietsch T, Bader G, Yaspo ML, von Deimling A, Lichter P, Taylor MD, Gilbertson R, Ellison DW, Aldape K, Korshunov A, Kool M, Pfister SM (2015) Molecular classification of ependymal tumors across all CNS compartments, histopathological grades, and age groups. Cancer Cell 27:728–743

46. Parsa AT, Fiore AJ, McCormick PC, Bruce JN (2000) Genetic basis of intramedullary spinal cord tumors and therapeutic implications. J Neurooncol 47:239–251

47. Patel U, Pinto RS, Miller DC, Handler MS, Rorke LB, Epstein FJ, Kricheff II (1998) MR of spinal cord ganglioglioma. AJNR Am J Neuroradiol 19:879–887

48. Payer S, Mende KC, Westphal M, Eicker SO (2015) Intramedullary spinal cord metastases: an increasingly common diagnosis. Neurosurg Focus 39:E15

49. Pompili A, Crispo F, Raus L, Telera S, Vidiri A (2011) Symptomatic spinal cord necrosis after irradiation for vertebral metastatic breast cancer. J Clin Oncol 29:e53–e56

50. Prayson RA (1999) Clinicopathologic study of 61 patients with ependymoma including MIB-1 immunohistochemistry. Ann Diagn Pathol 3:11–18

51. Redmond KJ, Robertson S, Lo SS, Soltys SG, Ryu S, McNutt T, Chao ST, Yamada Y, Ghia A, Chang EL, Sheehan J, Sahgal A (2017) Consensus contouring guidelines for postoperative stereotactic body radia-

tion therapy for metastatic solid tumor malignancies to the spine. Int J Radiat Oncol Biol Phys 97:64–74

52. Richard S, Campello C, Taillandier L, Parker F, Resche F (1998) Haemangioblastoma of the central nervous system in von Hippel-Lindau disease. French VHL Study Group. J Intern Med 243:547–553

53. Sahgal A, Chou D, Ames C, Ma L, Lamborn K, Huang K, Chuang C, Aiken A, Petti P, Weinstein P, Larson D (2007) Image-guided robotic stereotactic body radiotherapy for benign spinal tumors: the University of California San Francisco preliminary experience. Technol Cancer Res Treat 6:595–604

54. Saleh J, Afshar F (1987) Spinal cord astrocytoma with intracranial spread: detection by magnetic resonance imaging. Br J Neurosurg 1:503–508

55. Sarikaya S, Acikgoz B, Tekkok IH, Gungen YY (2007) Conus ependymoma with holocord syringohydromyelia and syringobulbia. J Clin Neurosci 14:901–904

56. Schwartz TH, McCormick PC (2000) Intramedullary ependymomas: clinical presentation, surgical treatment strategies and prognosis. J Neurooncol 47:211–218

57. Seki T, Hida K, Yano S, Aoyama T, Koyanagi I, Houkin K (2015) Surgical outcomes of high-grade spinal cord gliomas. Asian Spine J 9:935–941

58. Stupp R, Mason WP, van den Bent MJ, Weller M, Fisher B, Taphoorn MJ, Belanger K, Brandes AA, Marosi C, Bogdahn U, Curschmann J, Janzer RC, Ludwin SK, Gorlia T, Allgeier A, Lacombe D, Cairncross JG, Eisenhauer E, Mirimanoff RO (2005) Radiotherapy plus concomitant and adjuvant temozolomide for glioblastoma. N Engl J Med 352:987–996

59. Sun B, Wang C, Wang J, Liu A (2003) MRI features of intramedullary spinal cord ependymomas. J Neuroimaging 13:346–351

60. Tampieri D, Leblanc R, TerBrugge K (1993) Preoperative embolization of brain and spinal hemangioblastomas. Neurosurgery 33:502–505.; ; discussion 505

61. van den Bent MJ (2004) Diagnosis and management of oligodendroglioma. Semin Oncol 31:645–652

62. Van Velthoven V, Reinacher PC, Klisch J, Neumann HP, Glasker S (2003) Treatment of intramedullary hemangioblastomas, with special attention to von Hippel-Lindau disease. Neurosurgery 53:1306–1313.; ; discussion 1304–1313

63. Viljoen S, Hitchon PW, Ahmed R, Kirby PA (2014) Cordectomy for intramedullary spinal cord glioblastoma with a 12-year survival. Surg Neurol Int 5:101

64. Wang C, Zhang J, Liu A, Sun B (2001) Surgical management of medullary hemangioblastoma. Report of 47 cases. Surg Neurol 56:218–226; discussion 217–226

65. Westphal M, Koch C (1999) Management of spinal dural arteriovenous fistulae using an interdisciplinary neuroradiological/neurosurgical approach: experience with 47 cases. Neurosurgery 45:451–457.; ; discussion 457–458

66. Wong CS, Fehlings MG, Sahgal A (2015) Pathobiology of radiation myelopathy and strategies to mitigate injury. Spinal Cord 53:574–580

67. Xia L, Lin S, Wang ZC, Li SW, Xu L, Wu J, Hao SY, Gao CC (2009) Tumefactive demyelinating lesions: nine cases and a review of the literature. Neurosurg Rev 32:171–179.; ; discussion 179

68. Yeh JS, Sgouros S, Walsh AR, Hockley AD (2001) Spinal sagittal malalignment following surgery for primary intramedullary tumours in children. Pediatr Neurosurg 35:318–324

Intradural Extramedullary Tumors

35

Roland Goldbrunner and Volker Neuschmelting

35.1 Epidemiology

Spinal intradural tumors are uncommon lesions with a fivefold smaller incidence than intracranial neoplasms. The total incidence of spinal intradural tumors varies from 3 to 10 per 100,000 population [1, 2]. In adults, about one third of these lesions are located within the spinal cord itself; two thirds are found extramedullary. In children, the ratio of intra-/extramedullary tumors is approximately 50% [2]. Respecting the intramedullary location, astrocytomas and ependymomas are the most common entities, whereas nerve sheath tumors (NST), such as schwannomas and neurofibromas, as well as meningiomas, are the most frequent extramedullary tumors. The incidence of meningiomas and NST is about equal in the Western population (25–35% of all intraspinal tumors); however, in Asian populations, spinal schwannomas are much more frequent than meningiomas with ratios of almost 4:1 in China and Japan [3].

Within the vertebral canal, intradural extramedullary tumors generally are most often encountered in the thoracic region, followed by the cervical section. Accordingly, 80% of meningiomas are thoracic; meningioma growth caudal to the level of the conus medullaris is very uncommon. Also, NSTs predominantly grow in the thoracic area. In contrast to meningiomas, the lumbosacral region seems to be affected with a similar incidence as the cervical section.

There is a strong female predominance in spinal meningiomas with 75–85% of meningiomas arising in women. They are found in any age group, but most occur between the fifth and eighth decades of life. In spinal nerve sheath tumors, there is no sex predilection in contrast to intracranial NST, which has a female to male ratio of 2:1. All ages are affected, but a peak incidence can be evaluated between the fourth and sixth decades of life.

35.2 Symptoms and Clinical Signs

Pain is the most common and usually the first symptom produced by extramedullary spinal tumors. It may precede the diagnosis of the (usually benign) tumor by about 2 years. Particularly in schwannomas affecting single nerve roots, the pain has a radicular character and may be indicative for the site of the lesion. Many intraspinal tumors create signs and symptoms with a combination of segmental and distant features. Segmental signs and symptoms comprise motor neuron defects one level lower by affection of the anterior roots or compression of the anterior horn cells as well as specific sensory losses by

R. Goldbrunner (✉) · V. Neuschmelting
Klinik für Allgemeine Neurochirurgie, Zentrum für Neurochirurgie, Uniklinikum Köln, Köln, Germany
e-mail: Roland.Goldbrunner@uk-koeln.de; volker.neuschmelting@uk-koeln.de

© Springer Nature Switzerland AG 2019
J.-C. Tonn et al. (eds.), *Oncology of CNS Tumors*, https://doi.org/10.1007/978-3-030-04152-6_35

659

involvement of the dorsal roots. Distant signs and symptoms are caused by affection of the ascending or descending longitudinal tracts, interrupting function below the level of the lesion. In case of the corticospinal tract, upper motor neuron deficits with spastic paresis may occur; in case of compression of the spinothalamic tract, pain and temperature sensation are decreased. If the dorsal tracts are affected, positional sense and vibration are disturbed, resulting in gait ataxia as a very common symptom. In case of extramedullary tumors, the affection of longitudinal tracts is caused by external compression, which often is unilateral. This explains the higher incidence of Brown-Sequard-like signs in extramedullary tumors compared to intramedullary tumors. Sympathetic and parasympathetic signs, which are caused by involvement of descending autonomic pathways, are more uncommon in extramedullary tumors compared to intramedullary lesions. However, large lumbar schwannomas or other mass lesions compressing the conus medullaris may present with bladder or bowel dysfunction as a first symptom.

Interpretation of the symptoms and clinical signs that may be produced by extradural mass lesions has to take into consideration that not every symptom is indicative of the level of spinal cord or root compression. An important factor to be deliberated is a potential vascular affection. Compression of radicular arteries or the anterior spinal artery may produce complex and unexpected signs and symptoms. Spinal cord regions located in the watershed zone between the large radicular arteries usually are the first regions to suffer when the vascular supply is compromised. These watershed-related symptoms may precede the symptoms of direct root or cord affection for months, leading to an incorrect clinical diagnosis. A third factor that might cause or aggravate unexpected signs and symptoms is tethering of the spinal cord or nerve roots by the tumor. The main symptom of tethering in adults is pain. Tethering as a primary symptom is a rare feature in extramedullary tumors; however, it might play a role if a recurrence is suspected and postoperative alterations of the arachnoid have to be differentiated from a real tumor recurrence.

35.3 Diagnostics

35.3.1 Synopsis

Magnetic resonance imaging (MRI) is the method of choice for visualization of intradural tumors. Contrast-enhanced T1-weighted images, T2-weighted images, and particularly constructive interference in steady-state (CISS) sequences provide data about exact localization, size, and relations to adjacent structures as well as fat-saturated sequences providing information about the fat content of the tissue (e.g., short-tau inversion recovery (STIR)). Therefore, MRI offers clues for the differential diagnosis of the most common extramedullary tumors (NST and meningiomas) from other lesions like myxopapillary filum terminale ependymomas, intradural lipoma, and others and provides crucial information needed for surgical planning [4].

Imaging of the spinal canal has been performed by myelography and computed tomography (CT) for many years; since the late 1980s, MRI has become the method of choice. Detailed MRI of the spine requires the use of dedicated surface coils, which improve the signal-to-noise ratio, provide greater tissue contrast resolution and greater spatial resolution, and make thinner slices possible. The sagittal plane provides the most diagnostic information and presents an overview over large areas of the spinal canal. Axial slices, more than coronal slices, offer additional anatomical information that might be necessary for surgical planning.

From the almost infinite number of options MRI offers to the investigator, several sequences have proven to be the most valuable in providing information about the tumor of interest. Routinely, T1-weighted (with and without application of the contrast medium gadolinium) and T2-weighted images are obtained with and without fat saturation. At many institutions, CISS sequences are also employed. CISS sequences have ultrashort repetition times (TR) and echo times (TE), providing the best contrast resolution of all sequences available. Therefore, these sequences contribute information about intratumoral cysts and involvement of nerve roots or even denticulate ligaments within the tumor mass. Additionally, they can display CSF signal between well-demarcated tumors and the cord parenchyma, allowing proper surgical planning.

There are very few indications for myelography or CT scans in the diagnostics of spinal tumors. In patients with contraindications for MRI, e.g., electronic implants like pacemakers, contrast-enhanced, high-resolution CT, in some cases also CT-myelography, is used to determine the level and the size of the tumor. CT may also be useful and provides additional information for surgical planning (e.g., dumbbell nerve sheath tumors).

35.3.2 Meningiomas

Spinal meningiomas are isointense to the spinal cord or slightly hyperintense on T2-weighted imaging and iso- or hypointense on T1-weighted images. They have a broad contact to the dura

and characteristically display a strong and homogeneous enhancement with gadolinium. Similar to intracranial meningiomas, contrast uptake may be seen beyond the solid tumor along the dural adhesion site, which is known as the "dural tail." These tumors are well circumscribed and delineated from the spinal cord. Calcified areas are dark on all MRI sequences and lack any contrast uptake. These calcified areas also can be detected by high-resolution CT (Fig. 35.1).

35.3.3 Nerve Sheath Tumors

Schwannomas are the most common nerve sheath tumors, followed by neurofibromas. Malignant NSTs are very rare entities within the spinal canal. Schwannomas are usually diagnosed as solitary. Since neurofibromas are associated with neurofibromatosis type I (von Recklinghausen's disease), these tumors are often found to be mul-

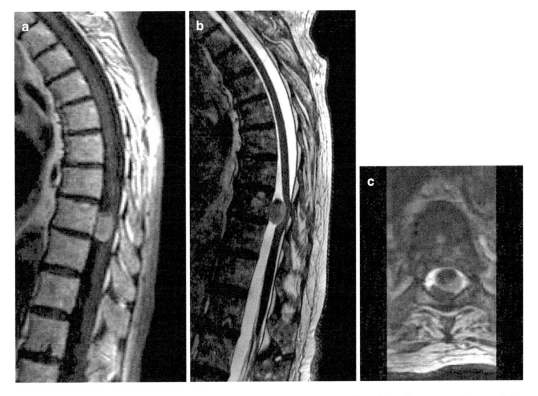

Fig. 35.1 (**a**) Sagittal T1-weighted MRI showing homogeneous contrast uptake and broad contact to the ventral dura. (**b**) Sagittal CISS sequence and (**c**) axial CISS sequence revealing clear demarcation between tumor and myelon

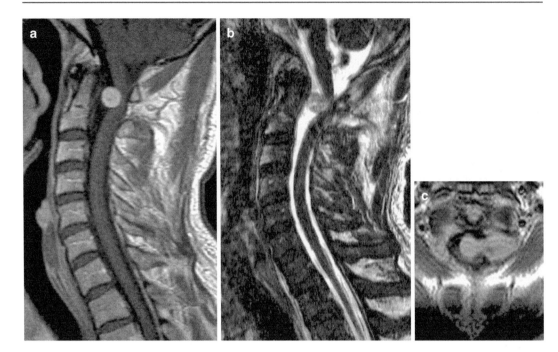

Fig. 35.2 (**a**) T1-weighted MRI showing a round, well-demarcated tumor with intense contrast uptake. (**b**) Sagittal CISS sequences imaging the compression of the myelon by the well-confined tumor. (**c**) Contrast-enhanced, axial T1 images displaying the typical dumbbell shape

tiple. Similar to meningiomas, both NST entities are isointense on T1-weighted images and hyperintense on T2-weighted imaging. Contrast enhancement is variable and can be very intense and homogeneous—like in meningiomas—while others display inhomogeneous or only faint enhancement at the periphery of the tumor (Fig. 35.2). The nerve root sleeve is often found to be enlarged as they arise from the nerve root. Neurofibromas occasionally show low signal areas within the tumor mass, representing dense areas of collagenous stroma. However, a clear distinction between schwannoma and neurofibroma is not reliable by neuroradiological means.

35.4 Staging and Classification

35.4.1 Synopsis

Nerve sheath tumors, comprising schwannomas and neurofibromas, and meningiomas are the most common intradural extramedullary tumors. These tumors are benign except for rare cases of malignant NST or anaplastic meningioma. There are a few malignant entities found in the intradural extramedullary site, e.g., drop metastases. There is a significant correlation of NST with neurofibromatosis type I, type II, or spinal schwannomatosis.

In 2016, the World Health Organization's (WHO) classification of tumors of the nervous system was updated [5]. This WHO classification and grading should be the basis for description and grading of intradural extramedullary tumors. As stated above, meningiomas and NST, comprising schwannomas, neurofibromas, and hybrid nerve sheath tumors, are the most common entities, having a very similar incidence [6]. The hybrid nerve sheath tumor is a newly defined entity and shows a combination of features of neurofibroma, schwannoma, or perineurioma. It most commonly occurs as a schwannoma/perineurioma or neurofibroma/schwannoma hybrid subtype. The melanotic schwannoma is also separated from the other schwannomas as a distinct entity according to the 2016 WHO classification. All those entities are benign (WHO grade I) in most cases. Other tumor entities found within the intradural extramedullary space are lipomas, dermoids, epidermoids, teratomas, hemangioblastomas, and paragangliomas. All these entities are very uncommon; there are only few case reports in the literature (reviewed in [7]). Also, these rare entities are benign; the only malignant tumor types in the intradural extramedullary space are malignant nerve sheath tumors (WHO grades III or IV), anaplastic meningiomas (WHO grade III), and hematogenous metastases or drop metastases, e.g., from medulloblastomas (WHO grade IV).

Meningiomas arise from arachnoid cluster cells and therefore are located preferably at the exit zones of nerve roots or entry zones of arteries in the spinal canal. They have a rubbery or firm consistency and are rounded or lobulated in most cases. In almost any case, they have a broad attachment to the dura, which can be used for diagnostics (see Sect. 35.3). Most meningiomas are purely intradural, but they also may grow intra- and extradurally. There are also reports about purely extradural spinal meningiomas as well as intramedullary meningioma growth [2]. Meningiomas usually are well vascularized and may show intense calcifications, which can be visible on CT. These calcifications may increase the consistency of the tumor and could influence the surgical strategy in case of a ventrally located, large, and highly calcified meningioma, which cannot be debulked due to its consistency. Atypical meningiomas (WHO grade II) constitute between 4.7 and 7.2% of all meningiomas; anaplastic meningiomas (WHO grade III) account for 1.0–2.8% of all meningiomas [8]. The percentage of these grades seems to occur even less often in the spine than intracranially, and thus, data on atypical meningioma in the spine are extremely scarce [9].

Schwannomas are derived from differentiated neoplastic Schwann cells nearly exclusively of the posterior sensory root; neurofibromas are composed of Schwann cells, perineurial-like cells, fibroblasts, and cells with intermediate features. Schwannomas are globoid, encapsulated masses with thick-walled, hyalinized tumor vessels and a lack of necrosis or calcifications. They are composed of Antoni A areas with closely packed tumor cells presenting nuclear palisades and Antoni B areas with loosely arranged tumor cells and clusters of lipid-laden cells. In both areas, so-called Verocay bodies can be found formed by roughly parallel arrays of tumor cell nuclei separated by dense, hypereosinophilic tissue. Neurofibromas have a firm consistency and often present a plexiform or multinodular shape. They may or may not be confined to a single nerve, surrounded by thickened epineurium. Typically the cells are surrounded by collagen fibers and a myxoid matrix; this is the reason for the firm consistency. Neurofibromas may contain atypical nuclei and show increased cellularity and mitotic figures, which can be interpreted as the basis for malignant progression [10]. Hybrid nerve sheath tumors contain features of both schwannoma and neurofibroma and/or perineurioma. However, in contrast to peripheral nerves, where malignant peripheral nerve sheath tumors (MPNST, WHO grade III or IV) are a well-defined entity representing 5% of all soft tissue tumors, malignant NSTs in the spinal canal are extremely rare. Most NSTs grow within the intradural extramedullary space but may extend via the nerve root sleeve, the intervertebral foramen into the extraspinal region (e.g., as dumbbell tumors) where they can reach enormous sizes. There are also reports about intramedullary schwannomas or neurofibromas, which can be explained by tumor growth originating from aberrant nerve roots. In case of association with neurofibromatosis type 1 or 2 (NF1 or NF2), multiple tumors may be present at different levels of the spinal cord. Neurofibromas and neurofibroma/perineurioma hybrid nerve sheath tumors are more common in NF1; schwannomas and neurofibroma/schwannoma hybrid nerve sheath tumors are typical for NF2 [5, 11]. However, the presence of multiple NSTs is not automatically indicative of the classical neurofibromatosis variants NF1 or NF2. Patients with multiple spinal schwannomas without bilateral vestibular neoplasms may have schwannomatosis, an autosomal dominantly inherited tumor suppressor syndrome with reduced penetrance linked to a germline SMARCB1 or LZTR1 pathogenic variants [12]. Individuals with familial schwannomatosis usually present within the second to fourth decade of life, while the sporadic form presents later in life [13]. Loss of heterozygosity and mutations of the NF-2 gene can occasionally be demonstrated in tumor specimens. However, there are no systemic alterations of the NF-2 gene on chromosome 22 excluding a germline mutation [14–17].

35.5 Treatment

35.5.1 Synopsis

Surgery is the method of choice for treatment of intradural extramedullary tumors. The uppermost cases of these tumors can be removed totally by surgical means and do not need further treatment. Electrophysiological monitoring of motor and sensory functions increases the safety of intraoperative procedures. Ultrasonography allows intraoperative imaging for exact approaching and provides information about tumor morphology transdurally. The approaches through the bony structures considering appropriate exposure and postoperative stability (laminectomy, laminoplasty) are discussed. Finally, the most advantageous ways of incision and closure of the dura and the techniques for debulking and complete resection of these tumors are shown.

35.5.2 Surgery

Since the vast majority of intradural extramedullary tumors are benign and since most of them are well circumscribed and show a clear demarcation to spinal cord tissue, surgery offers excellent chances for total removal and, thus, must be considered the therapy of choice for these lesions.

35.5.2.1 Preparation and Positioning
Patients should be informed about the high probability of a benign nature of these lesions once diagnosed by MRI. However, the risk of paraparesis or paraplegia during surgery by vascular irritation or direct affection of the spinal cord has

to be discussed. This risk may be significant in elderly patients or patients with a severe neurological deficit preoperatively. To minimize the risk of intramedullary edema and consequent neurological deterioration, steroids (methylprednisolone 8–16 mg/day) are routinely administered preoperatively. In case of intraoperative irritation of the spinal cord, additional steroid doses, up to 1000 mg methylprednisolone, are administered.

In thoracic and lumbosacral tumor locations, patients are positioned in a prone position. In cervical locations, also the sitting position may be chosen with the head fixed in the Mayfield clamp. Sitting position has the advantage of increased venous drainage to minimize congestion in the operated area. On the other hand, extensive CSF drainage possibly leading to intracranial subdural hematoma and the risk of air embolism are significant disadvantages of the sitting position. Additionally, in the prone position, the assistant, who is standing opposite to the surgeon, can work much more effectively than in the sitting position, which usually only allows one-handed assistance.

35.5.2.2 Monitoring
To assess neurological functions during surgery, electrophysiological monitoring is a standard procedure in intramedullary tumors. In extramedullary neoplasms, surgery for small and dorsally located tumors does not need electrophysiologic monitoring since the risk of harming the spinal cord is minimal. However, in large or ventrally located tumors, electrophysiologic monitoring may be very useful for intraoperative decision-making and for the prediction of neurologic outcome. The function of the dorsal columns is easily monitored by somatosensory evoked potentials (SSEP), which are bilaterally induced at the tibial nerve. In case of cervical tumors, these potentials also can be evoked by stimulation of the median nerve, which leads to more stable responses with shorter latencies. Motor-evoked potentials (MEP) by transcranial electrical or magnetic stimulation of the motor cortex allow monitoring of the function of the corticospinal tract. However, since MEP monitoring leads to mass movements of the stimulated

Table 35.1 Monitoring strategy depending on tumor location

	Cervical	Thoracic	Lumbosacral	Conus medullaris
SEP	++	++	(+)	++
EMG	++	−	++	++
MEP (ventral locations)	+	+	(+)	++

++ important, + helpful, − unnecessary

musculature, it only can be applied discontinuously, in contrast to SSEP. In extramedullary tumors, MEP monitoring may be helpful in ventral locations. An important method for monitoring nerve root function during surgery of a cervical or cauda equina NST is electromyographic (EMG) recording by single muscle electrodes, which allows (1) identification of single nerve roots and (2) monitoring of the current functional status of the nerve. Analogous to intramedullary tumors, special care is taken in tumors compressing the conus medullaris. In these cases, any of the electrophysiological methods could be very helpful. An overview of the monitoring strategy for large tumors dependent on the tumor location is shown in Table 35.1.

35.5.2.3 Approach

Most intradural extramedullary tumors can be operated on via the standard postero- or posterolateral approach. Before skin incision, the level of the lesion is marked under fluoroscopy. A midline skin incision is performed, and the laminae covering the spinal canal are exposed at the level of the pathologic process. Choosing the appropriate approach through the bony structures, optimal exposure of the tumor, and spinal stability are the most important concerns. The dural exposure should encompass the area of the tumor, leaving a space of some millimeters at the cranial and caudal margin of the process to allow for tumor mobilization and a watertight dural suture after the removal. For most tumor sizes and locations, one- or two-level laminectomy, which also may be partial laminotomy, is sufficient. In case of small lateral tumors, a hemilaminectomy is performed. If an intraforaminal NST is operated on, hemilaminectomy or laminectomy is combined with partial or total facetectomy. This approach also allows exposure of large, cervical dumbbell schwannomas

reaching several centimeters lateral to the level of the dura. In some cases of large lateroventral or ventral NST, an even more lateral approach may be necessary. This strategy requires a long midline or paramedian incision. The muscle masses are dissected far laterally and maintained by a retractor. The patient is tilted to the contralateral side to expose the posterolateral side of the spinal canal to the surgeon. After hemilaminectomy, one or two pedicles are drilled off subtotally providing adequate exposure of the ventrally located tumor. If this lateral approach is not sufficient for safe removal of large, ventral, and cervical tumors without traction of the spinal cord, a ventral approach performing a corpectomy with reconstruction is the safest choice [18]. Large dumbbell schwannomas may require a combined or a two-stage procedure. Thoracic or thoracolumbar dumbbell tumors are best exposed via the lateral extracavitary approach, which allows a combination of posterior midline access to the spinal canal and lateral access to the spine after complete mobilization of the paravertebral muscle mass [19]. The pleura is not opened during this approach; ribs do not necessarily have to be resected. Alternatively, a two-stage procedure may be chosen with resection of the intraspinal part via a posterior or posterolateral approach at the first and resection of the extraspinal part via a lateral approach at the second stage. For large ventrally located tumors, e.g., meningiomas, the best and safest exposure is via a transthoracic approach with vertebrectomy and reconstruction. The risk of procedure-related paraparesis is least using this approach. In large cervical dumbbell schwannomas, which cannot be resected by a posterolateral approach alone, an anterolateral cervicotomy via the lateral aspect of the carotid sheath is performed, permitting wide exposure of the extraspinal portion of the spinal roots.

If a multilevel approach is necessary (laminectomy over more than two levels), we prefer performing a laminoplasty with refixation of the incised lamina by nonresorbable sutures. This has been proven to avoid kyphosis and subluxation in children [20, 21]. Since instability is a common problem after multiple laminectomies in adults, this procedure has been introduced as a standard at our institution.

35.5.2.4 Ultrasonography

Ultrasonography has been employed for spinal diseases like dysraphism in infants for many years. Intraoperative sonography during spinal procedures—particularly during surgery of spinal tumors—is a relatively new indication. Transdural ultrasonography allows localization of the pathologic process precisely and in real time. Particularly cauda equina tumors might migrate cranially depending on the position of the patient [22]. Therefore, surgical planning with preoperative scans alone might not be sufficient. When the dura is exposed, ultrasound scanning of the myelon and the adjacent tumor is performed in the sagittal and transversal plane. Transdural visualization of the tumor makes sure that the exposure is sufficient and that there is enough space left rostrally and caudally of the tumor (see Sect. 35.5.2.3). Further removal of bone or ligaments after opening of the dura, usually leading to bleeding into the intradural space, is avoided. Ultrasonography also provides anatomical data of the tumor itself (cysts, hyperechoic areas) in real time and permits resection control; however, this information is much more valuable in intramedullary than in extramedullary processes.

35.5.2.5 Tumor Resection

In contrast to intramedullary lesions, where a median durotomy is by far the most frequent approach, in extramedullary tumors, dural incision has to be modified depending on the anatomical relation of the tumor and the myelon. In lateral tumors, the durotomy should be lateralized or slightly curved to choose the shortest way to the tumor without unnecessary exposure of the myelon. In ventrally located tumors, which have to be approached from a dorsolateral or ventrolateral direction, transverse cutting of the dura may be combined with a median or paramedian longitudinal incision. In NST extending into the intervertebrate foramen, the transverse dura incision parallels the dural root sleeve.

The vast majority of extramedullary tumors possess a clear demarcation toward the spinal cord, which facilitates preparation. Small tumors can be removed in toto after preparation of the tumor surface with standard microsurgical techniques. Large tumors have to be debulked first to avoid traction or pressure to the medulla. The safest way to perform debulking is the use of an ultrasonic aspirator. After that, the tumor surface can be prepared and the tumor mass removed as in smaller tumors.

In meningiomas, which may be strongly vascularized, the same strategy is used as in intracranial locations: The first step is to identify and dissect the area of dural attachment and primary vascular supply in order to avoid bleeding into the intradural and subarachnoidal space during further preparation. To keep the intradural space free of blood is one of the major concerns of the surgeon and one of the major tasks for the assistant. Simpson grade I resection and, thus, excision of the tumor adjacent dura are only recommended whenever practicable in posteriorly or posterolaterally located tumors in younger patients or dumbbell-type meningiomas.

The strategy in NST is to identify the nerve root of origin first (Fig. 35.3). In large tumor masses, debulking may be necessary to get a sufficient overview. Preservation of the motor root and most sensory fascicles is usually possible with dorsal root NST. When the intraspinal tumor mass is removed, the dural sleeve of the root is opened. In nearly all cases of NST, the tumor originates from a dorsal root; therefore, motor function can be preserved (with valuable aid of EMG monitoring). If root preservation seems possible, an intrafascicular tumor dissection has to be performed. However, if the tumor extends into the nerve root sleeve beyond the dorsal root ganglion, total extirpation is only

Fig. 35.3 Dumbbell schwannoma of the right C2 dorsal nerve root. The dura has been opened in a T-shaped fashion to expose the myelon (*M*) as well as the tumor (*T*) along the root

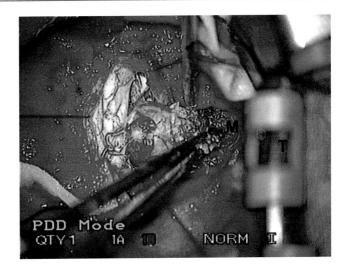

possible if the entire nerve is sacrificed. Therefore, this situation has to be discussed with the patient, and the decision for radical resection versus preservation of function has to be made prior to the procedure. If the nerve root is dissected, a complete separation of all nerve root and dural tissue from the intraspinal dura has to be carried out to make a watertight closure of the dura possible using autologous grafts, lyophilized fascia lata, or artificial compounds containing fibrin. If the root is preserved, the use of fibrin glue or analogous compounds is encouraged, since a complete dural reconstruction by suture is difficult to perform intraforaminally.

There are no additional considerations for surgery of benign extramedullary neoplasms other than meningioma or NST except for the filum terminale myxopapillary ependymomas: In the latter the integrity of the tumor capsule in an en bloc resection approach reduces the risk of local recurrence due to minimizing the risk of CSF seeding ependymoma cell in cases of capsule opening [23]. Lipomas, dermoids, epidermoids, or teratomas may occur in combination with dysraphism. In these cases, clinical investigation, and X-ray of the spine may provide additional information. Surgery usually is not the first option for systemic metastases or drop metastases of medulloblastomas. In these cases, radiotherapy and/or chemotherapy is the first choice.

35.6 Radiotherapy and Chemotherapy

Since the vast majority of intradural extramedullary tumors are benign and can be removed completely by surgical means, radio- and chemotherapy only play a marginal role in these entities. Recurrent meningiomas or NSTs usually occur in case of subtotal removal. In these tumors, repeated surgery offers a good chance of total or subtotal resection without adding to the patient's neurological deficit. In case of anaplastic meningiomatosis or malignant NST, adjuvant irradiation of the spine may be indicated after surgery. Many patients suffering from medulloblastoma present with spinal tumor manifestation. In these patients, irradiation and chemotherapy within a therapeutic concept (e.g., HIT regimen) are performed. The role of spinal radiosurgery, an upcoming technique, still has to be determined and is performed in patients with recurrent or residual disease or in cases where surgery in contraindicated. Satisfactory short-term results have been reported in a case series of 103 patients with only one tumor progression within the 33 months follow-up period [24]. However, dealing with benign lesions in most cases, long-term data about radiosurgery-associated toxicity on the spinal cord are still lacking, and because the therapeutic effect of radiosurgery requires time to settle in, radiosurgery remains a therapeutic option only in a distinct subset of patients.

35.7 Prognosis and Functional Outcome

The overall prognosis of patients with intradural extramedullary tumors is excellent. The majority of these tumors are benign, and if the tumor has been removed thoroughly, the patient is cured from the oncological point of view. Total removal is accomplished in 89–98% of patients in larger series [25–28]. Data about recurrence rates differ widely from 1 to 14.4% in the same series; there is no significant difference between meningiomas and NST. In a long-term retrospective case series of 64 patients, however, meningiomas WHO I recurred in approximately 30% of patients who underwent Simpson grade II resection 12 years thereafter on average [29]. In atypical meningioma of the spine, a case series of 17 patients found the 5-year overall and progression-free survival rate to be approximately 84% and 85%, respectively [9].

The functional outcome is dependent on the preoperative neurological status. Thus, surgery performed at an early stage of the disease provides the best results. In our series of 40 intradural extramedullary tumors, operated on within 2 years, patients were graded according to the McCormick score (Table 35.2 [30]) preoperatively and 6 months after surgery. Of 35 patients with grades I and II preoperatively, 27 showed improvement of the neurological status for at least 1 grade, with 14 patients remaining without any neurological deficit (grade 0) 6 months postoperatively. There was no deterioration to grades III and IV in these patients. Among the small group of preoperative grades III and IV patients, three patients improved to grades 0 and I, and two patients stayed unchanged at grade IV. Similar data are presented in other series [25–28] with even better

Table 35.2 Functional classification scheme [30]

Grade	Definition
0	No deficit
1	Mild focal deficit not significantly affecting function of involved limb; mild spasticity or reflex abnormality; normal gait
2	Presence of sensorimotor deficit affecting function of involved limb; mild to moderate gait difficulty; severe pain or dysesthetic syndrome impairing patient's quality of life; still functions and ambulates independently
3	More severe neurological deficit; requires cane/brace for ambulation; may or may not function independently
4	Severe deficit; major sensorimotor deficit of more than one limb; patient functionally fully dependent

outcomes at later follow-up stages. It has to be kept in mind that in patients with a poor neurological status, recovery might take 2 years or even longer and that intense physiotherapeutic effort can be regarded as very beneficial for these patients [31].

The anatomical location of the tumor has been identified as a prognostic factor for neurological outcome: tumors of the upper anterior thoracic spine cause the highest rate of surgical complications [32].

35.8 Follow-Up/Specific Problems and Measures

In benign extramedullary tumors without suspected neurofibromatosis, there is no need for a regular follow-up during a patient's lifetime. If the tumor is resected completely, we recommend a clinical and MRI control 1 year after surgery with another follow-up after 3 years. In case of incomplete resection or malignancies, a follow-up dependent on the histology and growth characteristics of the tumor is performed. In patients with different types of neurofibromatosis or schwannomatosis, MRI is performed annually. In these patients, we recommend a conservative attitude operating only on progressive or symptomatic lesions.

35.9 Future Perspectives

Surgery at early stages of the disease provides the best outcomes. Since first symptoms usually precede the diagnosis by about 2 years, efforts have to be made to perform MRI as the most sensitive diagnostic tool as soon as possible. Significant progress has been made within recent years in improving surgical approaches to the spine. However, further optimization of small-sized approaches and more refined surgical techniques may allow better function preservation rates despite radical tumor resection. Further development of spinal radiosurgery using linear accelerators including the CyberKnife technique or the gamma knife may lead to a valuable addition to the treatment options for complex intradural, extramedullary tumors.

References

1. Sloof JL, Kernohan JW, MacCarthy CS (1964) Primary intramedullary tumors of the spinal cord and filum terminale. W.B. Saunders, Philadelphia
2. Stein BM, McCormick PC (1996) Spinal intradural tumors. In: Wilkins RH, Rengachary SS (eds) Neurosurgery. McGraw-Hill, New York, pp 1769–1781
3. Cheng MK (1982) Spinal cord tumors in the People's Republic of China: a statistical review. Neurosurgery 10:22–24
4. Abul-Kasim K, Thurnher MM, McKeever P, Sundgren PC (2008) Intradural spinal tumors: current classification and MRI features. Neuroradiology 50:301–314
5. Sahm F, Reuss ED, Giannini C (2018) WHO 2016 classification: changes and advancements in the diagnosis of miscellaneous primary CNS tumours. Neuropathol Appl Neurobiol 44:163–171
6. Traut D, Shaffrey ME, Schiff D (2007) Part I: spinal-cord neoplasms—intradural neoplasms. Lancet Oncol 8:35–45
7. Van Goethem JW, van den HL, Ozsarlak O, De Schepper AM, Parizel PM (2004) Spinal tumors. Eur J Radiol 50:159–176
8. Louis DN, Budka H, von Deimling A (2000) Meningeal tumours. In: Kleihues P, Cavenee WK (eds) Tumours of the nervous system. International Agency for Research on Cancer (IARC), Lyon, pp 133–152
9. Noh SH, Kim KH, Shin DA, Park JY, Yi S, Kuh SU, Kim KN, Chin DK, Kim KS, Yoon DH, Cho YE (2018) Treatment outcomes of 17 patients with atypical spinal meningioma, including 4 with metastases: a retrospective observational study. Spine J. [Epub ahead of print]
10. Woodruff JM, Kourea HP, Louis DN (2000) Tumours of cranial and peripheral nerves. In: Kleihues P, Cavenee WK (eds) Tumours of the nervous system. International Agency for Research on Cancer (IARC), Lyon, pp 125–132
11. Mautner VF, Schroder S, Pulst SM, Ostertag H, Kluwe L (1998) Neurofibromatosis versus schwannomatosis. Fortschr Neurol Psychiatr 66:271–277
12. Merker VL, Esparza S, Smith MJ, Stemmer-Rachamimov A, Plotkin SR (2012) Clinical features of schwannomatosis: a retrospective analysis of 87 patients. Oncologist 17:1317–1322
13. Koontz NA, Wiens AL, Agarwal A, Hingtgen CM, Emerson RE, Mosier KM (2013) Schwannomatosis: the overlooked neurofibromatosis? AJR Am J Roentgenol 200:W646–W653
14. Kaufman DL, Heinrich BS, Willett C, Perry A, Finseth F, Sobel RA et al (2003) Somatic instability of the NF2 gene in schwannomatosis. Arch Neurol 60:1317–1320
15. Leverkus M, Kluwe L, Roll EM, Becker G, Brocker EB, Mautner VF et al (2003) Multiple unilateral schwannomas: segmental neurofibromatosis type 2 or schwannomatosis? Br J Dermatol 148:804–809
16. MacCollin M, Willett C, Heinrich B, Jacoby LB, Acierno JS Jr, Perry A et al (2003) Familial schwannomatosis: exclusion of the NF2 locus as the germline event. Neurology 60:1968–1974
17. Seppala MT, Sainio MA, Haltia MJ, Kinnunen JJ, Setala KH, Jaaskelainen JE (1998) Multiple schwannomas: schwannomatosis or neurofibromatosis type 2? J Neurosurg 89:36–41
18. O'Toole JE, McCormick PC (2003) Midline ventral intradural schwannoma of the cervical spinal cord resected via anterior corpectomy with reconstruction: technical case report and review of the literature. Neurosurgery 52:1482–1485
19. McCormick PC, Torres R, Post KD, Stein BM (1990) Intramedullary ependymoma of the spinal cord. J Neurosurg 72:523–532
20. Abbott R, Feldstein N, Wisoff JH, Epstein FJ (1992) Osteoplastic laminotomy in children. Pediatr Neurosurg 18:153–156
21. Raimondi AJ, Gutierrez FA, Di Rocco C (1976) Laminotomy and total reconstruction of the posterior spinal arch for spinal canal surgery in childhood. J Neurosurg 45:555–560
22. Friedman JA, Wetjen NM, Atkinson JL (2003) Utility of intraoperative ultrasound for tumors of the cauda equina. Spine 28:288–290

23. Nakamura M, Ishii K, Watanabe K, Tsuji T, Matsumoto M, Toyama Y, Chiba K (2009) Long-term surgical outcomes for myxopapillary ependymomas of the cauda equina. Spine (Phila Pa 1976) 34:E756–E760

24. Sachdev S, Dodd RL, Chang SD, Soltys SG, Adler JR, Luxton G, Choi CY, Tupper L, Gibbs IC (2011) Stereotactic radiosurgery yields long-term control for benign intradural, extramedullary spinal tumors. Neurosurgery 69:533–539

25. Conti P, Pansini G, Mouchaty H, Capuano C, Conti R (2004) Spinal neurinomas: retrospective analysis and long-term outcome of 179 consecutively operated cases and review of the literature. Surg Neurol 61:34–43

26. King AT, Sharr MM, Gullan RW, Bartlett JR (1998) Spinal meningiomas: a 20-year review. Br J Neurosurg 12:521–526

27. Klekamp J, Samii M (1999) Surgical results for spinal meningiomas. Surg Neurol 52:552–562

28. Solero CL, Fornari M, Giombini S, Lasio G, Oliveri G, Cimino C et al (1989) Spinal meningiomas: review of 174 operated cases. Neurosurgery 25:153–160

29. Nakamura M, Tsuji O, Fujiyoshi K et al (2012) Long-term surgical outcomes of spinal meningiomas. Spine 37:E617–E623

30. McCormick PC (1996) Surgical management of dumbbell and paraspinal tumors of the thoracic and lumbar spine. Neurosurgery 38:67–74

31. Eriks IE, Angenot EL, Lankhorst GJ (2004) Epidural metastatic spinal cord compression: functional outcome and survival after inpatient rehabilitation. Spinal Cord 42:235–239

32. Mehta AI, Adogwa O, Karikari IO, Thompson P, Verla T, Null UT, Friedman AH, Cheng JS, Bagley CA, Isaacs RE (2013) Anatomical location dictating major surgical complications for intradural extramedullary spinal tumors: a 10-year single-institutional experience. J Neurosurg Spine 19:701–707

Epidural Tumors and Metastases

36

Krisztina Moldovan, Jared Fridley,
Thomas Kosztowski, and Ziya Gokaslan

36.1 Introduction

Tumors originating from the spinal column can be categorized into either primary or metastatic tumors. Primary spinal tumors are relatively rare, comprising less than 10% of all spinal neoplasms, while metastatic spine disease is quite common [1, 2]. Cancer was the second most common cause of death in the United States in 2016 [3]. Complications from metastatic disease are one of the major causes of morbidity and mortality in cancer patients [4]. The skeletal system follows the lung and liver as the third most commonly affected by metastatic disease, and within the skeletal system, the spine is the most frequently involved bone structure [5–8]. Autopsy studies have reported vertebral metastases in 90% of patients with prostate cancer, 74% of those with breast cancer, 45% with lung cancer, and 29% with lymphoma or renal cell carcinoma [9]. Vertebral metastases are a significant cause of pain and suffering in cancer patients, as they can affect neurological function, mobility, and quality of life [10, 11]. Studies have shown that up to half of patients with spinal metastases end up needing some kind of treatment for their symptoms, and 5–10% require surgical intervention [1, 4, 12, 13]. Improving systemic treatments for cancer and lengthened overall survival for cancer patients continue to improve, which has led to an increased overall incidence of spinal metastases [3].

Treatment of primary and metastatic spinal disease can be challenging and requires a multidisciplinary approach to management. While the goal of treatment for primary spinal tumors is often obtaining a cure, treatment for spinal metastases is palliative in nature, focused on improvement in neurologic function, pain, and overall quality of life. Differentiation between primary and metastatic tumors pathologically is key to optimal patient treatment outcomes.

36.2 Epidemiology

36.2.1 Metastatic Tumors

The most common etiologies of spinal metastatic disease are breast, lung, prostate, and renal malignancies [4, 14]. Breast cancer is the most common of these with up to 85% of patients developing bone metastases during the course of their illness [15]. Most spinal metastases are found in the thoracic spine (45–70%), followed by lumbar spine (20–35%) and the cervical spine (10–20%).These percentages loosely correlate

K. Moldovan · J. Fridley · T. Kosztowski
Z. Gokaslan (✉)
Department of Neurosurgery, Warren Alpert Medical School of Brown University, Providence, RI, USA
e-mail: kmoldovan@Lifespan.org;
Jared.Fridley@lifespan.org;
Ziya.Gokaslan@Lifespan.org

© Springer Nature Switzerland AG 2019
J.-C. Tonn et al. (eds.), *Oncology of CNS Tumors*, https://doi.org/10.1007/978-3-030-04152-6_36

Table 36.1 Primary tumors of the spine

Intramedullary
Astrocytoma
Ependymoma
Hemangioblastoma
Intradural extramedullary
Schwannoma
Neurofibroma
Meningioma
Extradural tumors
Metastases
Benign primary spinal tumors
Hemangiomas, osteoid osteoma, osteoblastoma, giant-cell tumor, osteochondroma, aneurysmal bone cyst, eosinophilic granuloma
Malignant primary spinal tumors: solitary plasmacytoma, chordoma, chondrosarcoma, osteosarcoma

with the combined volumes of the vertebral bodies in each region [2, 4, 16–18].

When considering primary spine tumors, one can classify them into three general categories: (1) intramedullary, (2) intradural extramedullary, and (3) extradural tumors (Table 36.1). Extradural tumors, which primarily are metastases, are the most common tumors of the spine. Primary spinal neoplasms comprise less than 10% of all spinal epidural tumors [1, 2]. Their pathology correlates with the age at presentation, with younger patients more likely to have benign lesions compared to the older population. The mean age at diagnosis for benign lesions is 21 years old compared with 49 years old for malignant tumors [19, 20]. Benign primary tumors include hemangiomas, osteoid osteoma, osteoblastoma, giant-cell tumor, osteochondroma, aneurysmal bone cyst, and eosinophilic granuloma. Malignant primary epidural spinal tumors include solitary plasmacytoma, chordoma, chondrosarcoma, and osteosarcoma.

36.2.2 Benign Primary Tumors

Hemangiomas are the most common benign primary spinal tumor and are typically diagnosed incidentally on spinal imaging. They are relatively common, with nearly 11% of people found to harbor these on autopsy [21]. Hemangiomas

originate in the vertebral body in nearly all patients; rarely are they seen in the posterior elements (10%). Imaging characteristics are pathognomonic, and only rarely is tissue required for diagnosis. Computed tomography (CT) of the spine reveals a characteristic "polka dot" appearance. They are mostly asymptomatic and rarely (<1% of cases) can cause pain or neurological deficit if they expand and fracture the vertebral body, potentially causing cord compression [22].

Osteoid osteomas have a peak age of 10–20 years with a male predominance; they are most frequently detected in long bones, but in 10% of cases, they can involve the spine [23–25]. They are usually found in the neural arch, rarely in the body of the vertebra, and frequently in the lumbar spine. Radiographs show a central lucent area with variable amount of mineralization and surrounding sclerosis. This central area of lucency represents the nidus which is less than 2 cm in size [26]. Presenting symptoms include scoliosis and pain, worse at night, which responds to nonsteroidal anti-inflammatory drugs (NSAIDs) or aspirin [20].

Osteoblastomas are similar to osteoid osteoma, with a male predominance and age of presentation in the second decade, but in contrast to osteoid osteomas are greater than 2 cm in size. They are most frequently found in the posterior elements of the cervical spine and cause pain which is less readily responsive to anti-inflammatory medications than in the case of osteoid osteoma [27, 28].

Giant-cell tumors have a peak age of 10–40 years with a female predominance; although they are usually found in the long bones, in rare instances, they can occur in the sacrum or elsewhere in the spine. These are lytic, expansile lesions which are locally aggressive with destruction of the bone; they frequently hemorrhage, recur, and rarely can undergo malignant transformation (5–10% of cases) or even metastasize (2–3% of cases) [1, 29].

Aneurysmal bone cysts are benign lytic vascular lesions consisting of thin-walled blood cavities without endothelium. They are found frequently in females and often present prior to the second decade. These lesions are frequently found in the long bones, but in 20% of cases, they are found in the spine. Within the spine, they are typically found in the posterior elements of the cervical and thoracic segments [15, 20, 30]. Presenting symptoms include pain, swelling, fracture, and compression [31–33].

Eosinophilic granulomas (Langerhans cell histiocytosis of the bone) are benign lytic lesions of unknown etiology presenting in the first decade of life, more commonly in males. They are often found in the skull, but can be seen in the spine as well, predominantly in the thoracic and lumbar segments. Within the spine, they are classically diagnosed on imaging as a single collapsed vertebral body (vertebrae plana) [22, 34–38].

36.2.3 Malignant Primary Tumors

Solitary plasmacytomas are the most common primary malignancy of the spine, seen in patients in their fifth to sixth decades of life, more commonly in men than women [15, 22]. Plasma cell neoplasms are characterized by the neoplastic proliferation of a single clone of plasma cells, which produce a monoclonal immunoglobulin. In the case of solitary plasmacytoma, they present as a single lesion, while in the case of multiple myeloma, they present as multiple lesions [39, 40].

Chordomas are the second most common primary malignancy of the spine with a peak age of 50–60 and 2:1 male predominance [41]. These lesions derive from notochord remnants and are found at the ends of the spinal axis, in the sacrum (50%), clivus (35%), and less often vertebral bodies (15%) [42]. They are locally aggressive lesions which destroy surrounding bone and can be very difficult to resect. They can metastasize and 2–8% may transform into sarcoma [43, 44].

Chondrosarcomas are rare malignant neoplasms which comprise approximately 10% of malignant primary spinal tumors [15, 20]. Their histologic appearance can range from a benign-appearing round cell tumor to a more malignant-appearing spindle cell sarcoma. These tumors have no sex predilection, have a propensity to appear in the thoracic spine, and appear in a middle-aged population with the median age of 45 [45].

Osteosarcomas are rare, primary bone neoplasms most commonly seen in the metaphysis of the long bones. They do rarely occur in the spine as well with an incidence of 0.85–2% [20, 46]. Up to 30% of spinal osteosarcomas are reported to be secondary radiation-induced tumors following treatment for Paget's disease. Patients affected by radiation-induced osteosarcomas tend to be significantly older than those with primary osteosarcoma [15, 20].

36.3 Clinical Presentation

The most common presenting complaint for patients with metastatic lesions in the spine is pain. The type of pain that a patient experiences depends on extent and location of metastatic lesions in the spine. Patients can experience radicular pain, which is usually described as a sharp, shooting, or burning pain which radiates down the arms or legs (or in a band-like distribution across the chest and abdomen in the thoracic spine) in a dermatomal distribution. Patients with spinal tumors can experience this type of pain when tumor extends into the neural foramen causing nerve root compression or when the neural foramen is narrowed due to vertebral body collapse as a result of pathological fracture. Patients can also suffer from mechanical back pain, which is described as pain worsened with standing/weight-bearing, ambulation, and improved in the recumbent position. Mechanical pain results from loss of integrity of the spinal column and inability of the spine to provide the structural stability it was designed for. Tumors can infiltrate and replace vertebral bodies and posterior elements, oftentimes leading to compression fractures or vertebral body collapse, weakening the support structure of the spinal column and leading to mechanical pain. Mechanical pain rarely responds to pain medications or palliative radiation, and patients frequently require bracing or surgical stabilization to achieve pain relief. Lastly, patients with metastatic spine lesions can also experience oncologic or biological pain, which is said to result from periosteal stretching and inflammation. This pain is often nocturnal and has a deep aching quality; unlike mechanical pain, it responds to anti-inflammatory medications and palliative radiation.

Neurological dysfunction is the second most common presenting symptom for patients affected by metastatic spine tumors. Neurological deficits most often result from epidural extension of tumors which can result in nerve root, cord, or cauda equina compression. Pathological fractures resulting from tumor invasion of vertebral bodies can also cause bony retropulsion into the spinal canal leading to compression or irritation of neural elements. Depending on the degree of tumor invasion and the levels involved, neurologic deficits can range from radiculopathy with sensory or focal motor weakness due to nerve root impingement to myelopathy (with weakness of proximal muscle groups, difficulty ambulating, hyperreflexia, and ataxia) from spinal cord compression or cauda equina syndrome with urinary/bowel dysfunction, saddle anesthesia, and sexual dysfunction.

Early recognition of the above symptoms is helpful to guide treatment and accurately gauge patient prognosis. The prevalence of degenerative back pain in the general population can pose a problem to clinicians in recognizing which patients to work up more thoroughly vs. treat conservatively. Back pain in any patient with a history of malignancy should prompt clinicians to perform an expedited workup for metastatic disease of the spine with MRI of the affected region.

36.4 Diagnostic Workup

Performing a detailed history and physical exam is perhaps the most vital step in ultimately diagnosing a neoplastic spinal process. Patients with a past medical history of cancer; systemic signs of malignancy such as unintended weight loss, night sweats, etc.; or cancer risk factors such as tobacco use should have an expedited workup. In patients with known cancer history and new back pain, imaging should be obtained even in the absence of neurological dysfunction.

36.4.1 Laboratory Tests

Laboratory serum studies, such as a complete blood cell count (CBC), can reveal abnormalities that raise suspicion for malignancy. Anemia, thrombocytopenia, and neutropenia/leukocytosis can all be associated with malignancy. More specific serum studies such as prostate-specific antigen (PSA) can point to specific pathology. If multiple myeloma is suspected, a serum protein electrophoresis (SPEP) and urine protein electrophoresis (UPEP) can be useful. A bone marrow biopsy is used to confirm suspicion of a hematologic malignancy such as multiple myeloma.

36.4.2 Imaging

36.4.2.1 Plain Radiographs

Plain film radiographs often serve as the initial imaging modality in the evaluation of patients with back pain due to their low cost and widespread availability. Despite their many limitations, plain films can help identify abnormalities such as compression fractures with significant loss of height or scoliosis/deformity as a result of large lytic lesions. Plain films can reveal a metastatic tumor in 85% of patients presenting with symptomatic epidural compression [4]. They can also sometimes point to metastatic tumor involvement through subtler signs such as loss of a pedicle on the AP view if the tumor spreads toward the posterior elements [47]. In the event of mechanical neck or back pain, dynamic flexion-extension plain films can be helpful in determining if there is associated radiographic instability. However, despite their ability to identify significant profound pathology, plain films are a poor screening tool for visualizing metastatic lesions of the spine and are unable to reliably detect subtler findings that are of clinical significance. Metastases would have to be large and cause a significant amount of deformity for them to be reliably identified; usually at least 50% loss of vertebral body height is necessary to identify the fracture [12, 48, 49]. For this reason, they should not be relied upon in the workup of patients with known malignancy or with high suspicion of metastatic lesions. As will be discussed, CT and MRI are the most commonly used imaging modalities when assessing spinal tumors and determining treatment plans.

36.4.2.2 Technetium 99 (Tc-99) Bone Scan

A nuclear bone scan can detect osseous metastatic lesions by identifying areas of increased osteoblastic activity in the skeleton. 99 m Tc-methylene diphosphonate tracer (Tc-99) accumulates in areas of increased bone turnover ("hot spots") and can detect lesions as small as 2 cm [4]. A Tc-99 study can be an excellent screening modality in that the entire skeletal system can be evaluated at once for osseous lesions. In patients with known cancer-producing osteoblastic or mixed lytic/blastic lesions, a bone scan is useful in evaluating the extent of skeletal metastatic disease. In patients with a variety of malignancies, Tc-99 has reasonable sensitivity (79–86%) and specificity (81–88%) for diagnosing bone metastases [50–53]. Limitations of this diagnostic tool include that it cannot usually identify lesions with little or no osteoblastic activity such as multiple myeloma (MM); in the case of MM lesions, for example, bone scan is positive only 20% of the time [51–53]. Furthermore, bone scan cannot differentiate between benign and malignant lesions; lesions positive on bone scan can reflect a neoplastic process, but the differential also includes infectious, inflammatory, or traumatic etiologies.

36.4.2.3 Positron Emission Tomography Scanning (PET)

PET imaging detects increased metabolic activity by identifying the uptake of fluorine-18 deoxyglucose in metabolically active tissues. 18-FDG-PET/CT is frequently used in clinical staging for metastatic disease, and for certain malignancies (lung, breast cancer), PET is more specific,

although less sensitive, in detecting lesions compared to a Tc-99 bone scan. In a meta-analysis of 13 studies of patients with metastatic breast cancer, on a per-patient basis, PET had sensitivity and specificity of 53% and 100% vs. 88% and 96% for bone scan, whereas on a per-lesion basis, the sensitivity and specificity of PET were 83% and 95% compared to 87% and 88% for a Tc-99 scan [54]. PET has the advantage of screening tissues other than bone for metastatic lesions, and in the skeletal system, it can detect lytic lesions, whereas a Tc-99 scan is less reliable in patients whose tumors do not have a significant component of osteoblastic activity [55]. The National Comprehensive Cancer Network (NCCN) recommends PET for evaluation of patients with newly diagnosed lung cancer, anaplastic thyroid, and some head and neck cancers.

36.4.2.4 Computed Tomography (CT)

Multidetector CT scanners obtain rapid, high resolution images of the spine and surrounding structures with excellent bony detail, enabling accurate assessment of bony integrity and detection of both osteolytic and osteoblastic lesions [56, 57]. Both osteolytic and osteoblastic metastases can be visualized on CT. Malignancy-producing osteolytic lesions include lung, GI, renal cell, melanoma, and multiple myeloma. Osteoblastic metastases include breast, prostate, and medullary thyroid carcinomas and appear as sclerotic and hyperdense. CT is useful in assessing the structural integrity of the spinal column and in planning any surgical stabilization procedures.

Although CT is cheaper and more easily obtainable than MRI, it has far less soft tissue resolution and therefore cannot assess spinal cord or nerve root compression as accurately as MRI in cases where involvement of neural elements is suspected. CT myelography may be useful in determining the presence of epidural tumor compression in patients unable to undergo MRI such as those patients with pacemakers and claustrophobia or in patients in which there is significant imaging artifact on MRI due to previously placed hardware.

36.4.2.5 Magnetic Resonance Imaging (MRI)

MRI is the gold standard imaging modality for evaluating spinal tumors due to its superior ability to visualize tumor and adjacent soft tissue or neural element involvement [51, 58]. In a meta-analysis of multiple imaging modalities for diagnosis of vertebral metastases, MRI was superior to both CT and PET scan on a per-lesion basis with a sensitivity and specificity of 94% [59].

Metastatic vertebral lesions are identified on MRI by comparing bone marrow density to normal parameters based on the patient's age. On T1-weighted imaging, bone marrow usually appears hypointense in children, transitioning to isointense and finally to hyperintense in adults. Metastatic lesions to the bone are T1 hypointense due to the replacement of bone marrow with tumor. In patients with pathologic spinal fractures, T1 hypointensity can often be detected around the fracture [60]. On T2-weighted imaging, the signal characteristics of metastatic lesions are less predictable. Although metastatic bony lesions are often easily identified on non-contrast MRI studies, intravenous gadolinium administration significantly improves the detection of extra-vertebral tumor and is therefore very important in evaluating for epidural extension of disease [47]. It is important to note that when patients are found to have a metastatic lesion in the spine, complete contrast-enhanced MRI imaging of the spinal axis should be completed to rule out additional areas of involvement.

As for primary spinal neoplasms, in the benign category, osteoid osteomas usually have a hypointense nidus on T1W images and variable signal on T2W with contrast enhancement. MRI can sometimes show edema in surrounding bone and soft tissue, which can mimic infectious etiologies, but these changes spare the disk space in contrast to infectious processes. The MRI appearance of osteoblastomas is similar to osteoid osteoma, with the exception of the larger size of these lesions as previously discussed. Osteochondromas have central fatty marrow which appears hyperintense on both T1W and T2W images with a peripheral hypointense rim which represents the cortex. T2W hyperintensity beyond the cortex demarcates the cartilaginous cap [26]. A cap which is thicker than 1 cm in an adult patient can signify sarcomatous degeneration.

Hemangiomas show avid contrast enhancement on MRI and are overall T1 and T2 hyperintense with occasional thick low intensity bony struts interspersed in the lesion. Giant-cell tumors appear overall hypointense on T1W images, with occasional areas of T1 hyperintensity which demarcate areas of hemorrhage. On T2W images giant-cell tumors appear low to intermediate intensity due to hemosiderin deposits and high collagen content. MRI can also reveal cystic areas and fluid-fluid levels in these lesions [26].

In the category of malignant primary spinal tumors, osteosarcomas can also have fluid-fluid levels present on MRI imaging. Chondrosarcomas have frequent signal voids on MRI due to matrix mineralization. The non-mineralized parts of the tumor can have high signal intensity due to high water content in cartilaginous portions and can also demonstrate nodular or diffuse enhancement [26]. Plasmacytomas have high signal intensity on T2W images and low intensity on T1W images; these lesions also have occasional T1/T2 hypointense bony struts interspersed in the lesion [26]. Chordomas have large soft tissue components with calcifications seen in 40% of lesions. They can have T1 high signal intensity due to hemorrhagic components or high protein content of mucinous portions of the lesions. T2W images often reveal hypointense portions which can demarcate hemosiderin or fibrous tissue. Hypointense fibrous septations are interspersed in the lesions [26].

36.4.2.6 Biopsy

Biopsy can be an essential part of the diagnosis and staging of spinal tumors. In patients with no known primary tumor who are found to have likely metastatic spinal disease, this will allow the treatment team to establish a diagnosis and plan further treatment approaches. Biopsy can be performed on the spinal lesion itself, but if another more accessible lesion is found on workup, biopsy of the least risky site is undertaken. It is important to note that when performing a biopsy of a spinal lesion, the biopsy site and biopsy tract should be planned in such a way that this may be excised en bloc at the time of surgical intervention if definitive surgical treatment is planned. For example, in cases of chordoma, seeding of a biopsy tract with tumor cells could lead to tumor recurrence, and thus en bloc resection of the biopsy tract along with the tumor is critical.

36.5 Treatment Approaches

The treatment goal for metastatic tumors of the spine is palliative in nature, specifically relief of pain, improvement or preservation of neurological functioning, and maintenance of mechanical stability of the spine. Unlike metastases, treatment of primary spinal tumors is often focused either on cure or reduction in the local recurrence rate. We must also take under consideration the fact that over the past couple of decades the treatment options available for the management of spinal metastatic disease have changed drastically. Whereas, in the past, the treatment options largely comprised of surgical decompression versus conventional external beam radiation therapy, today there are a multitude of treatment options available including minimally invasive surgical approaches, stereotactic radiosurgery, endovascular options, and new chemotherapeutic agents just to name a few. Considering the wide array of treatment modalities available to clinicians, it is important to have a decision paradigm available for choosing the right approach for each patient. One of the most commonly used decision paradigms was developed at Memorial Sloan Kettering Cancer Center referred to as the NOMS framework, which consists of neurologic, oncologic, mechanical, and systemic considerations to aid in determining optimal multidisciplinary therapy for patients suffering from metastatic spinal disease [61]. The NOMS paradigm aims to integrate radiation oncology, medical oncology, surgical approaches, and interventional radiology to come up with the most suitable treatment for patients based on their specific tumor histology and stage of disease.

36.6 Neurologic Assessment

The neurologic assessment portion of the decision framework takes into consideration the degree of epidural spinal cord compression (ESCC) and myelopathy/radiculopathy through clinical and radiological evaluation. For the radiographic assessment, the Spine Oncology Study Group (SOSG) designed and validated a 6-point grading scale for the degree of ESCC. Axial T2 images at the site of the most severe compression are used, and based on this, a grade of 0, 1a, 1b, 2, or 3 is given; grade 0 refers to metastatic lesions confined to the bone, grade 1 means tumor extension into the epidural space without compression of the spinal cord, grade 2 refers to cases with spinal cord compression where cerebrospinal fluid is still visible, and grade 3 refers to those cases where there is complete CSF obstruction due to the degree of tumor compression. Grade 1 is further subdivided into 1a, cases with epidural impingement but no thecal sac abutment; 1b, where there is deformation of the thecal sac but no abutment of the spinal cord; and 1c where there is abutment of the spinal cord without obvious degree of spinal cord compression [62]. Grades 0 through 1b correspond to lower-grade ESCC, and for these patients, radiation is usually sufficient as an initial treatment option. Patients with high-grade ESCC of grade 2 or 3 frequently require operative decompression in combination with radiation therapy, unless their tumor histology is highly radiosensitive [61].

36.7 Oncologic Assessment

The oncologic assessment portion of the NOMS framework examines the responsiveness of tumors depending on histology to currently available treatment options, primarily focusing on tumor response to radiation therapy, currently the least invasive and most effective approach to local tumor control. Tumors are categorized as radiosensitive or radioresistant based on their degree of response to conventional external beam radiation therapy (cEBRT). In general, nonsolid tumors including lymphoma, seminoma, and myeloma are considered to be radiosensitive, which means they respond readily to cEBRT and should be treated with first-line radiation therapy regardless of the degree of ESCC or neurological deficits that patients experience [61]. Solid tumors have more variability in their response to radiation therapy with breast, prostate, ovarian, and neuroendocrine tumors generally considered more sensitive and renal, thyroid, hepatocellular, colon, non-small cell lung cancer, sarcoma, and melanoma considered resistant tumor types [12, 63–69]. Radioresistant tumor types usually require stereotactic radiosurgery rather than cEBRT for successful local control. Patients presenting with high-grade ESCC or neurological compromise with radioresistant tumor histologies also require surgical decompression to halt progression of disease and symptoms in addition to radiation therapy.

36.8 Mechanical Assessment

The mechanical assessment portion of NOMS takes spinal stability into consideration as an independent predictor of whether a patient with metastatic spinal disease may benefit from surgical stabilization. Spinal instability due to a neoplastic process is defined by the SOSG as loss of the spine's ability to maintain its role as support structure for the spinal cord and nerve roots under physiological stress without resulting in movement related pain, progressive deformity or neurological deficits. Patients with certain pathological fractures or certain degree of bony invasion by a tumor can suffer from significant pain, worse with standing or movement, and/or develop spinal deformity. Pain and neurological compromise due to mechanical instability do not respond to radiation therapy or steroid medications [70]. For this reason, independent of the degree of ESCC or tumor radiosensitivity, mechanical instability can be an indication for surgical intervention. The SOSG has developed a tool to help clinicians make the determination of whether or not a patient with spinal metastases has mechanical instability requiring surgical sta-

bilization. The Spinal Instability Neoplastic Score (SINS) is an 18-point system which takes into consideration both clinical and radiological criteria, specifically tumor location (junctional, mobile, semirigid, or rigid segments of the spine), presence of mechanical pain, alignment, degree of vertebral body collapse, osteolysis, and posterior element involvement, to grade the degree of mechanical instability [71] (Table 36.2). The SINS scoring system has been shown to have good inter-observer reliability [72, 73]. Patients with lesions scoring 0–6 are generally considered stable without the need for surgical fixation, while those with SINS scores 13–18 usually need surgical stabilization. Patients with intermediate scores can fall into either category based on further clinical assessments.

Table 36.2 SINS criteria

	Score
Location	
Junctional (Occiput-C2, C7-T2, L11-L1, L5-S1)	3
Mobile (C3–C6, L2–L4)	2
Semirigid	1
Rigid	0
Pain	
Yes—mechanical	3
Yes/occasional—not mechanical	1
No	0
Type of bony lesion	
Lytic	2
Mixed	1
Blastic	0
Spinal alignment on imaging	
Subluxation/translation	4
De novo kyphosis/scoliosis	2
Normal alignment	0
Presence of compression of affected vertebral body	
>50% collapse	3
<50% collapse	2
No collapse; >50 VB involvement	1
None	0
Posterior element involvement	
Bilateral	3
Unilateral	1
None	0
Total score	
Stable	0–6
Indeterminate	7–12
Unstable	13–18

36.9   Systemic Assessment

Lastly, the systemic assessment portion of the NOMS framework sets out to determine the ability of individual patients to tolerate different treatment modalities based on their extent of metastatic disease, their systemic illnesses/comorbidities, and their tumor histology. Systemic assessment is especially important when considering invasive treatment approaches such as open surgery, which come with multiple perioperative risks and often require prolonged hospital stays and additional postoperative rehabilitation with physical and occupational therapy. In cases such as this, the surgeon has to have a good understanding of the patient's overall disease status and prognosis to determine if the proposed treatment can be administered with an acceptable level of risk for the patient. For one, tumor histology is again an important factor in understanding prognosis. Certain histologies in the setting of spinal metastatic disease have shortened survival times—colon, non-small cell lung cancer, and carcinoma of unknown primary origin, for example, have a median survival of 4 months from the time of surgery, making it difficult to justify highly invasive approaches which may require prolonged and painful recovery [74].

There have been multiple scoring systems devised to help clinicians predict survival in patients with metastatic spinal disease [75–79]. The most well-known of these is the Tokuhashi score, with a predictive value which has been validated in multiple cohorts [80–85]. This scoring system provides clinicians with an estimated survival time for patients based on six categories: Karnofsky performance status, number of extraspinal bone metastases, number of vertebral levels involved, presence of metastases to major organ systems, type of primary tumor, and neurological status based on Frankel grading system [76, 77]. A score of 0–8 suggests a survival time of 6 months or less and 9–11 of 6–12 months and a score of 12–15 predicts survival of greater than 1 year. The primary histology of the metastatic lesion as part of the Tokuhashi score weighs heavily on predicting survival, with lung, stomach, bladder, pancreas, esophageal, and liver primaries predicting a mean survival of less than 6 months, while renal, uterine, thyroid, prostate, and breast primaries have somewhat improved survival (Table 36.3). Although grading systems to predict survival are available, because systemic assessment is so dependent on individual patient characteristics, it is best to work with the patient's medical oncology team or primary care provider to determine the answer to the above questions.

36.10   Radiation Therapy

As previously mentioned, with a limited number of available treatment modalities, conventional external beam radiation therapy (cEBRT) was the historic standard of care for patients

Table 36.3 Tokuhashi revised evaluation system for prognosis of metastatic spine tumors

Characteristic	Score
General condition/Karnofsky performance score	
Poor (10–40%)	0
Moderate (50–70%)	1
Good (80–100%)	2
Number of extraspinal bone metastases	
3 or greater	0
1–2	1
1	2
Metastases to major internal organs	
Nonremovable	0
Removable	1
None	2
Cancer primary site	
Lung, osteosarcoma, stomach, bladder, esophagus, pancreas	0
Liver, gallbladder, unknown	1
Others	2
Kidney, uterus	3
Rectum	4
Thyroid, breast, prostate, carcinoid tumor	5
Palsy	
Complete (Frankel A, B)	0
Incomplete (Frankel C, D)	1
None	2
Prognosis based on total score	
6 months or less	0–8
6 months or greater	9–11
1 year or greater	12–15

with spinal metastases. The drawbacks of cEBRT include lack of precision, and as a result, higher concern for radiotoxicity to the spinal cord and other surrounding vital structures, limiting the overall dose that can be administered to tumors. With recent technological advances and the advent of stereotactic radiosurgery (SRS), however, a lot of these concerns have been overcome. Stereotactic radiosurgery allows for image-guided delivery of conformal radiation doses with high spatial precision, allowing appropriate dosing of radiation to malignant tissue even in close proximity to the spinal cord [61]. With SRS even radioresistant tumors became treatable with improved outcomes.

For pain symptoms associated with metastatic spinal lesions, cEBRT has a reported pain control rate of 60% [86], whereas pain control with SRS is considerably higher at 80–90% with improved durability, reduced narcotic and steroid dependence, and overall improved quality of life [87–91]. Recalling that pain is the most common presenting symptom of metastatic disease to the spine, the ability of SRS to relieve pain is of great importance. Given the noninvasive nature of this treatment modality and its low morbidity, SRS can be used for palliation purposes even in the setting of extensive spinal and extraspinal metastatic disease, in patients who would otherwise not qualify for more invasive operative treatments.

But the role of radiation therapy, and specifically of stereotactic radiosurgery, is not limited to palliation and pain control. Local control of disease is an important treatment goal, even in patients with extensive systemic malignancy, but even more so in patients with oligometastatic disease where successful treatment with SRS can lead to oncological benefits. For example, a large case series of solitary spinal metastases showed a long-term control rate in 90% of lesions primarily treated by radiosurgery [90]. This effect was most impressive in radiosensitive tumors (100% local control in the breast and NSCLC) but was also noteworthy in more radioresistant tumors such as renal cell carcinoma with 87% and melanoma with 75% control rate.

The decision between conventional external beam radiation and stereotactic radiosurgery depends on the patient's tumor histology (whether the tumor is radiosensitive or radioresistant) and also on the patient's degree of ESCC. For patients with radiosensitive lesions, the literature supports the use of cEBRT even in cases of high-grade ESCC [12, 66]. A prospective study by Maranzano and Latini showed that in patients suffering from myeloma, breast, and prostate cancer spinal metastases, patients had response duration of 16, 12, and 10 months respective of histology. Furthermore, in patients with breast metastases, 67% of nonambulatory patients regained ambulation after radiation treatment [66]. In patients with radioresistant tumor histologies and low-grade ESCC (0, 1a, and 1b), because tumors do not have acceptable response rate to cEBRT, SRS can usually be employed as a first line of treatment, avoiding the need for surgical intervention [66, 67]. By utilizing high-dose SRS, durable local tumor control can be achieved regardless of tumor histology in greater than 85% of patients [63]. In a study by Yamada et al., SRS was used in 103 patients with resistant tumor histologies with a local control rate of 92% at a 16-month follow-up [92].

The excellent response to SRS has shifted the conventional treatment of radioresistant tumors from surgical interventions to utilizing radiotherapy as a first line of treatment [93]. SRS is especially appealing in patients who would be poor surgical candidates due to systemic illnesses or comorbidities but who are able to tolerate the generally mild side effects of SRS [89, 92, 94, 95].

In patients suffering from radioresistant metastatic spinal disease who also have high-grade ESCC, surgical decompression is usually necessary, followed by postoperative radiation. While conventional radiation therapy after surgical intervention has poor long-term control rates (31% at 1 year), postoperative SRS provides long-term local tumor control similar to SRS for low-grade ESCC [96]. Rock et al. showed greater than 92% local control rate in patients treated with SRS following surgical intervention [97]. Moulding et al. found 1-year progression risk after 24 Gy radiation dose to be 6.3% in 21 patients with radioresistant metastases with high-grade ESCC after decompression and fusion procedure [98]. Another study involving 186 patients undergoing radiation after separation surgery found 1-year progression rate of 4.1% for high-dose single-fraction SRS. Such high rates of local tumor control make extensive tumor resections unnecessary in patients who may not be ideal surgical candidates due to comorbidities/prognosis, etc.

In cases where post-SRS failure with tumor recurrence is observed, the failure usually occurs at the epidural margin, where radiation for the tumor may be underdosed due to fear of radiotoxicity to the spinal cord. To combat this phenomenon, utilizing the multidisciplinary approach to metastatic lesions, the concept of separation surgery was developed. Here, prior to radiation therapy, the surgeon would decompress around the spinal cord to create a buffer zone, so the appropriate radiation dose could be applied to the tumor being targeted, with lessened concern for toxicity to neural structures. In a study by Laufer et al. of 186 patients treated in this manner, local progression was noted in only 18.3% of patients within a 5-month follow-up window [99].

36.11 Surgery

Historically, the surgical treatment of spinal metastatic lesions was limited by a lack of variety in approaches and mostly consisted of laminectomy, which, in most cases, could only provide indirect decompression of the neural elements. These limitations frequently failed to establish improvements in neurological function and added to patients' degree of spinal instability and pain. In recent years, more sophisticated surgical approaches with multiple strategies to access the ventral spinal canal have greatly improved the treatment options for patients with metastases with mechanical instability or neural compression.

Before discussing specific surgical approaches, it is important to consider the indications for surgery; in the case of metastatic lesions, the overall goal of surgery is palliative, attempting to alleviate pain due to mechanical instability or restore or prevent further deterioration of neurological function due to spinal cord or nerve root compression. For patients with primary tumors of the spine, the goal of surgery can be quite different, aiming for complete en bloc resection with avoidance of violation of tumor margins to achieve a cure or decrease the chances of recurrence and prolong survival (Figs. 36.1 and 36.2).

When discussing metastatic disease, the goal of surgery is often pain relief, which can be achieved by restoring stability to the spine and thereby decreasing mechanical spine pain (Fig. 36.3). Classically, this is accomplished through spinal instrumentation which provides a rigid construct to stabilize the spine and allow for bony fusion. In the past this had been in large part achieved through open pedicle screw instrumentation. Although this is still a proven and safe approach, it carries certain limitations including a large incision with extensive dissection through posterior musculature and at times considerable blood loss, postoperative pain, and the need for rehabilitation. Many of these patients will need to undergo postoperative radiation and/or chemotherapy, which can impair wound healing. For this reason, less invasive approaches have been developed aimed at restoring stability and relieving mechanical back pain.

Percutaneous vertebroplasty is an example of a minimally invasive procedure in which the surgeon or interventionalist injects acrylic bone cement into the vertebral body under fluoroscopic image guidance with the patient under light sedation and/or utilizing only local anesthetic. Kyphoplasty is a variation of this procedure where a balloon is inflated in the cancellous bone of the vertebral body into which cement is injected. These minimally invasive procedures are used to restore bony integrity to vertebral bodies affected by osteoporotic or pathological compression fractures. The procedures are advantageous because they can be done without general anesthesia and require no large incision/tissue dissection or prolonged recovery time. Complications are relatively few and include possible leakage of cement outside of the

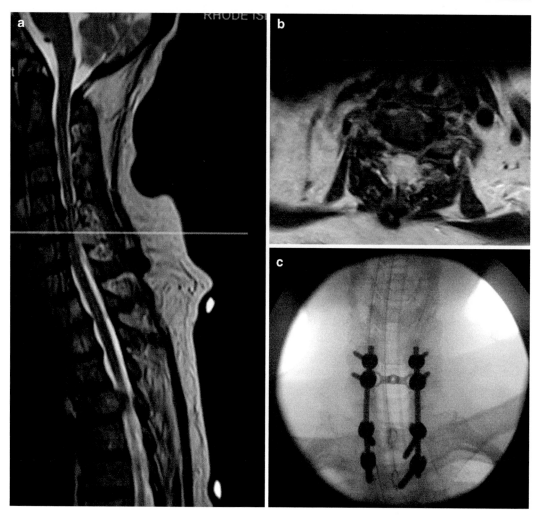

Fig. 36.1 A 70-year-old woman with a history of leio-myosarcoma presented with 1 week of worsening leg numbness and weakness (3/5 strength). MRI found spinal cord compression at the C7 level and severe myelopathy from epidural tumor compression at C7 (**a**, **b**). Surgery was recommended, and she underwent a C5-T2 instrumented fusion and C5–C7 laminectomies for decompression of a C7 tumor (**c**)

vertebral body (to disk space, venous plexus, epidural space) which can rarely lead to neurologic deficits from compression. For this reason, it is important to ensure that the posterior longitudinal ligament (PLL) is not disrupted from the pathologic fracture before injecting cement. Sequential fluoroscopic images should be obtained as the cement is being injected to monitor for extravasation of cement into the spinal canal. Two randomized controlled trials failed to show improvement in pain symptoms compared to placebo in patients with osteoporotic compression fractures treated with vertebroplasty, but some smaller series looking at pathological fractures from metastatic disease did show benefit from these procedures with regard to pain [100]. Specifically, in cohort studies, pain relief was achieved in 90% of patients [101, 102]. Vertebroplasty has been used in combination with SRS for even greater benefit in patients with metastatic spine lesions. Vertebral body compression fractures are a frequent complication of stereotactic radiosurgery (SRS). Cement augmentation prior to SRS may help prevent this complication or treat this complication after it has occurred [103]. In patients who received a

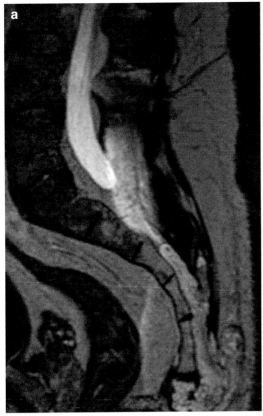
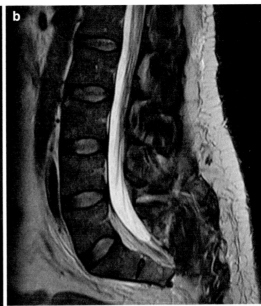

Fig. 36.2 This 47-year-old man presented with sacral pain. MRI found a T2-hyperintense lesion spanning from S3-coccyx with epidural extension (**a**). The patient was neurologically intact but had admitted some gradually worsening urinary incontinence. The tumor was entirely in the canal and dorsal to the canal, except for coccyx where it replaces the coccyx completely. CT-guided biopsy confirmed it was a chordoma. S2 and S3 rostral laminectomies were performed, and mobilization of both the S2 and S3 nerve roots bilaterally was performed. En bloc high sacral amputation at S2–S3 with removal of S3, S4, S5 vertebral bodies and coccyx was accomplished with the aid of general surgery to separate the tumor for the rectum (**b**). Plastic surgery was crucial in the complex closure of the wound

combination of these two therapies, there was 92% pain improvement, and prevention of progressive deformity was in 95% [104]. This combination of treatments appears most appropriate in patients without significant epidural tumor involvement or neurologic compression and with an intact PLL.

While vertebroplasty and kyphoplasty are useful tools in relieving mechanical back pain in patients with pathological fractures, this approach cannot be used when the degree of spinal instability is more significant thus requiring fixation of the spine across multiple levels. In such cases, multilevel rigid fixation can be accomplished through percutaneous

pedicle screw placement under fluoroscopic guidance. This is another minimally invasive strategy that allows for small incisions, decreased tissue dissection, and a smaller surgical cavity [105]. Case series have shown greater than 90% pain reduction in patients with mechanical back pain treated with this intervention [106]. It is important to note, however, that while percutaneous screws allow for rigid fixation across multiple levels, this intervention does not lead to arthrodesis. If the patient has a prognosis of several more years of life, this may lead to ultimate instrumentation failure. However, if the patient has a more limited prognosis of about a year, then it is much

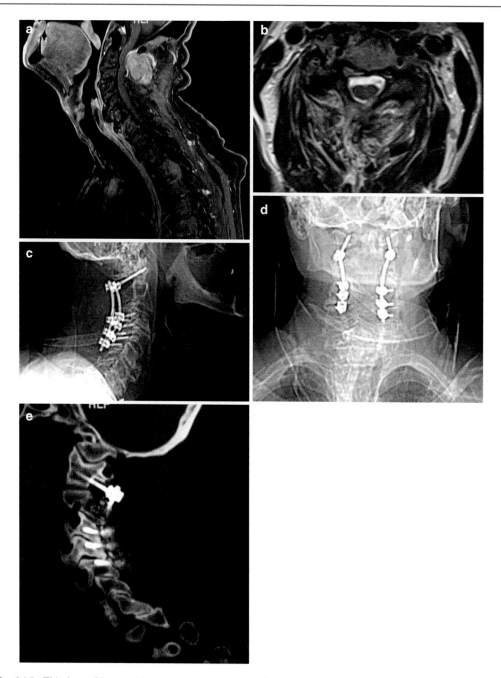

Fig. 36.3 This is an 82-year-old male who was transferred to the hospital with severe mechanical neck pain. The patient's imaging studies, including MRI and the CT scan, both revealed a large destructive lesion dorsally situated at C2, C3, and C4 (**a, b**). There was significant radiographic compression of the spinal cord. However, the patient was neurologically intact and had no myelopathic signs. The patient also had cervical instability with mechanical neck pain, and given his highly functional status, the patient wanted surgical intervention to improve his pain. A CT-guided biopsy of this patient was performed that found a non-small cell lung carcinoma. The patient also had an MRI scan of the brain, which showed 13 metastases. Given the patient's severe mechanical neck pain and impending neurological injury, decision was made to proceed with the surgical intervention. The patient C2–C4 laminectomy with C3/C4 and C4/C5 facetectomies to remove the lesion en bloc. Posterior cervical segmental fixation using C1 cervical lateral mass screws and lateral mass screws at C3, C4, and C5 (**c, d, e**)

less likely that the instrumentation will fail during the patient's lifetime. Percutaneous instrumentation is also limited in that it does not provide any decompression of the spinal cord or nerve roots. Therefore, it is not an appropriate approach in cases where compression of neural elements is a concern. Percutaneous screw placement can however be combined with other surgical approaches, such as minimally invasive transpedicular vertebrectomy or decompression through tubular retractors, which provide targeted decompression of neural elements [107–110], allowing for shortened operative time, improved postoperative pain, decreased blood loss, and faster recovery [111].

Minimally invasive strategies are not adequate in patients with a significant degree of mechanical spinal instability/deformity or in patients with significant epidural compression from metastatic tumors. The Patchell study in 2005 was the first randomized controlled trial to demonstrate the importance of circumferential surgical decompression and mechanical stabilization of the spinal cord in patients suffering from metastases and presenting with weakness or myelopathy due to epidural compression [112]. Patients were randomized to external beam radiation versus early surgical intervention with circumferential decompression of the spinal cord followed by adjuvant radiation therapy. Of note, patients with anticipated survival under 3 months and those with highly radiosensitive tumors (lymphoma, leukemia, multiple myeloma, germ cell tumors) were excluded from the study. The study showed that 85% of the operative group regained ambulatory function versus 57% of the radiation only group and retained the ability to walk longer.

When the goal of surgery is decompression of the spinal cord and nerve roots, the surgical approach depends on the levels of the spine involved and the location of compression. When there is posterior element involvement or posterior compression, a posterior midline approach with laminectomy is suitable. If the tumor is ventrolateral, a transpedicular approach or costotransversectomy can be performed (Fig. 36.4). Posterior bilateral transpedicular corpectomies allow for achieving anterior decompression and reconstruction of the spinal column with an expandable interbody cage, with positive outcomes reported through several case series [113–117]. With anteriorly located lesions, the surgical approach depends on the level of spine involvement (Fig. 36.5). For lesions at the occipitocervical junction, a transoral, extended open door maxillofacial or transmandibular circumglossal approach would be necessary. It is important to consider that patients undergoing an anterior approach to the craniocervical junction will frequently need tracheostomy and gastrostomy tube placement, often pre-emptively before surgery, due to the increased risk of airway compromise, infection, pharyngeal dehiscence, and swallowing dysfunction. For lesions in the mid- to lower-cervical spine, a standard anterolateral approach will allow for anterior decompression of the canal and anterior reconstruction. When lesions are located in the low cervical or high thoracic spine, a median sternotomy or partial sternotomy and ventrolateral thoracotomy may be performed [118]. For lower thoracic lesions, dorsolateral thoracotomy is the approach utilized, whereas for thoracolumbar lesions, thoracoabdominal approaches are utilized. In the lumbosacral spine, direct ventral decompression can be done through retroperitoneal or transperitoneal approaches [119]. The minimally invasive direct lateral approach offers an alternative approach for decompressing the lower thoracic and lumbar spinal canal while avoiding extensive disruption of posterior ligamentous structures and musculature. In the minimally invasive direct lateral approach, a distractable tubular retractor system is used through a retroperitoneal or retropleural approach to gain access to the anterior column of the spinal canal. The approach for the thoracic spine is transpleural or retropleural, while that for the lumbar spine is retroperitoneal transpsoas. Of note, this approach was originally developed for discectomy and interbody fusion but has been used in some cases for patients with tumors [120–122].

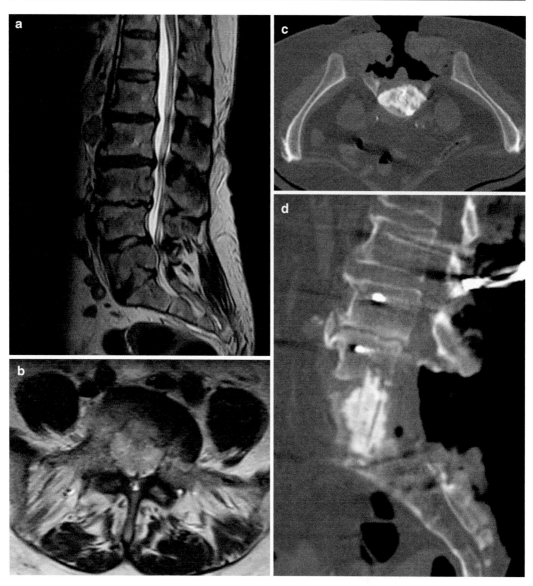

Fig. 36.4 This is a 67-year-old woman who presented with new-onset severe mechanical low back pain and right lower extremity pain. The patient had right lower extremity pain that was in the L5 distribution. The patient subsequently had an MRI scan of the lumbar spine which showed pathological L5 vertebral body fracture with compression of the cauda equina as well as right-sided L5 nerve root with what appeared to be because of the retropulsed bone fragment and tumor (**a, b**). CT of the chest, abdomen, and pelvis was also performed. The CT of the abdomen demonstrated a kidney mass suggestive of a renal cell carcinoma. The patient subsequently had a CT-guided biopsy which proved this to be a renal cell carcinoma. Given the patient's severe right lower extremity pain and mechanical back pain and pathological fracture, decision was made to proceed with the surgical procedure described above. The patient also underwent a preoperative embolization of L5 vertebral body lesion using direct puncture with methyl methacrylate injection. Soon after the injection, the patient's right lower extremity pain worsened with some additional numbness. She was taken to surgery for L2-S2AI pelvic fusion with corpectomy of L5 and reconstruction with chest tube and cement (**c, d, e**). The construct was reinforced with quad rods

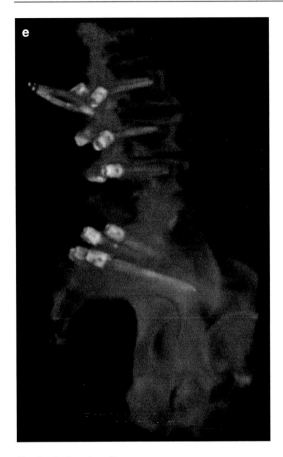

Fig. 36.4 (continued)

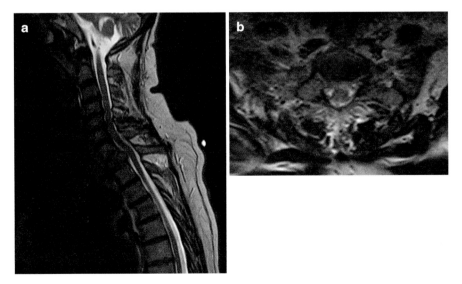

Fig. 36.5 A 71-year-old man presented to the hospital with tingling in his right hand and weakness in his right hand. MRI showed a compressive pathological fracture at T1 indenting on the spinal cord (**a**, **b**). Preoperative CT-guided biopsy revealed the lesion to be urothelial carcinoma. Cement was injected into T1 preoperatively as an alternative to embolization. The patient was then taken to surgery for a posterior cervicothoracic decompression and fusion instrumenting C5-T5 with a T1 corpectomy with cage (**c**, **d**, **e**). The patient also required cement augmentation of several of the thoracic screws given the extensive metastatic disease and the weak bone

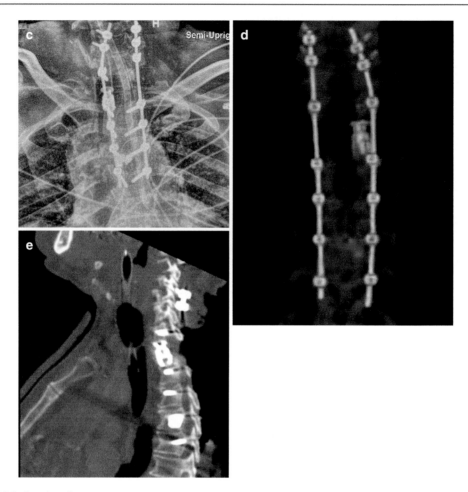

Fig. 36.5 (continued)

36.12 Conclusion

Over the last couple of decades, the approach to treatment and available treatment options for epidural tumors of the spine have changed significantly. Especially when it comes to epidural metastases, which make up a majority of pathology in this location, treatment approach has changed from limited surgical options and external beam radiation to a multimodality, multidisciplinary view of the disease process. As made evident in this chapter, successful treatment of patients with metastatic epidural disease requires careful consideration of the neurologic, oncologic, mechanical, and systemic status of the patient and is based on the situation involvement of medical and radiation oncology, surgery, and interventional radiology teams. Lastly, when evaluating any patient with an epidural tumor, the specific disease process at play is of utmost importance, as treatment approaches and goals of therapy vary widely depending on the pathology. The goal of intervention in primary tumors is often achieving a cure, whereas in the case of metastatic disease it is palliation, with decrease in pain and improved quality of life for patients.

References

1. Bell GR (1997) Surgical treatment of spinal tumors. Clin Orthop Relat Res 335:54–63

2. Weinstein JN, McLain RF (1987) Primary tumors of the spine. Spine (Phila Pa 1976) 12(9):843–851

3. Siegel RL, Miller KD, Jemal A (2016) Cancer statistics, 2016. CA Cancer J Clin 66(1):7–30

4. York JE, Wildrick DM, Gokaslan ZL (1999) Metastatic tumors. In: Benzel EC, Stillerman C (eds) The thoracic spine. Quality Meidcal Publishing, St. Louis, pp 392–411

5. Bubendorf L, Schöpfer A, Wagner U, Sauter G, Moch H, Willi N et al (2000) Metastatic patterns of prostate cancer: an autopsy study of 1,589 patients. Hum Pathol 31(5):578–583

6. Lee YT (1983) Breast carcinoma: pattern of metastasis at autopsy. J Surg Oncol 23(3):175–180

7. Ortiz Gómez JA (1995) The incidence of vertebral body metastases. Int Orthop 19(5):309–311

8. Black P (1979) Spinal metastasis: current status and recommended guidelines for management. Neurosurgery 5(6):726–746

9. Posner JB (1978) Neurologic complications of systemic cancer. Dis Mon 25(2):1–60

10. Coleman RE (2006) Clinical features of metastatic bone disease and risk of skeletal morbidity. Clin Cancer Res 12(20 Pt 2):6243s–6249s

11. Pockett RD, Castellano D, McEwan P, Oglesby A, Barber BL, Chung K (2010) The hospital burden of disease associated with bone metastases and skeletal-related events in patients with breast cancer, lung cancer, or prostate cancer in Spain. Eur J Cancer Care (Engl) 19(6):755–760

12. Bilsky MH, Lis E, Raizer J, Lee H, Boland P (1999) The diagnosis and treatment of metastatic spinal tumor. Oncologist 4(6):459–469

13. Walsh GL, Gokaslan ZL, McCutcheon IE, Mineo MT, Yasko AW, Swisher SG et al (1997) Anterior approaches to the thoracic spine in patients with cancer: indications and results. Ann Thorac Surg 64(6):1611–1618

14. Brihaye J, Ectors P, Lemort M, Van Houtte P (1988) The management of spinal epidural metastases. Adv Tech Stand Neurosurg 16:121–176

15. Cahill DW (1996) Surgical management of malignant tumors of the adult bony spine. South Med J 89(7):653–665

16. Cole JS, Patchell RA (2008) Metastatic epidural spinal cord compression. Lancet Neurol 7(5):459–466

17. Ibrahim A, Crockard A, Antonietti P, Boriani S, Bünger C, Gasbarrini A et al (2008) Does spinal surgery improve the quality of life for those with extradural (spinal) osseous metastases? An international multicenter prospective observational study of 223 patients. Invited submission from the Joint Section Meeting on Disorders of the Spine and Peripheral Nerves, March 2007. J Neurosurg Spine 8(3):271–278

18. Abdu WA, Provencher M (1998) Primary bone and metastatic tumors of the cervical spine. Spine (Phila Pa 1976) 23(24):2767–2777

19. Berenson JR, Lichtenstein A, Porter L, Dimopoulos MA, Bordoni R, George S et al (1996) Efficacy of pamidronate in reducing skeletal events in patients with advanced multiple myeloma. Myeloma Aredia Study Group. N Engl J Med 334(8):488–493

20. Boriani SWJ (1997) Differential diagnosis and surgial treatment of primary benign and malignant neoplasms. In: Freid J (ed) The adult spine: principles and practice. Lippincott-Raven, Philadelphia, pp 951–987

21. Doppman JL, Oldfield EH, Heiss JD (2000) Symptomatic vertebral hemangiomas: treatment by means of direct intralesional injection of ethanol. Radiology 214(2):341–348

22. Burger P, Scheithauer BW, Vogel F (2002) Surgical pathology of the nervous system and its coverings. Churchill Livingstone, Philadelphia

23. Kaweblum M, Lehman WB, Bash J, Grant AD, Strongwater A (1993) Diagnosis of osteoid osteoma in the child. Orthop Rev 22(12):1305–1313

24. Orlowski JP, Mercer RD (1977) Osteoid osteoma in children and young adults. Pediatrics 59(4):526–532

25. Cohen MD, Harrington TM, Ginsburg WW (1983) Osteoid osteoma: 95 cases and a review of the literature. Semin Arthritis Rheum 12(3):265–281

26. Patnaik S, Jyotsnarani Y, Uppin SG, Susarla R (2016) Imaging features of primary tumors of the spine: a pictorial essay. Indian J Radiol Imaging 26(2):279–289

27. Copley L, Dormans JP (1996) Benign pediatric bone tumors. Evaluation and treatment. Pediatr Clin North Am 43(4):949–966

28. de Andrea CEBJ, Schiller A (2013) Osteoblastoma. In: Fletcher CD, Bridge JA, Hogendoorn PC, Mertens F (eds) WHO classification of tumors of soft tissue and bone, 4th edn. International Agency for Research on Cancer, Lyon, p 279

29. Balke M, Schremper L, Gebert C, Ahrens H, Streitbuerger A, Koehler G et al (2008) Giant cell tumor of bone: treatment and outcome of 214 cases. J Cancer Res Clin Oncol 134(9):969–978

30. Ameli NO, Abbassioun K, Saleh H, Eslamdoost A (1985) Aneurysmal bone cysts of the spine. Report of 17 cases. J Neurosurg 63(5):685–690

31. Yildiz C, Erler K, Atesalp AS, Basbozkurt M (2003) Benign bone tumors in children. Curr Opin Pediatr 15(1):58–67

32. Biermann JS (2002) Common benign lesions of bone in children and adolescents. J Pediatr Orthop 22(2):268–273

33. Nielsen GPFJ, Oliveira AM (2013) Aneurysmal bone cyst. In: Fletcher CD, Bridge J, Hogendoorn PC, Mertens F (eds) WHO classification of tumors

of soft tissue and bone, 4th edn. International Agency for Research on Cancer, Lyon, p 348

34. Aricò M, Nichols K, Whitlock JA, Arceci R, Haupt R, Mittler U et al (1999) Familial clustering of Langerhans cell histiocytosis. Br J Haematol 107(4):883–888

35. Shahla A, Parvaneh V, Hossein HD (2004) Langerhans cells histiocytosis in one family. Pediatr Hematol Oncol 21(4):313–320

36. Bhatia S, Nesbit ME, Egeler RM, Buckley JD, Mertens A, Robison LL (1997) Epidemiologic study of Langerhans cell histiocytosis in children. J Pediatr 130(5):774–784

37. Nicholson HS, Egeler RM, Nesbit ME (1998) The epidemiology of Langerhans cell histiocytosis. Hematol Oncol Clin North Am 12(2):379–384

38. Milne P, Bigley V, Bacon CM, Néel A, McGovern N, Bomken S et al (2017) Hematopoietic origin of Langerhans cell histiocytosis and Erdheim-Chester disease in adults. Blood 130(2):167–175

39. Soutar R, Lucraft H, Jackson G, Reece A, Bird J, Low E et al (2004) Guidelines on the diagnosis and management of solitary plasmacytoma of bone and solitary extramedullary plasmacytoma. Clin Oncol (R Coll Radiol) 16(6):405–413

40. Swerdlow SH, Campo E, Pileri SA, Harris NL, Stein H, Siebert R et al (2016) The 2016 revision of the World Health Organization classification of lymphoid neoplasms. Blood 127(20):2375–2390

41. York JE, Kaczaraj A, Abi-Said D, Fuller GN, Skibber JM, Janjan NA et al (1999) Sacral chordoma: 40-year experience at a major cancer center. Neurosurgery 44(1):74–79; discussion 9–80

42. Heffelfinger MJ, Dahlin DC, MacCarty CS, Beabout JW (1973) Chordomas and cartilaginous tumors at the skull base. Cancer 32(2):410–420

43. Meis JM, Raymond AK, Evans HL, Charles RE, Giraldo AA (1987) "Dedifferentiated" chordoma. A clinicopathologic and immunohistochemical study of three cases. Am J Surg Pathol 11(7):516–525

44. Hruban RH, Traganos F, Reuter VE, Huvos AG (1990) Chordomas with malignant spindle cell components. A DNA flow cytometric and immunohistochemical study with histogenetic implications. Am J Pathol 137(2):435–447

45. York JE, Berk RH, Fuller GN, Rao JS, Abi-Said D, Wildrick DM et al (1999) Chondrosarcoma of the spine: 1954 to 1997. J Neurosurg 90(Suppl 1): 73–78

46. Cohen ZR, Fourney DR, Marco RA, Rhines LD, Gokaslan ZL (2002) Total cervical spondylectomy for primary osteogenic sarcoma. Case report and description of operative technique. J Neurosurg 97(3 Suppl):386–392

47. Guillevin R, Vallee JN, Lafitte F, Menuel C, Duverneuil NM, Chiras J (2007) Spine metastasis imaging: review of the literature. J Neuroradiol 34(5):311–321

48. Galasko CS (1975) The value of scintigraphy in malignant disease. Cancer Treat Rev 2(4):225–272

49. Muindi J, Coombes RC, Golding S, Powles TJ, Khan O, Husband J (1983) The role of computed tomography in the detection of bone metastases in breast cancer patients. Br J Radiol 56(664):233–236

50. Peterson JJ, Kransdorf MJ, O'Connor MI (2003) Diagnosis of occult bone metastases: positron emission tomography. Clin Orthop Relat Res (Suppl 415):S120–S128

51. Yang HL, Liu T, Wang XM, Xu Y, Deng SM (2011) Diagnosis of bone metastases: a meta-analysis comparing ^{18}FDG PET, CT, MRI and bone scintigraphy. Eur Radiol 21(12):2604–2617

52. Qu X, Huang X, Yan W, Wu L, Dai K (2012) A meta-analysis of ^{18}FDG-PET-CT, ^{18}FDG-PET, MRI and bone scintigraphy for diagnosis of bone metastases in patients with lung cancer. Eur J Radiol 81(5):1007–1015

53. Shen G, Deng H, Hu S, Jia Z (2014) Comparison of choline-PET/CT, MRI, SPECT, and bone scintigraphy in the diagnosis of bone metastases in patients with prostate cancer: a meta-analysis. Skelet Radiol 43(11):1503–1513

54. Liu T, Cheng T, Xu W, Yan WL, Liu J, Yang HL (2011) A meta-analysis of 18FDG-PET, MRI and bone scintigraphy for diagnosis of bone metastases in patients with breast cancer. Skelet Radiol 40(5):523–531

55. Peterson JJ (2007) F-18 FDG-PET for detection of osseous metastatic disease and staging, restaging, and monitoring response to therapy of musculoskeletal tumors. Semin Musculoskelet Radiol 11(3):246–260

56. Rybak LD, Rosenthal DI (2001) Radiological imaging for the diagnosis of bone metastases. Q J Nucl Med 45(1):53–64

57. Mahnken AH, Wildberger JE, Gehbauer G, Schmitz-Rode T, Blaum M, Fabry U et al (2002) Multidetector CT of the spine in multiple myeloma: comparison with MR imaging and radiography. AJR Am J Roentgenol 178(6):1429–1436

58. Frank JA, Ling A, Patronas NJ, Carrasquillo JA, Horvath K, Hickey AM et al (1990) Detection of malignant bone tumors: MR imaging vs scintigraphy. AJR Am J Roentgenol 155(5):1043–1048

59. Liu T, Wang S, Liu H, Meng B, Zhou F, He F et al (2017) Detection of vertebral metastases: a meta-analysis comparing MRI, CT, PET, BS and BS with SPECT. J Cancer Res Clin Oncol 143(3):457–465

60. Fayad LM, Kamel IR, Kawamoto S, Bluemke DA, Frassica FJ, Fishman EK (2005) Distinguishing stress fractures from pathologic fractures: a multimodality approach. Skelet Radiol 34(5):245–259

61. Laufer I, Rubin DG, Lis E, Cox BW, Stubblefield MD, Yamada Y et al (2013) The NOMS framework: approach to the treatment of spinal metastatic tumors. Oncologist 18(6):744–751

62. Bilsky MH, Laufer I, Fourney DR, Groff M, Schmidt MH, Varga PP et al (2010) Reliability analysis of the epidural spinal cord compression scale. J Neurosurg Spine 13(3):324–328

63. Gerszten PC, Mendel E, Yamada Y (2009) Radiotherapy and radiosurgery for metastatic spine disease: what are the options, indications, and outcomes? Spine (Phila Pa 1976) 34(Suppl 22):S78–S92

64. Gilbert RW, Kim JH, Posner JB (1978) Epidural spinal cord compression from metastatic tumor: diagnosis and treatment. Ann Neurol 3(1):40–51

65. Maranzano E, Bellavita R, Rossi R, De Angelis V, Frattegiani A, Bagnoli R et al (2005) Short-course versus split-course radiotherapy in metastatic spinal cord compression: results of a phase III, randomized, multicenter trial. J Clin Oncol 23(15):3358–3365

66. Maranzano E, Latini P (1995) Effectiveness of radiation therapy without surgery in metastatic spinal cord compression: final results from a prospective trial. Int J Radiat Oncol Biol Phys 32(4):959–967

67. Katagiri H, Takahashi M, Inagaki J, Kobayashi H, Sugiura H, Yamamura S et al (1998) Clinical results of nonsurgical treatment for spinal metastases. Int J Radiat Oncol Biol Phys 42(5):1127–1132

68. Rades D, Fehlauer F, Schulte R, Veninga T, Stalpers LJ, Basic H et al (2006) Prognostic factors for local control and survival after radiotherapy of metastatic spinal cord compression. J Clin Oncol 24(21):3388–3393

69. Rades D, Fehlauer F, Stalpers LJ, Wildfang I, Zschenker O, Schild SE et al (2004) A prospective evaluation of two radiotherapy schedules with 10 versus 20 fractions for the treatment of metastatic spinal cord compression: final results of a multicenter study. Cancer 101(11):2687–2692

70. Fisher CG, DiPaola CP, Ryken TC, Bilsky MH, Shaffrey CI, Berven SH et al (2010) A novel classification system for spinal instability in neoplastic disease: an evidence-based approach and expert consensus from the Spine Oncology Study Group. Spine (Phila Pa 1976) 35(22):E1221–E1229

71. Fourney DR, Frangou EM, Ryken TC, Dipaola CP, Shaffrey CI, Berven SH et al (2011) Spinal instability neoplastic score: an analysis of reliability and validity from the spine oncology study group. J Clin Oncol 29(22):3072–3077

72. Fisher CG, Versteeg AL, Schouten R, Boriani S, Varga PP, Rhines LD et al (2014) Reliability of the spinal instability neoplastic scale among radiologists: an assessment of instability secondary to spinal metastases. AJR Am J Roentgenol 203(4):869–874

73. Campos M, Urrutia J, Zamora T, Román J, Canessa V, Borghero Y et al (2014) The Spine Instability Neoplastic Score: an independent reliability and reproducibility analysis. Spine J 14(8):1466–1469

74. Wang JC, Boland P, Mitra N, Yamada Y, Lis E, Stubblefield M et al (2004) Single-stage posterolateral transpedicular approach for resection of epidural metastatic spine tumors involving the vertebral body with circumferential reconstruction: results in 140 patients. Invited submission from the Joint Section Meeting on Disorders of the Spine and Peripheral Nerves, March 2004. J Neurosurg Spine 1(3):287–298

75. Bauer HC, Wedin R (1995) Survival after surgery for spinal and extremity metastases. Prognostication in 241 patients. Acta Orthop Scand 66(2):143–146

76. Tokuhashi Y, Matsuzaki H, Oda H, Oshima M, Ryu J (2005) A revised scoring system for preoperative evaluation of metastatic spine tumor prognosis. Spine (Phila Pa 1976) 30(19):2186–2191

77. Tokuhashi Y, Matsuzaki H, Toriyama S, Kawano H, Ohsaka S (1990) Scoring system for the preoperative evaluation of metastatic spine tumor prognosis. Spine (Phila Pa 1976) 15(11):1110–1113

78. Tomita K, Kawahara N, Kobayashi T, Yoshida A, Murakami H, Akamaru T (2001) Surgical strategy for spinal metastases. Spine (Phila Pa 1976) 26(3):298–306

79. van der Linden YM, Dijkstra SP, Vonk EJ, Marijnen CA, Leer JW, Group DBMS (2005) Prediction of survival in patients with metastases in the spinal column: results based on a randomized trial of radiotherapy. Cancer 103(2):320–328

80. Yilmazlar S, Dogan S, Caner B, Turkkan A, Bekar A, Korfali E (2008) Comparison of prognostic scores and surgical approaches to treat spinal metastatic tumors: a review of 57 cases. J Orthop Surg Res 3:37

81. Leithner A, Radl R, Gruber G, Hochegger M, Leithner K, Welkerling H et al (2008) Predictive value of seven preoperative prognostic scoring systems for spinal metastases. Eur Spine J 17(11):1488–1495

82. Wang M, Bünger CE, Li H, Wu C, Høy K, Niedermann B et al (2012) Predictive value of Tokuhashi scoring systems in spinal metastases, focusing on various primary tumor groups: evaluation of 448 patients in the Aarhus spinal metastases database. Spine (Phila Pa 1976) 37(7):573–582

83. Quraishi NA, Manoharan SR, Arealis G, Khurana A, Elsayed S, Edwards KL et al (2013) Accuracy of the revised Tokuhashi score in predicting survival in patients with metastatic spinal cord compression (MSCC). Eur Spine J 22(Suppl 1):S21–S26

84. Lee CH, Chung CK, Jahng TA, Kim KJ, Kim CH, Hyun SJ et al (2015) Which one is a valuable surrogate for predicting survival between Tomita and Tokuhashi scores in patients with spinal metastases? A meta-analysis for diagnostic test accuracy and individual participant data analysis. J Neuro-Oncol 123(2):267–275

85. Petteys RJ, Spitz SM, Rhee J, Goodwin CR, Zadnik PL, Sarabia-Estrada R et al (2015) Tokuhashi score is predictive of survival in a cohort of patients undergoing surgery for renal cell carcinoma spinal metastases. Eur Spine J 24(10):2142–2149

86. Wu JS, Wong R, Johnston M, Bezjak A, Whelan T, Group CCOPGISC (2003) Meta-analysis of dose-fractionation radiotherapy trials for the palliation of painful bone metastases. Int J Radiat Oncol Biol Phys 55(3):594–605

87. Ryu S, Fang Yin F, Rock J, Zhu J, Chu A, Kagan E et al (2003) Image-guided and intensity-modulated

radiosurgery for patients with spinal metastasis. Cancer 97(8):2013–2018

88. Ryu S, Jin R, Jin JY, Chen Q, Rock J, Anderson J et al (2008) Pain control by image-guided radiosurgery for solitary spinal metastasis. J Pain Symptom Manag 35(3):292–298

89. Degen JW, Gagnon GJ, Voyadzis JM, McRae DA, Lunsden M, Dieterich S et al (2005) CyberKnife stereotactic radiosurgical treatment of spinal tumors for pain control and quality of life. J Neurosurg Spine 2(5):540–549

90. Gerszten PC, Burton SA, Ozhasoglu C, Welch WC (2007) Radiosurgery for spinal metastases: clinical experience in 500 cases from a single institution. Spine (Phila Pa 1976) 32(2):193–199

91. Gagnon GJ, Nasr NM, Liao JJ, Molzahn I, Marsh D, McRae D et al (2009) Treatment of spinal tumors using cyberknife fractionated stereotactic radiosurgery: pain and quality-of-life assessment after treatment in 200 patients. Neurosurgery 64(2):297–306; discussion 7

92. Yamada Y, Bilsky MH, Lovelock DM, Venkatraman ES, Toner S, Johnson J et al (2008) High-dose, single-fraction image-guided intensity-modulated radiotherapy for metastatic spinal lesions. Int J Radiat Oncol Biol Phys 71(2):484–490

93. Bilsky MH, Laufer I, Burch S (2009) Shifting paradigms in the treatment of metastatic spine disease. Spine (Phila Pa 1976) 34(Suppl 22):S101–S107

94. Benzil DL, Saboori M, Mogilner AY, Rocchio R, Moorthy CR (2004) Safety and efficacy of stereotactic radiosurgery for tumors of the spine. J Neurosurg 101(Suppl 3):413–418

95. Chang EL, Shiu AS, Mendel E, Mathews LA, Mahajan A, Allen PK et al (2007) Phase I/II study of stereotactic body radiotherapy for spinal metastasis and its pattern of failure. J Neurosurg Spine 7(2):151–160

96. Klekamp J, Samii H (1998) Surgical results for spinal metastases. Acta Neurochir 140(9):957–967

97. Rock JP, Ryu S, Shukairy MS, Yin FF, Sharif A, Schreiber F et al (2006) Postoperative radiosurgery for malignant spinal tumors. Neurosurgery 58(5):891–898; discussion 8

98. Moulding HD, Elder JB, Lis E, Lovelock DM, Zhang Z, Yamada Y et al (2010) Local disease control after decompressive surgery and adjuvant high-dose single-fraction radiosurgery for spine metastases. J Neurosurg Spine 13(1):87–93

99. Laufer I, Iorgulescu JB, Chapman T, Lis E, Shi W, Zhang Z et al (2013) Local disease control for spinal metastases following "separation surgery" and adjuvant hypofractionated or high-dose single-fraction stereotactic radiosurgery: outcome analysis in 186 patients. J Neurosurg Spine 18(3):207–214

100. Buchbinder R, Golmohammadi K, Johnston RV, Owen RJ, Homik J, Jones A et al (2015) Percutaneous vertebroplasty for osteoporotic verte-

bral compression fracture. Cochrane Database Syst Rev 4:CD006349

101. Cotten A, Dewatre F, Cortet B, Assaker R, Leblond D, Duquesnoy B et al (1996) Percutaneous vertebroplasty for osteolytic metastases and myeloma: effects of the percentage of lesion filling and the leakage of methyl methacrylate at clinical follow-up. Radiology 200(2):525–530

102. Weill A, Chiras J, Simon JM, Rose M, Sola-Martinez T, Enkaoua E (1996) Spinal metastases: indications for and results of percutaneous injection of acrylic surgical cement. Radiology 199(1):241–247

103. Ryu S, Rock J, Rosenblum M, Kim JH (2004) Patterns of failure after single-dose radiosurgery for spinal metastasis. J Neurosurg 101(Suppl 3):402–405

104. Gerszten PC, Germanwala A, Burton SA, Welch WC, Ozhasoglu C, Vogel WJ (2005) Combination kyphoplasty and spinal radiosurgery: a new treatment paradigm for pathological fractures. J Neurosurg Spine 3(4):296–301

105. Foley KT, Gupta SK (2002) Percutaneous pedicle screw fixation of the lumbar spine: preliminary clinical results. J Neurosurg 97(Suppl 1):7–12

106. Park HY, Lee SH, Park SJ, Kim ES, Lee CS, Eoh W (2015) Minimally invasive option using percutaneous pedicle screw for instability of metastasis involving thoracolumbar and lumbar spine: a case series in a single center. J Korean Neurosurg Soc 57(2):100–107

107. Huang TJ, Hsu RW, Li YY, Cheng CC (2006) Minimal access spinal surgery (MASS) in treating thoracic spine metastasis. Spine (Phila Pa 1976) 31(16):1860–1863

108. Tancioni F, Navarria P, Pessina F, Marcheselli S, Rognone E, Mancosu P et al (2012) Early surgical experience with minimally invasive percutaneous approach for patients with metastatic epidural spinal cord compression (MESCC) to poor prognoses. Ann Surg Oncol 19(1):294–300

109. Zairi F, Arikat A, Allaoui M, Marinho P, Assaker R (2012) Minimally invasive decompression and stabilization for the management of thoracolumbar spine metastasis. J Neurosurg Spine 17(1):19–23

110. Rao PJ, Thayaparan GK, Fairhall JM, Mobbs RJ (2014) Minimally invasive percutaneous fixation techniques for metastatic spinal disease. Orthop Surg 6(3):187–195

111. Miscusi M, Polli FM, Forcato S, Ricciardi L, Frati A, Cimatti M et al (2015) Comparison of minimally invasive surgery with standard open surgery for vertebral thoracic metastases causing acute myelopathy in patients with short- or mid-term life expectancy: surgical technique and early clinical results. J Neurosurg Spine 22(5):518–525

112. Patchell RA, Tibbs PA, Regine WF, Payne R, Saris S, Kryscio RJ et al (2005) Direct decompressive surgical resection in the treatment of spinal cord com-

pression caused by metastatic cancer: a randomised trial. Lancet 366(9486):643–648

113. Chou D, Lu D, Chi J, Wang V (2008) Rib-head oste-otomies for posterior placement of expandable cages in the treatment of metastatic thoracic spine tumors. J Clin Neurosci 15(9):1043–1047

114. Chou D, Lu DC (2011) Mini-open transpedicular corpectomies with expandable cage reconstruction. Technical note. J Neurosurg Spine 14(1):71–77

115. Shen FH, Marks I, Shaffrey C, Ouellet J, Arlet V (2008) The use of an expandable cage for cor-pectomy reconstruction of vertebral body tumors through a posterior extracavitary approach: a mul-ticenter consecutive case series of prospectively fol-lowed patients. Spine J 8(2):329–339

116. Metcalfe S, Gbejuade H, Patel NR (2012) The pos-terior transpedicular approach for circumferential decompression and instrumented stabilization with titanium cage vertebrectomy reconstruction for spi-nal tumors: consecutive case series of 50 patients. Spine (Phila Pa 1976) 37(16):1375–1383

117. Jandial R, Kelly B, Chen MY (2013) Posterior-only approach for lumbar vertebral column resection and expandable cage reconstruction for spinal metasta-ses. J Neurosurg Spine 19(1):27–33

118. Nazzaro JM, Arbit E, Burt M (1994) "Trap door" exposure of the cervicothoracic junction. Technical note. J Neurosurg 80(2):338–341

119. Gokaslan ZL, York JE, Walsh GL, McCutcheon IE, Lang FF, Putnam JB et al (1998) Transthoracic verte-brectomy for metastatic spinal tumors. J Neurosurg 89(4):599–609

120. Ozgur BM, Aryan HE, Pimenta L, Taylor WR (2006) Extreme Lateral Interbody Fusion (XLIF): a novel surgical technique for anterior lumbar inter-body fusion. Spine J 6(4):435–443

121. Karikari IO, Nimjee SM, Hardin CA, Hughes BD, Hodges TR, Mehta AI et al (2011) Extreme lateral interbody fusion approach for isolated thoracic and thoracolumbar spine diseases: initial clinical expe-rience and early outcomes. J Spinal Disord Tech 24(6):368–375

122. Rodgers WB, Gerber EJ, Patterson J (2011) Intraoperative and early postoperative complications in extreme lateral interbody fusion: an analysis of 600 cases. Spine (Phila Pa 1976) 36(1):26–32

Spinal Robotic Radiosurgery

Alexander Muacevic, Arjun Sahgal, and Jörg-Christian Tonn

37.1 Introduction

Spinal radiosurgery is a new class of procedures designed for primary or adjuvant treatment of certain spinal disorders [4, 7, 8, 10, 26, 27]. Because such large doses of radiation are administered, spinal radiosurgery, similar to its intracranial predecessor, requires extremely accurate targeting. In contrast, the lack of precision inherent in conventional external beam radiation therapy and the limitations of target immobilization techniques generally preclude large single-fraction irradiation near radiosensitive structures such as the spinal cord [6, 10, 11]. The frameless CyberKnife radiosurgery system has overcome these problems by using real-time image guidance which allows the spinous/paraspinous target to be tracked even in the presence of occasional

A. Muacevic (✉)
CyberKnife Zentrum München, München, Germany
e-mail: alexander.muacevic@cyber-knife.net

A. Sahgal
University of Toronto, Toronto, ON, Canada

Department of Radiation Oncology, Odette Cancer Centre, Sunnybrook Health Sciences Centre, Toronto, ON, Canada
e-mail: Arjun.Sahgal@sunnybrook.ca

J.-C. Tonn
Department of Neurosurgery, University Hospital Ludwig Maximilian University Munich, Munich, Germany
e-mail: joerg.christian.tonn@med.uni.muenchen.de

patient movement [12, 18, 26]. Continuous tracking and correction for motion of the spine throughout treatment are prerequisite for spinal radiosurgery, because patients do move after setup is complete [20, 25]. In the past, clinicians surgically implanted fiducials into the spine to track the movement of the lesion during treatment [10, 27]. In the first reported use of image-guided robotics to perform spinal radiosurgery, Ryu and co-workers demonstrated the safety and short-term efficacy for a variety of neoplastic and vascular lesions [27]. Surgical implantation of fiducials into adjacent vertebral segments was necessary for tracking the ablated spinal lesion. However, this step introduces the added surgical risks associated with an invasive surgery, lengthens treatment time, and reduces patient comfort. Recently, a fiducial-free spinal tracking system has been introduced (Xsight Spine Tracking System, Accuray Incorporated) [15, 26, 30].

Despite being frameless, the CyberKnife emulates an important feature of the Gamma Knife, its ability to deliver many beams from many non-coplanar orientations [1, 24]. Unlike the Gamma Knife, however, the CyberKnife is not restricted to treating isocenters; instead, at each position of the robot, the beam is directed toward a different area of the target region. This design feature enables the treating surgeon to select from a large array of non-isocentric and noncoplanar beams during the process of constructing a treatment plan, creating dose distributions that conform to

© Springer Nature Switzerland AG 2019
J.-C. Tonn et al. (eds.), *Oncology of CNS Tumors*, https://doi.org/10.1007/978-3-030-04152-6_37

even irregularly shaped lesion volumes (Fig. 37.1). In contrast, conventional radiosurgical devices are capable of constructing only spherical dose distributions around a discrete isocenter.

37.2 Fiducial-Free Spinal Tracking

The Xsight fiducial-free localization process is performed in several stages, beginning with image enhancement, in which digital reconstructed radiographs (DRRs) and intra-treatment radiographs undergo processing to improve the visualization of skeletal structures. Prior to treatment, a region of interest (ROI) surrounding the target volume is selected based on an initial user-defined position, which is refined automatically by an algorithm that seeks to maximize the image entropy within the ROI. The resulting optimal ROI typically includes one to two vertebral bodies which form the basis of patient motion tracking and alignment. Two dimensional-three dimensional (2D-3D) image registration uses similarity measures to compare the

X-ray images and DRRs and a spatial transformation parameter search method to determine changes in patient position. A mesh is overlaid in the ROI, and local displacements in the mesh nodes are estimated individually, constrained by displacement smoothness. Nodal displacements in the two images within the mesh form two 2D displacement fields. 3D displacements of the targets and global rotations of spinal structures within the ROI can then be calculated from the two 2D displacement fields by interpolation. A screen shot from an Xsight treatment session shows that the overlaid mesh technique is successful even in the presence of spinal instrumentation (Fig. 37.2) [20, 26].

The main advantages of the fiducial-free system are (1) the ability to account for non-rigid deformation, thereby improving the targeting accuracy in the situation that a patient pose change occurs subsequent to the CT scan, and (2) no risk of complication and increased convenience for both the patient and the clinician. The fiducial-free tracking system of the CyberKnife has been proven in end-to-end phantom tests and simulations, using existing

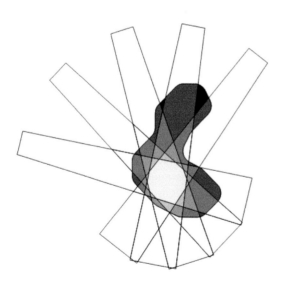
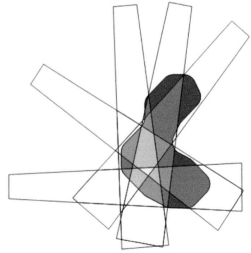
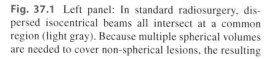

Fig. 37.1 Left panel: In standard radiosurgery, dispersed isocentrical beams all intersect at a common region (light gray). Because multiple spherical volumes are needed to cover non-spherical lesions, the resulting dose distribution tends to be inhomogeneous. Right panel: Non-isocentric beams from various directions do not all cross a single point, and the dose is more homogeneous

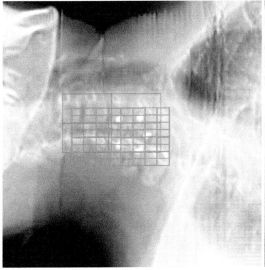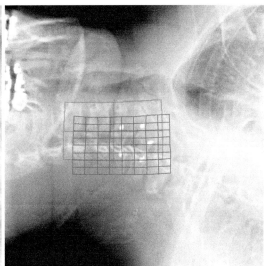

Fig. 37.2 The hierarchical mesh tracking procedure. Registration is performed using a hierarchical mesh technique, where the calculation is made at a series of discrete points within the ROI. The process is iterative, with additional registration points added at each step in order to improve the spatial resolution of the result. This approach generates a deformable registration model, which can account for nonrigid changes in the patient pose between pre-treatment and intra-treatment imaging. The deformation is apparent in the mesh in the X-ray panel

CT image sets of the spine, to be accurate to within about 0.5 mm [20, 26, 32]. Fürweger et al. evaluated the clinical targeting precision and assessed patient movement data during fiducial-free, single-fraction spinal radiosurgery with the CyberKnife [12]. Image-guided spine tracking accuracy was tested using two phantoms. Movement patterns from the three translations axes (X, Y, and Z) and three rotational axes (pitch, roll, and yaw) were obtained from log files of 260 patient treatments (47 cervical, 89 thoracic, 90 lumbar, and 34 pelvic/sacral). Phantom spine position was registered with an accuracy of <0.2 mm for translational and <0.3 for rotational directions. Residual patient motion yielded mean targeting errors per beam of 0.28 ± 0.13 mm (X), 0.25 ± 0.15 mm (Y), 0.19 ± 0.11 mm (Z) and 0.40 ± 0.20 (roll), 0.20 ± 0.08 (pitch), and 0.19 ± 0.08 (yaw). The spine region had little influence on overall targeting error, which was <1 mm for more than 95% of treatments (median, 0.48 mm). In the maximum motion case, target coverage decreased by 1.7% (from 92.1% to 90.4%) for the 20-Gy prescription isodose. Spinal cord volume receiving more than 8 Gy increased

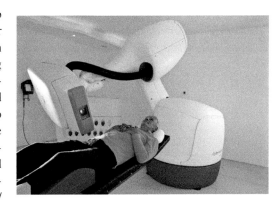

Fig. 37.3 Patient position during spinal radiosurgery for a lumbar lesion. The patient lies on the treatment couch without any vacuum bags or fixation devices. A cushion is placed under the legs for patient comfort. The pre-treatment CT scan was performed in the same position. The head of the robot shows the new Micro-Multi-Leaf Collimator (InCise, Accuray Inc.) which shows significant treatment time reduction in spinal radiosurgery [23]

slightly, from 2.41 to 2.46 cm³. The authors concluded that submillimeter targeting precision was obtained for fiducial-free spinal radiosurgery despite patient motion. Patient motion has little effect on the delivered dose distribution when image-guided correction of beam aiming is employed (Fig. 37.3).

37.3 Clinical Data

Prospective and multiple retrospective studies have established the safety and efficacy of spinal SBRT; however, as yet no randomized trials have been reported to confirm superior outcomes [2, 13, 14, 16, 19, 29–32]. The first report of the Spine response assessment in Neuro-Oncology (SPINO) group of the Response Assessment in Neuro-Oncology (RANO) working group established recommendations with respect to imaging and technical requirements for delivery and provided recommendations for outcome definitions for local control and pain control [28]. The key recommendations include the use of thin-slice CT and MRI for SBRT planning, follow-up MRI imaging in order to assess for tumor response and diagnose toxicities including vertebral compression fracture (VCF), and utilization of Brief Pain Inventory (BPI) and International Consensus Pain Response Endpoints (ICPRE) for assessment of pain response. Recently, postoperative SBRT has been implemented in spine treatment protocols which directly changed the pattern of practice of spinal surgery for metastatic disease. There has been a shift in surgical indications, surgical goals, and expected outcomes for patients with spinal metastases as a direct consequence of spine SBRT. Future publications will need to standardize the metrics used to determine surgical candidacy and outcome assessment that ensure utility of this intervention.

37.4 Munich Outcome Data

In the Munich center within the first 10 years, 560 patients with a total of 717 spinal lesions were treated using the described fiducial-free spinal tracking method [26, 30] (Fig. 37.4). All treatments were performed using single-session spinal radiosurgery (Fig. 37.5). For ablation of spinal metastases, a median marginal dose of 19.4 Gy (range 15–24 Gy) was delivered to the 70% (range 50–85%) isodose. The dose level did not differ between patients with and without spinal pain syndromes. The median tumor volume for all patients was 29.7 cm^3. There was one patient with a spinal myelopathy, three patients with a segmental instability, and one intratumoral bleeding after radiosurgery requiring surgical evacuation. No acute side effects were observed except for nausea in 8% of treated patients. The local tumor control rate after a median follow-up of 36 months was 92% (Fig. 37.6). Pain relief occurred as early as 1 h and within 7 days after radiosurgery. Statistical analysis identified the initial pain score as the

Fig. 37.4 Tumor histologies/treated lesions

Tumor histologies	Percentage
Metastatic lesions	**85%**
UGT	44%
GIT	14%
lung	11%
breast	16%
Melanoma	3%
Sarcoma	1%
Prostate	10%
Others	11%
Spinal AVM	**2%**
Benign lesions	**14%**
Neurinoma	8%
Meningeoma	3%
Cordoma	3%
Ependymoma	1%

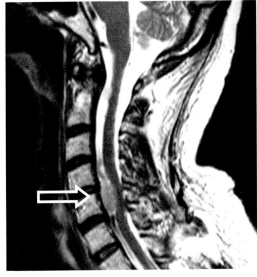
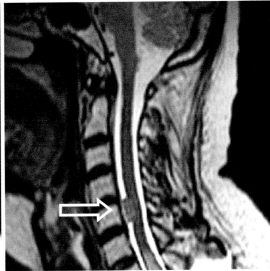

Fig. 37.5 The left image shows a T2 sagittal MRI scan of a patient undergoing surgery and conventional radiation therapy for a malignant peripheral nerve sheath tumor at the level of C6 (open arrow). The recurrent tumor was compressing the spinal cord from ventral. Instead of repeat surgery, CyberKnife radiosurgery was performed using fiducial-free tracking. On the right image, the result after spinal radiosurgery is depicted. The tumor shrank significantly (open arrow), and ventral compression to the spinal cord was eliminated

Fig. 37.6 Cumulative local tumor control in patients ($\underline{n} = 540$) with malignant spinal tumors after CyberKnife radiosurgery (Kaplan-Meier method)

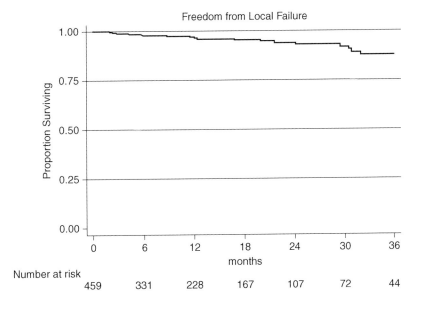

only significant variable to predict pain reduction after spinal radiosurgery ($p < 0.03$). No radiation damage of the spinal cord or the spinal nerve roots was observed. Gerszten et al. presented the largest published series (500 spinal lesions) treated in a single fraction using fiducial tracking [18]. Long-term pain improvement occurred in 290 of 336 cases (86%). Long-term tumor control was demonstrated in 90% of lesions treated with radiosurgery as a primary treatment modality and in 88% of lesions treated for radiographic tumor progression. In both the Gerszten study and our investigation, treatment-related toxicity was very low.

The classic single-fraction definition of radiosurgery, proposed by Leksell [24], has been expanded recently to include up to five fractions of focused radiation delivered to relatively small and well-defined targets in the brain and the spine [1, 3, 5]. This updated definition reflects, in part, the fact that frameless delivery of high-dose radiation has made possible the treatment, with ablative intent, of lesions in more than one fraction, a procedure that was impractical when lesion targeting was accomplished using stereotactic frames. Whether it is clinically advisable to treat in more than one fraction is another matter, however, clearly the intent of treating in multiple fractions is to reduce the likelihood of damage to nearby critical structures. For example, Degen et al. treated 51 patients with various metastatic lesions [9]. A local control rate of 100% in patients who had not been previously irradiated was observed, but there were three recurrences among the patients who had undergone irradiation before radiosurgery. Only minor and transient side effects from radiosurgery were observed during a 3-month follow-up period. The authors also found that CyberKnife radiosurgery resulted in rapid and durable pain control and maintained pre-treatment quality of life. Thus, hypofractionated treatment of spine lesions is also feasible and locally effective [21, 22].

CyberKnife radiosurgery has been combined with kyphoplasty to address pathological compression fractures [17]. This is a new treatment paradigm for metastatic spinal tumors. Even more integrated radiosurgical approaches are likely to emerge in the future which will further change the classic surgical management of many spinal lesions.

37.5 CyberKnife Team

High-quality radiosurgical applications are getting increasingly complex; thus, different treatment applications require different medical professionals, such as surgeons, radiation oncologists, or radiologists, as well as specially trained medical physicists to achieve the most effective and safe treatment results. Intracranial and spinal treatments should be reviewed by experienced neurosurgeons capable of understanding the complex topographical relationships of cranial and spinal anatomy and pathology. Orthopedic surgeons may also be helpful to support spinal treatments. The contribution of experienced imaging experts for optimal selection and interpretation of imaging studies will enhance the quality of the radiosurgical application significantly. Noninvasive robotic radiosurgery, nowadays, is a truly interdisciplinary field and opens new horizons in the area of cancer treatment.

37.6 Conclusions

Single-fraction spinal radiosurgery with the CyberKnife is a completely noninvasive, safe, and effective treatment method for selected cancer patients. Patients with limited spinal disease and a comparatively long cancer survival time are particularly suited for this type of therapy. The short amount of time required to deliver this outpatient procedure allows it to fit well into oncological treatment concepts. Furthermore, in patients with tumor-associated pain syndromes, the method provides significant pain reduction.

References

1. Adler JR Jr, Chang SD, Murphy MJ, Doty J, Geis P, Hancock SL (1997) The Cyberknife: a frameless robotic system for radiosurgery. Stereotact Funct Neurosurg 69:124–128
2. Al-Omair A, Masucci L, Masson-Cote L et al (2013) Surgical resection of epidural disease improves local control following postoperative spine stereotactic body radiotherapy. Neuro-Oncology 15(10):1413–1419
3. Barnett GH, Linskey ME, Adler JR et al (2007) Stereotactic radiosurgery—an organized neurosurgery-sanctioned definition. J Neurosurg 106:1–5
4. Benzil DL, Saboori M, Mogilner AY, Rocchio R, Moorthy CR (2004) Safety and efficacy of stereotactic radiosurgery for tumors of the spine. J Neurosurg 101(Suppl 3):413–418
5. Bhatnagar AK, Gerszten PC, Ozhasaglu C et al (2005) CyberKnife frameless radiosurgery for the treatment of extracranial benign tumors. Technol Cancer Res Treat 4:571–576
6. Bilsky MH, Yamada Y, Yenice KM et al (2004) Intensity-modulated stereotactic radiotherapy of

paraspinal tumors: a preliminary report. Neurosurgery 54:823–830; discussion 821–830

7. Buatti JM, Friedman WA, Meeks SL, Bova FJ (1998) The radiobiology of radiosurgery and stereotactic radiotherapy. Med Dosim 23:201–207

8. Chang EL, Shiu AS, Lii MF et al (2004) Phase I clinical evaluation of near-simultaneous computed tomographic image-guided stereotactic body radiotherapy for spinal metastases. Int J Radiat Oncol Biol Phys 59:1288–1294

9. Degen JW, Gagnon GJ, Voyadzis JM et al (2005) CyberKnife stereotactic radiosurgical treatment of spinal tumors for pain control and quality of life. J Neurosurg Spine 2:540–549

10. Dodd RL, Ryu MR, Kamnerdsupaphon P, Gibbs IC, Chang SD Jr, Adler JR Jr (2006) CyberKnife radiosurgery for benign intradural extramedullary spinal tumors. Neurosurgery 58:674–685; discussion 674–685

11. Eble MJ, Eckert W, Wannenmacher M (1995) Value of local radiotherapy in treatment of osseous metastases, pathological fractures and spinal cord compression. Radiologe 35:47–54

12. Fürweger C, Drexler C, Kufeld M, Muacevic A, Wowra B, Schlaefer A (2010) Patient motion and targeting accuracy in robotic spinal radiosurgery: 260 single-fraction fiducial-free cases. Int J Radiat Oncol Biol Phys 78(3):937–945. https://doi.org/10.1016/j.ijrobp.2009.11.030

13. Garg AK, Wang XS, Shiu AS et al (2011) Prospective evaluation of spinal reirradiation by using stereotactic body radiation therapy: the University of Texas MD Anderson Cancer Center experience. Cancer 117(15):3509–3516

14. Gerszten PC, Ozhasoglu C, Burton SA, Kalnicki S, Welch WC (2002) Feasibility of frameless single-fraction stereotactic radiosurgery for spinal lesions. Neurosurg Focus 13:e2

15. Gerszten PC, Ozhasoglu C, Burton SA et al (2003) Cyberknife frameless real-time image-guided stereotactic radiosurgery for the treatment of spinal lesions. Int J Radiat Oncol Biol Phys 57:S370–S371

16. Gerszten PC, Ozhasoglu C, Burton SA et al (2003) Evaluation of CyberKnife frameless real-time image-guided stereotactic radiosurgery for spinal lesions. Stereotact Funct Neurosurg 81:84–89

17. Gerszten PC, Germanwala A, Burton SA, Welch WC, Ozhasoglu C, Vogel WJ (2005) Combination kyphoplasty and spinal radiosurgery: a new treatment paradigm for pathological fractures. Neurosurg Focus 18(3):e8

18. Gerszten PC, Burton SA, Ozhasoglu C, Welch WC (2007) Radiosurgery for spinal metastases: clinical experience in 500 cases from a single institution. Spine 32:193–199

19. Guckenberger M, Mantel F, Gerszten PC et al (2014) Safety and efficacy of stereotactic body radiotherapy as primary treatment for vertebral metastases: a multi-institutional analysis. Radiat Oncol 9:226

20. Ho AK, Fu D, Cotrutz C, Hancock SL et al (2007) A study of the accuracy of Cyberknife spinal radiosurgery using skeletal structure tracking. Neurosurgery 60:147–156

21. Kanda M, Matsuhashi M, Sawamoto N et al (2002) Cortical potentials related to assessment of pain intensity with visual analogue scale (VAS). Clin Neurophysiol 113:1013–1024

22. Kelly AM (2001) The minimum clinically significant difference in visual analogue scale pain score does not differ with severity of pain. Emerg Med J 18:205–207

23. Kim N, Lee H, Kim JS, Baek JG, Lee CG, Chang SK, Koom WS (2017) Clinical outcomes of multileaf collimatorbased CyberKnife for spine stereotactic body radiation therapy. Br J Radiol 90(1079):20170523. https://doi.org/10.1259/bjr.20170523

24. Leksell L (1951) The stereotaxic method and radiosurgery of the brain. Acta Chir Scand 102:316–319

25. Ma L, Sahgal A, Hossain S, Chuang C, Descovich M, Huang K, Gottschalk A, Larson DA (2009) Nonrandom intrafraction target motions and general strategy for correction of spine stereotactic body radiotherapy. Int J Radiat Oncol Biol Phys 75(4):1261–1265

26. Muacevic A, Staehler M, Drexler C, Wowra B, Reiser M, Tonn JC (2006) Technical description, phantom accuracy, and clinical feasibility for fiducial-free frameless real-time image-guided spinal radiosurgery. J Neurosurg Spine 5:303–312

27. Ryu SI, Chang SD, Kim DH et al (2001) Image-guided hypo-fractionated stereotactic radiosurgery to spinal lesions. Neurosurgery 49:838–846

28. Thibault I, Chang EL, Sheehan J et al (2015) Response assessment after stereotactic body radiotherapy for spinal metastasis: a report from the SPIne response assessment in Neuro-Oncology (SPINO) group. Lancet Oncol 16(16):e595–e603

29. Wang XS, Rhines LD, Shiu AS et al (2012) Stereotactic body radiation therapy for management of spinal metastases in patients without spinal cord compression: a phase 1-2 trial. Lancet Oncol 13(4):395–402

30. Wowra B, Zausinger S, Drexler C, Kufeld M, Muacevic A, Staehler M, Tonn JC (2008) Cyberknife radiosurgery for malignant spinal tumors: characterization of well-suited patients. Spine 33(26):2929–2934

31. Yamada Y, Lovelock DM, Yenice KM et al (2005) Multifractionated image-guided and stereotactic intensity-modulated radiotherapy of paraspinal tumors: a preliminary report. Int J Radiat Oncol Biol Phys 62:53–61

32. Yu C, Main W, Taylor D, Kuduvalli G, Apuzzo ML, Adler JR Jr (2004) An anthropomorphic phantom study of the accuracy of Cyberknife spinal radiosurgery. Neurosurgery 55:1138–1149

Peripheral Nerve Sheath Tumors

38

Suganth Suppiah, Shirin Karimi, and Gelareh Zadeh

38.1 Overview

Peripheral nerve sheath tumors (PNST) are a relatively uncommon soft tissue neoplasm that can arise from anywhere on the body and range from benign tumors, such as schwannomas and cutaneous neurofibromas, to high-grade malignant tumors referred to as malignant peripheral nerve sheath tumors (MPNST). These tumors often result in severe physical disfigurement, especially in the context of genetic disorders, and cause debilitating pain and neurological disability. Majority of peripheral nerve tumors are solitary and sporadic; however, multiple lesions are a common occurrence in the setting of tumor predisposing syndromes, such as neurofibromatosis type 1 (NF1), neurofibromatosis type 2 (NF2), and schwannomatosis.

There are major challenges in the diagnosis and management of PNSTs, as these tumors are assessed by a variety of medical and surgical specialties, due to its non-specific symptoms and ubiquitous presentations. Optimal management requires a multidisciplinary team of surgeons, radiologists, neuropathologists, and medical oncologists with expertise in PNSTs, at a special-ized center. Not all patients with a suspected diagnosis of PNST require surgical intervention. PNSTs that are asymptomatic or minimally symptomatic with imaging features suggestive of a benign lesion can often be clinically and/or radiologically monitored. However, tumors that demonstrate local compressive symptoms or develop signs suspicious of malignant transformation, such as increased growth rate, require surgical intervention. The goals of surgery may be to obtain biopsy for pathological confirmation of tumor, debulking to decrease mass effect or complete tumor excision. The surgical options available to a patient are dictated by the tumor histopathology and location. Although preoperative MRI often suggests the optimal surgical goal, the final decision is made intraoperatively depending on the evaluation of the risks of tumor removal versus associated neurological deficits. Therefore, it is important to establish the expectations of surgery with the patient prior to surgery.

Schwann cells are the cell of origin in PNSTs, although the histopathological appearance and clinicopathological behavior vary significantly among the different types [1–3]. Schwannomas, the most common PNST, are sporadic in 90% of cases with the remaining occurring in the context of NF2 and schwannomatosis [4]. These tumors are encapsulated and grow extrafascicular, making them amenable to gross total surgical resection. In contrast, neurofibromas are difficult to

S. Suppiah · S. Karimi · G. Zadeh (✉)
MacFeeters-Hamilton Centre for Neuro-Oncology Research, Toronto Medical Discovery Tower, University of Toronto, Toronto, ON, Canada
e-mail: suganth.suppiah@mail.utoronto.ca; shirin.karimi@uhnresearch.ca; Gelareh.zadeh@uhn.ca

© Springer Nature Switzerland AG 2019
J.-C. Tonn et al. (eds.), *Oncology of CNS Tumors*, https://doi.org/10.1007/978-3-030-04152-6_38

completely resect without causing iatrogenic neurological injury due to its intrafascicular growth. Neurofibromas, also, develop sporadically in majority of cases and are the most common tumor type associated with NF1. Plexiform neurofibromas, pathognomonic for NF1, carry a 5–10% lifetime risk of malignant transformation [5]. Despite aggressive surgical and adjuvant oncological therapy, MPNST portend a poor prognosis with 23–52% 5-year disease-specific mortality [6–8]. Primarily peripheral nerve sheath tumors will be discussed further, with a brief overview of other nonneural peripheral nerve tumors.

38.2   Symptoms and Clinical Signs

Due to the PNSTs' ability to develop anywhere in the body, these tumors present with a wide range of symptoms and clinical signs. For tumors within the cranial vault, such as acoustic schwannomas, patients can present with cranial nerve dysfunction, obstructive hydrocephalus (headaches, nausea/vomiting), and cerebellar dysfunction. Peripheral nerve tumors within the spinal canal can present with neuropathic pain, weakness, numbness, myelopathy, and bowel/bladder dysfunction. A palpable growing mass, focal pain, neuropathic pain, and neurological symptoms can accompany a tumor within the extremities. A focused history should be directed toward the onset, duration, and progression of symptoms and any palpable masses. It is imperative to perform a review of symptoms when assessing a patient with a focal peripheral nerve tumor, to rule out additional lesions that may be indicative of an underlying genetic predisposition. A family history for NF1, NF2, or schwannomatosis should be interrogated as a significant number of PNSTs occur in the context of these genetic disorders.

The physical exam should be focused on any palpable masses, with comments on its consistency (firm vs. soft), mobility (mobile vs. adhered to soft tissue), pulsatility (pulsatile vs. nonpulsatile), and tenderness. Although majority of PNSTs do not present with neurological symptoms, the presence of signs and symptoms such as neuropathic pain, weakness, numbness, or Tinel's sign may help localize the nerve of origin. In addition, a complete systemic examination with a focus on identifying clinical manifestations of NF1 and NF2, such as café au lait spots, axillary freckling, and other signs, is listed in Table 38.1.

38.3   Diagnostics

Additional investigations are warranted in the workup of a suspected peripheral nerve tumor to help guide clinicians in the optimal management plan. Magnetic resonance imaging (MRI) is the imaging modality of choice to investigate these lesions. A combination of clinical history and imaging features can be highly suggestive of a benign lesion, although serial clinical and radiographical follow-up is required to confirm diagnosis. Furthermore, the MRI features are not diagnostic of the benign PNST subtype (neurofibroma vs. schwannoma) but can provide the clinician with clues to help infer the diagnosis. Both schwannomas and neurofibromas appear hypointense on T1 and hyperintense on T2 (Figs. 38.1 and 38.2). However, schwannomas tend to have intense homogenous contrast enhancement compared to heterogenous contrast enhancement in neurofibromas. Further, schwannomas are well-defined and demonstrate adjacent bone remodeling on computed tomography (CT) scans. Neurofibromas are more fusiform or multinodular due to their intrafascicular growth. The presence of a target sign, a hyperintense rim and central area of low signal, is suggestive of a neurofibroma but is occasionally, also, observed in schwannomas and MPNSTS.

Based on current technology, it is difficult to reliably differentiate between a benign and malignant peripheral nerve sheath tumor, as there is significant overlap in radiological features. There are no definitive radiological features on an MRI that define an MPNST. However, lesions that have demonstrated rapid growth (clinical and or radiographical) or have irregular

Table 38.1 Diagnostic criteria for neurofibromatosis type 1 and 2 and schwannomatosis [21, 23, 26]

Neurofibromatosis type 1
- **NIH criteria are met if ≥2 of the following are present**
- ≥6 café au lait spots (diameter >5 mm in prepubertal patients and >15 mm in post pubertal patients)
- ≥2 neurofibromas of any type or 1 plexiform neurofibroma
- Freckling of axillary or inguinal regions
- Optic gliomas
- ≥Lisch nodules (iris hamartomas)
- Distinctive osseous lesions (such as sphenoid wing dysplasia or apparent thinning of long-bone cortex with or without pseudarthrosis)
- First degree relative with NF1 (by above criteria)

Neurofibromatosis Type 2
- **Clinical diagnosis is based on meeting ONE of the following criteria:**
- Bilateral vestibular schwannomas before age 70
- Unilateral vestibular schwannoma before age 70 AND first-degree relative with NF2
- Any two of the following: meningioma, non-vestibular schwannoma, neurofibroma, glioma, cerebral calcification, cataract; AND
  - First degree relative with NF2 OR
    - Unilateral vestibular schwannoma AND negative LZTR1 testing
- Multiple meningiomas AND
  - Unilateral vestibular schwannoma OR
    - Any two of the following: non-vestibular schwannoma, neurofibroma, glioma, cerebral calcification, cataract
- Constitutional or mosaic pathogenic NF2 gene mutation form blood or identification of identical mutation from two separate tumors in the same individual

Schwannomatosis
- **Definite diagnosis of schwannomatosis based on meeting ONE of the following criteria:**
- Age >30 and all of the following:
  - Two or more nonintradermal schwannomas, at least one with histologic confirmation
  - Diagnostic criteria for NF2 not fulfilled
  - No evidence of vestibular schwannoma on high-quality MRI scan
  - No first-degree relative with NF2
  - No known constitutional NF2 mutation
- One pathologically confirmed nonvestibular schwannoma plus a first degree relative who meets the above criteria
- **Possible diagnosis of schwannomatosis based on meeting any of the following circumstances**
- Age <30 and all of the following:

Table 38.1 (continued)
- Two or more nonintradermal schwannomas, at least one with histologic confirmation
- Diagnostic criteria for NF2 not fulfilled
- No evidence of vestibular schwannoma on high-quality MRI scan
- No first-degree relative with NF2
- No constitutional NF2 mutation
- Age >45 years; no symptoms of eighth cranial nerve dysfunction; and all of the following:
  - Two or more intradermal schwannomas, at least one with histologic confirmation
  - Diagnostic criteria for NF2 are not fulfilled
  - No first-degree relative with NF2
  - No known constitutional NF2 mutation
- Radiographic evidence of a schwannoma and first-degree relative meeting criteria for definitive schwannomatosis

borders are more likely to be malignant. In addition, 18-fluorodeoxyglucose (FDG) positron-emission tomography (PET) imaging may have utility in differentiation of benign and malignant tumors, with increased uptake in MPNSTs [9]. However, the sensitivity of FDG PET ranges from 89 to 100% and specificity ranges from 72 to 95% [10–12]. As a result, tumors that demonstrate growth over serial imaging or progression of symptomology pose a management dilemma, often requiring surgical biopsy for confirmation of malignant transformation.

38.4 Pathological Classification

Histopathological analysis of tumor sample obtained through surgery is the gold standard for diagnosis and classification of peripheral nerve tumors. Broadly speaking, peripheral nerve tumors are classified into neural and nonneural tumors based on the cell of origin. Firstly, the most common neural tumors are schwannomas, neurofibromas and malignant peripheral nerve sheath tumors, arising from the nerve sheath. Other rare neural tumors include perineuromas, ganglioneuromas, ganglioneuroblastomas, and primary peripheral nerve lymphomas. Within the second category, tumors with nonneural sheath origin include

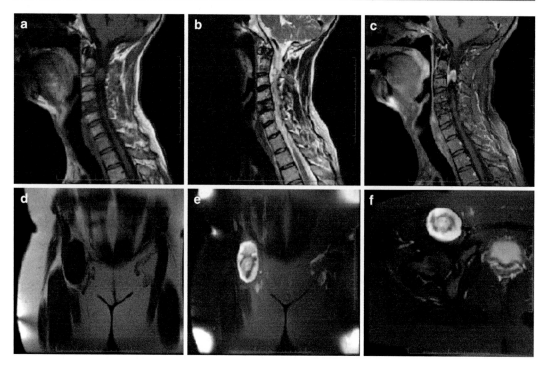

Fig. 38.1 (**a–c**) Neurofibroma arising from C2 nerve root within the cervical spine. The neurofibroma appears hypointense on T1-weighted (**a**) and hyperintense on T2-weighted (**b**) MRI sequences. There is also diffuse contrast enhancement on T1 + gadolinium sequence (**c**). (**d**) Neurofibroma arising from the femoral nerve. Again, the neurofibroma is hypointense on T1-weighted and hyperintense on T2-weighted sequences. The target sign is also present in this neurofibroma (**e + f**)

ganglion cysts, lipomas, desmoids, and neuromas.

Although schwannomas and neurofibromas are characterized by neoplastic proliferation of Schwann cells, they differ vastly based on histopathological features and growth patterns. For instance, neurofibromas also incorporate multiple other cell types within the tumor and grow in an extrafascicular fashion, as compared to a well-encapsulated and intrafascicular schwannoma. The reason for the difference in histopathological characteristics of these Schwann cell-derived neoplasms is unclear. Schwann cells are a diverse group of cells that develop from neural crest cells, and perhaps the biological subtype that is transformed drives tumor growth behavior. Schwannomas could represent a proliferation of a more mature Schwann cell, while neurofibromas and MPNSTs originate from a Schwann cell progenitor (Fig. 38.3). Animal models and in vitro studies support this hypothesis by dem-

onstrating that plexiform neurofibromas can develop from progenitor Schwann cells [1, 13, 14]. However, cutaneous neurofibromas may develop from a neural crest like stem cell, named skin-derived precursors (SKPs), that can differentiate along neuronal and glial lineages, with loss of NF1 giving rise to neurofibromas [14]. Ultimately, the timing of the primary molecular alteration in the maturity of the Schwann cell is important in determining the type of PNST to develop.

As previously noted, neurofibromas primarily consist of Schwann cells but also have proliferation of all elements of the peripheral nerve including perineural cells and fibroblasts. On gross examination, neurofibromas are nonencapsulated lesions with tan-white glistening surfaces and intrafascicular growth pattern. Although the nerve is frequently not grossly identifiable, pathologically, neurofibromas are composed of spindle cells that are elongated,

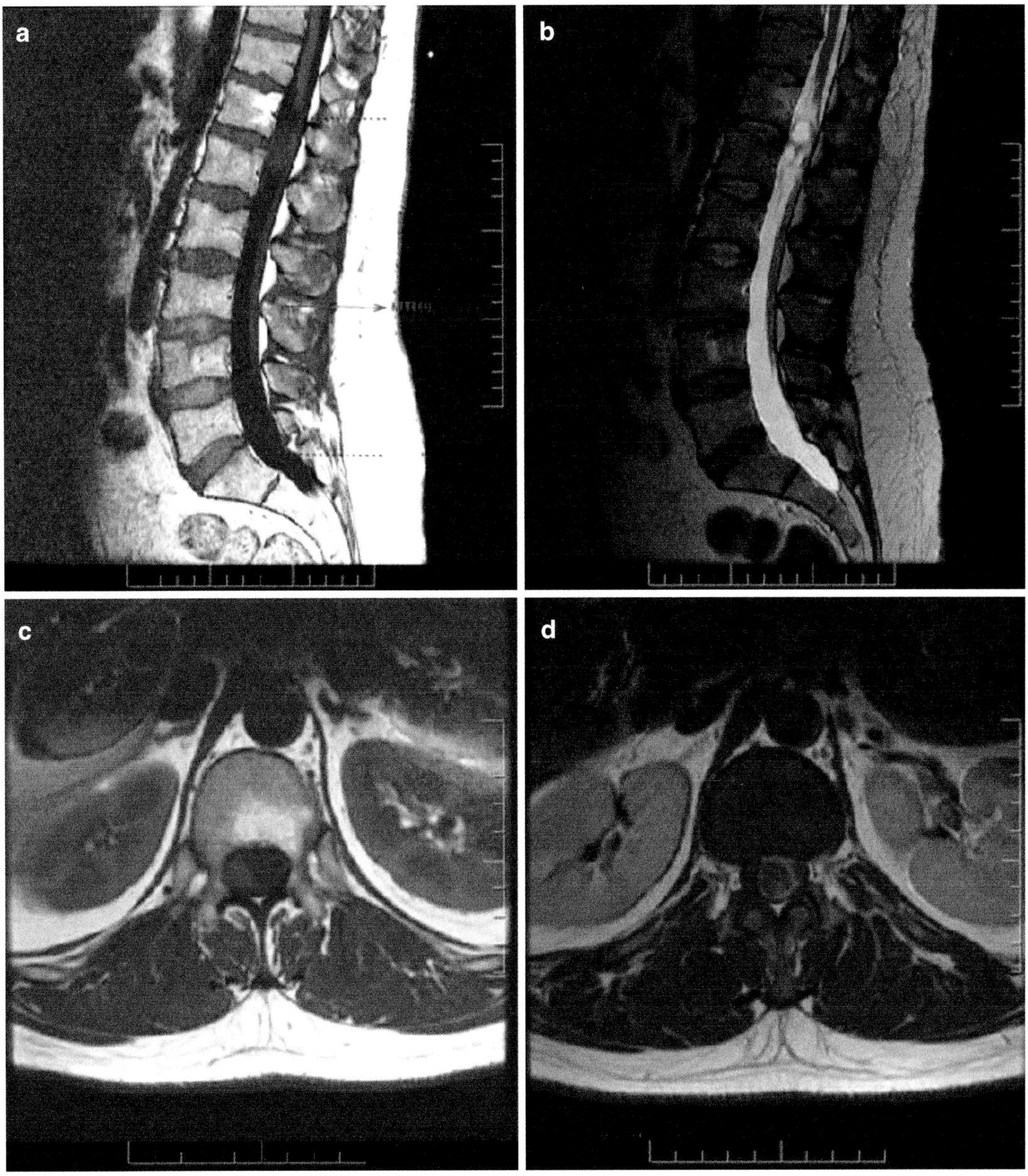

Fig. 38.2 (a–d) Schwannoma arising from the L1 nerve root on the left. Schwannoma appears hypointense on T1-weighted and hyperintense on T2-weighted MRI sequences. (c, d) Demonstrates diffuse contrast enhancement within the schwannoma on T1 + gadolinium sequence

wavy, and hyperchromatic in a loose myxoid background. Pathologists often describe a "shredded carrot collagen" appearance with thin and thick collagen strands (Fig. 38.4). Immunostaining for S-100 is variable, ranging from 30 to 40%. SOX10 a pan-schwannic marker is diffusely positive in neurofibroma [3, 15]. In addition, CD34 positivity is sometimes present and EMA is negative [3].

Neurofibromas are categorized into subtypes based on growth patterns and locations of tumors. Cutaneous, localized intraneural, diffuse, melanotic, and plexiform neurofibromas are common subtypes. Cutaneous neurofibromas are circum-

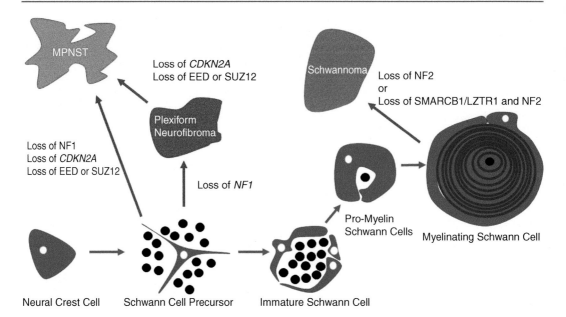

Fig. 38.3 Schwann cell lineage with a neural crest cell differentiating into a mature myelinating schwann cell. It is hypothesized that genomic alterations leading to loss of NF1, CDKN2A, and/or EED/SUZ12 can lead to the development of neurofibromas and MPNSTs [1, 16, 18]. Loss of NF2/SMARCB1/LZTR1 in mature schwann cells leads to the development of schwannomas [26, 32]

scribed lesions that are found in the dermis and subcutis and arise from small cutaneous nerves. Localized neurofibromas result in segmental and fusiform nerve enlargement with axons traversing through the lesion. In contrast, diffuse neurofibromas are ill-defined and grow diffusely along a nerve with infiltration of subcutaneous tissues. Melanotic neurofibromas are melanin-bearing pigmented tumors, which is usually only appreciated microscopically. Notably, malignant transformation is rare in these subtypes. The most worrisome subtype is the plexiform neurofibroma, which is exclusively found in patients with NF1. Macroscopically, plexiform neurofibromas distort the nerve to resemble a "bag of worms" and carries a 5–10% risk of malignant transformation [3].

In addition, there is a nebulous entity of atypical neurofibromas and low-grade MPNSTS that are "intermediate" peripheral nerve sheath tumor that fall in between benign neurofibromas and MPNSTs in the tumor spectrum. Atypical neurofibromas are characterized by marked nuclear atypia, loss of architecture, hypercellularity, increased mitotic activity, and high proliferation

index by Ki67. These tumors are believed to be premalignant and often have increased glucose uptake on 18-FDG PET scan [16]. It is hypothesized that benign neurofibromas undergo malignant transformation toward a MPNST through an intermediate atypical neurofibroma stage.

On the other hand, schwannomas are wellencapsulated lesions with an extrafascicular growth pattern. Schwannomas are firm gray masses that may have cystic and hemorrhagic regions. The nerve is usually attached but can be separated from the tumor. Histologically, schwannomas consist of densely cellular Antoni A regions, with spindle-shaped cells forming palisading rows of nuclei aligned parallel to each other called Verocay bodies (Fig. 38.4). These regions are usually accompanied by alternating Antoni B regions of hypocellular degenerative tissue rich in macrophages and collagen fibers. Schwannomas typically demonstrate diffuse and strong S100 and SOX10 protein expression. Also, CD34-positive cells are found in Antoni B areas and calretinin-positive cells in Antoni A areas [3].

Schwannomas are classified into five subtypes: epithelioid, plexiform, cellular, ancient,

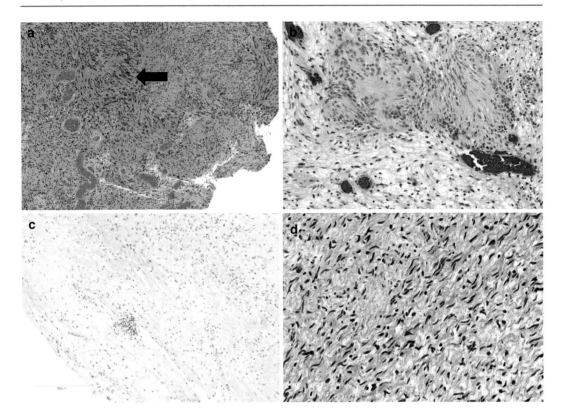

Fig. 38.4 H and E stains at 20×. (**a**) Schwannoma: Biphasic tumor growth pattern with hypercellular Antoni A (arrow) and myxoid hypocellular Antoni B areas. Several vascular channels with thickened hyalinized walls are also seen. (**b**) Schwannoma: Verocay body is visualized. (**c**) Schwannoma: Appearance of thick fibrous capsule with subcapsular perivascular inflammatory cell infiltration. (**d**) Neurofibroma: Diffuse proliferation of bland-looking spindle cells with wavy serpentine nuclei and interspersed wire collagen fibers

and melanotic schwannomas. Epithelioid schwannomas consist primarily of round, epithelioid Schwann cells arranged in clusters. Antoni A and B areas may be absent or present focally. This subtype is often found in subcutaneous tumors. Epithelioid tumors can be difficult to differentiate with MPNSTs, but the small cellular size, sharp circumscription, and low proliferative activity favor schwannomas. Plexiform schwannomas often have intraneural growth, with majority Antoni A and infrequent Antoni B areas. Unlike its neurofibroma counterpart, plexiform schwannomas have no significant risk of malignant transformation. Ancient schwannomas (also known as schwannomas with degenerative changes) have marked degenerative atypia but lack mitotic activity, while cellular schwannomas are composed predominantly of Antoni A areas without Verocay bodies and may have mild

mitotic activity. Cellular schwannomas have an increased risk of recurrence but no malignant behavior. Finally, melanotic schwannomas are partially encapsulated grossly pigmented tumors which are immunoreactive with melanocytic markers (HMB-45). This tumor subtype often lacks clear Antoni A/B areas and Verocay bodies. Other melanin-producing neoplasms, specifically melanomas, are the main differential diagnosis for melanotic schwannomas. Of note, melanotic schwannomas have malignant potential and require long-term follow-up.

Hybrid benign nerve sheath tumor is a newly described entity with variable components of schwannoma, neurofibroma, and perineurioma. Since the first description of hybrid PNST in a review of nine cases by Feany et al. in 1998, several publications have explored this pathology [3, 17]. The most common types are schwannoma/

perineurioma and neurofibroma/schwannoma, which occur in the sporadic and neurofibromatosis settings, respectively. Neurofibroma/perineurioma is a rare hybrid tumor that has been observed in NF1 patients. To date, there is only one reported case of a malignant transformation of a hybrid PNST (neurofibroma/perineurioma); however, larger longitudinal studies need to be conducted to better understand its malignant potential.

MPNSTs account for 3–10% of all soft tissue sarcomas, with half of these cases occurring in NF1 patients. The diagnosis of MPNST can be difficult due to the lack of specific histopathological criteria and ancillary immunohistochemical tests. These tumors are notably hypercellular, with nuclear enlargement and hyperchromasia, compared to benign PNST (Fig. 38.5). The mitotic rate is over 5 per 10 high power field (hpf). The gross appearance of a tumor arising from a peripheral nerve tumor or pre-existing plexiform neurofibroma helps differentiate MPNSTs from other sarcomas. In addition, correlation with clinical history including presence of NF1 syndrome provides diagnostic clues. MPNSTs have variable S100 and SOX10 positivity, since approximately half of the tumors have dedifferentiated to lose their Schwann cell signature [3, 6, 8]. Recently, the complete loss of trimethylation at lysine 27 of histone h3 (H3K27me3) has been described as a relatively sensitive and specific marker for diagnosis of MPNST [18, 19].

Adding to the complexity of diagnosis, sampling bias plays a major role in MPNST biopsies. These tumors are heterogenous and often arise

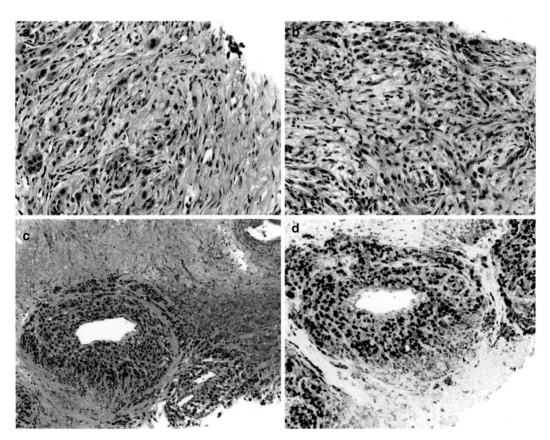

Fig. 38.5 H and E stains 20× of MPNST. (**a, b**) illustrate malignant proliferation of spindle, plump, and serpentine tumor cells with atypical mitotic figures. (**c**) Geographic necrosis and perivascular plump tumor cells are seen. (**d**) Immunohistochemistry staining of SOX10 of the corresponding case demonstrates diffuse strong nuclear positivity in the tumor cells

from a plexiform neurofibroma, and therefore it is imperative to get samples from an area representative of the MPNST. At specialized centers, a percutaneous Tru-Cut needle biopsy is performed with a multidisciplinary team of surgeons, radiologists, and pathologists. However, the gold standard remains an open incision biopsy with four-quadrant sampling to overcome sampling inefficiencies.

38.5 Tumor Predisposition Syndromes

As mentioned previously, majority of PNSTs occur sporadically in patients. However, PNSTs are also a major component of neurocutaneous tumor predisposing syndromes such as NF1, NF2, and schwannomatosis. Diagnostic criteria for the three genetic diseases are summarized in Table 38.1.

NF1, first described by Friedrich von Recklinghausen in 1882, is an autosomal dominant neurocutaneous disorder affecting 1 in 2500 births [20]. Individuals with NF1 harbor a mutation in the NF1 gene, which encodes a protein called neurofibromin, located on chromosome 17q11.2. This functions as a tumor suppressor by reducing cell proliferation through inactivation of the proto-oncogene p21-ras. Diagnosis can be made by genetic testing; however, family history and physical examination are often enough to diagnose NF1 based on the National Institute of Health (NIH) diagnostic criteria.

Clinically, the defining features of NF1 are the development of multiple neurofibromas and cutaneous pigmentary abnormalities. According to the NIH criteria, established in 1987, NF1 can be diagnosed if an individual presents with two or more of the following features: (1) six or more café au lait macule (CALMs) (greater than or equal to 5 mm in diameter before puberty or 1.5 mm in diameter after puberty); (2) axillary (Crowe sign) or inguinal skinfold freckling; (3) two or more dermal neurofibromas or one plexiform neurofibroma; (4) two or more iris hamartomas (Lisch nodules); (4) optic pathway glioma; (5) distinctive osseous dysplasia, such as sphe-

noid wing dysplasia or thinning of the long bone cortex with or without pseudarthrosis; or (6) a first-degree relative with NF1 [5, 9].

However, clinical diagnosis can be difficult in young children, less than 6 years of age, or children who present with only CALMs. Genetic testing is recommended in these cases and in individuals who present with a phenotype that does not satisfy the NIH diagnostic criteria. Prenatal genetic testing is also offered, as NF1 is an autosomal dominant genetic disorder which is fully penetrant. The risk of having a child with NF1 is 50% in families with one parent who has the condition. Although genetic testing can identify NF1 mutations in the prenatal stage, it cannot predict the severity of the clinical phenotype.

NF1 patients require close clinical and radiological observations as they are prone to develop multiple complications from their genetic disease. The plexiform neurofibromas that develop in NF1 patients harbor a 5–10% risk of malignant transformation into a MPNST [9]. In addition, patients can develop optic pathway gliomas, brainstem gliomas, and pilocytic astrocytomas. Other malignancies that can also develop in this population are pheochromocytomas, juvenile chronic myelogenous leukemia, juvenile myelomonocytic leukemia, and gastrointestinal stromal tumors (GIST). Other non-oncological manifestations include juvenile xanthogranulomas and vasculopathies, which can lead to systematic hypertension, cerebrovascular events, or peripheral vascular insufficiency [5, 21].

Similarly, NF2 is an autosomal dominant disorder caused by a mutation in a tumor suppressor gene located on chromosome 22q12.2, encoding a protein called Merlin (or Schwannomin). NF2 is a rarer genetic condition compared to NF1, affecting 1 in 25,000 people [22]. Among the de novo cases, 60% of mutations develop after conception and later in embryogenesis, leading to a mosaic NF2 [22, 23]. Mosaic individuals are less severely affected as a smaller subset of their cells harbor a NF2 mutation.

The hallmark of NF2 is the presence of bilateral acoustic schwannomas. However, there are multiple other clinical diagnostic criteria in individuals with family history of NF2 or unilateral acoustic schwannomas. NF2 patients are, also, prone to developing meningiomas, gliomas, neurofibromas, and ependymomas. Due to the higher prevalence of CNS tumors, the morbidity and mortality encountered by NF2 patients are higher than in NF1 patients [22, 23].

Schwannomatosis is another rare genetic disorder, originally described in Japanese patients, characterized by the development of multiple cutaneous and peripheral nerve schwannomas. This condition afflicts 1 in 40,000 individuals [24–26]. Schwannomatosis was previously believed to be an attenuated type of NF2, due to the absence of bilateral acoustic schwannomas, but now is recognized as a separate syndrome. Although schwannomatosis and NF2 both result in the development of multiple schwannomas, germline NF2 gene mutations are not identified in this population. Molecular studies have identified that schwannomatosis is a heterogenous disease, with a subset of individuals patients with SMARCB1 mutations and another subset with LZTR1 mutations, both found on chromosome 22 [26].

38.6 Management

Not all patients suspected of harboring a benign PNST warrant surgical intervention. For example, a patient with a clear history, examination, and imaging suggesting a benign lesion, with minimal or no symptoms, can be monitored with serial MRIs and clinical follow-up. However, there is minimal data on the incidence of neurological progression or malignant transformation in observed tumors. In patients with local compressive symptoms or suspected malignant conversion, preoperative goals of surgery can vary from gross total excision to subtotal excision or biopsy. Although preoperative imaging may suggest the optimal surgical plan based on radiological features of the tumor and its relationship to nearby neurovascular structures, the management plan is finalized intraoperatively with assistance from electrophysiology and tumor pathology.

The surgical principles guiding the resection of benign PNSTs are (1) microsurgical technique to preserve functional nerve fascicles, (2) intraoperative electrophysiology to distinguish between functional and nonfunctional fascicles, (3) appropriate positioning and draping of the affected limb to allow for intraoperative evaluation of muscles innervated by nerve in question by direct palpation of electrical stimulation, (4) appropriate exposure of nerve-tumor complex to identify normal nerve proximal and distal to the tumor, (5) use of short-acting neuromuscular paralysis (or short-acting) to allow intraoperative monitoring, and (6) incisions made along flexor or extensor creases and prophylactic decompression of nearby entrapment points, such as carpal tunnel or fibular head, to prevent delayed compression syndromes. The overall goal of surgical management of benign PNSTs is to remove the lesion with minimal morbidity.

In contrast, the goal of surgery for MPNSTs is the complete removal of the lesion with tumor-free margins, which is not always possible. There are many different approaches to MPNSTs, with many surgeons opting for a staged surgical procedure. The surgical resection of MPNSTs may require sacrifice of vital nerves and soft tissue structures, and thus a surgical biopsy is often performed prior to definitive surgery. Fine needle biopsy remains controversial in MPNSTs as there is a risk of missing the malignant cells since MPNSTs are a heterogenous tumor that often develops from a bed of plexiform neurofibroma. Inadequate sampling can lead to misdiagnosis and suboptimal management. A modification to this approach is to perform an open biopsy with four-quadrant sampling, which allows surgeons to sample tissue from representative areas. Others advocate for a gross total resection of the tumor, without violating the tumor capsule, and full pathological analysis of the entire tumor. If the diagnosis of MPNST is confirmed on histopathology, a second procedure is undertaken to explore the margins around the resected tumor and sent for frozen sectioning until a clear 2 cm margin is obtained on all sides of the tumor.

Adjuvant radiotherapy is recommended for patients with high-grade tumors greater than

5 cm in size or with positive margins. In clinical trials, adjuvant radiotherapy has been shown to improve local recurrence, but no effect on overall survival has been demonstrated to date [6, 27]. The role of chemotherapy is, also, debated in management of MPNSTs. Various combinations of chemotherapy agents (vincristine, doxorubicin, cyclophosphamide, dactinomycin, ifosfamide, and etoposide) have been trialed to treat MPNST with results ranging from modest to disappointing [8]. Some studies have also suggested that patients with NF1 are less responsive than patients with sporadic disease. Adjuvant chemotherapy, in most practices, has been reserved for patients with high-grade tumors, in which metastatic disease is likely. Currently, targeted therapies are in various stages of drug development with mixed results. Trials for epidermal growth factor receptor (EGFR) inhibitor (erlotinib) have shown no effect, despite promising results in preclinical studies [8]. Mechanistic target of rapamycin (mTOR) inhibitors and tyrosine kinase inhibitors has also failed to show clinical effects [8, 28]. Despite the failure of bringing bench to bedside, it is important to continue with molecular research in MPNSTs to identify potential targetable molecules that can advance our current oncological treatment paradigm.

38.7   Outcome

At our institution, the recurrence rates for schwannomas and neurofibromas were 5.3% and 8.2%, respectively [29]. Previous literature has reported a recurrence rate of 1.3–35.9%. The extent of resection is a major predictor of recurrence in BPNST, and in our series, we achieved gross total resection (GTR) less frequently in neurofibromas compared to schwannomas. As previously discussed, the growth patterns of neurofibromas (intrafascicular growth) makes it difficult to completely resect safely. GTR was achieved in 76.7% of schwannomas and 44.9% of neurofibromas. In schwannomas, the location of the tumor affected the ability to achieve GTR, with schwannomas in the extremities easier to completely resect compared to plexal tumors [29].

Preservation of neurological function is the main goal during surgical resection of BPNST. However, surgery in NF1 patients for neurofibromas has a higher likelihood of pain and neurologic deficits compared to sporadic patients. In one series, resection of sporadic neurofibromas resulted in better neurological and pain outcomes compared to NF1-associated neurofibromas [30]. Similarly, neurofibromas in the brachial plexus are associated with higher postoperative morbidity [30]. Schwannomas, on the other hand, have a better prognosis after surgery compared to neurofibromas [29, 30].

Despite the aggressive neuro-oncological management of MPNSTS, the overall prognosis remains grim. Poor prognostic signs include high-grade tumor, size greater than 5 cm, association with NF1, positive surgical margins, and distant metastases. In meta-analyses of 1800 patients, a significantly higher overall survival and disease-specific survival were observed in sporadic MPNSTs compared to NF1-associated MPNSTs. However, in the past decade, the survival in the NF1 group has improved. The 5-year overall survival in all patients with MPNST ranged from 20 to 50% [31].

38.8   Conclusion

Peripheral nerve tumors present a wide range of clinical and pathological behaviors that warrant specialized and individualized management strategies. Although complete surgical resection is curative in benign PNST, this option may not always be feasible considering tumor location and pathology. In addition, MPNSTs have poor prognosis despite aggressive surgical and oncological treatment that is available. This highlights the importance of better understanding the molecular and genomic drivers of oncogenesis in these tumors to early detection of high grade tumors, better screening program, and uncover novel therapeutic targets and lead to development of novel treatment strategies. Patients with genetic tumor predisposing syndromes, specifically the neurofibromatosis family of syndromes, can potentially develop tens to hundreds of

peripheral nerve tumor will benefit from a targeted therapy to ease their pain and morbidity.

References

1. Zhu Y, Ghosh P, Charnay P, Burns DK, Parada LF (2002) Neurofibromas in NF1: schwann cell origin and role of tumor environment. Science 296:920–922

2. Agnihotri S et al (2017) Therapeutic radiation for childhood cancer drives structural aberrations of NF2 in meningiomas. Nat Commun 8:186

3. Rodriguez FJ, Folpe AL, Giannini C, Perry A (2012) Pathology of peripheral nerve sheath tumors: diagnostic overview and update on selected diagnostic problems. Acta Neuropathol (Berl) 123:295–319

4. Antinheimo J et al (2000) Population-based analysis of sporadic and type 2 neurofibromatosis-associated meningiomas and schwannomas. Neurology 54:71–76

5. Ward BA, Gutmann DH (2005) Neurofibromatosis 1: from lab bench to clinic. Pediatr Neurol 32:221–228

6. Anghileri M et al (2006) Malignant peripheral nerve sheath tumors. Cancer 107:1065–1074

7. Baehring JM, Betensky RA, Batchelor TT (2003) Malignant peripheral nerve sheath tumor the clinical spectrum and outcome of treatment. Neurology 61:696–698

8. Farid M et al (2014) Malignant peripheral nerve sheath tumors. Oncologist 19:193–201

9. Ferner RE, Gutmann DH (2002) International consensus statement on malignant peripheral nerve sheath tumors in neurofibromatosis 1. Cancer Res 62:1573–1577

10. Ferner RE et al (2000) Evaluation of 18fluorodeoxyglucose positron emission tomography (18FDG PET) in the detection of malignant peripheral nerve sheath tumours arising from within plexiform neurofibromas in neurofibromatosis 1. J Neurol Neurosurg Psychiatry 68:353–357

11. Ferner RE et al (2008) [18F]2-fluoro-2-deoxy-D-zglucose positron emission tomography (FDG PET) as a diagnostic tool for neurofibromatosis 1 (NF1) associated malignant peripheral nerve sheath tumours (MPNSTs): a long-term clinical study. Ann Oncol 19:390–394

12. Warbey VS, Ferner RE, Dunn JT, Calonje E, O'Doherty MJ (2009) [18F]FDG PET/CT in the diagnosis of malignant peripheral nerve sheath tumours in neurofibromatosis type-1. Eur J Nucl Med Mol Imaging 36:751–757

13. Le LQ et al (2011) Susceptible stages in schwann cells for NF1-associated plexiform neurofibroma development. Cancer Res 71:4686–4695

14. Le LQ, Shipman T, Burns DK, Parada LF (2009) Cell of origin and microenvironment contribution for NF1-associated dermal neurofibromas. Cell Stem Cell 4:453–463

15. Bhatheja K, Field J (2006) Schwann cells: origins and role in axonal maintenance and regeneration. Int J Biochem Cell Biol 38:1995–1999

16. Beert E et al (2011) Atypical neurofibromas in neurofibromatosis type 1 are premalignant tumors. Genes Chromosomes Cancer 50:1021–1032

17. Feany, Anthony, Fletcher (1998) Nerve sheath tumours with hybrid features of neurofibroma and schwannoma: a conceptual challenge. Histopathology 32:405–410

18. Miettinen MM et al (2017) Histopathologic evaluation of atypical neurofibromatous tumors and their transformation into malignant peripheral nerve sheath tumor in patients with neurofibromatosis 1—a consensus overview. Hum Pathol 67:1–10

19. Pekmezci M, Cuevas-Ocampo AK, Perry A, Horvai AE (2017) Significance of H3K27me3 loss in the diagnosis of malignant peripheral nerve sheath tumors. Mod Pathol 30:1710–1719

20. From Recklingausen FD. Berlin: A. Hirschwald; 1882. [Cited by: Sakorafas GH, et al. JOP. J Pancreas (Online) 2008; 9 (5): 633–639. (Reference 15)]. http://www.joplink.net.myaccess.library.utoronto.ca/prev/200809/ref/07-015.html. Accessed 4 Jan 2018

21. Gutmann DH et al (2017) Neurofibromatosis type 1. Nat Rev Dis Primers 3:17004

22. Asthagiri AR et al (2009) Neurofibromatosis type 2. Lancet 373:1974–1986

23. Evans GR, Lloyd SKW, Ramsden RT (2011) Neurofibromatosis type 2. Adv Otorhinolaryngol 70:91–98

24. Hans VH (2009) Schwannomatosis. Neurology 72:1188–1189

25. MacCollin M et al (2005) Diagnostic criteria for schwannomatosis. Neurology 64:1838–1845

26. Plotkin SR et al (2013) Update from the 2011 International schwannomatosis workshop: from genetics to diagnostic criteria. Am J Med Genet A 161:405–416

27. Wong WW, Hirose T, Scheithauer BW, Schild SE, Gunderson LL (1998) Malignant peripheral nerve sheath tumor: analysis of treatment outcome. Int J Radiat Oncol Biol Phys 42:351–360

28. James AW, Shurell E, Singh A, Dry SM, Eilber FC (2016) Malignant peripheral nerve sheath tumor. Surg Oncol Clin 25:789–802

29. Guha D et al (2017) Management of peripheral nerve sheath tumors: 17 years of experience at Toronto Western Hospital. J Neurosurg 128(4):1–9. https://doi.org/10.3171/2017.1.JNS162292

30. Kim DH, Murovic JA, Tiel RL, Moes G, Kline DG (2005) A series of 397 peripheral neural sheath tumors: 30-year experience at Louisiana State University Health Sciences Center. J Neurosurg 102:246–255

31. Kolberg M et al (2013) Survival meta-analyses for >1800 malignant peripheral nerve sheath tumor patients with and without neurofibromatosis type 1. Neuro Oncol 15:135–147

32. Agnihotri S et al (2016) The genomic landscape of schwannoma. Nat Genet 48:1339–1348

Part V

Aspects of General Care in Neurooncology

David A. Reardon

Epilepsy and Anticonvulsant Therapy in Brain Tumor Patients

Sylvia C. Kurz, David Schiff, and Patrick Y. Wen

39.1 Seizures and Epilepsy in Patients with Brain Tumors

Seizures are common in patients with brain tumors, represent an important factor of morbidity, and require appropriate management. It has been estimated that in 30–50% of glioma patients, seizures are the initial presenting symptom leading to subsequent brain tumor diagnosis [1]. It is further estimated that 40–80% of patients will experience a seizure over the course of their disease [2]. About 10–15% of patients who undergo craniotomy and glioma surgery will experience a seizure perioperatively [3].

S. C. Kurz
Brain Tumor Center, Laura and Isaac Perlmutter Cancer Center, New York University Langone Health, New York, NY, USA
e-mail: Sylvia.Kurz@nyulangone.org

D. Schiff
Department of Neurology, University of Virginia, Charlottesville, VA, USA

Department of Neurological Surgery, University of Virginia, Charlottesville, VA, USA

Department of Medicine, University of Virginia, Charlottesville, VA, USA
e-mail: ds4jd@virginia.edu

P. Y. Wen (✉)
Center For Neuro-Oncology, Dana-Farber Cancer Institute, Boston, MA, USA
e-mail: pwen@partners.org

It is important to note that these estimates are derived from studies focusing on patients with gliomas. The actual seizure risk in brain tumor patients depends on the underlying histology and tumor location (Table 39.1). The highest seizure risk has been described for patients with glioneuronal tumors including gangliogliomas and dysembryoplastic neuroepithelial tumors (DNET). Approximately 74–86% of these patients will have an epileptic event during the course of their illness [4–6]. Patients with low-grade gliomas also have a higher risk of experiencing seizures (60–85%) [7, 8]. In contrast, the seizure risk is relatively low in patients with glioblastoma (28–49%) [9–11]. The seizure risk in patients with meningiomas varies greatly across studies and ranges from 12 to 76% based on a recent systematic review [12]. Seizure risk is higher with convexity-based tumors and peritumoral edema [12, 13]. Patients with brain metastases appear to have the lowest seizure risk overall (20–35%) although there is significant variation based on tumor histology, hemorrhagic component, tumor location, and associated edema [14, 15]. Seizure risk from brain metastases is lowest in patients with breast cancer (16%) and highest in patients with melanoma (67%) [14, 16].

These differences in seizure risk have been explained by the predilection of DNETs, gangliogliomas, and low-grade gliomas for the temporo-

Table 39.1 Seizure frequency in brain tumor patients depends on tumor type

Tumor type	Seizure frequency (%)	References
Glioneuronal tumors	74–86	[4–6]
Low-grade gliomas	60–85	[7, 8]
High-grade gliomas	28–49	[9–11]
Meningiomas	12–76	[12]
Metastases	20–35	[14, 15]

insular and frontal regions as well as the predominant involvement or associated disorganization of the cerebral cortex. In contrast, high-grade gliomas and brain metastases more commonly are located in the subcortical white matter or at the gray to white matter junction [17, 18]. In addition, patients with low-grade gliomas, in particular *IDH*-mutant gliomas, tend to have a longer overall survival seen in patients, therefore allowing more time for seizures to occur [19].

Changes on a molecular and cellular level within the cerebral tumor microenvironment may be important factors that contribute to seizure risk. The cortical dysplasia and structural abnormalities associated with glioneuronal tumors (DNETs, gangliogliomas) may increase epileptogenicity [20, 21]. Tissue irritation due to hypoxia, changes in local pH levels within the tumor microenvironment, and the hemosiderin deposition seen in hemorrhagic tumors may further lower the seizure threshold [22–24]. In addition, alterations in inhibitory (γ-amino-butyric acid (GABA)) and excitatory (glutamate) transmitter levels have been described in patients with low-grade and high-grade gliomas and may correlate with seizure risk [25–29]. Most recently, it has been proposed that 2-hydroxy-glutarate (2-HG), which accumulates in tumor cells that harbor an *IDH* mutation, may mimic the excitatory function of glutamate at the N-methyl-D-aspartate (NMDA) receptor, resulting in increased seizure frequency in patients with *IDH*-mutated gliomas [30].

39.1.1 The Prognostic Significance of Seizures in Patients with Gliomas

Seizures at time of diagnosis or early on appear to be associated with an overall survival benefit in patients with low-grade and high-grade gliomas [11, 31–33]. This may be attributable to the fact that cortically based and therefore epileptogenic tumors are discovered earlier and may be more amenable to surgical resection due to the preferential location in the frontal, temporal, and parietal lobes. In addition, low-grade gliomas are often characterized by an *IDH* mutation, which represents both a prognostic biomarker conferring a more favorable prognosis and a predictive biomarker of treatment response to radiation and chemotherapy [34–37]. Moreover, presence of an *IDH* mutation appears to be associated with increased seizure risk independent of tumor location and tumor grade, perhaps due to the glutaminergic effects of 2-HG, a by-product of the abnormal function of *IDH* in affected glioma cells [30, 38–40].

In contrast to the favorable prognostic associations with seizures that occur early in the disease course, recurrent or worsening seizures following tumor-directed therapy in both low-grade and high-grade gliomas portend a poor prognosis because this frequently heralds progression of the underlying tumor [17, 32, 41].

39.2 Seizure Management in Brain Tumor Patients

Seizures and epilepsy due to underlying brain tumors have significant impact on quality of life in affected patients. In addition to the morbidity caused by the seizures themselves, the side effects from antiepileptic medications frequently further aggravate the neurocognitive impairment already present due to the underlying brain tumor [42–45]. Therefore, care should be undertaken when considering the indication for and choice of antiepileptic drugs. Studies have demonstrated that in the absence of seizures or other neurological symptoms, the side effects from antiepileptic drugs represent the single most important factor influencing quality of life in this patient population [46].

39.2.1 Tumor-Directed Therapies and Seizure Control

If possible, the first step in management with tumor-associated epilepsy is maximal safe resection of the tumor. This is particularly critical in patients with slow-growing tumors associated with a high seizure risk. It has been demonstrated that seizure freedom can be achieved by gross-total tumor resection in 80–90% of glioneuronal tumors [5, 47–51] and up to 64–82% of low-grade gliomas [8, 52, 53], respectively. Similarly, durable seizure control can be achieved in up to 62–83% of patients with meningiomas after a gross-total tumor resection [54, 55] and in up to 98% of patients who undergo resection of brain metastases [15]. In high-grade gliomas, maximal safe resection followed by treatment with combined radiation and temozolomide leads to seizure control in up to 77% of patients [41].

Based on retrospective studies, radiotherapy appears to have an independent effect on seizure control in gliomas. It has been demonstrated that up to 38% of patients are seizure-free and 75–77% achieve reduction in seizure frequency after radiation alone [56–59]. Similarly, treatment with the alkylating agents temozolomide and the combination of procarbazine, CCNU, and vincristine (PCV) may contribute to seizure control [60–66]. Based on the recent evidence of a possible excitatory effect of 2-HG at the glutaminergic N-methyl-D-aspartate (NMDA) receptor and subsequent increase in seizure frequency in patients with *IDH*-mutated gliomas, it has now been hypothesized that IDH-targeting agents may indirectly contribute to seizure control [30]. However, this information is preliminary at this time and primarily based on retrospective or preclinical studies. Prospective studies will be necessary to confirm the correlation of antitumor treatments and seizure control.

39.2.2 Antiepileptic Drug Therapy in Brain Tumor Patients

The prophylactic use of anticonvulsive agents in patients with brain tumors who never had a seizure has been controversial. Several studies investigating the utility of perioperative seizure prophylaxis in patients undergoing brain tumor surgery have led to conflicting results with regard to preventing perioperative seizures [3, 67–70]. A double-blind placebo-controlled study demonstrated significant reduction in postoperative seizure frequency in patients treated with phenytoin, in particular during the first two postoperative weeks [71]. Based on these results, it has become common practice to begin antiepileptic drugs prior to craniotomy and tumor resection [72, 73]. However, several recent meta-analyses not only concluded that the prophylactic use of antiepileptic drugs fails to reliably prevent seizures in brain tumor patients but that the side effects from anti-seizure medications may have important implications on quality of life in this patient population [74–77]. These studies support the published American Academy of Neurology Practice Parameter guidelines which recommend discontinuing prophylactic antiepileptic drugs 1–2 weeks after brain tumor surgery in patients who never had a clinical seizure [78, 79]. Nevertheless, these guidelines are primarily based on studies that are limited by their retrospective design, small sample size, or small proportion of brain tumor patients in the overall study population. To more conclusively answer the question of whether antiepileptic drug therapy reduces perioperative seizures, prospective randomized trials evaluating the role of prophylactic antiepileptic drugs in patients with brain tumors should be conducted. Unfortunately, these studies have been difficult to carry out, and several trials were closed prematurely due to poor accrual.

In patients who have experienced a seizure, antiepileptic therapy is generally recommended. Seizures in patients with brain tumors are considered symptomatic and can be classified as either simple or complex focal seizures with or without secondary generalization. The selection of the antiepileptic agent therefore should follow published guidelines for patients with focal epilepsy [80, 81]. The choice of the antiepileptic drug (AED) is influenced by individual patient factors such as age, sex, comorbidities, and co-medications. Antiepileptic drugs that are known to alter the function of hepatic cytochrome P450 (CYP450) co-enzymes (e.g., phenytoin, carbamazepine, oxcarbazepine, etc.) are generally avoided in patients with brain tumors given the potential for drug-drug interactions with concurrent chemotherapies. CYP450 enzyme-inducing antiepileptic drugs may accelerate metabolism and decrease the efficacy of corticosteroids and chemotherapeutic agents including nitrosoureas, paclitaxel, cyclophosphamide, etoposide, topotecan, irinotecan, thiotepa, doxorubicin, and methotrexate [82–88]. AEDs interacting with the CYP450 system may also alter the serum levels of tyrosine kinase inhibitors such as imatinib [89–91]. If antiepileptic drugs with potential CYP450 interactions have to be considered, the antiepileptic agent with the best efficacy-toxicity profile should be selected based on patient- and treatment-related factors (Fig. 39.1).

Levetiracetam and valproic acid are the most commonly used antiepileptic drugs in patients with brain tumors [92–94]. Lamotrigine may represent a reasonable alternative due to its favorable side effect profile, but its use is limited because it requires slow up-titration to therapeutic dose levels given the risk of skin rash and the rare but life-threatening complication of Stevens-Johnson syndrome. Lacosamide is another antiepileptic drug that appears to be effective, is well tolerated, and has little drug-drug interactions [95, 96]. The characteristics of the AEDs commonly used in neuro-oncology are outlined in the following section and in Table 39.2.

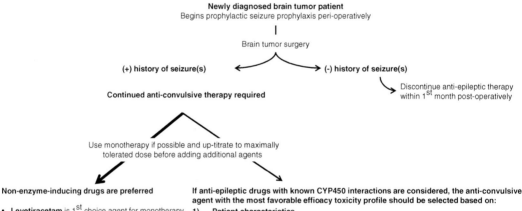

Fig. 39.1 Approach to anti-epileptic drug use in patients with brain tumors

Table 39.2 Antiepileptic drugs commonly used in neuro-oncology

Drug	Mechanism of action	Typical dosing	Route	Metabolism and excretion	Common and important side effects
No effect on CYP450 enzymes					
Brivaracetam	Suspected binding to SV2A vesicle	50–200 mg/day	po, iv	Hepatically metabolized, >95% renally excreted	Adverse effect on mood
Lacosamide	Blocks Na⁺-channels	200–400 mg/day	po, iv	Hepatic metabolism, ~40% renally excreted	Dizziness, headache, diplopia, blurred vision, cognitive dysfunction, skin reactions
Lamotrigine	Blocks Na⁺-channels	200–600 mg/day	po only	Mostly hepatic metabolism, ~10% renally excreted	Drowsiness, dizziness, fatigue, headache, ataxia, rash, SJS/TEN, DRESS
Levetiracetam	Suspected binding to SV2A vesicles	1000–3000 mg/day	po, iv	Hydrolization in blood, renal excretion	Somnolence, 5–10%: increased irritability, anxiety, psychosis
Topiramate	Na⁺-channel blocker, GABA-receptor agonist, NMDA receptor blocker	200–400 mg/day	po only	Not metabolized, mainly renally excreted	Drowsiness, impaired cognition, weight loss, kidney stones, hepatotoxicity
CYP450-inducing agents					
Carbamazepine	Na⁺-channel blocker	400–1600 mg/day	po, iv	Hepatic metabolism	Drowsiness, dizziness, diplopia, hyponatremia, hepatotoxicity, leukopenia, SJS/TEN
Clobazam	Potentiates GABAergic neurotransmission		po only	Hepatic metabolism	Somnolence, pyrexia, irritability, ataxia, hepatotoxicity
Eslicarbazepine	Suspected to block voltage-gated Na⁺ channels	800–1200 mg/day	po only	Hepatic metabolism, 90% renally excreted	Dizziness, somnolence, nausea, diplopia
Oxcarbazepine	Na⁺-channel blocker	900–2400 mg/day	po only	Hepatic metabolism	Drowsiness, dizziness, diplopia, headache, hyponatremia, bone marrow suppression, hepatotoxicity, SJS
Perampanel	Inhibits the AMPA receptor	8–12 mg/day at bedtime	po only	Hepatic metabolism	Fatigue, weight gain, irritability/mood changes including suicidal and homicidal ideations
Phenytoin, fosphenytoin	Na⁺-channel blocker	150–400 mg/day	po, iv (fosphenytoin preferred when given iv)	Hepatic metabolism	Drowsiness, dizziness, bone marrow suppression, gingival hyperplasia, hirsutism, skin sensitivity to light (lupus-like reactions), cerebellar degeneration, SJS

(continued)

Table 39.2 (continued)

Drug	Mechanism of action	Typical dosing	Route	Metabolism and excretion	Common and important side effects
Zonisamide	Blocks Na$^+$- and Ca^{2+}-channels	200–600 mg/day	po only	Hepatic metabolism (~20%), renal excretion (~30%)	Somnolence, ataxia, dizziness, kidney stones
CYP450-inhibiting agents					
Valproic acid	GABA-receptor agonist, Na+-channel blocker, glutaminergic inhibitor	500–2500 mg/day		Hepatic metabolism	Hepatotoxicity, thrombo- and neutropenia, tremor, weight gain, hair loss, PCOS

Abbreviations: *CYP450* cytochrome P450 co-enzymes, *Na$^+$* sodium, *Ca^{2+}* calcium, *K$^+$* potassium, *AMPA* amino-OH-methyl-isoxazolepropionic-acid, *NMDA* N-methyl-D-aspartate, *GABA* γ-amino butyric acid, *SV2A* synaptic vesicle protein, *SJS* Stevens-Johnson Syndrome, *TEN* toxic epidermal necrolysis, *DRESS* drug reactions with eosinophilia and systemic symptoms, *PCOS* polycystic ovarian syndrome, *po* per os (oral), *iv* intravenously
Adapted from Drappatz et al., *Neurol Clin* 25 (2007) 1035–1071 and Englot et al., *Handb Clin Neurol* Vol 134, Chapter 16 (2016)

39.2.2.1 Levetiracetam and Brivaracetam

The precise mechanism of action of levetiracetam is not known, but it likely acts by binding to synaptic vesicle protein 2 (SV2A) on the neuron and thereby enhancing GABA release and stabilizing the neuronal cell membrane. Levetiracetam is available in intravenous and oral formulations, and therapeutic drug levels can be achieved quickly. In general, levetiracetam is well tolerated although 5–10% of patients develop increased irritability, anxiety, and depression requiring transition to alternative AED. Levetiracetam is renally cleared, and lower maintenance doses may be necessary in patients with renal dysfunction. There are no known interactions with the hepatic CYP450 co-enzymes or other frequently administered drugs. Brivaracetam is a newer analogue to levetiracetam with similar efficacy but perhaps less severe effects on mood [97, 98].

39.2.2.2 Valproic Acid

Valproic acid (VPA) stabilizes neuronal membranes by its Na$^+$-channel blocking and GABA-receptor agonistic properties. Its efficacy in controlling partial and generalized epilepsy is well established. However, it is also characterized by its extensive hepatic metabolism and inhibition of the CYP450 co-enzymes. This may potentially lead to increased serum levels of other drugs including chemotherapeutic agents. Although well tolerated overall, it can cause thrombocytopenia and neutropenia, tremor, weight gain, and hair loss. VPA has been described to have histone deacetylase-inhibiting properties, and an anti-glioma effect synergistic with tumor-directed therapies therefore has been postulated. However, based on information from a recent meta-analysis, there appears to be no benefit on survival, and the utility of VPA as first-line antiepileptic therapy in patients with high-grade glioma is now being questioned.

39.2.2.3 Lacosamide

Lacosamide is a newer antiepileptic agent and acts as a Na$^+$-channel blocker. It is available in intravenous and oral formulations and is gaining popularity as an adjunct antiepileptic agent in neuro-oncology patients. In general, it has a favorable side effect profile but can cause dizziness, headaches, diplopia, or blurry vision in some patients. Although metabolized in the liver, it does not interact with the hepatic CYP450 enzymes and has no significant drug-drug interactions, including chemotherapeutic agents.

39.2.2.4 Lamotrigine

Lamotrigine acts by modulating Na$^+$-channels and has an established track record as add-on medication with efficacy in partial epilepsy. In addition, it acts as a mood stabilizer. Overall, side effects are infrequent, but skin rashes and in particular Stevens-Johnson syndrome (SJS) or toxic epidermal necrolysis are feared complications. Because the risk of developing these adverse reactions is reduced with slow up-titration of the drug, it may take several weeks until a therapeutic dose is achieved. This in turn limits the utility when treating patients with active seizures. Lamotrigine is subject to hepatic metabolism, and drug availability may therefore be altered when combined with CYP450 inhibiting (i.e., VPA) or inducing agents (e.g., phenytoin, carbamazepine, oxcarbazepine, phenobarbital, etc.).

39.2.2.5   Eslicarbazepine

Eslicarbazepine is a newer antiepileptic drug and is structurally related to carbamazepine and oxcarbazepine; it is suspected to act through inhibition of voltage-gated sodium channels (VGSC) thereby reducing neuronal excitability. FDA approval was granted in 2013 based on several phase III clinical studies that demonstrated efficacy in reducing seizure frequency in adults with refractory partial-onset epilepsy. Overall, the drug appears to be well tolerated although dizziness, somnolence, nausea, and diplopia can occur. Hyponatremia appears to be less common compared to carbamazepine or oxcarbazepine. Eslicarbazepine is predominantly hepatically metabolized and induces enzymes of the CYP450 family. Therefore, caution is warranted when used in brain tumor patients who undergo treatment with chemotherapy [99].

39.2.2.6   Perampanel

Perampanel is a novel anticonvulsive agent that acts via selective inhibition of the AMPA-type glutamate receptor that has been demonstrated to be effective as add-on therapy for treatment-refractory partial-onset epilepsy. The drug is hepatically metabolized, primarily by oxidation and glucuronidation, but oxidative metabolism via CYP enzymes has also been described. Drug-drug interactions have been described, in particular when used with other CYP enzyme-inducing antiepileptic drugs. Side effects include dizzi-

ness, somnolence, fatigue, and irritability. In some cases, aggressive behaviors including those with suicidal and homicidal intent have been reported [100–103]. Given the extensive drug-drug interactions, caution is warranted when using perampanel in patients with brain tumors undergoing therapy.

39.3   Special Considerations: Do Valproic Acid and Levetiracetam Have Potential Antitumor Effects?

39.3.1   Valproic Acid

Valproic acid has histone-deacetylase-inhibiting properties, and the changes in histone acetylation/deacetylation may change the methylation of important DNA promoter regions thereby inducing apoptosis. This potentially increases the efficacy of radiation or chemotherapy on glioma cells *in vitro* [104–106]. Several retrospective clinical studies and post hoc analyses of clinical trials have investigated the potential synergistic effect of VPA in glioma patients treated with radiation and chemotherapy [94, 107, 108]. Based on the possible survival benefit in glioma patients seen in these studies, VPA has long been postulated to be the AED of choice in glioma patients although clinical evidence from a large randomized and blinded clinical study confirming this benefit was lacking. Most recently, Happold et al. analyzed this question in a large patient cohort ($n = 1869$) pooled from several prospective phase III clinical studies. The information regarding AED use was prospectively collected in these patients treated with radiation and temozolomide for high-grade glioma. In this analysis, early use of VPA (prior to start of chemoradiation) had no impact on progression-free survival or overall survival [109]. Information regarding VPA use was only available for the duration of chemoradiation, and, therefore, this study could not evaluate a potential synergistic benefit attributable to long-term use of VPA. Nevertheless, based on these data, VPA should no longer be considered as first-line antiepileptic drug in patients with malignant gliomas.

39.3.2 Levetiracetam

Levetiracetam was found to negatively affect expression of the DNA repair enzyme methylene-guanine-methyl transferase (MGMT) and thereby was postulated to enhance the efficacy of temozolomide in patients with high-grade gliomas [110, 111]. In the study by Happold et al., the possible beneficial effect of levetiracetam use in patients treated with radiation and chemotherapy for high-grade gliomas was also evaluated but did not reveal a benefit on progression-free or overall survival [109].

39.4 Conclusions

Seizures are common in patients with brain tumors and may have a significant impact on quality of life. The actual seizure risk varies significantly based on tumor histology and tumor location. While antiepileptic therapy is indicated in patients with a history of seizure, it remains unclear if the prophylactic perioperative use of AEDs reduces seizure frequency. In brain tumor patients that require anticonvulsant treatment, the choice of AED follows the principles of treatment for focal symptomatic epilepsy, but AEDs that interact with the hepatic CYP450 co-enzymes should be avoided due to potential interactions with other drugs and in particular chemotherapeutic agents. Levetiracetam is the antiepileptic drug of choice in patients with brain tumors with a large body of evidence supporting its efficacy, favorable side effect profile, and no significant drug-drug interactions. Although a potential antitumor effect of valproic acid has been suspected based on retrospective studies, this has not been supported by a recent meta-analysis evaluating prospectively obtained information on antiepileptic drug use and outcome in patients with high-grade gliomas.

References

1. Lote K, Stenwig AE, Skullerud K, Hirschberg H (1998) Prevalence and prognostic significance of epilepsy in patients with gliomas. Eur J Cancer 34:98–102
2. Herman ST (2002) Epilepsy after brain insult: targeting epileptogenesis. Neurology 59:S21–S26
3. De Santis A, Villani R, Sinisi M, Stocchetti N, Perucca E (2002) Add-on phenytoin fails to prevent early seizures after surgery for supratentorial brain tumors: a randomized controlled study. Epilepsia 43:175–182
4. Southwell DG, Garcia PA, Berger MS, Barbaro NM, Chang EF (2012) Long-term seizure control outcomes after resection of gangliogliomas. Neurosurgery 70:1406–1413; discussion 1413–1404
5. Chang EF, Christie C, Sullivan JE et al (2010) Seizure control outcomes after resection of dysembryoplastic neuroepithelial tumor in 50 patients. J Neurosurg Pediatr 5:123–130
6. Tomita T, Volk JM, Shen W, Pundy T (2016) Glioneuronal tumors of cerebral hemisphere in children: correlation of surgical resection with seizure outcomes and tumor recurrences. Childs Nerv Syst 32:1839–1848
7. Pallud J, Audureau E, Blonski M et al (2014) Epileptic seizures in diffuse low-grade gliomas in adults. Brain 137:449–462
8. Chang EF, Potts MB, Keles GE et al (2008) Seizure characteristics and control following resection in 332 patients with low-grade gliomas. J Neurosurg 108:227–235
9. Moots PL, Maciunas RJ, Eisert DR, Parker RA, Laporte K, Abou-Khalil B (1995) The course of seizure disorders in patients with malignant gliomas. Arch Neurol 52:717–724
10. Flanigan PM, Jahangiri A, Kuang R et al (2017) Improved survival with decreased wait time to surgery in glioblastoma patients presenting with seizure. Neurosurgery 81(5):824–833
11. Toledo M, Sarria-Estrada S, Quintana M et al (2017) Epileptic features and survival in glioblastomas presenting with seizures. Epilepsy Res 130:1–6
12. Englot DJ, Magill ST, Han SJ, Chang EF, Berger MS, McDermott MW (2016) Seizures in supratentorial meningioma: a systematic review and meta-analysis. J Neurosurg 124:1552–1561
13. Lieu AS, Howng SL (2000) Intracranial meningiomas and epilepsy: incidence, prognosis and influencing factors. Epilepsy Res 38:45–52
14. Oberndorfer S, Schmal T, Lahrmann H, Urbanits S, Lindner K, Grisold W (2002) [The frequency of seizures in patients with primary brain tumors or cerebral metastases. An evaluation from the Ludwig Boltzmann Institute of Neuro-Oncology and the Department of Neurology, Kaiser Franz Josef Hospital, Vienna]. Wien Klin Wochenschr 114:911–916

15. Wu A, Weingart JD, Gallia GL et al (2017) Risk factors for preoperative seizures and loss of seizure control in patients undergoing surgery for metastatic brain tumors. World Neurosurg 104:120–128

16. Lynam LM, Lyons MK, Drazkowski JF et al (2007) Frequency of seizures in patients with newly diagnosed brain tumors: a retrospective review. Clin Neurol Neurosurg 109:634–638

17. You G, Sha ZY, Yan W et al (2012) Seizure characteristics and outcomes in 508 Chinese adult patients undergoing primary resection of low-grade gliomas: a clinicopathological study. Neuro Oncol 14:230–241

18. Lee JW, Wen PY, Hurwitz S et al (2010) Morphological characteristics of brain tumors causing seizures. Arch Neurol 67:336–342

19. Englot DJ, Chang EF, Vecht CJ (2016) Epilepsy and brain tumors. Handb Clin Neurol 134:267–285

20. Fish DR, Spencer SS (1995) Clinical correlations: MRI and EEG. Magn Reson Imaging 13:1113–1117

21. Spencer S, Huh L (2008) Outcomes of epilepsy surgery in adults and children. Lancet Neurol 7:525–537

22. Schaller B (2005) Influences of brain tumor-associated pH changes and hypoxia on epileptogenesis. Acta Neurol Scand 111:75–83

23. Wolf HK, Roos D, Blumcke I, Pietsch T, Wiestler OD (1996) Perilesional neurochemical changes in focal epilepsies. Acta Neuropathol 91:376–384

24. Beaumont A, Whittle IR (2000) The pathogenesis of tumour associated epilepsy. Acta Neurochir (Wien) 142:1–15

25. Yuen TI, Morokoff AP, Bjorksten A et al (2012) Glutamate is associated with a higher risk of seizures in patients with gliomas. Neurology 79:883–889

26. Rosati A, Poliani PL, Todeschini A et al (2013) Glutamine synthetase expression as a valuable marker of epilepsy and longer survival in newly diagnosed glioblastoma multiforme. Neuro Oncol 15:618–625

27. Pallud J, Capelle L, Huberfeld G (2013) Tumoral epileptogenicity: how does it happen? Epilepsia 54(Suppl 9):30–34

28. Aronica E, Yankaya B, Jansen GH et al (2001) Ionotropic and metabotropic glutamate receptor protein expression in glioneuronal tumours from patients with intractable epilepsy. Neuropathol Appl Neurobiol 27:223–237

29. Bateman DE, Hardy JA, McDermott JR, Parker DS, Edwardson JA (1988) Amino acid neurotransmitter levels in gliomas and their relationship to the incidence of epilepsy. Neurol Res 10:112–114

30. Chen H, Judkins J, Thomas C et al (2017) Mutant IDH1 and seizures in patients with glioma. Neurology 88:1805–1813

31. Blumcke I, Luyken C, Urbach H, Schramm J, Wiestler OD (2004) An isomorphic subtype of long-term epilepsy-associated astrocytomas associated with benign prognosis. Acta Neuropathol 107:381–388

32. Danfors T, Ribom D, Berntsson SG, Smits A (2009) Epileptic seizures and survival in early disease of grade 2 gliomas. Eur J Neurol 16:823–831

33. Berendsen S, Varkila M, Kroonen J et al (2016) Prognostic relevance of epilepsy at presentation in glioblastoma patients. Neuro Oncol 18:700–706

34. Yan H, Parsons DW, Jin G et al (2009) IDH1 and IDH2 mutations in gliomas. N Engl J Med 360:765–773

35. Hartmann C, Hentschel B, Wick W et al (2010) Patients with IDH1 wild type anaplastic astrocytomas exhibit worse prognosis than IDH1-mutated glioblastomas, and IDH1 mutation status accounts for the unfavorable prognostic effect of higher age: implications for classification of gliomas. Acta Neuropathol 120:707–718

36. Buckner JC, Shaw EG, Pugh SL et al (2016) Radiation plus procarbazine, CCNU, and vincristine in low-grade glioma. N Engl J Med 374:1344–1355

37. Cairncross JG, Wang M, Jenkins RB et al (2014) Benefit from procarbazine, lomustine, and vincristine in oligodendroglial tumors is associated with mutation of IDH. J Clin Oncol 32:783–790

38. Stockhammer F, Misch M, Helms HJ et al (2012) IDH1/2 mutations in WHO grade II astrocytomas associated with localization and seizure as the initial symptom. Seizure 21:194–197

39. Liubinas SV, D'Abaco GM, Moffat BM et al (2014) IDH1 mutation is associated with seizures and protoplasmic subtype in patients with low-grade gliomas. Epilepsia 55:1438–1443

40. Neal A, Kwan P, O'Brien TJ, Buckland ME, Gonzales M, Morokoff A (2017) IDH1 and IDH2 mutations in postoperative diffuse glioma-associated epilepsy. Epilepsy Behav 78:30–36

41. Chaichana KL, Parker SL, Olivi A, Quinones-Hinojosa A (2009) Long-term seizure outcomes in adult patients undergoing primary resection of malignant brain astrocytomas. Clinical article. J Neurosurg 111:282–292

42. Sheth RD (2002) Adolescent issues in epilepsy. J Child Neurol 17(Suppl 2):2S23–22S27

43. Klein M, Engelberts NH, van der Ploeg HM et al (2003) Epilepsy in low-grade gliomas: the impact on cognitive function and quality of life. Ann Neurol 54:514–520

44. Taphoorn MJ, Klein M (2004) Cognitive deficits in adult patients with brain tumours. Lancet Neurol 3:159–168

45. Batchelor TT, Byrne TN (2006) Supportive care of brain tumor patients. Hematol Oncol Clin North Am 20:1337–1361

46. Auriel E, Landov H, Blatt I et al (2009) Quality of life in seizure-free patients with epilepsy on monotherapy. Epilepsy Behav 14:130–133

47. Giulioni M, Galassi E, Zucchelli M, Volpi L (2005) Seizure outcome of lesionectomy in glioneuronal tumors associated with epilepsy in children. J Neurosurg 102:288–293

48. Giulioni M, Gardella E, Rubboli G et al (2006) Lesionectomy in epileptogenic gangliogliomas: seizure outcome and surgical results. J Clin Neurosci 13:529–535

49. Giulioni M, Rubboli G, Marucci G et al (2009) Seizure outcome of epilepsy surgery in focal epilepsies associated with temporomesial glioneuronal tumors: lesionectomy compared with tailored resection. J Neurosurg 111:1275–1282

50. Bonney PA, Glenn CA, Ebeling PA et al (2015) Seizure freedom rates and prognostic indicators after resection of gangliogliomas: a review. World Neurosurg 84:1988–1996

51. Bonney PA, Boettcher LB, Conner AK et al (2016) Review of seizure outcomes after surgical resection of dysembryoplastic neuroepithelial tumors. J Neurooncol 126:1–10

52. Englot DJ, Han SJ, Berger MS, Barbaro NM, Chang EF (2012) Extent of surgical resection predicts seizure freedom in low-grade temporal lobe brain tumors. Neurosurgery 70:921–928; discussion 928

53. Bonney PA, Boettcher LB, Burks JD et al (2017) Rates of seizure freedom after surgical resection of diffuse low-grade gliomas. World Neurosurg 106:750–756

54. Chaichana KL, Pendleton C, Zaidi H et al (2013) Seizure control for patients undergoing meningioma surgery. World Neurosurg 79:515–524

55. Chen WC, Magill ST, Englot DJ et al (2017) Factors associated with pre- and postoperative seizures in 1033 patients undergoing supratentorial meningioma resection. Neurosurgery 81(2):297–306

56. Ruda R, Magliola U, Bertero L et al (2013) Seizure control following radiotherapy in patients with diffuse gliomas: a retrospective study. Neuro Oncol 15:1739–1749

57. Rogers LR, Morris HH, Lupica K (1993) Effect of cranial irradiation on seizure frequency in adults with low-grade astrocytoma and medically intractable epilepsy. Neurology 43:1599–1601

58. Chalifoux R, Elisevich K (1996) Effect of ionizing radiation on partial seizures attributable to malignant cerebral tumors. Stereotact Funct Neurosurg 67:169–182

59. Taphoorn MJ, Stupp R, Coens C et al (2005) Health-related quality of life in patients with glioblastoma: a randomised controlled trial. Lancet Oncol 6:937–944

60. Koekkoek JA, Kerkhof M, Dirven L, Heimans JJ, Reijneveld JC, Taphoorn MJ (2015) Seizure outcome after radiotherapy and chemotherapy in low-grade glioma patients: a systematic review. Neuro Oncol 17:924–934

61. Kaloshi G, Benouaich-Amiel A, Diakite F et al (2007) Temozolomide for low-grade gliomas: predictive impact of 1p/19q loss on response and outcome. Neurology 68:1831–1836

62. Pace A, Vidiri A, Galie E et al (2003) Temozolomide chemotherapy for progressive low-grade glioma: clinical benefits and radiological response. Ann Oncol 14:1722–1726

63. Koekkoek JA, Dirven L, Heimans JJ et al (2015) Seizure reduction in a low-grade glioma: more than a beneficial side effect of temozolomide. J Neurol Neurosurg Psychiatry 86:366–373

64. Soffietti R, Ruda R, Bradac GB, Schiffer D (1998) PCV chemotherapy for recurrent oligodendrogliomas and oligoastrocytomas. Neurosurgery 43:1066–1073

65. Lebrun C, Fontaine D, Bourg V et al (2007) Treatment of newly diagnosed symptomatic pure low-grade oligodendrogliomas with PCV chemotherapy. Eur J Neurol 14:391–398

66. Frenay MP, Fontaine D, Vandenbos F, Lebrun C (2005) First-line nitrosourea-based chemotherapy in symptomatic non-resectable supratentorial pure low-grade astrocytomas. Eur J Neurol 12:685–690

67. Wu AS, Trinh VT, Suki D et al (2013) A prospective randomized trial of perioperative seizure prophylaxis in patients with intraparenchymal brain tumors. J Neurosurg 118:873–883

68. Franceschetti S, Binelli S, Casazza M et al (1990) Influence of surgery and antiepileptic drugs on seizures symptomatic of cerebral tumours. Acta Neurochir (Wein) 103:47–51

69. Forsyth PA, Weaver S, Fulton D et al (2003) Prophylactic anticonvulsants in patients with brain tumour. Can J Neurol Sci 30:106–112

70. Dewan MC, White-Dzuro GA, Brinson PR et al (2017) The influence of perioperative seizure prophylaxis on seizure rate and hospital quality metrics following glioma resection. Neurosurgery 80:563–570

71. North JB, Penhall RK, Hanieh A, Frewin DB, Taylor WB (1983) Phenytoin and postoperative epilepsy. A double-blind study. J Neurosurg 58:672–677

72. Chang SM, Parney IF, Huang W et al (2005) Patterns of care for adults with newly diagnosed malignant glioma. JAMA 293:557–564

73. Dewan MC, Thompson RC, Kalkanis SN, Barker FG II, Hadjipanayis CG (2017) Prophylactic antiepileptic drug administration following brain tumor resection: results of a recent AANS/CNS section on tumors survey. J Neurosurg 126:1772–1778

74. Sirven JI, Wingerchuk DM, Drazkowski JF, Lyons MK, Zimmerman RS (2004) Seizure prophylaxis in patients with brain tumors: a meta-analysis. Mayo Clin Proc 79:1489–1494

75. Pulman J, Greenhalgh J, Marson AG (2013) Antiepileptic drugs as prophylaxis for postcraniotomy seizures. Cochrane Database Syst Rev 2:CD007286

76. Kuijlen JM, Teernstra OP, Kessels AG, Herpers MJ, Beuls EA (1996) Effectiveness of antiepileptic prophylaxis used with supratentorial craniotomies: a meta-analysis. Seizure 5:291–298

77. Weston J, Greenhalgh J, Marson AG (2015) Antiepileptic drugs as prophylaxis for post-craniotomy seizures. Cochrane Database Syst Rev 3:CD007286

78. Glantz MJ, Cole BF, Forsyth PA et al (2000) Practice parameter: anticonvulsant prophylaxis in patients

with newly diagnosed brain tumors. Report of the Quality Standards Subcommittee of the American Academy of Neurology. Neurology 54:1886–1893

79. Soffietti R, Baumert BG, Bello L et al (2010) Guidelines on management of low-grade gliomas: report of an EFNS-EANO task force. Eur J Neurol 17:1124–1133

80. Glauser T, Ben-Menachem E, Bourgeois B et al (2013) Updated ILAE evidence review of anti-epileptic drug efficacy and effectiveness as initial monotherapy for epileptic seizures and syndromes. Epilepsia 54:551–563

81. Crepeau AZ, Sirven JI (2017) Management of adult onset seizures. Mayo Clin Proc 92:306–318

82. Gilbert MR, Supko JG, Batchelor T et al (2003) Phase I clinical and pharmacokinetic study of irinotecan in adults with recurrent malignant glioma. Clin Cancer Res 9:2940–2949

83. Maschio M, Albani F, Baruzzi A et al (2006) Levetiracetam therapy in patients with brain tumour and epilepsy. J Neurooncol 80:97–100

84. Vecht CJ, Wagner GL, Wilms EB (2003) Interactions between antiepileptic and chemotherapeutic drugs. Lancet Neurol 2:404–409

85. Oberndorfer S, Piribauer M, Marosi C, Lahrmann H, Hitzenberger P, Grisold W (2005) P450 enzyme inducing and non-enzyme inducing antiepileptics in glioblastoma patients treated with standard chemotherapy. J Neurooncol 72:255–260

86. Neef C, de Voogd-van der Straaten I (1988) An interaction between cytostatic and anticonvulsant drugs. Clin Pharmacol Ther 43:372–375

87. Ruegg S (2002) Dexamethasone/phenytoin interactions: neurooncological concerns. Swiss Med Wkly 132:425–426

88. Lackner TE (1991) Interaction of dexamethasone with phenytoin. Pharmacotherapy 11:344–347

89. Pursche S, Schleyer E, von Bonin M et al (2008) Influence of enzyme-inducing antiepileptic drugs on trough level of imatinib in glioblastoma patients. Curr Clin Pharmacol 3:198–203

90. Raymond E, Brandes AA, Dittrich C et al (2008) Phase II study of imatinib in patients with recurrent gliomas of various histologies: a European Organisation for Research and Treatment of Cancer Brain Tumor Group Study. J Clin Oncol 26:4659–4665

91. Wen PY, Yung WK, Lamborn KR et al (2006) Phase I/II study of imatinib mesylate for recurrent malignant gliomas: North American Brain Tumor Consortium Study 99-08. Clin Cancer Res 12:4899–4907

92. Maschio M, Dinapoli L, Sperati F et al (2011) Levetiracetam monotherapy in patients with brain tumor-related epilepsy: seizure control, safety, and quality of life. J Neurooncol 104:205–214

93. Usery JB, Michael LM II, Sills AK, Finch CK (2010) A prospective evaluation and literature review of levetiracetam use in patients with brain tumors and seizures. J Neurooncol 99:251–260

94. Kerkhof M, Dielemans JC, van Breemen MS et al (2013) Effect of valproic acid on seizure control and on survival in patients with glioblastoma multiforme. Neuro Oncol 15:961–967

95. Maschio M, Zarabla A, Maialetti A et al (2017) Quality of life, mood and seizure control in patients with brain tumor related epilepsy treated with lacosamide as add-on therapy: a prospective explorative study with a historical control group. Epilepsy Behav 73:83–89

96. Maschio M, Dinapoli L, Mingoia M et al (2011) Lacosamide as add-on in brain tumor-related epilepsy: preliminary report on efficacy and tolerability. J Neurol 258:2100–2104

97. Brodie MJ, Whitesides J, Schiemann J, D'Souza J, Johnson ME (2016) Tolerability, safety, and efficacy of adjunctive brivaracetam for focal seizures in older patients: a pooled analysis from three phase III studies. Epilepsy Res 127:114–118

98. Moseley BD, Sperling MR, Asadi-Pooya AA et al (2016) Efficacy, safety, and tolerability of adjunctive brivaracetam for secondarily generalized tonic-clonic seizures: pooled results from three phase III studies. Epilepsy Res 127:179–185

99. Elger C, Koepp M, Trinka E et al (2017) Pooled efficacy and safety of eslicarbazepine acetate as add-on treatment in patients with focal-onset seizures: data from four double-blind placebo-controlled pivotal phase III clinical studies. CNS Neurosci Ther 23:961–972

100. Plosker GL (2012) Perampanel: as adjunctive therapy in patients with partial-onset seizures. CNS Drugs 26:1085–1096

101. French JA, Krauss GL, Biton V et al (2012) Adjunctive perampanel for refractory partial-onset seizures: randomized phase III study 304. Neurology 79:589–596

102. French JA, Krauss GL, Steinhoff BJ et al (2013) Evaluation of adjunctive perampanel in patients with refractory partial-onset seizures: results of randomized global phase III study 305. Epilepsia 54:117–125

103. Krauss GL, Serratosa JM, Villanueva V et al (2012) Randomized phase III study 306: adjunctive perampanel for refractory partial-onset seizures. Neurology 78:1408–1415

104. Van Nifterik KA, Van den Berg J, Slotman BJ, Lafleur MV, Sminia P, Stalpers LJ (2012) Valproic acid sensitizes human glioma cells for temozolomide and gamma-radiation. J Neurooncol 107:61–67

105. Hosein AN, Lim YC, Day B et al (2015) The effect of valproic acid in combination with irradiation and temozolomide on primary human glioblastoma cells. J Neurooncol 122:263–271

106. Chie EK, Shin JH, Kim JH, Kim HJ, Kim IA, Kim IH (2015) In vitro and in vivo radiosensitizing effect of valproic acid on fractionated irradiation. Cancer Res Treat 47:527–533

107. Weller M, Gorlia T, Cairncross JG et al (2011) Prolonged survival with valproic acid use in the EORTC/NCIC temozolomide trial for glioblastoma. Neurology 77:1156–1164

108. Barker CA, Bishop AJ, Chang M, Beal K, Chan TA (2013) Valproic acid use during radiation therapy for glioblastoma associated with improved survival. Int J Radiat Oncol Biol Phys 86:504–509

109. Happold C, Gorlia T, Chinot O et al (2016) Does valproic acid or levetiracetam improve survival in glioblastoma? A pooled analysis of prospective clinical trials in newly diagnosed glioblastoma. J Clin Oncol 34:731–739

110. Bobustuc GC, Baker CH, Limaye A et al (2010) Levetiracetam enhances p53-mediated MGMT inhibition and sensitizes glioblastoma cells to temozolomide. Neuro Oncol 12:917–927

111. Kim YH, Kim T, Joo JD et al (2015) Survival benefit of levetiracetam in patients treated with concomitant chemoradiotherapy and adjuvant chemotherapy with temozolomide for glioblastoma multiforme. Cancer 121:2926–2932

Hydrocephalus Related to CNS Malignancies in Adults

40

Emilie Le Rhun, Jörg-Christian Tonn, and Michael Weller

40.1 General Presentation and Pathogenesis of Hydrocephalus

Hydrocephalus is defined as a nonphysiological accumulation of cerebrospinal fluid (CSF) in the ventricles. It is usually divided into two categories: obstructive hydrocephalus and communicative hydrocephalus. Obstructive hydrocephalus is related to a mechanical block of CSF drainage by a space-occupying lesion or congenital or acquired aqueductal stenosis. Communicative hydrocephalus is related to an increased production or decreased resorption of CSF, e.g., after

subarachnoid hemorrhage or acute or chronic meningitis [1] or after radiotherapy [2], or to a modification of CSF composition, e.g., increased protein level and presence of malignant cells, resulting in CSF malabsorption. Overall, central nervous system tumors represent the main cause of hydrocephalus [3], and approximately 5–10% of patients with glioblastoma develop hydrocephalus [4–7] as do 6–24% of patients with central nervous system metastases [8–12]. The incidence may be higher, up to 23% at presentation, in the adult population of patients with posterior fossa tumors [13].

Symptoms and signs of hydrocephalus include headache, nausea and vomiting, gait disorders, vertigo, dizziness, cognitive disorders, visual disturbances, urinary incontinence, and decreased level of consciousness. However, these symptoms and signs may be also related to expansive posterior fossa lesions [4, 8, 11, 14]. A risk of acute obstructive hydrocephalus does exist for posterior fossa lesions, eventually leading to sudden coma and death. This risk requires to manage such lesions as neurosurgical emergencies as outlined below. Conversely, symptoms and signs of hydrocephalus depend on the kinetics of its evolution, and hydrocephalus can also be largely asymptomatic when developing slowly and may be detected only by neuroimaging.

MRI with contrast enhancement is the gold standard for the diagnosis of brain tumors. In the context of hydrocephalus, it may show enlarged

E. Le Rhun (✉)
Neuro-Oncology Department of Neurosurgery, University Hospital Lille, Salengro Hospital, Lille, France

Neurology Department of Medical Oncology, Oscar Lambret Center, Lille, France

Inserm U-1192, Villeneuve d'Ascq, France

Department of Neurology, University Hospital and University of Zurich, Zurich, Switzerland
e-mail: emilie.lerhun@chru-lille.fr

J.-C. Tonn
Department of Neurosurgery, University Hospital Ludwig Maximilian University Munich, Munich, Germany
e-mail: joerg.christian.tonn@med.uni-muenchen.de

M. Weller
Department of Neurology, University Hospital and University of Zurich, Zurich, Switzerland
e-mail: michael.weller@usz.ch

© Springer Nature Switzerland AG 2019
J.-C. Tonn et al. (eds.), *Oncology of CNS Tumors*, https://doi.org/10.1007/978-3-030-04152-6_40

ventricles proximal to a CSF blockade in case of obstruction or throughout the ventricular system in case of communicating hydrocephalus. The Evans' index defined as the largest width between the lateral part of the frontal horns divided by the largest internal cranial diameter, measured on the same neuroimaging plane [15], has been proposed to aid in the diagnosis of normal pressure hydrocephalus, and a ventricular enlargement was defined by an index of 0.3 or more. However, significant differences can be observed depending on the level of the plane used to obtain this measure. In addition, the patient's age has to be considered—children and adolescents have narrow ventricles, and a size being enlarged in a young patient may be a normal width in the aged population. Volumetric assessment of the ventricles can also be used for the follow-up of hydrocephalus [16].

In case of newly developed or progressive clinical symptoms of raised intracranial pressure, a computed tomography (CT) scan is a widely available and quick to perform imaging modality to diagnose or rule out an acute hydrocephalus which might need immediate treatment.

40.2 Therapeutic Options

Several options are available for the management of hydrocephalus: direct surgical removal of the responsible lesion or endoscopic third ventriculostomy (ETV) for obstructive hydrocephalus, shunting either ventriculoperitoneal (VPS) or ventriculoatrial (VA) for both obstructive and communicative hydrocephalus, and external ventricular drainage as a transient emergency measure. Symptomatic pharmacological treatments such as steroids or analgesics usually have limited efficacy [14].

40.2.1 ETV

ETV is an endoscopic minimal invasive technique which involves creation of a small hole at the floor of the third ventricle to obtain a diversion of CSF into the interpeduncular cistern. ETV can help to control intracranial pressure, avoid a procedure inserting an implant and creating a potential entry for a CSF infection, both risks associated with an EVD, and help to perform definitive surgery in better general and neurological condition [13, 17].

In a systematic literature review on 130 studies on ETV including 11,952 cases, brain tumors and cysts were the most frequent indications. The ETV failure rate was estimated at 34.7% and was higher in the first months. Complications were observed in approximately 8% and included meningitis, ventriculitis, CSF leaks, and second brain surgery [3].

Several cohorts of adult patients with posterior fossa tumors have reported success rates of an ETV between 70 and 90% [13, 18–21]. In case of persisting hydrocephalus after surgery due to a partial resection or due to failure of initial ETV mostly related to hemorrhage, a second ETV or an EVD worked [17, 22].

However, with a history of central nervous system infection, ventricular hemorrhage, high CSF protein level, or leptomeningeal metastasis, VPS or VA shunt should be used rather than an ETV [11, 23–25]. In these situations, one factor for hydrocephalus might be a block of CSF absorption on the pial surface or arachnoid granulations outside the ventricles; thus the concept of "circumventing a CSF block distal to the third ventricle" does not work [25]. Also, unfavorable anatomy for ETV (e.g., too short distance between floor of the third ventricle and the basilar tip) or any obstruction at the level of the lateral ventricles (with block of Monroe's foramen) or of the third ventricle demands a shunt procedure.

40.2.2 VPS

VPS consists in the implantation of a catheter connecting the cerebral ventricles and the peritoneal cavity. Different types of valves, either programmable or not, can be used. Improvement occurs within the first days after surgery [14]. In a cohort of 417 patients with VPS implantation for hydrocephalus, 62 fixed shunts (15%) and

355 programmable shunts (85%) were implanted. Shunt revision rates were similar between groups: 22% for programmable pressure valves and 21% for fixed pressure valves. Complications of VPS were observed in approximately 12% of the patients [26] and include infection, obstruction, bleeding, shunt malfunction, overdrainage, and formation of cystic fluid collection in the abdominal cavity sometimes referred to as abdominal "pseudocysts" [14, 26, 27]. The latter usually indicates the malposition of the distal catheter outside the peritoneal cavity and requires revision.

40.2.3 Ventriculoatrial Shunt (VAS)

VA shunt consists in the implantation of a catheter from the cerebral ventricles into the right cardiac atrium. VAS is usually considered as more challenging than VPS due to potential severe cardiopulmonary and renal complications. However, VPA represents an option for patients with contraindication to a VPS, such as multiple prior abdominal surgeries, cirrhosis with ascites, peritoneal infection, and prior severe abdominal complications of VPS. In a retrospective analysis of 496 patients presenting with idiopathic normal pressure hydrocephalus (NPH), 150 received a VAS and 346 a VPS. Post-surgery complications were observed in 36% of VAS and 42.5% of VPS. Overdrainage was the main complication observed (27.4% for VAS, 19.8% for VPS) [28]. It remains uncertain in how far such data for NPH can be extrapolated to brain tumor patients. However, in the absence of severe contraindications, currently shunting into the peritoneum (VPS) is widely preferred over VAS.

40.2.4 External Ventricular Drainage (EVD)

An EVD is a temporary measure and usually indicated as an acute emergency procedure in patients with an acutely evolving clinical deterioration due to increased intracranial pressure on the basis of a hydrocephalus. Besides the controlled release of CSF, it allows to monitor the intracranial pressure. The main complication is infection. In a contemporary prospective cohort of 187 patients treated with an EVD and hospitalized in an intensive care unit, 31 related infections (16.6%) were observed [29]. Serum and CSF biomarkers have been shown useful to early detect infectious complications of EVD in patients with subarachnoid hemorrhage; whether this can be expanded on tumor patients is yet unclear [30].

40.2.5 Choice of Indications

The management of hydrocephalus depends on its cause and on the neurological condition. In a cohort of 243 adult patients with posterior fossa tumors, 52 patients (21.4%) had hydrocephalus at the time of admission: 39 of 52 patients had an early tumor resection, 11 of 52 patients had an ETV prior to resection, and 2 of 52 received an external ventricular drainage (EVD) initially [13]. The incidence of hydrocephalus prior to surgery was thus lower than for the pediatric population with posterior fossa tumors, where figures of 76% have been reported [31]. The risk of persistent hydrocephalus after surgery was 5.7%. Of the 191 patients without hydrocephalus prior to surgery, 4 patients (2.1%) developed post-surgery hydrocephalus. A risk factor for the need of a permanent CSF shunting procedure could not be identified [13].

In other cohorts of 36 patients treated with VPS and 16 patients treated with ETV, the efficacy was similar, 75% success rate for VPS and 69% success rate for ETV. Efficacy was higher in patients with severe symptoms. Complication rates were 19.4% for VPS and 12.6% for ETV [24]. In another report of 159 patients with hydrocephalus (123 patients treated with VPS and 36 patients treated with VTE), no revision was necessary in 69% of patients in the VPS group and 86% of patients in the ETV group. However, the complication rate was 42.7% in the VPS group versus only 9.4% in the ETV group [32]. In case of symptomatic hydrocephalus requiring CSF diversion prior to surgery, ETV should be considered as procedure of first choice as it has the same efficacy with less morbidity and is only transient and less costly than VPS or VA shunt [21, 23, 24, 33–35]. Even more, tissue detritus and blood being spilled into the CSF during surgery of intraventricular tumors leads with a high likelihood to an obstruction of a permanent shunt system with subsequent necessity of revision—another strong argument for EVD instead of shunting in this situation [13, 23]. ETV is associated with lower rates of perioperative complications and persistent hydrocephalus after tumor resection in children; however, in adult patients, this correlation has been less well studied [17, 36].

40.3 Primary Brain Tumors

40.3.1 Glioblastoma

In a report about 841 glioblastoma patients, 64 patients (8%) underwent a VPS for symptomatic hydrocephalus [4]. Fifteen patients presented with radiographic signs of hydrocephalus at diagnosis. Symptomatic hydrocephalus was observed during the course of the disease in 49 additional patients. VPS was performed after a median of 0.4 months (range 0–25.6 months) after glioblastoma diagnosis in patients with obstructive hydrocephalus (34% of patients with symptomatic hydrocephalus) and after a median of 10.6 (0.3–461) months after glioblastoma diagnosis in patients with communicative hydrocephalus (66%). In other smaller glioblastoma cohorts, communicative hydrocephalus was observed in 5–10% during the course of disease [5–7]. Risk factors for communicative hydrocephalus include ventricular opening during surgical procedures and leptomeningeal tumor cell dissemination [6, 7]. Radiotherapy may also contribute to the development of hydrocephalus in these patients, probably by inducing fibrosis of arachnoid granulations [2].

Out of 64 patients treated by shunt, a clinical improvement was noted after CSF diversion in 61% of the patients, independent of the type of hydrocephalus: 62% of the patients with communicative hydrocephalus improved and 59% of the patients with obstructive hydrocephalus improved [4]. In another cohort of 41 patients with WHO grade III and IV glioma receiving a shunt, clinical improvement was observed in 75% [37].

In patients with glioma-associated hydrocephalus, prognostic factors for longer survival were improvement of symptoms after shunt insertion, short time between initial tumor diagnosis and shunt, and, in case of communicative hydrocephalus, later onset of symptoms during the course of the disease [4]. Complications requiring a shunt revision have been reported in 17–29% of patients [4, 37]. The administration of bevacizumab prior to the surgical procedure may be associated with a somewhat higher bleeding rate ($p = 0.026$) [37].

40.3.2 Other Primary Brain Tumors

A rate of 27–58% of hydrocephalus has been reported in adult patients with hemangioblastomas prior to surgery [38, 39], and up to 14% of patients with preoperative hydrocephalus may require a VPS for persistent hydrocephalus after surgery [38]. The rate of hydrocephalus varies from 13.7 to 32.5% in vestibular schwannomas [13, 40–43]. In a cohort of 77 patients with small-to-medium vestibular schwannomas, the rate of hydrocephalus was 11.6% [42]. In this cohort no shunt was required after surgery, whereas 16 of 49 patients (32.5%) with large vestibular schwannomas underwent VPS for persistent hydrocephalus [43]. Especially in vestibular schwannomas, an increased CSF protein level might be found which is associated with a higher risk of shunt obstruction. Thus, and since in many cases enlargement of the ventricles resumes after surgical removal of the schwannoma, upfront shunting is seldom indicated. However, in elderly and frail patients with vestibular schwannoma and concomitant hydrocephalus, it is highly recommendable to check whether the symptoms are more likely derived from the hydrocephalus. In these patients, a shunting procedure might resolve the symptoms and avoid a more risky surgical procedure since surgical morbidity is closely linked to age in this entity [44].

In meningioma, age greater than 65 years, posterior fossa tumor location, tumor size greater than 5 cm, and Simpson resection grade II to IV were identified as risk factors of requiring a CSF diversion. In a cohort of 48 patients with meningiomas requiring a CSF shunt, the shunt failure rate was 27%, with single revision in 16.7% and multiple revisions in 10.4% [45]. Medulloblastoma and ependymoma are commonly observed in the fossa posterior, especially in the fourth ventricle, and may require postsurgical shunting due to hydrocephalus also in adult patients [13].

40.4 Brain Metastases

40.4.1 Posterior Fossa Metastasis

The incidence of brain metastases is increasing due to an improvement of therapeutic strategies which lead to improved systemic tumor control and increased overall survival in several types of common cancer. Posterior fossa metastases represent 27% of brain metastases [46]. The main tumor histology for posterior fossa metastases includes lung, breast, gastrointestinal, gynecological, and renal tumors and melanoma [11, 12]. In a cohort of 92 consecutive patients with posterior fossa metastases, 7.6% developed obstructive hydrocephalus requiring an emergency CSF shunt prior to surgical resection, and 7.1% required a CSF diversion after tumor surgery [11]. In another cohort of 50 patients, up to 24% of patients with posterior fossa metastasis presenting with symptomatic hydrocephalus required a permanent CSF drainage after resection of the metastases [12]. The risk of leptomeningeal tumor spread with potentially subsequent hydrocephalus is significantly higher with piecemeal tumor resection than with other either en bloc resection or stereotactic radiosurgery [47].

In a cohort of patients presenting with hydrocephalus related to brain metastases, 16 ETV and 36 VPS were performed [24]. In this cohort no ETV was performed in patients with prior history of CNS infection or bleeding or with leptomeningeal metastases. A comparable efficacy on symptoms was obtained after ETV (69%) and VPS (75%). While the precise prognosis of asymptomatic or symptomatic obstructive hydrocephalus is unknown [48], surgical resection or at least biopsy of identified lesions can be recommended with the aims to obtain a pathological diagnosis and to improve local control [48].

40.4.2 Leptomeningeal Metastases

Communicating hydrocephalus has been reported in 5–17% of patients with leptomeningeal metastases [9, 10, 25]. Obstructive hydrocephalus related to a block of CSF flow by metastatic nodules may also be observed. The goal of the treatment of hydrocephalus in this situation is to improve symptoms and quality of life. Adequate treatment of hydrocephalus may also help to administer other therapies which may improve the prognosis of the patients [25]. Several retrospective studies have shown 77–88% of improvement of neurological symptoms related to hydrocephalus and of the general condition after shunt placement in patients with leptomeningeal metastases [8, 33, 49]. The quality of life is usually improved [14, 24, 49]. The greatest improvements are usually seen for headache and nausea but less so for cognitive disorders, urinary incontinence, or gait disturbance [8, 24, 33, 49]. The main complications of VPS in patients with leptomeningeal metastases include infection, bleeding, obstruction or malfunction, and subdural hematoma, with an overall complication rate estimated between 9 and 15% [8]. Peritoneal dissemination of tumor cells has been reported [50–52] but seems to be rare [8, 24, 33].

Repeated CSF depletion by lumbar puncture or through a ventricular device can be an option in patients with a-/pauci-symptomatic hydrocephalus treated with intra-CSF pharmacotherapy. However, intra-CSF pharmacotherapy is usually not recommended in case of symptomatic hydrocephalus which requires a VPS, especially in the absence of a valve with an on/off option. Complications of ventricular devices include obstruction, malposition, leukoencephalopathy, and infection, although the revision rates are below 8% [53–55].

ETV represents an option for patients with obstructive hydrocephalus, e.g., secondary to brain metastases [56], but should be avoided in patients with communicative hydrocephalus as efficacy cannot be expected in these situations.

40.5 Conclusions

CSF diversion may have a role in the early diagnostic setting, sometimes as an emergency measure, or during the course of the disease in patients with primary and secondary central nervous system tumors. The method for CSF diversion should be determined according to the type of hydrocephalus (obstructive vs. communicative), the clinical presentation of the patient, and the overall medical history. CSF shunting may allow for rapid improvement of clinical symptoms and quality of life with an acceptable rate of complications and may provide the opportunity to apply further oncologic treatments. The option of CSF diversion appears to be undervalued in neuro-oncology and should be considered in patients with central nervous system tumors.

References

1. Lam S, Harris DA, Lin Y, Rocque BG, Ham S, Pan I-W (2016) Outcomes of endoscopic third ventriculostomy in adults. J Clin Neurosci 31:166–171
2. Perrini P, Scollato A, Cioffi F, Mouchaty H, Conti R, Di Lorenzo N (2002) Radiation leukoencephalopathy associated with moderate hydrocephalus: intracranial pressure monitoring and results of ventriculoperitoneal shunting. Neurol Sci 23(5):237–241
3. Madsen PJ, Mallela AN, Hudgins ED, Storm PB, Heuer GG, Stein SC (2018) The effect and evolution of patient selection on outcomes in endoscopic third ventriculostomy for hydrocephalus: a large-scale review of the literature. J Neurol Sci 385:185–191
4. Castro BA, Imber BS, Chen R, McDermott MW, Aghi MK (2017) Ventriculoperitoneal shunting for glioblastoma: risk factors, indications, and efficacy. Neurosurgery 80(3):421–430
5. Inamasu J, Nakamura Y, Saito R, Kuroshima Y, Mayanagi K, Orii M et al (2003) Postoperative communicating hydrocephalus in patients with supra-

tentorial malignant glioma. Clin Neurol Neurosurg 106(1):9–15
6. Montano N, D'Alessandris QG, Bianchi F, Lauretti L, Doglietto F, Fernandez E et al (2011) Communicating hydrocephalus following surgery and adjuvant radiochemotherapy for glioblastoma. J Neurosurg 115(6):1126–1130
7. Fischer CM, Neidert MC, Péus D, Ulrich NH, Regli L, Krayenbühl N et al (2014) Hydrocephalus after resection and adjuvant radiochemotherapy in patients with glioblastoma. Clin Neurol Neurosurg 120:27–31
8. Omuro AMP, Lallana EC, Bilsky MH, DeAngelis LM (2005) Ventriculoperitoneal shunt in patients with leptomeningeal metastasis. Neurology 64(9):1625–1627
9. Niwińska A, Rudnicka H, Murawska M (2013) Breast cancer leptomeningeal metastasis: propensity of breast cancer subtypes for leptomeninges and the analysis of factors influencing survival. Med Oncol 30(1):408
10. Lee SJ, Lee J-I, Nam D-H, Ahn YC, Han JH, Sun J-M et al (2013) Leptomeningeal carcinomatosis in non-small-cell lung cancer patients: impact on survival and correlated prognostic factors. J Thorac Oncol 8(2):185–191
11. Sunderland GJ, Jenkinson MD, Zakaria R (2016) Surgical management of posterior fossa metastases. J Neuro-Oncol 130(3):535–542
12. Ghods AJ, Munoz L, Byrne R (2011) Surgical treatment of cerebellar metastases. Surg Neurol Int 2:159
13. Marx S, Reinfelder M, Matthes M, Schroeder HWS, Baldauf J (2018) Frequency and treatment of hydrocephalus prior to and after posterior fossa tumor surgery in adult patients. Acta Neurochir 160(5):1063–1071
14. Nigim F, Critchlow JF, Kasper EM (2015) Role of ventriculoperitoneal shunting in patients with neoplasms of the central nervous system: an analysis of 59 cases. Mol Clin Oncol 3(6):1381–1386
15. Relkin N, Marmarou A, Klinge P, Bergsneider M, Black PM (2005) Diagnosing idiopathic normal-pressure hydrocephalus. Neurosurgery 57(Suppl 3):S4–S16; discussion ii–v
16. Toma AK, Holl E, Kitchen ND, Watkins LD (2011) Evans' index revisited: the need for an alternative in normal pressure hydrocephalus. Neurosurgery 68(4):939–944
17. Di Rocco F, Jucá CE, Zerah M, Sainte-Rose C (2013) Endoscopic third ventriculostomy and posterior fossa tumors. World Neurosurg 79(Suppl 2):S18.e15–S18.e19
18. Di Vincenzo J, Keiner D, Gaab MR, Schroeder HWS, Oertel JMK (2014) Endoscopic third ventriculostomy: preoperative considerations and intraoperative strategy based on 300 procedures. J Neurol Surg A Cent Eur Neurosurg 75(1):20–30
19. Grand W, Leonardo J, Chamczuk AJ, Korus AJ (2016) Endoscopic third ventriculostomy in 250 adults with hydrocephalus: patient selection, outcomes, and complications. Neurosurgery 78(1):109–119

20. Isaacs AM, Bezchlibnyk YB, Yong H, Koshy D, Urbaneja G, Hader WJ et al (2016) Endoscopic third ventriculostomy for treatment of adult hydrocephalus: long-term follow-up of 163 patients. Neurosurg Focus 41(3):E3

21. Nguyen TT, Smith MV, Rodziewicz GS, Lemke SM (1999) Hydrocephalus caused by metastatic brain lesions: treatment by third ventriculostomy. J Neurol Neurosurg Psychiatry 67(4):552–553

22. Marx S, El Damaty A, Manwaring J, El Refaee E, Fleck S, Fritsch M et al (2018) Endoscopic third ventriculostomy before posterior fossa tumor surgery in adult patients. J Neurol Surg A Cent Eur Neurosurg 79(2):123–129

23. Chen CC, Kasper E, Warnke P (2011) Palliative stereotactic-endoscopic third ventriculostomy for the treatment of obstructive hydrocephalus from cerebral metastasis. Surg Neurol Int 2:76

24. Gonda DD, Kim TE, Warnke PC, Kasper EM, Carter BS, Chen CC (2012) Ventriculoperitoneal shunting versus endoscopic third ventriculostomy in the treatment of patients with hydrocephalus related to metastasis. Surg Neurol Int 3:97

25. Jung T-Y, Chung W-K, Oh I-J (2014) The prognostic significance of surgically treated hydrocephalus in leptomeningeal metastases. Clin Neurol Neurosurg 119:80–83

26. Agarwal N, Kashkoush A, McDowell MM, Lariviere WR, Ismail N, Friedlander RM (2018) Comparative durability and costs analysis of ventricular shunts. J Neurosurg 11:1–8

27. Anwar R, Sadek A-R, Vajramani G (2017) Abdominal pseudocyst: a rare complication of ventriculoperitoneal shunting. Pract Neurol 17(3):212–213

28. Hung AL, Vivas-Buitrago T, Adam A, Lu J, Robison J, Elder BD et al (2017) Ventriculoatrial versus ventriculoperitoneal shunt complications in idiopathic normal pressure hydrocephalus. Clin Neurol Neurosurg 157:1–6

29. Berger-Estilita J, Passer M, Giles M, Wiegand J, Merz TM (2018) Modalities and accuracy of diagnosis of external ventricular drainage-related infections: a prospective multicentre observational cohort study. Acta Neurochir 160(10):2039–2047

30. Lenski M, Huge V, Schmutzer M, Ueberschaer M, Briegel J, Tonn J-C et al (2018) Inflammatory markers in serum and cerebrospinal fluid for early detection of external ventricular drain-associated ventriculitis in patients with subarachnoid hemorrhage. J Neurosurg Anesthesiol

31. Sainte-Rose C, Cinalli G, Roux FE, Maixner R, Chumas PD, Mansour M et al (2001) Management of hydrocephalus in pediatric patients with posterior fossa tumors: the role of endoscopic third ventriculostomy. J Neurosurg 95(5):791–797

32. Gliemroth J, Käsbeck E, Kehler U (2014) Ventriculocisternostomy versus ventriculoperitoneal shunt in the treatment of hydrocephalus: a retrospective, long-term observational study. Clin Neurol Neurosurg 122:92–96

33. Lee SH, Kong DS, Seol HJ, Nam D-H, Lee J-I (2011) Ventriculoperitoneal shunt for hydrocephalus caused by central nervous system metastasis. J Neuro-Oncol 104(2):545–551

34. de Lima BO, Pratesi R (2014) Endoscopic third ventriculostomy has no higher costs than ventriculoperitoneal shunt. Arq Neuropsiquiatr 72(7):524–527

35. Reddy GK, Bollam P, Caldito G, Willis B, Guthikonda B, Nanda A (2011) Ventriculoperitoneal shunt complications in hydrocephalus patients with intracranial tumors: an analysis of relevant risk factors. J Neuro-Oncol 103(2):333–342

36. Lin C-T, Riva-Cambrin JK (2015) Management of posterior fossa tumors and hydrocephalus in children: a review. Childs Nerv Syst 31(10):1781–1789

37. Rinaldo L, Brown D, Lanzino G, Parney IF (2017) Outcomes following cerebrospinal fluid shunting in high-grade glioma patients. J Neurosurg 22:1–13

38. Fukuda M, Takao T, Hiraishi T, Yoshimura J, Yajima N, Saito A et al (2014) Clinical factors predicting outcomes after surgical resection for sporadic cerebellar hemangioblastomas. World Neurosurg 82(5):815–821

39. Niu L, Zhang Y, Li Q, Dai J, Yin H, Duan L et al (2016) The analysis of correlative factors affecting long-term outcomes in patients with Solid Cerebellar Hemangioblastomas. Clin Neurol Neurosurg 150:59–66

40. Atlas MD, Perez de Tagle JR, Cook JA, Sheehy JP, Fagan PA (1996) Evolution of the management of hydrocephalus associated with acoustic neuroma. Laryngoscope 106(2 Pt 1):204–206

41. Pirouzmand F, Tator CH, Rutka J (2001) Management of hydrocephalus associated with vestibular schwannoma and other cerebellopontine angle tumors. Neurosurgery 48(6):1246–1253; discussion 1253–1254

42. Taniguchi M, Nakai T, Kohta M, Kimura H, Kohmura E (2016) Communicating hydrocephalus associated with small- to medium-sized vestibular schwannomas: clinical significance of the tumor apparent diffusion coefficient map. World Neurosurg 94:261–267

43. Harati A, Scheufler K-M, Schultheiss R, Tonkal A, Harati K, Oni P et al (2017) Clinical features, microsurgical treatment, and outcome of vestibular schwannoma with brainstem compression. Surg Neurol Int 8:45

44. McClelland S, Kim E, Murphy JD, Jaboin JJ (2017) Operative mortality rates of acoustic neuroma surgery: a national cancer database analysis. Otol Neurotol 38(5):751–753

45. Bir SC, Sapkota S, Maiti TK, Konar S, Bollam P, Nanda A (2017) Evaluation of ventriculoperitoneal shunt-related complications in intracranial meningioma with hydrocephalus. J Neurol Surg B Skull Base 78(1):30–36

46. Ghia A, Tomé WA, Thomas S, Cannon G, Khuntia D, Kuo JS et al (2007) Distribution of brain metastases in relation to the hippocampus: implications for neurocognitive functional preservation. Int J Radiat Oncol Biol Phys 68(4):971–977

47. Suki D, Hatiboglu MA, Patel AJ, Weinberg JS, Groves MD, Mahajan A et al (2009) Comparative risk of leptomeningeal dissemination of cancer after surgery or stereotactic radiosurgery for a single supratentorial solid tumor metastasis. Neurosurgery 64(4):664–674; discussion 674–676

48. Roux A, Botella C, Still M, Zanello M, Dhermain F, Metellus P et al (2018) Posterior fossa metastasis-associated obstructive hydrocephalus in adult patients: literature review and practical considerations from the Neuro-Oncology Club of the French Society of Neurosurgery. World Neurosurg 117:271–279

49. Murakami Y, Ichikawa M, Bakhit M, Jinguji S, Sato T, Fujii M et al (2018) Palliative shunt surgery for patients with leptomeningeal metastasis. Clin Neurol Neurosurg 168:175–178

50. Narayan A, Jallo G, Huisman TAGM (2015) Extracranial, peritoneal seeding of primary malignant brain tumors through ventriculo-peritoneal shunts in children: case report and review of the literature. Neuroradiol J 28(5):536–539

51. Rickert CH (1998) Abdominal metastases of pediatric brain tumors via ventriculo-peritoneal shunts. Childs Nerv Syst 14(1–2):10–14

52. Jamjoom ZA, Jamjoom AB, Sulaiman AH, Naim-Ur-Rahman null, al Rabiaa A (1993) Systemic metastasis of medulloblastoma through ventriculoperitoneal shunt: report of a case and critical analysis of the literature. Surg Neurol 40(5):403–410

53. Zairi F, Le Rhun E, Bertrand N, Boulanger T, Taillibert S, Aboukais R et al (2015) Complications related to the use of an intraventricular access device for the treatment of leptomeningeal metastases from solid tumor: a single centre experience in 112 patients. J Neuro-Oncol 124(2):317–323

54. Kennedy BC, Brown LT, Komotar RJ, McKhann GM (2016) Stereotactic catheter placement for Ommaya reservoirs. J Clin Neurosci 27:44–47

55. Morgenstern PF, Connors S, Reiner AS, Greenfield JP (2016) Image guidance for placement of ommaya reservoirs: comparison of fluoroscopy and frameless stereotactic navigation in 145 patients. World Neurosurg 93:154–158

56. Volkov AA, Filis AK, Vrionis FD (2017) Surgical treatment for leptomeningeal disease. Cancer Control 24(1):47–53

Gliomas and Pregnancy

41

Jacob J. Mandel, Akash Patel,
and Shlomit Yust-Katz

41.1 Introduction

The decision to have a child is a complex one that often takes multiple factors into consideration including the ethical, philosophical, and religious influences of the mother and/or her partner. Being diagnosed with a brain tumor prior to a pregnancy or while pregnant can further complicate the situation for the patient and their family. However, due to the recent improvement in prognosis of brain tumor patients, young women with glial brain tumors are now more likely to consider pregnancy.

Additionally, the care of a pregnant patient with a glioma also presents distinct dilemmas for physicians. Treatment decisions often can have possible consequences on the health of the mother and/or the baby.

Management of these cases should involve a large multidisciplinary group of physicians including a neuro-oncologist, neurosurgeon, neuroradiologist, radiation oncologist, obstetrician/

gynecologist, anesthesiologist, neonatologist, and medical ethicist.

This chapter will examine the incidence, presentation, diagnosis, treatments, prognosis, and management of this unique quandary.

41.2 Incidence

The occurrence of a primary brain tumor is rare. The incidence rate of all primary malignant and nonmalignant brain and other CNS tumors is 22.36 cases per 100,000 for a total count of 368,117 incident tumors (7.18 per 100,000 for malignant and 15.18 per 100,000 for nonmalignant tumors). The rate is higher in females (24.46 per 100,000) than in males (20.10 per 100,000) [1]. Despite the rarity, brain tumors are the fifth leading cause of cancer-related death in women aged 20–39 years [2]. Glial neoplasms are the most common histological type of malignant primary brain tumor in adults and are more common among males [1]. The incidence of maternal malignant brain tumors has been reported at 3.6 per 1,000,000 live births [3]. A study using a probability-based calculation estimated that around 90 women each year have a brain tumor during pregnancy in the United States [4]. The stated incidence of primary brain tumors in pregnant women is marginally lower compared with age-matched women [5]. The incidence of a brain

J. J. Mandel · A. Patel
Department of Neurology and Neurosurgery, Baylor College of Medicine, Houston, TX, USA
e-mail: Jacob.mandel@bcm.edu; Akash.Patel@bcm.edu

S. Yust-Katz (✉)
Rabin Medical Center, Neuro-Oncology Unit, Davidoff Cancer Center and Tel-Aviv University, Petah Tikva, Israel

© Springer Nature Switzerland AG 2019
J.-C. Tonn et al. (eds.), *Oncology of CNS Tumors*, https://doi.org/10.1007/978-3-030-04152-6_41

tumor presenting during pregnancy is in the range of about 1 in 20,000–40,000 [6, 7]. Additionally, the relative frequencies of each brain tumor type appear to be similar for pregnant and nonpregnant women [5].

41.3 Pathogenesis/Pathophysiology

Numerous hypotheses have been offered to explain the development and possible progression of brain tumors in pregnancy. One proposed mechanism is that a change in hormonal factors during the pregnancy can increase the growth rate in brain tumors with progesterone and estrogen receptors [8, 9]. Another possible method of tumor growth is the rise of angiogenic factors such as vascular endothelial growth factor and placental growth factor during pregnancy. Elevated levels of these angiogenic factors have been well identified in malignant glioma and targeted for potential therapeutics in these tumors [10, 11]. Additionally, patients may become symptomatic secondary to an increase in blood volume during pregnancy resulting in worsening of peritumoral edema [12–14].

41.4 Clinical Presentation

Brain tumors can present with one or several different symptoms depending on the location of the tumor. Many of these symptoms such as headaches, nausea/vomiting, visual changes, and seizures may occur during pregnancy secondary to pregnancy-related factors. This can make it a difficult decision when to pursue further work-up of these symptoms with imaging studies.

Headaches are particularly common among women in their childbearing years. In a large Norwegian, population-based study, 60% of women ≤40 years of age reported experiencing a headache within the previous year [15]. Another study asking 430 postpartum women about headache symptoms during their preceding pregnancy found that 35% of women reported suffering some type of headache [16]. A recent 5-year, single-center, retrospective study of consecutive pregnant women presenting to acute care with headache reported that women most often (56.4%) presented in the third trimester [17]. Regarding pregnant women undergoing inpatient neurologic consultation, greater than one-third can have a secondary headache [17]. Additionally, a prospective cohort study estimated that 40% of postpartum women have headaches typically transpiring within the first week after delivery [18].

Seizures can also arise as a presenting symptom in 32% of patients with glioma [19]. Seizures due to tumors are often focal in nature at onset but may secondarily generalize. Preeclampsia is a unique condition in pregnant women distinguished by the inception of hypertension and either proteinuria or end-organ dysfunction later than 20 weeks of gestation. Eclampsia is the occurrence of new-onset, generalized, tonic-clonic seizures or coma in a woman with preeclampsia. Eclampsia appears in 2–3% of women with severe features of preeclampsia not receiving anti-seizure prophylaxis and up to 0.6% of women with preeclampsia without severe features [20].

Nausea and vomiting have been reported to occur in 13% of glioma patients as a presenting symptom [19]. Nausea is also extremely common in pregnancy, with up to 90% of pregnancies describing some degree of nausea with or without vomiting. The severity of nausea can vary in pregnancy with hyperemesis gravidarum being a serious condition with weight loss exceeding 5% of prepregnancy body weight.

Indications for neuroimaging in pregnant women are akin to those in nonpregnant adults. Patients with new headaches, sudden onset of a severe headache, worsening headaches, or qualities different from usual headaches warrant urgent neurological evaluation and imaging [21]. Additionally, headaches with altered mental status, seizures, papilledema, changes in vision, stiff neck, or focal neurological signs/symptoms should also prompt urgent neuroimaging [21].

41.5 Diagnostic Tests

Exposure to ionizing radiation from CT (computed tomography) and strong magnetic fields from MRI (magnetic resonance imaging), with or without the use of contrast, might carry potential risks to the pregnant patient and her fetus. The choice of diagnostic modality to evaluate neurologic disorders in the pregnant patient should aim to provide the patient with the standard of care for diagnosis and treatment while minimizing potential risks to her fetus.

Several studies have demonstrated that CT head scanning is safe for the fetus, particularly in the venue of abdominal lead shielding practices [4]. The estimated fetal exposure from indirect radiation disseminated through the mother's body from a head CT is very low (less than 0.1 rad) [22]. No conclusive association between radiation exposure of less than 5 rad (50 mGy) and an increased risk of spontaneous abortion, fetal anomalies, developmental malformations, or mental retardation has been established [23]. However, the use of contrast with a head CT should be avoided unless absolutely necessary as iodinated contrast is classified by the US Food and Drug Administration (FDA) in the class B category for pregnancy. This is because the majority of CT contrast agents contain iodine by-products, and neonatal hypothyroidism has been associated with various iodinated agents taken in early pregnancy [12].

While CT scans are routinely used as a screening tool because of its low cost and prevalent obtainability, magnetic resonance imaging (MRI) is the favored imaging technique for brain tumors. This is because the information present on MR images can reveal a tumor's detailed location and even help a physician appraise the tumor grade and histology based upon the location and contrast enhancement pattern seen on the scan. In pregnant patients, MRI is especially advantageous because no ionizing radiation is involved. MR scanners using a magnetic field from 1.5 to 3.0 T in strength have demonstrated no harmful effects on human tissue [24]. MRI uses gadolinium-based contrast agents that are paramagnetic and do not contain iodine. Gadolinium contrast though has been classified by the FDA as class C due to animal studies (using concentrations of gadolinium higher than normally given in humans) associating it's use with abortion and developmental malformations [25]. Additionally, recent studies revealing the detection of gadolinium deposition in the brain (most notably in the dentate nuclei and globus pallidus) have been reported [26]. Another study evaluating the long-term safety of exposure to MRI in the first trimester of pregnancy or to gadolinium at any time during pregnancy found that exposure to MRI during the first trimester of pregnancy compared with no exposure was not associated with increased risk of harm to the fetus or in early childhood [27]. Gadolinium MRI at any time during pregnancy was associated with an increased risk of a broad set of rheumatological, inflammatory, or infiltrative skin conditions and for stillbirth or neonatal death [27]. However, it has been suggested that the results of this study are prejudiced by the data being established in part with older unstable gadolinium-based contrast agents [28]. These older gadolinium-based contrast agent chelates were linear molecules and are essentially not in use anymore as newer chelates have been shown to be more stable with little free gadolinium release [28].

The use of gadolinium should therefore be given if needed to evaluate a tumor appropriately and if its presence or absence could change management, treatment, or prognosis. Routine radiographic surveillance in pregnant patients with a known history of a brain tumor should proceed regularly with MRI scans without contrast, as disease progression can occur prior to the development of new clinical signs or symptoms.

41.6 Treatment

Treatments used for brain tumors include surgical resection, radiation therapy and chemotherapy, and symptomatic treatment that includes anti-epileptic drugs and steroids. Important issues to consider when evaluating the pregnant patient for possible treatments include neurological stability of the patient, assumed grade and histology of tumor, intracranial location of the tumor, and the gestational age/viability of the fetus [29]. Although countries and states have differing laws regarding termination of the fetus, if the pregnancy is discovered early in the first trimester, the benefits/risks of this option should be discussed.

41.6.1 Surgery

There currently is no clear evidence to determine the optimal timing of neurosurgical intervention in pregnant patients with brain tumors. Authors of case series and reviews have offered different recommendations based upon their experiences. One proposed algorithm recommended for neurologically stable patients in their first and early second trimesters that gestational advancement should be allowed until the early second trimester prior to neurosurgery [6]. However, due to the perceived high risk of intracranial hemorrhage with increased maternal intravascular volume in the late second and third trimester, neurosurgical procedure was not recommended at this time [6]. For patients in the late second and third trimester with a progressive focal neurologic deficit, radiation treatment was recommended, but if there was concern for possible pending brain herniation, then delivery by C-section followed by subsequent neurosurgical decompression was advised [6].

Other authors have suggested that anytime a malignant glioma is presumed, a surgical removal should be done immediately regardless of gestational age [30, 31]. This was recommended in an attempt to maximize the extent of resection possible as pregnancy should not prevent them from receiving the best treatment for their glioma [30, 31]. Yet, others have cautioned against this approach recommending to delay neurosurgery until the early second trimester whenever feasible due to the possibility of an elevated risk of miscarriage and birth defects associated with a surgery in the first trimester [32, 33].

41.6.2 Radiotherapy

Data on the use of radiotherapy during pregnancy is also limited. Doses of 0.1–0.5 Gy during the first trimester of pregnancy have noteworthy risks of toxicity including microcephaly, organ malformations, and growth and mental retardation [34]. Doses of 0.5 Gy remain a high risk for toxicity in the second and third trimesters. Additionally, the potential for radiation-induced malignancy exists with an estimate of the lifetime risk of a radiation-induced fatal cancer at doses of 0.01 Gy at around 1 in 1700 (0.06%) [35].

Radiation therapy dosing for gliomas can often limit fetal exposure to below 0.1 Gy [36]. Furthermore, the use of abdominal shielding devices and adjustment of radiation beam angles to limit fetal dose to as low as possible is recommended [37]. Case reports of radiation treatment of gliomas during pregnancy have been reported without subsequent deleterious effects on the fetus [36, 37]. Irradiation of large tumors can sometimes cause increased intracranial edema and inflammation. Caution may be warranted in certain incidences of large or subcortical tumors in order to prevent increased risk of cerebral herniation with radiation.

41.6.3 Chemotherapy

Chemotherapy use during pregnancy can pose significant dangers to the fetus and mother. The potential harmful effects of chemotherapy treatment in pregnancy include congenital malformations, developmental delay, carcinogenesis, organ toxicity, premature delivery, spontaneous abortion, and intrauterine demise [38, 39]. Systemic chemotherapy should not be electively started during the first trimester as most cases of toxicity were reported during embryogenesis [40]. While certain chemotherapies (mainly for breast cancer) appear to be safe to be administered in the second and third trimester, it has been recommended that chemotherapeutic agents that cross the placenta at increased levels should be postponed until after delivery [40, 41]. Among the chemotherapeutic drugs, antimetabolites and alkylating agents are the most frequent drugs noted to induce malformation or to exert teratogenic effects [39, 42].

The most common chemotherapeutic regimens used in treatment of gliomas are temozolomide and PCV (procarbazine, lomustine, and vincristine) [43, 44]. Concurrent chemoradiation with temozolomide followed by adjuvant temozolomide is the current standard of care for newly diagnosed glioblastoma [43]. Additionally, preliminary results of the CATNON trial also suggest benefit with the use of adjuvant temozolomide in addition to radiation in newly diagnosed anaplastic gliomas with 1p/19q intact chromosomes. Adjuvant PCV following radiation treatment recently has been found to improve overall survival in newly diagnosed "high"-risk low-grade gliomas and 1p/19q co-deleted oligodendrogliomas [45–47].

Temozolomide is a prodrug which is quickly and nonenzymatically transformed to the active alkylating metabolite MTIC [(methyl-triazene-1-yl)-imidazole-4-carboxamide]. The cytotoxic results of MTIC are established through alkylation (methylation) of DNA at the O6, N7 guanine positions which initiate DNA double-strand breaks and apoptosis. Temozolomide is categorized by the US Food and Drug Administration (FDA) in the class D for pregnancy.

The three drug regimen PCV consists of procarbazine, lomustine, and vincristine. Procarbazine is also an alkylating agent that impedes DNA, RNA, and protein synthesis by inhibiting transmethylation of methionine into transfer RNA [38]. Procarbazine is categorized by the US Food and Drug Administration (FDA) in the class D for pregnancy as well. Lomustine is a nitrosourea that hinders DNA, RNA, and protein synthesis via alkylation and carbamylation of DNA and RNA. Adverse effects with lomustine use have been reported in animal reproduction studies. Vincristine is a vinca alkaloid that binds to tubulin and inhibits microtubule formation and is similarly in the class D for pregnancy according to the US Food and Drug Administration (FDA) [48].

While the most commonly used chemotherapeutic agents used to treat malignant gliomas cross the placenta and are not recommended to be administered during pregnancy, there have been several case reports of patients who were discovered to be pregnant during treatment with temozolomide or PCV [38]. Uncomplicated pregnancies and healthy live births can occur despite chemotherapy exposure with temozolomide or PCV use early during an unplanned pregnancy in patients with gliomas [29, 38]. Additionally, a case has been reported of a successful pregnancy and delivery after concurrent chemoradiation in a patient who was newly diagnosed with a glioblastoma while 14 weeks pregnant [49]. However, another case of a pregnant patient on temozolomide prior to discovering her pregnancy was reported where the child subsequently was born with a neural tube defect and cerebral palsy [14].

Gliadel (carmustine polymer) wafers implanted at the time of surgical resection for local drug delivery have been examined in clinical trials and approved for use in patients with newly diagnosed or recurrent gliomas [50–52]. It has been suggested, since the implantable wafers in the surgical cavity site have demonstrated no carmustine in the systemic circulation, that these wafers may be safe in pregnant patients with gliomas undergoing a resection [38]. However, no cases have been reported describing their use or safety in pregnant patients.

Bevacizumab is a recombinant humanized monoclonal antibody that hinders the biologic activity of vascular endothelial growth factor (VEGF) and currently is approved by the FDA for use in recurrent glioblastoma [10, 53–55]. VEGF binding initiates angiogenesis (endothelial proliferation and the formation of new blood vessels) and in animal studies has resulted in adverse fetal outcomes including fetal death [56]. No cases of cancer patients treated with bevacizumab during pregnancy have been reported. However, pregnant patients have been exposed to intravitreal injection of bevacizumab. A number of patients treated during the first trimester have been reported to have had spontaneous miscarriages, whereas treatment during the second and third trimesters has not been associated with adverse events [57–59]. Bevacizumab should not be administered in pregnancy [60].

41.7 Anti-epileptic Drugs (AEDs)

Seizures have been estimated to occur as the presenting symptom in 30–50% of patients with brain tumors, and another 10–30% of patients can develop seizures later in the disease course [61]. Studies have reported the incidence of seizures in pregnant patients with gliomas to be at least 24% of patients [13, 29]. Uncontrolled seizures during pregnancy can be potentially harmful for both the mother and the fetus [62]. Furthermore, it remains unclear if pregnancy increases seizure frequency in brain tumor patients, and an association of low-grade gliomas with epilepsy during pregnancy was noted in a recent Norwegian study [63]. Therefore, AEDs should not be discontinued to pregnant patients with known seizures [6]. Despite earlier retrospective data that valproic acid may have antitumor effect and possibly prolong survival, a subsequent pooled analysis of four prospective clinical trials in newly diagnosed glioblastoma found no association with valproic acid or levetiracetam use and improved outcomes [64–66]. Additionally, due to the increased risk for fetal malformations with valproic acid, it should be avoided, and newer AEDs like lamictal or levetiracetam are preferred [33]. Additionally, plasma drug levels of AEDs need to be monitored, supplemental folic acid should be given, and monotherapy with lowest dose possible to control tonic-clonic and/or complex partial seizures is recommended for pregnant patients with seizures [67]. Debate remains on the need for prophylactic AEDs in brain tumor patients without a history of seizures, but the current recommendation is to withhold routine AEDS per the American Academy of Neurology [68, 69]. An epileptologist should be included in the multidisciplinary care of any pregnant brain tumor patient with seizures.

41.8 Prognosis

Debate remains whether pregnancy may lead to an increased risk of glial brain tumor progression or malignant transformation and thus ultimately poorer overall survival (Table 41.1). A retrospective study at MDACC noted that of 18 patients with grade 2 or 3 gliomas prior to pregnancy, 8 (44%) had tumor progression during pregnancy or within 8 weeks following pregnancy [14]. Five patients in this study with grade 1 gliomas prior to pregnancy had stable disease during and following pregnancy [14]. A recent case series also reported three low-grade gliomas with progression and transformation in the setting of pregnancy to higher-grade tumors [70]. A Dutch study found that of seven women with low-grade gliomas prior to pregnancy, two (29%) had disease progression during the pregnancy [29]. The same study also reported that on literature review, 5 out of 20 patients (25%) with a known low-grade glioma prior to pregnancy had deterioration during pregnancy [29]. A retrospective review of all observed pregnancies in the adult female population of supratentorial hemispheric gliomas diagnosed by a French glioma study group between 1992 and 2007 identified 443 women of which 5 had a glioma diagnosis prior to a pregnancy [71]. Three (60%) of these patients were found to have worsening of their disease during the pregnancy [71]. Another retrospective French study found 52 pregnancies in 50 women diagnosed with a glioma of which 24 pregnancies, occurred in 22 women after glioma diagnosis [72]. This study reported that nine patients (37.5%) experienced clinical deterioration while pregnant. Additionally, quantitative imaging follow-up before and during pregnancy was available in 15 cases of which imaging progression determined by an increase in the velocity of diametric expansion (VDE) was observed during pregnancy in 13 cases (86.7%) [72]. An additional French retrospective study of 11 women with low-grade tumors known prior to pregnancy reported VDE was significantly increased during pregnancy as compared to prepregnancy and to postdelivery periods [73]. Furthermore, an

Table 41.1 Retrospective studies or case series of patients with gliomas prior to pregnancy

Name of study	Number of patients	Grade/histology	% of patients who progressed clinically or had tumor growth during pregnancy
Tumor progression and transformation of low-grade glial tumors associated with pregnancy [70]	3	2 low-grade astrocytoma, 1 low-grade oligodendroglioma	100%
Influence of pregnancy in the behavior of diffuse gliomas: clinical cases of a French glioma study group [51]	5	4 low-grade oligodendroglioma, 1 low-grade astrocytoma	60%
Management of malignant gliomas during pregnancy: a case series [38]	6	2 anaplastic astrocytoma, 1 anaplastic oligodendroglioma, 1 glioblastoma, 1 low-grade oligodendroglioma, 1 low-grade oligoastrocytoma	0%
Pregnancy in women with gliomas: a case series and review of the literature [29]	7 (case series), 28 (literature review)	3 astrocytoma, 1 pleomorphic xanthoastrocytoma, 1 oligoastrocytoma, 1 ependymoma, 1 anaplastic oligoastrocytoma (case series), 20 low grade and 8 high grade (literature review)	29% (case series), 21% (literature review)
Obstetric outcomes of women with intracranial neoplasms [74]	9 (gliomas) 13 (intracranial tumors)	5 astrocytic tumors, 2 oligodendrogliomas, 2 mixed gliomas, 2 meningiomas, 1 ependymoma, 1 acoustic neuroma	0% (gliomas), 23% (intracranial tumors)
Pregnancy increases the growth rates of World Health Organization grade II gliomas [73]	11	7 low-grade oligodendrogliomas, 2 low-grade mixed gliomas, and 1 low-grade astrocytoma	100% (imaging), 40% (clinical)
Interactions between glioma and pregnancy: insight from a 52 case multicenter series [72]	22 (24 pregnancies)	18 WHO grade II, 4 WHO grade III, and 2 WHO grade IV	37.5%
Pregnancy and glial brain tumors [38]	23	5 grade I, 9 grade II, 9 grade III	35%

increase in seizure frequency was noted in 40% of cases, and oncological treatment was commenced following delivery in 25% of cases [73].

In contrast to the studies described above, a recent population-based Norwegian study including patients from two large, prospectively maintained registries concluded that pregnancy does not seem to have an impact on the survival of female patients with LGG [63]. The study identified 346 women with low-grade gliomas from January 1, 1970, to December 31, 2008, of which 65 patients gave birth to children after tumor diagnosis [63]. The median survival was 14.3 years for the entire study population and found that the effect of pregnancy was insignificant in the multivariate model [63]. Additionally, a small case series of six patients reported uneventful pregnancies with no glioma-related complications [38]. A retrospective study of two major Canadian referral institutions for perinatal medicine and neurologic disorders in Ontario discovered 13 patients with intracranial neoplasms prior to pregnancy of which 3 patients (23%) had tumor growth or recurrence during pregnancy [74]. However, the recurrences were in patients with a meningioma, ependymoma, and acoustic neuroma with 0/9 glioma patients exhibiting tumor growth during pregnancy [74].

41.9 Delivery

The timing and type of delivery for the baby should be tailored to each individual patient depending on the neurologic status of the mother, age and development of the fetus, and suspected tumor histology/grade (based upon the history as well as most recent imaging characteristics) [30]. Whenever possible, delivery should be delayed at least until the fetus weighs 1 kg (corresponding to 26th–30th week of the gestational period) because after this period there is a 90% chance that the infant will be born healthy [30]. A recent retrospective Swedish study found that maternal cancer during pregnancy was associated with elevated risks of infrequent but deadly outcomes, including stillbirth and neonatal mortality [75]. These fatal outcomes were suspected to be related to situations associated with fetal growth restriction and iatrogenic preterm birth [75]. Vigilant observation of fetal growth and careful decision-making on preterm delivery are warranted.

A single course of steroids can be given in preterm pregnant patients to accelerate delivery by stimulating fetal lung development and help with cerebral edema if necessary [33]. The benefit/risk of repeated antenatal steroid courses is less clear with decreased birth weight, length, and head circumference in babies who had repeated courses of steroids noted in a randomized trial comparing mothers receiving either multiple or a single dose of corticosteroids [76, 77].

Patients with low-grade tumors that are neurologically stable without any evidence of increased intracranial pressure can be followed by close monitoring with periodic clinical exams and MR scans during pregnancy. As long as they remain without evidence of disease progression, delivery can be based upon obstetric criteria [78].

For pregnant patients with clinical or radiographic progression of the brain tumor, it remains uncertain the optimal management strategy. A prior management algorithm has suggested that patients with symptomatic tumors in the first and early second trimesters be allowed gestational advancement until the second trimester prior to neurosurgical intervention and subsequent radiation [6]. Regarding patients in the late second and third trimesters with symptomatic tumors, radiation was endorsed for a progressive neurological deficit. Additionally, if pregnant patients were at risk for cerebral herniation, then a cesarean section followed by a neurosurgical decompression under the same general anesthetic was recommended [6]. Others have recommended surgical intervention for all cases of suspected malignant glioma regardless of gestation period [49].

Pregnant patients with stable tumors may be able to deliver safely with vaginal or cesarean approaches (Table 41.2). However, in patients where there is a concern for potential increased intracranial pressure induced by a vaginal delivery, then a cesarean section is generally preferred.

41.10 Conclusion

Many of the decisions involving a pregnant patient with a glioma are very complex in nature and require individualized treatment plans tailored to that specific situation. It is imperative that these decisions be made in a multidisciplinary setting involving input from a large group of physicians including a neuro-oncologist, neurosurgeon, neuroradiologist, radiation oncologist, obstetrician/gynecologist, anesthesiologist, neonatologist, and medical ethicist in conjunction with the patient and her family members' wishes. Due to the relative rarity of this situation and inability to perform randomized prospective clinical trials in this patient population for ethical reasons, many questions still remain open to debate. Currently, there is no clear answer whether becoming pregnant increases the risk of tumor progression or effects overall survival in patients previously diagnosed with gliomas. It is therefore imperative that an international prospective registry be formed to improve our knowledge of the situation. Hopefully, a registry would better enable us to more accurately counsel our patients regarding the potential risks/benefits of the many difficult yet necessary decisions made in this intricate scenario.

Table 41.2 Delivery outcomes in retrospective studies or case series of pregnant patients with gliomas

Study	Number of patients with newly diagnosed glioma during pregnancy	Method of delivery–vaginal/C-sections	Deaths prior to or during delivery–fetal/maternal	Number of patients with previously diagnosed glioma in pregnancy	Method of delivery–vaginal/C-sections	Deaths prior to or during delivery–fetal/maternal
Primary brain tumors manifesting during pregnancy: presentation of six cases and a review of the literature [78]	2 (1 anaplastic astrocytoma, 1 pilocytic astrocytoma)	0/2	0/0	n/a	n/a	n/a
Brain tumor and pregnancy [7]	2 (2 astrocytoma)	1/0 (1-IUD)	1/0	n/a	n/a	n/a
Glioma in the third trimester of pregnancy: two cases and a review of the literature [79]	2 (anaplastic astrocytoma, anaplastic oligodendroglioma)	0/2	0/0	n/a	n/a	n/a
Influence of pregnancy in the behavior of diffuse gliomas: clinical cases of a French glioma study group [71]	3 (anaplastic astrocytoma, anaplastic oligodendroglioma, unknown)	2/1	0/0	5 (4 low-grade oligodendroglioma, 1 low-grade astrocytoma)	4/1	0/0
Management strategy for brain tumor diagnosed during pregnancy [30]	4 (3 low-grade astrocytoma, 1 low-grade oligodendroglioma)	0/4	0/0	n/a	n/a	n/a
Obstetric emergencies precipitated by malignant brain tumors [6]	6 (4 glioblastoma, 2 anaplastic astrocytoma)	0/6	0 / 2	1 (anaplastic astrocytoma)	0/1	1/ 1
Obstetric outcomes of women with intracranial neoplasms [74]	9 (5 astrocytic tumors, 2 oligodendroglioma, 2 mixed gliomas)	Unknown/unknown	Unknown/unknown	2 (glioblastoma, low-grade oligoastrocytoma)	2/0	0/0
Primary brain tumors, meningiomas, and brain metastases in pregnancy: report on 27 cases and review of literature [80]	14 (6 glioblastoma, 3 anaplastic astrocytoma, 2 low-grade astrocytoma)	4/8 1-TOP, 1-IUD)	2/1	2 (1 anaplastic astrocytoma, 1 low-grade astrocytoma)	0/1 (1-TOP)	1/0

(continued)

Table 41.2 (continued)

Study	Number of patients with newly diagnosed glioma during pregnancy	Method of delivery–vaginal/C-sections	Deaths prior to or during delivery–fetal/maternal	Number of patients with previously diagnosed glioma in pregnancy	Method of delivery–vaginal/C-sections	Deaths prior to or during delivery–fetal/maternal
Pregnancy and glial brain tumors [38]	15 (6 grade II, 6 grade III, 3 grade IV)	3/7 (2-TOP, 3- unknown)	2/0	18 (9 grade II, 9 grade III)	Unknown/unknown (5-TOP, 1-IUD)	6/0
Interactions between glioma and pregnancy: insight from a 52 case multicenter series [72]	28 (14 WHO grade II, 10 WHO grade III, and 4 WHO grade IV)	8/8 (1-TOP, 11-unknown)	1/0	22 (24 pregnancies) 18 WHO grade II, 4 WHO grade III, and 2 WHO grade IV	8/10 (1-TOP, 5-unknown)	1/0
Pregnancy in women with gliomas: a case series and review of the literature [29]	75 (literature review) 33 low grade and 42 high grade	20/38 (9-TOP, 8-IUD)	17/12	7 (case series), 28 (literature review) 3 astrocytoma, 1 pleomorphic xanthoastrocytoma, 1 oligoastrocytoma, 1 ependymoma, 1 anaplastic oligoastrocytoma (case series), 20 low grade and 8 high grade (literature review)	3/2 (2-TOP), 16/11, (1 unknown)	2/0
Tumor progression and transformation of low-grade glial tumors associated with pregnancy [70]	n/a	n/a	n/a	3 (2 low-grade astrocytoma, 1 low-grade oligodendroglioma)	1/1 (1-TOP)	1/0
Management of malignant gliomas during pregnancy: a case series [38]	n/a	n/a	n/a	6 (2 anaplastic astrocytoma, 1 anaplastic oligodendroglioma, 1 glioblastoma, 1 low-grade oligodendroglioma, 1 low-grade oligoastrocytoma)	4/2	0/0
The effect of pregnancy on survival in a low-grade glioma cohort [63]	n/a	n/a	n/a	65 (95 births) (37 low-grade astrocytoma, 12 pilocytic astrocytoma, 11 low-grade oligodendroglioma, 5 low-grade oligoastrocytoma)	64/30	1/0

Abbreviations: *IUD* intrauterine demise, *TOP* termination of pregnancy

References

1. Ostrom QT, Gittleman H, Xu J et al (2016) CBTRUS statistical report: primary brain and central nervous system tumors diagnosed in the United States in 2009-2013. Neuro-Oncology 18(s5):iv1–iv76

2. Jemal A, Siegel R, Ward E, Hao Y, Xu J, Thun MJ (2009) Cancer statistics, 2009. CA Cancer J Clin 59(4):225–249. https://doi.org/10.3322/caac.20006

3. Haas JF, Janisch W, Staneczek W (1986) Newly diagnosed primary intracranial neoplasms in pregnant women: a population-based assessment. J Neurol Neurosurg Psychiatry 49(8):874–880

4. Simon RH (1988) Brain tumors in pregnancy. Semin Neurol 8(3):214–221. https://doi.org/10.1055/s-2008-1041380

5. Roelvink NC, Kamphorst W, van Alphen HA, Rao BR (1987) Pregnancy-related primary brain and spinal tumors. Arch Neurol 44(2):209–215

6. Tewari KS, Cappuccini F, Asrat T, Flamm BL, Carpenter SE, Disaia PJ et al (2000) Obstetric emergencies precipitated by malignant brain tumors. Am J Obstet Gynecol 182(5):1215–1221

7. Isla A, Alvarez F, Gonzalez A, Garcia-Grande A, Perez-Alvarez M, Garcia-Blazquez M (1997) Brain tumor and pregnancy. Obstet Gynecol 89(1):19–23

8. DeAngelis LM (1994) Central nervous system neoplasms in pregnancy. Adv Neurol 64:139–152

9. Wahab M, Al-Azzawi F (2003) Meningioma and hormonal influences. Climacteric 6(4):285–292

10. de Groot JF, Mandel JJ (2014) Update on antiangiogenic treatment for malignant gliomas. Curr Oncol Rep 16(4):380. https://doi.org/10.1007/s11912-014-0380-6

11. McNamara MG, Mason WP (2012) Antiangiogenic therapies in glioblastoma multiforme. Expert Rev Anticancer Ther 12(5):643–654. https://doi.org/10.1586/era.12.35

12. Stevenson CB, Thompson RC (2005) The clinical management of intracranial neoplasms in pregnancy. Clin Obstet Gynecol 48(1):24–37

13. Terry AR, Barker FG II, Leffert L, Bateman BT, Souter I, Plotkin SR (2012) Outcomes of hospitalization in pregnant women with CNS neoplasms: a population-based study. Neuro-Oncology 14(6):768–776. https://doi.org/10.1093/neuonc/nos078

14. Yust-Katz S, de Groot JF, Liu D, Wu J, Yuan Y, Anderson MD et al (2014) Pregnancy and glial brain tumors. Neuro-Oncology 16(9):1289–1294. https://doi.org/10.1093/neuonc/nou019

15. Aegidius K, Zwart JA, Hagen K, Stovner L (2009) The effect of pregnancy and parity on headache prevalence: the head-HUNT study. Headache 49(6):851–859. https://doi.org/10.1111/j.1526-4610.2009.01438.x

16. Maggioni FAC, Maggino T et al (1997) Headache during pregnancy. Cephalalgia 17:765–769

17. Robbins MS, Farmakidis C, Dayal AK, Lipton RB (2015) Acute headache diagnosis in pregnant women: a hospital-based study. Neurology 85(12):1024–1030. https://doi.org/10.1212/wnl.0000000000001954

18. Goldszmidt E, Kern R, Chaput A, Macarthur A (2005) The incidence and etiology of postpartum headaches: a prospective cohort study. Can J Anaesth 52(9):971–977. https://doi.org/10.1007/bf03022061

19. Chang SM, Parney IF, Huang W, Anderson FA Jr, Asher AL, Bernstein M et al (2005) Patterns of care for adults with newly diagnosed malignant glioma. JAMA 293(5):557–564. https://doi.org/10.1001/jama.293.5.557

20. Sibai BM (2004) Magnesium sulfate prophylaxis in preeclampsia: lessons learned from recent trials. Am J Obstet Gynecol 190(6):1520–1526. https://doi.org/10.1016/j.ajog.2003.12.057

21. Edlow JA, Caplan LR, O'Brien K, Tibbles CD (2013) Diagnosis of acute neurological emergencies in pregnant and post-partum women. Lancet Neurol 12(2):175–185. https://doi.org/10.1016/s1474-4422(12)70306-x

22. Brent RL (2009) Saving lives and changing family histories: appropriate counseling of pregnant women and men and women of reproductive age, concerning the risk of diagnostic radiation exposures during and before pregnancy. Am J Obstet Gynecol 200(1):4–24. https://doi.org/10.1016/j.ajog.2008.06.032

23. Bove RM, Klein JP (2014) Neuroradiology in women of childbearing age. Continuum (Minneapolis, Minn) 20(1 Neurology of Pregnancy):23–41. https://doi.org/10.1212/01.CON.0000443835.10508.2b

24. Kanal E, Shellock FG, Talagala L (1990) Safety considerations in MR imaging. Radiology 176(3):593–606. https://doi.org/10.1148/radiology.176.3.2202008

25. Nelson JA, Livingston GK, Moon RG (1982) Mutagenic evaluation of radiographic contrast media. Investig Radiol 17(2):183–185

26. Malayeri AA, Brooks KM, Bryant LH, Evers R, Kumar P, Reich DS et al (2016) National Institutes of Health perspective on reports of gadolinium deposition in the brain. J Am Coll Radiol 13(3):237–241. https://doi.org/10.1016/j.jacr.2015.11.009

27. Ray JG, Vermeulen MJ, Bharatha A, Montanera WJ, Park AL (2016) Association between MRI exposure during pregnancy and fetal and childhood outcomes. JAMA 316(9):952–961. https://doi.org/10.1001/jama.2016.12126

28. Symons SP, Heyn C, Maralani PJ (2016) Magnetic resonance imaging exposure during pregnancy. JAMA 316(21):2275. https://doi.org/10.1001/jama.2016.17296

29. Zwinkels H, Dorr J, Kloet F, Taphoorn MJ, Vecht CJ (2013) Pregnancy in women with gliomas: a case-series and review of the literature. J Neuro-Oncol 115(2):293–301. https://doi.org/10.1007/s11060-013-1229-9

30. Lynch JC, Gouvea F, Emmerich JC, Kokinovrachos G, Pereira C, Welling L et al (2011) Management strategy for brain tumour diagnosed during pregnancy. Br J Neurosurg 25(2):225–230. https://doi.org/10.3109/02688697.2010.508846

31. Ducray F, Colin P, Cartalat-Carel S, Pelissou-Guyotat I, Mahla K, Audra P et al (2006) Management of malignant gliomas diagnosed during pregnancy. Rev Neurol 162(3):322–329

32. Cohen-Kerem R, Railton C, Oren D, Lishner M, Koren G (2005) Pregnancy outcome following non-obstetric surgical intervention. Am J Surg 190(3):467–473. https://doi.org/10.1016/j.amjsurg.2005.03.033

33. Jayasekera BA, Bacon AD, Whitfield PC (2012) Management of glioblastoma multiforme in pregnancy. J Neurosurg 116(6):1187–1194. https://doi.org/10.3171/2012.2.jns112077

34. Kal HB, Struikmans H (2005) Radiotherapy during pregnancy: fact and fiction. Lancet Oncol 6(5):328–333. https://doi.org/10.1016/s1470-2045(05)70169-8

35. Doll R, Wakeford R (1997) Risk of childhood cancer from fetal irradiation. Br J Radiol 70:130–139. https://doi.org/10.1259/bjr.70.830.9135438

36. Sneed PK, Albright NW, Wara WM, Prados MD, Wilson CB (1995) Fetal dose estimates for radiotherapy of brain tumors during pregnancy. Int J Radiat Oncol Biol Phys 32(3):823–830. https://doi.org/10.1016/0360-3016(94)00456-u

37. Horowitz DP, Wang TJ, Wuu CS, Feng W, Drassinower D, Lasala A et al (2014) Fetal radiation monitoring and dose minimization during intensity modulated radiation therapy for glioblastoma in pregnancy. J Neuro-Oncol 120(2):405–409. https://doi.org/10.1007/s11060-014-1565-4

38. Blumenthal DT, Parreno MG, Batten J, Chamberlain MC (2008) Management of malignant gliomas during pregnancy: a case series. Cancer 113(12):3349–3354. https://doi.org/10.1002/cncr.23973

39. Pavlidis NA (2002) Coexistence of pregnancy and malignancy. Oncologist 7(4):279–287

40. Azim HA Jr, Peccatori FA, Pavlidis N (2010) Treatment of the pregnant mother with cancer: a systematic review on the use of cytotoxic, endocrine, targeted agents and immunotherapy during pregnancy. Part I: solid tumors. Cancer Treat Rev 36(2):101–109. https://doi.org/10.1016/j.ctrv.2009.11.007

41. Zagouri F, Dimitrakakis C, Marinopoulos S, Tsigginou A, Dimopoulos MA (2016) Cancer in pregnancy: disentangling treatment modalities. ESMO Open 1(3):e000016. https://doi.org/10.1136/esmoopen-2015-000016

42. Pentheroudakis G (2008) Cancer and pregnancy. Ann Oncol 19(Suppl 5):v38–v39. https://doi.org/10.1093/annonc/mdn307

43. Stupp R, Mason WP, van den Bent MJ, Weller M, Fisher B, Taphoorn MJ et al (2005) Radiotherapy plus concomitant and adjuvant temozolomide for glioblastoma. N Engl J Med 352(10):987–996. https://doi.org/10.1056/NEJMoa043330

44. Buckner JC, Shaw EG, Pugh SL, Chakravarti A, Gilbert MR, Barger GR et al (2016) Radiation plus procarbazine, CCNU, and vincristine in low-grade glioma. N Engl J Med 374(14):1344–1355. https://doi.org/10.1056/NEJMoa1500925

45. Buckner JC, Chakravarti A, Curran WJ Jr (2016) Radiation plus chemotherapy in low-grade glioma. N Engl J Med 375(5):490–491. https://doi.org/10.1056/NEJMc1605897

46. Cairncross G, Wang M, Shaw E, Jenkins R, Brachman D, Buckner J et al (2013) Phase III trial of chemoradiotherapy for anaplastic oligodendroglioma: long-term results of RTOG 9402. J Clin Oncol 31(3):337–343. https://doi.org/10.1200/jco.2012.43.2674

47. van den Bent MJ, Brandes AA, Taphoorn MJ, Kros JM, Kouwenhoven MC, Delattre JY et al (2013) Adjuvant procarbazine, lomustine, and vincristine chemotherapy in newly diagnosed anaplastic oligodendroglioma: long-term follow-up of EORTC brain tumor group study 26951. J Clin Oncol 31(3):344–350. https://doi.org/10.1200/jco.2012.43.2229

48. Voulgaris E, Pentheroudakis G, Pavlidis N (2011) Cancer and pregnancy: a comprehensive review. Surg Oncol 20(4):e175–e185. https://doi.org/10.1016/j.suronc.2011.06.002

49. McGrane J, Bedford T, Kelly S (2012) Successful pregnancy and delivery after concomitant temozolomide and radiotherapy treatment of glioblastoma multiforme. Clin Oncol 24(4):311. https://doi.org/10.1016/j.clon.2012.01.005

50. Kunwar S, Chang S, Westphal M, Vogelbaum M, Sampson J, Barnett G et al (2010) Phase III randomized trial of CED of IL13-PE38QQR vs Gliadel wafers for recurrent glioblastoma. Neuro-Oncology 12(8):871–881. https://doi.org/10.1093/neuonc/nop054

51. Valtonen S, Timonen U, Toivanen P, Kalimo H, Kivipelto L, Heiskanen O et al (1997) Interstitial chemotherapy with carmustine-loaded polymers for high-grade gliomas: a randomized double-blind study. Neurosurgery 41(1):44–48; discussion 8–9

52. Westphal M, Hilt DC, Bortey E, Delavault P, Olivares R, Warnke PC et al (2003) A phase 3 trial of local chemotherapy with biodegradable carmustine (BCNU) wafers (Gliadel wafers) in patients with primary malignant glioma. Neuro-Oncology 5(2):79–88. https://doi.org/10.1215/s1522-8517-02-00023-6

53. Cohen MH, Shen YL, Keegan P, Pazdur R (2009) FDA drug approval summary: bevacizumab (Avastin) as treatment of recurrent glioblastoma multiforme. Oncologist 14(11):1131–1138. https://doi.org/10.1634/theoncologist.2009-0121

54. Friedman HS, Prados MD, Wen PY, Mikkelsen T, Schiff D, Abrey LE et al (2009) Bevacizumab alone and in combination with irinotecan in recurrent glioblastoma. J Clin Oncol 27(28):4733–4740. https://doi.org/10.1200/jco.2008.19.8721

55. Kreisl TN, Kim L, Moore K, Duic P, Royce C, Stroud I et al (2009) Phase II trial of single-agent bevacizumab followed by bevacizumab plus irinotecan at tumor progression in recurrent glioblastoma. J Clin Oncol 27(5):740–745. https://doi.org/10.1200/jco.2008.16.3055

56. Kaygusuz I, Eser A, Inegol Gumus I, Kosus A, Yenidunya S, Namuslu M et al (2014) Effect of

anti-vascular endothelial growth factor antibody during early fetal development in rats. J Matern Fetal Nneonatal Med 27(17):1744–1748. https://doi.org/10.3109/14767058.2013.879645

57. Kianersi F, Ghanbari H, Naderi Beni Z, Naderi BA (2016) Intravitreal vascular endothelial growth factor (VEGF) inhibitor injection in unrecognised early pregnancy. Investig New Drugs 34(5):650–653. https://doi.org/10.1007/s10637-016-0361-8

58. Tarantola RM, Folk JC, Boldt HC, Mahajan VB (2010) Intravitreal bevacizumab during pregnancy. Retina (Philadelphia, Pa) 30(9):1405–1411. https://doi.org/10.1097/IAE.0b013e3181f57d58

59. Sullivan L, Kelly SP, Glenn A, Williams CP, McKibbin M (2014) Intravitreal bevacizumab injection in unrecognised early pregnancy. Eye (London, England) 28(4):492–494. https://doi.org/10.1038/eye.2013.311

60. Lambertini M, Peccatori FA, Azim HA Jr (2015) Targeted agents for cancer treatment during pregnancy. Cancer Treat Rev 41(4):301–309. https://doi.org/10.1016/j.ctrv.2015.03.001

61. van Breemen MS, Wilms EB, Vecht CJ (2007) Epilepsy in patients with brain tumours: epidemiology, mechanisms, and management. Lancet Neurol 6(5):421–430. https://doi.org/10.1016/s1474-4422(07)70103-5

62. Smith KC (2010) The management of seizures in brain tumor patients. J Neurosci Nurs 42(1):28–37; quiz 8–9

63. Ronning PA, Helseth E, Meling TR, Johannesen TB (2016) The effect of pregnancy on survival in a low-grade glioma cohort. J Neurosurg 125(2):393–400. https://doi.org/10.3171/2015.6.jns15985

64. Barker CA, Bishop AJ, Chang M, Beal K, Chan TA (2013) Valproic acid use during radiation therapy for glioblastoma associated with improved survival. Int J Radiat Oncol Biol Phys 86(3):504–509. https://doi.org/10.1016/j.ijrobp.2013.02.012

65. Happold C, Gorlia T, Chinot O, Gilbert MR, Nabors LB, Wick W et al (2016) Does valproic acid or levetiracetam improve survival in glioblastoma? A pooled analysis of prospective clinical trials in newly diagnosed glioblastoma. J Clin Oncol 34(7):731–739. https://doi.org/10.1200/jco.2015.63.6563

66. Kerkhof M, Dielemans JC, van Breemen MS, Zwinkels H, Walchenbach R, Taphoorn MJ et al (2013) Effect of valproic acid on seizure control and on survival in patients with glioblastoma multiforme. Neuro-Oncology 15(7):961–967. https://doi.org/10.1093/neuonc/not057

67. Borgelt LM, Hart FM, Bainbridge JL (2016) Epilepsy during pregnancy: focus on management strategies. Int J Women's Health 8:505–517. https://doi.org/10.2147/ijwh.s98973

68. Glantz MJ, Cole BF, Forsyth PA, Recht LD, Wen PY, Chamberlain MC et al (2000) Practice parameter: anticonvulsant prophylaxis in patients with newly diagnosed brain tumors. Report of the quality standards Subcommittee of the American Academy of neurology. Neurology 54(10):1886–1893

69. Sirven JI, Wingerchuk DM, Drazkowski JF, Lyons MK, Zimmerman RS (2004) Seizure prophylaxis in patients with brain tumors: a meta-analysis. Mayo Clin Proc 79(12):1489–1494. https://doi.org/10.4065/79.12.1489

70. Daras M, Cone C, Peters KB (2014) Tumor progression and transformation of low-grade glial tumors associated with pregnancy. J Neuro-Oncol 116(1):113–117. https://doi.org/10.1007/s11060-013-1261-9

71. Pallud J, Duffau H, Razak RA, Barbarino-Monnier P, Capelle L, Fontaine D et al (2009) Influence of pregnancy in the behavior of diffuse gliomas: clinical cases of a French glioma study group. J Neurol 256(12):2014–2020. https://doi.org/10.1007/s00415-009-5232-1

72. Peeters S, Pages M, Gauchotte G, Miquel C, Cartalat-Carel S, Guillamo JS et al (2018) Interactions between glioma and pregnancy: insight from a 52-case multicenter series. J Neurosurg 128(1):3–13. https://doi.org/10.3171/2016.10.jns16710

73. Pallud J, Mandonnet E, Deroulers C, Fontaine D, Badoual M, Capelle L et al (2010) Pregnancy increases the growth rates of World Health Organization grade II gliomas. Ann Neurol 67(3):398–404. https://doi.org/10.1002/ana.21888

74. Johnson N, Sermer M, Lausman A, Maxwell C (2009) Obstetric outcomes of women with intracranial neoplasms. Int J Gynaecol Obstet 105(1):56–59. https://doi.org/10.1016/j.ijgo.2008.11.037

75. Lu D, Ludvigsson JF, Smedby KE, Fall K, Valdimarsdottir U, Cnattingius S et al (2017) Maternal cancer during pregnancy and risks of stillbirth and infant mortality. J Clin Oncol 35(14):1522–1529. https://doi.org/10.1200/jco.2016.69.9439

76. Newnham JP, Jobe AH (2009) Should we be prescribing repeated courses of antenatal corticosteroids? Semin Fetal Neonatal Med 14(3):157–163. https://doi.org/10.1016/j.siny.2008.11.005

77. Murphy KE, Hannah ME, Willan AR, Hewson SA, Ohlsson A, Kelly EN et al (2008) Multiple courses of antenatal corticosteroids for preterm birth (MACS): a randomised controlled trial. Lancet (London, England) 372(9656):2143–2151. https://doi.org/10.1016/s0140-6736(08)61929-7

78. Nishio S, Morioka T, Suzuki S, Takeshita I, Ikezaki K, Fukui M et al (1996) Primary brain tumours manifesting during pregnancy: presentation of six cases and a review of the literature. J Clin Neurosci 3(4):334–337

79. Wu J, Ma YH, Wang TL (2013) Glioma in the third trimester of pregnancy: two cases and a review of the literature. Oncol Lett 5(3):943–946. https://doi.org/10.3892/ol.2013.1106

80. Verheecke M, Halaska MJ, Lok CA, Ottevanger PB, Fruscio R, Dahl-Steffensen K et al (2014) Primary brain tumours, meningiomas and brain metastases in pregnancy: report on 27 cases and review of literature. Eur J Cancer (Oxford, England: 1990) 50(8):1462–1471. https://doi.org/10.1016/j.ejca.2014.02.018

Delayed Neurologic Complications of Brain Tumor Therapy

42

Jörg Dietrich, Sebastian F. Winter, and Michael W. Parsons

42.1 Introduction

Delayed neurotoxic complications from radiation and chemotherapy are a major challenge in the management of brain tumor patients. Long-term survivors are especially affected, such as patients successfully treated for childhood brain tumors or adult brain cancer patients who outlive their disease for several years. Classic delayed treatment complications evident by neuroimaging include progressive brain atrophy, white matter disease (leukoencephalopathy), tissue necrosis, neurovascular complications, and secondary tumors.

Delayed complications can cause significant *functional* impairment, including cognitive decline, loss of motor function and coordination, visual impairment, and autonomic dysfunction.

It is important to note that *structural* brain changes detected on neuroimaging do not always correlate in extent and severity with the degree of functional impairment observed. For example, some patients may show clinical decline with progressive dementia even in the absence of any significant imaging abnormalities.

With improved efficacy of multimodal therapies for both primary and secondary brain tumors and longer patient survival, delayed treatment complications have been increasingly recognized. Moreover, the use of novel treatment approaches, such as targeted therapies, anti-angiogenic treatment, and immunotherapies, has been associated with a range of unique adverse events, and their long-term effects on patients remain largely unknown.

The present chapter will provide a review of well-known delayed neurological complications encountered in brain tumor patients following cranial irradiation and chemotherapy. Potential mechanisms of nervous system injury will be discussed and available treatment options highlighted.

J. Dietrich (✉) · M. W. Parsons
Department of Neurology, Center for Neuro-Oncology, Massachusetts General Hospital Cancer Center, Harvard Medical School, Boston, MA, USA
e-mail: Dietrich.Jorg@mgh.harvard.edu;
MWParsons@mgh.harvard.edu

S. F. Winter
Department of Neurosurgery, Charité – Universitätsmedizin Berlin, Corporate Member of Freie Universität Berlin, Humboldt-Universität zu Berlin and Berlin Institute of Health,
Berlin, Germany
e-mail: sebastian-friedrich.winter@charite.de

42.2 Cognitive Impairment

Neurocognitive function is frequently impaired in patients treated for brain cancer and has been shown to be a poor prognostic factor in malignant glioma [1]. The etiology and specific cause of cognitive dysfunction is usually difficult to ascertain in an individual patient. Numerous factors

© Springer Nature Switzerland AG 2019
J.-C. Tonn et al. (eds.), *Oncology of CNS Tumors*, https://doi.org/10.1007/978-3-030-04152-6_42

are known to contribute to cognitive impairment, such as the type of cancer-directed therapy (e.g., chemotherapy, radiation therapy, or biologic agents). Many other factors can contribute and exacerbate cancer therapy-induced cognitive deficits, such as medications (e.g., pain medications, long-term use of antiepileptic drugs and corticosteroids), genetic predispositions, comorbidities (e.g., anemia, renal insufficiency, or liver disease), pre-existing neurological deficits, mood alterations, and fatigue. Moreover, as further discussed below, the tumor itself may play a significant role in symptom presentation depending on tumor location and histology [2, 3].

Specific neurocognitive deficits may result in varying degrees of disability and impaired quality of life and the patient's ability to perform social and professional activities.

It should be noted that neurocognitive deficits can be detected even *prior to* tumor-directed therapies in some brain tumor patients [4, 5], and symptom manifestation may depend on the location, size, and biology of the underlying tumor [4, 6–8]. Cognitive dysfunction has been identified in up to 90% of patients with frontal or temporal gliomas prior to cancer therapy with measurable impairment of memory and attention in 60% and reduced executive function in up to 80% of patients [9]. Tumor-associated complications, such as cerebral edema, seizures, and associated use of edema- and seizure-controlling medications, are also known to influence neurocognitive function [10–14].

42.2.1 Radiation Therapy-Induced Cognitive Dysfunction

Radiation therapy is well known to cause cognitive decline both in children and adults treated for brain tumors [15–26]. The current literature suggests a prevalence of cognitive dysfunction in up to 85% of patients treated with cranial radiation therapy [27], though a wide range of reported frequencies is likely explained by variability in cognitive assessment methods, differences in patient populations, and treatment variables.

While the effects on cognitive function are perhaps most profound after whole brain radiation therapy (WBRT) [28], emerging data suggests that focal radiation therapy can also cause global structural brain changes with brain atrophy and cognitive decline with functional morbidity in a subset of patients [29, 30].

Radiation-induced cognitive decline is usually slowly progressive. Therefore, long-term survivors are at particular risk, such as children treated with prophylactic cranial radiation for childhood leukemia [31]. A number of risk factors are associated with radiation-induced neurotoxicity, such as young *and* old age (neurotoxic complications from cranial irradiation are more likely to occur at <5 years and >60 years of age), cumulative radiation dose, total volume of brain irradiated, a shorter overall treatment time, fractionation dose of >2 Gy, hyperfractionation treatment schedules, pre-existing cerebrovascular risk factors [17, 27, 32, 33], and genetic factors [34–36]. Concurrent (or sequential) chemotherapy is also known to increase the severity of radiation-induced toxicity [17]. For instance, patients treated with WBRT and chemotherapy for primary central nervous system lymphoma are at particularly high risk for cognitive impairment, brain volume loss, and leukoencephalopathy [37].

Radiation-associated neurotoxicity has generally been categorized in acute, early-delayed, and late-delayed side effects [27, 38], though a clear distinction between these phases cannot always be made in clinical practice.

Acute adverse effects from cranial irradiation occur within days to weeks of therapy. Symptoms are characterized by encephalopathy, fatigue, and worsening of pre-existing deficits and are mostly reversible with supportive management. It has been suggested that inflammation, neurovascular toxicity, blood-brain barrier disruption, and cerebral edema are the main mechanisms driving such acute adverse effects [39, 40].

Early-delayed radiation-associated adverse side effects occur within weeks to months and are characterized by fatigue and cognitive deficits, such as poor attention, short-term memory impairment, delayed processing speed, impaired word and memory retrieval, executive dysfunction, and impaired fine motor dexterity [17, 41–43]. Radiation-induced transient demyelination may be one of the main causes of early-delayed neurotoxic symptoms [44].

Perhaps most concerning are the late-delayed adverse effects from cranial irradiation, which typically develop months to years after treatment and are considered irreversible and often progressive. Symptoms include mild to moderate cognitive impairment and deficits in memory, attention, concentration, and executive function [45]. Although symptom severity does not correlate with abnormalities on cranial imaging [46], focal necrosis, leukoencephalopathy, and global brain atrophy can be evident on neuroimaging studies in severe cases [15, 37, 47–52].

Given the negative neurotoxic effects of large volume cranial irradiation, such as after WBRT, ongoing discussions have addressed the use of focal or stereotactic radiation versus WBRT [53–55]. With comparable survival data with either modality, the use of stereotactic radiation has been favored in patients with limited number of cerebral metastases [55–57].

Potential mechanisms of late-delayed radiation-induced neurologic complications include chronic inflammatory changes, toxic effects on neurovascular cells and the blood-brain barrier, and damage to various neural cell types [58–62]. Impairment of adult hippocampal neurogenesis is considered one of the key mechanisms to drive cognitive decline after cranial irradiation [62]. Consequently, increasing efforts have recently been made to minimize the negative impact of radiation on the hippocampus, and early studies suggest that conformal avoidance of the hippocampus during WBRT in patients with brain metastases may preserve cognitive function [63].

Besides efforts to avoid or delay radiation therapy and to spare eloquent brain areas from radiation exposure, various pharmacological interventions have been explored in clinical trials as therapeutic options for cognitive function in patients treated with cranial irradiation [64]. While treatment of memory impairment and other cognitive deficits has remained challeng-

ing, potential strategies include use of neurostimulants (e.g., methylphenidate, modafinil), acetylcholinesterase inhibitors, and other agents used in dementia patients (donepezil, memantine, gingko biloba) [65–72]. Recent preclinical studies suggest that bone marrow support with granulocyte colony-stimulating factor (G-CSF) may be a promising intervention to improve cognitive function and white matter integrity following radiation injury [73]. Non-pharmacological treatment strategies have also demonstrated benefit in management of cognitive dysfunction following cranial irradiation, including cognitive rehabilitation, exercise, and meditation [74–78].

42.2.2 Chemotherapy-Induced Cognitive Dysfunction

Most brain cancer patients are treated with a combination of cranial radiation therapy and chemotherapy. In clinical practice, it is therefore difficult to separate radiation effects from chemotherapy-induced effects on cognitive function.

There is mounting evidence that chemotherapy alone can result in cognitive impairment with negative effects on quality of life in cancer patients. Chemotherapy-associated cognitive impairment has been most convincingly demonstrated in patients treated for noncentral nervous system malignancies. The incidence of chemotherapy-associated cognitive dysfunction is reported in up to 90% of patients [79–83], though a wide range of incidences is reported, depending on study design, patient population, and methods of evaluation. The most frequently identified neurocognitive deficits in pediatric and adult cancer patients include impaired attention, concentration, learning, memory, information-processing speed, and executive function [15, 24, 25, 27, 80, 81, 84–95].

The impact of chemotherapy on cognition has been most extensively studied in breast cancer patients, revealing cognitive deficits after treatment in approximately 20–40% of patients [81, 95–104]. While symptoms may be transient, persistent deficits can be seen in 30–60% of those affected 1–2 years after treatment with high-dose chemotherapy [87, 104, 105]. In one of the largest long-term studies of nearly 200 breast cancer survivors, neurocognitive impairment was notable more than 20 years after initial treatment in the domains of verbal memory, processing speed, executive functioning, and psychomotor speed [106].

Neurotoxic adverse effects have been observed with virtually all categories of chemotherapeutic drugs, including alkylating agents, antimetabolites, mitotic inhibitors, anti-hormonal agents, anti-angiogenic drugs, and molecular-targeted therapies [107].

Potential mechanisms of chemotherapy-induced central nervous system toxicity include damage to neural progenitor cells, vascular injury, pro-oxidative changes, and inflammation [62, 107–113].

The etiology of cognitive dysfunction in cancer patient is usually multifactorial. It is therefore challenging to define the exact impact of chemotherapy alone on cognitive function.

Various risk factors for chemotherapy-induced neurotoxicity have been identified and include type and dose of chemotherapy, mode of administration (intravenous, intrathecal, intra-arterial), and concurrent or sequential radiation therapy. The manifestation of cognitive deficits is further influenced by patient age, genetic susceptibility, presence of metabolic dysfunction and hormonal imbalance, comorbidities, and the level of cognitive function prior to treatment [7, 27, 114–124].

Assessment of neurocognitive function in cancer patients requires reliable, quantifiable, and valid measures sensitive to cognitive domains. Longitudinal assessment has been considered most useful to monitor overall outcomes. There are accepted guidelines regarding the most appropriate selection of neuropsychological test batteries to measure cognitive function in cancer patients [95, 125–127]. Specific guidelines for the inclusion of neuropsychological outcomes in clinical studies have been published by the International Cognition and Cancer Task Force to provide relevant information regarding treatment outcomes [128].

Unfortunately, there are currently no standard treatment interventions for patients affected by chemotherapy-induced cognitive impairment. While some agents have shown promising results in initial studies, larger prospective and randomized clinical trials to demonstrate conclusive evidence for the usefulness of a specific treatment intervention are mostly lacking. Neurostimulants, such as methylphenidate and modafinil, and the reversible acetylcholinesterase inhibitor donepezil have shown some benefit [65, 68, 129–138]. In addition, cognitive and behavioral therapy [139, 140] and other non-pharmacological interventions such as meditation [141] and exercise [137, 142, 143] have been used in management of chemotherapy-associated cognitive impairment.

42.3   Leukoencephalopathy

White matter disease, or damage to myelinated fiber tracts, is one of the most common manifestations of delayed toxicity from cranial irradiation but can also be seen in patients treated with chemotherapy alone [52, 144]. Consequently, the combined use of radiation and chemotherapy appears to be associated with a higher risk of delayed white matter injury [30]. Leukoencephalopathy is usually of delayed onset and can be progressive [27], creating a major challenge to the management of long-term survivors.

The exact incidence of leukoencephalopathy in brain cancer patients is unknown. The literature suggests an incidence of approximately 30% in patients undergoing radiation therapy alone, but higher rates may be seen in patients receiving concurrent chemotherapy, or a combination of WBRT and stereotactic radiosurgery for treatment of metastatic disease [37, 47, 145].

White matter changes can be detected on magnetic resonance imaging (MRI) in nearly all patients who were treated with radiation doses of more than 20 Gy and who survive more than 1 year [56]. The risk of radiation therapy-induced leukoencephalopathy has been well recognized in long-time survivors treated for CNS metastatic disease [15]. In the study by DeAngelis et al., patients were treated for cerebral metastasis with WBRT and developed white matter disease after 5–36 months [15]. Imaging findings were associated with nonspecific symptoms including dizziness, fatigue, and headache, followed by memory impairment, gait difficulties, recurrent falls, and ultimately severe dementia. Urinary incontinence was found in half of the patients [15]. Other symptoms reported to be associated with radiation-induced leukoencephalopathy include personality changes, neuropsychiatric abnormalities, tremors, seizures, and secondary Parkinsonism [37, 56, 145–147].

Leukoencephalopathy appears on MRI as T2-weighted hyperintensity within the subcortical, periventricular, and deep white matter (Fig. 42.1). Early imaging changes may reveal T2-weighted hyperintensities restricted to the

frontal and occipital horns of the lateral ventricles before more confluent and patchy white matter changes evolve. In severe cases, white matter changes demonstrate scattered foci of contrast enhancement consistent with tissue necrosis. Patients with pre-existing white matter changes at the time of treatment are more likely to develop progressive white matter changes on MRI than patients without white matter changes at the time of treatment [148]. Moreover, it has been suggested that a pre-existing demyelinating disease, such as multiple sclerosis, may render a patient more vulnerable to radiation-induced neurotoxicity [149].

Histopathological correlates of radiographic white matter changes reveal demyelination, loss of blood-brain barrier integrity, increase in capillary permeability, vasogenic edema, spongiform vacuoles, and gliosis [15, 47, 150]. Necrotizing leukoencephalopathy can occur in severe cases [146].

White matter disease is frequently associated with some degree of brain atrophy and can be seen after both focal and WBRT [15, 30, 151]. Leukoencephalopathy can further be associated with progressive communicating hydrocephalus, characterized by an enlargement of the ventricular system out of proportion to cerebral atrophy, with evidence of increased periventricular edema secondary to trans-ependymal flow [147]. Clinically, hydrocephalus associated with chemoradiation-induced leukoencephalopathy appears to have overlapping features with the cardinal symptoms of *normal pressure hydrocephalus* – cognitive impairment, gait difficulties, and incontinence [37, 52, 56, 145–147, 152, 153].

In line with this observation, placement of a ventriculoperitoneal shunt (VPS) has been shown to improve symptoms in a subset of patients [145, 154]. Gait difficulties and incontinence are more likely to improve after shunting than cognitive deficits [15, 147].

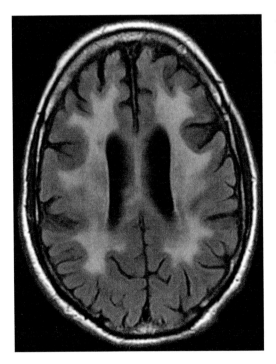

Fig. 42.1 Chemotherapy-induced leukoencephalopathy. Axial T2-FLAIR (fluid attenuation inversion recovery) image from an 80-year-old male treated for primary CNS lymphoma with eight cycles of high-dose methotrexate and rituximab and considered in complete remission. The MRI demonstrates diffuse subcortical and confluent white matter signal change in both hemispheres

42.4 Brain Atrophy

Progressive brain volume loss is considered a classic manifestation of radiation injury [155–159] (Fig. 42.2). While cerebral atrophy has

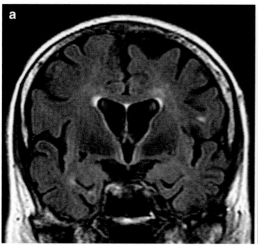
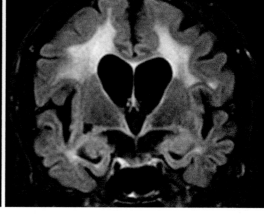

Fig. 42.2 Radiation-induced brain atrophy and leukoencephalopathy. A 71-year-old male presents with cognitive impairment and gait difficulties and recurrent falls 3 years after prophylactic whole brain radiation therapy for a neu- roendocrine tumor. (**a**) Coronal T2-FLAIR images at the time of radiation therapy and (**b**) at the time of onset of neurologic symptoms, demonstrating brain atrophy and dif- fuse subcortical and periventricular leukoencephalopathy

previously been recognized as a *late effect* of radi- ation-induced injury [58], more recent studies in patients treated for malignant glioma demonstrate *early-onset* and progressive global brain atrophy following standard involved field radiation ther- apy in combination with temozolomide [30] and after standard chemoradiation in combination with upfront anti-angiogenic therapy [160]. In severe cases, ventricular volumes expand to as much as double their pretreatment volume. Both loss of white and gray matter contribute to the decrease in total brain volume [30, 156, 160].

Of note, chemotherapy alone, in the absence of radiation therapy, can result in delayed brain atrophy but is usually associated with leukoen- cephalopathy [37, 161–163]. Numerous advanced imaging studies using structural and functional MRI and PET imaging have demonstrated chemotherapy-related brain changes [164, 165]. While imaging findings do not always correlate with the degree of cognitive impairment, advanced neuroimaging studies are emerging as a powerful tool in patient evaluation and in clinical studies with neurocognitive endpoints.

The exact mechanism of global brain atrophy following cranial irradiation and chemotherapy remains poorly understood. Vascular injury to distal perforating arteries, radiation-induced demyelination with spongiform vacuolization, and injury to neural progenitor cells with gliosis and contraction of the white matter space have been suggested [150]. Recent studies further reveal preferential vulnerability of the hippocam- pus [166] and of cortical areas relevant for higher cognitive function to radiation therapy [167]. Elderly patients appear particularly vulnerable to accelerated brain volume loss and associated cognitive symptoms, presumably as a result of premorbid age-related degenerative brain changes, such as microvascular disease and pre- existing brain atrophy [47].

Brain volume loss is considered irreversible, and patient management is usually supportive.

Both pharmacotherapy and neurocognitive rehabilitation have been incorporated in patient management but are generally of limited success. The same treatment principles apply as discussed for patients with neurocognitive impairment fol- lowing cancer therapy (see above).

While the therapeutic benefit from neurostim- ulants and anti-dementia agents has been dis- cussed controversially, such medications are generally well tolerated and may be reasonable to consider in selected patients.

42.5 Treatment-Induced Necrosis

Treatment-induced tissue necrosis (aka "radiation necrosis") is a common delayed complication of cerebral irradiation. The exact incidence of radiation necrosis in brain cancer patients is unknown and ranges between 5 and 50% [168, 169]. While approximately 5–10% of patients with malignant gliomas will develop treatment-related brain tissue necrosis after combined chemoradiation [170], the incidence is considered higher with up to 40% in patients treated for nasopharyngeal carcinoma [171, 172].

Radiation necrosis is usually seen 6–12 months after radiation therapy; however, onset may be quite variable and can occur more than 10 years after initial therapy [170, 173].

The mechanisms of radiation necrosis include vascular endothelial cell damage, resulting in small vessel fibrinoid necrosis, capillary leakage, inflammation, and subsequent demyelination. Vascular toxicity may be driven by local tissue ischemia and the release of vascular endothelial growth factor (VEGF) [174] in response to hypoxic changes. In support of a role of VEGF in the pathogenesis of radiation necrosis is the observation that VEGF blockade by the monoclonal antibody bevacizumab has been of benefit in patients with radiation necrosis and attenuates radiographic abnormalities [175].

Risk factors of radiation necrosis include type and modality of radiation (e.g., brachytherapy and stereotactic radiosurgery due to a higher focal radiation dose), the total radiation dose and volume, fractionation size, concurrent and/or adjuvant chemotherapy, and presence of vascular comorbidities [171, 176–182].

Radiation necrosis commonly develops at or adjacent to the original tumor site and within brain areas that received the highest radiation dose. Imaging findings on MRI demonstrate focal areas of abnormal contrast enhancement on T1-weighted images and increase in T2/FLAIR hyperintensities (Fig. 42.3).

The radiographic appearance of radiation necrosis mimics progressive or recurrent tumor and is therefore a major challenge to patient management. Unfortunately, a reliable distinction between radiation necrosis and progressive tumor is usually not possible by conventional MRI [177, 183, 184], and a surgical biopsy may be necessary in some patients to establish the correct diagnosis.

Various advanced imaging modalities are currently being investigated in an attempt to differentiate radiation necrosis from recurrent tumor [185].

Perfusion-weighted MRI, such as dynamic susceptibility contrast-enhanced MRI (DSC-MRI), may be useful to distinguish tumor recurrence from treatment-related effects based on elevated relative cerebral blood volume (rCBV) which is more frequently seen in active tumors [186–189].

Other modalities include MR spectroscopy (MRS) [190–192] and advanced positron emission tomography (PET) applications [185, 193–197]. Despite these diagnostic efforts, there are currently no uniformly established imaging modalities with high enough sensitivity or specificity to reliably differentiate between progressive tumor and treatment-related changes.

42.6 Neurovascular Complications

The risk of cerebrovascular complications, including mortality from stroke and intracerebral hemorrhage, is increased in patients treated with cranial irradiation [198–200]. As discussed above in the section on radiation necrosis, mechanisms implicated in the development of vascular complications include vascular endothelial cell damage and endothelial cell apoptosis, neuro-inflammation, small vessel fibrinoid necrosis, capillary leakage, edema, spongiosis, and demyelination [47, 201].

Patient-specific factors also appear to be important predictors of neurovascular toxicity following radiation therapy. Particularly vulnerable to late injury are young patients, presumably due to disruption of normal neurodevelopmental processes and neural networks that rely on rapid cell division and progenitor cell function [27]. In a recent study in medulloblastoma patients

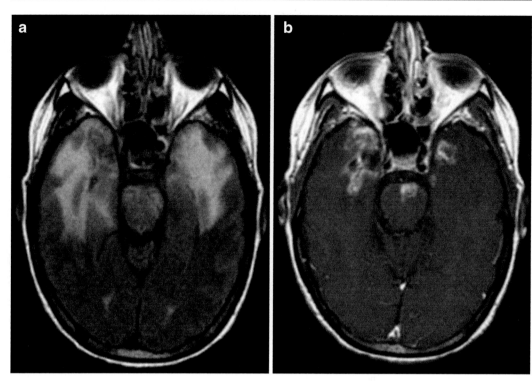

Fig. 42.3 Radiation-induced tissue necrosis. A 52-year-old female with nasopharyngeal carcinoma underwent photon beam radiation therapy and 3–4 years later develops cognitive impairment and behavioral abnormalities. Axial MRI of the brain reveals T2-FLAIR hyperintensi- ties in both temporal lobes consistent with cerebral edema (**a**). Corresponding axial T1-post contrast images (**b**) demonstrate scattered foci of abnormal enhancement con- sistent with treatment effects and radiation-induced tissue necrosis

treated with cranio-spinal irradiation, the cumu- lative incidence of neurovascular injury, as deter- mined by cerebral microbleeds, was highest in patients treated at younger age (<20), and evolu- tion of microbleeds followed a progressive pat- tern over time in the absence of additional treatment [202].

Management of patients with vascular com- plications from cranial irradiation is similar to management of non-cancer patients.

42.7 Secondary Tumors

Long-term survivors of cranial irradiation are at risk for the development of secondary neoplasms. This risk was carefully demonstrated in an epide- miologic study of Israeli children treated with radiation for tinea capitis in the 1940s and 1950s [203]. Compared with nonirradiated control sub- jects, those who had been treated (mean dose of 1.5 Gy) had 8.4 times greater risk of developing a head or neck neoplasm. The most common tumor types associated with irradiation were meningio- mas, nerve sheath tumors, gliomas, and other neural tumors. There was a clear dose-response relationship, with those receiving >2 Gy being at 20 times greater risk of developing a tumor in the radiation field, a finding that is consistent with the dose-response relationship seen in studies of other mechanisms of radiation exposure (e.g., radiation exposure from an atomic bomb).

Radiation-induced meningiomas occur with increased frequency after treatment with cranial or cranio-spinal irradiation for other malignan- cies, such as lymphoblastic leukemia or medul- loblastoma (Fig. 42.4). Because these treatments have improved overall survival rates and are typically administered to children, incidence of radiation-induced meningioma is increasing.

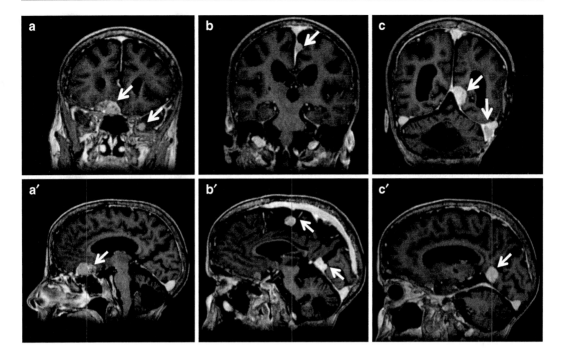

Fig. 42.4 Radiation-induced secondary tumors. A 35-year-old female with history of posterior fossa medulloblastoma treated at age 7 with cranio-spinal radiation therapy presents with new-onset seizure disorder, headaches, and irritability. MRI of the brain identifies multiple extra-axial and dura-based enhancing lesions, consistent with meningiomas. T1-post contrast coronal (upper panel, **a**–**c**) and corresponding sagittal (lower panel, **a′**–**c′**) MRI scans demonstrate multiple dura-based enhancing tumors (arrows)

The majority of these meningiomas are grade 1 tumors (68%) [204], though grade 2 and 3 tumors also occur (27% and 5%, respectively). There is a notable delay in the development of secondary tumors after radiation therapy. The median time from initial radiation treatment to diagnosis of secondary tumors has been characterized in meningiomas as 25 years in grade 1, 22 years for grade 2, and 13 years for grade 3 tumors [204].

Latency of onset also appears to be related to radiation dose, with those receiving >15 Gy having more rapid onset than those who received a lower-dose treatment. A genetic predisposition to tumor syndromes (e.g., retinoblastoma, neurofibromatosis) may contribute to more rapid onset than experienced by those without a known genetic risk factor. Yamanaka and colleagues cited 5- and 10-year survival rates in patients diagnosed with secondary tumors in the range of 78% and 61%, respectively, and median survival was not reached.

Treatment of these radiation-induced tumors includes surgery and stereotactic radiosurgery. Rates of recurrence of radiation-induced tumors are not well documented in the literature, which consists largely of case studies, small series, and reviews.

Sarcomas also occur after brain irradiation at an increased frequency. A single-institution case series conducted at MD Anderson demonstrated that 9% of all osteosarcomas seen over a 40-year period were likely radiation induced [205]. Although these tumors are rare, their aggressive behavior and treatment resistance is associated with dismal outcomes [206]. Radiation dose is related to the latency of onset, with moderate- to high-dose radiation (e.g., >15 Gy) having a median latency of 11 years postradiation and low-dose radiation having a median latency of 27.5 years. Median survival was 11 months from diagnosis, with 5-year survival rate of <15% and 10-year survival of 10% [206].

As with management of other sarcomas, treatment options include surgery, radiosurgery, and chemotherapy, with some modest improvement in median survival to 24 months in the subset of patients who receive multimodal therapy.

In summary, radiation therapy can be associated with secondary neoplasms, which are considered a late-onset complication of treatment. Although their occurrence appears fairly rare in the literature to date, it is likely that the incidence will increase as survivors of childhood radiation treatment age over the next few decades.

42.8   Conclusions

Collectively, both radiation and chemotherapy remain key treatment modalities in brain cancer patients to prolong survival and improve overall outcomes. Various delayed neurologic complications from brain cancer therapy have been recognized and are challenging to patient management. With prolonged survival due to the success of novel and combined anticancer therapies, delayed neurotoxic effects have been recognized with increasing frequency and compromise quality of life in survivors.

Complications include cognitive impairment, white matter disease, brain atrophy, tissue necrosis, and vascular complications. An increased understanding of risk factors and mechanisms that drive such delayed treatment complications will be essential to develop neuroprotective and neural repair strategies to improve overall patient outcome.

References

1. Johnson DR, Sawyer AM, Meyers CA, O'Neill BP, Wefel JS (2012) Early measures of cognitive function predict survival in patients with newly diagnosed glioblastoma. Neuro Oncol 14:808–816
2. Wefel JS, Noll KR, Rao G, Cahill DP (2016) Neurocognitive function varies by IDH1 genetic mutation status in patients with malignant glioma prior to surgical resection. Neuro Oncol 18:1656–1663
3. Kayl AE, Meyers CA (2003) Does brain tumor histology influence cognitive function? Neuro Oncol 5:255–260
4. Wu AS, Witgert ME, Lang FF et al (2011) Neurocognitive function before and after surgery for insular gliomas. J Neurosurg 115:1115–1125
5. Racine CA, Li J, Molinaro AM, Butowski N, Berger MS (2015) Neurocognitive function in newly diagnosed low-grade glioma patients undergoing surgical resection with awake mapping techniques. Neurosurgery 77:371–379; discussion 9
6. Wefel JS, Kayl AE, Meyers CA (2004) Neuropsychological dysfunction associated with cancer and cancer therapies: a conceptual review of an emerging target. Br J Cancer 90:1691–1696
7. Wefel JS, Witgert ME, Meyers CA (2008) Neuropsychological sequelae of non-central nervous system cancer and cancer therapy. Neuropsychol Rev 18(2):121–131
8. Noll KR, Sullaway C, Ziu M, Weinberg JS, Wefel JS (2015) Relationships between tumor grade and neurocognitive functioning in patients with glioma of the left temporal lobe prior to surgical resection. Neuro Oncol 17:580–587
9. Tucha O, Smely C, Preier M, Lange KW (2000) Cognitive deficits before treatment among patients with brain tumors. Neurosurgery 47:324–333; discussion 33–4
10. Shields LB, Choucair AK (2014) Management of low-grade gliomas: a review of patient-perceived quality of life and neurocognitive outcome. World Neurosurg 82:e299–e309
11. Guerrini R, Rosati A, Giordano F, Genitori L, Barba C (2013) The medical and surgical treatment of tumoral seizures: current and future perspectives. Epilepsia 54(Suppl 9):84–90
12. Heimans JJ, Reijneveld JC (2012) Factors affecting the cerebral network in brain tumor patients. J Neurooncol 108:231–237
13. van Breemen MS, Wilms EB, Vecht CJ (2007) Epilepsy in patients with brain tumours: epidemiology, mechanisms, and management. Lancet Neurol 6:421–430
14. Bosma I, Vos MJ, Heimans JJ et al (2007) The course of neurocognitive functioning in high-grade glioma patients. Neuro Oncol 9:53–62
15. DeAngelis LM, Delattre JY, Posner JB (1989) Radiation-induced dementia in patients cured of brain metastases. Neurology 39:789–796
16. Moore BD 3rd, Copeland DR, Ried H, Levy B (1992) Neurophysiological basis of cognitive deficits in long-term survivors of childhood cancer. Arch Neurol 49:809–817
17. Crossen JR, Garwood D, Glatstein E, Neuwelt EA (1994) Neurobehavioral sequelae of cranial irradiation in adults: a review of radiation-induced encephalopathy. J Clin Oncol 12:627–642
18. Roman DD, Sperduto PW (1995) Neuropsychological effects of cranial radiation:

current knowledge and future directions. Int J Radiat Oncol Biol Phys 31:983–998

19. Abayomi OK (1996) Pathogenesis of irradiation-induced cognitive dysfunction. Acta Oncol 35:659–663

20. Keime-Guibert F, Napolitano M, Delattre JY (1998) Neurological complications of radiotherapy and chemotherapy. J Neurol 245:695–708

21. Anderson VA, Godber T, Smibert E, Weiskop S, Ekert H (2000) Cognitive and academic outcome following cranial irradiation and chemotherapy in children: a longitudinal study. Br J Cancer 82:255–262

22. Surma-aho O, Niemela M, Vilkki J et al (2001) Adverse long-term effects of brain radiotherapy in adult low-grade glioma patients. Neurology 56:1285–1290

23. Laack NN, Brown PD (2004) Cognitive sequelae of brain radiation in adults. Semin Oncol 31:702–713

24. Duffner PK (2004) Long-term effects of radiation therapy on cognitive and endocrine function in children with leukemia and brain tumors. Neurologist 10:293–310

25. Perry A, Schmidt RE (2006) Cancer therapy-associated CNS neuropathology: an update and review of the literature. Acta Neuropathol 111:197–212

26. Edelstein K, Spiegler BJ, Fung S et al (2011) Early aging in adult survivors of childhood medulloblastoma: long-term neurocognitive, functional, and physical outcomes. Neuro Oncol 13:536–545

27. Dietrich J, Monje M, Wefel J, Meyers C (2008) Clinical patterns and biological correlates of cognitive dysfunction associated with cancer therapy. Oncologist 13:1285–1295

28. Tallet AV, Azria D, Barlesi F et al (2012) Neurocognitive function impairment after whole brain radiotherapy for brain metastases: actual assessment. Radiat Oncol 7:77

29. Gondi V, Hermann BP, Mehta MP, Tome WA (2013) Hippocampal dosimetry predicts neurocognitive function impairment after fractionated stereotactic radiotherapy for benign or low-grade adult brain tumors. Int J Radiat Oncol Biol Phys 85:348–354

30. Prust MJ, Jafari-Khouzani K, Kalpathy-Cramer J et al (2015) Standard chemoradiation for glioblastoma results in progressive brain volume loss. Neurology 85:683–691

31. Krull KR, Zhang N, Santucci A et al (2013) Long-term decline in intelligence among adult survivors of childhood acute lymphoblastic leukemia treated with cranial radiation. Blood 122:550–553

32. Lee AW, Kwong DL, Leung SF et al (2002) Factors affecting risk of symptomatic temporal lobe necrosis: significance of fractional dose and treatment time. Int J Radiat Oncol Biol Phys 53:75–85

33. Lawrence YR, Li XA, el Naqa I et al (2010) Radiation dose-volume effects in the brain. Int J Radiat Oncol Biol Phys 76:S20–S27

34. Andreassen CN, Alsner J (2009) Genetic variants and normal tissue toxicity after radiotherapy: a systematic review. Radiother Oncol 92:299–309

35. Barnett GC, West CM, Dunning AM et al (2009) Normal tissue reactions to radiotherapy: towards tailoring treatment dose by genotype. Nat Rev Cancer 9:134–142

36. West CM, Barnett GC (2011) Genetics and genomics of radiotherapy toxicity: towards prediction. Genome Med 3:52

37. Lai R, Abrey LE, Rosenblum MK, DeAngelis LM (2004) Treatment-induced leukoencephalopathy in primary CNS lymphoma: a clinical and autopsy study. Neurology 62:451–456

38. Sheline GE (1977) Radiation therapy of brain tumors. Cancer 39:873–881

39. Rubin P, Gash DM, Hansen JT, Nelson DF, Williams JP (1994) Disruption of the blood-brain barrier as the primary effect of CNS irradiation. Radiother Oncol 31:51–60

40. Behin A, Delattre JY (2004) Complications of radiation therapy on the brain and spinal cord. Semin Neurol 24:405–417

41. Meyers CA, Geara F, Wong PF, Morrison WH (2000) Neurocognitive effects of therapeutic irradiation for base of skull tumors. Int J Radiat Oncol Biol Phys 46:51–55

42. Gregor A, Cull A, Traynor E, Stewart M, Lander F, Love S (1996) Neuropsychometric evaluation of long-term survivors of adult brain tumours: relationship with tumour and treatment parameters. Radiother Oncol 41:55–59

43. Armstrong CL, Gyato K, Awadalla AW, Lustig R, Tochner ZA (2004) A critical review of the clinical effects of therapeutic irradiation damage to the brain: the roots of controversy. Neuropsychol Rev 14:65–86

44. Wong CS, Van der Kogel AJ (2004) Mechanisms of radiation injury to the central nervous system: implications for neuroprotection. Mol Interv 4:273–284

45. Strother DR (2002) Tumors of the central nervous system. In: PPA P, Poplack DG (eds) Principles and Practice of Pediatric Oncology. Lippincott, Williams and Wilkins, Philadelphia, pp 751–824

46. Dropcho EJ (1991) Central nervous system injury by therapeutic irradiation. Neurol Clin 9:969–988

47. Constine LS, Konski A, Ekholm S, McDonald S, Rubin P (1988) Adverse effects of brain irradiation correlated with MR and CT imaging. Int J Radiat Oncol Biol Phys 15:319–330

48. Oppenheimer JH, Levy ML, Sinha U et al (1992) Radionecrosis secondary to interstitial brachytherapy: correlation of magnetic resonance imaging and histopathology. Neurosurgery 31:336–343

49. Morris JG, Grattan-Smith P, Panegyres PK, O'Neill P, Soo YS, Langlands AO (1994) Delayed cerebral radiation necrosis. Q J Med 87:119–129

50. Chong VE, Fan YF (1997) Radiation-induced temporal lobe necrosis. AJNR Am J Neuroradiol 18:784–785

51. Fouladi M, Chintagumpala M, Laningham FH et al (2004) White matter lesions detected by magnetic resonance imaging after radiotherapy and high-dose chemotherapy in children with medulloblastoma or primitive neuroectodermal tumor. J Clin Oncol 22:4551–4560

52. Dietrich J, Klein JP (2014) Imaging of cancer therapy-induced central nervous system toxicity. Neurol Clin 32:147–157

53. Sneed PK, Suh JH, Goetsch SJ et al (2002) A multi-institutional review of radiosurgery alone vs. radiosurgery with whole brain radiotherapy as the initial management of brain metastases. Int J Radiat Oncol Biol Phys 53:519–526

54. Soffietti R, Ruda R, Trevisan E (2008) Brain metastases: current management and new developments. Curr Opin Oncol 20:676–684

55. McDuff SG, Taich ZJ, Lawson JD et al (2013) Neurocognitive assessment following whole brain radiation therapy and radiosurgery for patients with cerebral metastases. J Neurol Neurosurg Psychiatry 84:1384–1391

56. Monaco EA 3rd, Faraji AH, Berkowitz O et al (2013) Leukoencephalopathy after whole-brain radiation therapy plus radiosurgery versus radiosurgery alone for metastatic lung cancer. Cancer 119:226–232

57. Brown PD, Ballman KV, Cerhan JH et al (2017) Postoperative stereotactic radiosurgery compared with whole brain radiotherapy for resected metastatic brain disease (NCCTG N107C/CEC.3): a multicentre, randomised, controlled, phase 3 trial. Lancet Oncol 18:1049–1060

58. Belka C, Budach W, Kortmann RD, Bamberg M (2001) Radiation induced CNS toxicity—molecular and cellular mechanisms. Br J Cancer 85:1233–1239

59. Noble M, Dietrich J (2002) Intersections between neurobiology and oncology: tumor origin, treatment and repair of treatment-associated damage. Trends Neurosci 25:103–107

60. Monje ML, Palmer T (2003) Radiation injury and neurogenesis. Curr Opin Neurol 16:129–134

61. Fike JR, Rola R, Limoli CL (2007) Radiation response of neural precursor cells. Neurosurg Clin N Am 18:115–127

62. Monje M, Dietrich J (2012) Cognitive side effects of cancer therapy demonstrate a functional role for adult neurogenesis. Behav Brain Res 227:376–379

63. Gondi V, Pugh SL, Tome WA et al (2014) Preservation of memory with conformal avoidance of the hippocampal neural stem-cell compartment during whole-brain radiotherapy for brain metastases (RTOG 0933): a phase II multi-institutional trial. J Clin Oncol 32:3810–3816

64. Attia A, Page BR, Lesser GJ, Chan M (2014) Treatment of radiation-induced cognitive decline. Curr Treat Options Oncol 15:539–550

65. Shaw EG, Rosdhal R, D'Agostino RB Jr et al (2006) Phase II study of donepezil in irradiated brain tumor patients: effect on cognitive function, mood, and quality of life. J Clin Oncol 24:1415–1420

66. Conklin HM, Reddick WE, Ashford J et al (2010) Long-term efficacy of methylphenidate in enhancing attention regulation, social skills, and academic abilities of childhood cancer survivors. J Clin Oncol 28:4465–4472

67. Castellino SM, Tooze JA, Flowers L et al (2012) Toxicity and efficacy of the acetylcholinesterase (AChe) inhibitor donepezil in childhood brain tumor survivors: a pilot study. Pediatr Blood Cancer 59:540–547

68. Gehring K, Patwardhan SY, Collins R et al (2012) A randomized trial on the efficacy of methylphenidate and modafinil for improving cognitive functioning and symptoms in patients with a primary brain tumor. J Neurooncol 107:165–174

69. Attia A, Rapp SR, Case LD et al (2012) Phase II study of Ginkgo biloba in irradiated brain tumor patients: effect on cognitive function, quality of life, and mood. J Neurooncol 109:357–363

70. Brown PD, Pugh S, Laack NN et al (2013) Memantine for the prevention of cognitive dysfunction in patients receiving whole-brain radiotherapy: a randomized, double-blind, placebo-controlled trial. Neuro Oncol 15:1429–1437

71. Rapp SR, Case LD, Peiffer A et al (2015) Donepezil for irradiated brain tumor survivors: a phase III randomized placebo-controlled clinical trial. J Clin Oncol 33:1653–1659

72. Correa DD, Kryza-Lacombe M, Baser RE, Beal K, DeAngelis LM (2016) Cognitive effects of donepezil therapy in patients with brain tumors: a pilot study. J Neurooncol 127:313–319

73. Dietrich J, Baryawno N, Nayyar N et al (2018) Bone marrow drives central nervous system regeneration after radiation injury. J Clin Invest 128:281–293

74. Sahnoune I, Inoue T, Kesler SR et al (2018) Exercise ameliorates neurocognitive impairments in a translational model of pediatric radiotherapy. Neuro Oncol 20:695–704

75. Benzing V, Eggenberger N, Spitzhuttl J et al (2018) The Brainfit study: efficacy of cognitive training and exergaming in pediatric cancer survivors—a randomized controlled trial. BMC Cancer 18:18

76. Riggs L, Piscione J, Laughlin S et al (2017) Exercise training for neural recovery in a restricted sample of pediatric brain tumor survivors: a controlled clinical trial with crossover of training versus no training. Neuro Oncol 19:440–450

77. Bergo E, Lombardi G, Pambuku A et al (2016) Cognitive rehabilitation in patients with gliomas and other brain tumors: state of the art. Biomed Res Int 2016:3041824

78. Piil K, Juhler M, Jakobsen J, Jarden M (2016) Controlled rehabilitative and supportive care intervention trials in patients with high-grade gliomas

and their caregivers: a systematic review. BMJ Support Palliat Care 6:27–34

79. Moleski M (2000) Neuropsychological, neuroanatomical, and neurophysiological consequences of CNS chemotherapy for acute lymphoblastic leukemia. Arch Clin Neuropsychol 15:603–630

80. Ahles TA, Saykin A (2001) Cognitive effects of standard-dose chemotherapy in patients with cancer. Cancer Invest 19:812–820

81. Wefel JS, Lenzi R, Theriault RL, Davis RN, Meyers CA (2004) The cognitive sequelae of standard-dose adjuvant chemotherapy in women with breast carcinoma: results of a prospective, randomized, longitudinal trial. Cancer 100:2292–2299

82. Shilling V, Jenkins V, Morris R, Deutsch G, Bloomfield D (2005) The effects of adjuvant chemotherapy on cognition in women with breast cancer— preliminary results of an observational longitudinal study. Breast 14:142–150

83. Ahles TA, Saykin AJ, McDonald BC et al (2010) Longitudinal assessment of cognitive changes associated with adjuvant treatment for breast cancer: impact of age and cognitive reserve. J Clin Oncol 28:4434–4440

84. Butler RW, Haser JK (2006) Neurocognitive effects of treatment for childhood cancer. Ment Retard Dev Disabil Res Rev 12:184–191

85. Alvarez JA, Scully RE, Miller TL et al (2007) Long-term effects of treatments for childhood cancers. Curr Opin Pediatr 19:23–31

86. van Dam FS, Schagen SB, Muller MJ et al (1998) Impairment of cognitive function in women receiving adjuvant treatment for high-risk breast cancer: high-dose versus standard-dose chemotherapy. J Natl Cancer Inst 90:210–218

87. Schagen SB, van Dam FS, Muller MJ, Boogerd W, Lindeboom J, Bruning PF (1999) Cognitive deficits after postoperative adjuvant chemotherapy for breast carcinoma. Cancer 85:640–650

88. Brezden CB, Phillips KA, Abdolell M, Bunston T, Tannock IF (2000) Cognitive function in breast cancer patients receiving adjuvant chemotherapy. J Clin Oncol 18:2695–2701

89. Schagen SB, Muller MJ, Boogerd W et al (2002) Late effects of adjuvant chemotherapy on cognitive function: a follow-up study in breast cancer patients. Ann Oncol 13:1387–1397

90. Anderson-Hanley C, Sherman ML, Riggs R, Agocha VB, Compas BE (2003) Neuropsychological effects of treatments for adults with cancer: a meta-analysis and review of the literature. J Int Neuropsychol Soc : JINS 9:967–982

91. Tannock IF, Ahles TA, Ganz PA, Van Dam FS (2004) Cognitive impairment associated with chemotherapy for cancer: report of a workshop. J Clin Oncol 22:2233–2239

92. Schagen SB, Muller MJ, Boogerd W, Mellenbergh GJ, van Dam FS (2006) Change in cognitive function after chemotherapy: a prospective longitudinal study in breast cancer patients. J Natl Cancer Inst 98:1742–1745

93. Hurria A, Rosen C, Hudis C et al (2006) Cognitive function of older patients receiving adjuvant chemotherapy for breast cancer: a pilot prospective longitudinal study. J Am Geriatr Soc 54:925–931

94. Ahles TA, Saykin AJ (2007) Candidate mechanisms for chemotherapy-induced cognitive changes. Nat Rev Cancer 7:192–201

95. Vardy J, Wefel JS, Ahles T, Tannock IF, Schagen SB (2008) Cancer and cancer-therapy related cognitive dysfunction: an international perspective from the Venice cognitive workshop. Ann Oncol 19:623–629

96. Meyers CA, Abbruzzese JL (1992) Cognitive functioning in cancer patients: effect of previous treatment. Neurology 42:434–436

97. Heflin LH, Meyerowitz BE, Hall P et al (2005) Cancer as a risk factor for long-term cognitive deficits and dementia. J Natl Cancer Inst 97:854–856

98. Roe CM, Behrens MI, Xiong C, Miller JP, Morris JC (2005) Alzheimer disease and cancer. Neurology 64:895–898

99. Wefel JS, Meyers CA (2005) Cancer as a risk factor for dementia: a house built on shifting sand. J Natl Cancer Inst 97:788–789

100. Matsuda T, Takayama T, Tashiro M, Nakamura Y, Ohashi Y, Shimozuma K (2005) Mild cognitive impairment after adjuvant chemotherapy in breast cancer patients—evaluation of appropriate research design and methodology to measure symptoms. Breast Cancer 12:279–287

101. Hermelink K, Untch M, Lux MP et al (2007) Cognitive function during neoadjuvant chemotherapy for breast cancer: results of a prospective, multicenter, longitudinal study. Cancer 109:1905–1913

102. Vardy J, Rourke S, Tannock IF (2007) Evaluation of cognitive function associated with chemotherapy: a review of published studies and recommendations for future research. J Clin Oncol 25:2455–2463

103. Jansen CE, Dodd MJ, Miaskowski CA, Dowling GA, Kramer J (2008) Preliminary results of a longitudinal study of changes in cognitive function in breast cancer patients undergoing chemotherapy with doxorubicin and cyclophosphamide. Psychooncology 17:1189–1195

104. Wefel JS, Saleeba AK, Buzdar AU, Meyers CA (2010) Acute and late onset cognitive dysfunction associated with chemotherapy in women with breast cancer. Cancer 116:3348–3356

105. Hutchinson AD, Hosking JR, Kichenadasse G, Mattiske JK, Wilson C (2012) Objective and subjective cognitive impairment following chemotherapy for cancer: a systematic review. Cancer Treat Rev 38:926–934

106. Koppelmans V, Breteler MM, Boogerd W, Seynaeve C, Gundy C, Schagen SB (2012) Neuropsychological performance in survivors of breast cancer more than 20 years after adjuvant chemotherapy. J Clin Oncol 30:1080–1086

107. Seigers R, Schagen SB, Van Tellingen O, Dietrich J (2013) Chemotherapy-related cognitive dysfunction: current animal studies and future directions. Brain Imaging Behav 7:453–459

108. Dietrich J, Han R, Yang Y, Mayer-Proschel M, Noble M (2006) CNS progenitor cells and oligodendrocytes are targets of chemotherapeutic agents in vitro and in vivo. J Biol 5:22

109. Han R, Yang YM, Dietrich J, Luebke A, Mayer-Proschel M, Noble M (2008) Systemic 5-fluorouracil treatment causes a syndrome of delayed myelin destruction in the central nervous system. J Biol 7:12

110. Seigers R, Schagen SB, Beerling W et al (2008) Long-lasting suppression of hippocampal cell proliferation and impaired cognitive performance by methotrexate in the rat. Behav Brain Res 186:168–175

111. Winocur G, Vardy J, Binns MA, Kerr L, Tannock I (2006) The effects of the anti-cancer drugs, methotrexate and 5-fluorouracil, on cognitive function in mice. Pharmacol Biochem Behav 85:66–75

112. Fardell JE, Vardy J, Logge W, Johnston I (2010) Single high dose treatment with methotrexate causes long-lasting cognitive dysfunction in laboratory rodents. Pharmacol Biochem Behav 97:333–339

113. Dietrich J, Prust M, Kaiser J (2015) Chemotherapy, cognitive impairment and hippocampal toxicity. Neuroscience 309:224–232

114. Chen Y, Lomnitski L, Michaelson DM, Shohami E (1997) Motor and cognitive deficits in apolipoprotein E-deficient mice after closed head injury. Neuroscience 80:1255–1262

115. Hoffmeyer S, Burk O, von Richter O et al (2000) Functional polymorphisms of the human multidrug-resistance gene: multiple sequence variations and correlation of one allele with P-glycoprotein expression and activity in vivo. Proc Natl Acad Sci U S A 97:3473–3478

116. Ahles TA, Saykin AJ, Noll WW et al (2003) The relationship of APOE genotype to neuropsychological performance in long-term cancer survivors treated with standard dose chemotherapy. Psychooncology 12:612–619

117. McAllister TW, Ahles TA, Saykin AJ et al (2004) Cognitive effects of cytotoxic cancer chemotherapy: predisposing risk factors and potential treatments. Curr Psychiatry Rep 6:364–371

118. Okcu MF, Selvan M, Wang LE et al (2004) Glutathione S-transferase polymorphisms and survival in primary malignant glioma. Clin Cancer Res 10:2618–2625

119. Muramatsu T, Johnson DR, Finch RA et al (2004) Age-related differences in vincristine toxicity and biodistribution in wild-type and transporter-deficient mice. Oncol Res 14:331–343

120. Jamroziak K, Balcerczak E, Cebula B et al (2005) Multi-drug transporter MDR1 gene polymorphism and prognosis in adult acute lymphoblastic leukemia. Pharmacol Rep 57:882–888

121. Linnebank M, Pels H, Kleczar N et al (2005) MTX-induced white matter changes are associated with polymorphisms of methionine metabolism. Neurology 64:912–913

122. Krajinovic M, Robaey P, Chiasson S et al (2005) Polymorphisms of genes controlling homocysteine levels and IQ score following the treatment for childhood ALL. Pharmacogenomics 6:293–302

123. Largillier R, Etienne-Grimaldi MC, Formento JL et al (2006) Pharmacogenetics of capecitabine in advanced breast cancer patients. Clin Cancer Res 12:5496–5502

124. Fishel ML, Vasko MR, Kelley MR (2007) DNA repair in neurons: so if they don't divide what's to repair? Mutat Res 614:24–36

125. Abrey LE, Batchelor TT, Ferreri AJ et al (2005) Report of an international workshop to standardize baseline evaluation and response criteria for primary CNS lymphoma. J Clin Oncol 23:5034–5043

126. Correa DD, Maron L, Harder H et al (2007) Cognitive functions in primary central nervous system lymphoma: literature review and assessment guidelines. Ann Oncol 18:1145–1151

127. Krull KR, Okcu MF, Potter B et al (2008) Screening for neurocognitive impairment in pediatric cancer long-term survivors. J Clin Oncol 26:4138–4143

128. Wefel JS, Vardy J, Ahles T, Schagen SB (2011) International Cognition and Cancer Task Force recommendations to harmonise studies of cognitive function in patients with cancer. Lancet Oncol 12:703–708

129. Lawrence JA, Griffin L, Balcueva EP et al (2016) A study of donepezil in female breast cancer survivors with self-reported cognitive dysfunction 1 to 5 years following adjuvant chemotherapy. J Cancer Surviv 10:176–184

130. Iyer NS, Balsamo LM, Bracken MB, Kadan-Lottick NS (2015) Chemotherapy-only treatment effects on long-term neurocognitive functioning in childhood ALL survivors: a review and meta-analysis. Blood 126:346–353

131. Escalante CP, Meyers C, Reuben JM et al (2014) A randomized, double-blind, 2-period, placebo-controlled crossover trial of a sustained-release methylphenidate in the treatment of fatigue in cancer patients. Cancer J 20:8–14

132. Kohli S, Fisher SG, Tra Y et al (2009) The effect of modafinil on cognitive function in breast cancer survivors. Cancer 115:2605–2616

133. Lundorff LE, Jonsson BH, Sjogren P (2009) Modafinil for attentional and psychomotor dysfunction in advanced cancer: a double-blind, randomised, cross-over trial. Palliat Med 23:731–738

134. Lower EE, Fleishman S, Cooper A et al (2009) Efficacy of dexmethylphenidate for the treatment of fatigue after cancer chemotherapy: a randomized clinical trial. J Pain Symptom Manage 38:650–662

135. Conklin HM, Khan RB, Reddick WE et al (2007) Acute neurocognitive response to methylphenidate among survivors of childhood cancer: a randomized, double-blind, cross-over trial. J Pediatr Psychol 32:1127–1139

136. Mulhern RK, Khan RB, Kaplan S et al (2004) Short-term efficacy of methylphenidate: a randomized, double-blind, placebo-controlled trial among survivors of childhood cancer. J Clin Oncol 22:4795–4803

137. Schwartz AL, Thompson JA, Masood N (2002) Interferon-induced fatigue in patients with melanoma: a pilot study of exercise and methylphenidate. Oncol Nurs Forum 29:E85–E90

138. Meyers CA, Weitzner MA, Valentine AD, Levin VA (1998) Methylphenidate therapy improves cognition, mood, and function of brain tumor patients. J Clin Oncol 16:2522–2527

139. Ferguson RJ, Ahles TA, Saykin AJ et al (2007) Cognitive-behavioral management of chemotherapy-related cognitive change. Psychooncology 16:772–777

140. Evans JJ, Wilson BA, Needham P, Brentnall S (2003) Who makes good use of memory aids? Results of a survey of people with acquired brain injury. J Int Neuropsychol Soc JINS 9:925–935

141. Biegler KA, Chaoul MA, Cohen L (2009) Cancer, cognitive impairment, and meditation. Acta Oncol 48:18–26

142. Hsieh CC, Sprod LK, Hydock DS, Carter SD, Hayward R, Schneider CM (2008) Effects of a supervised exercise intervention on recovery from treatment regimens in breast cancer survivors. Oncol Nurs Forum 35:909–915

143. Mitchell SA (2010) Cancer-related fatigue: state of the science. PM R 2:364–383

144. Arrillaga-Romany IC, Dietrich J (2012) Imaging findings in cancer therapy-associated neurotoxicity. Semin Neurol 32:476–486

145. Perrini P, Scollato A, Cioffi F, Mouchaty H, Conti R, Di Lorenzo N (2002) Radiation leukoencephalopathy associated with moderate hydrocephalus: intracranial pressure monitoring and results of ventriculoperitoneal shunting. Neurol Sci 23:237–241

146. Cummings M, Dougherty DW, Mohile NA, Walter KA, Usuki KY, Milano MT (2016) Severe radiation-induced leukoencephalopathy: case report and literature review. Adv Radiat Oncol 1:17–20

147. Thiessen B, DeAngelis LM (1998) Hydrocephalus in radiation leukoencephalopathy: results of ventriculoperitoneal shunting. Arch Neurol 55:705–710

148. Sabsevitz DS, Bovi JA, Leo PD et al (2013) The role of pre-treatment white matter abnormalities in developing white matter changes following whole brain radiation: a volumetric study. J Neurooncol 114:291–297

149. Miller RC, Lachance DH, Lucchinetti CF et al (2006) Multiple sclerosis, brain radiotherapy, and risk of neurotoxicity: the Mayo Clinic experience. Int J Radiat Oncol Biol Phys 66:1178–1186

150. Valk PE, Dillon WP (1991) Radiation injury of the brain. AJNR Am J Neuroradiol 12:45–62

151. Harder H, Holtel H, Bromberg JE et al (2004) Cognitive status and quality of life after treatment for primary CNS lymphoma. Neurology 62:544–547

152. Douw L, Klein M, Fagel SS et al (2009) Cognitive and radiological effects of radiotherapy in patients with low-grade glioma: long-term follow-up. Lancet Neurol 8:810–818

153. Mamlouk MD, Handwerker J, Ospina J, Hasso AN (2013) Neuroimaging findings of the post-treatment effects of radiation and chemotherapy of malignant primary glial neoplasms. Neuroradiol J 26:396–412

154. Fischer CM, Neidert MC, Peus D et al (2014) Hydrocephalus after resection and adjuvant radiochemotherapy in patients with glioblastoma. Clin Neurol Neurosurg 120:27–31

155. Ailion AS, King TZ, Wang L et al (2016) Cerebellar atrophy in adult survivors of childhood cerebellar tumor. J Int Neuropsychol Soc JINS 22:501–511

156. Karunamuni R, Bartsch H, White NS et al (2016) Dose-dependent cortical thinning after partial brain irradiation in high-grade glioma. Int J Radiat Oncol Biol Phys 94:297–304

157. Omuro AM, Ben-Porat LS, Panageas KS et al (2005) Delayed neurotoxicity in primary central nervous system lymphoma. Arch Neurol 62:1595–1600

158. Shibamoto Y, Baba F, Oda K et al (2008) Incidence of brain atrophy and decline in mini-mental state examination score after whole-brain radiotherapy in patients with brain metastases: a prospective study. Int J Radiat Oncol Biol Phys 72:1168–1173

159. Swennen MH, Bromberg JE, Witkamp TD, Terhaard CH, Postma TJ, Taphoorn MJ (2004) Delayed radiation toxicity after focal or whole brain radiotherapy for low-grade glioma. J Neurooncol 66:333–339

160. Prust ML, Jafari-Khouzani K, Kalpathy-Cramer J et al (2018) Standard chemoradiation in combination with VEGF targeted therapy for glioblastoma results in progressive gray and white matter volume loss. Neuro Oncol 20:289–291

161. Dietrich J, Winter SF, Klein JP (2017) Neuroimaging of brain tumors: pseudoprogression, pseudo-response, and delayed effects of chemotherapy and radiation. Semin Neurol 37:589–596

162. Herrlinger U, Kuker W, Uhl M et al (2005) NOA-03 trial of high-dose methotrexate in primary central nervous system lymphoma: final report. Ann Neurol 57:843–847

163. Hertzberg H, Huk WJ, Ueberall MA et al (1997) CNS late effects after ALL therapy in childhood. Part I: neuroradiological findings in long-term survivors of childhood ALL—an evaluation of the interferences between morphology and neuropsychological performance. The German Late Effects Working Group. Med Pediatr Oncol 28:387–400

164. Kaiser J, Bledowski C, Dietrich J (2014) Neural correlates of chemotherapy-related cognitive impairment. Cortex 54:33–50

165. Horky LL, Gerbaudo VH, Zaitsev A et al (2014) Systemic chemotherapy decreases brain glucose metabolism. Ann Clin Transl Neurol 1:788–798

166. Seibert TM, Karunamuni R, Bartsch H et al (2017) Radiation dose-dependent hippocampal atrophy detected with longitudinal volumetric magnetic

resonance imaging. Int J Radiat Oncol Biol Phys 97:263–269

167. Seibert TM, Karunamuni R, Kaifi S et al (2017) Cerebral cortex regions selectively vulnerable to radiation dose-dependent atrophy. Int J Radiat Oncol Biol Phys 97:910–918

168. Rahmathulla G, Marko NF, Weil RJ (2013) Cerebral radiation necrosis: a review of the pathobiology, diagnosis and management considerations. J Clin Neurosci 20:485–502

169. Furuse M, Nonoguchi N, Kawabata S, Miyatake S, Kuroiwa T (2015) Delayed brain radiation necrosis: pathological review and new molecular targets for treatment. Med Mol Morphol 48:183–190

170. Eisele SC, Dietrich J (2015) Cerebral radiation necrosis: diagnostic challenge and clinical management. Rev Neurol 61:225–232

171. Lee AW, Foo W, Chappell R et al (1998) Effect of time, dose, and fractionation on temporal lobe necrosis following radiotherapy for nasopharyngeal carcinoma. Int J Radiat Oncol Biol Phys 40:35–42

172. Tuan JK, Ha TC, Ong WS et al (2012) Late toxicities after conventional radiation therapy alone for nasopharyngeal carcinoma. Radiother Oncol 104:305–311

173. Giglio P, Gilbert MR (2003) Cerebral radiation necrosis. Neurologist 9:180–188

174. Nordal RA, Nagy A, Pintilie M, Wong CS (2004) Hypoxia and hypoxia-inducible factor-1 target genes in central nervous system radiation injury: a role for vascular endothelial growth factor. Clin Cancer Res 10:3342–3353

175. Torcuator R, Zuniga R, Mohan YS et al (2009) Initial experience with bevacizumab treatment for biopsy confirmed cerebral radiation necrosis. J Neurooncol 94:63–68

176. Marks JE, Baglan RJ, Prassad SC, Blank WF (1981) Cerebral radionecrosis: incidence and risk in relation to dose, time, fractionation and volume. Int J Radiat Oncol Biol Phys 7:243–252

177. Kumar AJ, Leeds NE, Fuller GN et al (2000) Malignant gliomas: MR imaging spectrum of radiation therapy- and chemotherapy-induced necrosis of the brain after treatment. Radiology 217:377–384

178. Ruben JD, Dally M, Bailey M, Smith R, McLean CA, Fedele P (2006) Cerebral radiation necrosis: incidence, outcomes, and risk factors with emphasis on radiation parameters and chemotherapy. Int J Radiat Oncol Biol Phys 65:499–508

179. Brandsma D, Stalpers L, Taal W, Sminia P, van den Bent MJ (2008) Clinical features, mechanisms, and management of pseudoprogression in malignant gliomas. Lancet Oncol 9:453–461

180. Blonigen BJ, Steinmetz RD, Levin L, Lamba MA, Warnick RE, Breneman JC (2010) Irradiated volume as a predictor of brain radionecrosis after linear accelerator stereotactic radiosurgery. Int J Radiat Oncol Biol Phys 77:996–1001

181. Minniti G, Clarke E, Lanzetta G et al (2011) Stereotactic radiosurgery for brain metastases: analysis of outcome and risk of brain radionecrosis. Radiat Oncol 6:48

182. Fink J, Born D, Chamberlain MC (2012) Radiation necrosis: relevance with respect to treatment of primary and secondary brain tumors. Curr Neurol Neurosci Rep 12:276–285

183. Mullins ME, Barest GD, Schaefer PW, Hochberg FH, Gonzalez RG, Lev MH (2005) Radiation necrosis versus glioma recurrence: conventional MR imaging clues to diagnosis. AJNR Am J Neuroradiol 26:1967–1972

184. Dequesada IM, Quisling RG, Yachnis A, Friedman WA (2008) Can standard magnetic resonance imaging reliably distinguish recurrent tumor from radiation necrosis after radiosurgery for brain metastases? A radiographic-pathological study. Neurosurgery 63:898–903; discussion 4

185. Verma N, Cowperthwaite MC, Burnett MG, Markey MK (2013) Differentiating tumor recurrence from treatment necrosis: a review of neuro-oncologic imaging strategies. Neuro Oncol 15:515–534

186. Barajas RF Jr, Chang JS, Segal MR et al (2009) Differentiation of recurrent glioblastoma multiforme from radiation necrosis after external beam radiation therapy with dynamic susceptibility-weighted contrast-enhanced perfusion MR imaging. Radiology 253:486–496

187. Barajas RF, Chang JS, Sneed PK, Segal MR, McDermott MW, Cha S (2009) Distinguishing recurrent intra-axial metastatic tumor from radiation necrosis following gamma knife radiosurgery using dynamic susceptibility-weighted contrast-enhanced perfusion MR imaging. AJNR Am J Neuroradiol 30:367–372

188. Mitsuya K, Nakasu Y, Horiguchi S et al (2010) Perfusion weighted magnetic resonance imaging to distinguish the recurrence of metastatic brain tumors from radiation necrosis after stereotactic radiosurgery. J Neurooncol 99:81–88

189. Larsen VA, Simonsen HJ, Law I, Larsson HB, Hansen AE (2013) Evaluation of dynamic contrast-enhanced T1-weighted perfusion MRI in the differentiation of tumor recurrence from radiation necrosis. Neuroradiology 55:361–369

190. Zeng QS, Li CF, Zhang K, Liu H, Kang XS, Zhen JH (2007) Multivoxel 3D proton MR spectroscopy in the distinction of recurrent glioma from radiation injury. J Neurooncol 84:63–69

191. Smith EA, Carlos RC, Junck LR, Tsien CI, Elias A, Sundgren PC (2009) Developing a clinical decision model: MR spectroscopy to differentiate between recurrent tumor and radiation change in patients with new contrast-enhancing lesions. AJR Am J Roentgenol 192:W45–W52

192. Rock JP, Scarpace L, Hearshen D et al (2004) Associations among magnetic resonance spectroscopy, apparent diffusion coefficients, and image-guided histopathology with special attention to radiation necrosis. Neurosurgery 54:1111–1117; discussion 7–9

193. Ricci PE, Karis JP, Heiserman JE, Fram EK, Bice AN, Drayer BP (1998) Differentiating recurrent tumor from radiation necrosis: time for re-evaluation of positron emission tomography? AJNR Am J Neuroradiol 19:407–413

194. Chen W, Silverman DH, Delaloye S et al (2006) 18F-FDOPA PET imaging of brain tumors: comparison study with 18F-FDG PET and evaluation of diagnostic accuracy. J Nucl Med 47:904–911

195. Terakawa Y, Tsuyuguchi N, Iwai Y et al (2008) Diagnostic accuracy of 11C-methionine PET for differentiation of recurrent brain tumors from radiation necrosis after radiotherapy. J Nucl Med 49:694–699

196. Kim YH, Oh SW, Lim YJ et al (2010) Differentiating radiation necrosis from tumor recurrence in high-grade gliomas: assessing the efficacy of 18F-FDG PET, 11C-methionine PET and perfusion MRI. Clin Neurol Neurosurg 112:758–765

197. Lizarraga KJ, Allen-Auerbach M, Czernin J et al (2014) (18)F-FDOPA PET for differentiating recurrent or progressive brain metastatic tumors from late or delayed radiation injury after radiation treatment. J Nucl Med 55:30–36

198. Campen CJ, Kranick SM, Kasner SE et al (2012) Cranial irradiation increases risk of stroke in pediatric brain tumor survivors. Stroke 43:3035–3040

199. Mueller S, Fullerton HJ, Stratton K et al (2013) Radiation, atherosclerotic risk factors, and stroke risk in survivors of pediatric cancer: a report from the Childhood Cancer Survivor Study. Int J Radiat Oncol Biol Phys 86:649–655

200. Mueller S, Sear K, Hills NK et al (2013) Risk of first and recurrent stroke in childhood cancer survivors treated with cranial and cervical radiation therapy. Int J Radiat Oncol Biol Phys 86:643–648

201. Murphy ES, Xie H, Merchant TE, Yu JS, Chao ST, Suh JH (2015) Review of cranial radiotherapy-induced vasculopathy. J Neurooncol 122:421–429

202. Roongpiboonsopit D, Kuijf HJ, Charidimou A et al (2017) Evolution of cerebral microbleeds after cranial irradiation in medulloblastoma patients. Neurology 88:789–796

203. Ron E, Modan B, Boice JD Jr et al (1988) Tumors of the brain and nervous system after radiotherapy in childhood. N Engl J Med 319:1033–1039

204. Yamanaka R, Hayano A, Kanayama T (2017) Radiation-induced meningiomas: an exhaustive review of the literature. World Neurosurg 97:635–44 e8

205. Patel AJ, Rao VY, Fox BD et al (2011) Radiation-induced osteosarcomas of the calvarium and skull base. Cancer 117:2120–2126

206. Yamanaka R, Hayano A (2017) Radiation-induced sarcomas of the central nervous system: a systematic review. World Neurosurg 98:818–28 e7

Quality of Life and Cognition

43

Marijke B. Coomans, Linda Dirven,
and Martin J. B. Taphoorn

43.1 Introduction

Central nervous system (CNS) tumors can arise from any of the structures or cell types in or surrounding the brain and spinal cord, including the meninges and pituitary gland. The most common primary brain tumors are meningiomas, representing 36.4% of all primary CNS tumors. In contrast to several other types of brain tumors, up to 90% of the meningiomas are benign [1, 2]. Gliomas are the second most common primary brain tumors, arising from the glial cells and accounting for 80% of the malignant primary CNS tumors [3]. Among other primary brain tumors are nerve sheath tumors, pituitary tumors, and less common tumors such as primary CNS lymphomas [4, 5]. Brain metastases, or secondary brain tumors originating from distant primary cancers such as in the lung or breast, are the most prevalent CNS tumors with an incidence 3–10 times higher as compared to newly diagnosed

primary malignant brain tumors [6]. While patients treated for benign meningioma have a near-normal life expectancy [7], to date there is no cure for the majority of patients with a glioma or brain metastases. Median survival rates for patients with glioma range from only 15 months to over 15 years, depending on the histological subtype and genetic profile of the tumor [4, 8], while median survival rates of patients with brain metastases range from approximately 4 to 14 months, mainly depending on the primary tumor type, performance status, and first-line treatment modality [6, 9]. Despite the large variation in type, growth rate, location of the tumor, treatments, and prognosis, all brain tumor patients may suffer from impaired functioning and well-being. Patients may suffer from generic cancer symptoms such as fatigue and mood disorders but also CNS-specific symptoms such as seizures, signs of elevated intracranial pressure like headache, focal neurological deficits, personality changes, and cognitive deficits [4, 10]. These symptoms may subsequently impact activities in daily life, as well as the patient's well-being and social interactions.

Developing curative treatment options is the main challenge in neuro-oncology, for which purpose traditional endpoints such as (progression-free) survival and radiological response to treatment are used in clinical trials. However, the focus of healthcare has become more patient-centered in recent years, and as a

M. B. Coomans
Department of Neurology, Leiden University Medical Center, Leiden, The Netherlands
e-mail: M.B.Coomans@lumc.nl

L. Dirven · M. J. B. Taphoorn (✉)
Department of Neurology, Leiden University Medical Center, Leiden, The Netherlands

Department of Neurology, Haaglanden Medical Center, The Hague, The Netherlands
e-mail: L.Dirven@lumc.nl; m.j.b.taphoorn@lumc.nl; m.taphoorn@haaglandenmc.nl

© Springer Nature Switzerland AG 2019
J.-C. Tonn et al. (eds.), *Oncology of CNS Tumors*, https://doi.org/10.1007/978-3-030-04152-6_43

consequence, measures of patients' functioning and well-being have become more important. These measures are particularly important in patients with an (incurable) brain disease, for whom the quality of survival is at least as important as the duration of survival [11]. Functioning and well-being are broad concepts that entail a variety of domains, ranging from basic domains such as symptoms or impairments to complex and multidimensional concepts such as health-related quality of life (HRQoL). In neuro-oncology, HRQoL and cognitive functioning are two frequently used endpoints that are used to characterize patients' functioning and well-being. HRQoL is a multidimensional concept that refers to the patients' subjective perception of the effect of their disease and treatment on physical, psychological, and social aspects of daily life [12]. Many HRQoL questionnaires also cover symptoms caused by the disease and/or its treatment, such as cognitive symptoms. HRQoL is reflected at different levels of functioning (Fig. 43.1), according to the World Health Organization (WHO) International Classification of Functioning, Disability, and Health [13], as it measures on the level of impairment, activity limitations, as well as participation restrictions.

Cognitive functioning refers to the mental process of acquiring knowledge and understanding, the so-called "higher" cerebral functions, such as memory, attention, and processing speed, enabling us to participate in and function autonomously within society [14, 15]. Measurement of cognitive functioning is especially important in patients with a primary brain tumor, because the presence of the tumor directly threatens cognitive functioning. Cognitive functioning is measured at the level of impairment (Fig. 43.1). However, limitations at the level of activity limitations and participation restrictions may be present as a result of cognitive impairment. Objective cognitive functioning, such as memory or attentional impairment, is usually measured with standardized cognitive tests, thereby giving an impression of the objective cognitive functioning of the patient. Subjective cognitive complaints, i.e., how the patient perceives his or her cognitive functioning, entail a different concept that is typically measured with a patient-reported outcome (PRO) measure and are sometimes part of HRQoL questionnaires. Limitations in activities due to cognitive problems can be measured at the level of basic activities of daily living (BADL) and instrumental activities of daily living (IADL)

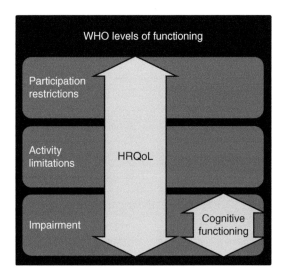

Fig. 43.1 Assessment of HRQoL and cognitive functioning based on the WHO levels of functioning. HRQoL is reflected at the three different levels of functioning, according to the World Health Organization (WHO) International Classification of Functioning, Disability, and Health [13], as it measures on the level of impairment, activity limitations, as well as participation restrictions. Cognitive functioning is measured at the level of impairment

[16, 17]. BADL are basic skills needed for self-maintenance, such as bathing, feeding, and dressing, while IADL includes cognitively complex activities, such as food preparation, handling finances, or using electronics. These latter may be particularly impaired in CNS tumor patients. Both BADL and IADL can be measured with a PRO or proxy-based measure. Lastly, participation restrictions caused by cognitive impairments can be measured with domains covered in HRQoL questionnaires.

This chapter will focus on HRQoL and cognition in patients with CNS tumors. First, we will discuss the assessment of HRQoL and cognition into more detail. Thereafter we will address the impact of the disease and treatment on these outcomes, and lastly, interventions for improving HRQoL and cognition will be discussed.

43.2 Assessment

43.2.1 HRQoL

Although quality of life (QoL) and HRQoL are often used interchangeably to refer to the same concept, they are different. QoL is a broad concept covering all aspects of human life, whereas HRQoL focuses specifically on the effects of illness and the impact of treatment on QoL [18]. As such, HRQoL is a double-sided concept that includes both negative and positive aspects of health [19]. HRQoL is a PRO measure, as it reflects the patient's perspective, and is therefore by definition subjective. The two most frequently used instruments to assess HRQoL are the European Organization for Research and Treatment of Cancer (EORTC) Quality of Life Questionnaire (QLQ-C30) combined with its specific brain tumor module QLQ-BN20 [20, 21] and the Functional Assessment of Cancer Therapy-General (FACT-G) in conjunction with the FACT-Brain (FACT-BR) specific subscale [22]. Both questionnaires are validated in brain cancer patients and have subscales that include measurements of functioning, for example, physical and emotional well-being, as well as symptoms, such as headaches and seizures [23].

Compared with the EORTC questionnaires, the FACT questionnaires are more focused on psychosocial aspects and less on symptoms. Another frequently used instrument to measure HRQoL in brain tumor patients is the MD Anderson Symptom Inventory-Brain Tumor (MDASI-BT) module [24, 25]. The MDASI-BT has similarities with the EORTC QLQ-BN20 as it focuses on symptoms. Besides these cancer- and brain tumor-specific questionnaires, also more generic questionnaires are used, such as the Short Form 36 (SF-36) health survey [26] and the EuroQol five dimensions (EQ-5D) questionnaire [27]. These questionnaires are typically short and easy to use. Nevertheless, disease-specific questionnaires such as the EORTC QLQ-BN20, the FACT-BR, and the MDASI-BT are most suitable to measure the different aspects of functioning and symptoms in patients with CNS tumors.

Electronic collection of HRQoL, which is fastly being developed in recent years, provides the opportunity of home-based and/or waiting room data collection, with the advantages of saving time during clinic visits, improving accuracy of symptom management, and improving the communication between patient and physician [28]. Also, less administrative faults and higher compliance rates might be achieved [29]. Consequently, home-based measurements of HRQoL in patients with a primary CNS tumor may provide opportunities to improve the quality of care and clinical decision-making, as well as the use of data for research purposes [30].

43.2.2 Cognition

Cognitive functioning measured with a standardized neuropsychological test battery can be classified as an objective measurement of the cognitive abilities of a patient. Various neuropsychological tests cover different domains of cognitive functioning, such as attention, memory, and executive functioning. Several tests are available, and the choice depends on the goal of assessment. When the primary goal is to gain insight in cognitive functioning in clinical practice, a test battery is typically designed for each individual patient, depending on the clinical problems and/or location of the tumor. In clinical trials, often a standard test battery is used that is typically short and easy to administer. Neuropsychological tests and subtests can cover multiple domains, and sometimes the distinction between the domains is not very clear. Fluency tests, for example, are sometimes classified as (part of) executive functioning or language functioning, but are sometimes also scored as a separate domain. Table 43.1 provides an overview of neuropsychological tests that are often used in or suggested for brain tumor patients, although this table is not exhaustive as more neuropsychological tests exist.

Besides standardized test batteries, also screening instruments that cover multiple domains are used to assess cognitive functioning, like the Mini-Mental State Examination (MMSE) [44] and the Montreal Cognitive Assessment (MoCA) [45]. These tests can be administered in approximately 5–10 min and are scored on a 0–30 scale, with a lower score indicating more cognitive problems. Although screening instruments are less time-consuming, they only provide a very general representation of the patients' cognitive problems (impaired versus not impaired). They may be too insensitive to detect subtle cognitive deficits and do

Table 43.1 Neuropsychological tests per cognitive domain

Test	Neuropsychological domain	Short description
Digit span [31]	Auditory attention/short-term memory	A sequence of digits is read aloud, and the patient is to repeat forward or backward
TMT A [32]	Attention/processing speed	Circles with numbers are to be connected in sequential order as quickly as possible while maintaining accuracy
Hopkins verbal learning test-revised [33]	Verbal memory	Words are read aloud, and the patient is to repeat in forward or reverse order
Rey auditory verbal learning test [34]	Verbal memory	Words are read aloud, and the patients is to repeat immediately and delayed
Rey-Osterrieth complex figure: Recall [35]	Visual memory	A previously drawn complex figure is to be drawn as precise as possible
Controlled oral word association test (COWAT) [36]	Fluency/executive functioning	Naming as many words as possible belonging to one category or beginning with a certain letter within 1 min
Rey-Osterrieth complex figure: Copy [35]	Visuoconstruction/executive functioning	A complex figure is to be copied as precise as possible
TMT B [32]	Mental flexibility/executive functioning	Circles with numbers and letters are to be connected in alternating order as quickly as possible while maintaining accuracy
Stroop color-word test [37]	Interference/executive functioning	Conflicting words and colors are to be read as precise and quickly as possible
Wisconsin card sorting test [38]	Executive functioning	Stimulus cards must be sorted according to color, shape, and number without explanation but with feedback (right or wrong)
Frontal assessment battery (FAB) [39]	Executive functioning	Test battery including several tasks that measure frontal lobe functions
Line bisection test [40]	Perception	A mark is to be placed precisely in the center of a horizontal line
Benton facial recognition test [41]	Perception	A photo of a face is to be matched with a series of faces
Judgement of line orientation test [42]	Perception	Line segments of varying spatial orientation must be matched with a set of longer lines
Digit symbol [31]	Perception/information processing	A corresponding symbol is to be written down as quickly as possible
Grooved pegboard test [43]	Psychomotor speed/visuospatial functioning	Placing pins in holes as quickly as possible in the right orientation, using the dominant, non-dominant, and both hands

not adequately discriminate between the different domains. As a consequence, they seem less appropriate to assess the impact of a specific brain tumor and its treatment [15]. Because testing with an extensive neuropsychological test battery is time-consuming and may fatigue the patient, a shorter, less comprehensive test battery might therefore be preferred in most situations.

In contrast to objectively measured cognitive functioning, self-perceived cognitive functioning or cognitive complaints can be assessed with PRO measures. The Medical Outcomes Study (MOS) Cognitive Functioning Scale is the most commonly used stand-alone questionnaire in glioma patients [46–48] to measure cognitive complaints. This six-item scale assesses everyday problems in cognitive functioning, including difficulty with reasoning and problem-solving, slowed reaction time, and problems with concentration [49]. The Cognitive Failure Questionnaire (CFQ) [50] is another stand-alone questionnaire used in glioma [50] and meningioma [51, 52] patients that measures cognitive failures in three domains: perception, motor functioning, and memory [53]. Besides these stand-alone questionnaires, HRQoL questionnaires may also cover cognitive functioning, for example, the cognitive functioning scale of the EORTC QLQ-C30 and the supplementary FACT Cognitive questionnaire (FACT-Cog) [54].

Studies on the congruence between subjectively and objectively measured cognitive functioning in glioma patients showed that the level of agreement was low [47, 55]. Patients might over- or underestimate their cognitive abilities, due to impaired judgment abilities or comorbidities such as mood disorders. Overestimating of cognitive abilities, i.e., underreporting of cognitive complaints, can occur in patients with more severe objective cognitive impairment, e.g., when a lack of insight is part of the cognitive deficits, which may occur in patients with a tumor in the frontal lobe [15, 47, 56, 57]. Underestimating of cognitive abilities, i.e., overreporting of cognitive complaints, can occur in patients with, for example, attentional and motivational problems in the context of

mood disorders [15, 47, 58]. Hence, clinicians need to be aware that patients who do not report cognitive problems may still have cognitive deficits and the other way around. Therefore, both subjective and objective cognitive functioning should be measured in patients with a CNS tumor.

Computerized neuropsychological testing is, like electronic collection of HRQoL data, recently being developed. A computerized test battery can be an adequate, time-efficient, and cost-effective clinical instrument to detect cognitive impairments in patients with a CNS tumor [59, 60]. Other advantages of computerized assessment of cognitive functions include improved standardization and increased reliability of response time variables [61]. Similar to electronic collection of HRQoL data, computerized neuropsychological testing might be used both in clinical practice and in clinical trials.

43.2.3 Assessment of HRQoL and Cognition in Daily Clinical Practice and Clinical Trials

In daily clinical practice, HRQoL and cognitive assessment can be used to monitor the patient's functioning during the course of disease. Regular assessment of HRQoL provides the physician with information on the impact of a specific treatment strategy. Intended and unintended adverse effects of the treatment can be monitored, and if these problems require follow-up, symptom treatment can be initiated, or patients can be referred to other relevant healthcare professionals. Also, regular HRQoL assessments can increase the physician's awareness of the patient's functioning and well-being [62, 63]. This may improve the communication between the patient and the physician during follow-up consultations [64, 65].

Because survival and patients' functioning and well-being are both of importance in patients with a CNS tumor, the benefit of a specific treatment strategy in terms of prolonged survival needs to be weighed against the possible adverse effects of a treatment on a patients' functioning and well-being [66]. This information can be derived from clinical trials that also include measurements of HRQoL and/or cognitive functioning, besides measures of survival and treatment response on MRI. However, it should be kept in mind that the HRQoL and cognition outcomes in clinical trials concern groups of patients and may not be directly applicable to the individual patient. Also, several issues should be considered in the interpretation of results derived from clinical trials, such as the timing of the HRQoL/cognition measurements, the amount of dropout in the treatment arms, and different statistical techniques that are used [67, 68]. Determining the clinical benefit of treatment can, however, result in a trade-off discussion. When functioning and overall survival (OS) are both of interest, several situations may arise when comparing an experimental treatment with a standard treatment (Fig. 43.2). Both survival and functioning outcomes may lead to three situations: survival or functioning can be better, similar, or worse in the experimental arm when compared to the standard treatment arm. The best possible outcome is that the experimental treatment strategy results in prolonged survival and better functioning compared to the standard treatment strategy. In this situation, one would definitely opt for the experimental treatment. Similarly, no discussion on the best treatment option arises when the experimental treatment strategy results in both worse survival and patients' functioning and well-being. In this case, the standard treatment would be the preferred option. In the situation where survival is similar in the experimental and standard treatment, but functioning is better in the experimental or treatment arm, measurement of functioning can be conclusive in treatment decision-making. However, a dilemma arises when a suggested treatment prolongs survival, but worsens functioning, or vice versa. In these situations, the patients' perspective, as well as patient- and tumor-related characteristics, would be conclusive in decision-making, which could be achieved by shared decision-making.

43.3 Factors Impacting Patients' HRQoL and Cognition

43.3.1 Impact of the Tumor

Cognitive deficits are common in patients with a CNS tumor and have been found in 91% of the patients before surgery [69], although prevalences vary with tumor type. Cognitive deficits may be the predominant clinical feature in patients with a primary CNS lymphoma or low-grade glioma, while signs of high intracranial pressure may be the main feature in rapidly growing tumors such as glioblastoma and brain metastasis [15]. Different cognitive domains can be impaired, depending on the location and size of the tumor. As such, greater deficits in verbally mediated cognitive functions are seen in patients with left hemisphere tumors compared to patients with right hemisphere tumors. However, when compared to stroke, more subtle and diffuse patterns of cognitive deficits are seen in brain tumor patients [14, 15, 70]. Cognitive impairment is related to a lower generic and disease-specific HRQoL in meningioma [51] and glioma patients [46]. Even mild cognitive deficits may affect a patient's ability to function independently, affecting their social and emotional functioning to a great extent. Long-term survivors and patients with a more favorable prognosis with subtle cognitive deficits may especially suffer from cognitive problems, as these patients are confronted with their cognitive impairment when trying to resume their personal and professional life after treatment [71, 72].

Furthermore, seizures are a common symptom of patients with a CNS tumor. They are a typical presenting symptom of the disease, occurring in 30–85% of the glioma patients with the highest incidence in slow-growing tumors compared to fast-growing tumors [73], in 40% of the meningioma patients [74], in 20% of the metastatic patients, and in 80–90% of the ganglioglioma patients [73, 74]. Seizures may also occur at a later disease stage and often persist during the end-of-life phase [75]. When uncontrolled, seizures may lead to morbidity as well as a negative impact on patients' HRQoL and cognition [76].

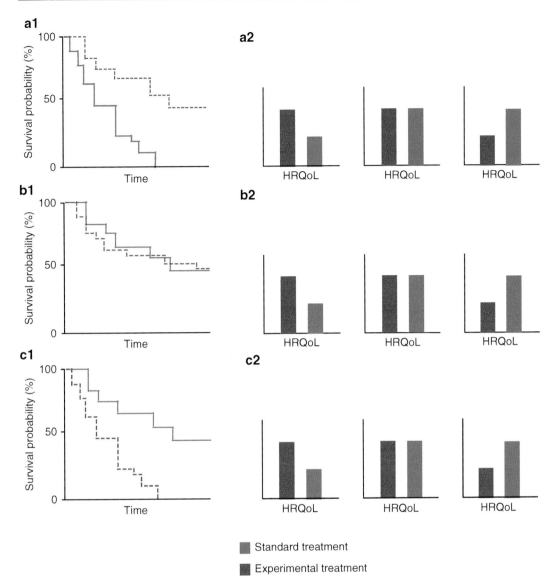

Fig. 43.2 Trade-off (reproduced from Dirven et al. [66]). Hypothetical scenarios for (overall or progression-free) survival and HRQoL outcomes when comparing experimental treatment (red, dotted line) with standard treatment (blue, solid line). Scenario A1 shows that the experimental treatment is superior to standard treatment in terms of survival probability. Scenario B1 shows that the experimental treatment and standard treatment are equal in terms of survival probability. Scenario C1 shows that the experimental treatment is inferior to standard treatment in terms of survival probability. Scenarios A2–C2 show that HRQoL is better for the experimental treatment (left panel), that HRQoL is equal for both treatment regimens (middle panel), or that HRQoL is worse for the experimental treatment (right panel). Trade-off is difficult when the survival probability of the experimental treatment is superior (scenario A1) but HRQoL worse (scenario A2, right panel) or when the survival probability is worse (scenario C1) but HRQoL better (scenario C2, left panel). The other scenarios do not result in difficult trade-off decisions

Other typical symptoms of patients with a CNS tumor are signs of intracranial pressure, such as headache and nausea and vomiting [77, 78]. Signs of intracranial pressure impacts function-ing directly but also indirectly by limiting patients' social life and serving as a psychosocial reminder of having a tumor [79]. Moreover, fatigue and sleep disorders [80–82]; focal symptoms such as hemiparesis, aphasia, or visual field deficits [83]; and psychiatric symptoms like mood and behavioral disorders [84, 85] are common in patients with a CNS tumor and have a negative impact on patients' HRQoL and cognition.

43.3.2 Impact of Antitumor Treatment

Besides the impact of the tumor, antitumor treatment in patients with a CNS tumor can also have an effect on the patients' functioning and well-being (Fig. 43.3).

43.3.2.1 Surgery

Maximal but safe resection or biopsy has been the standard treatment for decades for most tumors, whether or not combined with radiotherapy and/or chemotherapy in malignant tumors [4, 86]. In benign symptomatic tumors such as meningiomas, surgery can be curative if the tumor is completely removed [87]. In other tumors, such as primary CNS lymphoma that is an infiltrative tumor highly radiosensitive and chemosensitive, surgery is restricted to diagnostic biopsy, and in other cases surgery cannot be safely performed. In general, brain tumor patients experience less seizures, headache, and signs of intracranial pressure and report improved HRQoL after surgery [88–91]. However, surgery may also cause neurological deficits by damaging the surrounding tissue, for example, when

surgery is performed in eloquent areas, thereby impairing HRQoL and cognition. Despite an overall improvement of HRQoL, HRQoL after resection in meningioma patients was still found to be impaired compared to the general population [92, 93]. Nevertheless, HRQoL in glioma patients who underwent a gross total resection improved over time [94]. With respect to cognition, a large proportion of meningioma patients showed postoperative improvement on cognitive tests, but cognitive problems still existed [60]. In glioma patients, studies show a high percentage of postoperative cognitive deficits [95, 96]. These deficits may however be temporary, as cognitive functioning may improve over time due to the plasticity of the brain [97]. Hence, when possible to safely perform surgery, the relief of symptoms seems to outweigh the short-term side effects.

43.3.2.2 Radiotherapy

Radiotherapy, following surgery, is the standard treatment in many glioma subtypes and may be applied in combination with chemotherapy, depending on the type of tumor and clinical factors [98]. In patients with a meningioma [87], primary CNS lymphoma [99], and brain metastases [100], radiation may be administered as adjuvant treatment, or as an alternative to surgery in case of progression, clinical signs, and high-risk location, or when tumors are refractory to other treatments. Radiotherapy may stabilize the disease and delay tumor progression, thereby preserving HRQoL and cog-

Fig. 43.3 Impact of symptoms and treatment on functioning and well-being

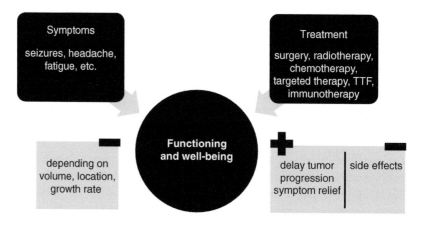

nition. However, radiotherapy may also have a negative impact on HRQoL and cognition. The neighboring tissue may be damaged by radiation, introducing neurotoxicity and encephalopathy. Radiotherapy can cause immediate side effects, such as fatigue or signs of increased intracranial pressure, and long-term side effects such as cognitive problems. Acute and short-term effects may occur directly up till months after radiotherapy but should diminish within 12 months, whereas long-term effects can occur many years after radiotherapy [101]. On the short term, radiotherapy was not associated with a decline in HRQoL in high-grade glioma patients [102–104]; however, a reduction in physical functioning was found in meningioma patients at the end of radiotherapy [105]. A transient cognitive impairment may occur consisting of short-term memory and attentional deficits [15]. Studies on the long-term effects of radiotherapy suggest that this treatment causes cognitive problems about 6 years after treatment in glioma patients [48, 106, 107]. Diffuse white matter encephalopathy, especially following whole-brain radiotherapy (WBRT), can occur on the long term and may progress to irreversible damage to the brain tissue, mainly characterized by cognitive decline. Ultimately, it may lead to dementia, severely impairing HRQoL [108, 109]. To minimize the negative effect of radiotherapy of HRQoL and cognition, less invasive techniques like lower fraction and overall dose instead of high dose and stereotactic radiotherapy (STR) instead of WBRT are administered when possible. Indeed, low-grade glioma patients who underwent high-dose radiotherapy reported worse HRQoL with respect to fatigue, malaise, and insomnia compared to patients who underwent low-dose radiation [15, 110]. Similarly, STR was found to be the preferred treatment compared to WBRT with better HRQoL and cognitive outcomes in brain metastasis patients [111]. STR may however cause (persistent) cerebral edema in combination with focal radiation necrosis in some patients [112, 113], which clearly may have a negative impact on HRQoL [114]. Thus, radiotherapy may have a (temporarily) negative impact on the short term by causing cerebral edema, and also long-term cognitive effects, especially in patients treated with WBRT and high-dose radiation, may occur. Nevertheless, treating the tumor by stabilizing the disease and delaying tumor progression and thereby preserving HRQoL and cognition outweighs the negative effects in most patients.

43.3.2.3 Chemotherapy

Systemic chemotherapy may be administered to patients with CNS tumors as primary treatment, in the adjuvant setting, concomitant to radiotherapy, or for tumor recurrence in patients with a glioma [98], meningioma [87], primary CNS lymphoma [115], brain metastases [10], and pituitary tumors [116]. Chemotherapy is aimed to postpone tumor progression or reduce tumor load, with the possibility of maintaining or even improving patients' functioning and well-being. However, the adverse effects of chemotherapy may result in a temporary deterioration of functioning. The effect of chemotherapy alone on HRQoL and cognition may be difficult to discern from other treatments, especially concomitant treatments [15]. In contrast to the late radiation encephalopathy, side effects of chemotherapy tend to arise during or shortly after chemotherapy [117]. For example, the administration of procarbazine, lomustine, and vincristine (PCV) following radiotherapy in anaplastic oligodendrogliomas resulted in increased nausea/vomiting, appetite loss, and drowsiness during and shortly after administration, but not on the long term [103]. Likewise, the addition of temozolomide (TMZ) to radiotherapy led to worse social functioning on the short term in glioblastoma patients, but no long-term differences between the treatment arms were found [118]. Cognitive deficits caused by PCV have only been reported with high-dose regimens [119], and chemotherapy often has little adverse neurocognitive effects when given in conventional doses [117]. For instance, the addition of PCV in low-grade glioma patients did not result in lower neurocognitive scores on the MMSE at 5-year follow-up [120]. Similarly, treatment with TMZ did not have a negative effect on HRQoL and cognition in patients with brain metastases [121, 122]. The effect of chemotherapy alone on cognition and HRQoL was found to be less detrimental compared to combined WBRT and chemotherapy in patients with primary CNS lymphoma, as 83% of the long-term survivors reported a good HRQoL and 95% of the patients showed preserved or improved cognitive functioning [123, 124]. Taken together, several aspects of HRQoL may deteriorate during and shortly after chemotherapy, but HRQoL and cognition remain more or less stable on the long term.

43.3.2.4 Targeted and Immunotherapy

The addition of angiogenesis inhibitors such as bevacizumab inhibits angiogenesis, thereby influencing tumor invasion and proliferation in highly vascular tumors like glioblastoma. In two trials where bevacizumab was added to the standard care for glioblastoma patients, a longer progression-free survival (PFS) time was found [102, 125]. HRQoL was found to be persevered in one study [102], while HRQoL and cognition were reported to deteriorate in the other study [125]. The addition of cilengitide, a selective inhibitor of two integrins that are thought to be important for angiogenesis of tumor cells [126], was not found to result in an improved OS or PFS in glioblastoma patients and did not negatively impact HRQoL [127, 128]. Targeted therapy including erlotinib [129] and gefitinib [121, 130] in patients with brain metastases originating from various primary cancers outside the CNS did not negatively impact HRQoL and/or cognition. On the contrary, HRQoL and cognition were improved in patients with a primary CNS lymphoma after administration of a combination of rituximab, TMZ, and high-dose methotrexate [131].

Immunotherapy, which gained attention in the treatment of patients with other tumor entities, also has been explored in patients with CNS tumors in the past few years [132, 133]. Trials in glioblastoma [132], anaplastic meningioma [134], and primary CNS lymphoma patients [135, 136] are ongoing, and the HRQoL and cognition results are to be awaited. All in all, the addition of targeted treatment so far does not seem to negatively impact HRQoL and cognition in patients with a CNS tumor, and the results of immunotherapy on HRQoL and cognition remain to be investigated.

43.3.2.5 New Treatment Modalities

Tumor-treating fields (TTFields) is a new therapeutic device being used for the treatment of glioblastoma, resulting in prolonged PFS and OS in newly diagnosed glioblastoma patients when administered together with adjuvant TMZ [137]. A first study in recurrent glioblastoma patients receiving chemotherapy or TTFields showed that physical functioning might be slightly worse with TTFields, while subjective cognitive functioning and emotional functioning favored TTFields [138]. However, only basic statistical methods were used, and more comprehensive analysis is required to understand the impact of TTFields on HRQoL [139]. Results in newly diagnosed glioma patients showed that only itchy skin, due to irritation of the skin beneath the electrodes, was related to TTFields, while other functioning and symptom scales of HRQoL neither deteriorated nor improved with TTFields [140]. Cognitive functioning was however not assessed.

43.4 Improving HRQoL and Cognition

43.4.1 Supportive Treatment

Supportive treatment improves HRQoL and cognition indirectly by reducing the signs and symptoms of the tumor. In addition to surgery, antiepileptic drugs (AEDs) are administered to patients to achieve sustained seizure control [88, 141]. Reducing the seizure burden with second-generation AEDs such as levetiracetam and oxcarbazepine minimalizes the negative impact of seizures on HRQoL and cognition [142, 143]. However, AEDs may also cause side effects, thereby directly deteriorating cognitive functioning and HRQoL [76, 144]. Therefore, AED withdrawal might be considered in selected patients who have achieved stable disease and long-term seizure freedom, but this should be carefully weighed against the risk of seizure recurrence [144].

Symptoms of elevated intracranial pressure, such as headache, nausea and vomiting, visual disturbances, drowsiness, and decreased consciousness, may be alleviated by corticosteroids [145]. The relief of these symptoms results in an improved HRQoL, while adverse effects such as weakness and gastrointestinal problems may decrease HRQoL. Side effects of corticosteroids can, however, be partly overcome by adjusting the dose [145].

Management of other symptoms such as fatigue, mood disorders, and anxiety can be pharmacological or non-pharmacological, including physical exercise and cognitive behavioral therapies. In general, some studies reported small success with pharmacological therapies, but no randomized trials showed beneficial effects on fatigue [146, 147] or mood disorders [148, 149]. Cognitive behavioral therapy [50], multimodal psychosocial interventions [150], acceptance and commitment therapy [151], Internet-based guided self-help course [152], and telephone-based support [153] might improve fatigue, depression, and/or anxiety in patients with a CNS tumor.

43.4.2 Improving HRQoL

In addition to antitumor treatment and supportive treatment, specific interventions to improve HRQoL in patients with a CNS tumor are warranted. First of all, routine measurement of HRQoL in itself is important to improve functioning and well-being in brain tumor patients since it may enhance the communication between patient and caregiver, identify problems, monitor changes, identify preferences, and subsequently improve HRQoL [154–156]. Improved functioning and well-being are also achieved by a multidisciplinary approach, often including a nurse practitioner who serves as an ongoing central point of contact between the patient and healthcare professionals [157].

43.4.3 Improving Cognition

Pharmacological intervention studies have investigated the use of methylphenidate [148], donepezil [158, 159], and a combination of methylphenidate and modafinil [160] to improve cognitive functioning. Although some studies have reported successes, limitations in the methods and study design, such as the lack of a control group, hamper generalizability of the results [71].

Non-pharmacological studies to improve cognition include cognitive rehabilitation programs, which are focused on improving attention, memory, and executive functioning in brain tumor patients [50]. A large invention study in mainly low-grade glioma patients [50] showed that immediate assessment after rehabilitation improved both cognitive complaints and cognitive deficits, and at 6 months after treatment, attention, verbal memory, and reduced mental fatigue were improved compared to the waiting-list group. Another randomized study in patients with primary brain tumors found an improved visual attention and verbal memory after cognitive training [161]. Results of other (pilot) studies including neurocognitive training [162, 163], exercise training [164–166], and virtual reality [167] suggest that rehabilitation programs have modest positive effects and are highly welcomed by patients and caregivers [162, 168]. Therefore, cognitive rehabilitation should be considered especially in young patients with a relatively favorable prognosis and in stable brain tumor patients with cognitive complaints or deficits.

43.5 Conclusions and Future Directions

Incorporating the patients' perspective on the impact of treatment in clinical practice and trials has become more important in recent years. HRQoL and cognition are two important endpoints to measure functioning and well-being, and several instruments are available that can be used for assessment. Both the tumor and its treatment can have an impact on HRQoL and cognition. Treatment and symptom management seem to have a positive effect on functioning and well-being by reducing signs and symptoms, while most side effects that negatively impact functioning and well-being are temporary. Altogether, antitumor treatment that prolongs (progression-free) survival seems to outweigh the (temporary) side effects that negatively impact functioning and well-being.

Although there are some interventions that may improve HRQoL and cognitive functioning somewhat in patients with a CNS tumor, these should be further developed. Multidisciplinary (home-based) rehabilitation programs that include physical exercise, cognitive rehabilitation, and/or therapy are promising in patients with a CNS tumor.

References

1. Wiemels J, Wrensch M, Claus EB (2010) Epidemiology and etiology of meningioma. J Neurooncol 99(3):307–314
2. Whittle IR, Smith C, Navoo P, Collie D (2004) Meningiomas. Lancet 363(9420):1535–1543
3. Ostrom QT, Gittleman H, Farah P, Ondracek A, Chen Y, Wolinsky Y et al (2013) CBTRUS statistical report: primary brain and central nervous system tumors diagnosed in the United States in 2006-2010. Neuro-Oncology 15(suppl_2):ii1–ii56
4. Ricard D, Idbaih A, Ducray F, Lahutte M, Hoang-Xuan K, Delattre J-Y (2012) Primary brain tumours in adults. Lancet 379(9830):1984–1996
5. Louis DN, Perry A, Reifenberger G, von Deimling A, Figarella-Branger D, Cavenee WK et al (2016) The 2016 World Health Organization classification of tumors of the central nervous system: a summary. Acta Neuropathol 131(6):803–820
6. Davis FG, Dolecek TA, McCarthy BJ, Villano JL (2012) Toward determining the lifetime occurrence of metastatic brain tumors estimated from 2007 United States cancer incidence data. Neuro-Oncology 14(9):1171–1177
7. van Alkemade H, de Leau M, Dieleman EM, Kardaun JW, van Os R, Vandertop WP et al (2012) Impaired survival and long-term neurological problems in benign meningioma. Neuro-Oncology 14(5):658–666
8. Ho VK, Reijneveld JC, Enting RH, Bienfait HP, Robe P, Baumert BG et al (2014) Changing incidence and improved survival of gliomas. Eur J Cancer 50(13):2309–2318
9. Barnholtz-Sloan JS, Sloan AE, Davis FG, Vigneau FD, Lai P, Sawaya RE (2004) Incidence proportions of brain metastases in patients diagnosed (1973 to 2001) in the metropolitan Detroit cancer surveillance system. J Clin Oncol 22(14):2865–2872
10. Patchell RA (2003) The management of brain metastases. Cancer Treat Rev 29(6):533–540
11. Efficace F, Taphoorn M (2012) Methodological issues in designing and reporting health-related quality of life in cancer clinical trials: the challenge of brain cancer studies. J Neurooncol 108(2):221–226
12. European Medicines Agency (2016) Appendix 2 to the guideline on the evaluation of anticancer medicinal products in man: the use of patient-reported outcome (PRO) measures in oncology studies. https://www.ema.europa.eu/documents/other/appendix-2-guideline-evaluation-anticancer-medicinal-productsman_en.pdf
13. World Health Organization (1980) International classification of impairments, disabilities, and handicaps: a manual of classification relating to the consequences of disease, published in accordance with resolution WHA29. 35 of the Twenty-ninth World Health Assembly, May 1976
14. Schagen S, Klein M, Reijneveld J, Brain E, Deprez S, Joly F et al (2014) Monitoring and optimising cognitive function in cancer patients: present knowledge and future directions. Eur J Cancer Suppl 12(1):29–40
15. Taphoorn MJ, Klein M (2004) Cognitive deficits in adult patients with brain tumours. Lancet Neurol 3(3):159–168
16. Overdorp EJ, Kessels RP, Claassen JA, Oosterman JM (2016) The combined effect of neuropsychological and neuropathological deficits on instrumental activities of daily living in older adults: a systematic review. Neuropsychol Rev 26(1):92–106
17. Sikkes S, De Lange-de Klerk E, Pijnenburg Y, Scheltens P (2009) A systematic review of instrumental activities of daily living scales in dementia: room for improvement. J Neurol Neurosurg Psychiatry 80(1):7–12
18. Guyatt GH, Ferrans CE, Halyard MY, Revicki DA, Symonds TL, Varricchio CG et al (eds) (2007) Exploration of the value of health-related quality-of-life information from clinical research and into clinical practice. Mayo Clinic proceedings. Elsevier, Amsterdam
19. World Health Organization (1948) Preamble to the Constitution of the World Health Organization, as adopted by the International Health Conference, New York, pp. 19–22 (June 1946): signed on 22 July 1946 by the Representatives of 61 States,(Official Records of the World Health Organization, No. 2 p. 100) and Entered into Force on 7 April 1948. http://www.who.int/abouwho/en/definition.html
20. Aaronson NK, Ahmedzai S, Bergman B, Bullinger M, Cull A, Duez NJ et al (1993) The European Organization for Research and Treatment of cancer QLQ-C30: a quality-of-life instrument for use in international clinical trials in oncology. J Natl Cancer Inst 85(5):365–376

21. Taphoorn MJ, Claassens L, Aaronson NK, Coens C, Mauer M, Osoba D et al (2010) An international validation study of the EORTC brain cancer module (EORTC QLQ-BN20) for assessing health-related quality of life and symptoms in brain cancer patients. Eur J Cancer 46(6):1033–1040

22. Cella DF, Tulsky DS, Gray G, Sarafian B, Linn E, Bonomi A et al (1993) The functional assessment of cancer therapy scale: development and validation of the general measure. J Clin Oncol 11(3):570–579

23. Chow R, Lao N, Popovic M, Chow E, Cella D, Beaumont J et al (2014) Comparison of the EORTC QLQ-BN20 and the FACT-Br quality of life questionnaires for patients with primary brain cancers: a literature review. Support Care Cancer 22(9):2593–2598

24. Cleeland CS, Mendoza TR, Wang XS, Chou C, Harle MT, Morrissey M et al (2000) Assessing symptom distress in cancer patients. Cancer 89(7):1634–1646

25. Armstrong TS, Mendoza T, Gring I, Coco C, Cohen MZ, Eriksen L et al (2006) Validation of the MD Anderson symptom inventory brain tumor module (MDASI-BT). J Neurooncol 80(1):27–35

26. Ware JE Jr, Sherbourne CD (1992) The MOS 36-item short-form health survey (SF-36): I. conceptual framework and item selection. Med Care 30:473–483

27. Rabin R, Charro FD (2001) EQ-5D: a measure of health status from the EuroQol group. Ann Med 33(5):337–343

28. Cella D, Gershon R, Lai J-S, Choi S (2007) The future of outcomes measurement: item banking, tailored short-forms, and computerized adaptive assessment. Qual Life Res 16(1):133–141

29. Stone AA, Shiffman S, Schwartz JE, Broderick JE, Hufford MR (2003) Patient compliance with paper and electronic diaries. Control Clin Trials 24(2):182–199

30. Dirven L, Groenvold M, Taphoorn MJ, Conroy T, Tomaszewski KA, Young T et al (2017) Psychometric evaluation of an item bank for computerized adaptive testing of the EORTC QLQ-C30 cognitive functioning dimension in cancer patients. Qual Life Res 26:2919–2929

31. Wechsler D (2008) Wechsler adult intelligence scale–Fourth Edition (WAIS–IV), vol 22. NCS Pearson, San Antonio, TX, p 498

32. Reitan RM (1958) Validity of the trail making test as an indicator of organic brain damage. Percept Mot Skills 8(3):271–276

33. Benedict RH, Schretlen D, Groninger L, Brandt J (1998) Hopkins verbal learning test–revised: normative data and analysis of inter-form and test-retest reliability. Clin Neuropsychol 12(1):43–55

34. Rey A (1958) L'examen clinique en psychologie. Presses Universitaries De France, Oxford

35. Meyers JE, Meyers KR (1995) Rey complex figure test and recognition trial professional manual. Psychological Assessment Resources, Odessa

36. Ruff R, Light R, Parker S, Levin H (1996) Benton controlled oral word association test: reliability and updated norms. Arch Clin Neuropsychol 11(4):329–338

37. Stroop JR (1935) Studies of interference in serial verbal reactions. J Exp Psychol 18(6):643

38. Nelson HE (1976) A modified card sorting test sensitive to frontal lobe defects. Cortex 12(4):313–324

39. Dubois B, Slachevsky A, Litvan I, Pillon B (2000) The FAB a frontal assessment battery at bedside. Neurology 55(11):1621–1626

40. Schenkenberg T, Bradford D, Ajax E (1980) Line bisection and unilateral visual neglect in patients with neurologic impairment. Neurology 30(5):509

41. Benton A, Van Allen M (1968) Impairment in facial recognition in patients with cerebral disease. Cortex 4(4):344–358

42. Benton A, Hannay HJ, Varney NR (1975) Visual perception of line direction in patients with unilateral brain disease. Neurology 25(10):907

43. Ruff RM, Parker SB (1993) Gender-and age-specific changes in motor speed and eye-hand coordination in adults: normative values for the finger tapping and grooved pegboard tests. Percept Mot Skills 76(3_suppl):1219–1230

44. Folstein MF, Folstein SE, McHugh PR (1975) "Mini-mental state": a practical method for grading the cognitive state of patients for the clinician. J Psychiatr Res 12(3):189–198

45. Nasreddine ZS, Phillips NA, Bédirian V, Charbonneau S, Whitehead V, Collin I et al (2005) The Montreal cognitive assessment, MoCA: a brief screening tool for mild cognitive impairment. J Am Geriatr Soc 53(4):695–699

46. Boele FW, Zant M, Heine EC, Aaronson NK, Taphoorn MJ, Reijneveld JC et al (2014) The association between cognitive functioning and health-related quality of life in low-grade glioma patients. Neurooncol Pract 1(2):40–46

47. Gehring K, Taphoorn MJ, Sitskoorn MM, Aaronson NK (2015) Predictors of subjective versus objective cognitive functioning in patients with stable grades II and III glioma. Neurooncol Pract 2(1):20–31

48. Aaronson NK, Taphoorn MJ, Heimans JJ, Postma TJ, Gundy CM, Beute GN et al (2011) Compromised health-related quality of life in patients with low-grade glioma. J Clin Oncol 29(33):4430–4435

49. Stewart AL, Ware JE (1992) Measuring functioning and Well-being: the medical outcomes study approach. Duke University Press, Durham, NC

50. Gehring K, Sitskoorn MM, Gundy CM, Sikkes SA, Klein M, Postma TJ et al (2009) Cognitive rehabilitation in patients with gliomas: a randomized, controlled trial. J Clin Oncol 27(22):3712–3722

51. Waagemans ML, van Nieuwenhuizen D, Dijkstra M, Wumkes M, Dirven CM, Leenstra S et al (2011) Long-term impact of cognitive deficits and epilepsy on quality of life in patients with low-grade meningiomas. Neurosurgery 69(1):72–79

52. van der Vossen S, Schepers VP, van der Sprenkel JWB, Visser-Meily J, Post MW (2014) Cognitive and emotional problems in patients after cerebral meningioma surgery. J Rehabil Med 46(5):430–437

53. Broadbent DE, Cooper PF, FitzGerald P, Parkes KR (1982) The cognitive failures questionnaire (CFQ) and its correlates. Br J Clin Psychol 21(1):1–16

54. Jacobs SR, Jacobsen PB, Booth-Jones M, Wagner LI, Anasetti C (2007) Evaluation of the functional assessment of cancer therapy cognitive scale with hematopoietic stem cell transplant patients. J Pain Symptom Manag 33(1):13–23

55. Klein M, Reijneveld JC, Heimans JJ (2008) Subjective ratings vs. objective measurement of cognitive function: in regard to Van Beek et al. (Int J Radiat Oncol Biol Phys 2007; 68: 986–991). Int J Radiat Oncol Biol Phys 70(3):961–962

56. Taphoorn M, Heimans J, Snoek F, Lindeboom J, Oosterink B, Wolbers J et al (1992) Assessment of quality of life in patients treated for low-grade glioma: a preliminary report. J Neurol Neurosurg Psychiatry 55(5):372–376

57. Schmidinger M, Linzmayer L, Becherer A, Fazeny-Doerner B, Fakhrai N, Prayer D et al (2003) Psychometric-and quality-of-life assessment in long-term glioblastoma survivors. J Neurooncol 63(1):55–61

58. Cull A, Hay C, Love S, Mackie M, Smets E, Stewart M (1996) What do cancer patients mean when they complain of concentration and memory problems? Br J Cancer 74(10):1674–1679

59. Tucha O, Smely C, Preier M, Becker G, Paul GM, Lange KW (2003) Preoperative and postoperative cognitive functioning in patients with frontal meningiomas. J Neurosurg 98(1):21–31

60. Meskal I, Gehring K, van der Linden SD, Rutten G-JM, Sitskoorn MM (2015) Cognitive improvement in meningioma patients after surgery: clinical relevance of computerized testing. J Neurooncol 121(3):617–625

61. Wilken J, Kane R, Sullivan C, Wallin M, Usiskin J, Quig M et al (2003) The utility of computerized neuropsychological assessment of cognitive dysfunction in patients with relapsing-remitting multiple sclerosis. Mult Scler J 9(2):119–127

62. Velikova G, Awad N, Coles-Gale R, Wright EP, Brown JM, Selby PJ (2008) The clinical value of quality of life assessment in oncology practice—a qualitative study of patient and physician views. Psychooncology 17(7):690–698

63. Taphoorn MJ, Sizoo EM, Bottomley A (2010) Review on quality of life issues in patients with primary brain tumors. Oncologist 15(6):618–626

64. Detmar SB, Muller MJ, Schornagel JH, Wever LD, Aaronson NK (2002) Health-related quality-of-life assessments and patient-physician communication: a randomized controlled trial. JAMA 288(23):3027–3034

65. Rodriguez KL, Bayliss NK, Alexander SC, Jeffreys AS, Olsen MK, Pollak KI et al (2011) Effect of patient and patient–oncologist relationship characteristics on communication about health-related quality of life. Psychooncology 20(9):935–942

66. Dirven L, Reijneveld JC, Taphoorn MJ (eds) (2014) Health-related quality of life or quantity of life: a difficult trade-off in primary brain tumors? Seminars in oncology. Elsevier, Amsterdam

67. Dirven L, Reijneveld JC, Aaronson NK, Bottomley A, Uitdehaag BM, Taphoorn MJ (2013) Health-related quality of life in patients with brain tumors: limitations and additional outcome measures. Curr Neurol Neurosci Rep 13(7):359

68. Bottomley A, Pe M, Sloan J, Basch E, Bonnetain F, Calvert M (2016) Setting international standards in analyzing patient-reported outcomes and quality of life endpoints data (SISAQOL) consortium. Analysing data from patient-reported outcome and quality of life endpoints for cancer clinical trials: a start in setting international standards. Lancet Oncol 17:e510–e5e4

69. Tucha O, Smely C, Preier M, Lange KW (2000) Cognitive deficits before treatment among patients with brain tumors. Neurosurgery 47(2):324–334

70. Anderson SW, Damasio H, Tranel D (1990) Neuropsychological impairments associated with lesions caused by tumor or stroke. Arch Neurol 47(4):397–405

71. Gehring K, Sitskoorn MM, Aaronson NK, Taphoorn MJ (2008) Interventions for cognitive deficits in adults with brain tumours. Lancet Neurol 7(6):548–560

72. Boele FW, Klein M, Reijneveld JC, Verdonck-de Leeuw IM, Heimans JJ (2014) Symptom management and quality of life in glioma patients. CNS Oncol 3(1):37–47

73. Kerkhof M, Vecht CJ (2013) Seizure characteristics and prognostic factors of gliomas. Epilepsia 54(s9):12–17

74. Xue H, Sveinsson O, Tomson T, Mathiesen T (2015) Intracranial meningiomas and seizures: a review of the literature. Acta Neurochir 157(9):1541–1548

75. Pace A, Dirven L, Koekkoek JA, Golla H, Fleming J, Rudà R et al (2017) European Association for Neuro-Oncology (EANO) guidelines for palliative care in adults with glioma. Lancet Oncol 18(6):e330–ee40

76. Klein M, Engelberts NH, van der Ploeg HM, Kasteleijn-Nolst Trenité DG, Aaronson NK, Taphoorn MJ et al (2003) Epilepsy in low-grade gliomas: the impact on cognitive function and quality of life. Ann Neurol 54(4):514–520

77. Kirby S, Purdy RA (2014) Headaches and brain tumors. Neurol Clin 32(2):423–432

78. Forsyth PA, Posner JB (1993) Headaches in patients with brain tumors a study of 111 patients. Neurology 43(9):1678

79. Bennett SR, Cruickshank G, Lindenmeyer A, Morris SR (2016) Investigating the impact of headaches on the quality of life of patients with glioblastoma multiforme: a qualitative study. BMJ Open 6(11):e011616

80. Armstrong TS, Gilbert MR (2012) Practical strategies for management of fatigue and sleep disorders in people with brain tumors. Neuro-Oncology 14(Suppl 4):iv65

81. Wellisch DK, Kaleita TA, Freeman D, Cloughesy T, Goldman J (2002) Predicting major depression in brain tumor patients. Psychooncology 11(3):230–238

82. Robertson ME, McSherry F, Herndon JE, Peters KB (2016) Insomnia and its associations in patients with recurrent glial neoplasms. Springerplus 5(1):1–5

83. DeAngelis LM (2001) Brain tumors. N Engl J Med 344(2):114–123

84. Arnold SD, Forman LM, Brigidi BD, Carter KE, Schweitzer HA, Quinn HE et al (2008) Evaluation and characterization of generalized anxiety and depression in patients with primary brain tumors. Neuro-Oncology 10(2):171–181

85. Madhusoodanan S, Ting MB, Farah T, Ugur U (2015) Psychiatric aspects of brain tumors: a review. World J Psychiatry 5(3):273

86. Asthagiri AR, Pouratian N, Sherman J, Ahmed G, Shaffrey ME (2007) Advances in brain tumor surgery. Neurol Clin 25(4):975–1003

87. Goldbrunner R, Minniti G, Preusser M, Jenkinson MD, Sallabanda K, Houdart E et al (2016) EANO guidelines for the diagnosis and treatment of meningiomas. Lancet Oncol 17(9):e383–ee91

88. Chozick BS, Reinert SE, Greenblatt SH (1996) Incidence of seizures after surgery for supratentorial meningiomas: a modern analysis. J Neurosurg 84(3):382–386

89. Englot DJ, Berger MS, Barbaro NM, Chang EF (2011) Predictors of seizure freedom after resection of supratentorial low-grade gliomas: a review. J Neurosurg 115(2):240–244

90. Jakola AS, Gulati M, Gulati S, Solheim O (2012) The influence of surgery on quality of life in patients with intracranial meningiomas: a prospective study. J Neurooncol 110(1):137–144

91. Brown PD, Ballman KV, Rummans TA, Maurer MJ, Sloan JA, Boeve BF et al (2006) Prospective study of quality of life in adults with newly diagnosed high-grade gliomas. J Neurooncol 76(3):283–291

92. Mohsenipour I, Deusch E, Gabl M, Hofer M, Twerdy K (2001) Quality of life in patients after meningioma resection. Acta Neurochir 143(6):547–553

93. Zamanipoor Najafabadi A, Peeters M, Dirven L, Broekman MD, Peul W, Taphoorn M et al (2016) P11.02 health-related quality of life in meningioma patients-a systematic review. Neuro-Oncology 18(suppl_4):iv65–iiv6

94. Brown PD, Maurer MJ, Rummans TA, Pollock BE, Ballman KV, Sloan JA et al (2005) A prospective study of quality of life in adults with newly diagnosed high-grade gliomas: the impact of the extent of resection on quality of life and survival. Neurosurgery 57(3):495–504

95. Reijneveld J, Sitskoorn M, Klein M, Nuyen J, Taphoorn M (2001) Cognitive status and quality of life in patients with suspected versus proven low-grade gliomas. Neurology 56(5):618–623

96. Talacchi A, Santini B, Savazzi S, Gerosa M (2011) Cognitive effects of tumour and surgical treatment in glioma patients. J Neurooncol 103(3):541–549

97. Duffau H, Capelle L, Denvil D, Sichez N, Gatignol P, Lopes M et al (2003) Functional recovery after surgical resection of low grade gliomas in eloquent brain: hypothesis of brain compensation. J Neurol Neurosurg Psychiatry 74(7):901–907

98. Weller M, van den Bent M, Tonn JC, Stupp R, Preusser M, Cohen-Jonathan-Moyal E et al (2017) European Association for Neuro-Oncology (EANO) guideline on the diagnosis and treatment of adult astrocytic and oligodendroglial gliomas. Lancet Oncol 18(6):e315–e329

99. Hoang-Xuan K, Bessell E, Bromberg J, Hottinger AF, Preusser M, Rudà R et al (2015) Diagnosis and treatment of primary CNS lymphoma in immunocompetent patients: guidelines from the European Association for Neuro-Oncology. Lancet Oncol 16(7):e322–e332

100. Soffietti R, Abacioglu U, Baumert B, Combs SE, Kinhult S, Kros JM et al (2017) Diagnosis and treatment of brain metastases from solid tumors: guidelines from the European Association of Neuro-Oncology (EANO). Neuro-Oncology 19(2):162–174

101. Sheline GE, Wara WM, Smith V (1980) Therapeutic irradiation and brain injury. Int J Radiat Oncol Biol Phys 6(9):1215–1228

102. Taphoorn MJ, Henriksson R, Bottomley A, Cloughesy T, Wick W, Mason WP et al (2015) Health-related quality of life in a randomized phase III study of bevacizumab, temozolomide, and radiotherapy in newly diagnosed glioblastoma. J Clin Oncol 33(19):2166–2175

103. Taphoorn MJ, van den Bent MJ, Mauer ME, Coens C, Delattre J-Y, Brandes AA et al (2007) Health-related quality of life in patients treated for anaplastic oligodendroglioma with adjuvant chemotherapy: results of a European Organisation for Research and Treatment of Cancer randomized clinical trial. J Clin Oncol 25(36):5723–5730

104. Ernst-Stecken A, Ganslandt O, Lambrecht U, Sauer R, Grabenbauer G (2007) Survival and quality of life after hypofractionated stereotactic radiotherapy for recurrent malignant glioma. J Neurooncol 81(3):287–294

105. Henzel M, Fokas E, Sitter H, Wittig A, Engenhart-Cabillic R (2013) Quality of life after stereotactic radiotherapy for meningioma: a prospective non-randomized study. J Neurooncol 113(1):135–141

106. Douw L, Klein M, Fagel SS, van den Heuvel J, Taphoorn MJ, Aaronson NK et al (2009) Cognitive and radiological effects of radiotherapy in patients with low-grade glioma: long-term follow-up. Lancet Neurol 8(9):810–818

107. Klein M, Heimans J, Aaronson N, Van der Ploeg H, Grit J, Muller M et al (2002) Effect of radiotherapy and other treatment-related factors on mid-term to

long-term cognitive sequelae in low-grade gliomas: a comparative study. Lancet 360(9343):1361–1368

108. Monje ML, Palmer T (2003) Radiation injury and neurogenesis. Curr Opin Neurol 16(2):129–134

109. Crossen JR, Garwood D, Glatstein E, Neuwelt EA (1994) Neurobehavioral sequelae of cranial irradiation in adults: a review of radiation-induced encephalopathy. J Clin Oncol 12(3):627–642

110. Kiebert G, Curran D, Aaronson N, Bolla M, Menten J, Rutten E et al (1998) Quality of life after radiation therapy of cerebral low-grade gliomas of the adult: results of a randomised phase III trial on dose response (EORTC trial 22844). Eur J Cancer 34(12):1902–1909

111. Habets EJ, Dirven L, Wiggenraad RG, Verbeek-de Kanter A, Lycklama à Nijeholt GJ, Zwinkels H et al (2015) Neurocognitive functioning and health-related quality of life in patients treated with stereotactic radiotherapy for brain metastases: a prospective study. Neuro-Oncology 18(3):435–444

112. Gazit I, Har-Nof S, Cohen ZR, Zibly Z, Nissim U, Spiegelmann R (2015) Radiosurgery for brain metastases and cerebral edema. J Clin Neurosci 22(3):535–538

113. Sheehan JP, Lee C-C, Xu Z, Przybylowski CJ, Melmer PD, Schlesinger D (2015) Edema following gamma knife radiosurgery for parasagittal and parafalcine meningiomas. J Neurosurg 123(5):1287–1293

114. Pan H-C, Sun M-H, Chen CC-C, Chen C-J, Lee C-H, Sheehan J (2008) Neuroimaging and quality-of-life outcomes in patients with brain metastasis and peritumoral edema who undergo gamma knife surgery. J Neurosurg 109(Suppl):90–98

115. Batchelor T, Loeffler JS (2006) Primary CNS lymphoma. J Clin Oncol 24(8):1281–1288

116. Almalki M, Aljoaib N, Alotaibi M, Aldabas B, Wahedi T, Ahmad M et al (2017) Temozolomide therapy for resistant prolactin-secreting pituitary adenomas and carcinomas: a systematic review. Hormones 16(2):139

117. Wen PY (2003) Central nervous system complications of cancer therapy. In: Cancer neurology in clinical practice. Springer, Berlin, pp 215–231

118. Stupp R, Mason WP, Van Den Bent MJ, Weller M, Fisher B, Taphoorn MJ et al (2005) Radiotherapy plus concomitant and adjuvant temozolomide for glioblastoma. N Engl J Med 352(10):987–996

119. Postma T, Van Groeningen C, Witjes R, Weerts J, Kralendonk J, Heimans J (1998) Neurotoxicity of combination chemotherapy with procarbazine, CCNU and vincristine (PCV) for recurrent glioma. J Neurooncol 38(1):69–75

120. Prabhu RS, Won M, Shaw EG, Hu C, Brachman DG, Buckner JC et al (2014) Effect of the addition of chemotherapy to radiotherapy on cognitive function in patients with low-grade glioma: secondary analysis of RTOG 98-02. J Clin Oncol 32(6):535–541

121. Pesce GA, Klingbiel D, Ribi K, Zouhair A, von Moos R, Schlaeppi M et al (2012) Outcome, quality of life and cognitive function of patients with brain metastases from non-small cell lung cancer treated with whole brain radiotherapy combined with gefitinib or temozolomide. A randomised phase II trial of the Swiss Group for Clinical Cancer Research (SAKK 70/03). Eur J Cancer 48(3):377–384

122. Addeo R, Caraglia M, Faiola V, Capasso E, Vincenzi B, Montella L et al (2007) Concomitant treatment of brain metastasis with whole brain radiotherapy [WBRT] and temozolomide [TMZ] is active and improves quality of life. BMC Cancer 7(1):18

123. Fliessbach K, Helmstaedter C, Urbach H, Althaus A, Pels H, Linnebank M et al (2005) Neuropsychological outcome after chemotherapy for primary CNS lymphoma a prospective study. Neurology 64(7):1184–1188

124. Doolittle ND, Korfel A, Lubow MA, Schorb E, Schlegel U, Rogowski S et al (2013) Long-term cognitive function, neuroimaging, and quality of life in primary CNS lymphoma. Neurology 81(1):84–92

125. Gilbert MR, Dignam JJ, Armstrong TS, Wefel JS, Blumenthal DT, Vogelbaum MA et al (2014) A randomized trial of bevacizumab for newly diagnosed glioblastoma. N Engl J Med 370(8):699–708

126. Desgrosellier JS, Cheresh DA (2010) Integrins in cancer: biological implications and therapeutic opportunities. Nat Rev Cancer 10(1):9–22

127. Stupp R, Hegi ME, Gorlia T, Erridge SC, Perry J, Hong Y-K et al (2014) Cilengitide combined with standard treatment for patients with newly diagnosed glioblastoma with methylated MGMT promoter (CENTRIC EORTC 26071-22072 study): a multicentre, randomised, open-label, phase 3 trial. Lancet Oncol 15(10):1100–1108

128. Reardon DA, Fink KL, Mikkelsen T, Cloughesy TF, O'Neill A, Plotkin S et al (2008) Randomized phase II study of cilengitide, an integrin-targeting arginine-glycine-aspartic acid peptide, in recurrent glioblastoma multiforme. J Clin Oncol 26(34):5610–5617

129. Lee SM, Lewanski CR, Counsell N, Ottensmeier C, Bates A, Patel N et al (2014) Randomized trial of erlotinib plus whole-brain radiotherapy for NSCLC patients with multiple brain metastases. J Natl Cancer Inst 106(7):dju151

130. Katz A, Zalewski P (2003) Quality-of-life benefits and evidence of antitumour activity for patients with brain metastases treated with gefitinib. Br J Cancer 89(Suppl 2):S15

131. Glass J, Won M, Schultz CJ, Brat D, Bartlett NL, Suh JH et al (2016) Phase I and II study of induction chemotherapy with methotrexate, rituximab, and temozolomide, followed by whole-brain radiotherapy and postirradiation temozolomide for primary CNS lymphoma: NRG oncology RTOG 0227. J Clin Oncol 34(14):1620–1625

132. Roth P, Preusser M, Weller M (2016) Immunotherapy of brain cancer. Oncol Res Treat 39(6):326–334

133. Weiss T, Weller M, Roth P (2015) Immunotherapy for glioblastoma: concepts and challenges. Curr Opin Neurol 28(6):639–646

134. Du Z, Abedalthagafi M, Aizer AA, McHenry AR, Sun HH, Bray M-A et al (2015) Increased expression of the immune modulatory molecule PD-L1 (CD274) in anaplastic meningioma. Oncotarget 6(7):4704

135. Rubenstein JL, Hsi ED, Johnson JL, Jung S-H, Nakashima MO, Grant B et al (2013) Intensive chemotherapy and immunotherapy in patients with newly diagnosed primary CNS lymphoma: CALGB 50202 (Alliance 50202). J Clin Oncol 31(25):3061–3068

136. Chamberlain MC (2014) Should dose-intense immunochemotherapy be the new standard of care for primary CNS lymphoma? J Clin Oncol 32(8):857–858

137. Stupp R, Wong E, Scott C, Taillibert S, Kanner A, Kesari S et al (2014) NT-40 interim analysis of the EF-14 trial: a prospective, multi-center trial of NovoTTF-100A together with temozolomide compared to temozolomide alone in patients with newly diagnosed GBM. Neuro-Oncology 16(suppl_5):v167–v16v

138. Stupp R, Wong ET, Kanner AA, Steinberg D, Engelhard H, Heidecke V et al (2012) NovoTTF-100A versus physician's choice chemotherapy in recurrent glioblastoma: a randomised phase III trial of a novel treatment modality. Eur J Cancer 48(14):2192–2202

139. Mehta M, Wen P, Nishikawa R, Reardon D, Peters K (2017) Critical review of the addition of tumor treating fields (TTFields) to the existing standard of care for newly diagnosed glioblastoma patients. Crit Rev Oncol Hematol 111:60–65

140. Taphoorn MJB et al (2018) Influence of treatment with tumor-treating fields on health-related quality of life of patients with newly diagnosed glioblastoma: a secondary analysis of a randomized clinical trial. JAMA Oncol. 4(4):495–504

141. Chang EF, Potts MB, Keles GE, Lamborn KR, Chang SM, Barbaro NM et al (2008) Seizure characteristics and control following resection in 332 patients with low-grade gliomas. J Neurosurg 108(2):227–235

142. Maschio M, Dinapoli L, Sperati F, Pace A, Fabi A, Vidiri A et al (2011) Levetiracetam monotherapy in patients with brain tumor-related epilepsy: seizure control, safety, and quality of life. J Neurooncol 104(1):205–214

143. Maschio M, Dinapoli L, Sperati F, Fabi A, Pace A, Vidiri A et al (2012) Oxcarbazepine monotherapy in patients with brain tumor-related epilepsy: open-label pilot study for assessing the efficacy, tolerability and impact on quality of life. J Neurooncol 106(3):651–656

144. Koekkoek JA, Dirven L, Taphoorn MJ (2017) The withdrawal of antiepileptic drugs in patients with low-grade and anaplastic glioma. Expert Rev Neurother 17(2):193–202

145. Kaal EC, Vecht CJ (2004) The management of brain edema in brain tumors. Curr Opin Oncol 16(6):593–600

146. Butler JM, Case LD, Atkins J, Frizzell B, Sanders G, Griffin P et al (2007) A phase III, double-blind, placebo-controlled prospective randomized clinical trial of d-threo-methylphenidate HCl in brain tumor patients receiving radiation therapy. Int J Radiat Oncol Biol Phys 69(5):1496–1501

147. Day J, Yust-Katz S, Cachia D, Rooney A, Katz LH, Wefel J et al (2016) Interventions for the management of fatigue in adults with a primary brain tumour. Cochrane Database Syst Rev 4:CD011376

148. Meyers CA, Weitzner MA, Valentine AD, Levin VA (1998) Methylphenidate therapy improves cognition, mood, and function of brain tumor patients. J Clin Oncol 16(7):2522–2527

149. Rooney A, Grant R (2010) Pharmacological treatment of depression in patients with a primary brain tumour. Cochrane Database Syst Rev (3):CD006932

150. Ownsworth T, Chambers S, Hawkes A, Walker DG, Shum D (2011) Making sense of brain tumour: a qualitative investigation of personal and social processes of adjustment. Neuropsychol Rehabil 21(1):117–137

151. Kangas M, McDonald S, Williams JR, Smee RI (2015) Acceptance and commitment therapy program for distressed adults with a primary brain tumor: a case series study. Support Care Cancer 23(10):2855–2859

152. Boele FW, Verdonck-de Leeuw IM, Cuijpers P, Reijneveld JC, Heimans JJ, Klein M (2014) Internet-based guided self-help for glioma patients with depressive symptoms: design of a randomized controlled trial. BMC Neurol 14(1):81

153. Mohr DC, Vella L, Hart S, Heckman T, Simon G (2008) The effect of telephone-administered psychotherapy on symptoms of depression and attrition: a meta-analysis. Clin Psychol Sci Pract 15(3):243–253

154. Luckett T, Butow P, King M (2009) Improving patient outcomes through the routine use of patient-reported data in cancer clinics: future directions. Psychooncology 18(11):1129–1138

155. Stewart MA (1995) Effective physician-patient communication and health outcomes: a review. Can Med Assoc J 152(9):1423

156. Rummans TA, Clark MM, Sloan JA, Frost MH, Bostwick JM, Atherton PJ et al (2006) Impacting quality of life for patients with advanced cancer with a structured multidisciplinary intervention: a randomized controlled trial. J Clin Oncol 24(4):635–642

157. Philip J, Collins A, Brand CA, Gold M, Moore G, Sundararajan V et al (2015) Health care professionals' perspectives of living and dying with primary malignant glioma: implications for a unique cancer trajectory. Palliat Support Care 13(6):1519–1527

158. Shaw EG, Rosdhal R, D'Agostino RB Jr, Lovato J, Naughton MJ, Robbins ME et al (2006) Phase II study of donepezil in irradiated brain tumor patients: effect on cognitive function, mood, and quality of life. J Clin Oncol 24(9):1415–1420

159. Rapp SR, Case LD, Peiffer A, Naughton MM, Chan MD, Stieber VW et al (2015) Donepezil for irradi-

ated brain tumor survivors: a phase III random-ized placebo-controlled clinical trial. J Clin Oncol 33(15):1653–1659

160. Gehring K, Patwardhan S, Collins R, Groves M, Etzel C, Meyers C et al (2012) A randomized trial on the efficacy of methylphenidate and modafinil for improving cognitive functioning and symptoms in patients with a primary brain tumor. J Neurooncol 107(1):165–174

161. Zucchella C, Capone A, Codella V, De Nunzio AM, Vecchione C, Sandrini G et al (2013) Cognitive reha-bilitation for early post-surgery inpatients affected by primary brain tumor: a randomized, controlled trial. J Neurooncol 114(1):93–100

162. Locke D, Cerhan JH, Wu W, Malec JF, Clark MM, Rummans TA et al (2008) Cognitive rehabilitation and problem-solving to improve quality of life of patients with primary brain tumors: a pilot study. J Support Oncol 6(8):383–391

163. Hassler MR, Elandt K, Preusser M, Lehrner J, Binder P, Dieckmann K et al (2010) Neurocognitive

training in patients with high-grade glioma: a pilot study. J Neurooncol 97(1):109–115

164. Han EY, Chun MH, Kim BR, Kim HJ (2015) Functional improvement after 4-week rehabilitation therapy and effects of attention deficit in brain tumor patients: comparison with subacute stroke patients. Ann Rehabil Med 39(4):560–569

165. Gomez-Pinilla F, Hillman C (2013) The influence of exercise on cognitive abilities. Compr Physiol 3:403–428

166. Hötting K, Röder B (2013) Beneficial effects of physical exercise on neuroplasticity and cognition. Neurosci Biobehav Rev 37(9):2243–2257

167. Yang S, Chun MH, Son YR (2014) Effect of virtual reality on cognitive dysfunction in patients with brain tumor. Ann Rehabil Med 38(6):726–733

168. Bergo E, Lombardi G, Pambuku A, Della Puppa A, Bellu L, D'Avella D et al (2016) Cognitive rehabilita-tion in patients with Gliomas and other brain tumors: state of the art. Biomed Res Int 2016:3041824

Palliative Care

44

C. Bausewein, S. Lorenzl, R. Voltz, M. Wasner,
and G. D. Borasio

44.1 Introduction

Patients with primary or secondary brain tumors have a limited life span and will most often die of their disease. Patients often suffer from neurological, psychological, and psychiatric symptoms as well as unpredictable personality changes with

C. Bausewein (✉)
Department of Palliative Medicine, Munich University Hospital, LMU Munich, Munich, Germany
e-mail: claudia.bausewein@med.uni-muenchen.de

S. Lorenzl
Department of Palliative Medicine, Munich University Hospital, LMU Munich, Munich, Germany

Department for Neurology, Krankenhaus Agatharied, Hausham, Germany

Institute of Nursing Science and Practice, Paracelsus Medical University, Salzburg, Austria
e-mail: Stefan.Lorenzl@khagatharied.de

R. Voltz
Department of Palliative Medicine, University Hospital of Cologne, Cologne, Germany
e-mail: raymond.voltz@uk-koeln.de

M. Wasner
Katholische Stiftungshochschule München, Munich, Germany
e-mail: maria.wasner@ksh-m.de

G. D. Borasio
Service of Palliative and Supportive Care, Department of Medicine, Lausanne University Hospital, Lausanne, Switzerland
e-mail: gian.borasio@chuv.ch

loss of autonomy. Compared to other malignant diseases, the main burden is often more related to the psychosocial rather than the physical dimension. The average life expectancy of most patients with glioblastoma (GBM) lies between several weeks and several months after postoperative radiotherapy, although recent advances in treatment have contributed to a better prognosis, especially for younger patients with good functional status. Given the lack of curative treatments and the short life expectancy of most patients, good palliative care is essential starting from the time of diagnosis.

44.2 Palliative Care

The multiple symptoms and psychosocial problems of patients with brain tumors and their families necessitate early integration of palliative care principles, in many cases from diagnosis onward. In many patients, the support of a multiprofessional and interdisciplinary team, including physiotherapy, occupational therapy, and speech therapy, is required to meet the multidimensional needs. This effort may be coordinated by the general practitioner, with the support of the neurologist or the palliative care specialist.

The WHO defines palliative care as "an approach that improves the quality of life of patients and their families facing the problem associated with life-threatening illness, through the

© Springer Nature Switzerland AG 2019

J.-C. Tonn et al. (eds.), *Oncology of CNS Tumors*, https://doi.org/10.1007/978-3-030-04152-6_44

prevention and relief of suffering by means of early identification and impeccable assessment and treatment of pain and other problems, physical, psychosocial and spiritual" [1]. Although in earlier times mainly related to care in the terminal phase, the WHO among others stresses now the importance of early integration in the course of a life-threatening illness, often in combination with disease-specific therapies intending to prolong life (e.g., chemotherapy or radiation). This is supported by evidence from other areas of oncology and supported by oncological and neuro-oncology guidelines [2–4]. Furthermore, families and relatives are seen as unit of care with the patients, acknowledging their needs during the illness of the patients. Especially in patients with brain tumors, this is highly important as a high burden of the relatives is reported consistently [5, 6].

Palliative care provision is not limited to specialist palliative care but includes primary and secondary levels of care, also described as generalist palliative care [7]. This indicates that it is the task of health-care providers such as general practitioners, hospital doctors and nurses, district nurses, etc. to integrate palliative approaches within the regular care plan to address unmet needs, particularly in the advanced stages of illness [8]. Specialist palliative care services are those where the *main activity* is the provision of palliative care for patients with complex and difficult clinical problems [9]. Specialist palliative care therefore requires a high level of palliative care education, appropriate staff, and other resources and is provided by multiprofessional teams [10] to provide in-depth pain and symptom management, communication regarding goals of care, and care coordination across settings and over time. For patients with brain tumors, an integrative approach from diagnosis to death could potentially reduce the care burden in the final period on the health-care system and the patient's family and improve access to a better place of death [11, 12].

44.3 Communication

Patients and families should be informed early in the course of the disease that the tumor—depending on its localization—will most probably lead to cognitive impairment, with the consequence of limitations in decision-making and legal capacity. Information about prognosis should be tailored to coping styles of individual patients and their relatives [13]. It has been recommended that clinicians seek patient preferences for the amount and type of information they require and that prognostic information should be individualized [14]. Patients with high-grade glioma expressed the following information needs: feelings of uncertainty around prognosis and quality of life, the need for individualized information, and communication with health-care professionals around prognostic uncertainty and disease progression despite communication barriers due to complex language deficits [15]. These relate mainly to dysphasia, confusion, or somnolence. Many brain tumor patients seem to be only partially informed about the negative prognosis [16], while their relatives appear more aware and more distressed [13, 17]. The complete appraisal of the diagnosis and prognosis has been reported to lead to an increased burden for the patients [13]. Nevertheless, anticipation regarding end-of-life issues, such as tube feedings, life-sustaining treatments, resuscitation, or discontinuation of steroids, is essential, and the patients should be encouraged to formulate an advance directive and name a health-care proxy within the time frame in which they can still make autonomous decisions [13, 18].

44.4 Psychosocial Burden of Patients and Relatives

Psychosocial issues play a major role in the care of brain tumor patients. At the time of diagnosis, most patients experience feelings of shock, anxiety, desperation, anger, and sadness [17]. During chemoradiotherapy, patients report a poor QOL, increased levels of distress, and high unmet needs [19]. The care needs of patients with glioma and their caregivers vary considerably in the different stages of disease [4].

Important issues for patients are the increasing dependency on external help, the change in body image (e.g., due to steroid-induced changes), and worries about the future, which are present in the majority of patients. The relatives feel progressively estranged from the patient and often experience the social death of the patient long before the actual death. Erratic emotional behavior is particularly difficult for the relatives to deal with, and they are often left to confront confusion, hallucinations, and violence alone.

One of the most important factors for the QoL of brain tumor patients is the family. However, the burden of carers of patients with glioblastoma is consistently reported as high with carers' quality of life strongly affected by the burden of care and the patient's mental state [5, 6]. Carers report moderate to high needs which are stable over time, but specific needs do change [20]. Most frequently reported carer needs include the impact of caring on the carer's working life or usual activities, finding more accessible parking, making life decisions in the context of uncertainty, reducing stress in the patient's life, and understanding the patient's experience [20]. Furthermore, carers express needs for information on adjusting to the patient's cognitive changes, managing difficult aspects of the patient's behavior, and adjusting to changes in the patient's personality [20]. Higher numbers of unmet needs were associated cross-sectionally with higher distress levels.

Therefore, early involvement of family members in medical decisions and care is mandatory, and family members need special attention, counseling, and care from the interdisciplinary team throughout the disease. Continuous re-evaluation of patients' and carers' needs should be implemented to detect unmet needs and adjust the care plan accordingly.

44.5 Physical Burden and Symptom Control

The disease-related symptoms experienced by patients with brain tumors usually are caused either by raised intracranial pressure or by direct impingement of the tumor on brain structures. Concurrent and interrelated causes of raised intracranial pressure include the expanding tumor mass, cerebral edema, and impaired absorption of cerebrospinal fluid.

44.5.1 Headache

In patients with brain tumors, headache is the predominant type of pain, occurring in 23–90% of patients, with an increase in frequency and severity over time [4]. Only a small group experiences the "classic" brain tumor headache, which is more severe on awakening, eases off after arising, and may be associated with nausea and vomiting [21, 22]. Most patients complain of a dull generalized headache of moderate intensity, and not specifically localized [22]. Headache pain mostly results from brain tumor growth or surrounding edema and indicates an increased intracranial pressure [4].

For the treatment of headaches, steroids are the drugs of choice as they reduce the raised intracranial pressure by decreasing vasogenic peritumoral edema. The effect of steroids on headache, reduced consciousness, nausea and vomiting, and neurological deficits is often dramatic, occurring within days. Depending on the extent and tempo of the disease, these benefits may not be long-lasting. This needs to be explained in advance to patients and relatives, together with the fact that steroids have no influence on tumor progression.

Dexamethasone is usually the drug of choice related to its side-effect profile with less mineralocorticoid effects [23]. Treatment is normally started with relatively high doses (12–16 mg/ day). Importantly, steroids should be given in the morning as a single dose—the biological half-life of dexamethasone is 36–72 h—and not in the evening, to reduce the risk of sleep disturbances [23]. The dosage should be left for 5 days and tapered when symptom control has been achieved to the lowest effective dose, which is often as low as 2 mg/day. In a randomized controlled trial in patients with brain tumors, doses of 4 mg dexamethasone/day were as effective as 16 mg/day but caused fewer side effects [24]. Prescription and dosage of steroids should be reviewed regularly. Many patients are given doses of steroids that are unnecessarily high, predisposing them to severe side effects, including Cushing's syndrome, psychosis, and myopathy. Alternatively, extract from *Boswellia serrata* (H15, 1200–3600 mg/day) can be used or combined with steroids to reduce edema. Based on clinical observation, about half of the patients report a positive effect, and the main side effects observed are nausea and vomiting [25].

In addition to the usual and well-recognized side effects from steroid drugs, the risk of drug–drug interactions must be noted. For example, the concomitant use of anticonvulsants, such as phenytoin, may decrease the blood levels of dexamethasone by as much as two thirds [26].

If steroids alone are not sufficient, analgesics and co-analgesics could also be considered in the treatment of headache (in accordance with the WHO cancer pain ladder) [4].

44.5.2 Dysphagia

Patients with primary brain tumors may develop dysphagia as a consequence of cranial nerve or bulbar palsy. In contrast to dysphagia due to obstruction, it is easier for patients with neurogenic dysphagia to swallow solids than fluids, which may necessitate dietary changes and thickening of fluids. Aspiration and malnutrition are the main complications of dysphagia. If appropriate, given the status of disease and the patient's wishes, placement of a feeding tube via percutaneous endoscopic gastrostomy may address these complications. Dysphagia was reported as one of the main symptoms in the last week of life occurring in relation to reduced consciousness [27].

44.5.3 Cognitive and Behavioral Dysfunction

Patients with brain tumors develop cognitive dysfunction much earlier than other patients with terminal illness. Fluctuation of these symptoms is common. The patients present with a variety of symptoms, ranging from attention deficit to personality changes and psychiatric problems. Brain

imaging and laboratory tests may be necessary to differentiate among the varied causes and assess the potential for reversibility with treatment. Steroid treatment has been associated with improvement in recognition memory. Other drugs, such as donepezil or psychostimulants (methylphenidate and modafinil), do not prevent cognitive decline [4]. Antiepileptic drugs, on the other hand, should be considered as a common cause of cognitive changes and have been shown to reduce working memory capacity in these patients [28, 29]. Risperidone, a neuroleptic with serotonin (5 HT$_2$) and dopamine (D$_2$) antagonist properties, seems to be more effective than haloperidol when the patient is aggressive, agitated, or confused [30]. Cognitive rehabilitation interventions aiming to improve cognitive functioning seem to be beneficial for patients [4].

44.5.4 Depression

The pooled prevalence of depression or depressive symptoms in patients with brain tumors was reported as 21.7% (95% confidence interval (CI) 18.2–25.2%) [31]. Diagnosis of depression is often difficult due to cognitive changes. Since depression is a major determinant of quality of life, it should be actively sought for and treated at all stages of the disease. A multimodal psychosocial intervention might improve depressive symptoms in patients with brain tumors [4, 32]. Unfortunately, there are no randomized studies evaluating the value of pharmacological treatment of depression in patients with a primary brain tumor [33]. However, for patients with physical disease and in palliative care, antidepressants have been shown to be effective [34, 35].

44.5.5 Speech and Language Problems

About one third of patients with high-grade gliomas have speech deficits at first presentation, requiring early access to speech therapy [36]. Comprehension of dysphasic patients is often worse than anticipated. Questions should be asked slowly and clearly. It is important to develop a yes/no code or to find alternative strategies like pointing, writing, or painting. Patients with fluent dysphasia should be taught to slow their speech, and those with hesitant speaking should be encouraged to speak nonetheless. Patience, time, and empathy are necessary to maintain communication, especially since the patients' communicative ability typically shows significant fluctuations. In patients with severe dysarthria, communication boards or electronic aids might be helpful.

44.5.6 Seizures

Seizures occur in up to 90% of glioma patients during the course of the disease depending on subtype, location, proximity to the cortex, and genetic factors [4, 37].

During the seizure, care must be taken that the patient does not get hurt. Epileptic seizures are typically brief and self-limited (usually 3–5 min) because of endogenous inhibitory mechanisms and therefore require no acute anticonvulsant therapy. However, status epilepticus (a seizure that persists more than 30 min or repeated seizures without return of consciousness between them) warrants aggressive therapy because of its high mortality rate.

Prophylactic anticonvulsant therapy is not recommended in newly diagnosed brain tumors as it does not provide substantial benefit and is associated with a higher incidence of side effects [38, 39]. However, long-term prophylaxis is necessary after a first seizure has occurred. Choosing the right drug depends on several considerations:

1. Time factor: If a rapid onset of effect is needed, benzodiazepines like lorazepam (also available as sublingual formulation) or midazolam may be best. Therapeutic valproate, phenytoin, or levetiracetam levels are reached within a short time, as they are available as intravenous preparations and can be administered in a regimen that includes a loading dose.

2. Drug interactions: Anticonvulsants such as phenytoin, valproic acid, and carbamazepine may lower serum levels of other medications, such as steroids or chemotherapy, and vice versa. This may be counteracted by increasing the doses of the medication. However, the danger of reaching toxic levels exists, especially with phenytoin, as this drug has nonlinear pharmacokinetics. Levetiracetam does not influence the steroid serum levels and shows less drug interactions [40] and may be preferred especially in the treatment of status epilepticus. Drug toxicity from anticonvulsants may mimic tumor symptoms, such as ataxia, double vision, gait disturbance, or cognitive impairment.

3. Efficacy and side effects: Anticonvulsant drug doses should be increased until no more seizures occur or side effects appear. Here, the upper limit of drug levels is of less clinical value than commonly believed. Some patients have side effects long before this "upper limit" is reached; others have no side effects even above it. The patient's response, and not the serum level, should guide treatment. Carbamazepine may be switched to oxcarbazepine on a milligram-to-milligram basis if side effects occur; oxcarbazepine may be further increased if necessary, as it is generally less toxic. Another severe side effect, especially relevant for brain tumor patients, is the so-called Stevens–Johnson syndrome (potentially lethal multiform exudating erythema) in patients receiving phenytoin, and sometimes carbamazepine, who have received cranial irradiation and are on decreasing doses of steroids. Levetiracetam may sometimes cause behavioral changes in brain tumor patients, mainly aggressive behavior, irritability, emotional lability, or hostility [41].

4. Route of administration: Once patients are no longer able to swallow, a parenteral route of application must be considered. Phenytoin, valproate, and levetiracetam are available as IV preparations, and lorazepam, midazolam, and levetiracetam can be given subcutaneously. Alternative routes of administration are sublingual lorazepam or intranasal midazolam.

44.5.7 Venous Thromboembolism

Compared to other malignancies, patients with brain tumors have a higher risk for venous thromboembolism, such as deep venous thrombosis or pulmonary embolism [4]. Anticoagulation, e.g., with low molecular weight heparin, is recommended in these patients, both prophylactically (when mobility is reduced) and when patients are symptomatic [42].

44.5.8 Mobility Problems

In patients with brain tumors, mobility may be impaired due to hemiplegia, increasing weakness, or obesity after long-term treatment with steroids. Problems with coordination may evolve from ataxia. Steroid myopathy affecting proximal muscles of legs and arms occurs frequently, may develop even after short-term treatment, and is often overlooked.

Since any gain in mobility decreases the need for care and increases the independence of the patient, physiotherapy and occupational therapy should be organized early on and adapted to the patient's actual situation, abilities, and skills.

44.5.9 Existential Distress

Existential distress has been reported in up to 50% of brain tumor patients [43], typically acute around diagnosis and again after initial treatment [44]. Correspondingly, maintaining a sense of hope and meaning in life has been shown to increase their quality of life [45]. Patients and families report a lack of support in this area, which may be due to the lack of training of the professional caregivers, most of whom feel uncomfortable in dealing with these questions.

44.5.10 Specific Issues in the Terminal Phase

Main symptoms in the terminal phase are decreased level of consciousness, dysphagia, fever, seizures, and headaches [46, 47]. With increasing weakness, dysphagia, or deteriorating consciousness, the patient will be unable to take medication orally. Therefore, alternative routes of drug administration, such as subcutaneous, intravenous, transdermal, or rectal administration, are necessary for symptom control and should be planned in advance of the terminal phase.

Discontinuation of steroid treatment: Most brain tumor patients receive long-term steroid therapy. When their condition deteriorates, it has to be decided whether to increase the dose or to discontinue the treatment. A raise in steroid dose should usually be limited to 5–7 days. If no effect is seen within that time, steroids should be reduced again. In dying patients who cannot take oral medication, continuation of steroids might prolong the dying phase, while discontinuation might lead to exacerbation of cerebral edema (unlikely if the fluid intake is reduced) and to adrenal insufficiency (unlikely to result in significant suffering). Thus, continuation of parenteral steroids in the dying phase is rarely appropriate or necessary. If steroids are discontinued, intensified symptom monitoring is required, and increases in analgesic, antiemetic, or anticonvulsant medication may be necessary.

Box 44.1 Nonconvulsive Status Epilepticus

The clinical presentation of nonconvulsive status epilepticus (NCSE) ranges from confusional state to coma. Automatisms may be present. In comatose patients, unilateral tonic head and eye movement is often observed. Other symptoms include myoclonic contractions of the angle of the mouth, mild clonus of an extremity, or, rarely, epileptic nystagmus. Typical signs of epileptic motor seizures (generalized tonic–clonic seizures) like tongue bite and urinary incontinence are usually missing. NCSE is an often unrecognized and potentially treatable complication in late-stage brain tumor patients [48].

References

1. Sixty-seventh World Health Assembly. Strengthening of palliative care as a component of comprehensive care throughout the life course. 2014 Ninth plenary meeting, 24 May 2014. Contract No.: A67/VR/9
2. Temel JS, Greer JA, Muzikansky A, Gallagher ER, Admane S, Jackson VA et al (2010) Early palliative care for patients with metastatic non-small-cell lung cancer. N Engl J Med 363(8):733–742
3. Ferrell BR, Temel JS, Temin S, Alesi ER, Balboni TA, Basch EM et al (2017) Integration of palliative care into standard oncology care: American Society of Clinical Oncology clinical practice guideline update. J Clin Oncol 35(1):96–112
4. Pace A, Dirven L, Koekkoek JAF, Golla H, Fleming J, Ruda R et al (2017) European Association for Neuro-Oncology (EANO) guidelines for palliative care in adults with glioma. Lancet Oncol 18(6):e330–ee40
5. Wasner M, Paal P, Borasio GD (2013) Psychosocial care for the caregivers of primary malignant brain tumor patients. J Soc Work End Life Palliat Care 9(1):74–95
6. Halkett GK, Lobb EA, Shaw T, Sinclair MM, Miller L, Hovey E et al (2017) Distress and psychological morbidity do not reduce over time in carers of patients with high-grade glioma. Support Care Cancer 25(3):887–893
7. Worldwide Palliative Care Alliance (WPCA) (2014) Global atlas of palliative care at the end of life. WPCA, London
8. Rocker GM, Simpson AC, Horton R (2015) Palliative care in advanced lung disease: the challenge of integrating palliation into everyday care. Chest 148(3):801–809
9. Radbruch L, Payne S (2009) White paper on standards and norms for hospice and palliative care in Europe: part 1. Eur J Palliat Care 16(6):278–289
10. Radbruch L, Payne S (2010) White paper on standards and norms for hospice and palliative care in Europe: part 2. Eur J Palliat Care 17(1):22–33
11. Alturki A, Gagnon B, Petrecca K, Scott SC, Nadeau L, Mayo N (2014) Patterns of care at end of life for people with primary intracranial tumors: lessons learned. J Neuro-Oncol 117(1):103–115
12. Sundararajan V, Bohensky MA, Moore G, Brand CA, Lethborg C, Gold M et al (2014) Mapping the patterns of care, the receipt of palliative care and the site of death for patients with malignant glioma. J Neuro-Oncol 116(1):119–126
13. Davies E, Higginson IJ (2003) Communication, information and support for adults with malignant cerebral glioma: a systematic literature review. Support Care Cancer 11(1):21–29
14. Lobb EA, Halkett GK, Nowak AK (2011) Patient and caregiver perceptions of communication of prognosis in high grade glioma. J Neuro-Oncol 104(1):315–322
15. Halkett GK, Lobb EA, Oldham L, Nowak AK (2010) The information and support needs of patients diagnosed with high grade glioma. Patient Educ Couns 79(1):112–119
16. Davies E, Clarke C, Hopkins A (1996) Malignant cerebral glioma—II: perspectives of patients and relatives on the value of radiotherapy. BMJ 313(7071):1512–1516
17. Adelbratt S, Strang P (2000) Death anxiety in brain tumour patients and their spouses. Palliat Med 14(6):499–507
18. Taillibert S, Laigle-Donadey F, Sanson M (2004) Palliative care in patients with primary brain tumors. Curr Opin Oncol 16(6):587–592
19. Halkett GK, Lobb EA, Rogers MM, Shaw T, Long AP, Wheeler HR et al (2015) Predictors of distress and poorer quality of life in high grade glioma patients. Patient Educ Couns 98(4):525–532
20. Halkett GKB, Lobb EA, Shaw T, Sinclair MM, Miller L, Hovey E et al (2018) Do carer's levels of unmet needs change over time when caring for patients diagnosed with high-grade glioma and how are these needs correlated with distress? Support Care Cancer 26(1):275–286
21. Nelson S, Taylor LP (2014) Headaches in brain tumor patients: primary or secondary? Headache 54(4):776–785
22. Schankin CJ, Ferrari U, Reinisch VM, Birnbaum T, Goldbrunner R, Straube A (2007) Characteristics of brain tumour-associated headache. Cephalalgia 27(8):904–911
23. Twycross R, Wilcock A, Howard P (2017) Palliative care formulary (PCF6), 6th edn
24. Vecht CJ, Hovestadt A, Verbiest HB, van Vliet JJ, van Putten WL (1994) Dose-effect relationship of dexamethasone on Karnofsky performance in metastatic brain tumors: a randomized study of doses of 4, 8, and 16 mg per day. Neurology 44(4):675–680
25. Winking M, Böker D, Simmet T (1996) Boswellic acid as an inhibitor of the perifocal edema in malignant glioma in man. J Neuro-Oncol 30:104
26. Chalk JB, Ridgeway K, Brophy T, Yelland JD, Eadie MJ (1984) Phenytoin impairs the bioavailability of dexamethasone in neurological and neurosurgical patients. J Neurol Neurosurg Psychiatry 47(10):1087–1090
27. Sizoo EM, Braam L, Postma TJ, Pasman HR, Heimans JJ, Klein M et al (2010) Symptoms and problems in the end-of-life phase of high-grade glioma patients. Neuro-Oncology 12(11):1162–1166
28. Klein M, Engelberts NH, van der Ploeg HM, Kasteleijn-Nolst Trenite DG, Aaronson NK, Taphoorn MJ et al (2003) Epilepsy in low-grade gliomas: the impact on cognitive function and quality of life. Ann Neurol 54(4):514–520
29. Taphoorn MJ, Klein M (2004) Cognitive deficits in adult patients with brain tumours. Lancet Neurol 3(3):159–168
30. Lee MA, Leng ME, Tiernan EJ (2001) Risperidone: a useful adjunct for behavioural disturbance in primary cerebral tumours. Palliat Med 15(3):255–256

31. Huang J, Zeng C, Xiao J, Zhao D, Tang H, Wu H et al (2017) Association between depression and brain tumor: a systematic review and meta-analysis. Oncotarget 8(55):94932–94943

32. Ownsworth T, Chambers S, Damborg E, Casey L, Walker DG, Shum DH (2015) Evaluation of the making sense of brain tumor program: a randomized controlled trial of a home-based psychosocial intervention. Psychooncology 24(5):540–547

33. Rooney A, Grant R (2013) Pharmacological treatment of depression in patients with a primary brain tumour. Cochrane Database Syst Rev 5:CD006932

34. Rayner L, Price A, Evans A, Valsraj K, Higginson IJ, Hotopf M (2010) Antidepressants for depression in physically ill people. Cochrane Database Syst Rev 3:CD007503

35. Rayner L, Price A, Evans A, Valsraj K, Hotopf M, Higginson IJ (2011) Antidepressants for the treatment of depression in palliative care: systematic review and meta-analysis. Palliat Med 25(1):36–51

36. Thomas R, O'Connor AM, Ashley S (1995) Speech and language disorders in patients with high grade glioma and its influence on prognosis. J Neuro-Oncol 23(3):265–270

37. Weller M, Stupp R, Wick W (2012) Epilepsy meets cancer: when, why, and what to do about it? Lancet Oncol 13(9):e375–e382

38. Glantz MJ, Cole BF, Forsyth PA, Recht LD, Wen PY, Chamberlain MC et al (2000) Practice parameter: anticonvulsant prophylaxis in patients with newly diagnosed brain tumors. Report of the Quality Standards Subcommittee of the American Academy of Neurology. Neurology 54(10):1886–1893

39. Froscher W, Kirschstein T, Rosche J (2014) [Anticonvulsant therapy for brain tumour-related epilepsy]. Fortschr Neurol Psychiatr 82(12):678–690

40. Ruegg S, Naegelin Y, Hardmeier M, Winkler DT, Marsch S, Fuhr P (2008) Intravenous levetiracetam: treatment experience with the first 50 critically ill patients. Epilepsy Behav 12(3):477–480

41. Brodie MJ, Besag F, Ettinger AB, Mula M, Gobbi G, Comai S et al (2016) Epilepsy, antiepileptic drugs, and aggression: an evidence-based review. Pharmacol Rev 68(3):563–602

42. Batchelor TT, Byrne TN (2006) Supportive care of brain tumor patients. Hematol Oncol Clin North Am 20(6):1337–1361

43. Pelletier G, Verhoef MJ, Khatri N, Hagen N (2002) Quality of life in brain tumor patients: the relative contributions of depression, fatigue, emotional distress, and existential issues. J Neuro-Oncol 57(1):41–49

44. Cavers D, Hacking B, Erridge SE, Kendall M, Morris PG, Murray SA (2012) Social, psychological and existential well-being in patients with glioma and their caregivers: a qualitative study. CMAJ 184(7):E373–E382

45. Salander P, Bergenheim T, Henriksson R (1996) The creation of protection and hope in patients with malignant brain tumours. Soc Sci Med 42(7):985–996

46. Thier K, Calabek B, Tinchon A, Grisold W, Oberndorfer S (2016) The last 10 days of patients with glioblastoma: assessment of clinical signs and symptoms as well as treatment. Am J Hosp Palliat Care 33(10):985–988

47. Bausewein C, Hau P, Borasio GD, Voltz R (2003) How do patients with primary brain tumours die? Palliat Med 17(6):558–559

48. Lorenzl S, Mayer S, Noachtar S, Borasio GD (2008) Nonconvulsive status epilepticus in terminally ill patients-a diagnostic and therapeutic challenge. J Pain Symptom Manag 36(2):200–205

Printed by Printforce, the Netherlands